Clinical Echocardiography Review

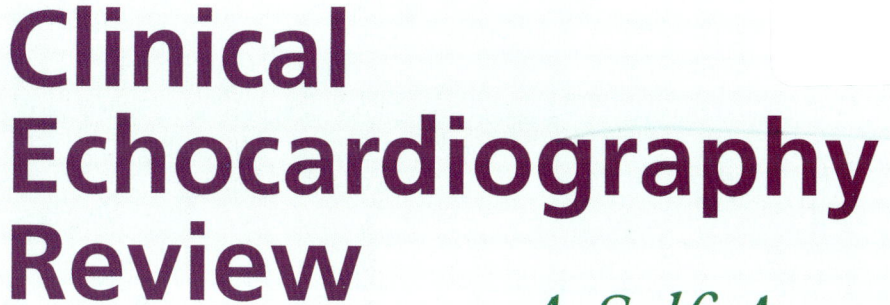

A Self-Assessment Tool

THIRD EDITION

Editors

Allan L. Klein, MD, FRCP(C), FACC, FAHA, FASE, FESC

Professor of Medicine
Cleveland Clinic Lerner College of Medicine of Case Western Reserve University
Director, Center for the Diagnosis and Treatment of Pericardial Diseases
Section of Cardiovascular Imaging
Department of Cardiovascular Medicine
Heart, Vascular and Thoracic Institute
Past-President of the American Society of Echocardiography
President-Elect of the National Board of Echocardiography
Cleveland Clinic
Cleveland, Ohio

Craig R. Asher, MD, FACC, FASE

Department of Cardiovascular Medicine
Heart, Vascular and Thoracic Institute
Director, Hypertrophic Cardiomyopathy Center
Past-Cardiology Fellowship Program Director
Cleveland Clinic Florida
Weston, Florida

Michael Chetrit, MD, FRCP(C), FACC

Assistant Professor of Medicine
Site Director, Echocardiography Lab, Montreal General Hospital
Director, McGill Amyloidosis Project
Clinical Director, Courtois Cardiac MRI Program
Vice President, Canadian Society of Cardiac MRI
Montreal, Canada

Wolters Kluwer

Philadelphia • Baltimore • New York • London
Buenos Aires • Hong Kong • Sydney • Tokyo

Acquisitions Editor: James Sherman
Senior Development Editor: Ashley Fischer
Editorial Coordinator: Sean Hanrahan
Marketing Manager: Kristin Watrud
Senior Production Project Manager: Catherine Ott
Manager, Graphic Arts & Design: Stephen Druding
Manufacturing Coordinator: Bernard Tomboc
Prepress Vendor: TNQ Tech

Third Edition

Copyright © 2025 Wolters Kluwer.

Copyright © 2017 Wolters Kluwer Copyright © 2011 by LIPPINCOTT WILLIAMS & WILKINS, a WOLTERS KLUWER business. All rights reserved. This book is protected by copyright. No part of this book may be reproduced or transmitted in any form or by any means, including as photocopies or scanned-in or other electronic copies, or utilized by any information storage and retrieval system without written permission from the copyright owner, except for brief quotations embodied in critical articles and reviews. Materials appearing in this book prepared by individuals as part of their official duties as U.S. government employees are not covered by the above-mentioned copyright. To request permission, please contact Wolters Kluwer at Two Commerce Square, 2001 Market Street, Philadelphia, PA 19103, via email at permissions@lww.com, or via our website at shop.lww.com (products and services).

9 8 7 6 5 4 3 2 1

Printed in Mexico

Library of Congress Cataloging-in-Publication Data

ISBN-13: 978-1-975211-89-9

Cataloging in Publication data available on request from publisher.

This work is provided "as is," and the publisher disclaims any and all warranties, express or implied, including any warranties as to accuracy, comprehensiveness, or currency of the content of this work.

This work is no substitute for individual patient assessment based upon healthcare professionals' examination of each patient and consideration of, among other things, age, weight, gender, current or prior medical conditions, medication history, laboratory data and other factors unique to the patient. The publisher does not provide medical advice or guidance and this work is merely a reference tool. Healthcare professionals, and not the publisher, are solely responsible for the use of this work including all medical judgments and for any resulting diagnosis and treatments.

Given continuous, rapid advances in medical science and health information, independent professional verification of medical diagnoses, indications, appropriate pharmaceutical selections and dosages, and treatment options should be made and healthcare professionals should consult a variety of sources. When prescribing medication, healthcare professionals are advised to consult the product information sheet (the manufacturer's package insert) accompanying each drug to verify, among other things, conditions of use, warnings and side effects and identify any changes in dosage schedule or contraindications, particularly if the medication to be administered is new, infrequently used or has a narrow therapeutic range. To the maximum extent permitted under applicable law, no responsibility is assumed by the publisher for any injury and/or damage to persons or property, as a matter of products liability, negligence law or otherwise, or from any reference to or use by any person of this work.

shop.lww.com

CONTRIBUTORS

Mohamed Al-Kazaz, MD, FACC
Section Chief, General Cardiology
Assistant Professor of Medicine
Division of Cardiology
Department of Medicine
Northwestern University Feinberg School of Medicine
Chicago, Illinois

Ben Alencherry, MD, MEd
Staff Cardiologist
Section of Cardiovascular Imaging
Department of Cardiovascular Medicine
Heart, Vascular, Thoracic Institute
Cleveland Clinic
Cleveland, Ohio

Bonita Anderson, DMU(Cardiac), MAppSc(MedUltrasound), ACS
Advanced Cardiac Scientist
Cardiac Sciences Unit
The Prince Charles Hospital
Brisbane, Australia

Edgar Argulian, MD, MPH
Associate Professor of Medicine
Department of Medicine
Icahn School of Medicine at Mount Sinai
New York, New York

Basant Arya, MD
Associate Professor
Section of Cardiology
Department of Medicine
Baylor College of Medicine
Houston, Texas

Craig R. Asher, MD, FACC, FASE
Department of Cardiovascular Medicine
Heart, Vascular and Thoracic Institute
Director, Hypertrophic Cardiomyopathy Center
Past-Cardiology Fellowship Program Director
Cleveland Clinic Florida
Weston, Florida

Gerard P. Aurigemma, MD
Professor Medicine and Radiology
UMass Chan Medical School
Worcester, Massachusetts

Daniel Bamira, MD
Assistant Professor
Leon H Charney Division of Cardiology
Department of Medicine
NYU Grossman School of Medicine
New York University Langone Health
New York, New York

Jeroen J. Bax, MD, PhD
Professor
Heart Lung Center
Leiden University Medical Center
Leiden, The Netherlands

Kwan Leung Chan, MD
Full Professor
Division of Cardiology
Department of Medicine
University of Ottawa
Ottawa, Ontario, Canada

Michael Chetrit, MD, FRCP(C), FACC
Assistant Professor of Medicine
Site Director, Echocardiography Lab, Montreal General Hospital
Director, McGill Amyloidosis Project
Clinical Director, Courtois Cardiac MRI Program
Vice President, Canadian Society of Cardiac MRI
Montreal, Quebec, Canada

Marie-Annick Clavel, DVM, PhD
Full Professor
Department of Medicine
Laval University
Quebec City, Quebec, Canada

Joshua A. Cohen, MD
Chief Fellow, Advanced Cardiac Imaging
Cleveland Clinic
Heart, Vascular, and Thoracic Institute
Cleveland, Ohio

Patrick H. Collier, MD, PhD, FASE, FESC, FACC
Associate Professor of Medicine
Cleveland Clinic Lerner College of Medicine of Case Western Reserve University
Staff, Section of Cardiovascular Imaging
Co-Director Cardio-Oncology Center
Deputy Director of the Echocardiographic Lab
Robert and Suzanne Tomsich Department of Cardiovascular Medicine
Cleveland Clinic
Cleveland, Ohio

Jordi S. Dahl, MD, PhD
Associate Professor
Department of Cardiology
Odense University Hospital
Odense, Denmark

Victoria Delgado, MD, PhD
Associate Professor
Department of Cardiology
University Hospital Germans Trias i Pujol
Barcelona, Spain

Milind Desai, MD, MBA
Professor of Medicine
Cleveland Clinic Lerner College of Medicine of Case Western Reserve University
Vice Chair, Heart, Vascular, and Thoracic Institute
Director, Center for Hypertrophic Cardiomyopathy
Medical Director, Aorta Center
Cleveland Clinic
Cleveland, Ohio

Tiffany Dong, MD
Advanced Imaging Fellow
Section of Cardiovascular Imaging
Heart, Vascular and Thoracic Institute
Cleveland Clinic
Cleveland, Ohio

Sasha-ann East, MD
Assistant Professor
Department of Cardiovascular Disease and Hypertension
Rutgers Robert Wood Johnson Medical School
New Brunswick, New Jersey

Benjamin W. Eidem, MD
Professor, Departments of Pediatrics & Cardiovascular Medicine
Mayo Clinic
Rochester, Minnesota

Maurice Enriquez-Sarano, MD, FACC, FAHA, FESC
Professor of Medicine
Senior Scientist
Minneapolis Heart Institute Foundation and the Valve Science Center
Minneapolis, Minnesota

Maria Fadous, MD, MHPE
Fellow
Harvard Medical School
Beth Israel Deaconess Medical Center
Boston, Massachusetts

Nadeen N. Faza, MD, FACC, FASE, FSCAI
Assistant Professor of Medicine
Weill Cornell Graduate School of Medical Sciences
New York, New York
Section of Cardiovascular Imaging
Department of Cardiology
Houston Methodist DeBakey Heart and Vascular Center
Houston, Texas

James M. Galas, MD
Associate Professor
Department of Pediatrics
Central Michigan University College of Medicine
Detroit, Michigan

Benjamin T. Galen, MD
Associate Professor
Department of Internal Medicine
Albert Einstein College of Medicine
Montefiore Medical Center
Bronx, New York

Linda D. Gillam, MD, MPH
Professor of Medicine
Sidney Kimmel Medical College/Thomas Jefferson University
Philadelphia, Pennsylvania
Chair
Department of Cardiovascular Medicine
Morristown Medical Center
Atlantic Health System
Morristown, New Jersey

Brian P. Griffin, MD, FACC
John and Rosemary Brown Chair of Cardiovascular Medicine
Section Head
Section of Cardiovascular Imaging
Department of Cardiovascular Medicine
Cleveland Clinic Lerner College of Medicine of Case Western Reserve University
Cleveland, Ohio

Pooja Gupta, MD, FASE, FACC
Associate Professor
Department of Pediatrics
Central Michigan University College of Medicine
Detroit, Michigan

Braeden Hill, BHSc
Department of Medicine
Queen's University
Kingston, Ontario, Canada

Diarmaid Hughes, MD
Fellow
Department of Cardiovascular Medicine
Cleveland Clinic
Cleveland, Ohio

Madeline Jankowski, RDCS, ACS, BS, FASE
Echocardiography Research Associate
Department of Medicine
Northwestern University Feinberg School of Medicine
Chicago, Illinois

Amer M. Johri, MD, MSc, FRCPC, FASE
Professor
Department of Medicine
Queen's University
Kingston, Ontario, Canada

Tahir S. Kafil, MD, FRCPC
Section of Cardiovascular Imaging
Department of Cardiovascular Medicine
Heart, Vascular and Thoracic Institute
Cleveland Clinic
Cleveland, Ohio

Allan L. Klein, MD, FRCP(C), FACC, FAHA, FASE, FESC
Professor of Medicine
Cleveland Clinic Lerner College of Medicine of Case Western Reserve University
Director, Center for the Diagnosis and Treatment of Pericardial Diseases
Section of Cardiovascular Imaging
Department of Cardiovascular Medicine
Heart, Vascular and Thoracic Institute
Past-President of the American Society of Echocardiography
President-Elect of the National Board of Echocardiography
Cleveland Clinic
Cleveland, Ohio

Srikanth Koneru, MD
Associate Professor
Section of Cardiology
Department of Medicine
Baylor College of Medicine
Director, Structural Heart Imaging and Valve Clinic
Texas Heart Institute at Baylor St Luke's Medical Center
Houston, Texas

Konstantinos P. Koulogiannis, MD
Director of Echocardiography
Morristown Medical Center
Morristown, New Jersey

Nakul S. Kumar, MD
Assistant Professor, Anesthesiology
Intensive Care and Resuscitation
Cleveland Clinic
Cleveland, Ohio

Roberto M. Lang, MD
Professor
Division of Internal Medicine
Division of Cardiovascular Medicine
University of Chicago
Chicago, Illinois

Lawrence Lau, MD
Assistant Professor
Department of Medicine, Division of Cardiology
University of Ottawa
Ottawa, Ontario, Canada

Antonio Lewis-Camarago, MD
Chief Fellow
Department of Cardiovascular Medicine
Heart, Thoracic and Vascular Institute
Cleveland Clinic Florida
Weston, Florida

Stephen H. Little, MD, FRCPC, FASE, FACC
Professor of Medicine, Weill Cornell Medicine
Director of Structural Heart Program, Houston Methodist System
Cardiovascular Imaging Section, Department of Cardiology
Houston Methodist DeBakey Heart and Vascular Center
Houston, Texas

Kameswari Maganti, MD, FACC, FASE
Professor of Medicine
Section Chief, Non-Invasive Cardiology
Director of Echocardiography Laboratory
Departmenet of Medicine
Rutgers University
New Brunswick, New Jersey

Sunil Mankad, MD, FACC, FCCP, FASE
Professor of Medicine
Division of Cardiovascular Diseases
Mayo Clinic
Rochester, Minnesota

Dimitrios Maragiannis, MD, PhD
Cardiologist
Director of Echocardiography at 401 Military Hospital of Athens, Greece
Director of Cardiovascular MRI Laboratory at 401 Military Hospital of Athens, Greece

Leo Marcoff, MD
Director of Interventional Echocardiography
Morristown Medical Center
Assistant Professor of Medicine
Thomas Jefferson University
Philadelphia, Pennsylvania

Thomas H. Marwick, MBBS, PhD, MPH
Professor, Head of Imaging Research Lab
Baker Heart and Diabetes Institute, Melbourne, Australia
Menzies Institute for Medical Research, Hobart, Australia
Hobart, Australia

Rhonda Miyasaka, MD
Director of Transesophageal Echocardiography
Section of Cardiovascular Imaging
Department of Cardiovascular Medicine
Cleveland Clinic
Cleveland, Ohio

Victor Mor-Avi, PhD
Research Professor
Director of Cardiac Imaging Research
Department of Medicine/Section of Cardiology
University of Chicago
Chicago, Illinois

Sherif F. Nagueh, MD
Professor of Cardiology at HM Academic Institute
Professor of Medicine at Weill Cornell Medicine
Medical Director of Echocardiography at Houston Methodist and the DeBakey Heart & Vascular Center
Houston, Texas

Gian M. Novaro, MD
Director, Echocardiography Laboratory
Department of Cardiovascular Medicine
Heart, Thoracic and Vascular Institute
Cleveland Clinic Florida
Weston, Florida

Mary Philip, MD
Department of Cardiology
La Timone Hospital, Aix-Marseille University
Marseille, France

Philippe Pibarot, DVM, PhD
Full Professor
Department of Medicine
Laval University
Quebec City, Quebec, Canada

Juan Carlos Plana, MD, FACC, FASE
Associate Professor of Medicine
Section of Cardiology
Department of Medicine
Baylor College of Medicine
Houston, Texas

Zoran B. Popovic, MD, PhD
Associate Professor of Medicine
Cleveland Clinic Lerner College of Medicine of Case Western Reserve University
Staff
Department of Cardiovascular Medicine
Cleveland Clinic
Cleveland, Ohio

Thomas R. Porter, MD
Professor of Medicine
Theodore F. Hubbard Distinguished Chair of Cardiology
Division of Cardiovascular Medicine
University of Nebraska Medical Center
Omaha, Nebraska

Nishath Quader, MD
Associate Professor of Medicine
Division of Cardiovascular Medicine
Washington University-St Louis
St. Louis, Missouri

L. Leonardo Rodriguez, MD
Program Director, Advanced Imaging
Section of Cardiovascular Imaging
Department of Cardiovascular Medicine
Cleveland Clinic
Cleveland, Ohio

Alejandro Sanchez-Nadales, MD
Fellow
Department of Cardiovascular Medicine
Heart, Thoracic and Vascular Institute
Cleveland Clinic Florida
Weston, Florida

Muhamed Saric, MD, PhD
Professor of Medicine
Leon H Charney Division of Cardiology
Department of Medicine
NYU Grossman School of Medicine
New York University Langone Health
New York, New York

Igal A. Sebag, MD, FRCPC, FACC, FASE
Associate Professor of Medicine
Department of Echocardiography and Non-Invasive Cardiology
McGill University
Montreal, Quebec, Canada

Partho P. Sengupta, MD, DM, FACC, FASE
Henry Rutgers Professor of Cardiology
Chief of Cardiovascular Disease and Hypertension
Rutgers Robert Wood Johnson Medical School
Chief of Cardiovascular Services
Robert Wood Johnson University Hospital
New Brunswick, New Jersey

Jeremy Slivnick, MD
Assistant Professor
Section of General Internal Medicine
Section of Cardiovascular Medicine
Deparment of Medicine
The University of Chicago Pritzker School of Medicine
Chicago, Illinois

Raymond F. Stainback, MD
Associate Professor
Section of Cardiology
Department of Medicine
Baylor College of Medicine
Houston, Texas

Jordan B. Strom, MD, MSc.
Assistant Professor of Medicine
Harvard Medical School
Director, Echocardiography Laboratory
Beth Israel Deaconess Medical Center
Boston, Massachusetts

Daniel Sykora, MD, MS
Resident
Department of Internal Medicine
Mayo Clinic
Rochester, Minnesota

James D. Thomas, MD, FASE, FACC, FESC
Professor of Medicine
Northwestern University Feinberg School of Medicine
Director, Center for Heart Valve Disease
Director, Academic Affairs
Bluhm Cardiovascular Institute
Northwestern Medicine
Lead Scientist for Ultrasound, NASA
Past-President, American Society of Echocardiography
Chicago, Illinois

Chrissy Thomson, DMU (Cardiac), BSc
Sessional Academic
Graduate Diploma in Cardiac Ultrasound
Queensland University of Technology
Brisbane, Australia

Dennis A. Tighe, MD
Professor
Department of Medicine
UMass Chan Medical School
Worcester, Massachusetts

Wendy Tsang, MD
Associate Professor
Division of Cardiology
University of Toronto
Toronto, Ontario, Canada

Dipan Uppal, MD
Fellow
Department of Cardiovascular Medicine
Heart, Thoracic and Vascular Institute
Cleveland Clinic Florida
Weston, Florida

Pieter van der Bijl, MD, PhD
Research Affiliate
Heart Lung Center
Leiden University Medical Center
Leiden, The Netherlands

Tom Kai Ming Wang, MBChB, MD
Assistant Professor
Cleveland Clinic Lerner College of Medicine of Case Western Reserve University
Staff Cardiologist
Section of Cardiovascular Imaging
Department of Cardiovascular Medicine
Heart, Vascular and Thoracic Institute
Cleveland Clinic
Cleveland, Ohio

Lynn Weinert, BS, RDCS
Section of Cardiology
Department of Medicine
The University of Chicago Pritzker School of Medicine
Chicago, Illinois

Terrence D. Welch, MD
Associate Professor of Medicine
Section of Cardiovascular Medicine
Heart and Vascular Center
Dartmouth-Hitchcock Medical Center
Lebanon, New Hampshire

Priscilla Wessly, MD, FACC
Structural Imaging, Department of Cardiology
Aurora St Luke's Medical Center
Advocate Aurora Health
Milwaukee, Wisconsin

Feng Xie, MD
Professor of Medicine
Division of Cardiovascular Medicine
Department of Medicine
University of Nebraska College of Medicine
University of Nebraska Medical Center
Omaha, Nebraska

FOREWORD

Beginning as A-mode vertical lines to depict cardiac structures in 1954, echocardiography now 70 years later has become an essential cardiac diagnostic and management tool by capturing 2D and 3D cardiovascular images and determining intracardiac as well as valvular hemodynamics. Once only as a tool for cardiologists, echocardiography is now performed by anesthesiologists, critical care providers, emergency room staff, cardiac radiologists, internists, trainees, and medical students for intraoperative study, interventional procedures, POCUS, and education as well as comprehensive diagnostic purposes.

There are many different ways to train or teach echocardiography. Since the ultimate goal of echocardiography study is to make a definitive diagnosis and to help manage patients, case-based approach is one of the most effective methods. *Clinical Echocardiography Review: A Self-Assessment Tool* by Drs. Klein, Asher, and Chetrit provides more than 1000 clinical cases of Echocardiography written by national and international experts in the field. Each case has a stepwise approach to help learners to understand the basic to the most challenging aspects of echocardiography.

Each chapter of the book was carefully designed and written to reflect the entire spectrum of echocardiography findings of unique, simple and challenging, cases pertaining to the chapter. Each case has clinical history and pertinent physical examination findings, followed by M-mode, 2D imaging, 3D imaging, and Doppler interpretation as necessary to make a correct diagnosis. Whenever appropriate, national and society guidelines are utilized to determine the severity of each condition and to provide teaching points. All case studies were obtained from responsible author's clinical experience or practice so that similar clinical echocardiographic scenarios will be encountered by the learners.

Echocardiography technology and its clinical applications continue to increase. Since the 2nd edition of this book, there has been an explosion of new interventional procedures requiring echocardiographic guidance as well as selection of patients and increasing use of strain imaging to detect early myocardial dysfunction and increased filling pressures. This 3rd edition dedicates several chapters to those new areas of clinical applications with illustrative cases.

Whether you are an experienced echocardiographer, a skillful sonographer, a medical professional interested in POCUS, a trainee, or a medical student, this *Clinical Echocardiography Review: A Self-Assessment Tool* will serve you well to understand echocardiography diagnostic features better, to expand your utilization of newer techniques, and to most of all provide a better care of your patients.

Jae K. Oh, MD
Samsung Professor of Cardiovascular Medicine
Mayo Clinic, Rochester, MN
President, Asian-Pacific Association of Echocardiography

FOREWORD

The publication of the 3rd edition of *Clinical Echocardiography Review* coincides with the 70th anniversary of the first published description of echocardiography by Drs. Inge Edler and Carl Hellmuth Hertz in 1954. Also, it is almost 60 years since Dr. Harvey Feigenbaums's publication describing diagnosis of pericardial effusion by echocardiography. Both events form the foundation for what has become the indispensable role of echocardiography for managing our patients.

Since those early descriptions of transthoracic M-mode echocardiography, the cardiac ultrasound technology has steadily evolved with the development of two-dimensional imaging, three-dimensional imaging, transesophageal imaging, contrast-enhanced imaging (including myocardial perfusion), Doppler assessment of intracardiac flow, hemodynamics and myocardial function, and, most recently, feature (speckle) tracking for assessment of myocardial mechanics. Miniaturization of devices has brought echocardiography to the point of care and even integration into the physical examination. Transmission of digital images (even wirelessly) allows experts to have access to the images and provide interpretations even when the studies are performed on the other side of the world. Artificial intelligence applications of machine learning algorithms and deep learning models can guide accurate image acquisition, perform near real-time measurements and diagnoses, and even identify features on echocardiograms not discernible to the human eye that are associated with specific diseases and prognosis. With all of these advances, the applications and the types of users of echocardiography continue to broaden.

While it remains important to have experts in echocardiographic performance and interpretation, given the wide use of echocardiography it has become important for all cardiologists and many in other disciplines of medicine to have a practical knowledge of the technique. This new edition of *Clinical Echocardiography Review* serves as an excellent tool for learning echocardiography for all these users of the technology. Dr. Allan Klein and his co-editors have assembled experts in the field to provide this education.

The approach of this book is unique in that the reader is introduced to each topic (and chapter) by a series of questions or cases that include high-quality still-frame and moving images. Comprehensive answers to each question provide a logical discussion of each topic. By answering the questions and reviewing the answers, the reader can quickly identify their areas of strengths and weaknesses. As stated in the subtitle of the book, Klein and colleagues provide an effective tool for self-assessment. The comprehensive answers to each question provide a strong resource to reinforce existing knowledge and fill in the readers' knowledge gaps. Key references are provided for those who wish more details on a topic.

This book is clinically oriented with a focus on disease diagnosis, patient management, and prognosis. Even the chapters on physics and artifacts are presented in a manner that enables the reader to understand how these technical issues impact image formation, which hopefully leads to improvements in image interpretation. New enhancements in this 3rd edition include more extensive chapters on individual valve diseases and interventional echo and a chapter on technologies that are new since the last edition.

I am sure that all users of echocardiography will enjoy interacting with this unique book.

Michael H. Picard, MD
Professor of Medicine, Harvard Medical School and Massachusetts General Hospital
Emeritus Editor in Chief, Journal of the American Society of Echocardiography
Boston, Massachusetts

PREFACE

We are delighted with the Third edition of this interactive and updated textbook entitled *Clinical Echocardiography Review: A Self-Assessment Tool*. In 2024, echocardiography continues to grow in technology, importance, volume, and diversity of users. In our contemporary era, point-of-care ultrasound, 3D and strain imaging, and structural interventional echocardiography have become mainstream tools. In addition, echocardiography has moved beyond the realm of the cardiologist and is performed regularly by emergency room physicians, intensivists, and anesthesiologists. The busy physician must keep up with the latest in the changing knowledge base of cardiac ultrasound. This book focuses on the time-tested way of "the Socratic method" to teach essential concepts in a multiple-choice question and answer format. The book emphasizes diagnostic interpretation rather than clinical management.

While the 1st edition of this text was 28 chapters, the Third edition has expanded to 35 chapters plus a tabular appendix ranging from fundamentals to new technologies and including a section of equations and formulas. The format of most chapters remains the same. There are multiple-choice questions followed by detailed answers, and then questions associated with a still-frame graphic and then answers. Finally, there are case-based questions associated with images and videos for which the online version will be required, but viewable on a mobile phone or computer. In the answer section, key points are highlighted as well as an increased number of figures and tables that summarize important clinical pearls. There are also key references and many guidelines-related algorithms. This format and emphasis on salient points mirror the way we teach our trainees to read echocardiograms. It also reminds the clinical cardiologist to look out for common and unusual findings (occasional "zebras") that will be encountered during echocardiography reads.

We have chosen leading national and international experts, also known educators in the field of echocardiography. We are delighted to have added a co-editor, Dr. Michael Chetrit, a younger-generation multimodality trained expert and leader in cardiovascular imaging, who assured we identified content that is important to trainees and recent graduates. We review the basics from physics (expanded from 1 to 2 chapters), artifacts, Doppler hemodynamics, chamber quantification, and ultrasound-enhancing agents to more clinically oriented topics including valvular heart disease, myocardial, pericardial and aortic disease, and coronary and congenital heart disease. Coverage of interventional echocardiography guiding structural heart disease and mechanical support therapies has broadened in scope, and new technologies including 3D echocardiography, strain, and cardio-oncology have been updated.

Clinical Echocardiography Review: A Self-Assessment Tool was among the first and most comprehensive echocardiographic review books available with over 1000 questions and answers. We hope you will find this hardcopy text and the online version enjoyable, instructive, user-friendly, and beneficial to your career in Cardiology.

Allan L. Klein, MD, FRCP(C), FACC,
FAHA, FASE, FESC
Craig R. Asher, MD, FACC, FASE
Michael Chetrit, MD, FRCP(C), FACC

ACKNOWLEDGMENTS

We would like to thank Marilyn, Jared, Lauren, Jordan, Jean and Sam Klein and Diann, Drew, Laura and George Asher and Laurel Levey as well as Laura Bendavid, in addition to Skylar and Kenzie Chetrit for their inspiration, encouragement, patience, and unwavering support of our careers and time editing this book. In addition, we would like to thank our leadership and colleagues at the Cleveland Clinic for their support and commitment to educational endeavors as one of the basic missions of our institution.

We would also like to thank Marie Phillips who assisted us with the preparation of the text beginning with the 1st edition. Finally, we would like to express gratitude to Wolters Kluwer, and in particular to Sean Hanrahan and Ashley Fischer for their assistance with the day-to-day work of communications with the authors, editing, and formatting the book and altogether striving to making it a great success.

CONTENTS

Contributors iii | Foreword ix | Foreword x | Preface xi | Acknowledgments xii

1 Physics: Fundamentals of Ultrasound Imaging and Instrumentation (Part 1) 1
Victor Mor-Avi, Lynn Weinert, and James D. Thomas

2 Physics: Basic Principles (Part 2) 17
Bonita Anderson and Chrissy Thomson

3 Cardiac Ultrasound Artifacts 34
Craig R. Asher, Zoran B. Popovic, and Bonita Anderson

4 M-Mode Echocardiography 57
Gerard P. Aurigemma and Dennis A. Tighe

5 Assessment of Chamber Quantification 76
Wendy Tsang, Jeremy Slivnick, and Roberto M. Lang

6 Three-Dimensional Echocardiography 104
Tiffany Dong and Rhonda Miyasaka

7 Transesophageal Echocardiography and Intraoperative Echocardiography 124
Ben Alencherry, Nakul S. Kumar, and L. Leonardo Rodriguez

8 Doppler and Hemodynamics 142
Daniel Bamira and Muhamed Saric

9 Tissue Doppler and Strain 198
Juan Carlos Plana and Srikanth Koneru

10 Contrast-Enhanced Ultrasound Imaging 212
Thomas R. Porter and Feng Xie

11 Systolic Function Assessment 227
Thomas H. Marwick

12 Diastology 248
Tahir S. Kafil, Patrick H. Collier, Tom Kai Ming Wang, and Allan L. Klein

13 Stress Echocardiography: Ischemic and Nonischemic 274
Edgar Argulian

14 Dyssynchrony Evaluation/Atrioventricular Optimization 298
Pieter van der Bijl, Victoria Delgado, and Jeroen J. Bax

15 Aortic Stenosis 323
Marie-Annick Clavel, Jordi S. Dahl, and Philippe Pibarot

16 Aortic Regurgitation 346
Joshua A. Cohen and Milind Desai

17 Mitral Regurgitation 360
Maurice Enriquez-Sarano

18 Mitral Stenosis 381
Mary Philip and Igal A. Sebag

19 Pulmonic and Tricuspid Valvular Disease 397
Diarmaid Hughes and Brian P. Griffin

20 Prosthetic Valves 414
Linda D. Gillam, Leo Marcoff, and Konstantinos P. Koulogiannis

21 Endocarditis 433
Lawrence Lau and Kwan Leung Chan

22 Interventional Echocardiography: Mitral, Aortic, and Prosthetic Valve Interventions 456
Stephen H. Little, Priscilla Wessly, and Nadeen N. Faza

23 Interventional Echocardiography: Tricuspid Valve, Septum, Left Atrial Appendage, and Hypertrophic Cardiomyopathy 477
Nishath Quader

24 Cardiomyopathies 496
Antonio Lewis-Camarago and Craig R. Asher

25 Durable and Temporary Left Ventricular Mechanical Circulatory Support Devices and Orthotopic Heart Transplantation 530
Basant Arya and Raymond F. Stainback

26 Systemic Disease 550
Daniel Sykora and Sunil Mankad

27 Pericardial Diseases 579
Terrence D. Welch

28 Aortic Diseases 598
Alejandro Sanchez-Nadales, Craig R. Asher, and Gian M. Novaro

29 Atrial Fibrillation 619
Maria Fadous and Jordan B. Strom

30 Right Ventricular Disease and Pulmonary Hypertension 632
Dimitrios Maragiannis and Sherif F. Nagueh

31 Tumors, Masses, and Source of Emboli 652
Mohamed Al-Kazaz, Madeline Jankowski, and Kameswari Maganti

32 Noncyanotic Congenital Heart Disease 671
Benjamin W. Eidem

33 Cyanotic Congenital Heart Disease 688
Pooja Gupta and James M. Galas

34 Cardiovascular Point-of-Care Ultrasound for the Noncardiologist 710
Amer M. Johri, Braeden Hill, and Benjamin T. Galen

35 New Technologies and Expanding Utility of Ultrasound 727
Sasha-ann East and Partho P. Sengupta

Appendix
Equations and Formulas 738
Dipan Uppal, Michael Chetrit, and Craig R. Asher

Index 746

CHAPTER 1

Physics: Fundamentals of Ultrasound Imaging and Instrumentation (Part 1)

Victor Mor-Avi, Lynn Weinert, and James D. Thomas

QUESTIONS

1. Sound waves cannot travel through which one of the following:
   A. Water.
   B. Air.
   C. Metal.
   D. Vacuum.

2. Ultrasound is a pressure wave with a frequency above the range of human hearing, which is:
   A. 200 Hz.
   B. 2 kHz.
   C. 20,000 Hz.
   D. 200 kHz.

3. The frequency of a sound wave is measured in hertz as the:
   A. Inverse of the wavelength.
   B. Maximal amplitude of particle vibration.
   C. Number of times particles vibrate each second in the direction perpendicular to wave propagation.
   D. Number of times particles vibrate each second in the direction of wave propagation.

4. Ultrasound imaging is usually performed using frequencies in the range of:
   A. 1 to 30 kHz.
   B. Below 5 MHz.
   C. Above 0.5 MHz.
   D. 1 to 30 MHz.

5. Assuming that sound velocity in muscle tissue is 1600 m/s, the wavelength of a sound wave with the frequency of 1.6 MHz is:
   A. 1 mm.
   B. 1 cm.
   C. 1 m.
   D. 0.1 mm.

6. As an ultrasound wave travels through the human body, the type of tissue that results in the fastest loss of its strength is:
   A. Fat.
   B. Bone.
   C. Lung.
   D. Blood.

7. The main goal of the gel used during ultrasound imaging is to:
   A. Disinfect the transducer.
   B. Cool the transducer.
   C. To numb the skin and thus reduce patient's discomfort caused by pressure.
   D. To improve the contact between transducer surface and the skin.

8. Materials that respond to acoustic waves by generating electric signals and vice versa are known as:
   A. Doppler crystals.
   B. Acoustic coupling gels.
   C. Piezoelectric crystals.
   D. Chronotropic agents.

9. Doppler effect refers to:
   A. Change in strength of a sound wave reflected by a moving target.
   B. Change in frequency of a sound wave reflected by a moving target.
   C. Change in shape of a sound wave reflected by a moving target.
   D. Loss of ultrasound energy as a result of wave dissipation by flow.

10. Doppler angle is the angle between:
    A. The flow and the long axis of the left ventricle.
    B. The ultrasound beam and the long axis of the left ventricle.
    C. The flow and the transmitted ultrasound beam.
    D. The flow and the central axis of the transducer.

11. A positive Doppler shift indicates that the reflector is moving:
    A. Faster than the sound wave propagates.
    B. Directly toward the transducer.
    C. Directly away from the transducer.
    D. Closer to the transducer, so that the angle between the direction of the beam and the direction of motion is >90°.

12. A Doppler shift of zero indicates that the reflector is stationary or:
    A. Moving in a direction perpendicular to the beam.
    B. Moving in a direction parallel to the beam.
    C. Moving in a direction perpendicular to the central axis of the transducer.
    D. Moving too fast to register.

13. Time gain compensation (**Figure 1.1**) is part of the ultrasound image formation aimed at correcting image intensity for variations in ultrasound _____ caused by different media.
    A. scattering
    B. absorption
    C. reflection
    D. attenuation

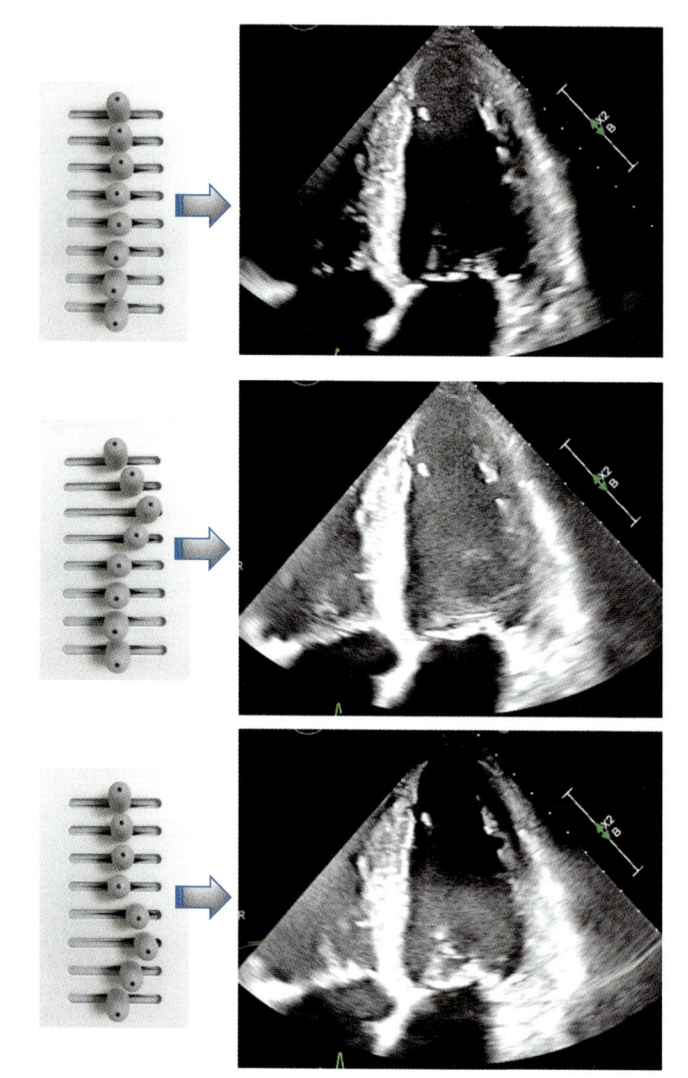

Figure 1.1

14. The strength of the transmitted ultrasound wave is controlled by adjusting the:
    A. Time gain compensation controls.
    B. Compression control.
    C. Power control.
    D. Overall gain control.

15. The spatial resolution of an ultrasound image is defined as the:
    A. Smallest distance between two objects that allows distinction between them.
    B. Size of the smallest object that can be clearly visualized in its entirety.
    C. Smallest cluster of pixels that can define a single object.
    D. Smallest difference in the size of an object that can be visually detected.

16. The spatial resolution of an ultrasound image is equal to the:
   A. Gap between two adjacent pixels.
   B. Twice the wavelength.
   C. Size of a pixel in the relevant direction.
   D. One-half of the wavelength.

17. The temporal resolution of a sequence of ultrasound images is defined by the:
   A. Shortest duration of an event that can be detected with confidence.
   B. Shortest time in which image information can change completely.
   C. Shortest time between two events that allows distinction between them.
   D. Shortest time in which pixel values can change.

18. Which of the following phrase is meaningless?
   A. Spatial resolution.
   B. Temporal resolution.
   C. Frequency resolution.
   D. Contrast resolution.

19. The temporal resolution of a sequence of ultrasound images is equal to the:
   A. Inverse of transducer frequency.
   B. Inverse of frame rate.
   C. One cycle of the ultrasound wave.
   D. Inverse of the number of frames in the sequence.

20. The dynamic range of echoes displayed on the screen is adjusted by the:
   A. Time gain compensation controls.
   B. Compression control.
   C. Transmit power control.
   D. Overall gain control.

21. As the frequency of ultrasound increases, the maximum imaging depth in the human body:
   A. Increases.
   B. Decreases.
   C. Remains unchanged.
   D. May increase or decrease depending on the mechanical index used.

22. Increasing which of the following can **BEST** compensate for image losses due to attenuation?
   A. Dynamic range.
   B. Gain.
   C. Frame rate.
   D. Depth.

23. Decreasing which of the following increases the contrast of the image?
   A. Dynamic range.
   B. Gain.
   C. Power.
   D. Baseline shift.

24. The energy of the transmitted ultrasound wave can be changed by adjusting which of the following?
   A. Gain.
   B. Dynamic range.
   C. Pulse repetition frequency.
   D. Power.

25. Filtering eliminates "ghosting" artifact by removing which of the following?
   A. Low-velocity signals.
   B. Acoustic shadowing.
   C. Mirroring.
   D. Aliasing.

26. With time gain compensation, the machine is generally preset to perform which of the following actions?
   A. Decrease signal in near field, increase signal in far field.
   B. Decrease signal in near field, decrease signal in far field.
   C. Increase signal in near field, increase signal in far field.
   D. Increase signal in near field, decrease signal in far field.

27. To better assess rapidly moving structures, a sonographer should perform which of the following actions?
  A. Narrow scan sector and decrease imaging depth.
  B. Narrow scan sector and increase imaging depth.
  C. Widen scan sector and decrease imaging depth.
  D. Widen scan sector and increase imaging depth.

28. To reduce aliasing on color flow Doppler, a sonographer should perform which of the following actions?
  A. Reduce the angle between the ultrasound beam and direction of flow.
  B. Reduce the color scale.
  C. Baseline shift away from the direction of flow.
  D. Increase the depth of the image.

29. If a rapidly moving structure such as a cardiac valve appears to be moving in slow motion, which one of the following may be set too high?
  A. Frame rate.
  B. Sector size.
  C. Nyquist limit.
  D. Persistence.

30. Image resolution for a region of interest can be improved by which of the following?
  A. Increasing the read zoom.
  B. Increasing the write zoom.
  C. Increasing the sector width.
  D. Increasing the dynamic range.

31. Increasing scan line density with a fixed sector width results in which of the following?
  A. Increase in frame rate.
  B. Increase in zoom.
  C. Increase in temporal resolution.
  D. Increase in spatial resolution.

32. After capturing the images shown in **Figure 1.2A**, another image was obtained by increasing imaging frequency in **Figure 1.2B**. The image in **Figure 1.2B** has:

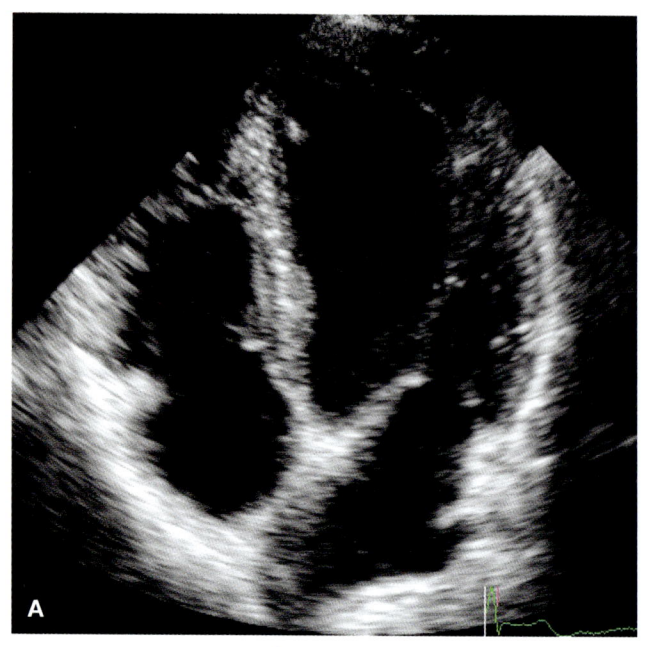

Figure 1.2A

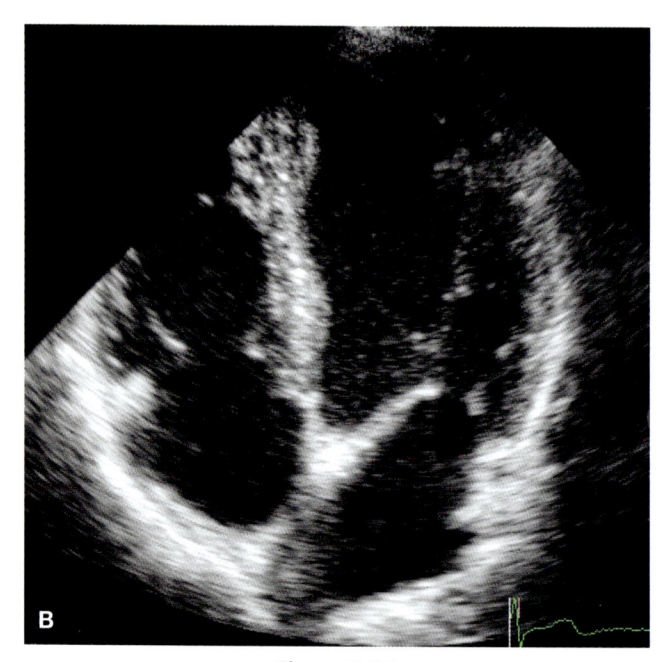

Figure 1.2B

  A. Bigger imaging depth.
  B. Better temporal resolution.
  C. Better spatial resolution.
  D. Less acoustic shadowing.

33. After capturing the image shown in **Figure 1.3A**, another image was obtained by switching to the harmonic mode in **Figure 1.3B**. **Figure 1.3B** was created from reflections of ultrasound of:
   A. Double the frequency of the transmitted waves.
   B. Half the frequency of the transmitted waves.
   C. Same frequency as the transmitted waves generated by resonating particles.
   D. Half the frequency of the transmitted waves generated by nonlinear reflectors.

34. After capturing the image shown in **Figure 1.4A**, another image was obtained by reducing imaging depth in **Figure 1.4B**. Which of the two images has lower frame rate?
   A. **Figure 1.4A**.
   B. **Figure 1.4B**.
   C. Both image sequences have identical frame rates.
   D. Impossible to determine without knowing how wavelength responded to the change.

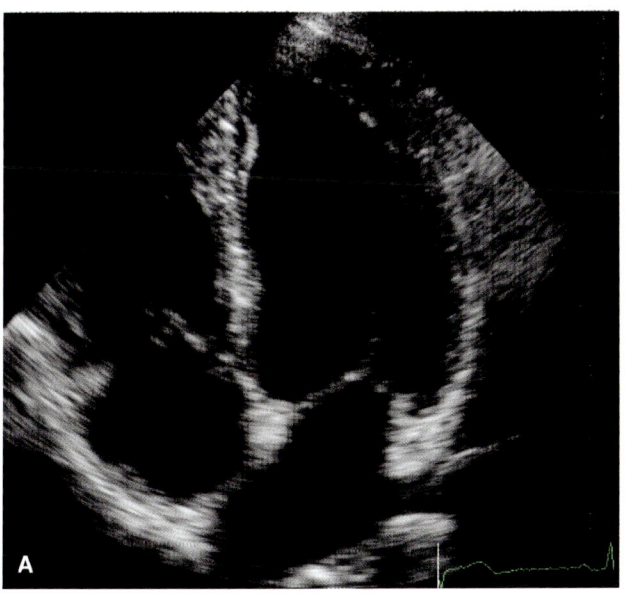

Figure 1.3A

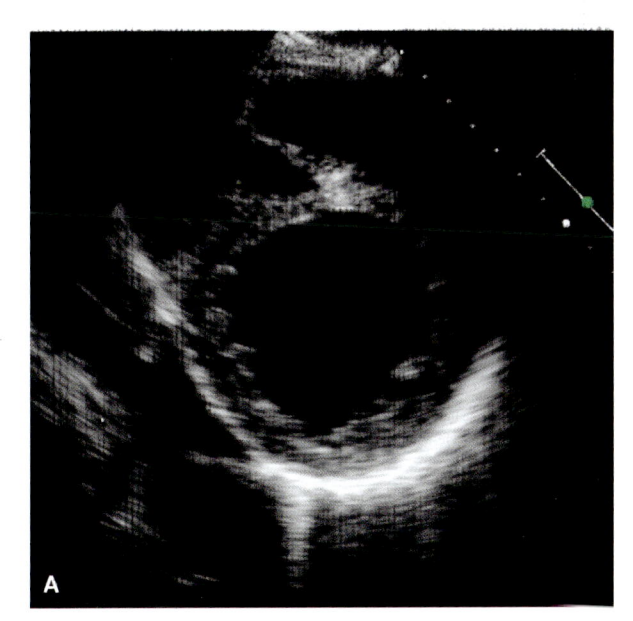

Figure 1.4A

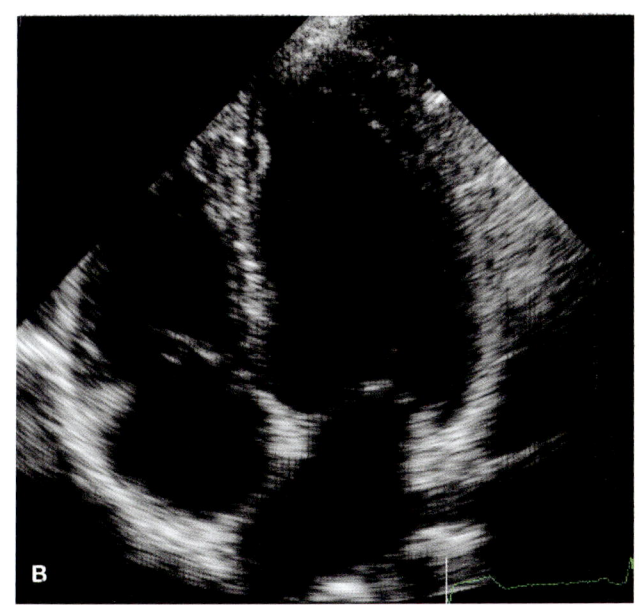

Figure 1.3B

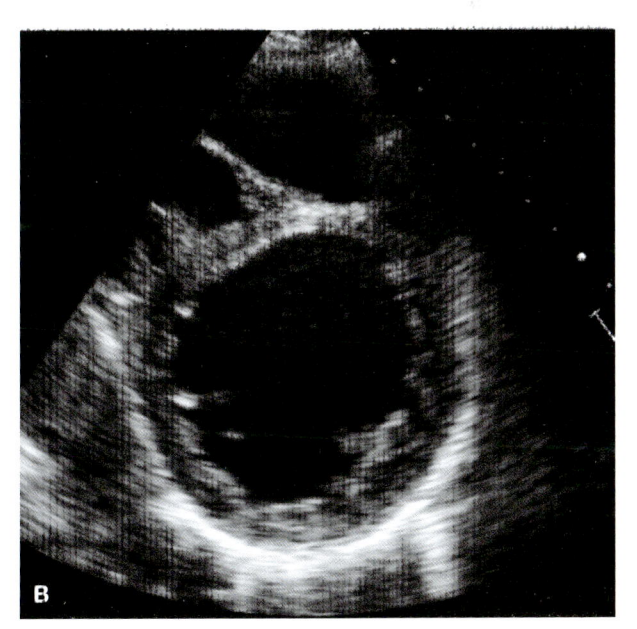

Figure 1.4B

35. After capturing the image sequence shown in **Figure 1.5A**, another sequence was obtained by reducing the sector angle in **Figure 1.5B**. The latter sequence has:
  A. Better spatial resolution.
  B. Lower temporal resolution.
  C. Higher frame rate.
  D. More scan lines per pixel.

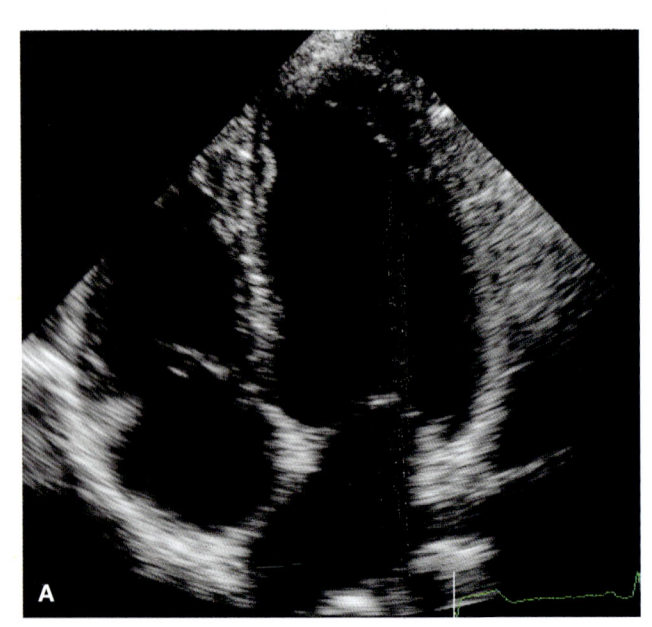

Figure 1.5A

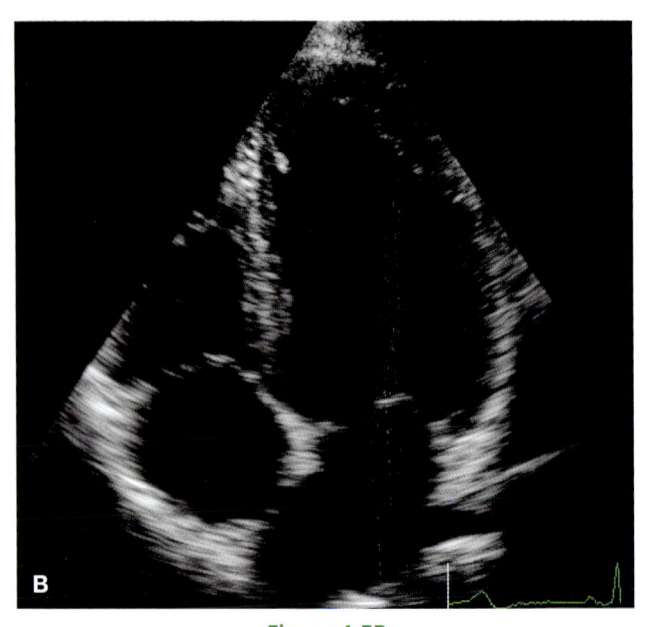

Figure 1.5B

36. Of the following statements, which one **DOES NOT** apply to **Figure 1.6**?
  A. It displays ultrasound reflections along a single scan line over time.
  B. It displays power spectrum of velocities measured along a single scan line over time.
  C. It has higher temporal resolution than two-dimensional imaging.
  D. It allows simultaneous visualization of different anatomical structures.

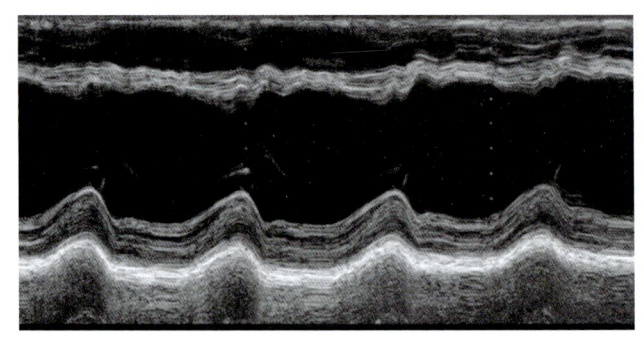

Figure 1.6

37. Of the following statements, which one **DOES NOT** apply to **Figure 1.7**?
  A. It displays ultrasound reflections along a single scan line over time.
  B. It displays power spectrum of velocities measured along a single scan line over time.
  C. It has higher temporal resolution than two-dimensional imaging.
  D. It is used to obtain information about distribution of flow velocities.

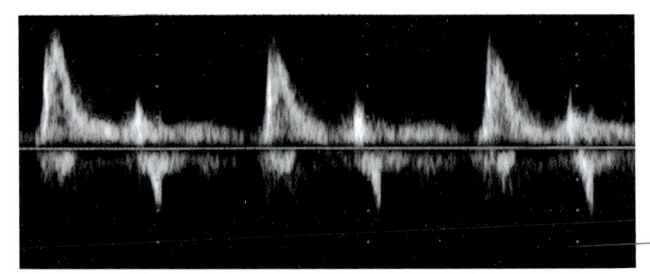

Figure 1.7

38. Continuous spectral Doppler image displays the strength of each velocity component by assigning to them:
  A. Different gray scale levels.
  B. Different height of the deflections.
  C. Different slopes of the deflections.
  D. Different colors in the color Doppler image.

39. The color pattern characterizing turbulent flow in the color flow Doppler image (**Figure 1.8**) can be described as:
   A. Disorganized.
   B. Spiral-shaped.
   C. Mosaic.
   D. Broken.

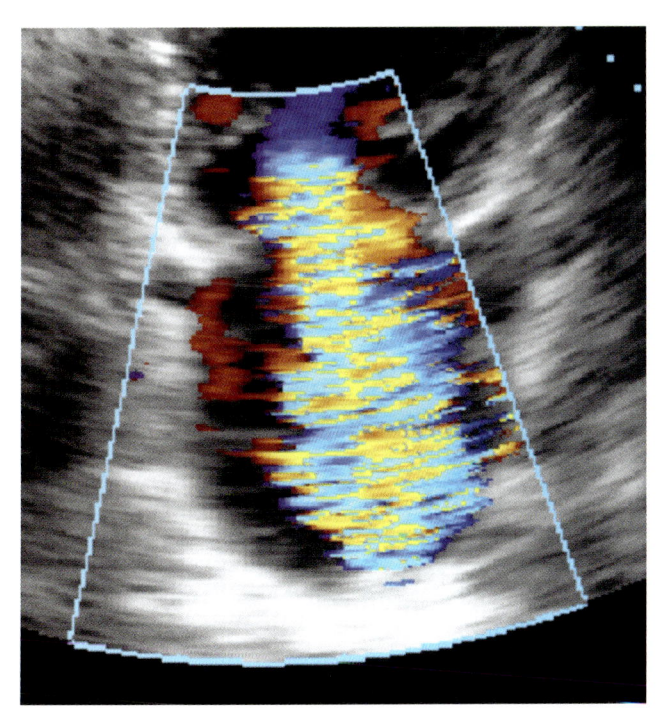

Figure 1.8

40. "Laminar flow" in a blood vessel means that flow velocities are:
   A. Completely disorganized and do not follow the laws of hydrodynamics.
   B. Highest along the central axis of the vessel and gradually decrease toward the walls.
   C. Low everywhere except the swirling around the central axis of the vessel.
   D. Same everywhere in the vessel.

41. Phased array transducers use differences in phase of pulses transmitted by individual elements to:
   A. Allow imaging the heart throughout the different phases of the cardiac cycle.
   B. Steer the ultrasound beam in different directions and thus scan a "slice" rather than a single line.
   C. Interrogate a range of flow velocities inside the heart by determining phase shifts caused by moving targets.
   D. Quickly switch the transducer between transmit and receive phases.

42. Echocardiographic contrast agents are based on the idea that ultrasound reflection is augmented by the:
   A. High content of gas in microbubbles.
   B. Added gas-liquid interface in the presence of microbubbles.
   C. High speed of sound waves in gas.
   D. Rapid motion of the microbubbles in blood.

43. One well-known artifact of ultrasound imaging is frequently referred to as "acoustic shadowing" depicted in **Figure 1.9**. The main cause of this artifact is the inability of the imaging system to accurately compensate for:
   A. Increased attenuation by a structure such as ventricular cavity.
   B. Reduced attenuation by structures such as ventricular cavity.
   C. Increased attenuation by structures such as contrast-filled ventricular cavity.
   D. Increased attenuation secondary to a temporary surge in frequency associated with the presence of contrast material.

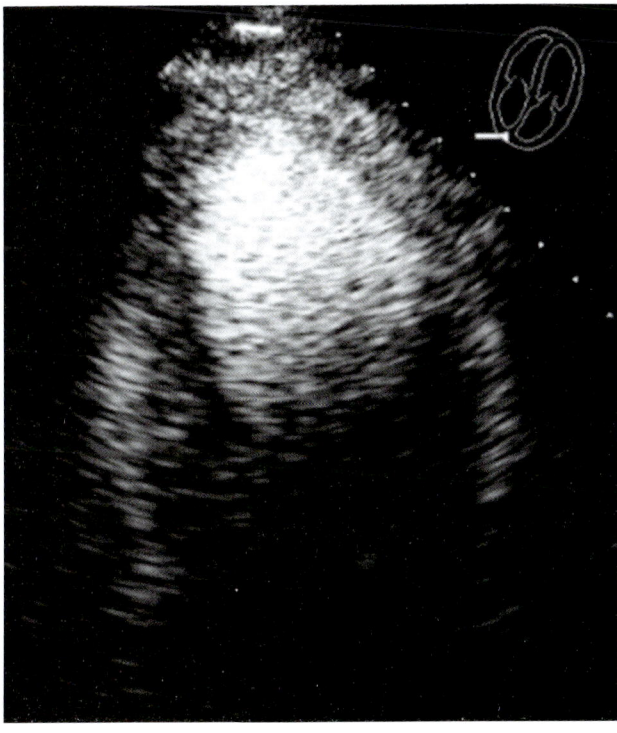

Figure 1.9

44. Shadowing artifacts (**Figure 1.10A**) can be effectively reduced as shown (**Figure 1.10B**) by using:
  A. Lower compression setting.
  B. Lower overall gain.
  C. Higher transmit power that destroys microbubbles.
  D. Less contrast material.

45. In **Figure 1.11A**, one of the following factors has been changed to improve resolution at the left ventricular apex, while in **Figure 1.11B**, it has been adjusted to improve resolution around the mitral valve. What factor is that?
  A. Dynamic range.
  B. Gain.
  C. Frame rate.
  D. Focus.

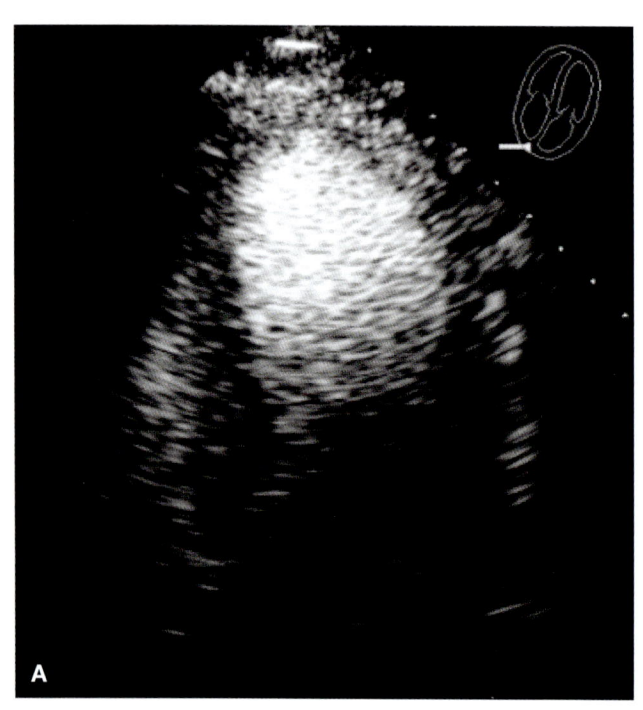

Figure 1.10A

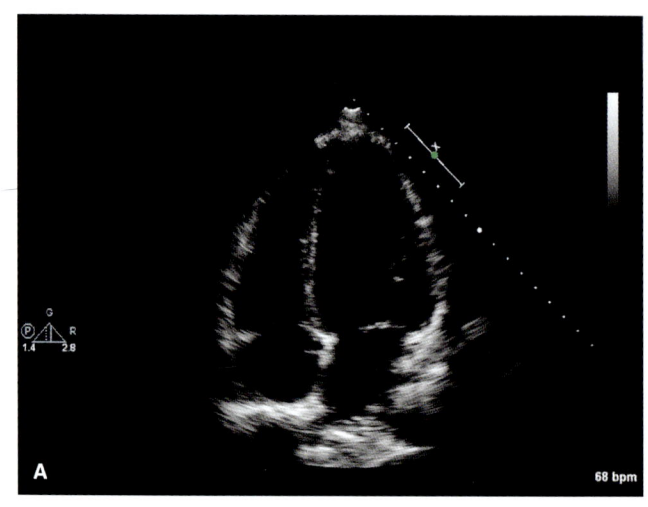

Figure 1.11A

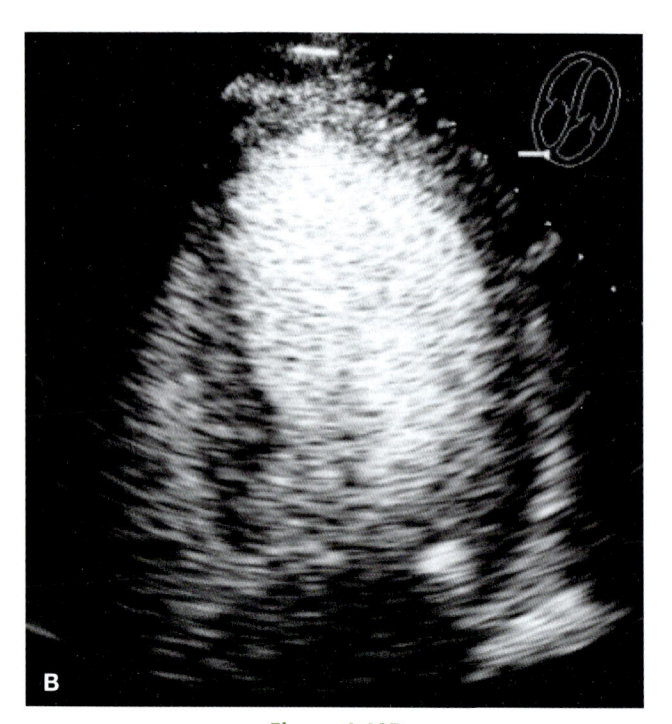

Figure 1.10B

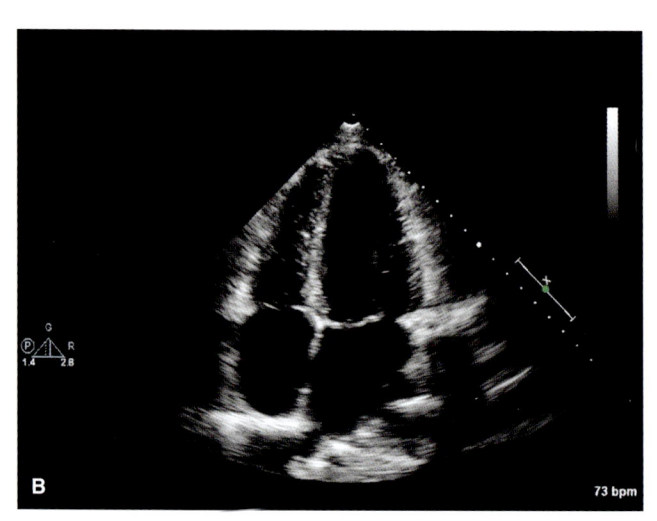

Figure 1.11B

46. Which of the following factors has been adjusted to result in greater contrast in **Figure 1.12B** compared with **Figure 1.12A**?
A. Compression.
B. Gain.
C. Sector width.
D. Power.

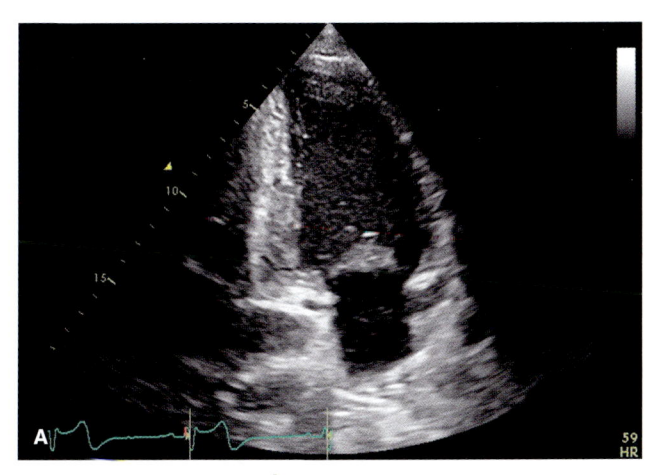

Figure 1.12A

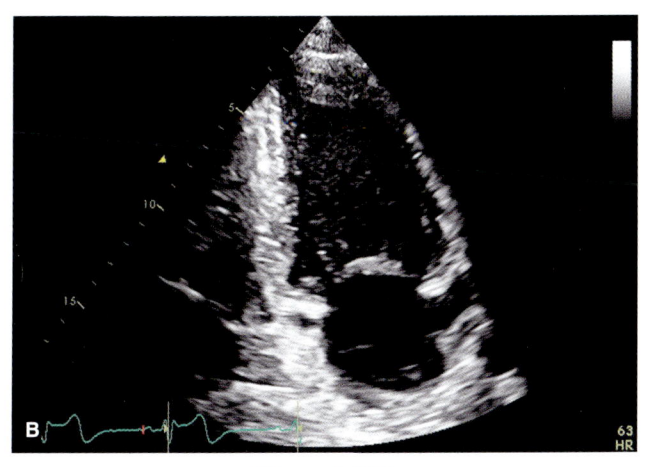

Figure 1.12B

47. In **Figure 1.13**, which of the following needs to be turned off to allow full visualization of the Doppler flow pattern?
A. Low-velocity filter.
B. High-velocity filter.
C. Persistence.
D. Compression.

48. What happened to the sweep speed to change the display from **Figure 1.14A** to **Figure 1.14B**?

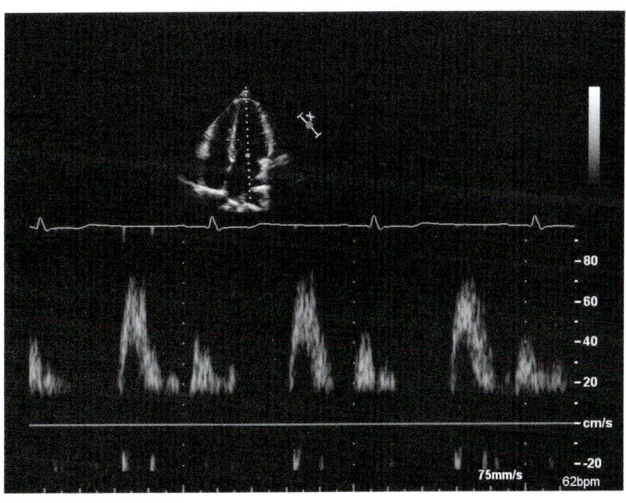

Figure 1.13

A. Increased.
B. Decreased.
C. Unchanged.
D. This change in appearance is due to a decrease in pulse repetition frequency.

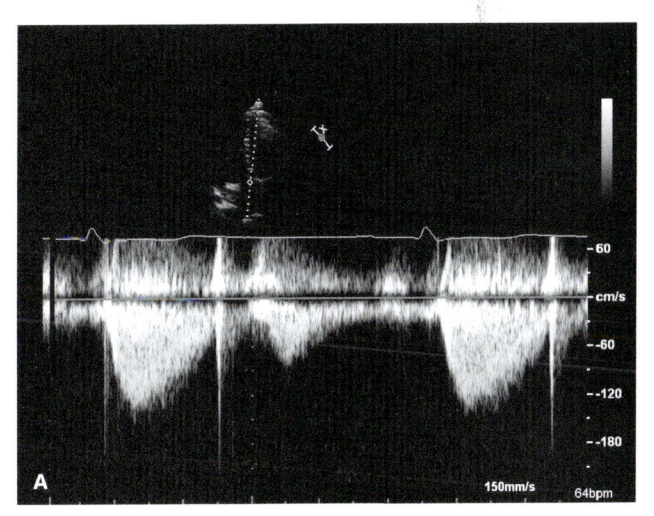

Figure 1.14A

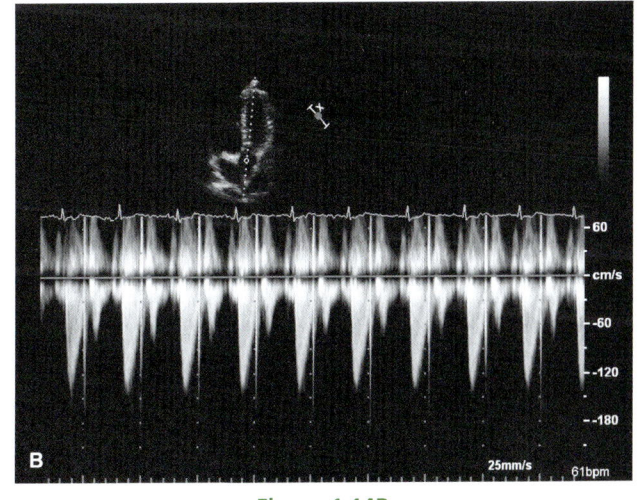

Figure 1.14B

10 / Clinical Echocardiography Review

49. In **Figure 1.15**, how should the time gain compensation (TGC) settings be adjusted in the near and far fields, respectively, to optimize the image?
   A. Decrease near field, decrease far field.
   B. Increase near field, increase far field.
   C. Decrease near field, increase far field.
   D. Increase near field, decrease far field.

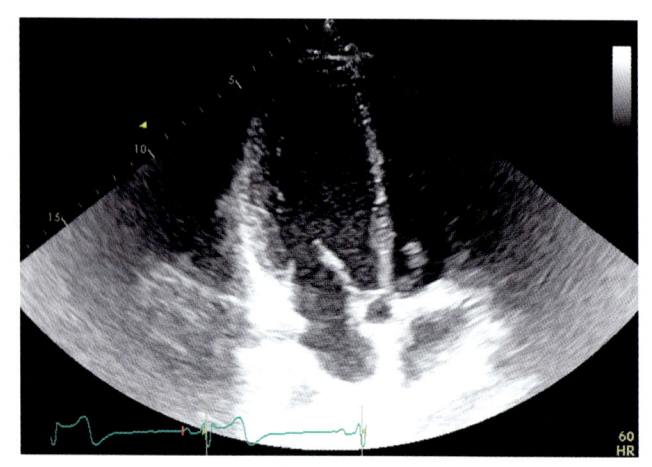

Figure 1.15

50. In ▶ **Video 1.1**, the color gain has been turned _____ resulting in _____ of the severity of the mitral regurgitation.
   A. too high, overestimation
   B. too high, underestimation
   C. too low, overestimation
   D. too low, underestimation

51. In ▶ **Video 1.2A** and **B**, the sonographer attempted to improve the _____ resolution of the valve, or the ability to observe for motion, by _____ the frame rate.
   A. temporal, increasing
   B. temporal, decreasing
   C. spatial, increasing
   D. spatial, decreasing

52. At the higher harmonics in the ▶ **Video 1.3**, typically proximal signals are _____ and deeper structures are _____.
   A. reduced, reduced
   B. enhanced, enhanced
   C. reduced, enhanced
   D. enhanced, reduced

53. In ▶ **Video 1.4**, color pixels have been averaged with adjacent pixels, producing more filling. This is called _____.
   A. inversion
   B. gain
   C. mapping
   D. smoothing

ANSWERS

1. **Answer: D.** Sound waves cannot travel in a vacuum, as pressure waves can be transmitted only through physical media consisting of molecules that interact with each other. Water, air, and metal are all such media and therefore sound waves can and indeed do travel in them.

2. **Answer: C.** The upper limit of the range of human hearing is 20,000 Hz or 20 kHz. There are animals that can hear sounds in different ranges than humans. For example, bats' hearing includes sounds in a much higher frequency range. This is known as supersonic hearing. They produce sound waves, which then echo back to them by bouncing off objects so that they know how far something is, just like a sonar on a submarine.

3. **Answer: D.** Frequency, in general, is measured in Hz (abbreviation for hertz), which is defined as 1/s. The frequency of a wave is defined as the number of times a particle in a conducting medium vibrates per unit time. Thus frequency is the inverse of the period. Since sound waves are pressure disturbance traveling in the medium in the direction of the particle vibrations, they are called longitudinal waves. In other words, sound waves are vibrations in the direction of wave propagation, and therefore this is the correct answer.

4. **Answer: D.** Ultrasound imaging is usually performed using frequencies in the range of 1 to 30 MHz (**Figure 1.16**). The lower frequencies in this range are used to image large organs or deeper structures that require significant penetration depth, while the higher frequencies are used for smaller and more superficial structures that require less depth but better spatial resolution.

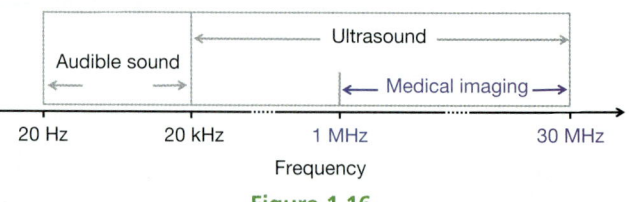

Figure 1.16

5. **Answer: A.** Wavelength, λ, is defined as the distance a wave travels during a single cycle. Wavelength can be calculated as the product of velocity, c, and the period, T, or alternatively the ratio of velocity and frequency, f:

$$\lambda = c \cdot T = \frac{c}{f} = \frac{1600 \text{ m/s}}{1.6 \text{ MHz}} = \frac{1.6 \cdot 10^3 \text{ m/s}}{1.6 \cdot 10^6 /\text{s}} = 10^{-3} = 1 \text{ mm}$$

Medium	Speed of Sound (m/s)
Blood	1560
Bone	4080
Fat	1460
Lung	600
Muscle	1600

6. **Answer: C.** Because of the high content of air and the abundance of highly reflective tissue/air interfaces, the sound waves dissipate in the lung so fast that the lungs are virtually opaque to ultrasound.
7. **Answer: D.** The main goal of the coupling gel is to improve the contact between transducer surface and the skin by eliminating any tissue/air interfaces, which are highly reflective and thus prevent ultrasound transmission into the body.
8. **Answer: C.** Piezoelectric crystals are materials that respond to electric signals by vibrating and generating acoustic waves and, vice versa, respond to acoustic waves by generating electric signals. These materials are the basis for medical ultrasound imaging, which relies on transmitting waves by "exciting" the crystals in the transducer by an electrical stimulus, and then receiving the ultrasound waves reflected by structures inside the body, and translating them back into electrical signals that are used to form an image of the reflecting structures.
9. **Answer: B.** Doppler effect refers to change in the frequency of a sound wave reflected by a moving target. The difference between the frequency of the sound wave received by the transducer (f_r) and the originally transmitted wave (f_t) signal can be calculated as:

$$\Delta f = f_r - f_t = 2f_t \frac{v \cos\theta}{c},$$

where v is the speed of the moving target, c is the speed of sound in the relevant media, and θ is the angle between the beam and the direction of the motion. Note that when the target moves toward the transducer, the angle θ is <90° and cos θ > 0, resulting in a positive change in frequency. In contrast, when the target moves away the transducer, the angle θ is >90° and cos θ < 0, resulting in a negative change in frequency. We are all familiar with the Doppler effect from our daily life: sound coming from a moving object has a higher pitch when the object approaches us than when the same object moves away from us. This is how we can tell if a train is approaching the station or leaving before we can actually see it (**Figure 1.17**). The factor of 2 in the equation above occurs because the ultrasound beam is actually Doppler shifted twice: once when absorbed by the moving red blood cells, then again when it is radiated back to the transducer.

10. **Answer: C.** Doppler angle is the angle between the direction of flow (in **Figure 1.18**, flow through the tricuspid valve indicated by the blue arrow) and that of the ultrasound beam (green line): angle "c". The orientation of either the ventricle relative to the flow (angle "a" between the flow direction and the long axis of the ventricle [pink line]; incorrect Answer A) or the transducer relative to the flow (angle "d" between the flow direction and the transducer's central axis [brown line]; incorrect Answer D) has no role in the interaction between ultrasound and moving blood cells that reflect ultrasound at a frequency that depends on the direction of blood flow along the beam. Clearly, the orientation of the ventricle relative to the beam (angle "b" between the beam and the long axis of the ventricle [pink line]; incorrect Answer B) has nothing to do with the flow and thus with the Doppler shift.

Like the train in Question 9, blood cells moving away from the transducer reflect sound with lower frequency than those moving toward the transducer. What determines whether the former or the latter is the case is the angle between the flow and the direction of the transmitted beam: when the angle

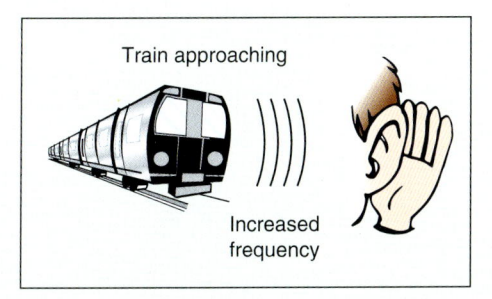

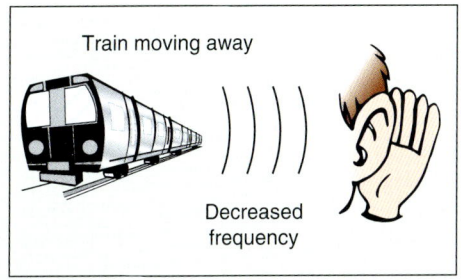

Figure 1.17

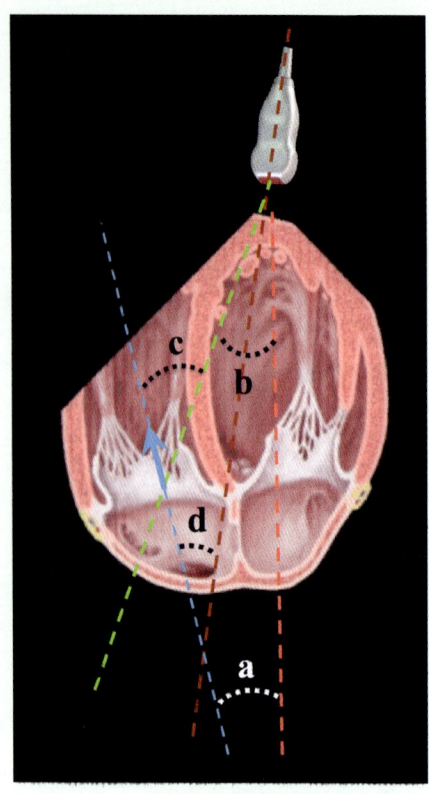

Figure 1.18

is >90°, then the flow is away from the transducer, and vice versa, when the angle is <90°, then the flow is toward the transducer.

11. **Answer: D.** A positive Doppler shift indicates that the reflector is moving so that the angle between the transmitted beam and the direction of flow is <90°; that is, the reflectors are getting closer, but not necessarily moving directly toward the transducer.

12. **Answer: A.** A Doppler shift of zero indicates that the reflector is stationary or moving in a direction perpendicular to the beam. Importantly, when the Doppler angle is 90°, the flow is neither toward nor away from the transducer; it is perpendicular to the beam and thus will produce no Doppler shift or, in other words, will reflect ultrasound at the same frequency that was transmitted. This reflects the fact that cos 90° = 0.

13. **Answer: D.** The combined result of ultrasound scattering, absorption, and reflection is attenuation. Time gain compensation aims at providing a correction for the loss of intensity (or attenuation) by all these different mechanisms. This is done assuming that attenuation in different types of tissue in the heart is the same, which is a reasonably accurate assumption. However, it may become quite inaccurate when there are materials with drastically different acoustic properties such as contrast agents that cause much stronger attenuation. This is the reason why acoustic shadowing artifacts are frequently seen distal to contrast-filled blood pools, such as ventricles or atria.

14. **Answer: C.** The strength of the transmitted ultrasound wave is controlled by adjusting the power control. Gain control determines to what extent the received signal is amplified, and the compression determines the dynamic range of received signals that are used to create the image. Time gain compensation has nothing to do with the strength of the transmitted power: it is part of postprocessing of the reflections designed to correct for beam attenuation as it travels through the body.

15. **Answer: A.** The spatial resolution of an ultrasound image is defined as the smallest distance between two objects that allows distinction between them. This is the definition of spatial resolution. Understandably, the spatial resolution also determines the size of the smallest object that can be visualized, but the change in the size of an object is certainly not the definition of resolution.

16. **Answer: C.** While spatial resolution along the ultrasound beam is directly related to wavelength, it is affected by other factors in other directions. However, it can be easily determined by the size of a pixel in the relevant direction, if that is known. The gap between two adjacent pixels is a nonsensical answer designed to confuse you, since there is no gap between adjacent pixels.

17. **Answer: C.** Similar to spatial resolution, temporal resolution of a sequence of ultrasound images is defined by the shortest time between two events that allows distinction between them. Similarly, temporal resolution determines the shortest duration of an event that can be detected, but "with confidence" is a subjective term that makes Answer A incorrect. Answers B and D are nonsense.

18. **Answer: C.** The meaningless phrase is "frequency resolution," while the other three phrases are legitimate, frequently used metrics of image quality that tell us the following (see **Table 1.1**):

Table 1.1. Types of Image Resolution

Spatial resolution	Minimal distance between two objects the image can depict
Temporal resolution	Minimal time between two events that dynamic images can depict
Contrast resolution	Minimal difference in the parameter displayed in the image as distinct pixel intensities (eg, reflection intensity in ultrasound images)

Chapter 1 Physics: Fundamentals of Ultrasound Imaging and Instrumentation (Part 1) / **13**

19. **Answer: B.** The temporal resolution of a sequence of ultrasound images is equal to the inverse of frame rate. For example, a rate of 20 frames/second corresponds to 1/20 second = 0.05 seconds = 50 ms. The inverse of the transducer frequency is a period (duration of a single cycle) of the ultrasound wave and is in the order of magnitude of microseconds. The temporal resolution of a sequence of images is nowhere near this: it is hundreds of thousands of times longer. Answer D is nonsense, as one can create a sequence of any number of frames, which has nothing to do with temporal resolution. Please note that a higher frame rate means that the minimum time between two events that the images can depict (see the previous answer) is shorter. In this regard, the definition of resolution is a bit deceiving (and potentially confusing), because smaller numbers mean better resolution, contrary to our intuition, which may lead us to think that bigger numbers should mean higher resolution. This is the case not only with temporal resolution (in this question), but resolution in general: it is better the smaller the number is. For instance, spatial resolution of 0.1 mm is better (or higher) than 10 mm. Similarly, for temporal resolution, 0.1 second is better (or higher) than 10 seconds.

20. **Answer: B.** The dynamic range of echoes displayed on the screen is adjusted by the compression control (**Figure 1.19**). This control can be used to enhance weak echoes by turning it clockwise (upper panel) or suppress them by turning it counterclockwise (lower panel).

21. **Answer: B.** Sound waves of higher frequencies dissipate in conducting media faster than those with lower frequencies, because of a variety of mechanisms. Thus, of two sound waves transmitted with identical intensities but at different frequencies, the intensity of the wave with the higher frequency that reaches a certain depth is smaller than that of the wave with the lower frequency. In other words, increased frequency translates into smaller imaging depth.

22. **Answer: B.** Attenuation is the loss of signal that can occur because of factors such as absorption with increasing depth and tissue density. Increasing the gain amplifies the return signal. The increase in amplification can come at the expense of greater noise.

23. **Answer: A.** Dynamic range, also called compression, describes the difference between the highest and lowest amplitude signals received. The differences in signals are fit into a grayscale range that is then displayed. Increasing the dynamic range results in more shades of gray, which, for instance, may be helpful in differentiating endocardial borders. At lower dynamic range, a higher black-white contrast is produced.

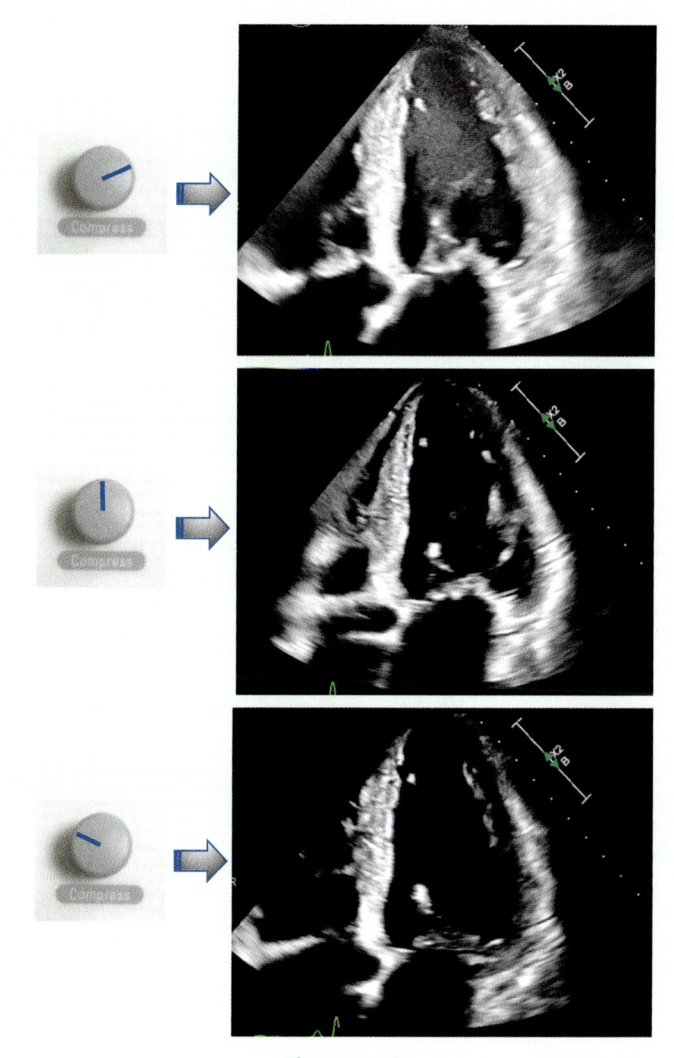

Figure 1.19

24. **Answer: D.** Increasing the power increases the energy delivered to the tissues. Visually, this can create similar changes compared to adjusting the gain, which increases the amplitude of the signal returning to the machine. However, unlike gain, increasing the power can result in more heat being transmitted to tissue.

25. **Answer: A.** When imaging higher-velocity regions, movement of cardiac structures produces low-velocity signals that appear on the screen as color and may make it harder to interpret the area of interest. Filtering can remove this artifact, called "ghosting," from the screen.

26. **Answer: A.** With increasing depth, a signal becomes increasingly attenuated. Time gain compensation accounts for this signal loss by effectively increasing gain in parallel with an increase in depth. Many modern systems automatically account for this and so the knobs should be left in the neutral position to start and then adjusted.

27. **Answer: A.** With moving structures, a higher frame rate is desired to improve temporal resolution. Some machines allow for a direct increase in frame rate, while with others, this can be achieved by narrowing the scan sector and decreasing the imaging depth.
28. **Answer: C.** Aliasing occurs when the Doppler shift of high-velocity flow exceeds the Nyquist limit (1/2 the pulse repetition frequency). Changing the baseline shifts the display scale to allow velocities to be displayed up to twice the original Nyquist limit. Increasing the angle between ultrasound beam and direction of flow can also reduce aliasing though at the expense of velocity underestimation. Imaging at an increased depth will decrease the pulse repetition frequency and increase aliasing. In addition, increasing the color scale can also reduce aliasing if it had previously been set lower than dictated by the imaging depth.
29. **Answer: D.** Images can be averaged together to create a smoothing effect by increasing persistence or they can be left unadjusted. Lower persistence maintains temporal resolution and can keep a structure from appearing as though it were moving in slow motion.
30. **Answer: B.** Increasing the write zoom improves image resolution by increasing both line density and the number of pixels in a given area. Read zoom, on the other hand, only magnifies the image without a change in resolution. Reducing the sector width while maintaining a fixed number of scan lines will also improve spatial resolution. Changing the dynamic range impacts how gray scale is presented on the display but not image resolution. Image resolution can also be improved for a given region by changing the focal point on the display.
31. **Answer: D.** Increasing line density improves spatial resolution but at the cost of a decrease in frame rate and temporal resolution. In addition, the number of scanning lines is increased within a given sector.
32. **Answer: C.** **Figure 1.2B** was obtained using higher frequency, which equates to smaller wavelength that allows differentiation between two distinct objects located closer to each other. Thus, this image has better spatial resolution.
33. **Answer: A.** Harmonic imaging (or more precisely, second harmonic imaging) uses ultrasound reflections that have twice the frequency of the transmitted waves (**Figure 1.20**). It is also possible to use higher harmonics such as third, fourth, and so on for image formation. Typically, only second harmonic imaging is available in commercial systems, because higher harmonic images are noisier and have not been shown useful.
34. **Answer: A.** To increase the frame rate, the operator should decrease imaging depth, as it takes less time for ultrasound waves to reach more superficial structures and return to the transducer. Thus, it takes less time to create and image with smaller depth and, consequently, more frames can be created every second, resulting in a higher frame rate.

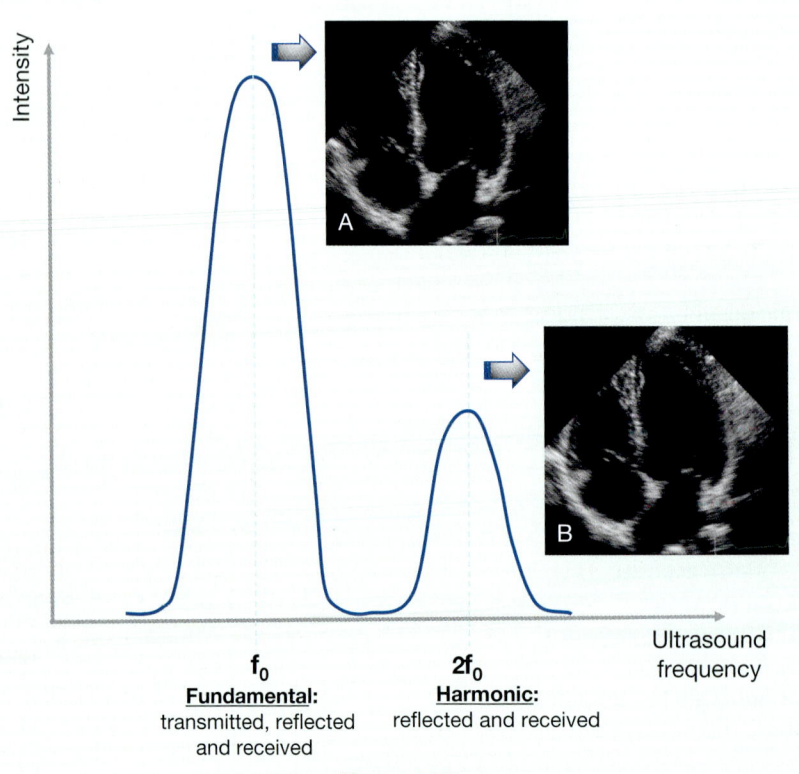

Figure 1.20

35. **Answer: C.** By reducing the sector angle, one reduces the number of scan lines used to generate an image. This results in shorter total time necessary to transmit waves and then receive and process the reflections from the scanned sector, that is, shorter time to create a single frame. This also translates into a larger number of frames per second, or a higher frame rate.
36. **Answer: B.** M-mode imaging does not display power spectrum of velocities measured along a single scan line over time, which can be obtained using the spectral Doppler mode. It does indeed display ultrasound reflections along a single scan line over time. It has higher temporal resolution than two-dimensional imaging because it is essentially one-dimensional: one scan line only which allows formation of a much larger number of lines per second than the number of full frames combined of hundreds of lines each in a two-dimensional image. M-mode does allow simultaneous visualization of different anatomical structures, as long as they can be connected by a straight line going through the transducer.
37. **Answer: A.** Spectral Doppler imaging does not display ultrasound reflections along a single scan line over time, which is what the M-mode does. It does indeed display the power spectrum of velocities measured along a single scan line over time, which provides information about the distribution of flow velocities.
38. **Answer: A.** Continuous spectral Doppler image displays the strength of each velocity component by assigning to them different grayscale levels. Each vertical line represents a power spectrum of the Doppler signal at one time point, while the x-axis represents time. The lowest velocities are shown closer to the base line, while higher velocities are shown farther away from the baseline. The brightness of each point indicates how predominant the specific velocity is at that moment. Thus, a higher deflection at a certain moment in time means that higher velocities were detected, and the brightest point along the deflection indicates the strongest, most predominant velocity.
39. **Answer: C.** Color pattern characterizing turbulent flow in color flow Doppler imaging can be described as mosaic. This is a common term used frequently by echocardiographers.
40. **Answer: B.** "Laminar" in Latin means "smooth" or "regular." "Laminar flow" in a blood vessel refers to a smooth flow pattern, where flow velocities are highest along the central axis of the vessel and gradually decrease toward the walls. In contrast, "turbulent flow" refers to a disorganized flow without any clear pattern, where particles appear to be moving at random speeds in random directions (see **Figure 1.21**).

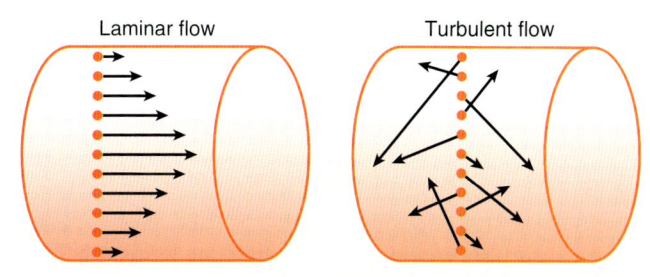

Figure 1.21

41. **Answer: B.** Phased-array transducers use differences in phase of pulses transmitted by individual elements to steer the ultrasound beam in different directions and thus scan a "slice" rather than a single line.
42. **Answer: B.** Echocardiographic contrast agents are based on the idea that ultrasound reflection is increased by the added gas-liquid interface in the presence of microbubbles.
43. **Answer: C.** The main source of acoustic shadowing is the inability of the imaging system to accurately compensate for increased attenuation by structures such as contrast-filled ventricular cavity.
44. **Answer: D.** Shadowing artifacts can be effectively reduced by using less contrast material.
45. **Answer: D.** Adjusting the focus knob can improve the resolution around a region of interest. In the images, the shift of focus is demonstrated on the right side of the screen where the focus, adjacent to the measurement lines, has been shifted downward from the apex in **Figure 1.11A** to the mitral valve level in **Figure 1.11B**.
46. **Answer: A.** Dynamic range, also called compression, describes the difference between the highest and lowest amplitude received signals that can be displayed. The differences in signals are fit into a grayscale range on the screen. Increasing the dynamic range allows echoes of higher and lower intensity to be displayed, which may be helpful in differentiating endocardial borders. At lower dynamic range, a more black-and-white high contrast is produced.
47. **Answer: A.** In this image, the velocities between 0 and 20 cm/s are not visible, indicating that the low-velocity filter is turned on. The higher velocities greater than 20 cm/s are still visible. This is also called the wall filter as it eliminates low-velocity but high-amplitude signals from the myocardium.
48. **Answer: B.** Sweep speed does not impact the ultrasound beam itself but rather the speed with which the Doppler spectrum moves across the screen. Higher sweep speeds can be useful in making detailed time estimates while lower sweep speeds, such as in the **Figure 1.14B**, allow for better appreciation of respiratory variation or other multicycle events.

49. **Answer: D.** In this image, the gain needs to be increased in the near field and decreased in the far field. The TGC settings allow for customization of the gain at different depths. For most images, attenuation has more of an impact at greater depths and gain may need to be increased to account for this. In this image though, the settings are overcorrecting for this phenomenon and need to be adjusted.
50. **Answer: A.** The color gain will reflect overall sensitivity to the Doppler flow. It should be increased until random pixels appear and then slightly reduced from that point. In this image, color is seen both in the chambers and in the tissue, suggesting that the color gain is too high, overestimating the appearance of regurgitation.
51. **Answer: A.** Temporal resolution refers to how well objects in motion can be assessed. The sonographer in this video increased the frame rate from ▶ **Video 1.2A** to **Video 1.2B** (seen as "FPS," or frames per second, in the upper corner) as one way to improve temporal resolution and generate an image with clearer valve motion. Improving the spatial resolution helps better delineate two adjacent structures but does not help better evaluate a rapidly moving area of interest. Typically, improvements in temporal resolution come at the expense of spatial resolution.
52. **Answer: C.** Sounds waves are distorted as they pass through tissue, generating higher frequency harmonics that can be isolated from the initial fundamental frequency when they are received by the transducer. These harmonic frequencies can produce an image with less noise and better clarity. The sound waves though need to travel a sufficient depth to be distorted and generate harmonics and so, as seen in the video, the far field structures at the bottom of the image benefit more from harmonic imaging relative to the near-field structures.
53. **Answer: D.** Smoothing refers to the process of averaging adjacent pixels to create a "smoother" image. Smoothing can be used to reduce the pixelated appearance of color packets in an image.

Acknowledgments: The authors thank and acknowledge Madeline Jankowski, RDCS; Brittney Guile, RDCS; and Roberto M. Lang, MD, for their assistance with this chapter. We gratefully acknowledge the contributions of previous edition author Rajesh Jaganath, as portions of their chapter have been retained in this revision.

SUGGESTED READINGS

Evans DH. *Doppler Ultrasound—Physics, Instrumentation and Clinical Applications.* John Wiley & Sons; 1989.
Gonzalez RC, Wintz P. *Digital Image Processing.* Addison Wesley; 1977.
Goss SA, Johnston RL, Dunn F. Comprehensive compilation of empirical ultrasonic properties of mammalian tissues. *J Acoust Soc Am.* 1978;64(2):423-457.
Hagen-Ansert L. *Textbook of Diagnostic Ultrasonography.* Mosby; 1995.
Hedrick WR, Hykes DL, Starchman DE. *Ultrasound Physics and Instrumentation.* Mosby; 1995.
Kremkau F. *Diagnostic Ultrasound—Principles, Instrumentation and Exercises.* Grune & Stratton; 1993.
Rumack CM, Wilson SR, Charboneau JW. *Diagnostic Ultrasound.* Mosby; 1991.
Smith H, Zagzebski JA. *Doppler Ultrasound.* Medical Physics Publishing; 1991.
Wells PNT. *Biomedical Ultrasonics.* Academic Press; 1977.
Zagzebski JA. *Essentials of Ultrasound Physics.* Mosby; 1996.

CHAPTER 2

Physics: Basic Principles (Part 2)

Bonita Anderson and Chrissy Thomson

QUESTIONS

1. **Figure 2.1** illustrates the "anatomy" of the ultrasound beam with tissue harmonic imaging. These components are identified as:
   A. 1 = grating lobe; 2 = fundamental frequency; 3 = second harmonic frequency.
   B. 1 = fundamental frequency; 2 = second harmonic frequency; 3 = grating lobe.
   C. 1 = grating lobe; 2 = second harmonic frequency; 3 = fundamental frequency.
   D. 1 = fundamental frequency; 2 = grating lobe; 3 = second harmonic frequency.

2. The acoustic impedance, or the resistance of a medium to the transmission of sound waves, determines the amount of reflection and transmission. Which two factors determine acoustic impedance?
   A. Tissue density and propagation speed.
   B. Transducer frequency and propagation speed.
   C. Transducer frequency and tissue density.
   D. Propagation speed and angle of incidence.

3. What does "X" measure on **Figure 2.2**?
   A. Pulse duration.
   B. Pulse repetition frequency.
   C. Pulse repetition period.
   D. Spatial pulse length.

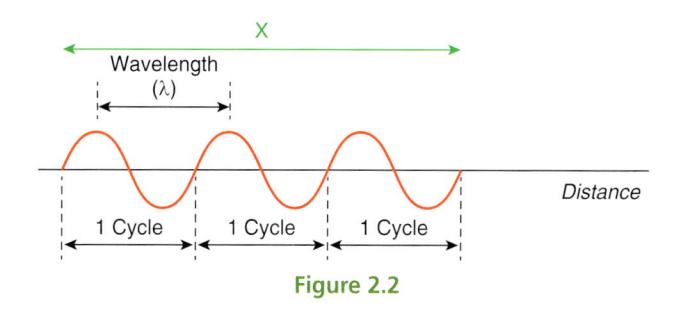

   Figure 2.2

4. Which of the following results in greater attenuation of the ultrasound beam?
   A. Decreasing the transducer frequency.
   B. Increasing image depth.
   C. Decreasing overall gain.
   D. Increasing compression.

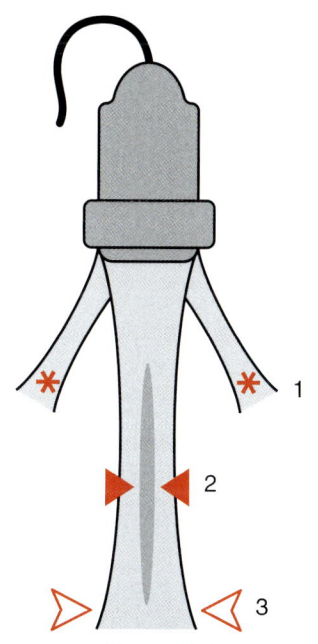

Figure 2.1

5. In ultrasound imaging, the attenuation coefficient describes the attenuation that occurs through 1 cm of soft tissue. What is the attenuation coefficient for a 5 MHz transducer?
   A. 0.5 dB/cm.
   B. 2.5 dB/cm.
   C. 5 dB/cm.
   D. 10 dB/cm.

6. Which of the following yields the lowest level of attenuation of reflectors arising from soft tissue?
   A. A 2.5 MHz transducer frequency and a total imaging depth of 15 cm.
   B. A 3 MHz transducer frequency and a total depth of 10 cm.
   C. A 5 MHz transducer frequency and a total depth of 12 cm.
   D. A 6 MHz transducer frequency and a total of 8 cm.

7. The "speckle" appearance seen in ultrasound images is caused by:
   A. Refraction.
   B. Absorption.
   C. Scattering.
   D. Diffraction.

8. Imaging of a specular reflector lying parallel to the ultrasound beam can be improved by:
   A. Off-axis imaging.
   B. Increasing transducer frequency.
   C. Decreasing transducer frequency.
   D. Narrowing the sector width.

9. Which of the following statements regarding axial resolution is correct?
   A. Axial resolution is defined as the ability to detect separate structures across the beam and to display these structures as being separate.
   B. Axial resolution is improved by moving the focus to narrow the beam width.
   C. Axial resolution is superior to lateral resolution.
   D. Axial resolution is the same as contrast resolution.

10. Which of the following statements regarding read zoom is correct?
   A. This is a preprocessing function.
   B. Spatial resolution is improved with this function.
   C. Frame rate remains the same with this function.
   D. There is an increase in the pixels per unit area with this function.

11. The equation "$C \div (2 \times d \times n)$," where C = propagation speed, d = depth, and n = number of scan lines calculates:
   A. Frame rate.
   B. Transducer frequency.
   C. Pulse repetition frequency.
   D. Wavelength.

12. What is the reflector depth in soft tissue when the elapsed time between the transmitted pulse and detected echo is 39 μs?
   A. 1 cm.
   B. 3 cm.
   C. 6 cm.
   D. 8 cm.

13. The velocity at which aliasing occurs with pulsed-wave Doppler will increase when:
   A. Transducer frequency is increased, and sample volume depth is decreased.
   B. Transducer frequency is increased, and sample volume depth is increased.
   C. Transducer frequency is decreased, and sample volume depth is increased.
   D. Transducer frequency is decreased, and sample volume depth is decreased.

14. Which of the following is correct in relation to high PRF mode?
   A. High PRF mode is used in continuous-wave Doppler to avoid aliasing.
   B. High PRF mode may result in range ambiguity artifacts.
   C. Multiple signals are transmitted from the transducer simultaneously to increase the PRF.
   D. High PRF mode uses multiple sample volumes to display high velocities while maintaining range resolution.

15. **Figure 2.3** is a still frame color Doppler image acquired from the suprasternal view.
   The area of black at the top of the aortic arch is due to:
   A. The absence of flow.
   B. The directional change in flow from toward to away from the transducer.
   C. The color Nyquist limit exceeding 78 cm/s.
   D. None of the above.

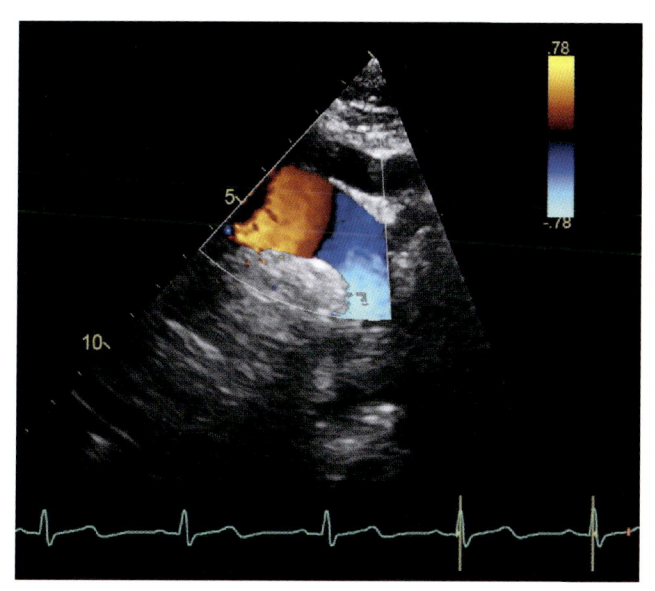

Figure 2.3. Color Doppler image acquired of the aortic arch during systole.

16. ▶ **Video 2.1** shows a color Doppler image acquired of the superior vena cava at the right supraclavicular fossa. The color Doppler signal can be better optimized by decreasing the:

   A. Image depth.
   B. Nyquist limit.
   C. Transducer frequency.
   D. All the above.

17. Compare the two images shown in **Figure 2.4** which were acquired in the operating room prior to mitral valve repair surgery for mitral regurgitation (MR). The change in the appearance of the MR jet in **Figure 2.4A** compared to **Figure 2.4B** is most likely due to:
   A. An increase in blood pressure.
   B. The operator decreasing the Nyquist limit.
   C. The operator increasing in the color gain.
   D. B and C.

18. Which of the following statements is correct in relation to color Doppler imaging?
   A. Lengthening the color Doppler box into the far field will increase the color Nyquist limit.
   B. Color Doppler is a pulsed-wave Doppler technique.
   C. The color Doppler Nyquist limit should be set to maximum for the interrogation of regurgitant jets.
   D. "Variance" on a color map reflects high-velocity flow.

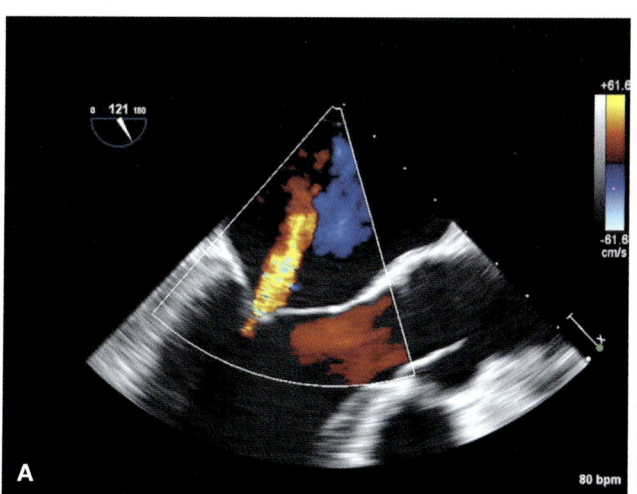

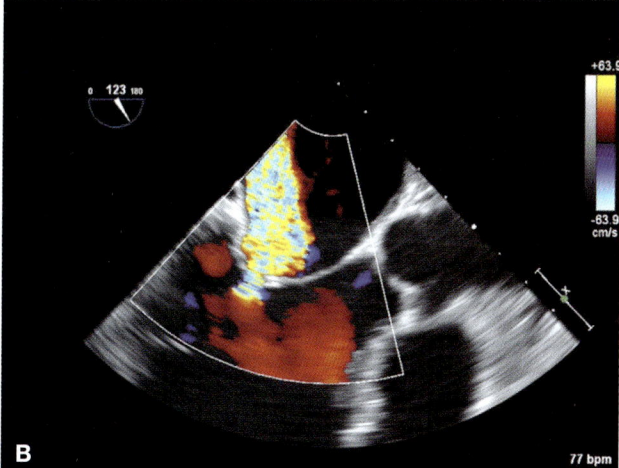

Figure 2.4. Transesophageal echocardiographic images of mitral regurgitation acquired from the same patient prior to mitral valve repair surgery.

19. The Bernoulli equation expresses the relationship between velocity and the pressure difference across a narrowing. This complex equation can be separated into three components. Considering **Figure 2.5**, these components are identified as:
A. 1 = flow acceleration; 2 = convective acceleration; 3 = viscous friction.
B. 1 = flow acceleration; 2 = viscous friction; 3 = convective acceleration.
C. 1 = viscous friction; 2 = convective acceleration; 3 = viscous friction.
D. 1 = convective acceleration; 2 = flow acceleration; 3 = viscous friction.

$$\Delta P = \underbrace{\tfrac{1}{2}\rho(V_2^2 - V_1^2)}_{\text{Component 1}} + \underbrace{\rho \int_1^2 \frac{d\vec{v}}{dt}\,d\vec{s}}_{\text{Component 2}} + \underbrace{\vec{R}(\eta)}_{\text{Component 3}}$$

Figure 2.5

20. The simplified Bernoulli equation $\Delta P = 4V^2$ is used to estimate the maximum instantaneous pressure gradient across a narrowing. Which of the following conditions will underestimate the pressure gradient using $4V^2$?
A. Long, tubular stenosis.
B. Severe anemia.
C. Decreased flow momentum across a prosthetic valve.
D. Increased velocity proximal to the narrowing.

21. An intercept angle between the Doppler beam and blood flow that will underestimate the true velocity by 6% or less is:
A. 10°.
B. 20°.
C. 30°.
D. 60°.

22. What is the relationship between the effective orifice area (EOA) derived via Doppler calculations compared with the geometric orifice area (GOA) measured via planimetry?
A. EOA is the same as the GOA in the absence of valvular stenosis.
B. EOA is always slightly smaller than the GOA.
C. EOA is always slightly larger than the GOA.
D. There is no relationship between the EOA and the GOA.

23. Angle correction for the effective regurgitant orifice area (EROA) via the PISA method may be required when there is flow constraint or a nonplanar flow convergence zone. The equation for the corrected EROA (EROAc) based on the angle α is:
A. EROAc = EROA × (α ÷ 180)
B. EROAc = EROA × (α × 180)
C. EROAc = EROA ÷ (α ÷ 180)
D. EROAc = EROA ÷ (α × 180)

24. For mitral regurgitation (MR), a simplified equation for calculating the effective regurgitant orifice area (EROA) via the PISA method is EROA = radius^2 ÷ 2. This simplified equation can be used when the aliased velocity is set to _____ and the peak MR velocity is assumed to be _____.
A. 40 cm/s; 5 m/s.
B. 30 cm/s; 5 m/s.
C. 40 cm/s; 4.5 m/s.
D. 35 cm/s; 4 m/s.

25. Based on the images provided in **Figure 2.6** and ▶ **Video 2.2**, and assuming that the left atrial pressure is 10 mm Hg, the estimated systolic blood pressure is:
A. 94 mm Hg.
B. 104 mm Hg.
C. 114 mm Hg.
D. 124 mm Hg.

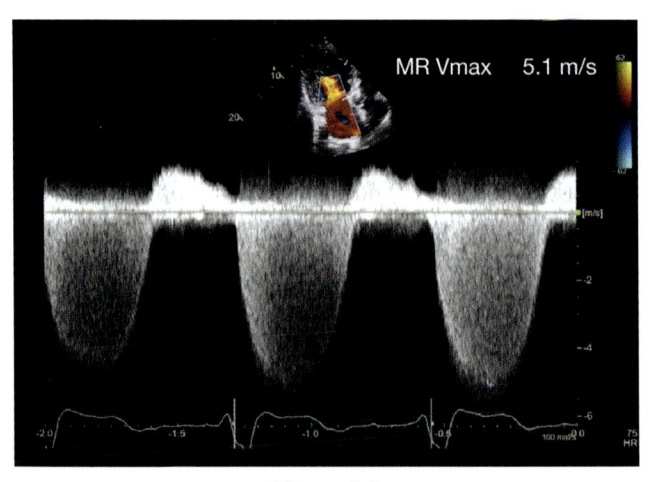

Figure 2.6

26. Calculation of the dP/dt using the mitral regurgitant (MR) Doppler signal can be used to:
    A. Assess the degree of MR.
    B. Evaluate left ventricular filling pressures.
    C. Assess left ventricular systolic function.
    D. Estimate the left ventricular systolic pressure.

27. In a patient with a systolic blood pressure of 130/85 mm Hg, a patent ductus arteriosus Doppler signal showing continuous flow over the cardiac cycle with a peak systolic velocity of 3.3 m/s suggests:
    A. Normal pulmonary pressures.
    B. Coexistent right ventricular outflow tract obstruction.
    C. At least moderate aortic stenosis.
    D. Pulmonary hypertension.

28. Which of the Doppler signals shown in **Figures 2.7A-2.7D** is most consistent with elevated pulmonary pressures in a patient with a normal systemic blood pressure and an estimated right atrial pressure of 8 mm Hg?
    A. **Figure 2.7A**.
    B. **Figure 2.7B**.
    C. **Figure 2.7C**.
    D. **Figure 2.7D**.

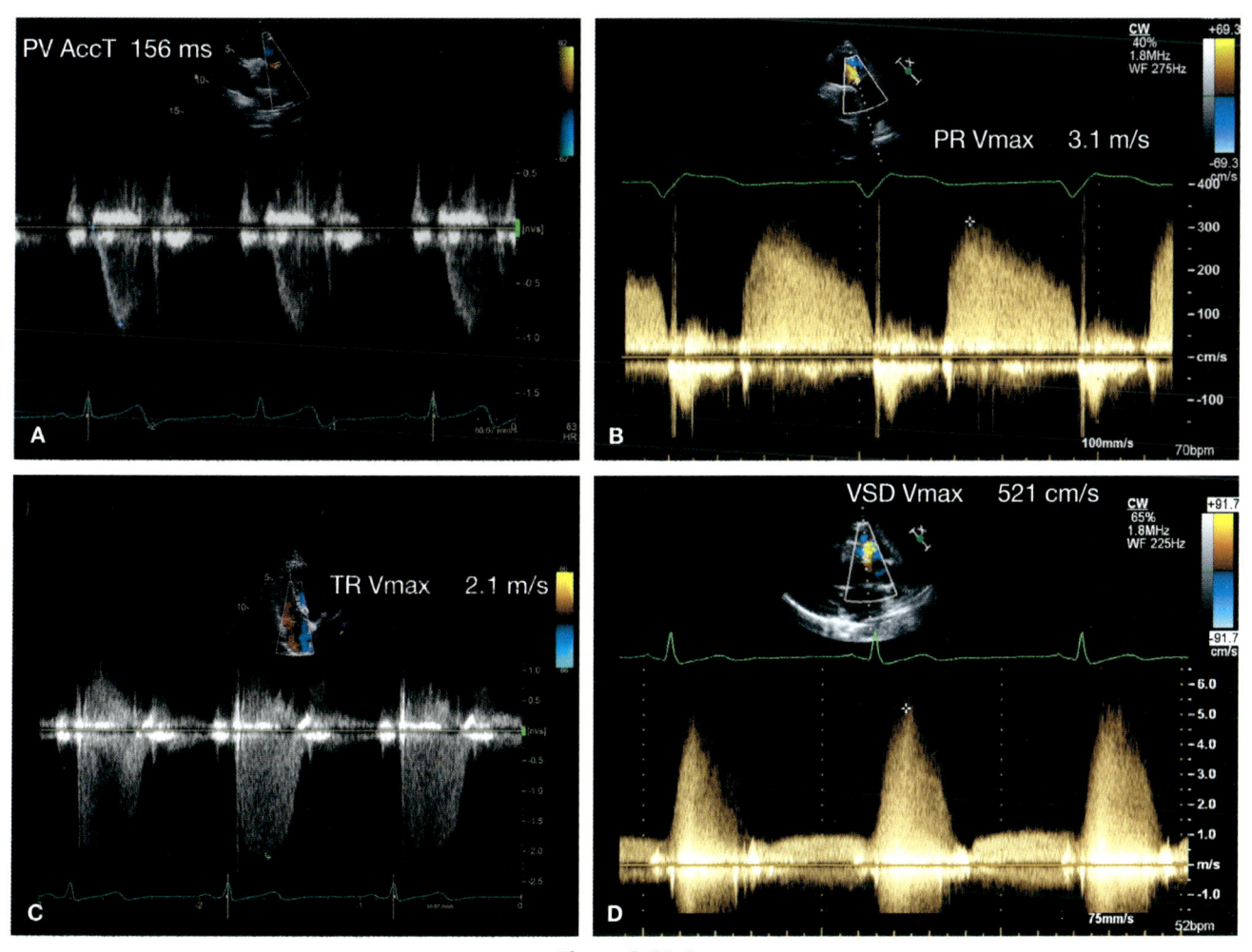

Figure 2.7A-D

22 / Clinical Echocardiography Review

29. Given the information provided in **Table 2.1** and assuming regurgitation of only one valve, there is:
  A. Mild aortic regurgitation.
  B. Moderate aortic regurgitation.
  C. Mild mitral regurgitation.
  D. Moderate mitral regurgitation.

30. Given the information provided in **Table 2.2**, and assuming normal pulmonary pressures and no valvular regurgitation, there is a:
  A. Ventricular septal defect.
  B. Patent ductus arteriosus.
  C. A or B.
  D. Neither A nor B.

Table 2.1

Measurement	Value
Mitral annular diameter	3.7 cm
Mitral annular VTI	13.5 cm
LVOT diameter	2.5 cm
LVOT VTI	20.3 cm

LVOT, left ventricular outflow tract; VTI, velocity time integral.

Table 2.2

Measurement	Value
RVOT diameter	2.6 cm
RVOT VTI	16 cm
LVOT diameter	2.4 cm
LVOT VTI	25 cm

LVOT, left ventricular outflow tract; RVOT, right ventricular outflow tract; VTI, velocity time integral

ANSWERS

1. **Answer: C.** The "anatomy" of the ultrasound beam with tissue harmonic imaging includes grating lobes (1), the second harmonic frequency profile (2), and the fundamental frequency (3) (**Figure 2.8**). Harmonic waves are generated when the normal sine wave becomes distorted in the central part of the beam as ultrasound travels through tissue. These additional waves resonate at multiples of the fundamental or transmitted frequency. This enables the ultrasound machine to transmit at lower frequencies—allowing increased depth penetration—and to receive the higher harmonic frequencies—allowing improved spatial and contrast resolution.

2. **Answer: A.** Acoustic impedance is dependent upon tissue density and the propagation speed through that tissue and is expressed as:

$$Z = \rho c$$

  where Z = acoustic impedance (kg/m²/s or Rayl), ρ = tissue density (kg/m³), and c = propagation speed (m/s).

  The amount of reflection and transmission is dependent upon the acoustic mismatch between two tissue interfaces, that is, the difference between Z_1 and Z_2. **Figure 2.9** illustrates the degree of transmission and reflection of ultrasound energy at tissue interfaces with similar and differing acoustic impedances.

  Calculation of the percentage ultrasound energy reflected and transmitted can be derived when the acoustic impedance of two tissues is known using the equation:

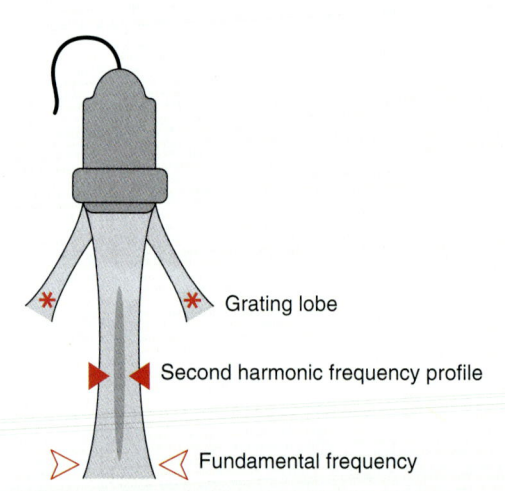

Figure 2.8. The "anatomy" of the ultrasound beam with tissue harmonic imaging includes grating lobes or secondary beams, the fundamental frequency, and the second harmonic frequency profile. Harmonic imaging improves the image quality in four primary ways: (1) grating lobe artifacts are eliminated because these extra beams are not sufficiently strong to generate the harmonics, (2) near-field artifacts are also eliminated because the harmonic beam is generated at a depth beyond where near-field artifactual problems occur, (3) the harmonic beam is much narrower because harmonics are generated only in the highest intensity portion of the beam and therefore lateral resolution is improved, and (4) the removal of much of the backscatter from the fundamental frequency improves the signal-to-noise ratio, thus improving contrast resolution.

$$\% \text{reflected} = \left[(Z_2 - Z_1) \div (Z_2 + Z_1) \right]^2 \times 100$$

$$\% \text{transmitted} = 100 - \% \text{reflected}$$

  where Z_1 = acoustic impedance in first tissue and Z_2 = acoustic impedance in second tissue.

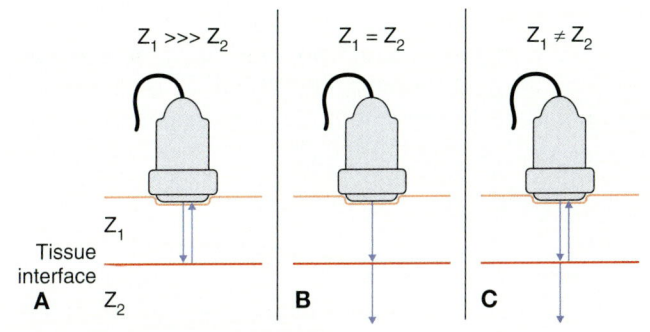

Figure 2.9. This schematic illustrates the effect of transmission and reflection of ultrasound energy at the tissue interface. **A:** When there is very large acoustic mismatch (eg, $Z_1 >> Z_2$), all the ultrasound energy is reflected at the tissue interface, and none is transmitted into the second tissue. **B:** When the acoustic impedance of two tissues is the same ($Z_1 = Z_2$), ultrasound energy is transmitted from the first tissue through to the second tissue without any reflection of the ultrasound beam at the tissue interface. **C:** When the acoustic impedances differ ($Z_1 \neq Z_2$), some of the ultrasound energy is reflected from the interface between the two media, and some of the energy is transmitted. The amount of ultrasound energy reflected and transmitted is dependent upon the acoustic mismatch between the two media.

Large differences in acoustic impedance occur at the bone and soft-tissue interface, and air and soft-tissue interface, resulting in poor transmission of ultrasound at these interfaces. This explains the need for acoustic windows to avoid the air-filled lung and the bony structures in the chest and supports the value of using a coupling medium such as ultrasound gel, which has low attenuation, and an acoustic impedance and propagation speed similar to soft tissue, thus enhancing the transmission of ultrasound.

3. **Answer: D.** The important clue to this answer is the x-axis, which is distance. What is measured by "X" is the distance from the start to the end of a pulse, which is the spatial pulse length (SPL) (**Figure 2.10**). SPL refers to the physical length of the pulse and is determined from the number of cycles in the pulse and the wavelength. SPL is important as this determines the axial resolution (AR):

$$AR(mm) = SPL(mm) \div 2$$

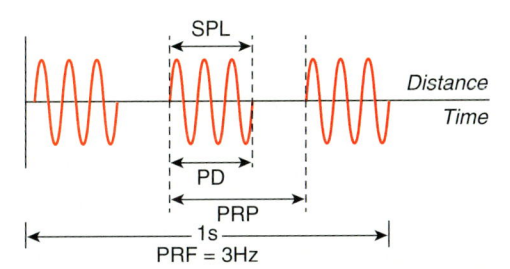

Figure 2.10. When time is on the x-axis, the pulse repetition period (PRP) is the time from the beginning of one pulse to the beginning of the next pulse; the pulse duration (PD) is the time during which the pulse occurs (the time from the start to the end of a pulse); the pulse repetition frequency (PRF) is the number of pulses emitted per second (in this example, the PRF is 3 Hz). When distance is on the x-axis, the spatial pulse length (SPL) is the length of the actual pulse; that is, the SPL is the distance from the start to the end of a pulse. Note: Each pulse contains several cycles. In this example, there are 3 cycles for each pulse.

4. **Answer: B.** Attenuation refers to the loss of intensity as the ultrasound beam passes through a medium. Attenuation is expressed in decibels (dB) and is derived as:

$$dB = f \times d \times \alpha$$

where f = transducer frequency (MHz), d = depth (cm), and α = attenuation coefficient of the medium (0.5 dB/cm/MHz in soft tissue).

It can be appreciated from this equation that attenuation is greater with increasing frequency and increasing depth. Therefore, answer B is correct.

Answer A is incorrect as decreasing the transducer frequency decreases attenuation.

Answer C is incorrect. Decreasing the overall gain simply decreases the amplification of the returning signals and does not directly influence attenuation.

Answer D is incorrect. Compression (or dynamic range) reflects the ratio of the maximum to minimum signal level or the strongest to the weakest echo in the image. Increasing the compression increases the range of echo intensities displayed so that weaker signals are included, and the image is softened. Decreasing compression eliminates weaker signals and reduces noise.

When selecting a transducer frequency, the sonographer should select the highest possible frequency that provides good spatial resolution while allowing adequate depth penetration.

5. **Answer: B.** The attenuation coefficient (a) in soft tissue is 0.5 dB/cm at 1 MHz, or 0.5 dB/cm/MHz. Therefore, the attenuation coefficient for a 5 MHz transducer is:

$$a = 0.5 \times 5 = 2.5 \text{ dB/cm}$$

As a result, higher frequency transducers result in greater attenuation (weakening) of the ultrasound beam as it travels through tissue.

6. **Answer: B.** As previously described in the answer outline for **Question 5**, the attenuation coefficient in soft tissue is 0.5 dB/cm at 1 MHz, or 0.5 dB/cm/MHz. Hence, greater attenuation (weakening) of the ultrasound beam occurs the further the sound wave travels and the higher the transducer frequency. In addition, the degree of attenuation is also dependent upon the distance that the ultrasound beam travels and is expressed by:

$$dB = a \times D$$

where dB = total attenuation, a = attenuation coefficient (dB/cm), and D = distance traveled in medium (cm).

When the transducer frequency and imaging depth are known, calculation of the attenuation coefficient is required to then calculate the total attenuation. **Table 2.3** displays the results of these calculations based on the information provided. Answer B is therefore correct as this yields the lowest value.

Table 2.3. Calculations Relating to Total Attenuation (dB) Based on the Transducer Frequency (F), Total Imaging Depth (D), and the Attenuation Coefficient (a)

F (MHz)	D	a	dB
2.5	15 cm	1.25	19
3	10 cm	1.5	15
5	12 cm	2.5	30
6	8 cm	3	24

where a = 0.5 × F and dB = a × D.

7. **Answer: C.** Scattering of the ultrasound beam produces the "speckle" appearance of an ultrasound image. Irregular reflectors that are small in comparison to the wavelength reflect the ultrasound beam in multiple directions resulting in weak reflections (**Figure 2.11**).

    Answer A is incorrect as refraction refers to bending of the ultrasound beam when the beam strikes an interface at an angle other than 90° and the propagation speeds of the two media are different. Absorption results in dissipation of the ultrasound beam into heat; therefore, Answer B is incorrect. Answer D is incorrect as diffraction describes the widening of the beam as it travels further from the sound source.

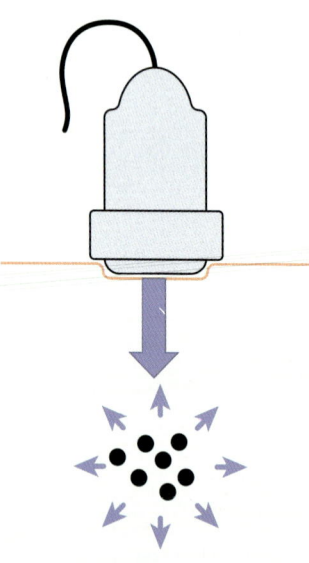

Figure 2.11. This schematic illustrates scattering of the ultrasound energy as it encounters rough or irregular surfaces that are small with respect to the wavelength. Scattering of the ultrasound energy produces the "speckle" appearance of an ultrasound image.

8. **Answer: A.** Specular reflectors are interfaces that present as large smooth surfaces. These reflectors act as a mirror and are highly angle dependent. When these reflectors are parallel to the ultrasound beam, dropout of echoes may occur as little, or no sound, is reflected from them. To optimize the ultrasound interrogation of specular reflectors, the incident angle between the ultrasound beam and these reflectors should be perpendicular. Therefore, the best way to optimize imaging of these reflectors is off-axis imaging to create nonparallel or perpendicular alignment. A classic example of a specular reflector is the interatrial septum. From the apical 4-chamber view, dropout is commonly seen at the fossa ovalis. Imaging of the septum from a para-apical view (ie, off-axis imaging) can eliminate this dropout (see **Figure 2.12** and ▶ **Video 2.3**).

9. **Answer: C.** Spatial resolution is defined as the ability of the ultrasound machine to detect anatomically separate structures and to display these structures as being separate. There are two types of spatial resolution: axial and lateral. Axial resolution is the ability of the ultrasound machine to detect separate structures along the beam path and then to display these structures as being separate. Lateral resolution is the ability of the ultrasound machine to detect structures across the beam and then to display these structures as being separate. Therefore, answer A is incorrect as this statement describes lateral and not axial resolution.

    Answer B is incorrect as narrowing the ultrasound beam improves lateral, not axial, resolution. Axial resolution (AR) is equal to half the spatial pulse length (SPL):

    $$AR(mm) = SPL(mm) \div 2$$

    When structures are separated by more than half the SPL, they will be resolved and will appear as separate structures. The SPL is equal to the wavelength (λ) multiplied by the number of cycles in the pulse (n):

    $$SPL(mm) = \lambda(mm) \times n$$

    Therefore, the shorter the wavelength, the smaller the SPL and the better the axial resolution. As the wavelength is inversely proportional to the frequency, the wavelength can be shortened by increasing the transducer frequency.

    Answer C is correct. Axial resolution is superior to lateral resolution. As shown in **Figure 2.13**, axial resolution is about four times better than lateral resolution.

    Answer D is incorrect. As stated above, axial resolution is a type of spatial resolution. Contrast resolution may be defined as the ability to detect subtle differences in soft-tissue echogenicity and to display these as being different and this is best achieved with harmonic imaging.

    As axial resolution is superior to lateral resolution, when measuring relatively small structures such as the LVOT diameter, measurements should be performed in the axial plane rather than in the

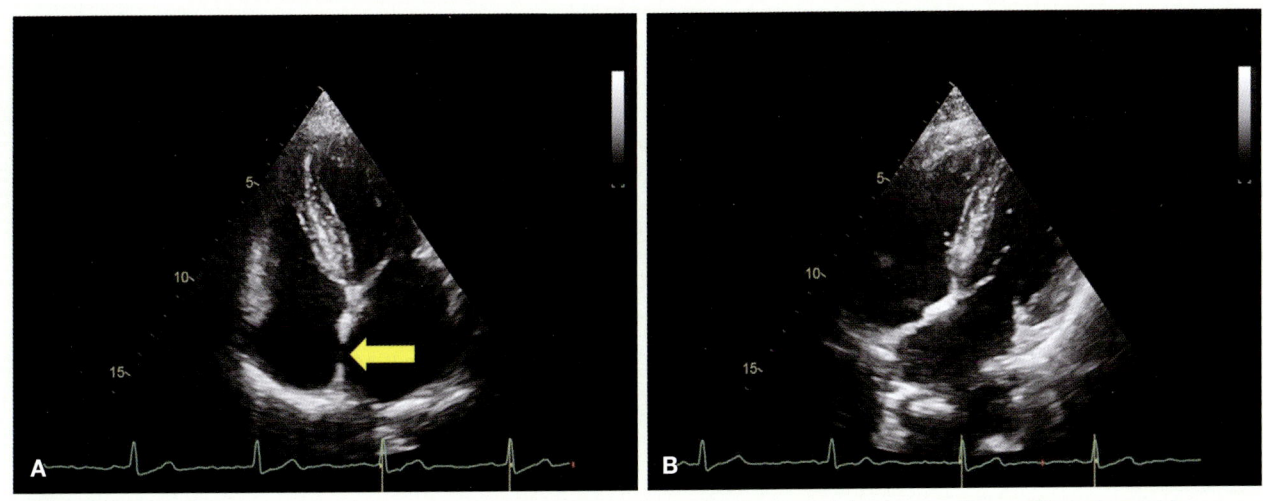

Figure 2.12. A: This is an on-axis apical 4-chamber view showing almost parallel alignment of the ultrasound beam with the interatrial septum. Note the dropout at the level of the fossa ovalis (arrow). **B:** Off-axis imaging from a para-apical view aligns the interatrial septum more perpendicular to the ultrasound beam, which eliminates the dropout artifact at the fossa ovalis. See ▶ **Video 2.3** for real-time images.

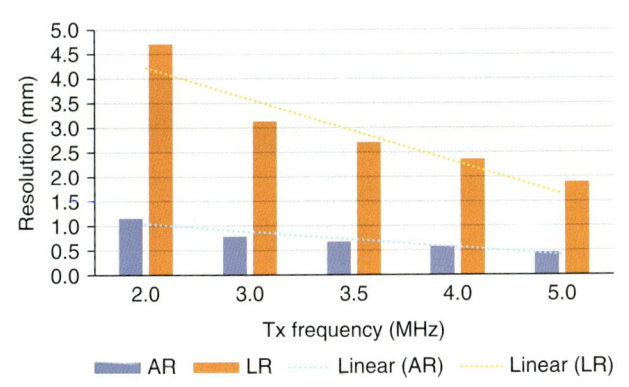

Figure 2.13. This graph compares axial resolution (AR) and lateral resolution (LR) values at different transducer frequencies, and assuming the number of cycles in the pulse is 3, the focal depth is set at 5 cm, and the aperture of the element is 2 cm. It can be appreciated that axial resolution is about 4 times superior to lateral resolution.

lateral plane. Hence, LVOT measurements should be performed in the parasternal long-axis view along the beam path rather than from the apical views where measurements would be made across the beam.

10. **Answer: C.** The zoom function can be used to magnify areas of interest. The two types of zoom function include read zoom and write zoom (**Figure 2.14** and ▶ **Video 2.4**). With read zoom, a defined area of the stored image in the image memory is selected and magnified to fill the entire display area and therefore the frame rate remains unchanged; therefore, answer C is correct. Read zoom is a postprocessing function and, therefore, magnification occurs after data collection; therefore, answer A is incorrect. As read zoom uses the same number of pixels per unit area, spatial resolution is not improved; therefore, answer D is incorrect.

Write zoom is a preprocessing function and, therefore, magnification occurs during data collection. As there is interrogation of only the area demarcated by the zoom box, there is an increase in the frame rate. Additionally, the entire storage matrix is used, providing an enlarged view of a specific anatomical area with an increase in the pixels per unit area and therefore write zoom also improves spatial resolution. The best zoom function to increase the frame rate and improve spatial resolution is write zoom.

11. **Answer: A.** Frame rate (FR) is calculated as:

$$FR(f/s) = C \div (2 \times d \times n)$$

where C = propagation speed (1540 m/s), d = depth to the reflector (m), n = number of scan lines per frame (lines/frame), and 2 = round-trip time.

From this equation, it can be appreciated that the frame rate can be increased by decreasing the imaging depth and/or by narrowing the sector width, which decreases the number of scan lines.

Answer B is incorrect. The operating transducer frequency depends on (1) the propagation speed within the piezoelectric crystal and (2) the thickness of the crystal and is expressed as:

$$F(MHz) = C_{crystal} \div (2 \times T_{crystal})$$

where $C_{crystal}$ = propagation speed within the crystal (mm/μs), 2 = accounts for the crystal thickness being half the wavelength, and $T_{crystal}$ = crystal thickness (mm).

Answer C is incorrect. Pulse repetition frequency (PRF) is the number of pulses emitted per second. PRF is inversely related to the pulse repetition period

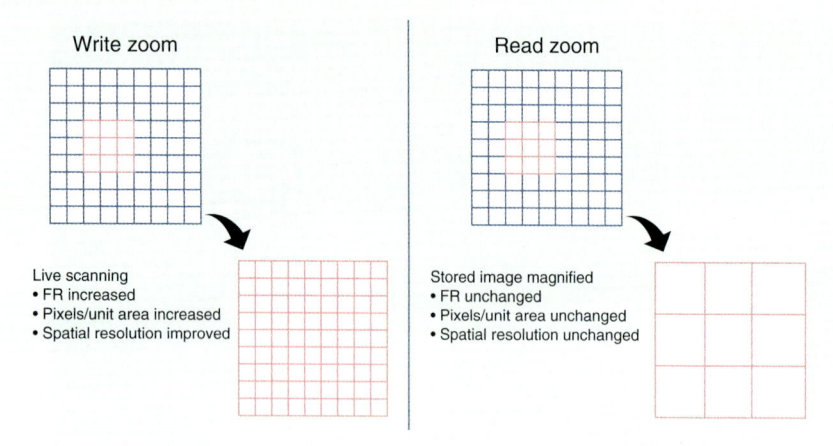

Figure 2.14. This schematic illustrates the differences between write zoom and read zoom. See answer text for further details. FR, frame rate.

(PRP), which is the time from the beginning of one pulse to the beginning of the next pulse:

$$PRF = 1 \div PRP$$

Answer D is incorrect. Wavelength refers to the distance occupied by one complete cycle when the amplitude is plotted against distance. Wavelength is an important component of the wave equation that describes the relationship between frequency, wavelength, and propagation speed:

$$F = c/\lambda$$

where F = frequency (MHz), λ = wavelength (mm), and c = propagation speed (mm/ms).

12. **Answer: B.** The depth position of a reflector is dependent upon the round-trip time of the pulse and the propagation speed through the medium and is expressed by the range equation:

$$D = (c \times t) \div 2$$

where D = depth to the reflector (m), c = propagation speed through tissue (m/s), t = time taken for the ultrasound signal to return to the transducer (s), and 2 = round-trip factor (accounts for pulse traveling from the transducer to the structure and then returning to the transducer from the structure).

By assuming that the propagation speed through soft tissue is 1540 m/s, then the round-trip time for a signal to travel 1 cm is 13 μs:

$$D = (c \times t) \div 2$$
$$t = (2 \times D) \div c$$
$$= (2 \times 0.01) \div 1540$$
$$= 13 \times 10^{-6} \text{ s}$$
$$= 13 \text{ μs}$$

This is known as the "13 μs/cm" rule. Based on this rule, the depth to a reflector is simply calculated as:

$$D(cm) = t(μs) \div 13 \text{ μs/cm}$$

Table 2.4 lists examples of the elapsed time, the reflector depth, and the total distance traveled based on the "13 μs/cm" rule.

Table 2.4. 13 μs/cm Rule

Elapsed Time	Reflector Depth	Total Distance Traveled
13 μs	1 cm	2 cm
26 μs	2 cm	4 cm
39 μs	3 cm	6 cm
52 μs	4 cm	8 cm
130 μs	10 cm	20 cm

13. **Answer: D.** The maximum Doppler shift (and therefore, the maximum velocity) that can be unambiguously displayed with pulsed-wave Doppler (PWD) is determined by the Nyquist limit. This limit is determined by the sampling rate or pulse repetition frequency (PRF) where:

$$\Delta f_{max} = PRF \div 2$$

where Δf_{max} = Nyquist limit (Hz) and PRF = pulse repetition frequency (Hz).

Then, based on the Doppler and PRF equations (see **Box 2.1**), the maximum velocity that can be unambiguously displayed by PWD can be derived as follows:

$$V_{max} = 1540^2 \div (8 \times f \times D)$$

where V_{max} = maximum velocity (m/s), 1540 = propagation speed in tissue (m/s), f = transducer frequency (Hz), and D = depth (m).

It can be appreciated from this equation that decreasing the transducer frequency and/or decreasing the sample volume depth will increase the maximum velocity that can be unambiguously displayed by PWD.

BOX 2.1

Doppler equation solved for velocity (assuming cos θ = 1 and can therefore be ignored):

$$V = (\Delta f \times c) \div (2 \times f)$$

PRF equation:

$$PRF = c \div (2 \times D)$$

where Δf = Doppler shift (Hz), f = transducer frequency (Hz), V = maximum velocity (m/s), c = propagation speed in tissue (1540 m/s), and D = depth (m).

14. **Answer: B.** The principal disadvantage of pulsed-wave Doppler (PWD) is the inability to display high-velocity blood flow without aliasing of the signal. As outlined in the answer to Question 13, a determinant of the maximum velocity that can be unambiguously displayed is the depth of the sample volume as the transducer waits until each pulse has been received before emitting the next pulse. By increasing the number of sample volumes, the Nyquist limit can be increased, thereby avoiding aliasing. This is known as high PRF mode. For example, by adding a second sample volume, the PRF is increased by two, which increases the Nyquist limit by a factor of two. This comes at the expense of range resolution whereby the signals from multiple sample volumes at different depths are received by the transducer at the same time and are superimposed on the PWD display. Therefore, answer D is incorrect.

    Answer A is incorrect as high PRF mode is not a continuous-wave Doppler technique.

    Answer C is incorrect as a single signal is still emitted by the transducer at any given time.

15. **Answer: B.** Recall that the basic principle of color Doppler imaging (CDI) is the detection of Doppler shifts, which are created by moving red blood cells (RBCs). When RBCs are moving toward the transducer, the received frequency is greater than the transmitted frequency resulting in a positive Doppler shift. When RBCs are moving away from the transducer, the received frequency is less than the transmitted frequency, resulting in a negative Doppler shift. When RBCs are moving perpendicular to the transducer, there is no Doppler shift. On CDI, positive Doppler shifts are shown in red, negative Doppler shifts are shown in blue, and zero Doppler shifts are shown in black (**Figure 2.15**).

    From this CDI of the aortic arch, flow toward the transducer in the upper ascending aorta is shown in red, while flow in the descending aorta is shown in blue. At the top of the arch, there is a directional change in flow from toward to away from the transducer. At the same time, flow is now perpendicular to the ultrasound beam. When the intercept angle is 90°, the value of cos 90 is zero

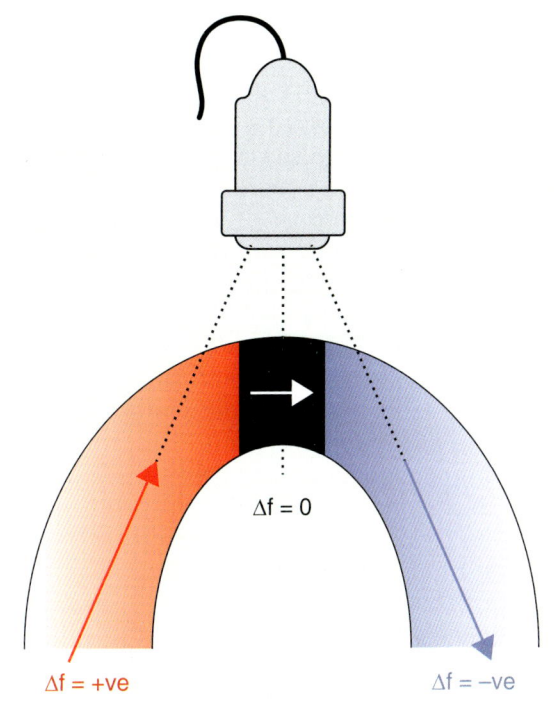

Figure 2.15. This schematic represents a color Doppler image of the aortic arch as seen from a suprasternal notch view. Observe that flow directed toward the transducer creates a positive Doppler shift (Δf = +ve) and is color-encoded red. Blood flow directed away from the transducer creates a negative Doppler shift (Δf = −ve) and is color-encoded blue. When flow is aligned perpendicular to the ultrasound beam, there is no Doppler shift (Δf = 0) and this region is devoid of color.

and there is no Doppler shift. Therefore, answer B is correct.

16. **Answer: B.** ▶ **Video 2.1** shows underfilling of the color box. Observe that the Nyquist limit (velocity scale) is set at 0.94 m/s (94 cm/s). This has resulted in underfilling of the color box. By lowering the Nyquist limit to 0.47 m/s (47 cm/s), low-velocity signals are enhanced and there is more filling of the color box (see ▶ **Video 2.5**). **Figure 2.16** explains how decreasing the color velocity scale enhances the detection of low velocity signals.

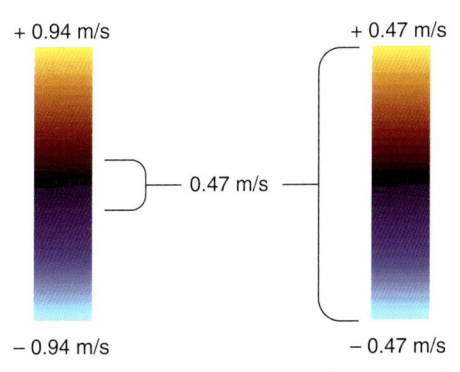

Figure 2.16. This figure illustrates the effect of decreasing the color velocity scale (Nyquist limit) to enhance the detection of low-velocity signals arising from blood flow. The color bar on the left shows the color velocity scale set to 0.94 m/s. It can be appreciated that the range of colors assigned for the detection of low-velocity flow (0.47 m/s) is relatively small. By decreasing the color velocity scale to 0.47 m/s as shown in the color bar on the right, the full range of colors is now assigned to the detection of lower velocity signals.

17. **Answer: A.** In these two images, the severity of mitral regurgitation via color Doppler is significantly different. The color gain in both images is the same at 59% and the difference in the color Nyquist limit is minimal (61.6 cm/s vs 63.9 cm/s). Therefore, answers B, C, and D are incorrect. Therefore, the correct answer must be answer A.

In fact, image 1 was acquired at a systolic blood pressure (SBP) of 109 mm Hg and image 2 was acquired after the administration of ephedrine with an increase in the SBP to 130 mm Hg. The increase in the SBP increases the size of the MR jet by effectively increasing the driving pressure across the valve (there is a higher momentum).

It is important to remember that the MR jet area via color Doppler imaging is dependent upon the driving pressure. For example, the jet area appears larger by increasing the driving pressure across the valve (higher momentum) or may appear smaller when the driving pressure is decreased. For this reason, it is important to measure the blood pressure for left heart lesions at the time of the study. This is especially important in the intraoperative setting or in a sedated patient.

18. **Answer: B.** Color Doppler imaging is a pulsed-wave Doppler technique. Spectral pulsed-wave Doppler uses a single sample volume to produce Doppler shift information from a specific site along a single scan line. Color Doppler images are produced by using multiple sample volumes from multiple scan lines, defined by the length and width of the color box. Therefore, answer B is correct.

Answer A is incorrect as lengthening the color Doppler box into the far field will reduce the color Nyquist limit. The Nyquist limit is equal to one-half the pulse repetition frequency (PRF), which is the number of pulses emitted per second from the transducer. The PRF is determined by the sample volume depth via the equation:

$$PRF_{max} = c \div 2D$$

where c = propagation speed of sound through tissue (m/s), D = sample volume depth (m), and 2 = return trip of the signal from the transducer to the sample volume location.

Therefore, by lengthening the color box into the far field, it will take longer to process the Doppler signals resulting in a lower PRF and lower Nyquist limit.

Answer C is incorrect. The recommended Nyquist limit for routine color Doppler imaging is 50 to 70 cm/s. This is important for comparison of serial studies as regurgitant lesions will appear larger at lower Nyquist limits and smaller at higher Nyquist limits.

Variance on a color map depicts turbulent flow, which represents a wide variability in Doppler shifts around the mean velocity, similar to spectral broadening in spectral pulsed-wave Doppler imaging. Therefore, answer D is incorrect.

19. **Answer: D.** As shown in **Figure 2.17**, the three important components to the complex Bernoulli equation include (1) convective acceleration which refers to the rate of change of velocity due to the change of position of fluid particles in a fluid flow, (2) flow acceleration which refers to the pressure drop required to overcome inertial forces between two points, and (3) viscous friction which refers to the loss of velocity due to friction between blood cells and vessel walls between two points.

$$\Delta P = \underbrace{\tfrac{1}{2}\rho(V_2^2 - V_1^2)}_{\text{Convective acceleration}} + \underbrace{\rho \int_1^2 \frac{d\vec{v}}{dt}\,d\vec{s}}_{\text{Flow acceleration}} + \underbrace{\vec{R}(\eta)}_{\text{Viscous friction}}$$

Figure 2.17

20. **Answer: A.** The simplified Bernoulli equation $\Delta P = 4V^2$ assumes that (1) flow acceleration is insignificant as at peak velocities acceleration is zero, (2) viscous friction is negligible as the flow profile within the center of the lumen is generally flat and losses are minimal toward the center of the vessel, (3) one-half of the mass density (ρ) for normal blood approximates 4, and (4) flow velocity proximal to a narrowed orifice (V_1) is insignificant.

In the presence of a significant, long, tubular stenoses where the cross-sectional area is less than or equal to 0.1 cm^2 and the length of the stenosis is greater than 10 mm, viscous friction is no longer negligible. In this case, the derived pressure gradient is underestimated by the simplified Bernoulli equation, $4V^2$.

Answer B is incorrect because in the presence of severe anemia, one-half of the mass density of blood may be significantly less than 4. In this case, the derived pressure gradient is overestimated by $4V^2$.

Answer C is incorrect. Increased, rather than decreased, momentum will underestimate the pressure gradient. An increase in the momentum of blood flow may be required to open certain prosthetic valves. In this case, flow acceleration is no longer negligible.

Answer D is incorrect. An increased velocity proximal to the narrowing will overestimate the pressure gradient. The simplified Bernoulli equation assumes that the velocity proximal to a fixed orifice (V_1) is much lower than the peak velocity across a fixed orifice and can therefore be disregarded. When V_1 is increased, the derived pressure gradient is overestimated by $4V^2$. In this situation, the expanded Bernoulli equation should be applied, where V_2 is the peak velocity across the narrowing and V_1 is the peak velocity proximal to the narrowing:

$$\Delta P = 4\left(V_2^2 - V_1^2\right)$$

21. **Answer: B.** The Doppler equation describes the relationship between (1) the transducer frequency, (2) propagation speed of sound in soft tissue, (3) blood flow velocity, and (4) the angle of intercept between the direction of blood flow and the ultrasound beam and is expressed by the following equation:

$$\pm\Delta f = \left(2 \times f_t \times V \times \cos\theta\right) \div c$$

where Δf = Doppler shift (Hz); 2 = the "double Doppler shift" (the change in the frequency between the stationary source and the moving receivers and the change in the frequency between the moving source and the stationary receiver); f_t = known transmitted frequency of the transducer (Hz); V = velocity of blood flow (m/s); θ = incident angle between the ultrasound beam and blood flow direction; and c = assumed propagation speed of sound in soft tissue (m/s).

This equation can be rearranged to solve for the velocity of blood flow as:

$$V = \left(\pm\Delta f \times c\right) \div \left(2 \times f_t \times \cos\theta\right)$$

When the ultrasound beam is aligned parallel with blood flow, the intercept angle is 0° and the value of cos at 0° is 1. Therefore, parallel alignment between the ultrasound beam and blood flow yields the most accurate Doppler shift and therefore velocity. However, as shown in **Figure 2.18**, when the incident angle between the ultrasound beam and blood flow is 20° or less, cos θ is close to 0° and the % error is 6% or less.

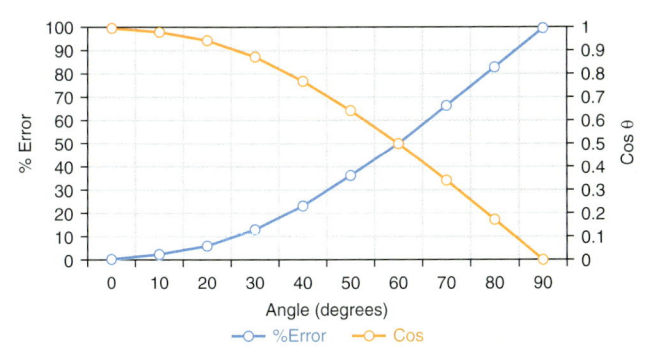

Figure 2.18. This dual-axis graph displays the % error on the left y-axis and the value of cos θ on the right y-axis with respect to the incident angle on the x-axis. It can be appreciated that the % error increases and the value of cos θ decreases as the incident angle increases. Note that as long as the incident angle between the ultrasound beam and blood flow is 20° or less, cos is close to 0° and the % error is 6% or less; therefore, the incident angle can be ignored.

22. **Answer: B.** Stenotic and prosthetic valve areas and regurgitant orifice areas derived via the stroke volume or PISA methods measure the effective orifice area (EOA). The EOA is slightly smaller than the geometric orifice area (GOA), which is derived via direct planimetry. This is because the EOA is calculated downstream from the GOA at the level of the vena contracta (**Figure 2.19**). The EOA, which is measured downstream from the GOA, is slightly smaller than the GOA.

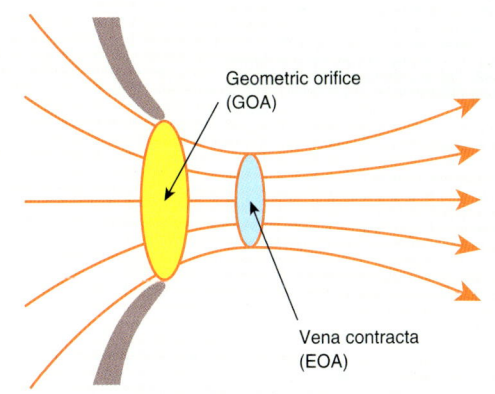

Figure 2.19. This schematic illustrates flow through a narrowed orifice. The vena contracta refers to the narrowest region of the jet, which is located downstream from the true anatomical orifice. The area at the vena contracta, which is the area derived via the stroke volume and proximal isovelocity surface area methods, correlates with the effective orifice area (EOA). Note that the EOA area is slightly smaller than the geometric orifice area (GOA), which is traced via direct planimetry of the valve orifice.

23. **Answer: A.** Calculation of the EROA via the proximal isovelocity surface area (PISA) method assumes that the flow convergence zone proximal to the narrowed orifice is flat with a flow convergence angle (α) of 180°. However, this angle may be less than 180° when there is flow constraint (eg, eccentric mitral regurgitation with mitral valve prolapse) or greater than 180° when there is an obtuse flow constraint (eg, ascending aortic aneurysm). In these cases, the PISA dome is no longer hemispherical and measurement of the PISA radius in this situation will lead to an overestimation of the EROA when the angle is <180° or an underestimation of the EROA when the angle is >180° (**Figure 2.20**).

24. **Answer: A.** EROA ≈ radius^2 ÷ 2 is the simplified equation for calculating the EROA via the proximal isovelocity surface area (PISA) method when the aliased velocity or Nyquist limit is set to 40 cm/s and when the peak MR velocity is assumed to be 5 m/s. Using the simplified Bernoulli equation, 4V^2, a peak MR velocity of 5 m/s equates to a pressure gradient of 100 mm Hg, which reflects the approximate LV-LA pressure gradient in a normotensive patient. The maths explaining this simplified equation is shown in **Figure 2.21**.

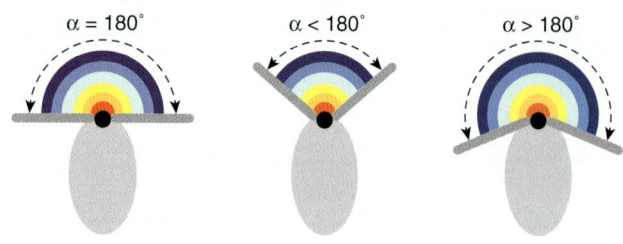

Figure 2.20. Calculation of the effective regurgitant orifice area (EROA) via the proximal isovelocity surface area method assumes that the flow convergence zone proximal to the regurgitant orifice is flat with a flow convergence angle (α) of 180° (left). However, when the flow convergence angle (α) is less than 180° (middle), there is "funneling" of the flow convergence zone due to flow constraint, which pushes the contours outward from the regurgitant orifice and increases the radius; calculation of the EROA in this situation will be overestimated. Conversely, the flow convergence zone may be obtuse with the flow convergence angle (α) exceeding 180° (right). This leads to "flattening" of the flow convergence zone decreasing the radius; in this situation, the EROA will be underestimated. When the flow convergence zone proximal to the regurgitant orifice is not flat (ie, angle is not 180°), the corrected EROA should be calculated by multiplying the EROA by $\alpha/180$.

$$EROA = \frac{2\pi \times r^2 \times V_a}{V_{max}}$$

V_a: Set to 40 cm/s
V_{max}: Assume 5 m/s (500 cm/s) $\approx \Delta P_{LV-LA}$ 100 mmHg

$$= \frac{6.28 \times r^2 \times 40}{500}$$

$$= \frac{251.2 \times r^2}{500}$$

$$\approx \frac{r^2}{2}$$

Figure 2.21. This figure explains how the simplified equation for estimating the mitral effective regurgitant orifice area (EROA = radius squared [r^2] divided by 2) is derived when the aliased velocity (V_a) is set to 40 cm/s and when the peak mitral regurgitant velocity (V_{max}) is assumed to be 5 m/s.

25. **Answer: C.** ▶ **Video 2.2** is a parasternal long-axis view and displays minor aortic valve thickening with good leaflet separation and no left ventricular outflow tract obstruction (LVOTO). **Figure 2.6** shows a continuous-wave Doppler signal of mitral regurgitation (MR) with a peak velocity of 5.1 m/s. From the peak MR velocity and an estimation of left atrial pressure (LAP), the left ventricular systole pressure (LVSP) can be estimated using the following equation:

$$LVSP = 4V_{MR}^2 + LAP$$

In the absence of aortic stenosis or LVOTO, the LVSP is approximately equal to the systolic blood pressure (SBP). Therefore, based on the information provided, the SBP is estimated as:

$$SBP = 4(5.1)^2 + 10$$
$$= 104 + 10 \text{ mm Hg}$$
$$= 114 \text{ mm Hg}$$

26. **Answer: C.** The dP/dt reflects the rate of left ventricular (LV) pressure rise during the isovolumic contraction period, where dP is the change in LV pressure and dt is the time taken for this change to occur. With normal LV systolic function, the left ventricle can produce a rapid rise in pressure, while in the setting of poor LV systolic function, the ventricle will take longer to generate pressure.

The dP/dt can be calculated by measuring two arbitrary points on the MR Doppler signal, typically between 1 and 3 m/s (**Figure 2.22**). dP, or change in pressure, is calculated from the velocities at 1 and 3 m/s using the simplified Bernoulli equation, $4V^2$, which equates to a pressure difference of 32 mm Hg. dt, or change in time, is the time interval between these two velocities. dP/dt is then calculated as:

$$dP/dt = 32 \div dt$$

With normal LV systolic function, the ventricle can generate 32 mm Hg of pressure during the isovolumic contraction phase very rapidly, while in the setting of LV systolic dysfunction, there is prolongation of dP/dt. With normal LV systolic function, dP/dt is >1200 mm Hg/s, with mild-moderate

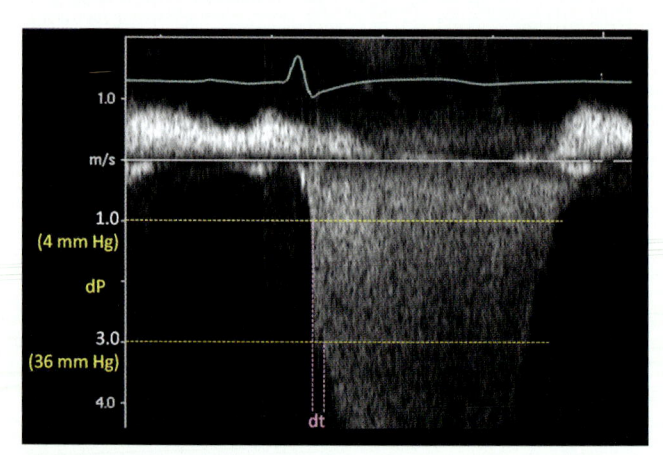

Figure 2.22. This schematic illustrates the measurement of the dP/dt from the continuous-wave Doppler signal of the mitral regurgitant signal. From velocity points at 1 m/s and 3 m/s, the time interval (dt) is measured. Using the simplified Bernoulli equation, $dP = 4V^2$, the pressure difference between these two points can be derived:

$$dP = \left[4 \times (3)^2\right] - \left[4 \times (1)^2\right]$$
$$= [4 \times 9] - [4 \times 1]$$
$$= 36 - 4$$
$$= 32 \text{ mm Hg}$$

Therefore, the change in pressure (dP) between 1 and 3 m/s is 32 mm Hg. dP/dt is then derived as $32 \div dt$.

LV systolic dysfunction, dP/dt is between 800 and 1200 mm Hg/s, and with severe LV systolic dysfunction, dP/dt is <800 mm Hg/s.

Answer A is incorrect. The intensity of the mitral regurgitant (MR) Doppler signal is useful in assessing the severity of MR.

Answer B is incorrect. The mitral inflow pulsed-wave Doppler spectrum can be used to assess LV filling pressures (in addition to other parameters). The peak MR velocity can also be used to estimate the left atrial pressure (LAP) using the following equation:

$$LAP = LVSP - 4V_{MR}^2$$

where LVSP = left ventricular systolic pressure, which can be assumed to be equal to the systolic blood pressure in the absence of aortic stenosis or LV outflow tract obstruction.

Answer D is incorrect. The peak velocity of the MR signal can be used to calculate the LVSP using the following equation:

$$LVSP = 4V_{MR}^2 + LAP$$

27. Answer: D. A patent ductus arteriosus (PDA) occurs when there is a persistent communication between the distal main pulmonary artery (near the origin of the left PA) and the descending aorta (just distal to the left subclavian artery). Because the pressure in the aorta is greater than the PA pressure throughout the cardiac cycle, flow through the PDA is directed left-to-right and is continuous throughout the cardiac cycle (▶ **Video 2.6** and **Figure 2.23**).

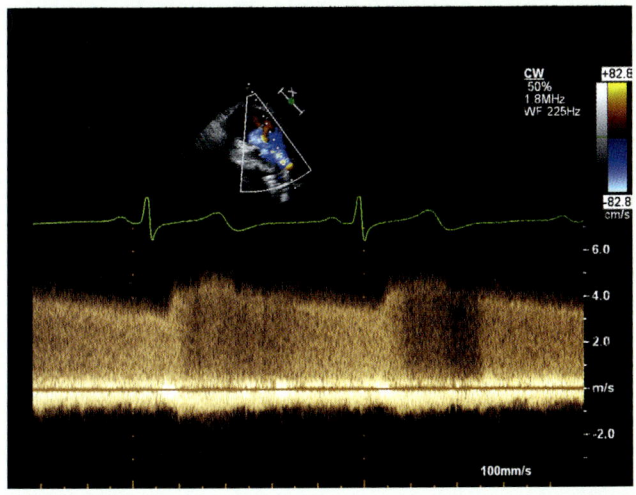

Figure 2.23. This continuous-wave Doppler trace acquired across a patent ductus arteriosus (PDA) demonstrates continuous flow across the PDA from the aorta to the pulmonary artery. Flow is continuous as the pressure in the aorta is greater than the pulmonary artery pressure over the cardiac cycle. The peak systolic velocity of this signal can be used to estimate the pulmonary artery systolic pressure.

From the peak PDA velocity and the systolic blood pressure (SBP), the pulmonary artery systolic pressure (PASP) can be estimated using the following equation:

$$PASP = SBP - 4V_{PDA}^2$$

Based on the information provided and using the above equation, the PASP is estimated as:

$$PASP = 130 - 4(3.3)^2$$
$$= 130 - 44$$
$$= 86 \text{ mm Hg}$$

Given a normal PASP is ≤ 35 mm Hg, a PASP of 86 mm Hg is consistent with pulmonary hypertension; therefore, answer D is correct and answer A is incorrect.

Answer B is incorrect. As the pulmonary arteries are downstream from the right ventricular outflow tract, obstruction at this level will not significantly affect the pressure in the pulmonary arteries (but will increase the pressure in the right ventricle).

Answer C is incorrect. As the aortic blood pressure is measured downstream from the aortic valve, aortic stenosis will not significantly affect the pressure in the aorta (but will increase the pressure in the left ventricle).

28. Answer: B. The pulmonary regurgitant (PR) early diastolic velocity can be used to estimate the mean pulmonary artery pressure (mPAP) using the following equation:

$$mPAP = 4VPR_{early}^2 + RAP$$

where RAP = right atrial pressure.

Therefore, given an early diastolic PR velocity of 3.1 m/s and an estimated RAP of 8 mm Hg, the mPAP is estimated as:

$$mPAP = 4(3.1)^2 + 8$$
$$= 38.4 + 8$$
$$= 46 \text{ mm Hg}$$

Given a normal mean PAP is ≤20 mm Hg, this is consistent with elevated pulmonary pressures.

Answer A is incorrect. The right ventricular outflow tract (RVOT) acceleration time (AT) can be used to estimate the mPAP using the following equation:

$$mPAP = 79 - (0.45 \times RVAT)$$

Therefore, given an RVAT of 156 ms, the mPAP is estimated as:

$$mPAP = 79 - (0.45 \times 156)$$
$$= 79 - 70.2$$
$$= 9 \text{ mm Hg}$$

Given a normal mPAP is ≤20 mm Hg, this is consistent with normal pulmonary pressures.

Answer C is incorrect. From the peak tricuspid regurgitant (TR) velocity, the right ventricular systolic pressure (RVSP) can be estimated using the following equation:

$$RVSP = 4 V_{TR}^2 + RAP$$

Therefore, given a peak TR velocity of 2.1 m/s and an estimated RAP of 8 mm Hg, the estimated RVSP is:

$$RVSP = 4(2.1)^2 + 8$$
$$= 17.6 + 8$$
$$= 26 \text{ mm Hg}$$

In the absence of pulmonary stenosis or RVOT obstruction, the RVSP is equivalent to the pulmonary artery systolic pressure (PASP). Given a normal PASP is ≤35 mm Hg, an RVSP of 26 mm Hg is consistent with normal pulmonary pressures.

Answer D is incorrect. From the peak systolic ventricular septal defect (VSD) velocity, and in the absence of LVOT obstruction or aortic stenosis, the RVSP can be estimated using the following equation:

$$RVSP = SBP - 4 V_{VSD}^2$$

where SBP = systolic blood pressure, which is assumed to be equivalent to the LVSP.

Therefore, given a peak VSD velocity of 521 cm/s or 5.21 m/s and assuming an SBP of 130 mm Hg, the estimated RVSP is:

$$RVSP = 130 - 4(5.21)^2$$
$$= 130 - 108.6$$
$$= 21 \text{ mm Hg}$$

In the absence of pulmonary stenosis or RVOT obstruction, the RVSP is equivalent to the PASP. Given a normal PASP is ≤35 mm Hg, an RVSP of 21 mm Hg is consistent with normal pulmonary pressures.

29. **Answer: D.** Based on the data provided, the stroke volume at the mitral annulus (SV_{MA}) and the left ventricular outflow tract (SV_{LVOT}) can be estimated:

$$SV_{MA} = CSA_{MA} \times VTI_{MA}$$
$$= (0.785 \times 3.7^2) \times 13.5 = 145 \text{ mL}$$
$$SV_{LVOT} = CSA_{LVOT} \times VTI_{LVOT}$$
$$= (0.785 \times 2.5^2) \times 20.3 = 100 \text{ mL}$$

As the SV_{MA} is >SV_{LVOT}, there is mitral regurgitation (MR). The mitral valve regurgitant volume (RVol) and regurgitation fraction (RF) are derived as follows:

$$RVol_{MR} = SV_{MA} - SV_{LVOT} = 145 - 100 = \textbf{45 mL}$$
$$RF_{MR} = RVol_{MR} \div SV_{MA} = 45 \div 145 = \textbf{31\%}$$

Based on these calculations, the MR severity is moderate.

30. **Answer: B.** The stroke volume (SV) across an outflow tract can be calculated from the diameter (D) and velocity time integral (VTI) as:

$$SV = (0.785 \times D^2) \times VTI$$

Based on the information, the stroke volumes across the RVOT (SV_{RVOT}) and LVOT (SV_{LVOT}) can be calculated.

$$SV_{RVOT} = (0.785 \times 2.6^2) \times 16 = 85 \text{ mL}$$
$$SV_{LVOT} = (0.785 \times 2.4^2) \times 25 = 113 \text{ mL}$$

From these calculations, it can be appreciated that the SV_{LVOT} is greater than the SV_{RVOT}. This suggests the presence of a patent ductus arteriosus (PDA) (see **Figure 2.24**).

Remember, in the case of a PDA, the SV_{LVOT} is the QP (pulmonary stroke volume) or the volume of blood flow returning from the lungs, while the SV_{RVOT} is the QS (systemic stroke volume) or the

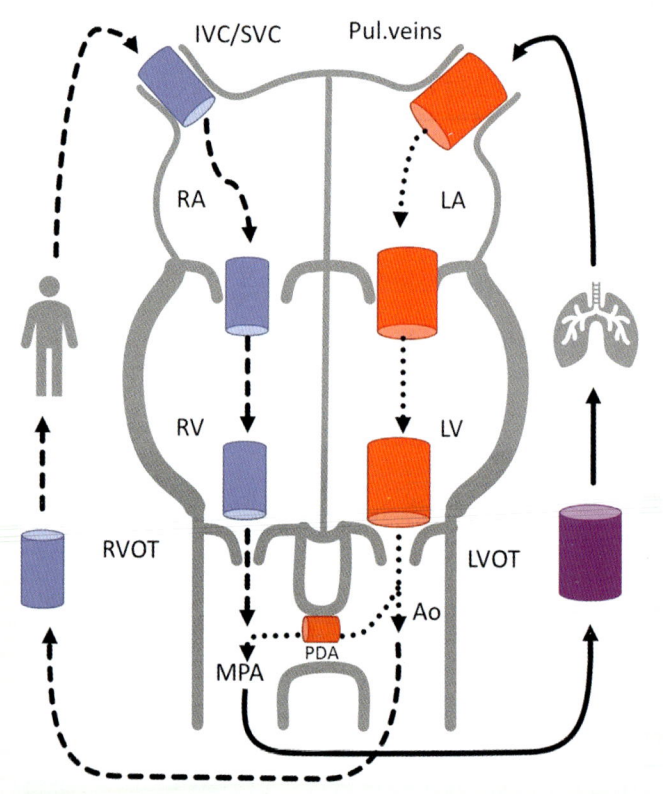

Figure 2.24. This schematic illustrates the volumetric flow through the systemic and pulmonary venous circulations in a patent ductus arteriosus (PDA). Volumetric flow is depicted as cylinders. Observe that there is shunting from the descending aorta (Ao) to the main pulmonary artery (MPA) via the PDA. This results in a greater volume of blood flow to the pulmonary circulation compared with that to the systemic circulation (QP > QS). Observe that the volumetric flow across the right ventricular outflow tract (RVOT) represents the volumetric flow returning from the body (QS), while the volumetric flow across the left ventricular outflow tract (LVOT) reflects the volumetric flow returning from the lungs (QP). IVC, inferior vena cava; LA, left atrium; LV, left ventricle; Pul. veins, pulmonary veins; RA, right atrium; RV, right ventricle; SVC, superior vena cava.

volume of blood flow returning from the body. This is opposite to the QP:QS calculation for a ventricular septal defect where the QP is calculated from the SV_{RVOT} and estimates the volume of blood flow to the lungs while QS is calculated from the SV_{LVOT} and estimates the volume of blood flow to the body.

SUGGESTED READINGS

Anderson B. *Chapter 1: introduction to basic haemodynamic calculations.* In: *A Sonographer's Guide to the Assessment of Heart Disease.* Echotext Pty Ltd; 2014:1-16.

Anderson B. *Chapter 1: basic principles of two-dimensional ultrasound imaging.* In: *Echocardiography: The Normal Examination and Echocardiographic Measurements.* Echotext Pty Ltd; 2017:1-31.

Anderson B. *Chapter 11: Doppler haemodynamic calculations.* In: *Echocardiography: The Normal Examination and Echocardiographic Measurements.* Echotext Pty Ltd; 2017:203-231.

Gill R. *The Physics and Technology of Diagnostic Ultrasound: A Practitioner's Guide.* 2nd ed. High Frequency Publishing; 2020.

Mitchell C, Rahko P, Blauwet L, et al. Guidelines for performing a comprehensive transthoracic echocardiographic examination in adults: recommendations from the American Society of Echocardiography. *J Am Soc Echocardiogr.* 2019;32(1):1-64.

Zoghbi W, Adams D, Bonow R, et al. Recommendations for non-invasive evaluation of native valvular regurgitation: a report from the American Society of Echocardiography developed in collaboration with the Society for Cardiovascular Magnetic Resonance. *J Am Soc Echocardiogr.* 2017;30(4):303-371.

CHAPTER 3

Cardiac Ultrasound Artifacts

Craig R. Asher, Zoran B. Popovic, and Bonita Anderson

QUESTIONS

1. Which of the following fundamental ultrasound principles is assumed to be **CORRECT** when interpreting an ultrasound image?
   A. All reflections are received from each pulse after the next pulse is sent.
   B. The distance to the reflecting object is inversely proportional to the round-trip travel time.
   C. The sound emitted by the transducer travels in straight lines.
   D. Sound travels in tissue at a speed of 900 m/s.

2. Which of the following statements regarding the Starr-Edwards mechanical valve (ball and cage) is **CORRECT**?
   A. The propagation speed of sound in the silastic ball is faster than the propagation speed of sound in soft tissue so that the shape of the ball appears distorted.
   B. The propagation speed of sound in the silastic ball is slower than the propagation speed of sound in soft tissue so that the shape of the ball appears distorted.
   C. Ball-and-cage valves cause a resolution-type artifact.
   D. The propagation speed of sound in soft tissue is assumed to be 13 microseconds to a depth of 1 mm.

3. Which of the following statements regarding the development of ascending aorta artifacts during transesophageal echocardiography (TEE) is **CORRECT**?
   A. Linear artifacts within the ascending aorta are most commonly caused by ultrasound refraction.
   B. Artifacts are more likely to appear when the aortic diameter is smaller than the left atrial diameter.
   C. A linear structure located at half the distance from the transducer as from the anterior aortic wall is most likely an artifact.
   D. M-mode echocardiography is useful in distinguishing artifacts from true aortic dissection flaps.

4. Which of the following statements regarding reverberation-type artifacts is **CORRECT**?
   A. They result from repeated reflections off the transducer or other strong reflectors.
   B. Reverberation lines are equally spaced and are located parallel to the main axis of the sound beam.
   C. Reverberation lines increase in intensity as their distance from the transducer increases.
   D. Reverberations occur when the acoustic impedance of two media through which sound is passing is similar.

5. Which of the following statements regarding comet-tail artifacts is **MOST ACCURATE**?
   A. They resemble reverberation artifacts with equidistant spaced lines of decreasing intensity associated with increased depth.
   B. They occur only with metallic objects.
   C. Common causes of comet-tail artifacts include mechanical valves.
   D. They cause hypoechoic artifacts that are located parallel to the sound beam.

6. Which of the following statements with respect to the echocardiographic appearance of beam width artifacts is **NOT CORRECT**?
   A. Reflectors producing the artifact lie behind or in front of the main beam plane.
   B. A single reflector appears wider than it really is.
   C. Strong reflectors at the edge of the beam appear within an echo-free space or cavity.
   D. Two separate reflectors lying side-by-side appear as one reflector.

7. Which of the following statements regarding Snell's law is **MOST ACCURATE**?
   A. It is the principle that explains the physics of reverberation artifacts.
   B. It requires information on the angle of incidence and transmit frequency of the transducer.
   C. It requires information on the propagation speed of ultrasound in two different media and the transmit frequency of the transducer.
   D. It requires information on the angle of incidence of the ultrasound beam and propagation speed of ultrasound in two different media.

8. Which of the following statements regarding side lobe artifacts is **CORRECT**?
   A. Side lobe artifacts are generated by a weakly reflective object that is close to the central ultrasound beam.
   B. In a side lobe artifact, additional echoes will appear lateral to the true object location.
   C. Side lobe artifacts are created after echoes are returned from highly reflective objects located within the pathway of the central ultrasound beam.
   D. All the energy emitted from an ultrasound transducer remains within the central (main) beam.

9. Which of the following statements regarding refraction artifacts is **NOT CORRECT**?
   A. Refraction of the ultrasound beam can result in misplacement of echoes.
   B. Refraction of the ultrasound beam can result in missing echoes.
   C. Refraction of the ultrasound beam can result in duplication of structures.
   D. Refraction of the ultrasound beam can result in distortion of structures.

10. Which of the following statements regarding range ambiguity is **TRUE**?
    A. Range ambiguity occurs when the propagation speed through a structure is lower than the assumed propagation speed.
    B. Range ambiguity occurs when echoes from deep structures created by a first pulse arrive at the transducer after the second pulse has been transmitted.
    C. Range ambiguity can be avoided by decreasing the image depth (field of view).
    D. Range ambiguity occurs when the ultrasound machine is operating at a low pulse repetition frequency (PRF).

11. Which of the following statements regarding mirror-image artifact in spectral Doppler echocardiography is **CORRECT**?
    A. This artifact usually appears when the Doppler gains are set too low.
    B. This artifact appears as symmetric spectral images on the opposite side of the baseline from the true signal.
    C. The mirror image is usually more intense but otherwise very similar to the true signal.
    D. This artifact can be reduced by increasing the power output and better alignment of the Doppler beam with the flow direction.

12. Which of the following techniques can help distinguish a left ventricular thrombus from a near-field clutter artifact?
    A. Increasing the depth.
    B. Decreasing the transducer frequency.
    C. Changing from fundamental to harmonic imaging.
    D. Increasing the mechanical index when giving an ultrasound-enhancing agent.

13. True structures, as opposed to artifacts, are characterized by which of the following features?
    A. Ill-defined borders.
    B. Visualization in a single view.
    C. Not crossing anatomical borders.
    D. Lack of attachments to nearby structures.

36 / Clinical Echocardiography Review

14. Which of the following artifacts **DOES NOT** result in a duplication of a structure?
   A. Mirror artifact.
   B. Refraction artifact.
   C. Reverberation artifact.
   D. Slice thickness artifact.

15. Which of the following statements is **CORRECT** regarding a ring-down artifact?
   A. This is a type of refraction artifact.
   B. This is a type of reverberation artifact.
   C. This is a type of ultrasound machine artifact caused when the transducer crystal is defective.
   D. This is a type of artifact that is not seen in cardiac imaging.

16. Which of the following statements regarding pseudomitral regurgitation is **CORRECT**?
   A. This artifact is related to a mechanical disc aortic valve prosthesis.
   B. This artifact is related to a mechanical disc mitral valve prosthesis.
   C. This artifact is seen with native mitral valve disease.
   D. This artifact is seen with metallic or nonmetallic reflectors such as pacemakers.

17. Figure 3.1 was acquired from an apical 4-chamber view of the left ventricle. The *arrow* points to an artifact in the left ventricle that is generated due to:
   A. Side lobes.
   B. Acoustic shadowing.
   C. Beam width.
   D. Range ambiguity.
   E. Refraction.

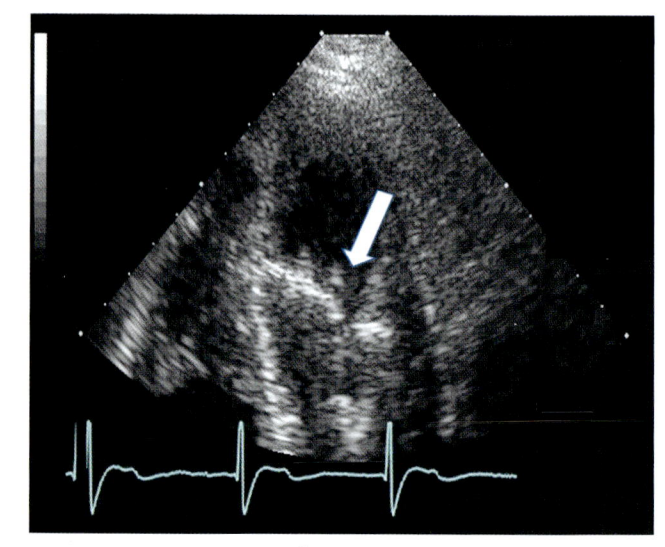

Figure 3.1

18. In a patient with normal left ventricular function and no regional abnormalities, the *arrow* in **Figure 3.2** (left [**A**] and right [**B**] panels) points to which of the following type of artifacts?
   A. Shadowing.
   B. Refraction.
   C. Near-field clutter.
   D. Beam width.
   E. Side lobes.

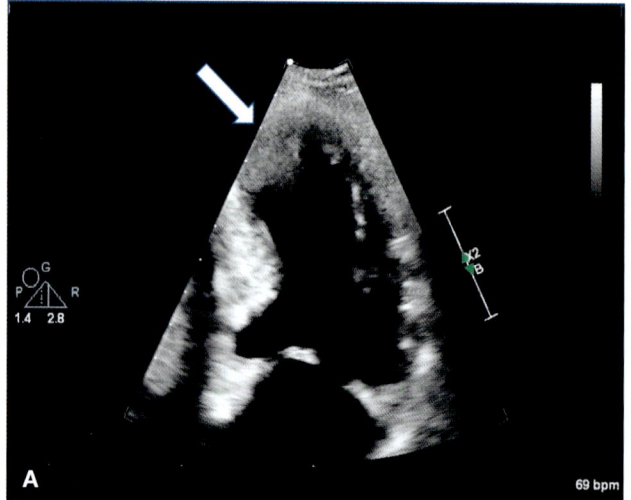

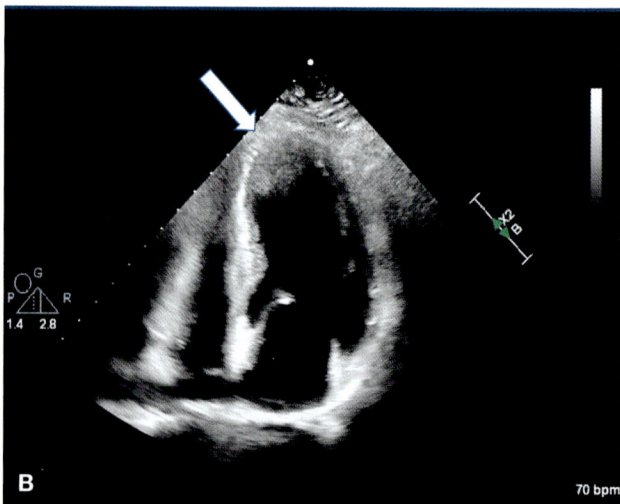

Figure 3.2

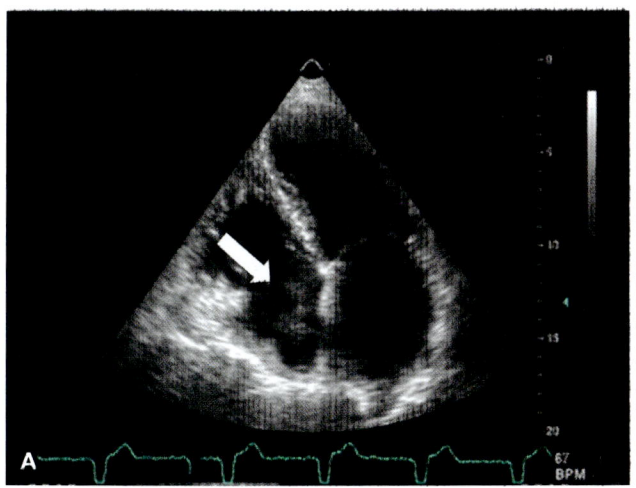

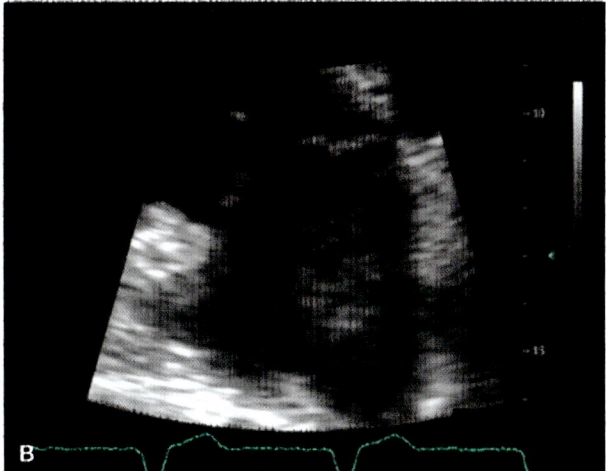

Figure 3.3

19. The artifact seen in **Figure 3.3** (left panel [**A**], *arrow*) corresponds to:
   A. Shadowing.
   B. Refraction.
   C. Near-field clutter.
   D. Range ambiguity.
   E. Beam dimension artifact.

20. The following TEE images of the aorta (**Figure 3.4A**, long-axis view at 83°, and corresponding **Figure 3.4B**, X-plane, **Figure 3.4C**, long-axis view with color Doppler Nyquist limit at 30.8 cm/s, and **Figure 3.4D**, M-mode) were obtained in a patient with a suspected acute aortic dissection. Which of the following statements is most accurate?
   A. The linear density seen in the aorta is most consistent with a dissection flap.
   B. The linear density seen in the aorta is a side lobe artifact.
   C. The linear density seen in the aorta is a reverberation artifact.
   D. The linear density seen in the aorta is a beam width artifact.

21. The numbered artifacts displayed on **Figure 3.5** are:
   A. (1) reverberation; (2) side lobe; (3) attenuation; (4) comet tail.
   B. (1) side lobe; (2) reverberation; (3) attenuation; (4) comet tail.
   C. (1) reverberation; (2) range ambiguity; (3) enhancement; (4) grating lobe.
   D. (1) mirror image; (2) side lobe; (3) enhancement; (4) grating lobe.

22. Which of the following statements is most accurate regarding the structure seen in the left atrium in **Figure 3.6** (see *arrow*)?
   A. There is an atrial septal aneurysm.
   B. The patient has undergone surgery for congenital heart disease.
   C. The patient has undergone an interventional procedure.
   D. The patient has Kawasaki disease.

38 / Clinical Echocardiography Review

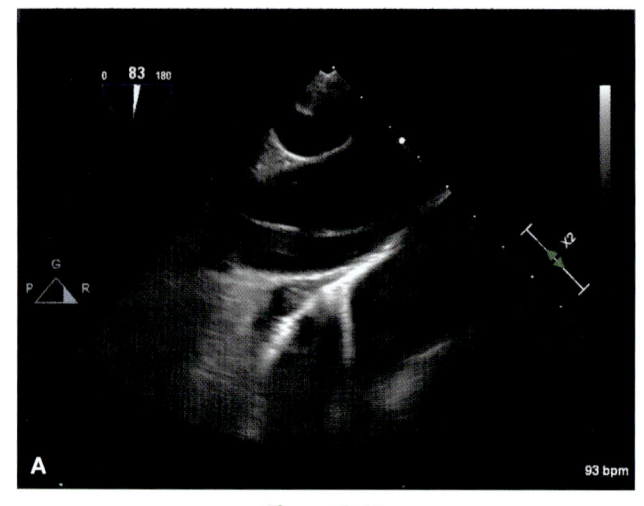

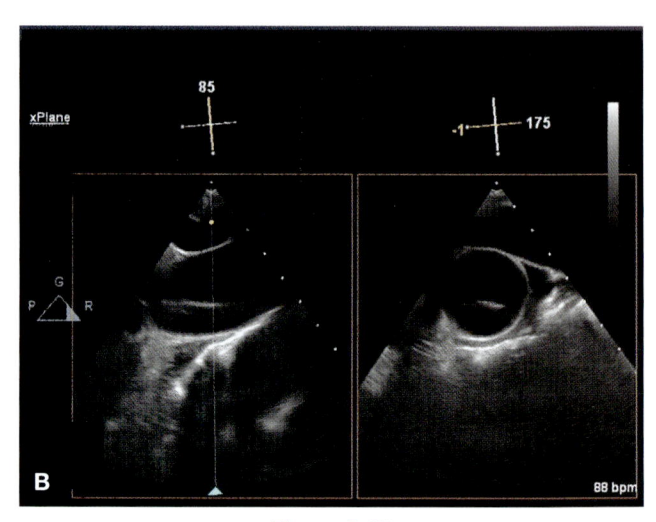

Figure 3.4A

Figure 3.4B

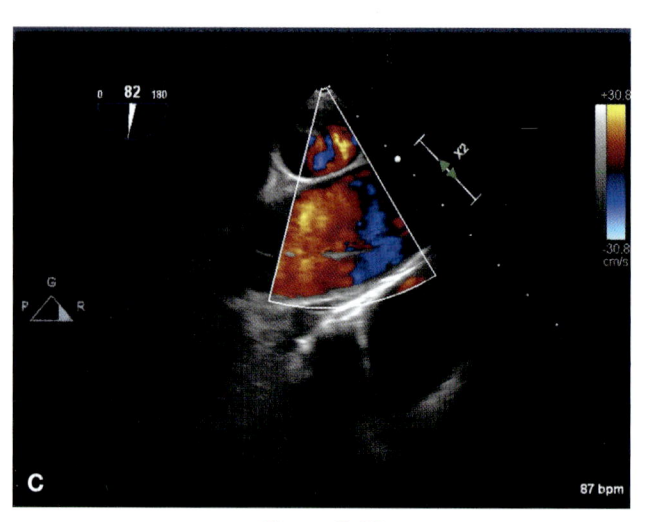

Figure 3.4C

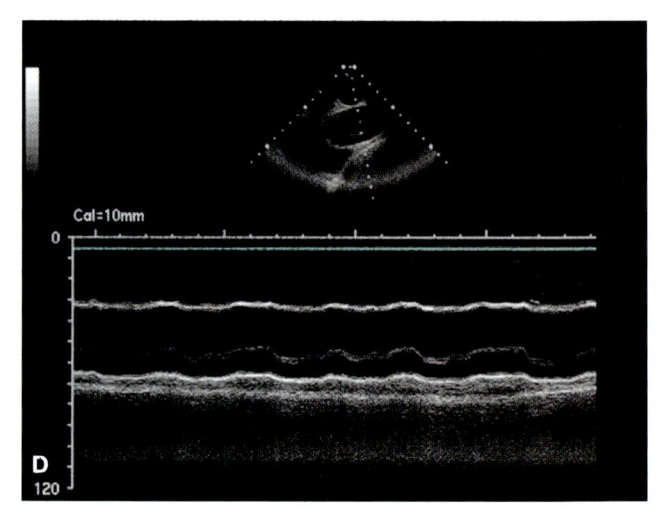

Figure 3.4D

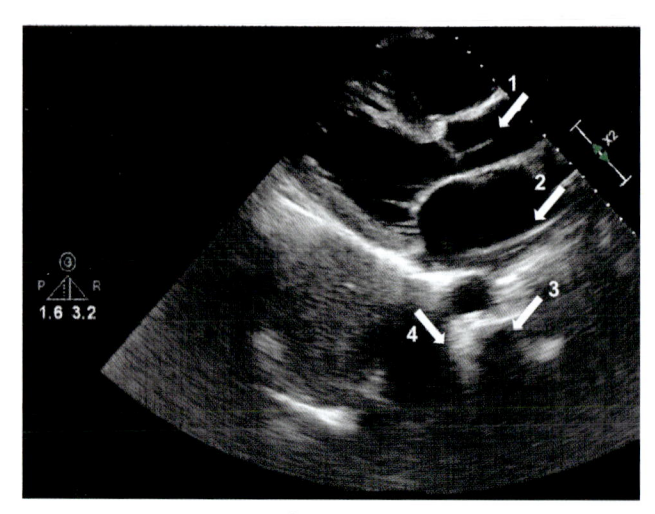

Figure 3.5

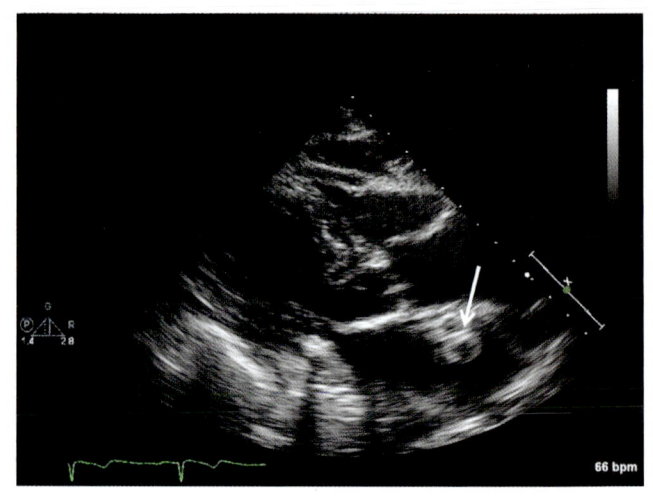

Figure 3.6

23. Which of the following types of artifacts are seen in the left atrium in this patient with a mechanical mitral prosthesis (**Figure 3.7**, see *arrows*)?
    A. Far-field clutter.
    B. Reverberation.
    C. Ring down.
    D. Refraction.

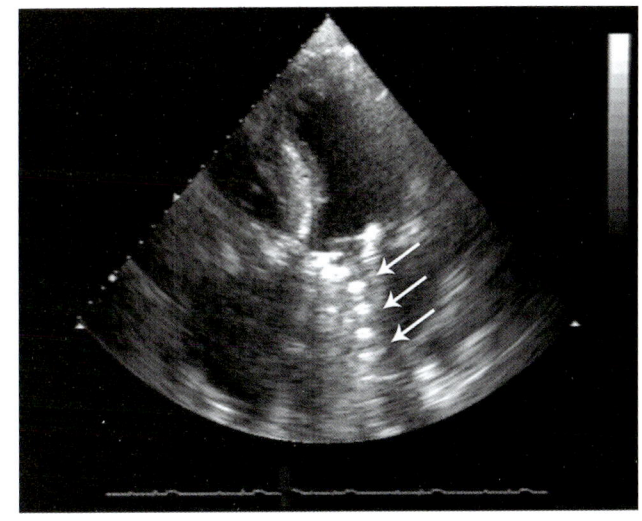

Figure 3.7

24. Identify the type of color Doppler artifact in this parasternal short-axis image acquired in a patient with a mechanical aortic valve prosthesis (**Figure 3.8**, *arrow* points to region of interest).
    A. Shielding.
    B. Refraction.
    C. Ghosting.
    D. Beam width.
    E. Side lobe.

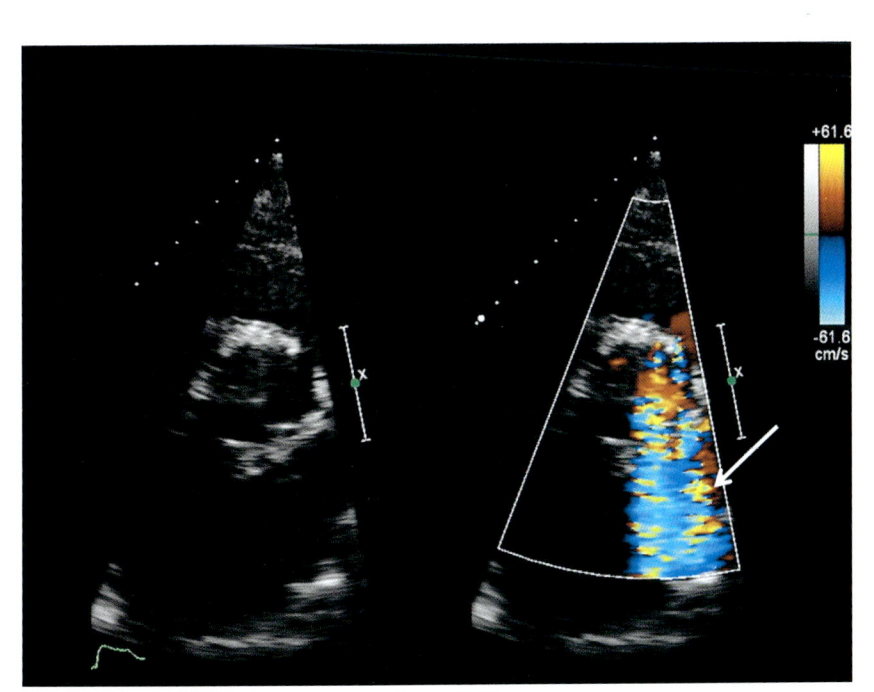

Figure 3.8

25. The following images (**Figure 3.9A-C**) were obtained in a patient with an Impella device implanted for the management of cardiogenic shock.
What conclusions can be made from the color mosaic appearance?

A. There is likely significant aortic regurgitation.
B. There is likely significant mitral regurgitation.
C. There is no significance.
D. There is likely normal Impella function.

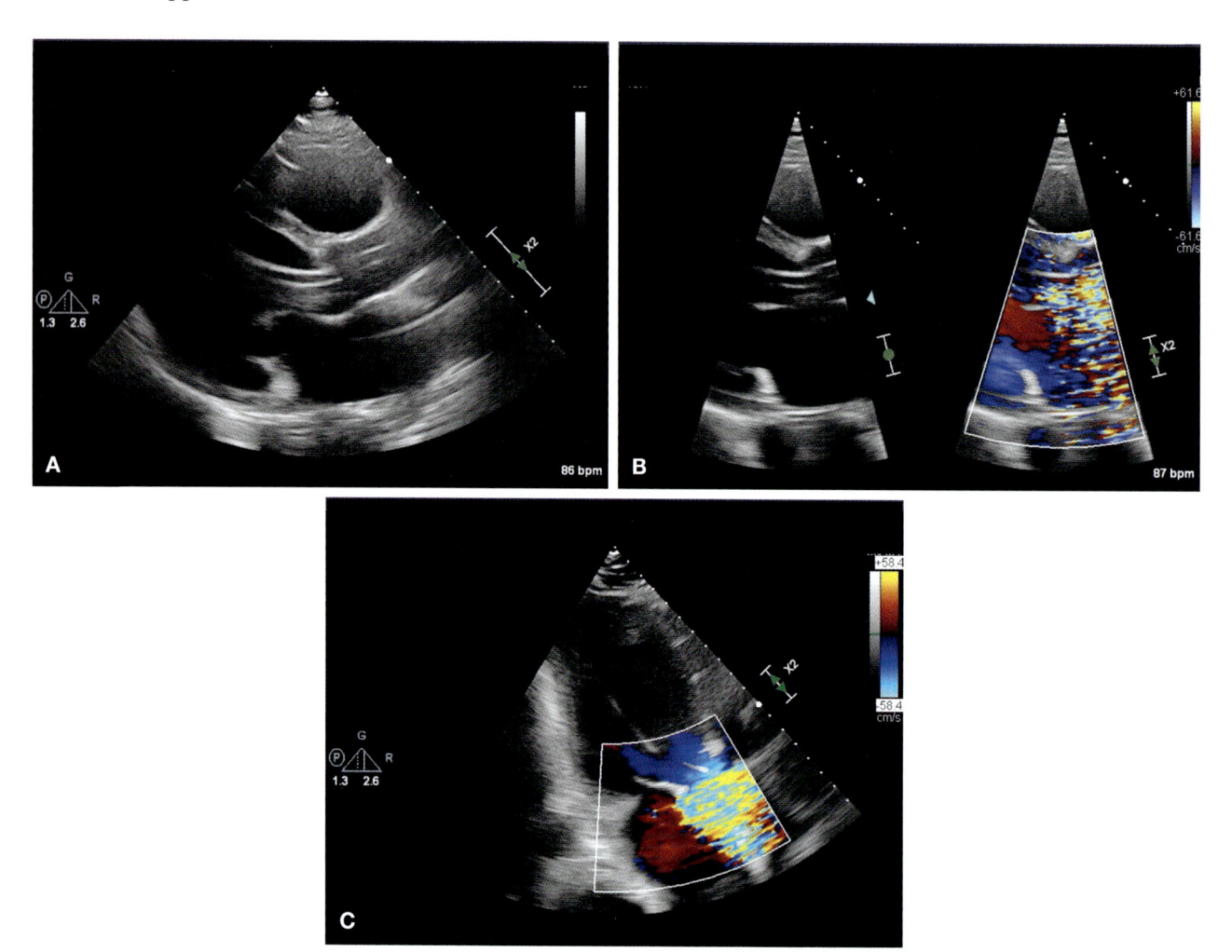

Figure 3.9

26. A young woman with dyspnea presents for an echocardiogram. Which of the following statements is **CORRECT** regarding the parasternal long-axis image (**Figure 3.10**)?

A. There is a left pleural effusion.
B. There is a pericardial cyst.
C. There is ascites.
D. This is a normal image.

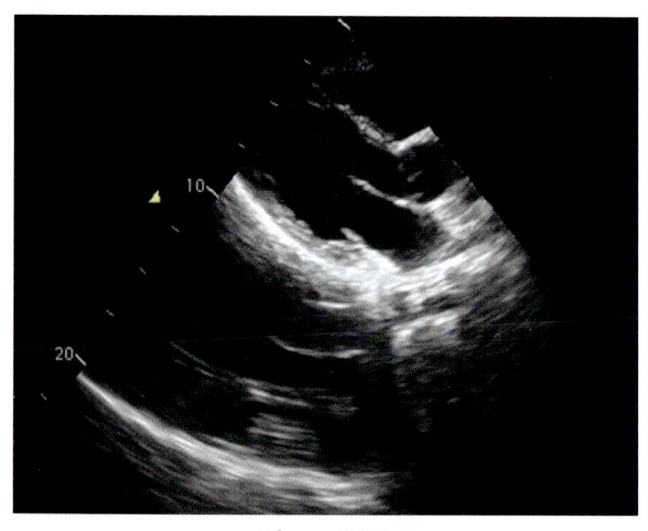

Figure 3.10

27. Which of the following statements best describes the findings seen in this continuous-wave Doppler trace of an aortic regurgitant jet (**Figure 3.11**)?
    A. There is an artifact created by mechanical interference from electrocautery (Bovie cautery) with the patient in the operating room.
    B. There is an artifact related to a tremor from Parkinson disease.
    C. There is no artifact.
    D. There is an artifact related to the aortic valve oscillations.

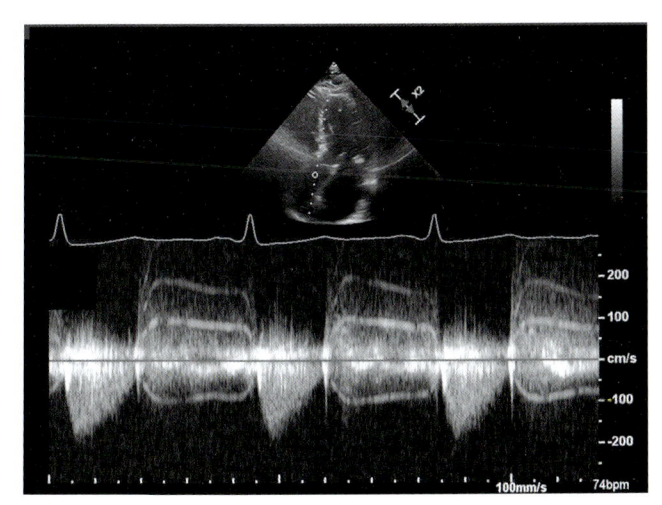

Figure 3.11

28. A continuous-wave Doppler profile was obtained by transesophageal echocardiography (TEE) in a patient with mitral stenosis (**Figure 3.12**). Which of the following statements is **CORRECT**?
    A. There is severe mitral stenosis with a peak gradient of at least 16 mm Hg.
    B. There is severe mitral stenosis with a peak velocity of near 4m/s.
    C. The severity of mitral stenosis cannot be determined since there are two levels of obstruction (valvular and subvalvular).
    D. The severity of mitral stenosis cannot be determined because there is a Doppler artifact that interferes with interpretation.

29. A young man with shortness of breath and a regurgitant systolic murmur has an echocardiogram performed with the following images shown: **Figure 3.13A** (apical long-axis) and **Figure 3.13B** (apical 4-chamber view, zoomed).
    Which of the following statements is most accurate?
    A. The images show a prominent region of flow convergence suggesting moderate to severe mitral regurgitation.
    B. The images show a prominent region of vena contracta suggesting moderate to severe mitral regurgitation.
    C. The images show a small jet area in the left atrium suggesting mild mitral regurgitation.
    D. The images show a region of color splay suggesting moderate to severe mitral regurgitation.

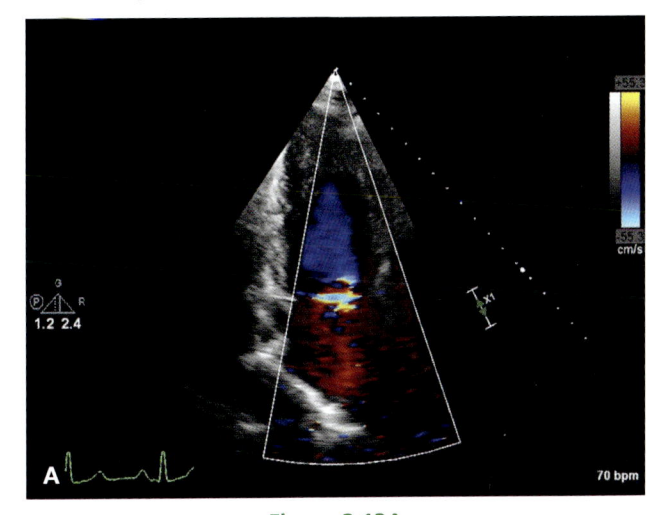

Figure 3.13A

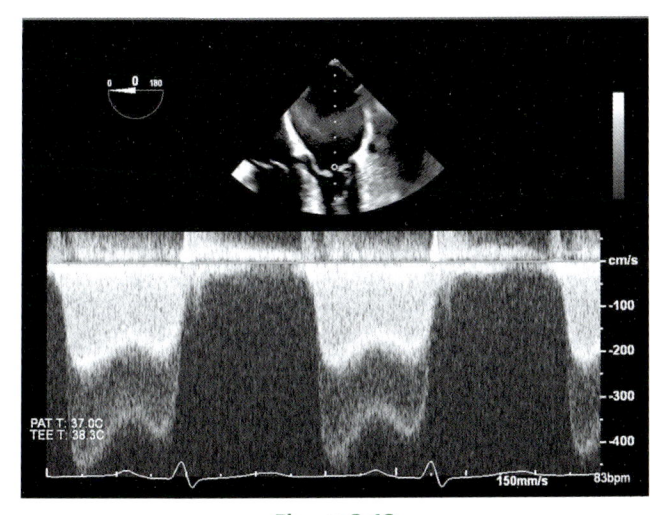

Figure 3.12

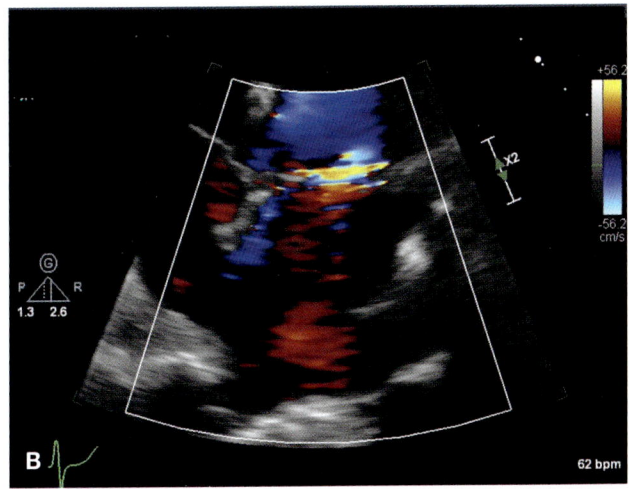

Figure 3.13B

30. After scanning the parasternal short axis at the level of the aortic valve, the sonographer calls you to help with the interpretation of this image (▶ **Video 3.1**). This finding corresponds to:
   A. A sinus of Valsalva aneurysm.
   B. A patient with a heterotopic heart transplant.
   C. A refraction artifact.
   D. A mirror-image artifact.
   E. A large mobile vegetation.

31. A routine echocardiogram to investigate a heart murmur is performed on a middle-aged woman who recently underwent cosmetic surgery. ▶ **Video 3.2** shows:
   A. A refraction artifact.
   B. An artifact secondary to breast implants.
   C. A near-field clutter artifact.
   D. A beam width artifact.

32. A 67-year-old man presented with congestive heart failure and aortic valve endocarditis. A continuous-wave spectral Doppler pattern is obtained from the apical long-axis view. Which of the following statements is correct regarding the image shown in **Figure 3.14**.

   A. Aortic regurgitation is present with an aliasing artifact.
   B. Aortic regurgitation is present with a range-ambiguity artifact.
   C. Aortic regurgitation is present with a mirror artifact.
   D. Aortic regurgitation is present with a beam width artifact along with pulmonary regurgitation.

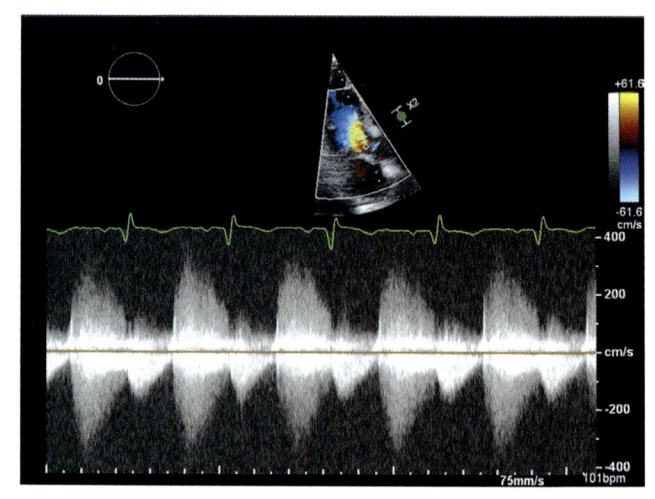

Figure 3.14

ANSWERS

1. **Answer: C.** The only statement that is correct regarding the assumed fundamentals of ultrasound is that sound travels in a straight line. The other statements are incorrect. Echocardiography is based on the physical principles of sound, which travels through a medium in the form of a propagating wave. There are several assumptions of ultrasound imaging that apply to echocardiography, and the violation of any of these can result in an artifact (**Tables 3.1** and **3.2**). Imaging artifacts are either not real; located in the wrong place; display an inappropriate brightness, shape, and size; or result in missing data.

   The key assumptions of ultrasound imaging include: (1) there is a constant rate of attenuation of 1 dB/cm/MHz, (2) all echoes arise from the center of a razor-thin beam, (3) the propagation speed of sound in soft tissue is 1540 m/s, (4) the distance to the reflecting object is directly related to the elapsed time between the transmitted pulse and the detected echo (this distance is proportional to the round-trip travel time), (5) the ultrasound beam travels in a straight line and reflects just once, and (6) the amplitude of returning echoes is related directly to the reflecting or scattering properties of distant objects.

2. **Answer: B.** The propagation speed of sound in the silastic ball is slower than the propagation speed of sound in soft tissue, so the shape of the ball appears distorted. One of the basic assumptions of ultrasound is that the propagation speed of sound in soft tissue is 1540 m/s. However, different tissues (air, fat, bone), depending on their density and stiffness properties, may speed up or slow down the propagation speed of sound. The silastic ball of a ball-cage valve (Starr-Edwards valve) slows the propagation speed (although this is dependent on the composition of the ball and is not true for all valves). This has the effect of distorting the appearance of the ball from a round to a more oval shape instead of affecting the depth of the ball (▶ **Video 3.3**). This type of artifact is referred to as a propagation

Table 3.1. Artifacts Occurring When Assumptions of Ultrasound Are Violated

Artifact	Violated Assumptions(s) Producing Artifact
Attenuation artifacts (improper brightness): include acoustic enhancement, acoustic shadowing	Constant rate of attenuation of 1 dB/cm/MHz
Beam dimension artifacts (added structures): include beam width, slice thickness, side lobe, or grating lobe	All echoes arise from the center of a razor-thin ultrasound beam
Depth of origin artifacts (wrong place or wrong size): include propagation speed or range ambiguity	Propagation speed in soft tissue is 1540 m/s Distance to the reflecting object is directly proportional to the round-trip travel time Ultrasound beam travels in a straight line and reflects just once
Beam path artifacts (duplication of structures or structures in the wrong place): include reverberation, mirror, refraction	Distance to the reflecting object is directly proportional to the round-trip travel time Ultrasound beam travels in a straight line and reflects just once

Reprinted with permission from Venkateshvaran A, Anderson B. Imaging artifacts. In: Anderson B, Park MM, eds. *Basic to Advanced Clinical Echocardiography*. Wolters Kluwer; 2021:60-77. Table 5.1.

Table 3.2. Two-Dimensional Imaging Artifacts

Artifact	Principle Assumption Violated	Mechanism of Formation	Overall Effect	Example	How to Minimize/Avoid
Acoustic enhancement	Attenuation of U/S beam = 1 dB/cm/MHz	Lower-than-expected attenuation of U/S beam	Improper brightness	Increased brightness posterior to PE	Decrease TGC in appropriate region Change Tx position to remove offending reflector from beam path Use alternative imaging plane
Acoustic shadow	Attenuation of U/S beam = 1 dB/cm/MHz	Higher-than-expected attenuation of U/S beam	Missing echoes	Absence of echoes distal to mitral annular calcification (**Figure 3.5(3)**)	Change Tx position to remove offending reflector from beam path Increase TGC in appropriate region Use alternative imaging plane
Beamwidth	All echoes arise from the central axis of U/S beam	Structures detected throughout full width of U/S beam	Wrong shape Wrong size Lateral extension	"Fuzziness" of atrial chamber walls	Move focal zone to area of interest Use alternative imaging plane
Comet tail	U/S beam travels in a straight line and is reflected only once	Close moving reflector(s)	Replication	Reverberation appearance without lines (**Figure 3.5(4)** and **Figure 3.18**)	Change Tx position to remove offending reflector from beam path Use alternative imaging plane

(Continued)

Table 3.2. Two-Dimensional Imaging Artifacts (Continued)

Artifact	Principle Assumption Violated	Mechanism of Formation	Overall Effect	Example	How to Minimize/Avoid
Grating/side lobe	All echoes arise from the central axis of U/S beam	Structures detected by secondary U/S beams	Replication	"Extra" echoes in RA arising from IVC (**Figure 3.5(1)**)	Decrease gain
Mirror	U/S beam travels in a straight line and is reflected only once	U/S beam interrogates the same structure twice	Duplication	"Two" mitral valves in the PLAX view (**Figure 3.10** and **Figure 3.27**)	Change Tx position to remove offending reflector from beam path. Use alternative imaging plane. Decrease TGC in appropriate region
Near-field clutter	All echoes arise from real structures	High amplitude of Tx oscillations	Added echoes Noise in the near field	LV apex pseudo mass (**Figure 3.2**)	Use alternative imaging plane
Range ambiguity	Round-trip time ∝ depth to reflector	Echo from pulse 1 is received after pulse 2 emitted	Improper depth	"Mass" within ventricular cavities in apical views (**Figure 3.1**)	Increase imaging depth
Refraction	U/S beam travels in a straight line and is reflected only once	Bending of U/S beam Improper placement	Duplication	Double aortic valve in SAX (▶ Video 3.1; **Figure 3.29**)	Change Tx position to remove offending structure from beam path. Use alternative imaging plane
Reverberation	U/S beam travels in a straight line and is reflected only once	Bouncing of U/S beam between two strongly reflective interfaces	Added echoes with equal spacing	Ladder appearance within LA from mechanical MVR (**Figure 3.4**, **Figure 3.5(2)**, and **Figure 3.7**)	Change Tx position to remove offending reflector from beam path. Use alternative imaging plane
Slice thickness	All echoes arise from the central axis of U/S beam	Structures detected in front of or behind main imaging plane	Added echoes	Apparent mass within chamber cavity (**Figure 3.3**)	Move focal zone to area of interest
Propagation speed	Round-trip time ∝ depth to reflector	Speed of sound ≠ 1540 m/s	Improper depth Wrong shape	Ball of Starr-Edwards MVR appears within LA cavity (▶ Video 3.3)	Change Tx position to remove offending reflector from beam path. Use alternative imaging plane

IVC, inferior vena cava; LA, left atrium; MVR, mitral valve replacement; PLAX, parasternal long axis; PE, pericardial effusion; RA, right atrium; SAX, short axis; TGC, time gain compensation; Tx, transducer; U/S, ultrasound.

Adapted from Anderson B. *Basic principles of two-dimensional ultrasound imaging.* In: *Echocardiography: The Normal Examination and Echocardiographic Measurements.* 3rd ed. Echotext Pty Ltd: 2016:20. Table 1.8. Reproduced with permission from Echotext Pty Ltd.

speed error artifact, not a resolution-type artifact. When the propagation speed is slower than expected by the ultrasound machine, the object imaged will be assumed to be farther from the transducer than it truly is (**Figure 3.15, left**). In contrast, when the propagation speed is faster than expected, the object imaged will be assumed to be closer to the transducer than it truly is (**Figure 3.15, right**).

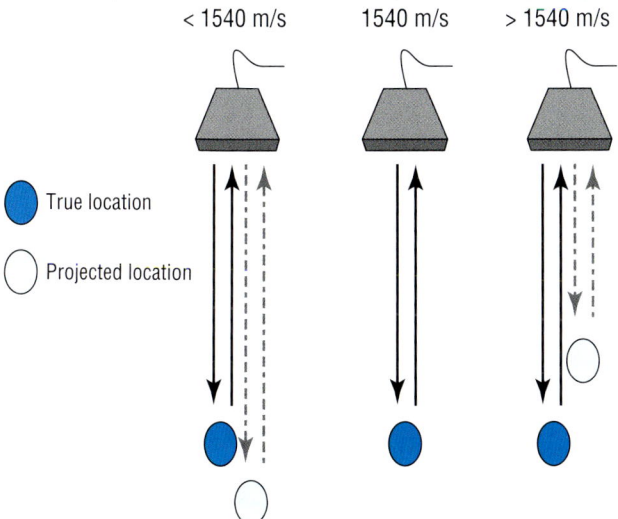

Figure 3.15

3. **Answer: D.** M-mode echocardiography remains a useful tool to distinguish ascending aortic artifacts from dissection flaps. Clinically, it is essential to be able to distinguish artifacts from a flap associated with an aortic dissection. The utilization of criteria to define artifacts in this scenario has been shown to improve the specificity of transesophageal echocardiography (TEE) for the diagnosis of aortic dissection.

There is in vivo and in vitro evidence to support that linear artifacts within the ascending aorta are caused by ultrasound reverberation. In a classic experiment by Appelbe et al, an ultrasound probe was introduced into a water tank containing two balloons placed in series: a "left atrial balloon" closest to the probe and an "aortic balloon" farther away from the probe. They observed that a linear image was consistently present within the aortic balloon when its diameter exceeded the diameter of the left atrial balloon, and since these contained only water, the image was by definition an artifact.

Evangelista et al described the utility of M-mode applied during TEE in recognizing artifacts as they evaluated patients with suspected aortic dissection. They distinguished several types of artifacts in the ascending aorta. The most common of which were type A and B artifacts. A type A artifact within the ascending aorta was defined as that located twice as far from the transducer as from the posterior aortic wall as shown in **Figure 3.16A**. By using M-mode echocardiography, they were able to show that dissection flaps have independent motion to the posterior aortic wall and that artifacts usually move parallel to the posterior aortic wall and therefore do not have independent motion, and also typically move with greater amplitude. Artifacts also lack rapid oscillatory movements, which are usually associated with dissection flaps. A type B artifact is located at twice the distance from the right pulmonary artery posterior wall as from the posterior aortic wall (**Figure 3.16B**).

Answer A is incorrect since these linear artifacts in the aorta are caused by reverberation, not refraction. Answer B is incorrect since artifacts in the aorta more typically appear when the aortic diameter is larger, not smaller, than the left atrial diameter as previously mentioned. Answer C is incorrect since artifacts are usually created at the posterior aortic wall interface with the left atrium (see **Figure 3.16A**). In addition, when applying color Doppler, artifacts usually do not produce turbulence or interruption in the pattern of blood flow as would be seen with the presence of a true and false lumen.

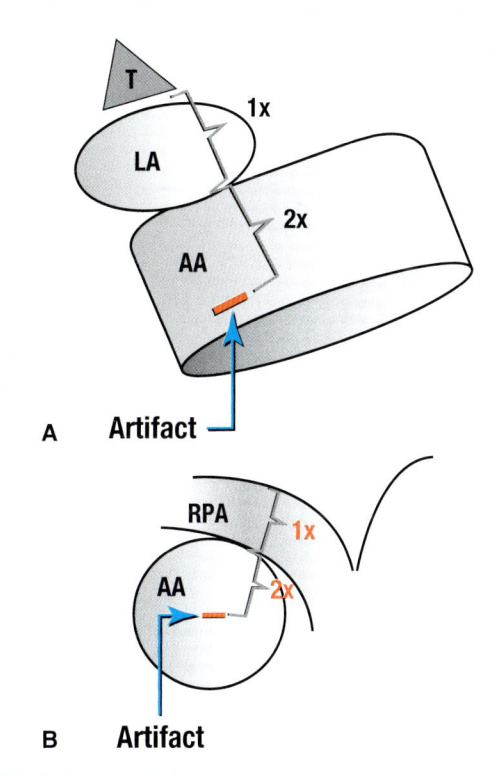

Figure 3.16. AA, ascending aorta; LA, left atrium; RPA, right pulmonary artery; T, transducer.

4. **Answer: A.** Reverberation-type artifacts occur because of multiple reflections between the transducer and other strongly reflective interfaces. The

amount of ultrasound energy reflected from an interface is primarily dependent upon the magnitude of the acoustic impedance mismatch at the interface. When the ultrasound beam encounters a strongly reflective interface, some energy returns to the transducer, some energy is re-reflected back into the patient, and it can be reflected again at the same interface. This second echo returns to the transducer at a later time, and will therefore be displayed farther away from the real structure since it is assumed to have arisen from a greater depth. Multiple reflections may occur when several interfaces are present for reflection, such as is the case of a mechanical valve disc. The intensity of reverberation lines decreases as the distance from the transducer increases. The reverberation lines are equally spaced and perpendicular to the main sound beam, often having the appearance of a ladder. Refraction artifacts, not reverberation artifacts, are affected by the difference in acoustic impedance between two media. **Figure 3.17** shows repeated "bouncing" of the ultrasound beam between two interfaces. Because the re-reflected echoes return to the transducer later, these structures will be placed deeper than the true reflector. The distance between reverberation artifacts is equal to the distance (d) between the two interfaces. Echoes produced from multiple reflections appear progressively weaker since the ultrasound intensity of reverberation artifacts decreases with each re-reflection.

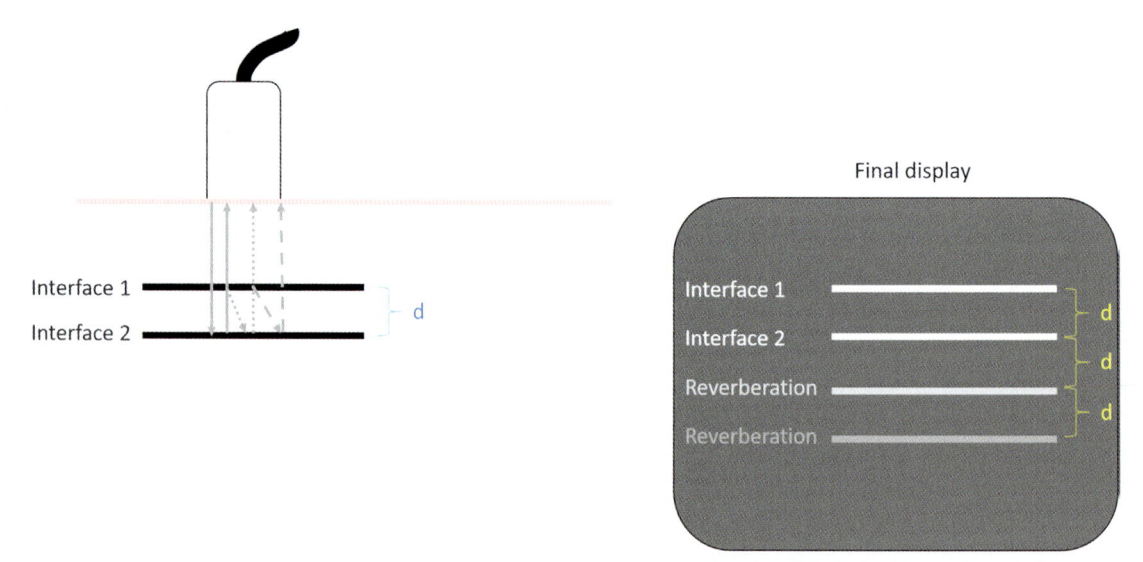

Figure 3.17. Reprinted with permission from Venkateshvaran A, Anderson B. Imaging artifacts. In: Anderson B, Park MM, eds. *Basic to Advanced Clinical Echocardiography*. Wolters Kluwer; 2021:60-77. Fig. 5.10.

5. **Answer: C.** Common causes of comet-tail artifacts include mechanical valves and pacemaker wires. Comet-tail artifacts occur with various metallic objects but can also occur without prosthetic materials with highly reflective interfaces such as the pericardium and small calcifications. These are reverberation-type artifacts where there is ringing of the transducer to create a solid hyperechoic beam of ultrasound distal to the creating object. The creation of a comet-tail artifact is similar to reverberation artifacts though the appearance differs in that the comet-tail artifact does not have equidistant spaced lines of decreasing intensity, and like the tail of a comet, these artifacts taper and fade with increasing depth (**Figure 3.18**).

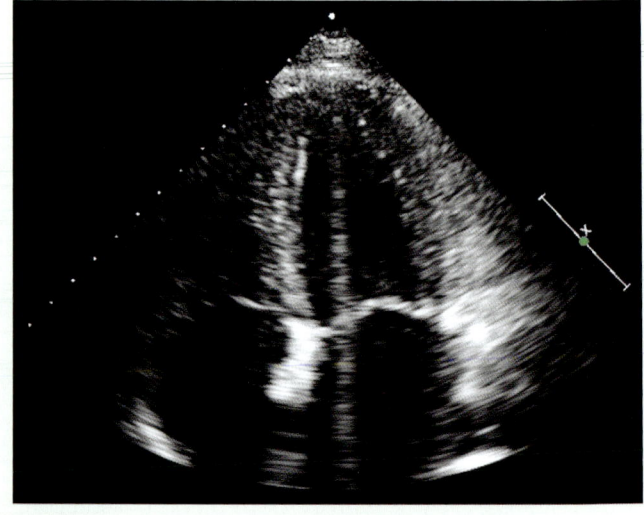

Figure 3.18

6. **Answer: A.** Reflectors producing a beam width artifact will always be imaged *adjacent* to the artifact, not behind or in front of the main beam plane. Therefore, Answer A is not correct. All other statements are true regarding the potential echocardiographic features of beam width artifacts. Recall that echoes are generated from reflectors lying within the full width of the ultrasound beam and echoes will continue to be generated if a reflector remains within the beam width. Therefore, beam width artifacts occur when: (1) two separate reflectors lying side-by-side within the ultrasound beam appear as one (**Figure 3.19**), (2) a narrow reflector within the ultrasound beam appears wider than it really is, and (3) a strong reflector to the side of an echo-free cavity appears within the cavity. Beam width artifacts are most apparent within echo-free cavities. **Figure 3.19** shows that two far-field objects at Depth B are encompassed within the ultrasound beam width beyond the focal zone and are therefore superimposed on the screen display, creating a beam width artifact. When the same two reflectors are separated by a distance greater than the ultrasound beam width, they are resolved and appear as two separate structures (Depth A).

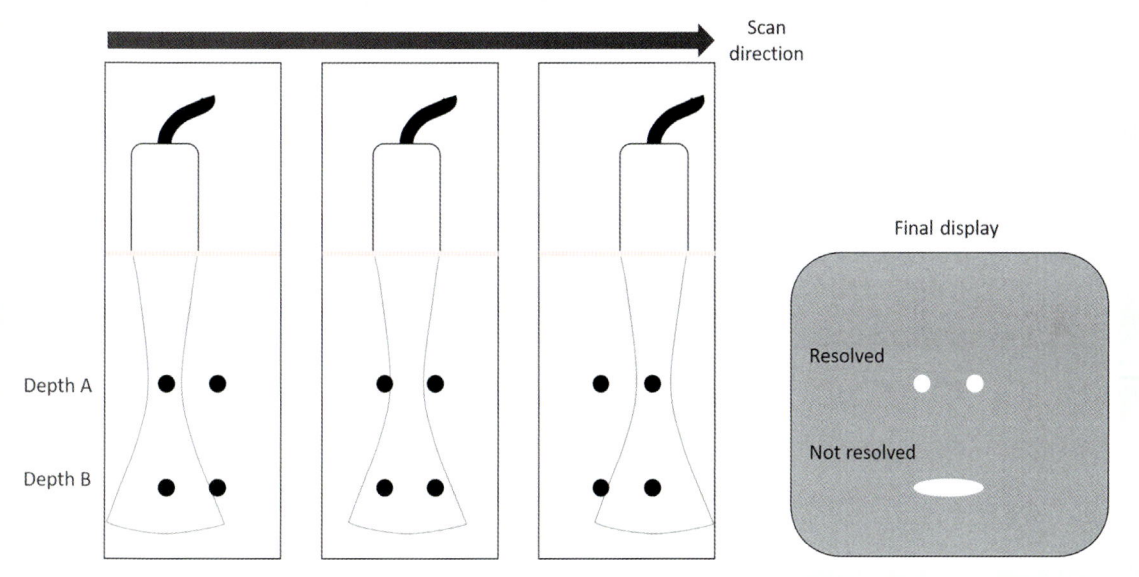

Figure 3.19. Reprinted with permission from Venkateshvaran A, Anderson B. Imaging artifacts. In: Anderson B, Park MM, eds. *Basic to Advanced Clinical Echocardiography*. Wolters Kluwer; 2021:60-77. Fig. 5.6.

7. **Answer: D.** Snell's law describes the principle by which refraction of the ultrasound beam occurs and contributes to the development of refraction-type artifacts. It requires information on the angle of incidence of the ultrasound beam and the propagation speed of ultrasound in two different media. Under normal conditions, if the propagation speed (c) is the same in two media, the transmission angle will equal the incident angle. However, if the c in medium 2 is greater than the c in medium 1, the transmission angle (or angle of refraction) in medium 2 will be greater than the incident angle in medium 1. In other words, refraction refers to the bending of an ultrasound beam as it passes from one media to another and requires different propagation speeds of ultrasound and an oblique angle of incidence to occur.

$$\text{Snell's Law}: \frac{\text{sin of incident angle}}{\text{c in medium 1}} = \frac{\text{sin of transmitted angle}}{\text{c in medium 2}}$$

8. **Answer: B.** In a side lobe artifact, additional echoes will appear lateral to the true object location. Most of the energy emitted by the ultrasound machine is concentrated along a central (main) beam. However, not all the energy arises from this central beam. Secondary beams of ultrasound energy exist outside of the central beam. These weaker secondary beams are caused by diffraction effects and have the capacity of transmitting and receiving ultrasound energy just like the central beam. These secondary beams are called side lobes (or grating lobes in the case of array transducers). If

a strong reflector is encountered by a side lobe, echoes will be produced and the machine will assume that these echoes originated from points along the central beam axis, and the echoes will be displayed as though they have arisen within the central beam. In **Figure 3.20**, as the ultrasound beam sweeps left to right, the structure is interrogated by side lobe beams (light blue) as well as by the main beam (dark blue). On the final image display, echoes originating from side lobe beams and the main beam are displayed with the weaker side lobe artifacts appearing lateral to the true structure. Most commonly, this artifact creates a linear "arclike" artifact at both sides of the strong reflector. These types of artifacts are most obvious in echo-free cavities.

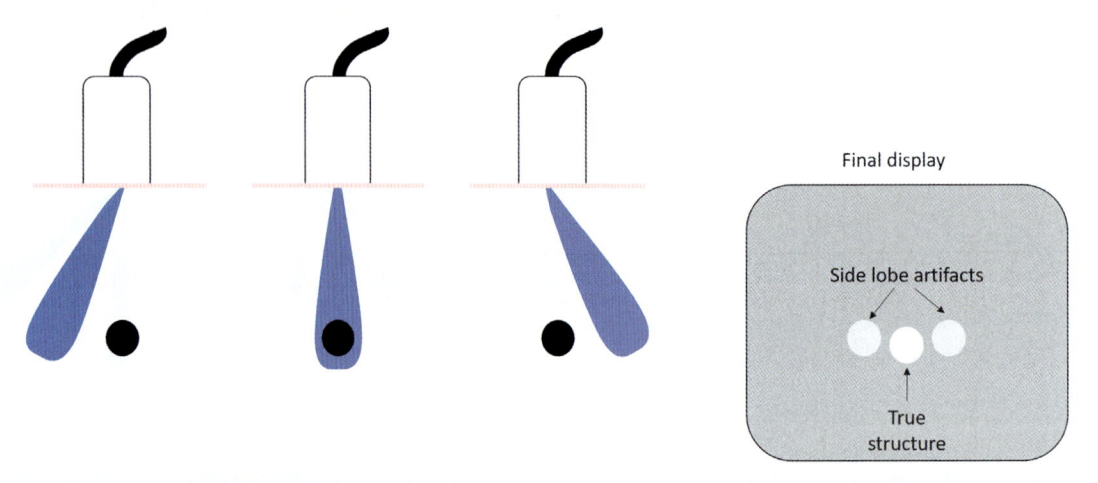

Figure 3.20. Reprinted with permission from Venkateshvaran A, Anderson B. Imaging artifacts. In: Anderson B, Park MM, eds. *Basic to Advanced Clinical Echocardiography*. Wolters Kluwer; 2021:60-77. Fig. 5.7.

9. **Answer: D.** Distortion of structures occurs when the propagation speed through a structure is not the assumed 1540 m/s; this is not a feature of refraction artifacts. Therefore, Answer D is correct as this is a false statement. Refraction or bending of the ultrasound beam occurs when an ultrasound beam strikes an interface at an angle other than 90° and when the propagation speeds of the two media at either side of the interface are different. This can result in (1) improper positioning or misplacement of structures (**Figure 3.21A**), (2) missing echoes or shadowing at the edge of curved structures (**Figure 3.21B**), or (3) duplication of structures (**Figure 3.21C**). Answers A, B, and C are true statements.

In **Figure 3.21A**, the propagation speed through media 1 (C_1) is less than the propagation speed through media 2 (C_2), resulting in bending of the beam away from the assumed path. This results in the misplacement of the structure on the final image display.

In **Figure 3.21B**, an edge shadowing is produced when the ultrasound beam strikes the edge of the circular structure. A combination of refraction and reflection occurs, causing the ultrasound beam to be deflected and broadened. This leads to a reduction on the beam intensity so that the echoes beyond the edge of the circular structure are reduced in amplitude. On a final image display, this results in a narrow shadow directly beneath the margins of the rounded structure.

In **Figure 3.21C**, duplication of a structure is produced when there is refraction of the ultrasound beam as it passess obliquely through the lens-shaped structure. As a result, the single structure (black circle) is interrogated twice: once by the refracted beam and once by the "normal" beam. On the final image display, the single structure is displayed twice as either two separate structures (as shown) or as two overlapping structures.

Figure 3.21D shows the subcostal 4-chamber view; solid white arrows point to right atrial and ventricular walls; dashed white arrows point to the refracted, "duplicated" right atrial and right ventricular wall.

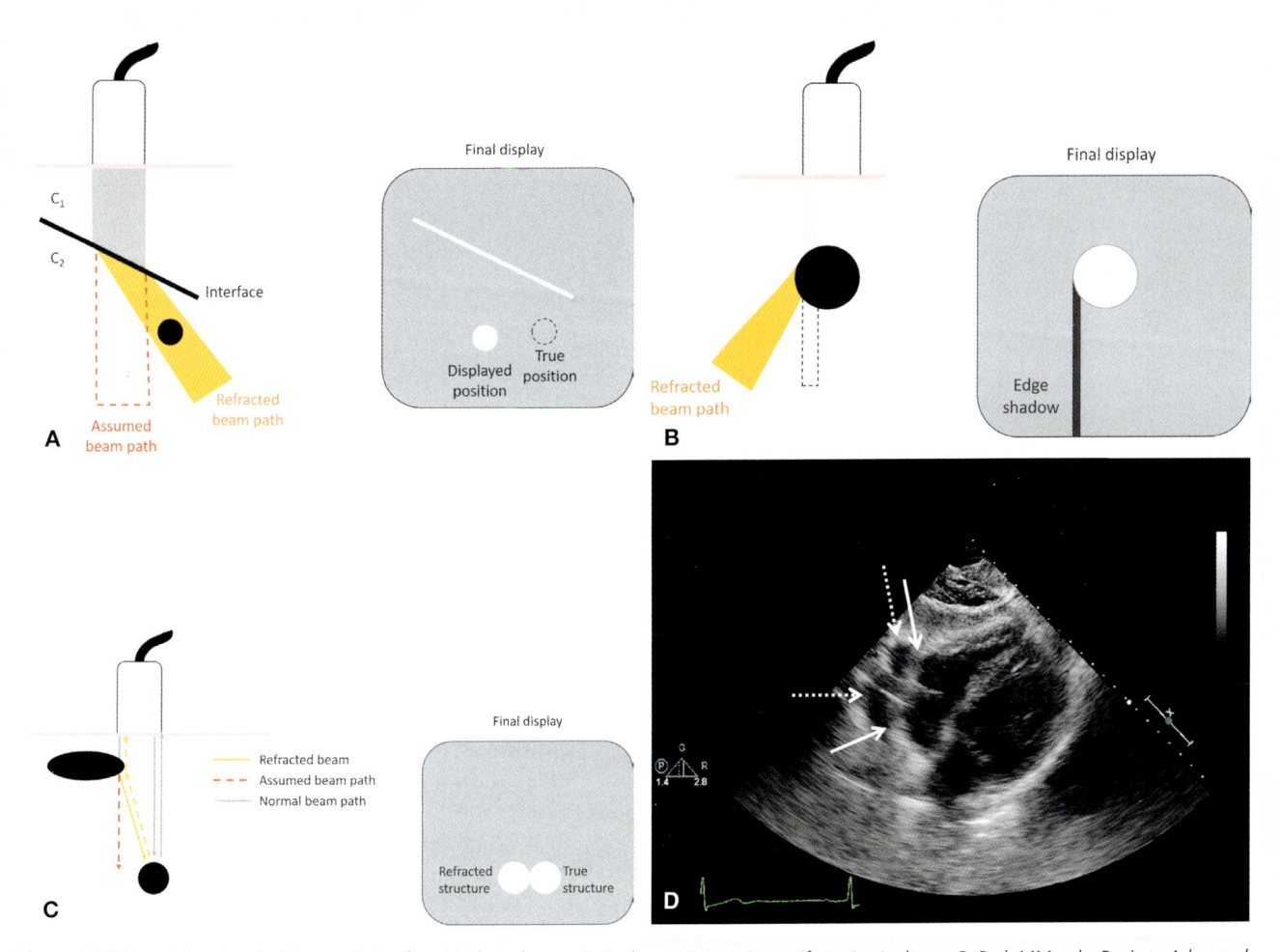

Figure 3.21. A-C, Reprinted with permission from Venkateshvaran A, Anderson B. Imaging artifacts. In: Anderson B, Park MM, eds. *Basic to Advanced Clinical Echocardiography*. Wolters Kluwer; 2021:60-77. Fig. 5.8.

10. **Answer: B.** Range ambiguity occurs when echoes from deep structures created by a first pulse arrive at the transducer after the second pulse has been transmitted. It is assumed that all received echoes are produced by the most recently sent pulse and the depth placement of received echoes is based on the return time of the transducer. Range-ambiguity artifacts may occur when a structure is detected outside the field of view by the first pulse. When the echoes generated from the first pulse arrive at the transducer after the second pulse has been emitted, the machine assumes that the returning echoes have originated from the second pulse and therefore incorrectly places the received echoes closer to the transducer than the actual location (**Figure 3.22**). These artifacts are especially apparent when the ultrasound beam passes through low-attenuating structures such as blood-filled cavities.

Answer A is not correct as propagation speed artifacts are not mechanistically the same as a range-ambiguity artifact. Propagation speed artifacts occur when the propagation speed is slower or faster than the assumed propagation speed of 1540 m/s.

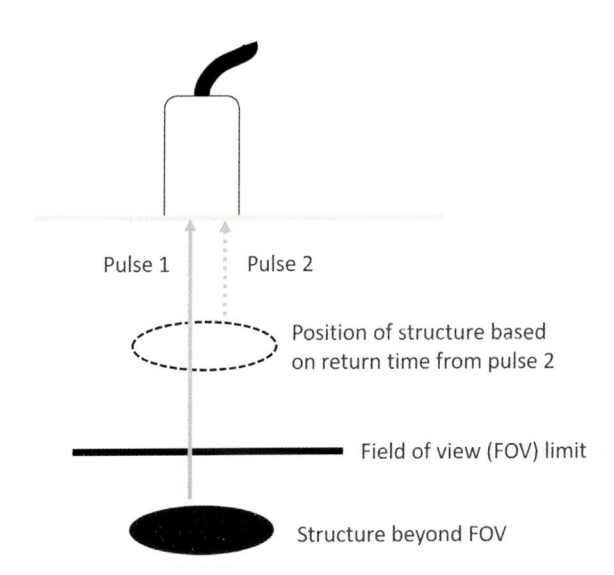

Figure 3.22. Reprinted with permission from Venkateshvaran A, Anderson B. Imaging Artifacts. In: Anderson B, Park MM, eds. *Basic to Advanced Clinical Echocardiography*. Wolters Kluwer; 2021:60-77. Fig. 5.12.

This results in the incorrect placement of echoes or the incorrect display of the size and shape of structures. Answer C is not correct as range ambiguity can be avoided by increasing the image depth or field of view, which effectively lowers the PRF. Therefore, echoes from deep structures created by the first pulse arrive at the transducer before the second pulse has been transmitted. Answer D is not correct as range ambiguity occurs when the ultrasound machine is operating at a high PRF, not a low PRF. At a high PRF, echoes from deep structures created by the first pulse arrive at the transducer after the second pulse has been transmitted. Range-ambiguity artifacts are commonly seen within the left ventricular cavity from the apical views especially when image quality is very good, and the image depth is shallow.

11. **Answer: B.** Spectral Doppler mirror artifacts result in the duplication (mirror image) of Doppler shifts on the opposite side of the baseline to the actual unidirectional flow. Mirror artifacts are produced in several ways: (1) by interaction with a strong reflector (eg, duplication of the inferior vena cava from the subcostal view), (2) when the incident angle is near 90° (eg, eccentric mitral regurgitant jet as seen from the apical views), or (3) from "cross-talk" between the forward and reverse channels (ie, electronic duplication of a unidirectional signal above and below the zero baseline). These artifacts can be eliminated or reduced by decreasing the power output or gain and/or by optimizing the angle between the ultrasound beam and blood flow direction.

12. **Answer: C.** Most cardiac ultrasound machines have harmonic imaging and changing from fundamental to harmonic imaging is helpful in reducing several types of artifacts such as side lobes, grating lobes, reverberations, and near-field clutter. Several structures can mimic a thrombus in the left ventricle (**Table 3.3**). Increasing the transducer frequency, decreasing the depth, using multiple views, moving the focal zone to the apex, or the utilization of ultrasound-enhancing agents (UEAs) can all help distinguish a left ventricular (LV) thrombus from an artifact. LV thrombus develops almost exclusively in the region of a wall motion abnormality and thrombi are most commonly seen in an akinetic, dyskinetic, or aneurysmal segment, usually at the apex. Thrombus is usually laminar, with discrete shape and borders, and may appear as protruding or mobile. Its motion is usually concordant with the LV wall. The mechanical index should be decreased when using UEAs to avoid excessive destruction of the bubbles.

13. **Answer: C.** True structures do not typically cross anatomic borders, may have independent motion, usually have well-defined borders and attachments to nearby structures, and can be visualized in multiple views. Artifacts may cross anatomic borders, have indistinct borders and no obvious attachments, and

Table 3.3. Differential of Structures/Artifacts in the Left Ventricle

Normal Variants or Pathologic Structures
- False tendons
- Prominent trabeculations
- Prominent papillary muscles (accessory or aberrant papillary muscle)
- Tumors (fibroma, myxoma, rhabdomyoma, lipoma, etc.)
- Endomyocardial fibrosis
- Apical hypertrophy (Yamaguchi syndrome)
- Congenital diverticuli
- Thrombus
- Aneurysms/pseudoaneurysms/outpouchings
- Noncompaction cardiomyopathy/hypertrabeculations

Artifact Types
- Reverberation (near-field clutter, comet tail)
- Range ambiguity
- Beam dimension (slice thickness)

are not seen in multiple views. With color Doppler imaging, true structures will affect flow patterns, whereas artifacts will not affect the flow patterns.

14. **Answer: D.** Slice thickness artifacts occur when a structure is detected within the elevation plane of the ultrasound beam; that is, when the structure is detected in front or behind the main (central) beam. Illustrated in **Figure 3.23**, the slice thickness or elevation plane is shown from a side view of the transducer (left). When an echo-free structure within the main beam (middle) and a structure behind the main beam (right) are detected, echoes are generated from both structures and then "collapsed" to produce a 2D image. As a result, the displayed image is composed of echoes that have originated from the main imaging plane as well as those that have arisen from structures in front and behind the main imaging plane. Therefore, Answer D is correct as slice thickness artifacts are not duplications or copies of real structures.

Answers A-C are not correct since these artifacts do result in the duplication of real structures. Reverberation artifacts produce multiple reflections of the same structure when the ultrasound beam bounces between two or more strong reflectors that are positioned in close proximity. Mirror artifacts can produce duplication of structures when the ultrasound beam encounters a strongly reflecting interface that acts as a mirror. A refraction artifact can produce duplication of structures via the lens principle.

15. **Answer: B.** A ring-down artifact is a type of reverberation artifact. Ring down is caused by air or gas particles that continuously resonate or vibrate back to the transducer, creating a bright continuous

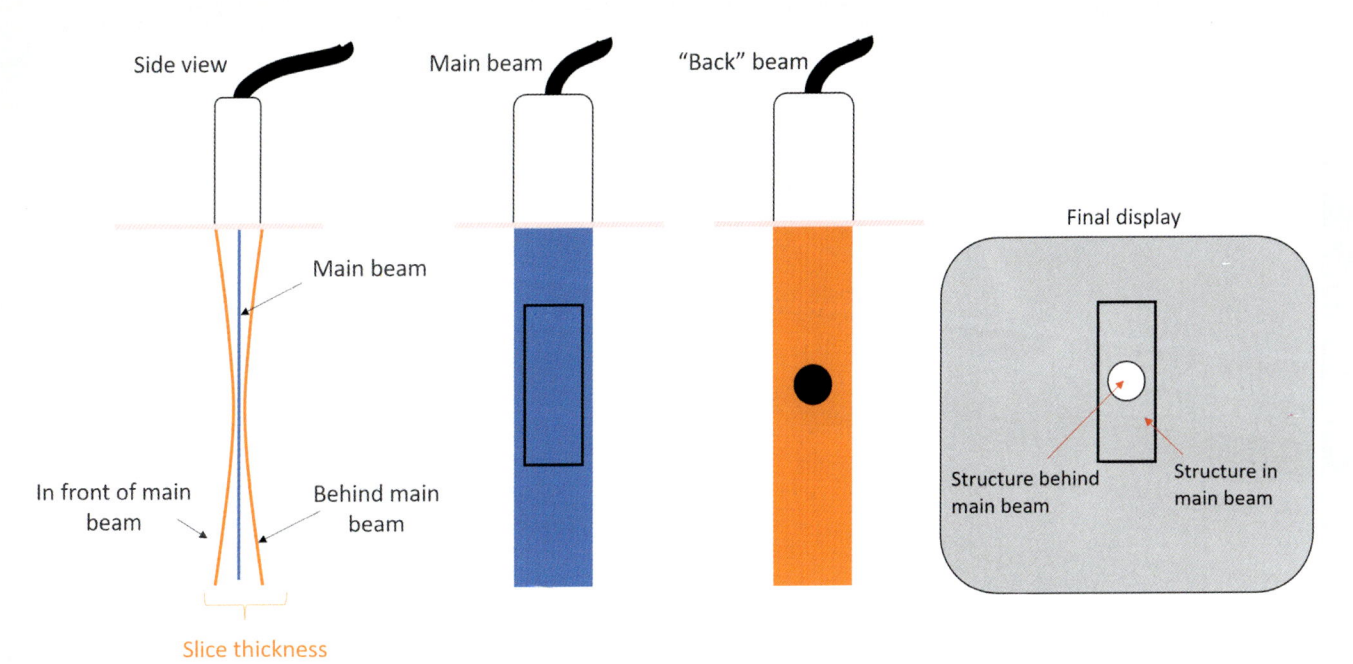

Figure 3.23. Reprinted with permission from Venkateshvaran A, Anderson B. Imaging artifacts. In: Anderson B, Park MM, eds. *Basic to Advanced Clinical Echocardiography*. Wolters Kluwer; 2021:60-77. Fig. 5.9.

streak distal to the reflector. In the gastrointestinal system, when a central fluid collection is trapped by a ring of air bubbles, the pocket of fluid and air may continuously resonate, reflecting back ultrasound and creating a bright reflector. Distal to this bright reflector of vibrating fluid and air is a linear beam of ultrasound, that is, the ring-down artifact. In cardiovascular imaging, ring-down artifact is similar to but appears mechanistically different than a comet-tail artifact. Strong repetitive reverberations cause ringing of the transducer crystal and thus the ring-down artifact. Unlike comet-tail artifacts, ring-down artifacts do not usually fade over the image depth.

16. **Answer: B.** Pseudomitral regurgitation refers to the artifact created by a mitral mechanical tilting disk prosthesis that mimics mitral regurgitation (MR). Evaluation of MR due to valvular dysfunction in mechanical mitral valves is difficult due to shadowing and shielding effects from the prosthesis, which obscure visualization of the left atrium (LA). A mirroring effect may occur with mechanical tilting disk mitral prostheses, whereby the left ventricular outflow tract (LVOT) Doppler flow is mirrored into the LA. While systolic flow in the LA would typically be MR, pseudo-MR may be seen on the color and spectral Doppler when LVOT flow is mirrored into the LA. This can be differentiated from the true MR via close observation of the timing and velocity of the spectral Doppler signal. See **Figure 3.24**, which shows the proposed mechanism of acoustic mirroring and artifact generation by the prosthetic mitral valve, whereby the ultrasound beam travels through left ventricular (LV) cavity and is reflected off the mitral prosthesis tilted toward LV outflow tract (LVOT) flow. Red blood cells passing through LVOT scatter some sound back toward prosthesis, where it is reflected back toward the transducer. Because of increased transit time taken, reflected LVOT flow is projected into left atrium (LA) as pseudomitral regurgitation signal.

17. **Answer: D.** The arrow in **Figure 3.1** points to a range-ambiguity artifact, which has the appearance

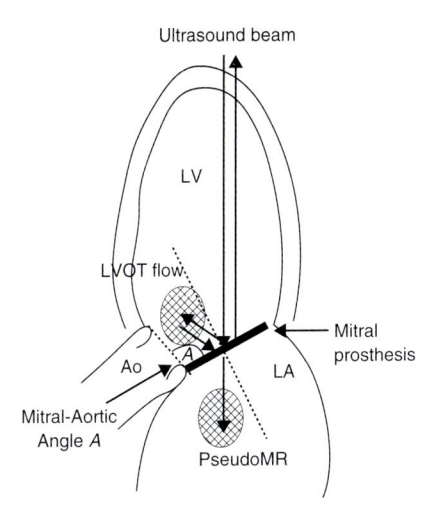

Figure 3.24. A, angle between aortic annulus and mitral prothesis; Ao, aorta; MR, mitral regurgitation. (Reprinted from Rudski LG, Chow CM, Levine RA. Prosthetic mitral regurgitation can be mimicked by Doppler color flow mapping: avoiding misdiagnosis. *J Am Soc Echocardiogr*. 2004;17(8):829-833. Copyright © 2004 American Society of Echocardiography. With permission.)

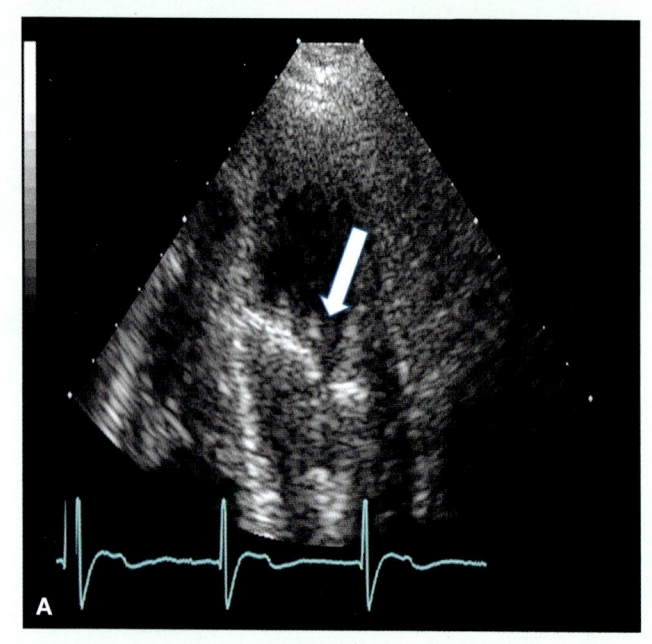

Figure 3.25A

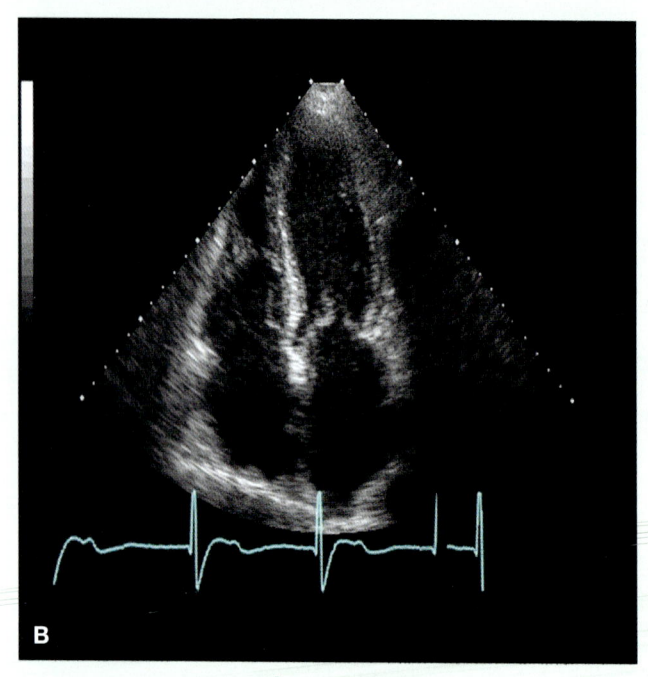

Figure 3.25B

of a "mass" within the left ventricle. This can be better visualized in **Figure 3.25** and in ▶ **Video 3.4A,B**. The arrow points to the range-ambiguity artifact in **Figure 3.25A**, and ▶ **Video 3.4A**. After increasing the imaging depth in **Figure 3.25B** and ▶ **Video 3.4B**, the artifact disappears. Range-ambiguity artifacts occur because objects outside of the field of view reflect ultrasound that is not received until early during the next transmit/listen cycle and therefore are thought to be closer to the transducer than they actually are (see **Figure 3.22**).

18. **Answer: C.** This type of artifact is known as near-field clutter or noise. The proposed mechanisms for this type of artifact include high-amplitude oscillations of the piezoelectric elements that affects the near field of the ultrasound beam, reverberation due to interaction with chest wall structures, and refraction from ribs. The appearance of additional echoes in the near field can mask weaker echoes of true anatomic structures. Improving the near-field resolution with higher-frequency transducers, decreasing the depth, changing the views, using ultrasound enhancing agents, and harmonic imaging can all help reduce or eliminate this type of artifact.

19. **Answer: E.** This is an example of a beam dimension artifact, which can create added echoes that appear in the wrong location. Reflectors displayed in the 2D image originate from the full width and thickness of a three-dimensional (3D) beam as well as from secondary beams (grating lobes). Therefore, when a structure is detected from anywhere within the 3D beam or from secondary beams, an echo will be produced and displayed as though it has originated from the central (main) beam. Therefore, the echocardiographic appearance of beam dimension artifact will be as (1) the merger of two separate objects so they appear as one (beam width artifact), (2) lateral smearing or extension of an object (side lobe or grating lobe artifact), and (3) a partial volume effect where a strong reflector appears within an echo-free space (slice thickness artifact see **Figure 3.23**). These artifacts are commonly seen in the apical views when trying to visualize structures in the far field, where the beam is the widest. In **Figure 3.3**, the specific type of beam dimension artifact is a slice thickness artifact secondary to a calcified aortic valve/ascending aorta that is out of plane with the anechogenic right atrial cavity, creating an appearance of a mass in the right atrium.

20. **Answer: C.** The linear density seen in the aorta is a reverberation artifact. This is an artifact (illustrated in **Figure 3.16B**), which is twice the distance from the PA posterior wall to aortic posterior wall. The movement of the artifact parallels the movement of the aortic posterior wall and does not have independent motion, whereas aortic dissection flaps would show independent motion. In addition, the linear density extends beyond anatomic borders, outside the boundaries of the aorta. Color Doppler imaging shows no disruption of flow, whereas aortic dissection flaps would show demarcation of flow between the true and false channels. The M-mode trace shows parallel motion of the artifact with the aortic wall with increased amplitude of the artifact relative to the aortic wall. Of note, these criteria are validated for acute dissection flaps that are typically

mobile and not chronic dissection flaps that may behave differently and may not have independent motion.

21. **Answer: B.** The initial scout view in the parasternal long-axis view is done to visualize structures below the heart. This view is plentiful with artifacts that we become skilled at filtering out during daily readings. Seen in this image are (1) side lobe artifact of the aortic valve seen in diastole demonstrating lateral extension of the coaptation zone; (2) reverberation artifact arising from the anterior aortic wall; (3) attenuation artifact due to acoustic shadowing beyond a region of calcification in the descending aorta; and (4) comet-tail artifact caused by the same aortic wall calcification.

22. **Answer: C.** The patient has undergone an interventional procedure. This patient has an atrial septal occluder device. The image seen in the left atrium is a "figure-of-8" artifact from the device. This artifact has been described with the Amplatzer closure device for left atrial appendage and atrial septal defect/patent foramen ovale closure. It is recognized on three-dimensional echocardiogram, TEE, and less frequently on the transthoracic echocardiogram. The ultrasound physics resulting in the "figure-of-8" appearance are complex and occur with disc occluders that have a specific epitrochoidal mesh configuration. The wires within the mesh cause reflection of ultrasound dependent on the angle of insonation of the beam. If the ultrasound beam strikes the wire perpendicularly, its energy is reflected directly to the transducer with the least amount of dissipation and creates the "figure-of-8" appearance.

23. **Answer: B.** The arrows point to echoes that appear in the left atrium in a patient with a mechanical prosthetic mitral valve. These are reverberations. They are characterized as multiple horizontal lines that are equidistant with decreasing intensity with increasing depth (see **Figure 3.17**). They are due to multiple reflections from the discs of the metallic prosthesis.

24. **Answer: C.** The image shows an example of ghosting, which is a type of artifact that can develop with color Doppler, often caused by a mechanical prosthesis or other strong, highly mobile reflectors. These artifacts are transient and do not correspond to expected blood flow. Ghosting refers to color Doppler that is distorted beyond anatomic borders due to multiple reflections with color appearing in adjacent regions with no actual flow. This can appear as brief flashes that are inconsistent with physiologic or pathologic jets of regurgitation. Other color Doppler artifacts along with the mechanism and typical appearance are summarized in **Table 3.4**.

Table 3.4. Color Doppler Artifacts

Artifact	Mechanism of Formation	Appearance	How to Minimize/Avoid
Aliasing	Velocities exceed Nyquist limit	Color reversal	Use lower Tx frequency Increase velocity scale Shift the zero baseline Decrease color box depth
Blooming (color bleeding)	Very high gain settings	Color extends beyond region of true blood flow	Decrease color gain
Flash/ghosting	Doppler shifts created by moving structure	Brief flashes of color overlaying anatomic structures	Change angle of interrogation Use off-axis imaging Reduce color box size
Mirror	Interaction with a strong reflector	Duplication of color outside of real structure	Change angle of interrogation Use off-axis imaging
Shadowing	Weakening of Doppler shifts beyond structure causing an acoustic shadow	Absence of color distal to structure creating shadow	Change angle of interrogation Use off-axis imaging
Twinkling	Strongly reflective structures/interfaces	Color "noise" Mosaic of rapidly changing colors around structures/interfaces	Decrease color gain Change angle of interrogation Use off-axis imaging
Color splay	Doppler side lobe at the level of vena contracta	Linear "arclike" color artifact at both sides of originating jet	Use off-axis imaging Change angle of interrogation

Tx, transducer.

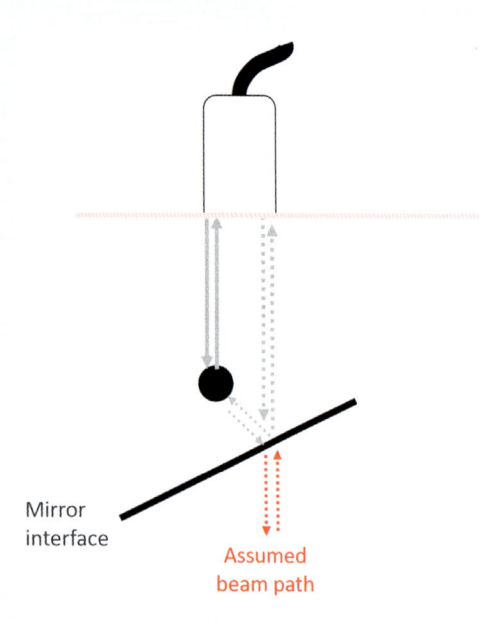

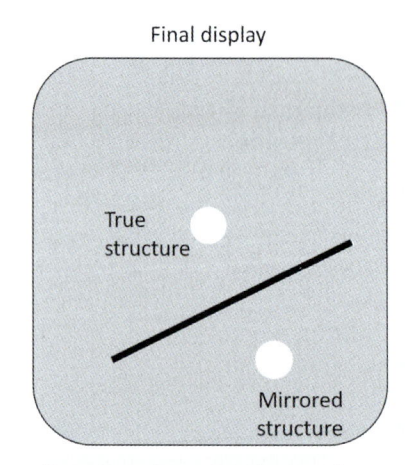

Figure 3.26. Reprinted with permission from Venkateshvaran A, Anderson B. Imaging artifacts. In: Anderson B, Park MM, eds. *Basic to Advanced Clinical Echocardiography*. Wolters Kluwer; 2021:60.77. Fig. 5.11.

25. **Answer: D.** Echocardiographic identification of proper Impella cannula location is essential to assure optimal hemodynamic support. Several different parameters can be useful to assess this positioning including the distance from the aortic valve/annulus to the inflow cannula, midcavitary positioning away from the subvalvular apparatus and mitral valve, and color Doppler mosaic identification. When the color Doppler mosaic occurs above the aortic valve, it identifies the outflow cannula in the optimal position. When the color Doppler mosaic occurs in the LVOT, it suggests the outflow cannula is below the aortic valve and not in the proper position. The color Doppler mosaic does not suggest aortic or mitral regurgitation, but rather is an artifact created by the outflow cannula. **Figure 3.9A** shows the Impella catheter and **Figure 3.9B** and **Figure 3.9C** show the color Doppler mosaic in reasonable position above the aortic valve.

26. **Answer: D.** This is a normal image. There is a mirror-image artifact posterior to the heart. A duplicate (mirror-image) mitral valve appears to be present within the echolucent region and confirms that this is not related to an effusion or other pathologies. The real mitral valve exists on one side of a strong (specular) reflector, which in this case is the pericardial interface where there is a large acoustic impedance mismatch. As seen in **Figure 3.26**, the true structure is interrogated twice by the transducer: once as the ultrasound beam travels straight to the structure and then straight back to the transducer (solid lines) and a second time when the beam hits a mirror interface. When the beam hits the mirror interface, it is reflected off the "mirror" to the structure and then echoes from the structure return along the same path back to the transducer (dashed lines). On the final image display, the real structure is displayed on the transducer side of the mirror interface, while the mirror artifact appears on the opposite side of the "mirror" because the return time to the transducer is longer. The true reflector and the artifact appear at equal distances from the mirror. **Figure 3.27** shows the "mirrored" anterior and posterior mitral leaflets.

27. **Answer: D.** The artifact seen is referred to as "tiger stripes." These high-amplitude bandlike signals correspond with the fundamental and harmonic frequencies, with the first band (lowest frequency on the Doppler recording) representing its fundamental frequency. These signals are thought to be caused by oscillating intracardiac structures such as the aortic valve. Although early descriptions were seen in flail bioprosthetic leaflets, "tiger stripes" are not necessarily a sign of valvular dysfunction. This finding is not rare, but commonly overlooked since

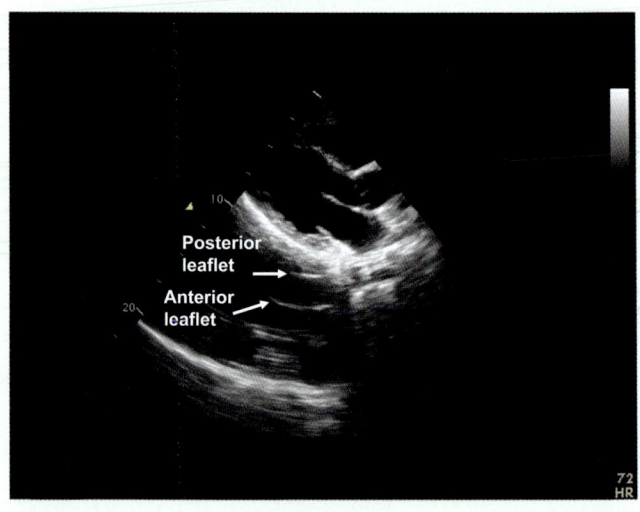

Figure 3.27

Table 3.5. Spectral Doppler Artifacts

Artifact	Mechanism of Formation	Appearance	How to Minimize/Avoid
Aliasing (PWD)	Velocities exceed Nyquist limit	Velocities displayed above and below the zero baseline	Use lower Tx frequency Shift the zero baseline Decrease sample volume depth Increase number of sample volumes (high PRF) Change to CWD
Beamwidth	Strong Doppler signal detected at edge of beam or detected by a grating/side lobe	Signal superimposed on trace as though it has originated from the center of main beam	Change angle of interrogation
Mirror	Interaction with a strong reflector Nonparallel incident angle (angle near 90°) "Cross-talk" between forward and reverse channels	Doppler shifts on opposite side of the baseline to actual unidirectional flow	Change angle of interrogation Reduce spectral gain or output power
Spectral Broadening (PWD)	Increased spectral width and/or absent spectral window	Filling of spectral window with variable velocities	Decrease sample volume size Decrease spectral Doppler gain

CWD, continuous-wave Doppler; PRF, pulse repetition frequency; PWD, pulsed-wave Doppler; Tx, transducer.

clinicians readily recognize that it is an artifact and may see no pertinent information related to this finding in the context of a comprehensive echocardiogram. Other spectral Doppler artifacts along with the mechanism and typical appearance are summarized in **Table 3.5**.

28. **Answer: A. Figure 3.12** shows a continuous-wave (CW) Doppler profile of mitral valve gradients obtained with transesophageal echocardiography. The spectral Doppler patterns shows a dense inner signal of peak velocity of 2.4 m/s or 23 mm Hg. In addition, there is a less dense outer signal with a peak velocity of near 4m/s or 64 mm Hg. This outer signal does not represent the true velocities of blood flow across the valve and is created as a form of Doppler artifact. The mechanism of this type of "double envelope" artifact is not agreed upon, but many hypotheses have been postulated including excess gain, reverberations, or a hydraulic phenomenon related to flow acceleration of the jet impinging on the interventricular septum. This later hydraulic phenomenon is similar to a pressure recovery phenomenon, where a narrow flow stream of the jet is created with acceleration of the velocity. Note in this example, the artifact resolved after adjustment of the imaging angle and without adjustment of the Doppler gain, wall filter, or the use of angle correction (**Figure 3.28**).

29. **Answer: D.** The images of a mitral regurgitant jet show an artifact referred to as "color Doppler splay." This is a horizontal arc of holosystolic or nonholosystolic color Doppler more often on the atrial side of the valve but also may be seen on the ventricular side. It is created from as a result of a color Doppler side lobe artifact. It may be present as the only color Doppler clue to severe mitral regurgitation (MR) and is not usually seen with mild MR. Color Doppler splay may be the only sign of significant MR in a given imaging plane and is more common with eccentric wall-hugging jets. In some cases of splay, the lateral sides of the Doppler profile may appear like "wings" with a thinner signal than the midportion.

30. **Answer: C.** This is an example (▶ **Video 3.1**) of a refraction artifact, which can create the appearance of a double image, which in this case is the aortic

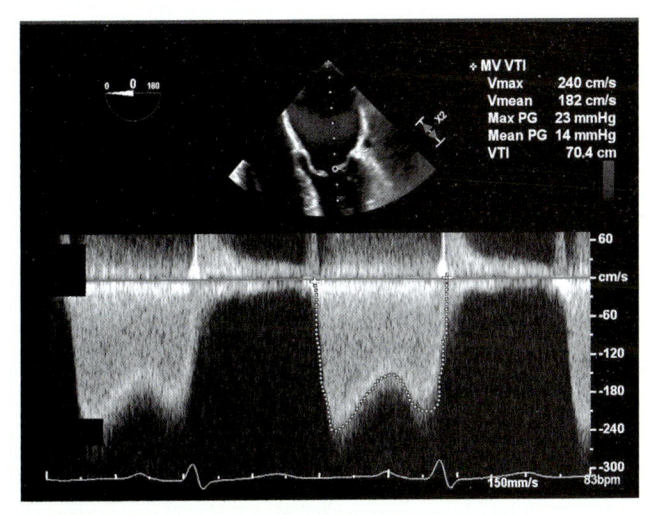

Figure 3.28

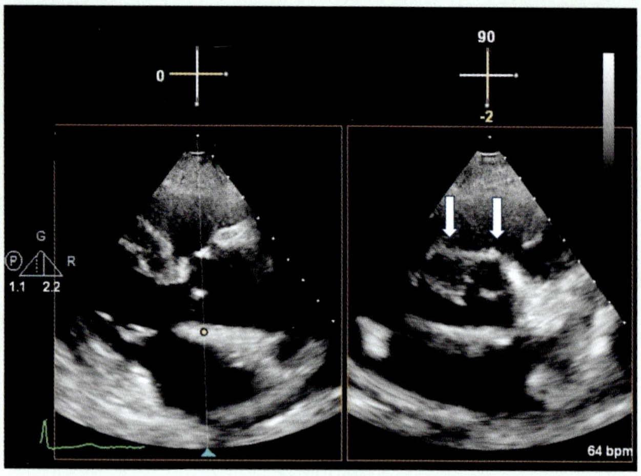

Figure 3.29

valve. Refraction, or bending, of the ultrasound beam occurs when the transmitted ultrasound beam is deviated from its straight path line (change in the angle of incidence) as it crosses the boundary between two media with different propagation speeds. Refraction of the ultrasound beam may cause duplication of structures (as in this example), displacement of structures laterally from their true location, or edge shadows (see **Figure 3.21A-C**). Refraction artifacts violate the assumption that ultrasound travels in straight lines and at a constant propagation speed. **Figure 3.29** shows another example of side-by-side aortic valves on parasternal short-axis view due to refraction artifact.

31. **Answer: B.** ▶ Video 3.2 shows an artifact secondary to breast implants. The artifacts caused by breast implants, either silicone or saline, are not well described. Breast implants may cause attenuation of ultrasound. Other bandlike artifacts and shadows occur in the field of view that obscure visualization of cardiac structures. Artifacts from breast implants can appear in both the parasternal and apical views, resulting in the need to acquire the images from off-axis positions. This often leads to suboptimal image quality and challenging interpretations. This study demonstrates a broad band of ultrasound artifacts extending around the heart in the parasternal long-axis view.

32. **Answer: C.** The continuous-wave Doppler (CWD) image obtained from the apical long-axis view shows an aortic regurgitation (AR) signal above the zero baseline in diastole with a rapid pressure half-time suggesting severe AR. There are two additional Doppler signals. In systole, there is a low-velocity profile below the zero baseline (<2 m/s), which is not consistent with aortic stenosis. In addition, there is a mirror-image signal in diastole below the zero baseline with similar shape, velocity, and intensity as the true AR signal above the zero baseline. Spectral Doppler mirror artifacts are produced in several ways: (1) by interaction with a strong reflector, (2) when the incident angle is near 90°, or (3) from "cross-talk" between the forward and reverse channels. In the example shown, the likely mirror signal is due to the AR jet direction being almost perpendicular to the Doppler beam (see ▶ **Video 3.5**), so Doppler shifts at one edge of the beam will be positive (signals are displayed above the zero baseline) and Doppler shifts at the opposite edge of the beam will be negative (signals are displayed below the zero baseline). Answers A and B are incorrect. Aliasing is a phenomenon particular to pulsed-wave Doppler (PWD) and occurs when the Nyquist limit is exceeded, so signals appear above and below the zero baseline. Range ambiguity is another type of artifact associated with PWD and occurs when multiple sample volumes are employed in an attempt to resolve higher velocity signals (high PRF mode). Because signals are received from multiple sample volumes at the same time, the precise location of the signal is unknown, which causes the range-ambiguity artifact. Answer D is incorrect, from the apical window, pulmonary regurgitation occurs in the same direction as AR; hence, would appear above the zero baseline.

SUGGESTED READINGS

Anderson B. *Echocardiography: The Normal Examination and Echocardiographic Measurements*. 3rd ed. Echotext Pty Ltd; 2017. Chapters 1, 5, and 7.

Appelbe AF, Walker PG, Yeoh JK, et al. Clinical significance and origin of artifacts in transesophageal echocardiography of the thoracic aorta. *J Am Coll Cardiol*. 1993;21(3):754-760.

Bertrand PB, Levine RA, Isselbacher EM, Vandervoort PM. Fact or artifact in two-dimensional echocardiography: avoiding misdiagnosis and missed diagnosis. *J Am Soc Echocardiogr*. 2016;29(5):381-391.

Edelman SK. *Understanding Ultrasound Physics*. 4th ed. Esp Inc; 2012.

Evangelista A, Garcia-del-Castillo H, Gonzalez-Alujas T, et al. Diagnosis of ascending aortic dissection by transesophageal echocardiography: utility of M-Mode in recognizing artifacts. *J Am Coll Cardiol*. 1996;27(1):102-107.

Feigenbaum H, Armstrong WF, Ryan T, eds. *Feigenbaum's Echocardiography*. 6th ed. Lippincott Williams & Wilkins; 2005.

Feldman MK, Katyal S, Blackwood MS. US artifacts. *Radiographics*. 2009;29(4):1179-1189.

Hedrick WR, Peterson CL. Image artifacts in real-time ultrasound. *J Diag Med Sonog*. 1995;11:300-308.

Kremkau FW. *Diagnostic Ultrasound Principles and Instruments*. Saunders Elsevier; 2006.

Rudski LG, Chow CM, Levine RA. Prosthetic mitral regurgitation can be mimicked by Doppler color flow mapping: avoiding misdiagnosis. *J Am Soc Echocardiogr*. 2004;17(8):829-833.

Weyman AE. *Principles and Practice of Echocardiography*. 2nd ed. Lippincott Williams & Wilkens; 1994.

CHAPTER 4

M-Mode Echocardiography

Gerard P. Aurigemma and Dennis A. Tighe

QUESTIONS

1. According to the 2015 Chamber Quantification Guidelines from the American Society of Echocardiography and the European Association of Cardiovascular Imaging, which of the following statements best describes the utility of M-mode echocardiography to assess left ventricular (LV) chamber size?
   A. M-mode echocardiography is the accepted technique to provide accurate measurements.
   B. M-mode echocardiography currently has no role to play in the assessment of LV chamber size.
   C. A two-dimensional echocardiography (2DE)–guided M-mode approach provides more accurate dimensions.
   D. Linear measurements obtained from 2DE images often provide oblique sections of the ventricle.

2. Calculation of left ventricular (LV) mass on the basis of M-mode echocardiography assumes that the geometry of the LV is?
   A. Spherical.
   B. Ellipsoid.
   C. Cylindrical.
   D. None of the above.

3. Which parameter of systolic function is independent of ventricular preload?
   A. Ejection fraction.
   B. Peak dP/dt.
   C. End-systolic volume.
   D. Fractional shortening.

4. In which of the following conditions would auscultation reveal a soft first heart sound?
   A. Mitral stenosis.
   B. Calcific aortic stenosis.
   C. Right bundle branch block.
   D. First-degree AV block.

5. According to the American Society of Echocardiography guidelines, LV chamber dimensions on two-dimensional echocardiography should be measured?
   A. Leading edge to leading edge.
   B. Trailing edge to leading edge.
   C. Trailing edge to trailing edge.
   D. None of the above.

6. In which condition would you expect to see normal motion of the interventricular septum (IVS) on M-mode?
   A. Right ventricular (RV) pacing.
   B. Severe tricuspid regurgitation.
   C. Atrial septal defect.
   D. Aortic valve replacement.
   E. Aortic insufficiency.

7. In which condition is LV mass index expected to be the lowest?
   A. Mitral stenosis.
   B. Ventricular septal defect with a significant left-to-right shunt.
   C. Chronic severe aortic regurgitation.
   D. Chronic severe mitral regurgitation due to mitral valve prolapse.

8. Which of the following statements is **TRUE**?
   A. The axial resolution of M-mode echocardiography is superior to that of two-dimensional echocardiography.
   B. The temporal resolution of M-mode echocardiography is superior to that of two-dimensional echocardiography.
   C. The axial resolution of M-mode echocardiography is inferior to that of two-dimensional echocardiography.
   D. The lateral resolution of M-mode echocardiography is superior to that of two-dimensional echocardiography.

9. Of the following M-mode signs, which is most specific to suggest the presence of cardiac tamponade?
   A. Right atrial inversion for less than one-third of the cardiac cycle.
   B. Plethora of the inferior vena cava.
   C. Rapid mitral E-F slope.
   D. Right ventricular diastolic collapse.

10. Which of the following statements concerning M-mode echocardiography is **TRUE**?
    A. It is a two-dimensional technique.
    B. Sampling rate exceeds 1000 samples per second.
    C. Sampling rate approaches 100 samples per second.
    D. Lateral resolution is superior to axial resolution.

11. According to the 2015 Chamber Quantification Guidelines from the American Society of Echocardiography and European Association of Cardiovascular Imaging, which of the following statement is **TRUE**?
    A. Measurements of LV dimensions and wall thickness by M-mode should preferentially be made at the level of the papillary muscles.
    B. M-mode echocardiography is the preferred method to assess LV volumes in order to estimate left ventricular ejection fraction (LVEF).
    C. LV dimensions and wall thickness should be measured at end-diastole and end-systole from two-dimensional or M-mode recordings.
    D. The M-mode or two-dimensional measurement of the left atrial anteroposterior dimension is the preferred method to assess size of this chamber.

12. This M-mode echocardiogram was taken from the study of a 48-year-old-man with dyspnea (**Figure 4.1**). His blood pressure is 120/90 mm Hg. What may be said about this patient's hemodynamic state?
    A. There is severe aortic regurgitation.
    B. The LV end-diastolic pressure is high.
    C. The stroke volume is normal.
    D. The stroke volume is low.

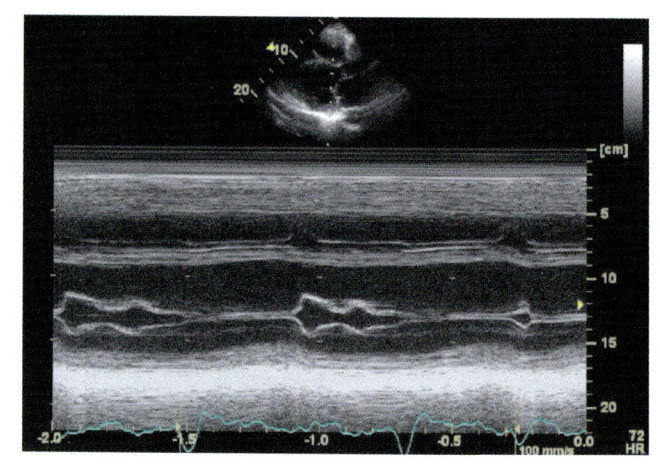

Figure 4.1

13. A 54-year-old man undergoes echocardiography (**Figure 4.2**). He has severe hypertension refractory to three drugs. He has no history of coronary or valvular heart disease. His septal and posterior wall thickness is 12 mm, and his end-diastolic dimension is 44 mm. His left ventricular (LV) mass index is 92 g/m^2. Which statement regarding this patient is least likely to be **TRUE**?
    A. He has concentric remodeling.
    B. He has diastolic dysfunction.
    C. LV mass index obtained by MRI would be less than that obtained by echocardiography.
    D. He has a normal ejection fraction.

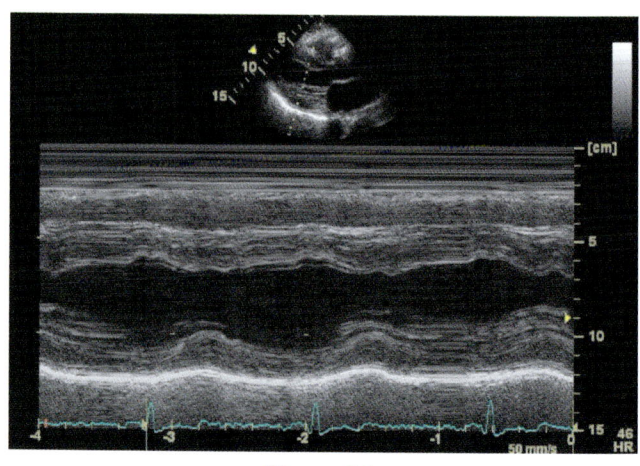

Figure 4.2

14. This M-mode is taken from the study of a 59-year-old man who presents with severe heart failure symptoms (**Figure 4.3**). You would expect his examination to show:
    A. An opening snap.
    B. Rales.
    C. An apical systolic murmur.
    D. A holodiastolic murmur.

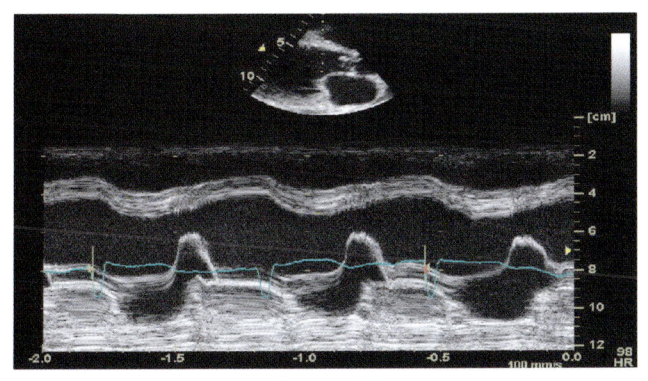

Figure 4.3

15. Which of the following statements best characterizes the utility of M-mode echocardiography in the assessment of right ventricular (RV) systolic function?
    A. Tricuspid annular plane systolic excursion (TAPSE) should be measured in the subcostal four-chamber view.
    B. Fractional shortening should be measured in the apical four-chamber view.
    C. The M-mode derived index of RV performance provides assessment of RV systolic and diastolic function.
    D. TAPSE < 17 mm is suggestive of RV systolic dysfunction.

16. Based on the parasternal long-axis two-dimensional (2D) clip shown in ▶ **Video 4.1**, which of the following findings would not be expected to be demonstrated on an M-mode examination?
    A. Mid-late systolic closure of the aortic valve.
    B. Eccentric position of the aortic closure line.
    C. High-frequency fluttering of the mitral valve.
    D. Early systolic beak in the M-mode of the interventricular septum.

17. A 56-year-old man presents to the hospital with progressive shortness of breath. Based on the results of the recorded M-mode echocardiogram (**Figure 4.4**), which of the following conclusions can be drawn?
    A. The left ventricular (LV) cavity size is normal, stroke volume is increased, and LV end-diastolic pressure is normal.
    B. The LV cavity is dilated, stroke volume is reduced, and the LV end-diastolic pressure is increased.
    C. The LV cavity is dilated, stroke volume is reduced, and LV end-diastolic pressure is normal.
    D. The LV cavity size is normal, stroke volume is increased, and mean left atrial pressure is increased.

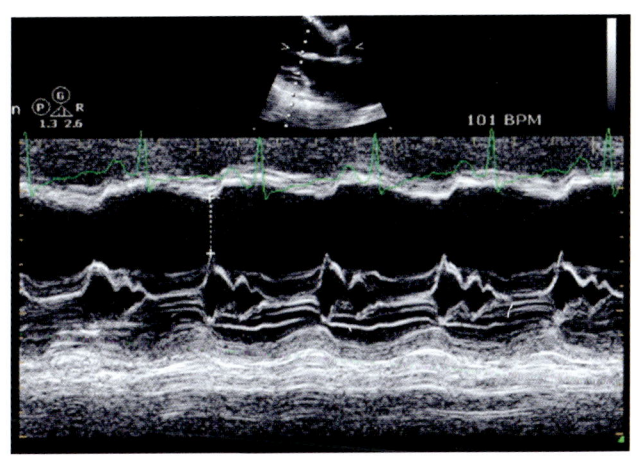

Figure 4.4

18. Based on this M-mode recording (**Figure 4.5**), which of the following statements most accurately characterizes LV wall motion (see also ▶ **Video 4.2**)?
    A. Acute infarction of the inferolateral wall.
    B. Paradoxical motion of the interventricular septum.
    C. Pseudodyskinesis.
    D. Septal bounce.

60 / Clinical Echocardiography Review

Figure 4.5

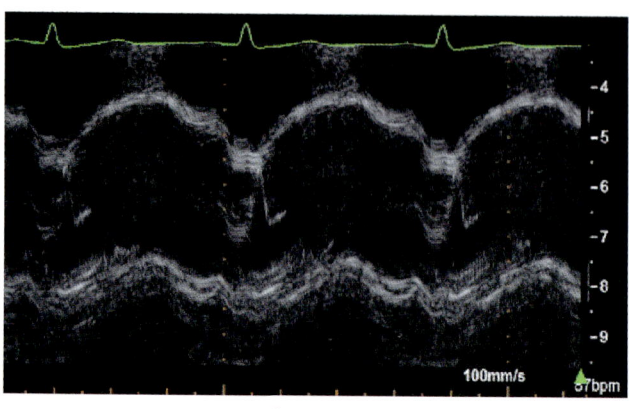

Figure 4.7

19. The condition most commonly associated with the M-mode finding in **Figure 4.6** is:
    A. Chronic severe pulmonary arterial hypertension.
    B. Severe pulmonary valve stenosis.
    C. Primary tricuspid valve regurgitation.
    D. Acute pulmonary emboli.

21. A 55-year-old woman is admitted to the hospital with syncope. Based on the M-mode in **Figure 4.8** what is your diagnosis?
    A. Hypertrophic obstructive cardiomyopathy.
    B. Acute severe mitral regurgitation due to flail mitral leaflet.
    C. Constrictive pericarditis.
    D. Aortic regurgitation, unknown severity.

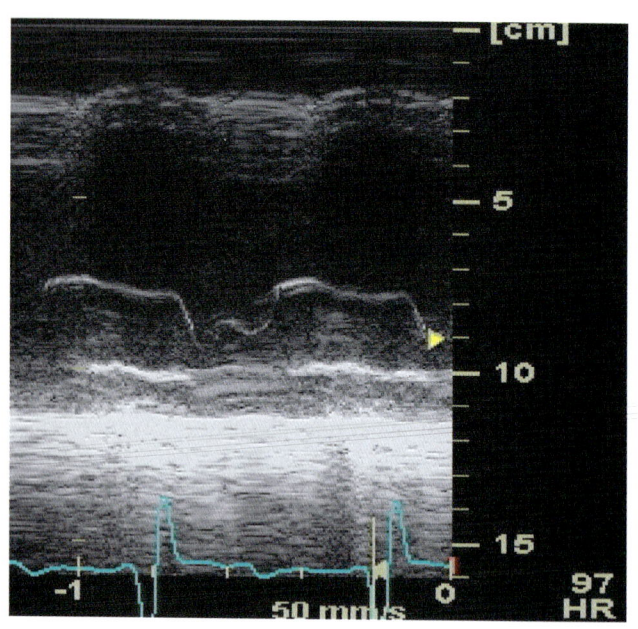

Figure 4.6

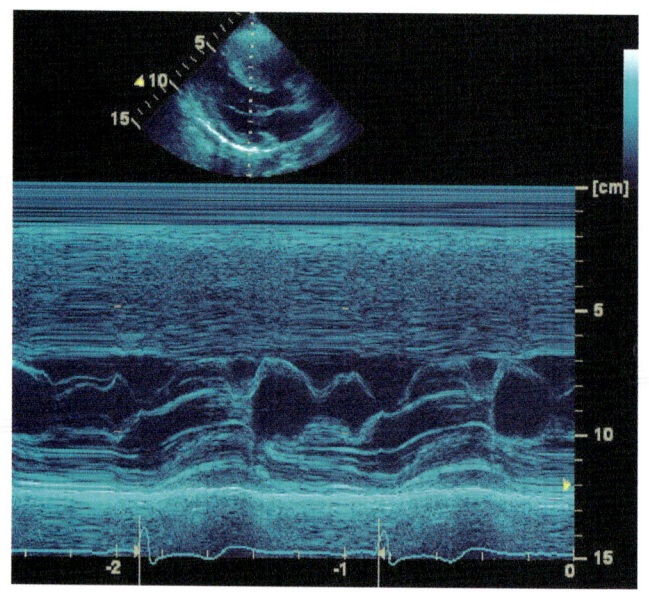

Figure 4.8

20. A 32-year-old woman is referred to you for a systolic murmur. She is completely asymptomatic. An echocardiogram is performed (**Figure 4.7**). Based on this M-mode recording through the aortic valve, what is your diagnosis?
    A. Bicuspid aortic valve.
    B. Subaortic membrane.
    C. Hypertrophic obstructive cardiomyopathy.
    D. Acute severe mitral regurgitation.

22. The M-mode in **Figure 4.9** is most consistent with what abnormality?
    A. Acute severe aortic regurgitation.
    B. Rheumatic mitral stenosis.
    C. Left atrial myxoma.
    D. Hypertrophic cardiomyopathy.

Figure 4.9

23. A 66-year-old woman with chest pain and shortness of breath presents to the hospital. A heart murmur is auscultated. The medical team caring for the patient requests an echocardiogram to evaluate her heart murmur. Based on the findings on this M-mode recording (**Figure 4.10**), which of the following descriptions would **BEST** characterize her heart murmur?
   A. Holosystolic murmur.
   B. Early diastolic murmur with soft S1.
   C. Diastolic rumble with prominent S1.
   D. Mid-late systolic murmur.

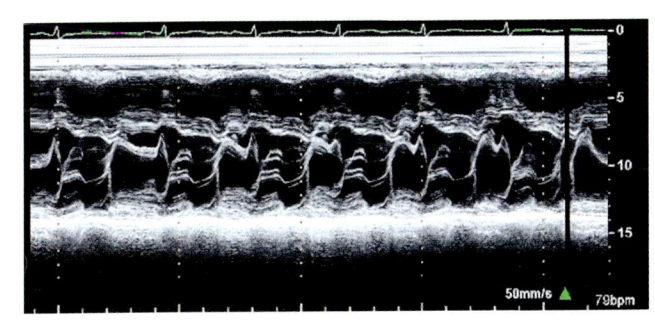

Figure 4.10

24. A 70-year-old woman collapses after a heated argument with her son. At presentation to the emergency room, she is complaining of chest pressure, is severely hypotensive, and has a loud holosystolic murmur. She is taken to the catheterization suite where she is found to have no obstructive coronary disease. A transesophageal echocardiography is performed, from which the following M-mode is obtained (**Figure 4.11**). What is the most likely explanation for her severe hypotension and systolic murmur?
   A. A flail aortic valve due to bacterial endocarditis.
   B. Dynamic LV outflow tract obstruction.
   C. Acute severe mitral regurgitation (MR) from papillary muscle rupture.
   D. A previously unrecognized subaortic membrane.

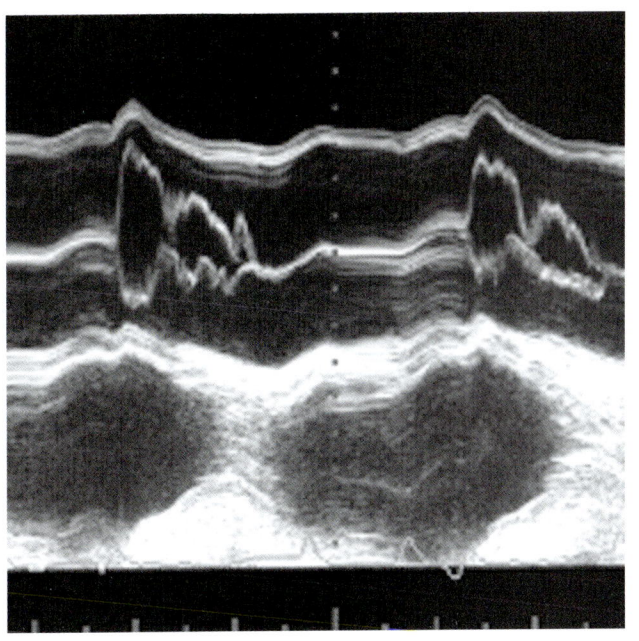

Figure 4.11

25. This M-mode (**Figure 4.12**) is taken from the study of an 86-year-old woman with shortness of breath and fatigue. She underwent a medical procedure approximately 4 months prior to her presentation with shortness of breath. What was the medical procedure?
   A. Drainage of an idiopathic pericardial effusion.
   B. Transcutaneous aortic valve implantation.
   C. Stent to the left anterior descending artery.
   D. Permanent pacemaker implantation.

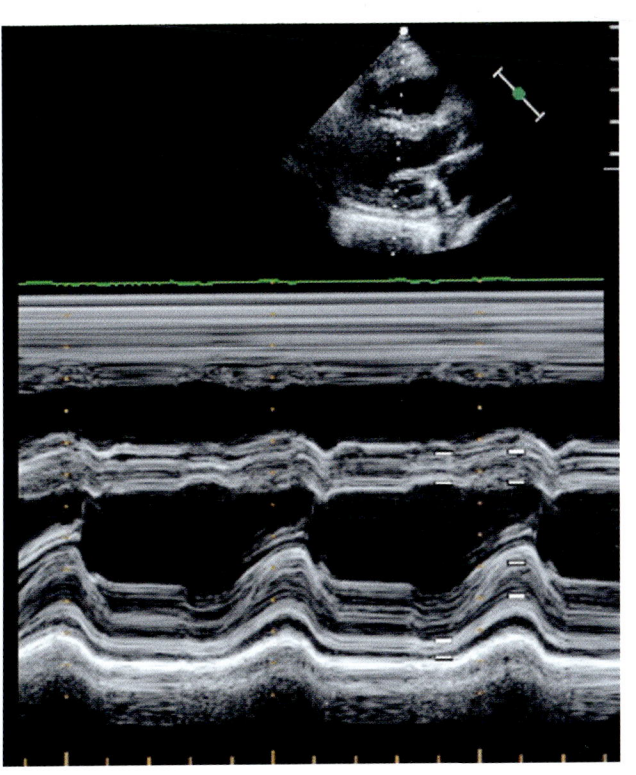

Figure 4.12

26. A 60-year-old woman with a history of rheumatic fever and progressive shortness of breath with exertion is seen in follow-up and the following M-mode images were obtained (**Figure 4.13A** and **B**). Which of the following findings are seen on these images?
  A. Reduced E-F slope.
  B. Reduced E-F slope and diastolic dip of the interventricular septum.
  C. Reduced E-F slope, diastolic dip of the interventricular septum, paradoxical anterior motion of the septum in systole.
  D. None of the above.

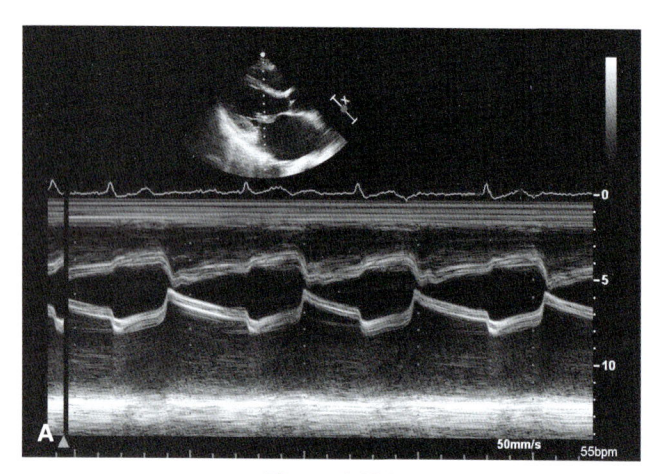

Figure 4.13A

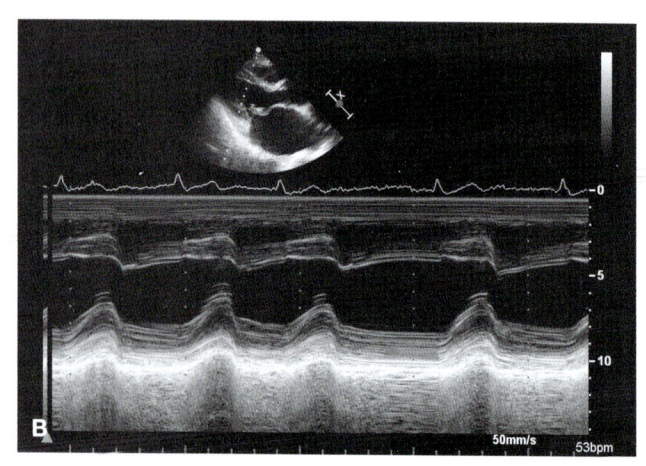

Figure 4.13B

27. A 72-year-old woman with breast cancer and with shortness of breath presents to the emergency room. M-mode images are obtained from the parasternal long-axis and subcostal views (**Figure 4.14A** and **B**). Which of the following statements are **CORRECT**?

  A. There is right atrial (RA) and RV chamber collapse consistent with cardiac tamponade.
  B. There is RV chamber collapse only consistent with cardiac tamponade.
  C. There is RA chamber collapse only consistent with cardiac tamponade.
  D. There is no RA or RV chamber collapse and therefore no cardiac tamponade.

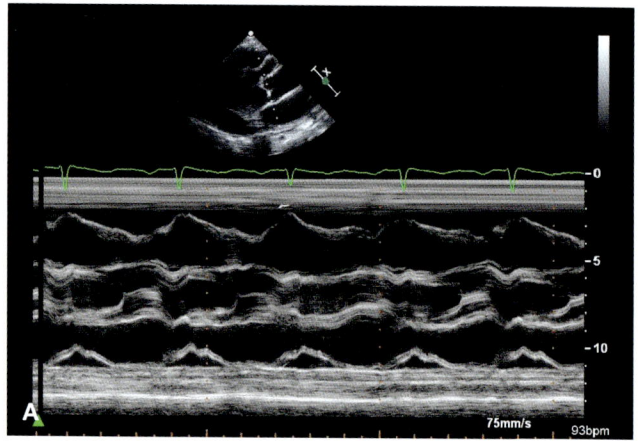

Figure 4.14A

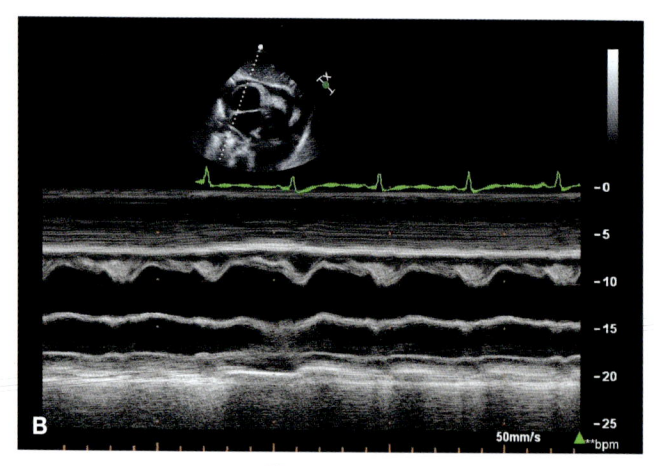

Figure 4.14B

28. A 74-year-old woman presents with edema and ascites 8 years following coronary artery bypass surgery. Which of the following statements are **CORRECT** regarding the following M-mode image (**Figure 4.15**)?
  A. There is a diastolic septal shudder.
  B. There is flattening of the posterior wall.
  C. There is pericardial thickening.
  D. All of the above are correct.

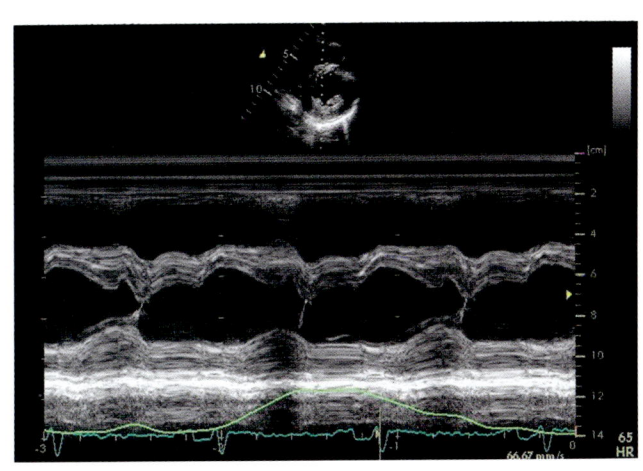

Figure 4.15. Reprinted from Klein AL, Abbara S, Agler DA, et al. American Society of Echocardiography clinical recommendations for multimodality cardiovascular imaging of patients with pericardial disease: endorsed by the Society for Cardiovascular Magnetic Resonance and Society of Cardiovascular Computed Tomography. *J Am Soc Echocardiogr.* 2013;26(9):965-1012.e15. Copyright © 2013 by the American Society of Echocardiography. With permission.

29. Which of the following findings is demonstrated on this M-mode tracing (**Figure 4.16**)?
    A. Prolapse of the mitral valve.
    B. Normal M-mode.
    C. Interrupted A-C closure.
    D. High-frequency fluttering.

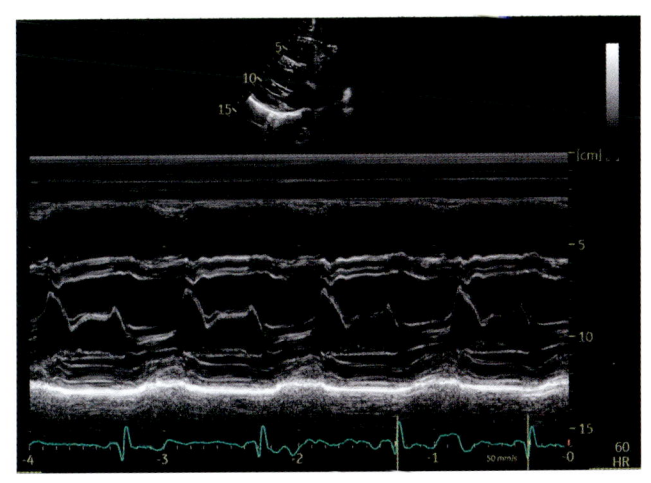

Figure 4.16

30. A 72-year-old man presents to hospital with progressive fatigue, shortness of breath, lower extremity edema, and a distended abdomen, and **Figure 4.17** panels A-C are taken from his 2D/Doppler echocardiographic study. Which of the following findings would be expected on M-mode echocardiography?
    A. Systolic anterior motion of the mitral valve.
    B. Reduced E-F slope.
    C. Reduced propagation velocity of early diastolic trans-mitral flow (color M-mode).
    D. Diastolic flattening of the LV posterior wall endocardium.

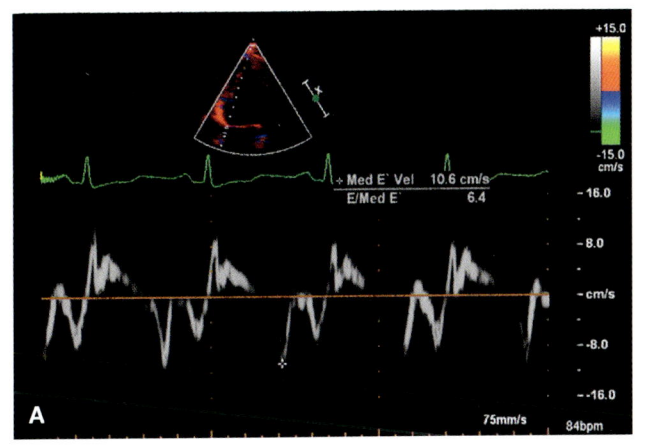

Figure 4.17A

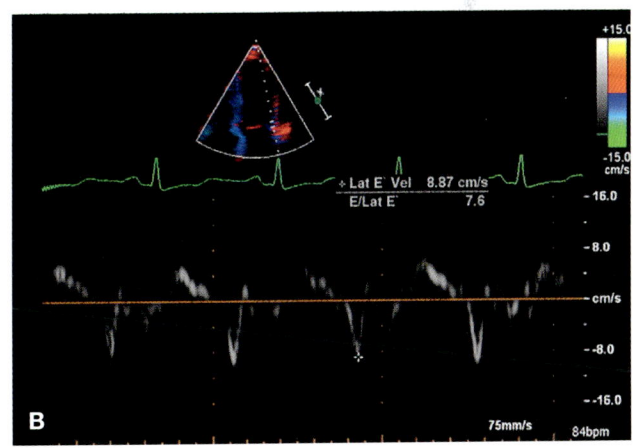

Figure 4.17B

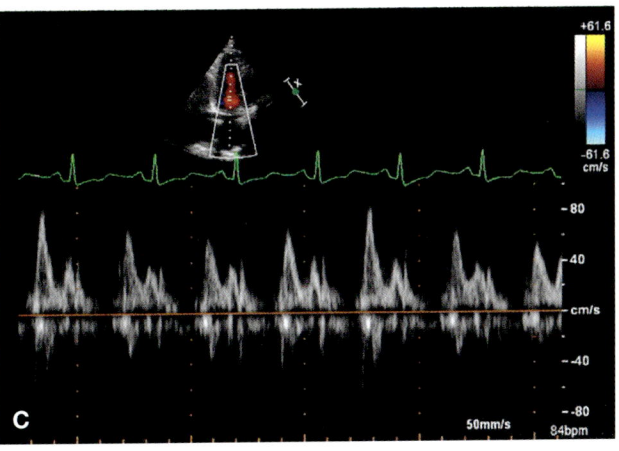

Figure 4.17C

31. A 43-year-old woman with an aneurysm of the ascending aorta (55 mm) undergoes an intraoperative TEE. While imaging the aorta, a linear echodensity is observed in the ascending aorta on 2D imaging. The aortic valve is found to be trileaflet, and only mild central aortic regurgitation is present. To further assess the nature of this linear echodensity, an M-mode echocardiogram is performed by the echocardiographer (**Figure 4.18**). Based on these images, what can be concluded about the echocardiographic findings?
    A. An aortic dissection flap is present.
    B. An intramural hematoma is present.
    C. Reverberation artifact is present.
    D. Mirror image artifact is present.

C. Holosystolic murmur.
D. Blowing diastolic murmur and late systolic murmur.

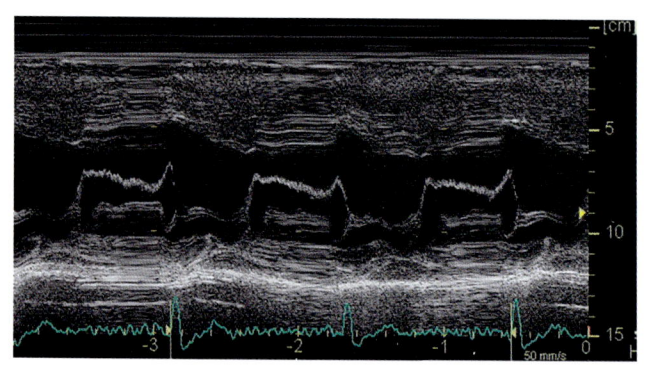

Figure 4.19

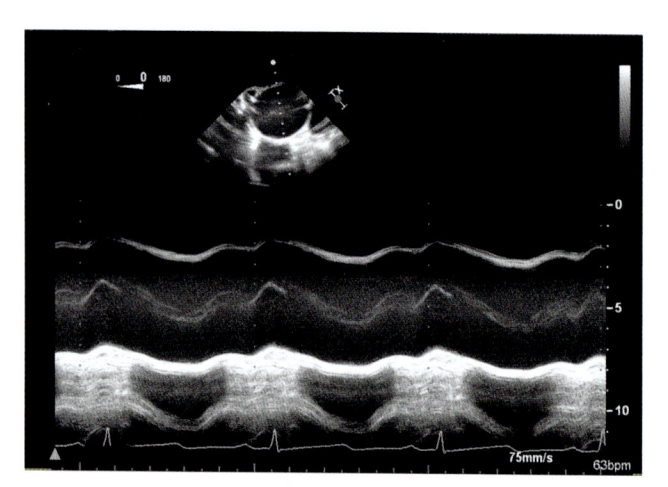

Figure 4.18

32. Based on this M-mode recording of the mitral valve (**Figure 4.19**), which of the following auscultatory findings could be expected on physical examination?
    A. Prominent S1, opening snap, and diastolic rumble.
    B. Harsh midsystolic murmur that is augmented by a Valsalva maneuver.

33. What is the cause of the wall motion abnormality seen on the M-mode (**Figure 4.20**)?
    A. Septal myocardial infarction.
    B. Left bundle branch block dyssynchrony.
    C. Tricuspid regurgitation.
    D. Ventricular pre-excitation.

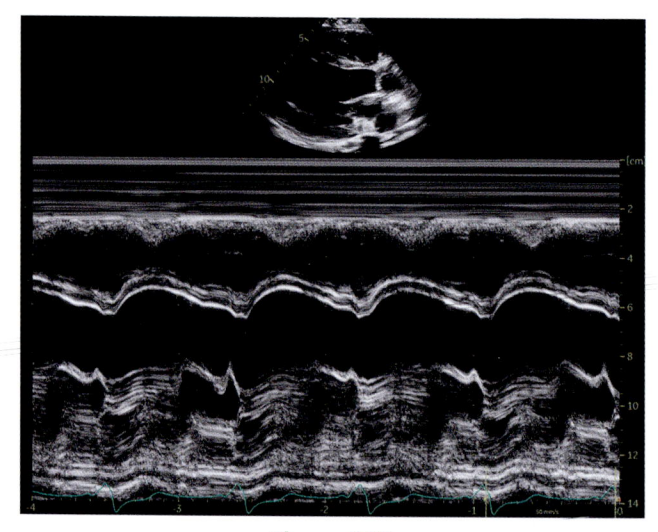

Figure 4.20

ANSWERS

1. **Answer: C.** The most used parameters to describe LV size include linear internal dimensions and volumes. Linear measurements should be obtained perpendicular to the long axis of the LV and measured at or immediately below the level of the mitral valve leaflet tips. Internal dimensions of the LV can be obtained with a 2DE-guided M-mode approach. The major limitation of M-mode echocardiography is beam orientation, which can provide off-axis cuts of the LV; thus, linear measurements obtained from 2D images are preferred to avoid oblique sectioning of the LV. M-mode echocardiography cannot provide an accurate volumetric assessment of the LV as the volume calculations derived from these linear measurements rely on the assumption of the chamber being a prolate ellipse, a shape that is not present in a variety of cardiac pathologies.

2. **Answer: B.** LV mass and LV volume measurements from M-mode and two-dimensional echocardiography are based on the geometric assumptions that the ventricle is an ellipsoid with a long-axis to short-axis ratio of 2:1. The mass formula, LV mass (g) = $0.8(1.04[(LVIDd + PWTd + SWTd)^3 - LVIDd^3]) + 0.6$ calculates the volumes of an inner and outer ellipsoid and subtracts the inner volume from the outer volume. The resulting volume is that of a "shell" of myocardium. The volume of this shell of myocardium is then multiplied by the specific gravity of myocardium, 1.04 g/m^2, to yield LV mass. This geometric assumption limits the applicability of the formula to normally shaped hearts.

3. **Answer: C.** Virtually all parameters of systolic function (ejection fraction, dP/dt, fractional shortening, and velocity of circumferential fiber shortening) depend on loading conditions. Preload is the force that acts to stretch the myocardial fibers at end-diastole and is related to end-diastolic volume. By the Starling law of the heart, increased preload will be associated with increased fiber stretch and increased force of contraction. Afterload is the force that opposes LV ejection.

   End-systolic volume is also a parameter of systolic function. A related concept is that, at any given contractile state, the LV will contract to the same end-systolic volume even as the LV diastolic volume increases.

4. **Answer: D.** The degree to which the mitral valve leaflets are separated when ventricular activation closes the mitral valve is an important determinant of the loudness of the mitral component of the S1. Accordingly, in a patient with a long PR interval (choice D), the mitral and tricuspid leaflets float into a semiclosed position because of the long period between atrial contraction and ventricular activation. Mitral stenosis is characterized by a loud first sound, if the leaflets are pliable, because the transmitral gradient at end-diastole prevents the leaflets from drifting close together. Calcific aortic stenosis (by itself) or right bundle branch block does not have much of an impact on the loudness of the S1.

5. **Answer: D.** According to the echocardiographic chamber quantification guidelines, two-dimensional echocardiographically derived linear dimensions overcome the common problem of oblique parasternal images, resulting in overestimation of cavity and wall dimensions from M-mode. The actual visualized thickness of the ventricular septum and other chamber dimensions can be measured as defined by the actual tissue-blood interface, rather than the distance between the leading edge echoes done by M-mode.

6. **Answer: E.** The IVS normally moves posteriorly (leftward) in early ventricular systole. Paradoxical septal motion is an early systolic anterior (rightward) motion of the septum. Thickening of the septum still occurs. Paradoxical septal motion is associated with conditions in which there is RV volume overload, or left bundle branch block, either developed or due to RV pacing. After aortic valve replacement, or any cardiac surgery, there is prominent translation of the heart that can give the appearance of paradoxical septal motion. Aortic insufficiency, a situation in which there is LV volume overload, would not be expected to be associated with paradoxical septal motion and is therefore the correct answer.

7. **Answer: A.** Mitral stenosis. Choices B–D will result in LV dilation, but choice A does not. Since the LV mass formula (Question 2) depends on chamber size, a large LV will usually be associated with a large LV mass index.

8. **Answer: B.** The temporal resolution of M-mode echocardiography is superior to that of two-dimensional echocardiography. The high temporal resolution of M-mode echocardiography is due to the fact that this technique has a much higher sampling rate compared with two-dimensional echocardiography. For both techniques, the axial resolution is similar since the same transducer frequency is used. Lateral resolution is superior with two-dimensional echocardiography because with the M-mode technique sampling occurs only along a single scan line.

9. **Answer: D.** Right ventricular diastolic collapse. Right atrial inversion and plethora of the inferior vena cava (IVC) are sensitive signs suggesting increased intrapericardial pressures, but they are not the most specific signs suggesting cardiac tamponade. When right atrial inversion extends for more than one-third of the cardiac cycle, however, the reported specificity is high. Plethora of the IVC is a nonspecific marker associated with increased right atrial pressures; plethora can be observed even when the right atrial pressure is not increased as is seen with certain highly trained athletes. With inspiration, the mitral E-F slope has been observed to diminish and, thus, is not rapid in the presence of cardiac tamponade. Of the choices available, right ventricular diastolic collapse is the most specific sign of cardiac tamponade.

10. **Answer: B.** The M-mode technique offers a unidimensional view of the heart. While dedicated M-mode transducers produced sampling rates of approximately 2000 Hz, current-generation transducers producing two-dimensional guided M-mode recordings sample at rates exceeding 1000 samples per second. Current-generation two-dimensional imaging systems can produce images at frame rates approaching 100 frames per second. With M-mode echocardiography, axial resolution exceeds lateral resolution.

11. **Answer: C.** When measuring LV dimensions and wall thickness, either two-dimensional or M-mode techniques can be used, although two-dimensional guided measurements are preferred to avoid issues

associated with oblique cuts. Measurements should be made at or immediately below the level of the tips of the mitral leaflets preferentially in the parasternal long-axis view as perpendicular to the major axis of the ventricle as possible. The Teichholz or Quinones method of calculating LVEF from LV linear dimensions can often result in considerable inaccuracies as a result of the geometric assumptions required to convert linear measurement to three-dimensional volumes; thus, the use of linear measurements to calculate LVEF is discouraged. The biplane method of discs (modified Simpson rule) is the recommended two-dimensional method for volumetric assessment of LVEF; alternatively three-dimensional echocardiography can be used for this purpose. As the left atrium is shown to have a complex shape, a single linear measurement of the anteroposterior dimension can lead to significant inaccuracy in assessing LA size. The currently recommended method to assess LA size is the biplane method of discs to determine volume.

12. **Answer: D.** This study was obtained in a patient with an idiopathic dilated cardiomyopathy. The M-mode echocardiogram shows marked LV dilation, with an end-diastolic dimension approaching 6 cm and an end-systolic dimension of 5.5 cm. The fractional shortening is therefore low. There is a large separation between the anterior leaflet of the mitral valve and the septum (the e-point septal separation, since the peak anterior position of the anterior leaflet is known as the e-point in M-mode parlance). This sign is associated with a low forward stroke volume. It is important to realize that LV dilation by itself does not lead to an abnormal e-point septal separation. An individual with severe aortic regurgitation might have a dilated LV but normal fractional shortening. In that case, the e-point septal separation would be normal.

As for the incorrect choices, while this patient might have high left ventricular end diastolic pressure (LVEDP), there is no definite evidence for this. The pathognomonic M-mode sign of this physiology, the so-called a-c shoulder or b-bump, is not present. **Figure 4.21** shows a prominent b-bump (see the arrow).

Finally, the etiology of the LV dysfunction shown in this case could have been chronic aortic regurgitation, with the development of contractile failure, but this M-mode tracing is not specific for such a cardiomyopathy. The lack of fluttering of the mitral leaflets provides some evidence against significant aortic regurgitation.

13. **Answer: A.** This patient's LV mass index is normal, by the partition values in the ASE quantitation guidelines, so he does not have left ventricular hypertrophy. According to the pioneering work of Ganau et al., and as recommended by the ASE quantitation guidelines, the combination of a high relative wall thickness with a normal LV mass index is termed concentric remodeling. This individual clearly has an elevated relative wall thickness, defined as (2 × PWTd)/LVIDd with the upper limit of normal 0.42 (for this patient 0.55). The term *concentric hypertrophy* refers to an elevated LV mass index (ie, greater than 95 g/m^2 in women, greater than 115 g/m^2 in men) and a high relative wall thickness.

According to the work by Wachtell and coworkers, most individuals with hypertension and evidence of remodeling, as the case with this individual, have abnormalities in diastolic filling.

The M-mode clearly shows normal fractional shortening; while this is not necessarily the same as a normal LV ejection fraction, the absence of coronary heart disease by history argues that global EF is normal.

14. **Answer: B.** The M-mode shows a classic example of early mitral valve closure, which is pathognomonic of acute severe aortic regurgitation. There is also LV dilation and a generous e-point septal separation. The early closure of the mitral valve is caused by the rapid equilibration of LV diastolic pressure and aortic diastolic pressure, and for this reason the murmur will not be holodiastolic. Patients with acute severe aortic regurgitation are likely to have evidence of elevated filling pressure and rales. An opening snap is heard in patients with rheumatic mitral stenosis with pliable leaflets. This is not the echocardiogram of such a patient. An apical systolic murmur implies mitral regurgitation, and there is no suggestion that this patient has coexisting mitral regurgitation.

15. **Answer: D.** According to the 2015 Chamber Quantification Guidelines from the American Society of Echocardiography and the European Association of Cardiovascular Imaging, use of several modalities is recommended to assess the RV systolic function due to its complex geometrical shape and inability to capture the entire chamber volume in any single imaging plane. Suggested 2DE, Doppler, and M-mode-derived parameters include fractional area change (FAC), Doppler tissue imaging–derived

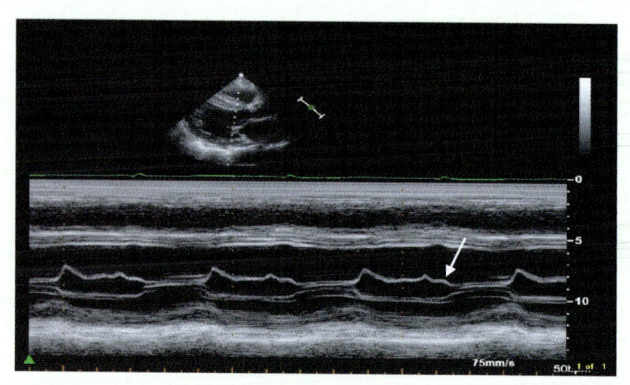

Figure 4.21

tricuspid lateral annular systolic velocity wave (s'), tricuspid annular plane systolic excursion (TAPSE), RV index of myocardial performance (RIMP), and RV longitudinal strain. Among these parameters, TAPSE is the only one that can be obtained using the M-mode technique. TAPSE is acquired by optimally aligning the M-mode cursor along the direction of the tricuspid lateral annulus in the apical four-chamber view. TASPE offers the advantage of being easily obtainable. While it provides only a measure of RV longitudinal function, it has shown good correlations with other parameters of global RV systolic function. TAPSE < 17 mm is considered highly suggestive of RV systolic dysfunction. Limitations of TAPSE to assess global RV function include angle dependency and providing only a regional assessment of longitudinal function. Fractional shortening is not a recommended parameter to assess RV systolic function. The RV performance index is reflective of global RV performance; however, it is derived from Doppler techniques and not M-mode echocardiography.

16. **Answer: A.** This single 2D parasternal long-axis clip (▶ **Video 4.1**) demonstrates three key findings: abnormal septal motion, eccentric position of the aortic closure line, and lack of apparent LV outflow tract obstruction. A key to test taking is always to use entirety of the information contained on the presented image(s). Note that, in the single-lead ECG, a wide QRS complex is present. In this case, the patient has a known left bundle branch block (LBBB) and a bicuspid aortic valve. Expected M-mode findings could include the characteristic diastolic dip found with LBBB (see **Answer 4.25,**

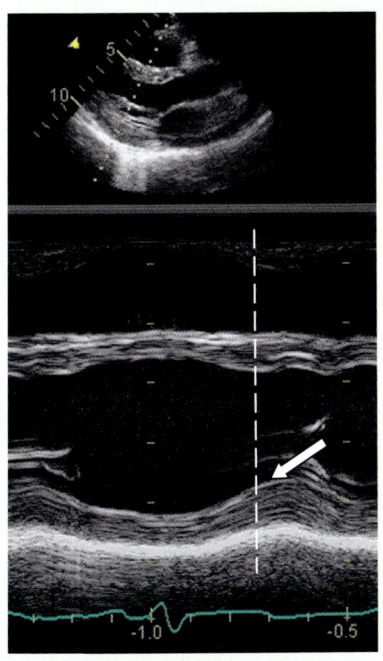

Figure 4.22. Normal M-mode. Dotted line shows synchronous inward septal and posterior wall motion.

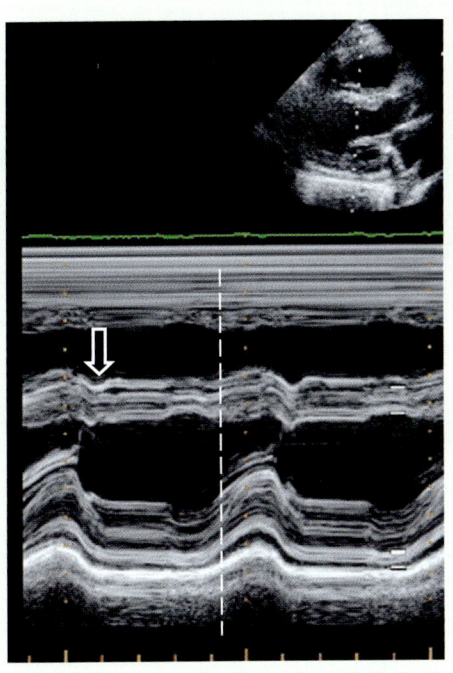

Figure 4.23. M-mode with LBBB and prominent diastolic dip (arrow), and paradoxical septal motion with inward posterior wall motion (dotted line).

and **Figures 4.22** and **4.23**), eccentric closure line that may accompany presence of a bicuspid aortic valve, and some degree of eccentrically directed aortic regurgitation that may strike the anterior leaflet of the mitral valve causing high-frequency fluttering. Mid to late systolic closure of the aortic valve M-mode would not be expected as dynamic LV outflow tract obstruction is not shown on this 2D clip. Of note, early systolic closure of the aortic valve shown on M-mode echocardiography is often associated with a fixed LV outflow tract obstruction. Regarding the eccentric closure line that has been associated with bicuspid aortic valve, valve anatomy plays a major role in whether this M-mode finding will be demonstrated. With a closure line that is "horizontal" (perpendicular to the direction of the ultrasonic beam), the M-mode echoes from the valve in diastole will appear to be centrally located within the aortic root (false-negative finding). When the closure line is "vertical" (parallel to the echo beam), the diastolic echoes will show the closure line to be eccentrically located. When the closure line is obliquely oriented, the ultrasonic images can demonstrate either a central or eccentric location.

17. **Answer: B.** This 56-year-old man presented with symptoms and signs of heart failure. This M-mode echocardiogram is recorded through the mitral leaflet tips (**Figure 4.24**). This recording shows significantly increased LV cavity dimensions in systole and diastole (stippled arrows), a significantly increased e-point septal-separation distance (stippled lines), and interrupted AC closure of the mitral valve echocardiogram. The findings of this M-mode

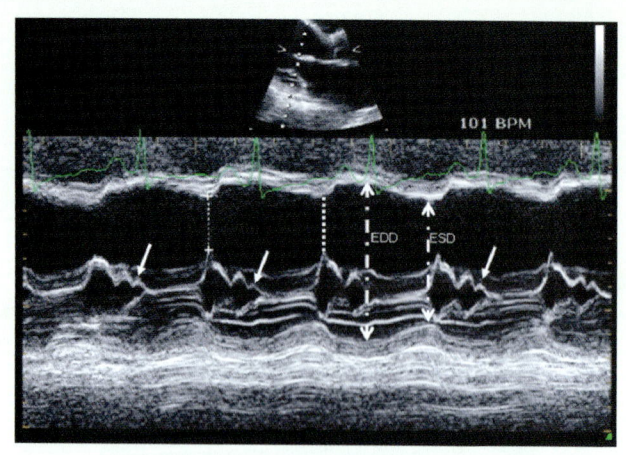

Figure 4.24. EDD, end-diastolic dimension; ESD, end-systolic dimension.

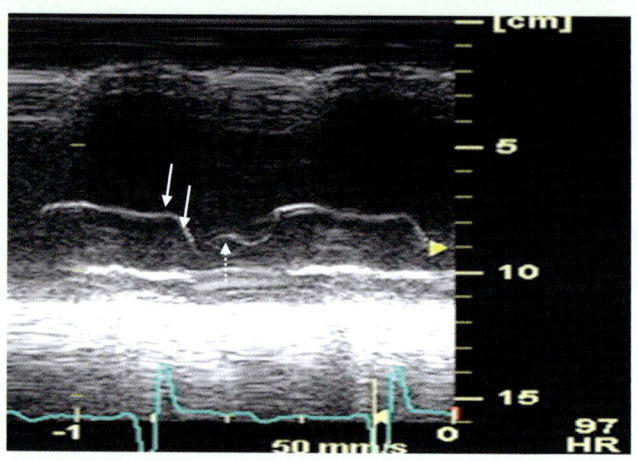

Figure 4.25

echocardiogram suggest that very poor systolic performance is present. The LV cavity is dilated and the LV ejection fraction is severely reduced. Stroke volume is severely reduced as indicated by the increased e-point septal-separation distance (normal <7 mm). The LV end-diastolic pressure is elevated as indicated by the presence of the interrupted AC closure (solid arrows) or "b-bump." The mean left atrial pressure, although likely elevated, cannot be derived from the information presented.

18. **Answer: C.** This two-dimensional video (▶ Video 4.2) and the accompanying M-mode recording illustrate findings of pseudodyskinesis, a condition that may be confused with infarction of the inferior/inferolateral wall. Pseudodyskinesis, in which systolic wall thickening (as shown by the M-mode recording and accompanying real-time video of the M-mode and two-dimensional images) is preserved, is characterized by diastolic flattening of the inferior/inferolateral wall followed by systolic rounding and again outward diastolic bulging caused by extrinsic compression. The LV will have a noncircular geometry at end-diastole consistent with the existence of extrinsic compression, while in systole the LV assumes a circular appearance. This circular appearance of the LV in systole would not be expected in the presence of a myocardial infarction. Paradoxical motion of the interventricular septum (IVS) occurs in the presence of RV volume overload; in this condition, echocardiography would show the IVS to flatten in diastole and assume a rounded contour in systole with motion toward the RV. A septal bounce, as occurs with constrictive pericarditis, is characterized by an early to mid-diastolic dip(s) in which the septal motion reflects right then LV filling in diastole. Dyssynergy, another condition in which an apparent wall motion abnormality may be confused with that caused by ischemic heart disease, occurs typically in the setting of LBBB and is characterized on the M-mode recording by an early systolic downward motion ("early systolic beak") during isovolumic contraction and paradoxical motion toward the RV during systole followed by an exaggerated "early diastolic dip". In this case study, motion of the IVS is normal as shown on the two-dimensional and M-mode recordings.

19. **Answer: A.** This M-mode recording of the pulmonary valve illustrates the "flying-W sign" (**Figure 4.25**). The normal pulmonary valve M-mode is characterized by presystolic a-wave with motion away from the transducer followed by further posterior motion of the valve leaflet during systole. With chronic severe pulmonary hypertension, a characteristic appearance to the M-mode tracing, termed the flying-W sign, may be generated. This tracing is characterized by the loss of the a-wave (solid arrows) and midsystolic notching (stippled arrow). With pulmonary valve stenosis, the a-wave is characteristically preserved, or even accentuated, and midsystolic notching is not observed. In a pure right-sided heart volume load state, such as occurs with primary tricuspid regurgitation, one would not expect pulmonary hypertension to be present and thus the pulmonary valve M-mode tracing should not be altered significantly. Among patients with acute pulmonary embolism, the level of elevation of the pulmonary artery pressure does not usually exceed 50 mm Hg and thus the M-mode findings of chronic severe pulmonary arterial hypertension would not be expected to be observed.

20. **Answer: B.** The image shown features an abrupt, very early posterior motion of the right cusp of the aortic valve, which is characteristic of the subaortic membrane. The mechanism for this finding is unclear. Bicuspid aortic valve motion features an eccentric closure line. Hypertrophic obstructive cardiomyopathy may have premature closure of the aortic valve on M-mode, but this tends to occur toward midsystole, rather than early systole.

21. **Answer: A.** This M-mode shows evidence of systolic anterior motion of the mitral valve, a sign that is usually pathognomonic for hypertrophic obstructive cardiomyopathy (**Figure 4.26**). Studies have shown

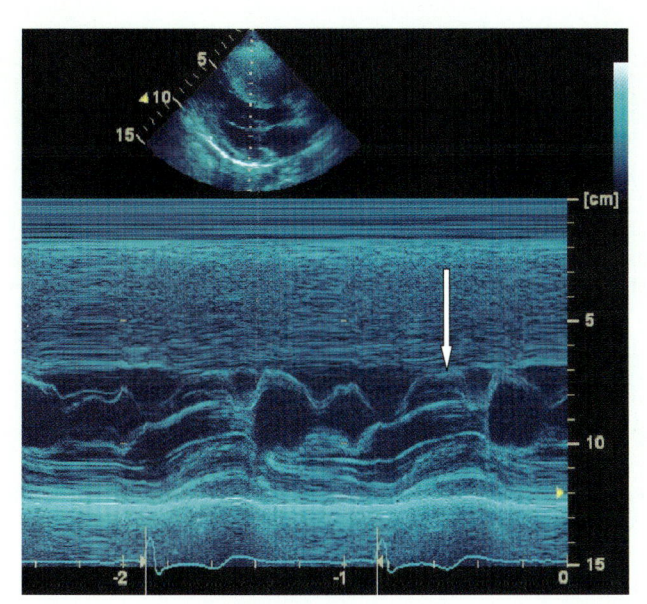

Figure 4.26

that 70% of patients with hypertrophic cardiomyopathy have obstruction either at rest or provoked by exercise. In hypertrophic obstructive cardiomyopathy, there is hyperdynamic systolic function, with low levels of wall stress; the LV outflow tract is narrowed by septal hypertrophy and, in some patients, by anterior displacement of the mitral valve. The arrow points to systolic anterior motion of the mitral valve with septal-mitral contact.

22. **Answer: C.** This M-mode recording illustrates a classic case of a left atrial myxoma prolapsing into the mitral orifice with valve opening (**Figure 4.27**). The tumor (Myx) appears as a mass of echoes behind the mitral valve during diastole. Note the echo free space behind the anterior leaflet at the onset of diastole (arrows). This echo free interval occurs because a time lag exists between the early diastolic opening of the valve and the subsequent movement of the tumor mass into the mitral orifice. This recording is not consistent with rheumatic mitral stenosis as the mitral leaflets are not thickened and the posterior leaflet appears to move normally (best illustrated in the last cardiac cycle). Findings consistent with the presence of acute severe aortic insufficiency,

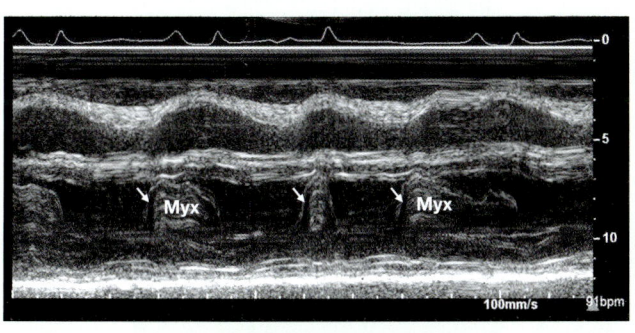

Figure 4.27

such as high-frequency diastolic fluttering of the mitral valve or, possibly, the interventricular septum (depending upon jet direction) and premature mitral valve closure, are not demonstrated. With hypertrophic obstructive cardiomyopathy, increased thickness of the interventricular septum and systolic anterior motion of the mitral apparatus would be expected; these findings are not demonstrated on this M-mode recording.

23. **Answer: D.** The M-mode recording (**Figure 4.28A**) demonstrates mid to late systolic prolapse of the mitral valve (arrow; solid line identifies onset of midsystole) consistent with mitral regurgitation occurring in mid to late systole as shown on the accompanying continuous wave Doppler spectral profile (**Figure 4.28B**; onset systole solid arrow; mitral regurgitation stippled arrow) and still frame color-flow Doppler images (**Figure 4.28C** and **D**) in early and late systole (note accompanying ECG recordings for timing), respectively. A holosystolic murmur would not be expected, given these M-mode findings. An early diastolic murmur with soft S1 would be expected with acute, severe aortic regurgitation; in this case, the M-mode recording does not show characteristic findings such as diastolic fluttering of the mitral leaflets or early closure of the mitral valve. With a diastolic rumble and prominent (loud) S1, mitral stenosis would be the expected pathology; findings of mitral stenosis are not demonstrated on this M-mode tracing. A characteristic finding with hypertrophic obstructive cardiomyopathy is a systolic ejection murmur that augments with performance of a Valsalva maneuver; characteristic findings such as systolic anterior motion of the anterior mitral leaflet and septal hypertrophy are not seen on this M-mode recording of the mitral valve.

24. **Answer: B.** Dynamic outflow tract obstruction. This patient had an acute stress cardiomyopathy with severe LV dysfunction (**Figure 4.29**) and developed acute LV outflow tract obstruction. The harsh murmur was due to either dynamic obstruction or mitral regurgitation, which itself resulted from systolic anterior motion of the mitral valve. The M-mode clearly demonstrates midsystolic closure of the aortic valve (arrow). This midsystolic closure is caused by obstruction to LV outflow. The base of the heart is not only involved in the stress cardiomyopathy-related LV dysfunction but, in fact, is hyperdynamic.

A is incorrect, as there is no evidence for a bacterial vegetation demonstrated on this still frame. C is also incorrect; while the aortic valve may close prematurely in acute severe mitral regurgitation, the clinical scenario fits better with dynamic outflow tract obstruction. Finally, D is incorrect; while fixed subaortic obstruction due to a subaortic membrane also features abnormality in the aortic

70 / Clinical Echocardiography Review

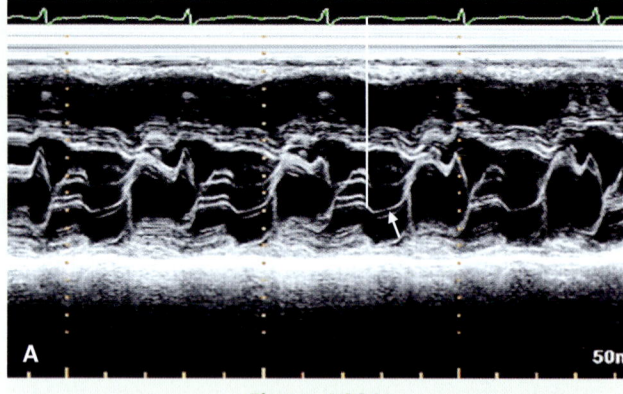

Figure 4.28A

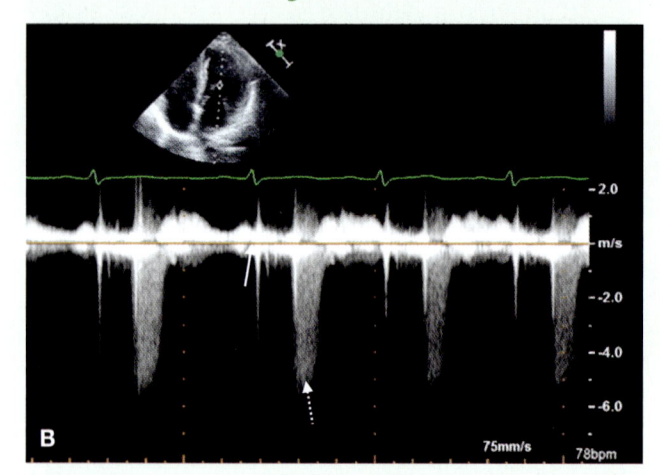

Figure 4.28B

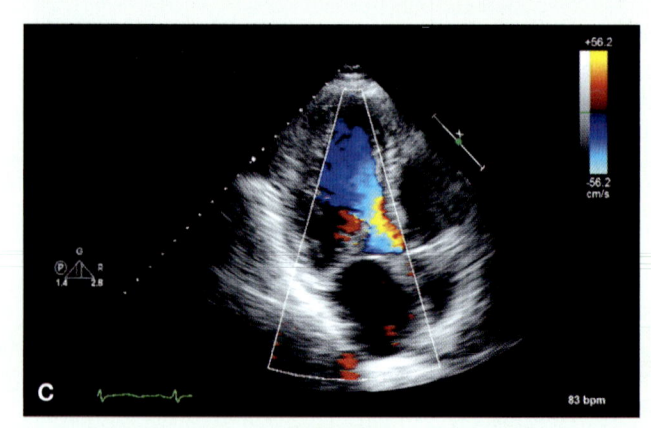

Figure 4.28C

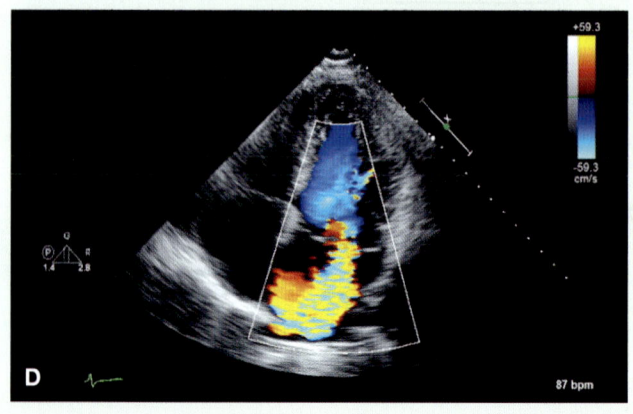

Figure 4.28D

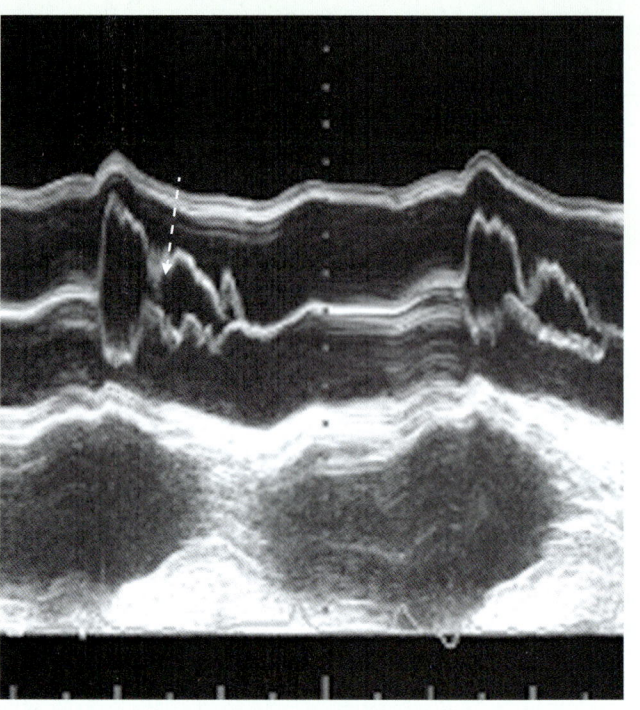

Figure 4.29

valve envelope, the opening and closing tend to be confined to the very early part of systole.

25. **Answer: D.** Insertion of a permanent pacemaker for chronotropic incompetence. This patient developed a pacemaker-related left bundle branch block. In normal activation, the normal downward motion of the septum slightly precedes the peak upward motion of the posterior wall. This is illustrated in **Figure 4.30**, on which is drawn a vertical dotted line, which illustrates that the peak downward or posterior motion of the interventricular septum is slightly earlier than the peak anterior motion of the posterior wall (arrow).

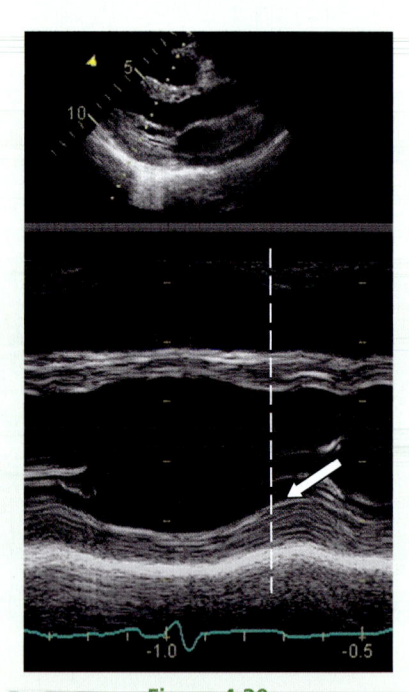

Figure 4.30

Chapter 4 M-Mode Echocardiography / 71

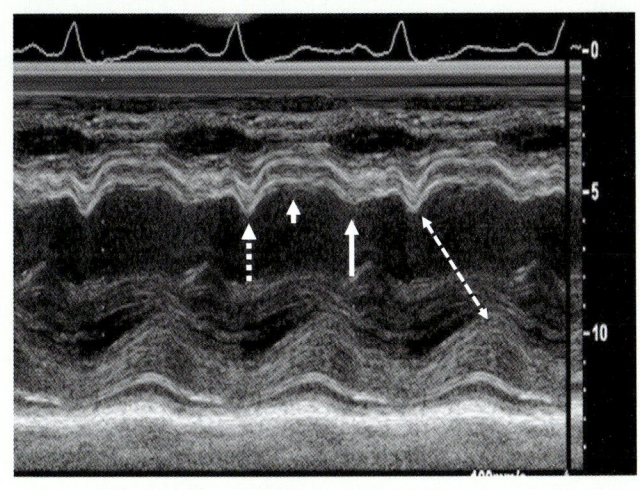

Figure 4.31

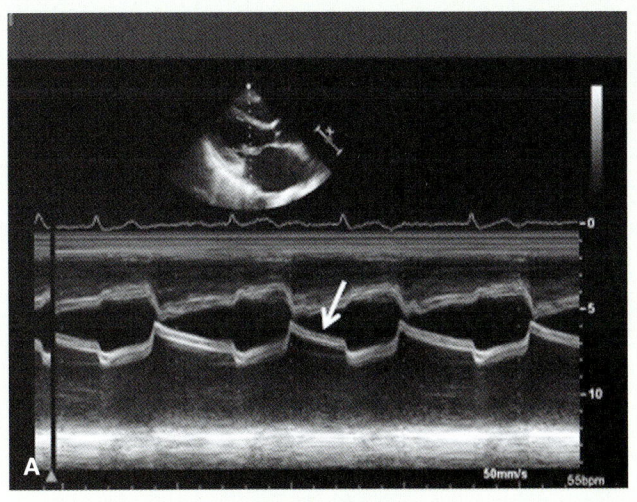

Figure 4.32A

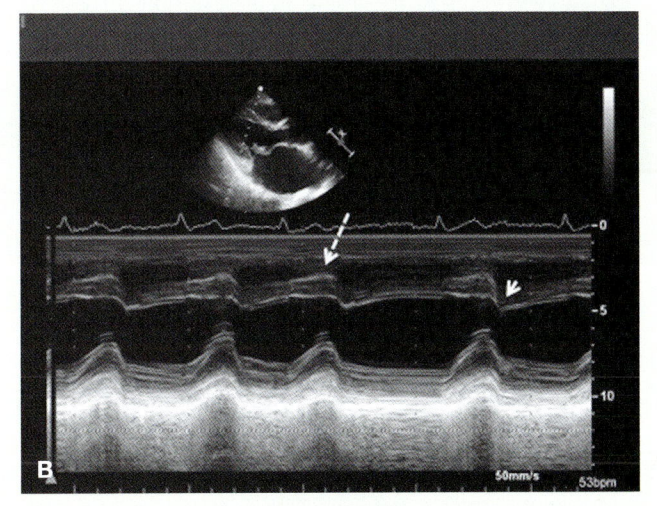

Figure 4.32B

By contrast, this M-mode (**Figure 4.31**) illustrates the classic features of left bundle branch block. In this instance, there is an early downward systolic movement "early systolic beak" (dashed white arrow), followed by paradoxical septal motion (white arrowhead), prolonged septal to posterior wall delay (dashed double headed arrow) and "diastolic dip" (solid white arrow). These finds predict an excellent response to resynchronization therapy.

26. **Answer: C.** The patient has rheumatic mitral stenosis. The most characteristic feature is a reduced E-F slope (**Figure 4.32A**; white arrow) seen on M-mode through the mitral valve. The normal mitral valve M-mode "M" shape is lost because of a reduction in early diastolic filling. In addition, as the M-mode cursor is moved to the LV cavity (**Figure 4.32B**), a characteristic prominent early diastolic dip (white arrow head) of mitral stenosis can be seen as well as paradoxical anterior motion of the septum in systole (dotted white arrow).

27. **Answer: B.** There is RV chamber collapse consistent with cardiac tamponade. M-mode of the RA and RV aids in the diagnosis of cardiac tamponade due to the high temporal resolution allowing for timing the duration of chamber collapse (**Figure 4.33**). Although RA chamber collapse >1/3 of the cardiac cycle is typically more sensitive than RV chamber collapse >1/3 of the cardiac cycle, the latter is much more specific. Therefore, although this patient has only a brief period of RA chamber collapse during systole, which is <1/3 of the cardiac cycle, there is prolonged RV chamber collapse >1/3 of the cardiac cycle (dotted arrow) consistent with cardiac tamponade.

28. **Answer: D.** The patient has constrictive pericarditis. Hallmark features on M-mode include a septal shudder (see smaller white arrow) in early diastole (equivalent to the pericardial knock on physical examination and the septal bounce seen on two-dimensional imaging) (**Figure 4.34**). There is flattening of the posterior wall in diastole (see larger white arrow pointing down) due to completion of most diastolic filling in early diastole and pericardial thickening or calcification (arrow pointing up). A respirometer is present, but LV and RV cavity sizes do not change significantly in the limited number of beats seen in this respiratory cycle. However, this would be expected in a more prolonged tracing of inspiratory and expiratory beats.

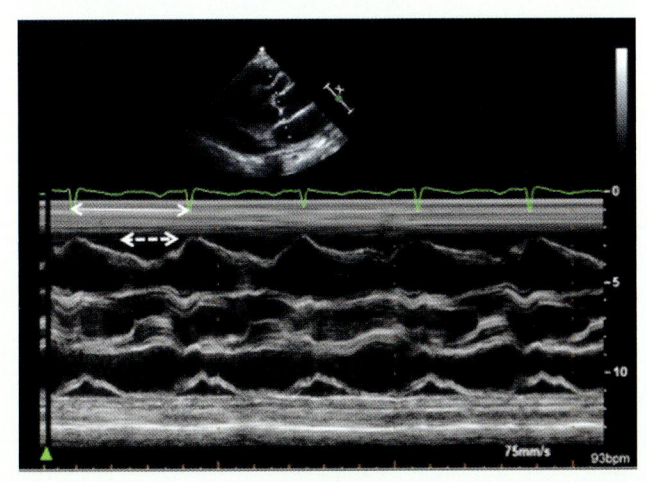

Figure 4.33

72 / Clinical Echocardiography Review

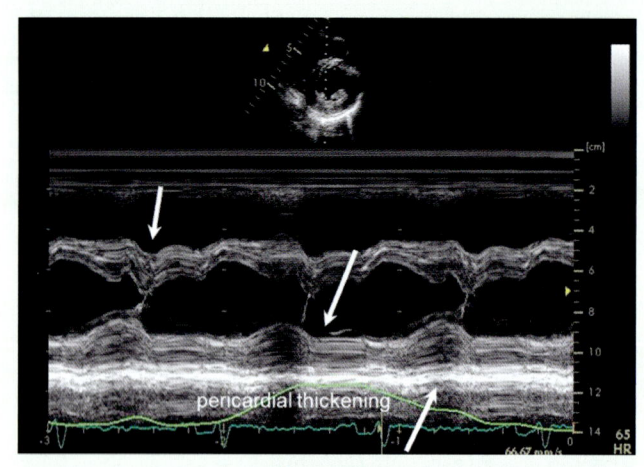

Figure 4.34

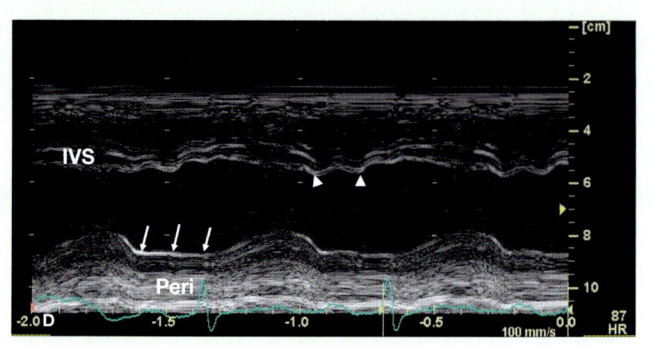

Figure 4.36

29. **Answer: B.** This recording is an example of a normal M-mode of the mitral valve. Parameters to note include a normal E-point septal separation (EPSS) distance (thin arrows), normal E-F slope, nonthickened mitral leaflets, no interruption of A-C closure, and normal motion of the systolic echoes (**Figure 4.35**). High-frequency fluttering of the anterior mitral leaflet, indicative of aortic regurgitation, is not present on this tracing. IVS, interventricular septum; LV, left ventricle; RV, right ventricle.

30. **Answer: D.** The patient presents with findings that are indicative of right-sided heart failure. **Review Figure 4.17**. The findings from the Doppler tissue imaging of the medial (panel A) and lateral (panel B) mitral annulus demonstrates annulus reversus, and the pulsed-wave interrogation of mitral inflow (panel C—showing a high E-wave velocity relative to the A-wave velocity and a shortened deceleration time; also note variation in E-wave velocity [without respirometer use]) raises suspicion for constrictive pericarditis (CP) in this clinical setting. Restrictive cardiomyopathy, which can present in a similar fashion, would not be expected as the annular velocities exceed 7 cm/s, and enhanced ventricular interaction (not expected with a restrictive cardiomyopathy) is suspected based on the presented Doppler tracings. M-mode findings reflect the hemodynamic characteristics of CP including enhanced ventricular interaction. Findings on M-mode echocardiography, which support the diagnosis of CP, include increased pericardial thickness, diastolic flattening of the LV posterior wall endocardium, abrupt posterior motion of the interventricular septum in early diastole with inspiration (septal shudder and bounce), and, on occasion, premature opening of the pulmonary valve. **Figure 4.36** shows an M-mode of a patient with surgery-proven constrictive pericarditis illustrating a thickened pericardium (Peri) and flattening of the LV posterior wall endocardium in diastole (arrows). Also illustrated on this tracing is abnormal motion of the interventricular septum (IVS) with prominent diastolic dips (arrow heads). On color M-mode echocardiography, the propagation velocity of early diastolic trans-mitral flow is found to be normal or increased (often >100 cm/s) reflecting the rapid, early diastolic filling of the LV characteristic of this condition. Reduced E-F slope for the reasons stated above and systolic anterior motion of the mitral apparatus would not be expected findings in this case. It must be emphasized that, while the M-mode recordings alone cannot establish this diagnosis, when coupled with the findings of 2DE and Doppler interrogation, strong evidence that CP may be present can be provided. Multimodality imaging may be necessary to firmly establish the diagnosis.

31. **Answer: C.** Imaging artifacts in the ascending aorta on transesophageal echocardiography (TEE) are common, especially in the setting of a dilated ascending aorta and when the size of the aorta exceeds that of the left atrium (as in this case). Failure to recognize this possibility may lead to a false-positive diagnosis of aortic dissection. In this case, a reverberation artifact is present. Note that on the M-mode examination (**Figure 4.37A**) the observed linear echodensity (Artifact) moves in a parallel fashion with the interface of the left atrium

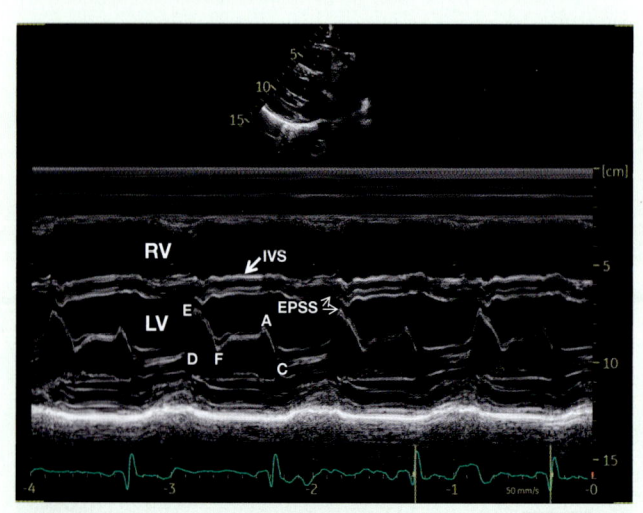

Figure 4.35

Figure 4.37A

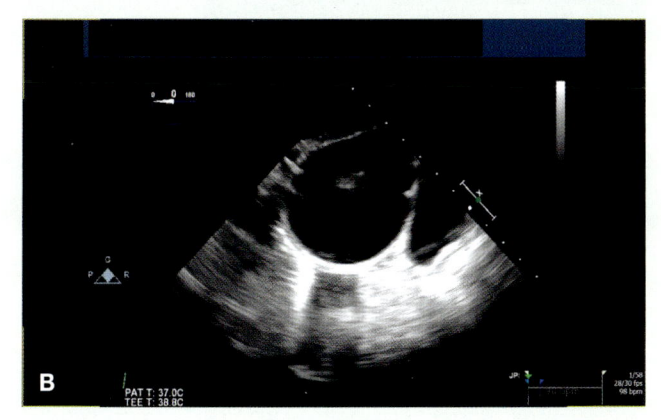

Figure 4.37B

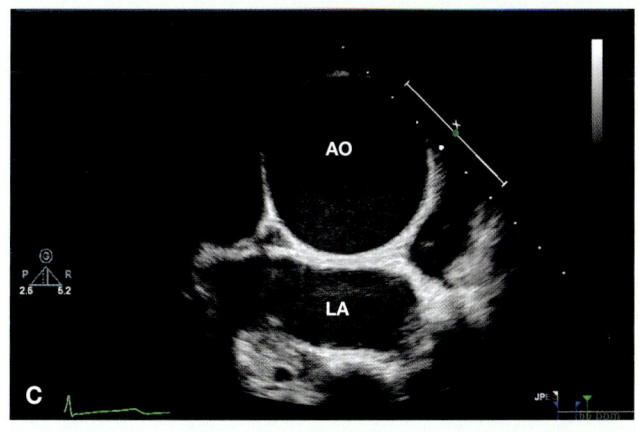

Figure 4.37C

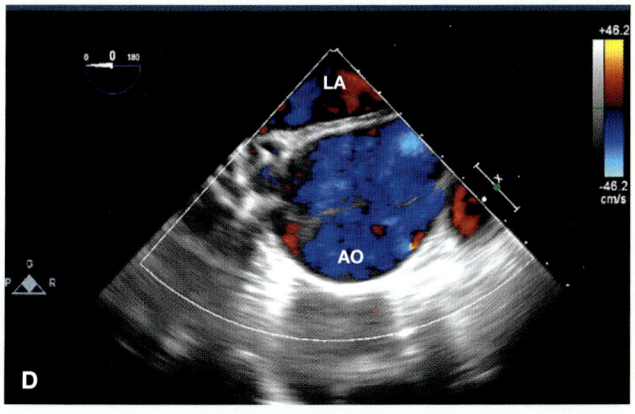

Figure 4.37D

Chapter 4 M-Mode Echocardiography / 73

(LA) and posterior wall of the ascending aorta (AO) and the leading edge is located at twice the distance from the transducer (double-headed arrows). An epiaortic ultrasound image is shown in **Figure 4.37B** where the transducer is placed directly on the ascending aorta (AO); as there is no intervening interface it shows no evident linear echodensity. Also note that, in this frame, the AO is larger in size than is the LA. It is hypothesized that such linear artifacts in the ascending aorta on TEE are the result of a multiple path effect in the left atrium or right pulmonary artery.

Other findings that may suggest artifact in the ascending aorta on TEE include presence of a thick linear image (>2.5 mm), fuzzy/indistinct borders, extension through the aortic wall, lack of color flow Doppler to respect the linear echodensity **(Figure 4.37C and D)**, similar blood flow velocities on both sides of the image, and no evident linear echodensity when an ultrasound enhancing agent is utilized.

Mirror image artifact, caused by reflection at the aorta-lung interface, produces a double image and is most frequently encountered in the descending thoracic aorta and transverse aortic arch.

An initial flap would not be expected to move in parallel with the posterior wall of the aorta.

An intramural hematoma typically does not present with an intimal flap; characteristic thickening of the aortic wall with a crescentic appearance or circumferential involvement is found.

32. **Answer: D.** Review **Figure 4.38**. This M-mode recording of the mitral valve (panel A) demonstrates high-frequency fluttering of the anterior

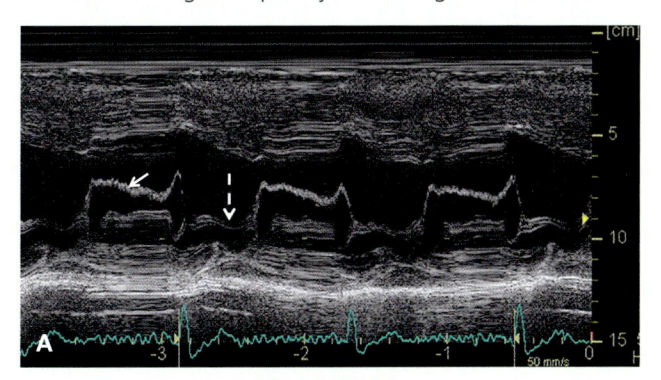

Figure 4.38A

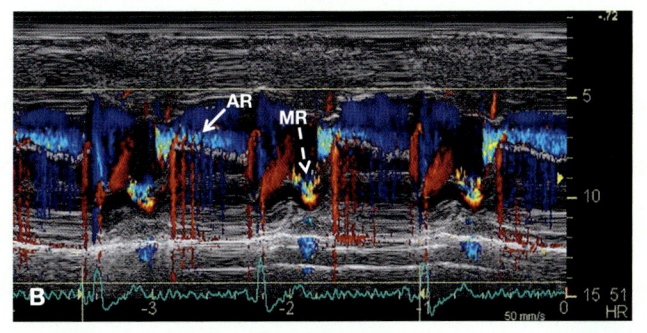

Figure 4.38B

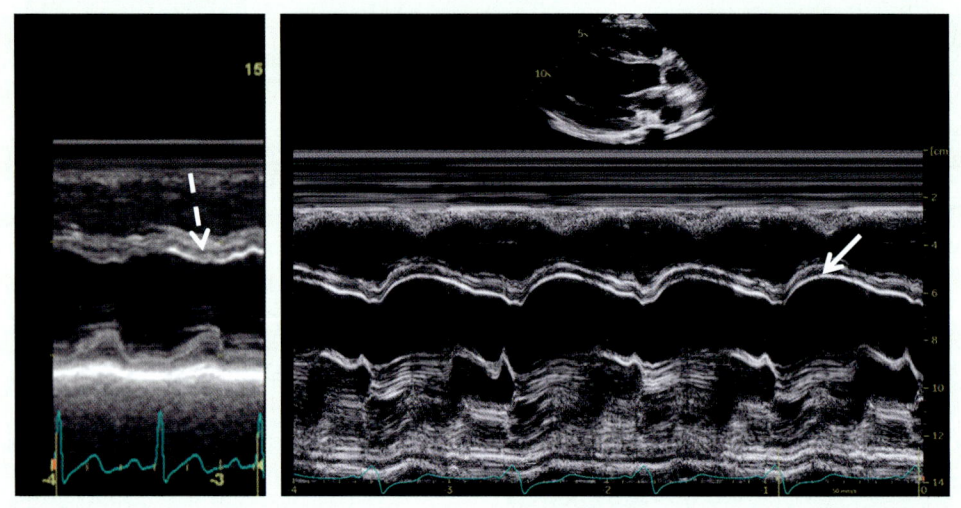

Figure 4.39. Left panel, normal motion of septum in systole (dotted arrow); Right panel, abrupt anterior motion of septum in systole due to preexcitation (solid arrow).

mitral leaflet (solid arrow) and late systolic prolapse (dashed arrow). On the color M-mode recording (panel B), both aortic regurgitation (AR; solid arrow) and late systolic mitral regurgitation (MR; dashed arrow) are demonstrated. A prominent S1, opening snap, and a diastolic rumble would be expected findings of mitral stenosis. On this M-mode recording the mitral leaflets are not shown to be thickened, the E-F slope is normal, and antiparallel motion of the valve leaflets in diastole is maintained. The tracing does not demonstrate systolic anterior motion of the mitral valve; thus, the finding of a harsh systolic murmur that augments with a Valsalva maneuver indicative of a dynamic LV outflow tract obstruction would not be an expected auscultatory finding. Finally, as this M-mode tracing shows only late systolic prolapse of the mitral valve, a holosystolic murmur would not be expected.

33. **Answer: D.** Review **Figure 4.39**. This M-mode shows abrupt anterior motion of the septum, as is pointed out by the solid white arrow on the right-hand panel. The left-hand panel shows the normal septal motion, by contrast (dotted white arrow). (This is also seen in **Figure 4.40**.) As is seen in the accompanying videos (▶ **Videos 4.3** and **4.4**), both parasternal long- and short-axis images, the anteroseptal wall is dyskinetic, but the wall is not thin in diastole. This would militate against a septal infarction—choice A. Incidentally, while isolated septal infarctions do occur, they are rare in the absence of prior percutaneous coronary intervention, where a septal branch might be occluded by a stent in the left anterior descending artery. The pattern of wall motion abnormality is also not typical for left bundle branch dyssynchrony, as is explained in the answer to question 25. Choice C is certainly a reasonable choice, and it would be hard to distinguish the two based on the M-mode alone; however, the presence of septal flattening, seen in the left-hand panel of **Figure 4.41** (dotted arrow) would help, as it is more abrupt and rapid than what is seen in the right-hand panel (solid arrow). (See accompanying ▶ **Video 4.5** for a 2D view of septal motion in a patient with severe tricuspid regurgitation).

The correct answer is choice D, conduction abnormality. This case illustrates a wall motion abnormality associated with a septal accessory pathway. This patient had Wolff-Parkinson-White syndrome (see ECG, **Figure 4.42**) with a right-sided septal accessory pathway leading to early activation of the interventricular septum. Such early activation causes septal dyskinesis, LV dysfunction (▶ **Video 4.6**), and adverse LV remodeling. Patients who undergo successful ablation of such an accessory pathway experience a diminution in dyssynchrony and improvement in left ventricular systolic function.

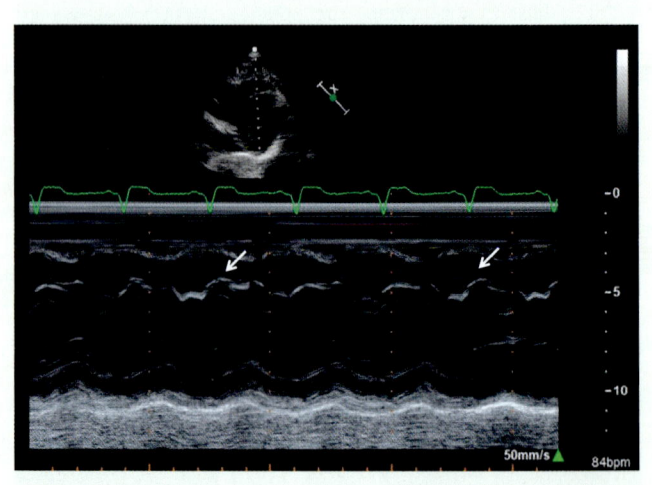

Figure 4.40. Abrupt anterior motion of the septum in systole (arrow) due to preexcitation.

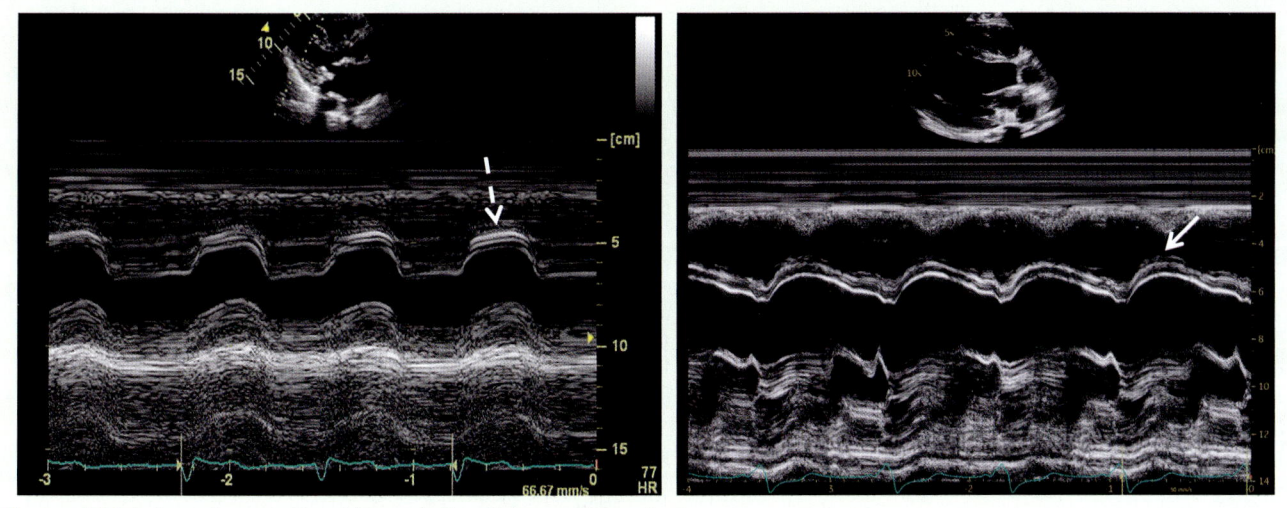

Figure 4.41. Left panel, severe tricuspid regurgitation; Right panel, preexcitation.

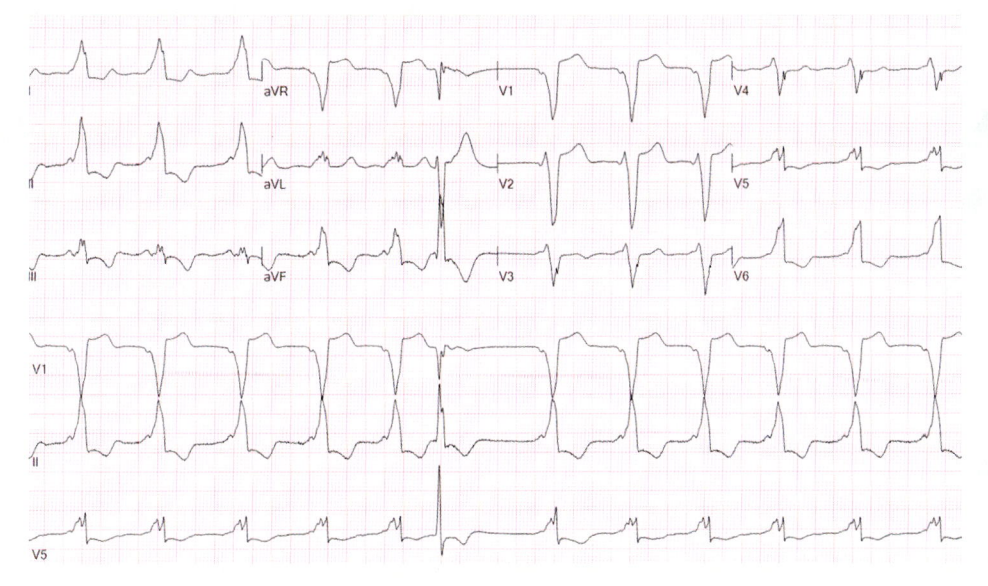

Figure 4.42

SUGGESTED READINGS

Alcini E, Monticelli M, Mottironi P, Anastasi R. Studio ecocardiografico mono e bidimensionale della valvola aortica bicuspide [Mono- and bi-dimensional echocardiographic study of a bicuspid aortic valve]. G Ital Cardiol. 1983;13(8):85-90. Italian.

Appelbe AF, Walker PG, Yeoh JK, Bonitatibus A, Yoganathan AP, Martin RP. Clinical significance and origin of artifacts in transesophageal echocardiography of the thoracic aorta. J Am Coll Cardiol. 1993;21(3):754-760.

Evangelista A, Garcia-del-Castillo H, Gonzalez-Alujas T, et al. Diagnosis of ascending aortic dissection by transesophageal echocardiography: utility of M-mode in recognizing artifacts. J Am Coll Cardiol. 1996;27(1):102-107.

Feigenbaum H. Role of m-mode technique in today's echocardiography. J Am Soc Echocardiogr. 2010;23:240-257.

Ganau A, Devereux RB, Roman MJ, et al. Patterns of left ventricular hypertrophy and geometric remodeling in essential hypertension. J Am Coll Cardiol. 1992;19(7):1550-1558.

Wachtell K, Smith G, Gerdts E, et al. Left ventricular filling patterns in patients with systemic hypertension and left ventricular hypertrophy (the LIFE study). Losartan intervention for endpoint. Am J Cardiol. 2000;85(4):466-472.

Kwon B, Bae E, Kim GB, Noh CI, Choi JY, Yun YS. Septal dyskinesia and global left ventricular dysfunction in pediatric Wolff-Parkinson-White syndrome with septal accessory pathway. J Cardiovasc Electrophysiol. 2010;21(3):290-295.

CHAPTER 5

Assessment of Chamber Quantification

Wendy Tsang, Jeremy Slivnick, and Roberto M. Lang

QUESTIONS

1. Which of the following statements regarding the left atrium is inaccurate?
   A. The left atrium functions as a contractile pump that delivers 15% to 30% of the entire LV filling.
   B. The left atrium functions as a reservoir that collects pulmonary venous return during ventricular systole.
   C. Left atrial dysfunction does not affect left ventricular function.
   D. The left atrium functions as a conduit for the passage of stored blood from the left atrium to the left ventricle during early ventricular diastole.

2. A 40-year-old woman is referred for assessment of diastolic function. As part of the evaluation, the echocardiogram report includes an assessment of left atrial size. Which of the following statements regarding left atrial size is **FALSE**?
   A. Left atrial size is best measured at left ventricular end-systole.
   B. Transesophageal echocardiography (TEE) provides more accurate measurements of left atrial size compared to transthoracic echocardiography.
   C. Left atrial volumes should be measured from dedicated left atrial views rather than using apical 4- and 2-chamber views acquired to measure left ventricular volumes.
   D. Left atrial anteroposterior measurement obtained from the parasternal window may underestimate left atrial size.

3. Which of the following statements regarding left atrial volume is **INCORRECT**?
   A. Left atrial volume is a superior to anteroposterior left atrial diameter because it accounts for alterations in left atrial chamber size in all directions.
   B. Left atrial volume has a stronger association with outcomes in cardiac patients compared to anteroposterior left atrial diameter.
   C. Left atrial volume is a powerful prognostic variable in disease states such as atrial fibrillation and diastolic heart failure.
   D. Left atrial volumes obtained from two-dimensional transthoracic echocardiography are similar to those reported on computed tomography and cardiac magnetic resonance imaging.
   E. Single-plane left atrial volume measurements obtained from the apical 4-chamber view are smaller than those obtained from the apical 2-chamber view.

4. Which of the following is not recommended in the American Society of Echocardiography guidelines as a method for measuring left atrial volume?
   A. Ellipsoid model using three linear measurements.
   B. Spherical model using two linear measurements.
   C. Disc summation method from single or biplane imaging assuming an oval shape.
   D. Biplane method using left atrial areas and lengths from the apical 4- and 2-chamber views.

5. Which of the following is recommended by the American Society of Echocardiography guidelines for reporting of left atrial size?
   A. Area-length method.
   B. Biplane disc summation method indexed for body surface area.
   C. Apical 4-chamber linear measurements.
   D. Left atrial area.

6. Which of the following is not an advantage of using three-dimensional echocardiography over two-dimensional echocardiography for measuring left atrial volume?
   A. It has a standardized methodology with ultrasound-enhancing agent use.
   B. It correlates better with computed tomography and cardiac magnetic resonance imaging.
   C. It is more accurate compared to the gold standard.
   D. It has better prognostic ability.

7. Which of the following characteristics of right atrial volume measurements is different from left atrial volume measurements?
   A. Right atrial volumes are more robust compared to right atrial linear dimensions.
   B. Right atrial volumes are more accurate compared to right atrial linear dimensions.
   C. Right atrial volumes cannot be calculated from biplane views.
   D. Right atrial volumes are underestimated on two-dimensional echocardiography compared to three-dimensional echocardiography.

8. Which of the following phases of right atrial strain would be expected to be absent in atrial fibrillation?
   A. Conduit strain
   B. Booster strain
   C. Conductive strain
   D. Reservoir strain

9. Which of the following statements is **FALSE** with respect to aortic root dilation?
   A. The presence of hypertension has little impact on aortic root diameter at the level of the sinuses of Valsalva.
   B. Aortic root diameter measurements at the level of the sinuses of Valsalva are closely related to age and body surface area.
   C. Aortic root dilatation at the sinuses of Valsalva is defined as an aortic root diameter above the upper limit of the 95% confidence interval of the distribution in a large reference population.
   D. Aortic regurgitation is not associated with aortic root dilation.

10. During a quality improvement exercise, it was discovered that there were systematic differences between echocardiographers in aortic root measurements. Which of the following statements could account for these differences?
   A. Measurements based on 2D images versus M-mode.
   B. Leading edge–to–leading edge versus inner edge–to–inner edge measurements.
   C. Measurements obtained from an image with an asymmetric aortic valve closure line in a patient with known tricuspid valve.
   D. Transesophageal versus transthoracic measurements.
   E. All of the above.

11. An 80-year-old woman with calcific aortic stenosis is referred for aortic annular measurement during evaluation for possible transcatheter aortic valve replacement. When measuring the aortic annulus, which of the following statements is **FALSE**?
   A. Calcium protuberances should be considered part of the lumen and not the aortic wall.
   B. Acoustic blooming due to calcium may affect accuracy of aortic annular measurements.
   C. The aortic annular diameter should be obtained from the parasternal long-axis view, which is a plane similar to the plane containing the long-axis of the left ventricle.
   D. The aortic annular diameter is measured in the parasternal long-axis view and is typically between the hinge points of the noncoronary cusp and right coronary cusp.
   E. 3D echocardiography may provide more accurate annular measurements compared to 2D methods due to lack of geometric assumptions.

12. Which of the following statements is **TRUE**?
   A. The aortic annulus should be measured in mid-systole.
   B. The aortic annulus should be measured in end-diastole.
   C. The aortic annulus should be measured during isovolumetric relaxation.
   D. The aortic annulus should be measured during isovolumetric contraction.

13. Which of the following statements is **FALSE**?
   A. An inferior vena cava measuring 1.0 cm with spontaneous collapse indicates the presence of intravascular volume depletion.
   B. Inferior vena cava diameters in mechanically ventilated patients are not reliable in the estimation of right atrial pressure.
   C. Inferior vena cava diameters in athletes are reliable estimates of right atrial pressure.
   D. The inferior vena cava is best assessed from the subcostal window.

14. A 50-year-old man is being evaluated in the intensive care unit. He is sedated and mechanically ventilated. The team has asked for an estimation of pulmonary artery pressures. Which of the following statements is **TRUE**?
   A. A dilated inferior vena cava indicates a high right atrial pressure in this patient.
   B. An inferior vena cava diameter <1.2 cm has a sensitivity of 100% for a right atrial pressure of <10 mm Hg.
   C. There is a better correlation between inferior vena cava diameter measured at end inspiration and end-diastole using M-mode echocardiography.
   D. None of the above.

15. Which of the following statements is **TRUE** with respect to estimating right atrial pressure to estimate pulmonary artery pressure based on tricuspid regurgitant jet velocity?
   A. When right atrial pressure is normal (0-5 mm Hg), there is a normal inspiratory collapse of 50% in an inferior vena cava with a normal diameter (<2.1 cm).
   B. When right atrial pressure is mildly elevated (6-10 mm Hg), a normal inspiratory collapse of greater than 50% is present even with a dilated (>2.1 cm) inferior vena cava.
   C. Right atrial pressure is around 15 mm Hg when the inferior vena cava is dilated (>2.1 cm) and there is less than 50% inspiratory collapse.
   D. Right atrial pressure is >15 mm Hg when the inferior vena cava is dilated (>2.1 cm) and there is no collapse.
   E. All of the above.

16. Which of the following is not a method for assessing right ventricular function?
   A. Fractional area change.
   B. Tissue Doppler imaging–derived tricuspid lateral annular systolic velocity wave (S′).
   C. Tricuspid annular plane systolic excursion (TAPSE).
   D. Right ventricular index of myocardial performance (RIMP).
   E. Biplane Simpson ejection fraction.

17. In the American Society of Echocardiography guidelines, right ventricular dimension and function cutoff values that do not account for gender or body surface area are provided. Application of such standard values without indexing may provide an inaccurate estimate of right ventricular size in all of the following populations **EXCEPT**:
   A. Athletes.
   B. Extremes of body surface area or height.
   C. Ventilated patients.
   D. Congenital heart disease patients.

18. You are asked to assess a 39-year-old woman with pulmonary regurgitation. Which of the following is not a **TRUE** statement about right ventricular ejection fraction?
   A. Right ventricular ejection fraction is higher in women than men.
   B. Normal right ventricular ejection fraction is lower than left ventricular ejection fraction.
   C. Right ventricular end-diastolic volume is larger than left ventricular end-diastolic volume.
   D. Right ventricular stroke volume is larger than left ventricular stroke volume.

19. Which of the following is **TRUE** regarding the use of three-dimensional echocardiography in the assessment of right ventricular function?
   A. Three-dimensional echocardiography–derived measurement of right ventricular ejection fraction has not been validated against the reference standard of cardiac magnetic resonance imaging.
   B. A manual tracing approach is the recommended method for measuring right ventricular ejection fraction.
   C. The three-dimensional right ventricle volume dataset should have a temporal resolution of 5 to 10 volumes per second.
   D. Right ventricular ejection fraction of <45% is considered abnormal.

20. Of the following descriptors regarding the right ventricle, which statement is **FALSE**?
   A. It has a complex crescentic shape.
   B. It is a thin-walled chamber.
   C. It is a low compliance and high afterload system.
   D. Its stroke volume is the same as the left ventricle.
   E. It uses 25% of the stroke work of the left ventricle.

21. Which of the following statements regarding measurements of right ventricular function is **INCORRECT**?
   A. Right ventricular index of myocardial performance can be falsely low in conditions associated with elevated right atrial pressures, which will shorten the isovolumic relaxation time.
   B. Tricuspid annular plane systolic excursion (TAPSE) and TDI-derived tricuspid lateral annular systolic velocity (S′) may over- or underestimate right ventricular function due to overall heart motion.
   C. A right ventricular fractional area change <40% indicates systolic dysfunction.
   D. To obtain TDI-derived tricuspid lateral annular systolic velocity, it is important to keep the basal segment and lateral annulus aligned with the Doppler cursor to avoid velocity underestimation.

22. Which of the following is the view recommended by the American Society of Echocardiography (ASE) for measuring right ventricular systolic function?
   A. Apical 4-chamber view.
   B. Right ventricular–focused apical 4-chamber view.
   C. Modified apical 4-chamber view.
   D. Modified apical 3-chamber view.

23. Which of the following statements is **TRUE** regarding the assessment of right ventricular systolic function?
   A. RV TAPSE and S′ provide accurate assessment of right ventricular function following sternotomy.
   B. RV ejection fraction by 3D is more accurate than RV TAPSE and S′ for predicting CMR-derived RVEF.
   C. RV TAPSE and S′ are less dependent on image acquisition angle compared to RV free wall strain.
   D. RV fractional area change is less prone to errors related to foreshortening compared to RV TAPSE and S′.

24. In which of the following views should right ventricular wall thickness be measured?
   A. Parasternal long axis.
   B. Parasternal short axis.
   C. Standard apical 4-chamber.
   D. RV-focused apical 4-chamber.
   E. Subcostal.

25. Which of the following statements regarding two-dimensional echocardiography and three-dimensional echocardiography in the assessment of left ventricular volumes is **TRUE**?
   A. Apical images are frequently foreshortened on two-dimensional echocardiography leading to overestimation of volumes.
   B. Three-dimensional echocardiography volumetric assessment avoids the geometric assumptions needed to calculate volumes on two-dimensional echocardiography.
   C. Two-dimensional echocardiographic volume measurements account for regional wall abnormalities.
   D. Three-dimensional echocardiography provides more accurate measurements when acoustic windows are poor compared to two-dimensional echocardiography.

26. Which of the follow statements regarding left ventricular volumetric measurements is **FALSE**?
   A. Left ventricular volume measurements can be obtained from two-dimensional or three-dimensional echocardiography.
   B. Volume calculations can be accurately derived from linear measurements.
   C. Contrast agents improve endocardial delineation and provide larger volumes than noncontrast images.
   D. Left ventricular volumes should be measured from the apical 2- and 4-chamber views.

27. Which of the following statements regarding two-dimensional echocardiography and three-dimensional echocardiography in the assessment of left ventricular volumes is **FALSE**?
   A. Apical images can be foreshortened on two-dimensional echocardiography leading to underestimation of volumes.
   B. Three-dimensional echocardiography volumetric assessment avoids the geometric assumptions needed to calculate volumes on two-dimensional echocardiography.
   C. Two-dimensional echocardiographic volume measurements cannot account for regional wall abnormalities.
   D. Three-dimensional echocardiography provides more accurate measurements when acoustic windows are poor compared to two-dimensional echocardiography.

28. Which of the following statements is **FALSE** regarding methods for assessing left ventricular systolic function?
   A. Fractional shortening is reliable when regional wall motion abnormalities are present.
   B. The biplane method of discs is also known as the modified Simpson rule.
   C. Three-dimensional left ventricular ejection fraction, when feasible, is recommended over two-dimensional left ventricular ejection fraction.
   D. Global longitudinal strain is abnormal when > –18%.

29. Which of the following is not included in the visual regional wall motion four grade scheme?
   A. Normal or hyperkinetic.
   B. Hypokinetic or reduced thickening.
   C. Akinetic or absent/negligible thickening.
   D. Dyskinetic or systolic thinning or stretching.
   E. Aneurysm or focal dilatation and thinning (remodeling) with either akinetic or dyskinetic systolic deformation.

30. Which of the following statements regarding left ventricular mass is **INCORRECT**?
   A. In a normally shaped left ventricle, both M-mode and two-dimensional echocardiography formulas to calculate LV mass can be used.
   B. Left ventricular mass is an important risk factor for and predictor of cardiovascular events.
   C. Three-dimensional echocardiography is the only echocardiographic method that directly measures myocardial volume.
   D. Left ventricular mass calculated using direct two-dimensional echocardiography is directly comparable to blind M-mode.

31. A 55-year-old man is undergoing transthoracic echocardiogram for pretransplant evaluation. The following values are noted on his examination:

- Septal wall thickness: 13 mm
- Posterior wall thickness: 13 mm
- LV end-diastolic diameter: 47 mm
- Indexed LV mass: 119 g/m^2

Which of the following best describes cardiac structure in this patient?
   A. Concentric hypertrophy.
   B. Eccentric hypertrophy.
   C. Concentric remodeling.
   D. Normal geometry.

32. Which of the following statements regarding left ventricular volumetric measurements is **TRUE**?
   A. LV volume calculations can be accurately derived from linear measurements.
   B. With 2D echocardiography, contrast agents improve endocardial delineation and provide smaller volumes than noncontrast images.
   C. Left ventricular volumes using three-dimensional echocardiography are larger than those obtained with CMR.
   D. Left ventricular volumes obtained with three-dimensional echocardiography are more accurate than those acquired with 2D echocardiography when compared to an MRI gold standard.

33. The following series of images (**Figure 5.1**) were obtained from a 38-year-old female.
   In which of the following images is the left atrium traced correctly?
   A. **Figure 5.1A**.
   B. **Figure 5.1B**.
   C. **Figure 5.1C**.
   D. **Figure 5.1D**.

34. The following series of images (**Figure 5.2**) is obtained from a 48-year-old woman.
   In which set of images is the left atrial volume measurements performed correctly?
   A. **Figure 5.2A**.
   B. **Figure 5.2B**.
   C. **Figure 5.2C**.
   D. **Figure 5.2D**.

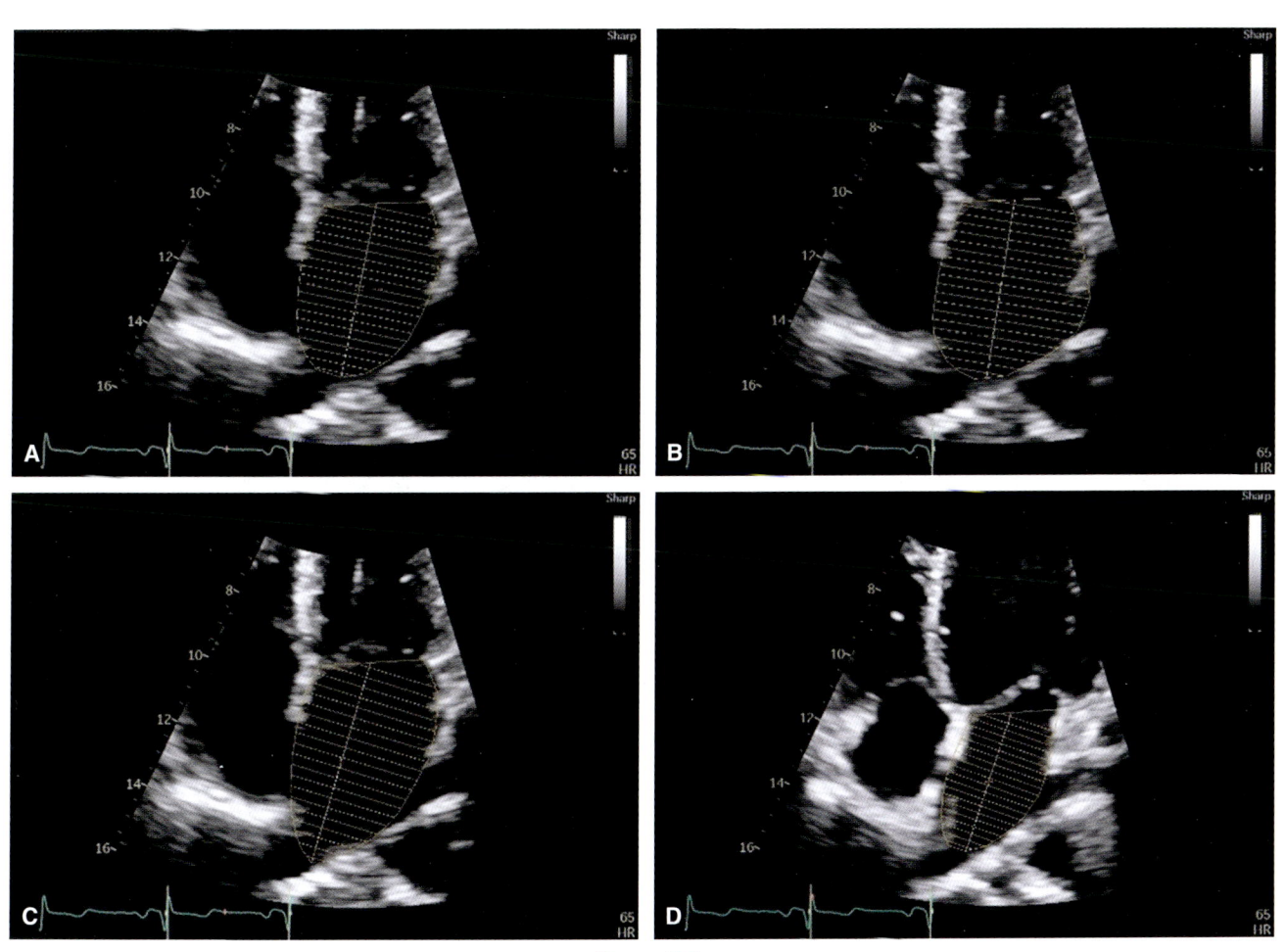

Figure 5.1

82 / Clinical Echocardiography Review

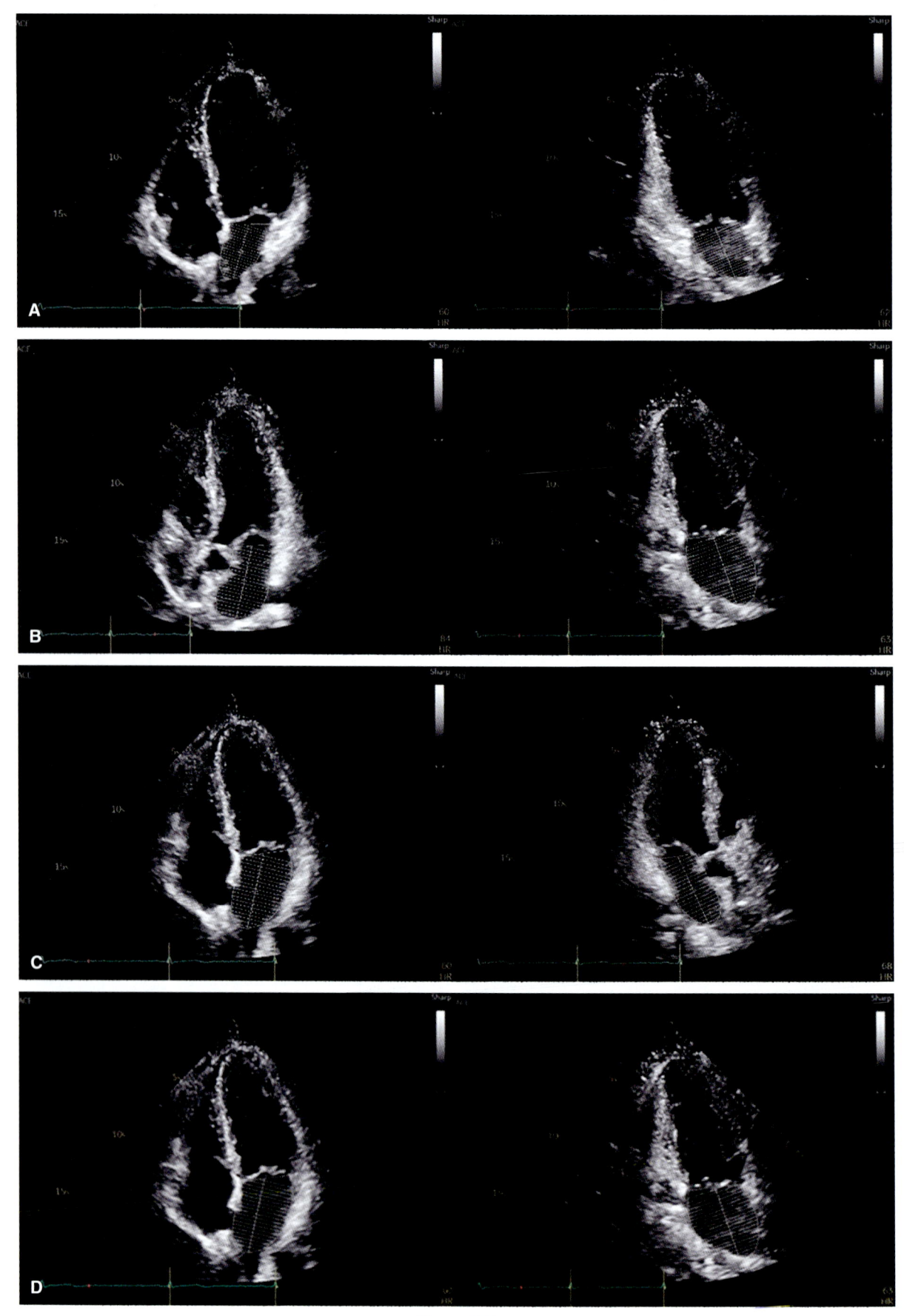

Figure 5.2

35. Which structure is **INCORRECTLY** labeled in **Figure 5.3** of the aortic root?
   A. Node of Arantius.
   B. Virtual aortic annulus.
   C. Sinus of Valsalva.
   D. Leaflet hinge point.

36. Which of the following measurements (shown in **Figure 5.4**) of LVOT is correct in this 75-year-old woman being evaluated for TAVR?
   A. Figure 5.4A.
   B. Figure 5.4B.
   C. Figure 5.4C.
   D. Figure 5.4D.

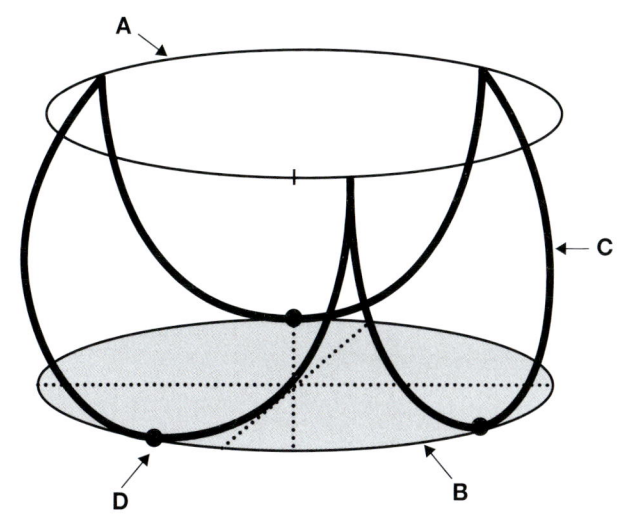

Figure 5.3. Illustration of aortic root anatomy. (Derived from Lang RM, Badano LP, Mor-Avi V, et al. Recommendations for cardiac chamber quantification by echocardiography in adults: an update from the American Society of Echocardiography and the European Association of Cardiovascular Imaging. *J Am Soc Echocardiogr.* 2015;28:1-39.e14.)

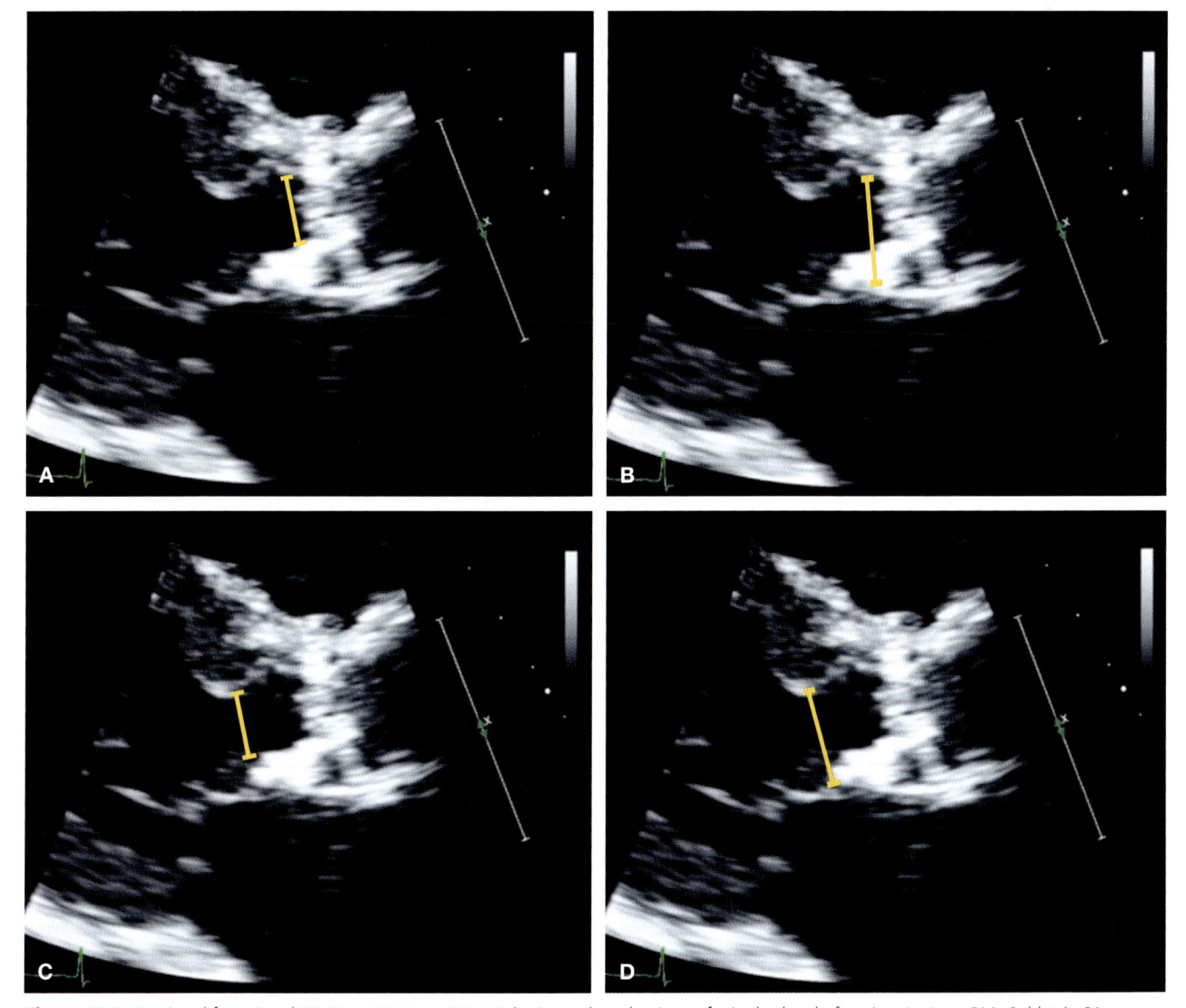

Figure 5.4. Reprinted from Freed BH, Tsang W, Lang RM. Etiologies and mechanisms of mitral valve dysfunction. In: Lang RM, Goldstein SA, Kronzon I, Khandheria B, Saric M, Mor-Avi V, eds. *ASE's Comprehensive Echocardiography*. 3rd ed. Philadelphia PA: Elsevier; 2022:521-523. Copyright © 2022 Elsevier. With permission.

84 / Clinical Echocardiography Review

37. You are asked to assess the inferior vena cava size from the patients shown in **Figure 5.5**.
Which image from **Figure 5.5** depicts a dilated inferior vena cava?
   A. **Figure 5.5A**.
   B. **Figure 5.5B**.
   C. **Figure 5.5C**.
   D. **Figure 5.5D**.

38. You are asked to assess right atrial pressure in the patients shown in **Figure 5.6**.
Which patient has an estimated right atrial pressure of 3 mm Hg?
   A. **Figure 5.6A**.
   B. **Figure 5.6B**.
   C. **Figure 5.6C**.
   D. **Figure 5.6D**.

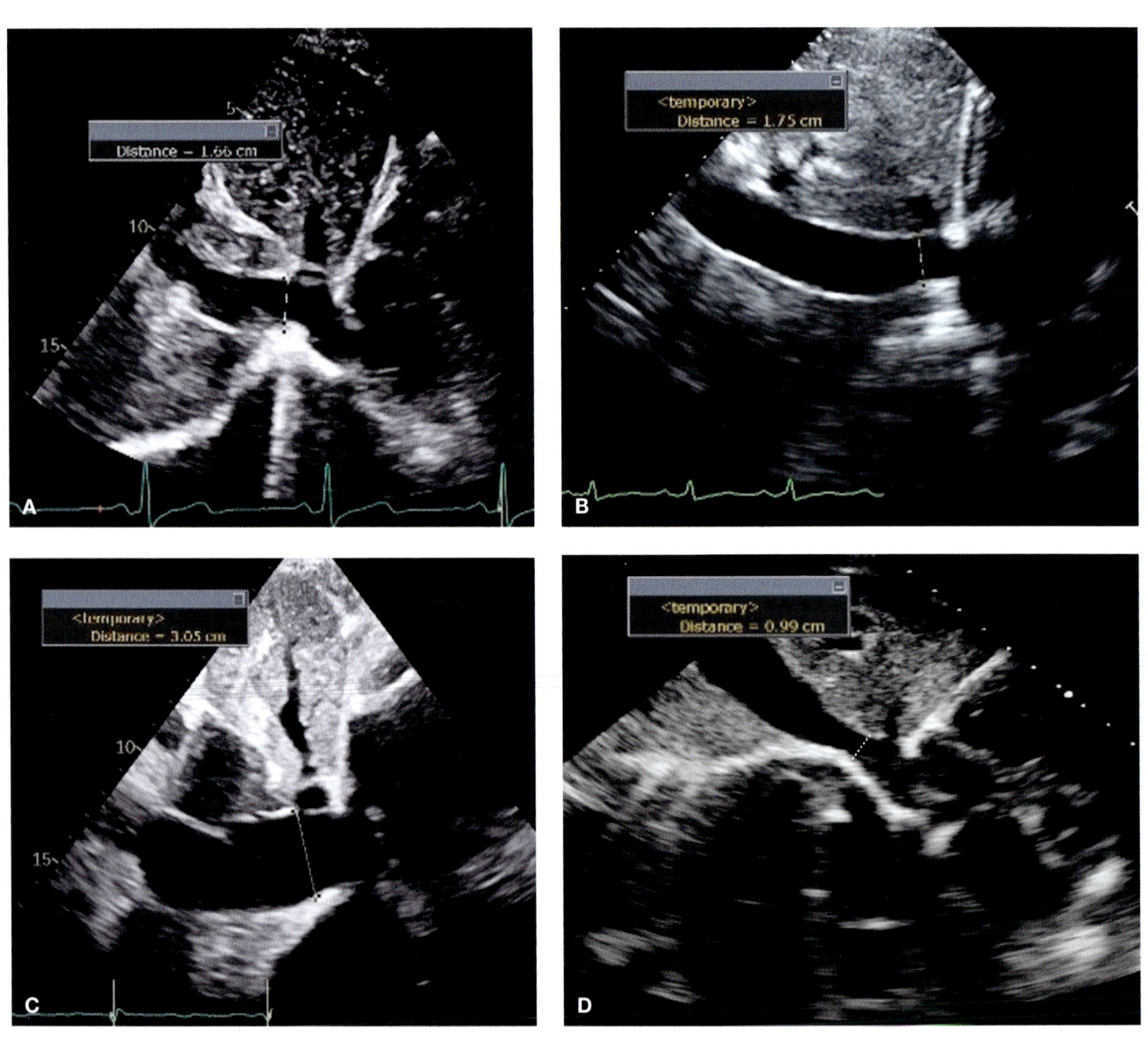

Figure 5.5

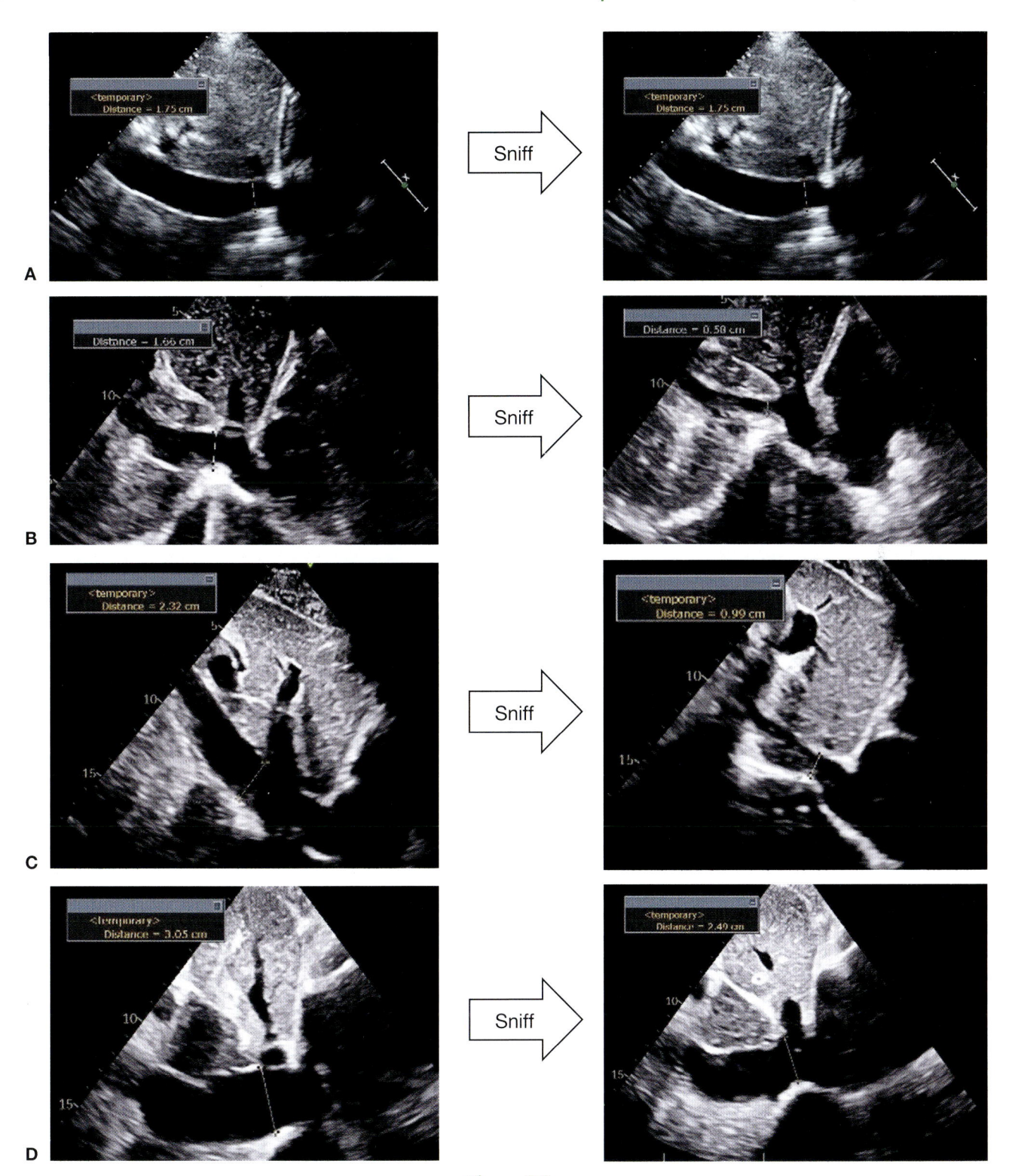

Chapter 5 Assessment of Chamber Quantification / 85

Figure 5.6

39. A 65-year-old female outpatient is suspected to have pulmonary hypertension. You have been asked to provide an estimation of systolic pulmonary artery pressure. Two-dimensional echocardiographic images of the inferior vena cava at rest and with sniffing are provided in **Figure 5.7A, B**. Continuous-wave Doppler of the tricuspid regurgitation jet is provided in **Figure 5.7C**.
What is the estimated systolic pulmonary artery pressure?

A. 35 to 39 mm Hg.
B. 30 to 34 mm Hg.
C. 24 to 29 mm Hg.
D. 40 mm Hg.

40. A 34-year-old man was referred for assessment of arrhythmogenic right ventricular cardiomyopathy. Which of the following views shown in **Figure 5.8** is not considered an essential view for visually assessing the right ventricle?

A. **Figure 5.8A**.
B. **Figure 5.8B**.
C. **Figure 5.8C**.
D. **Figure 5.8D**.

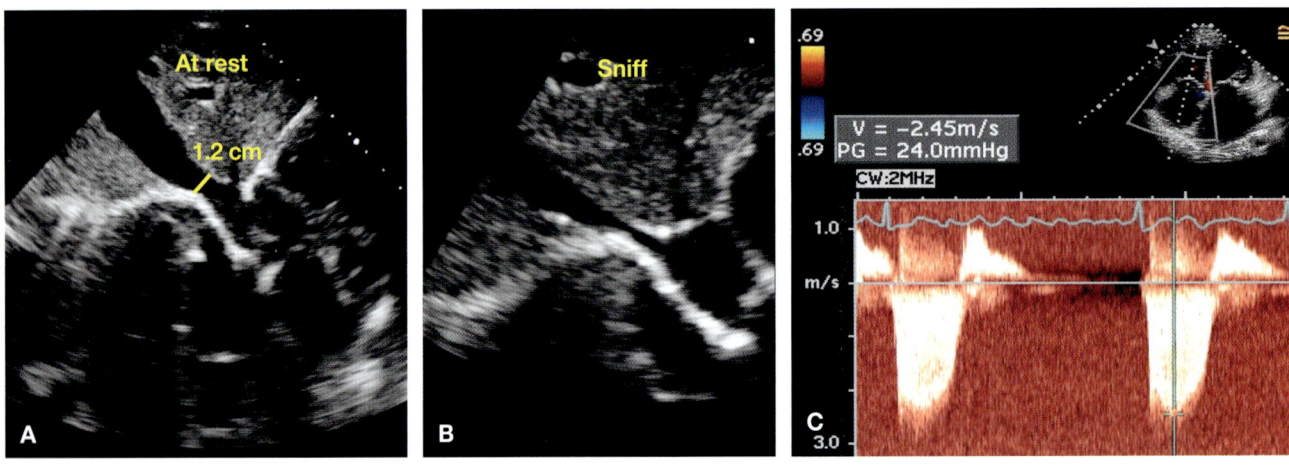

Figure 5.7

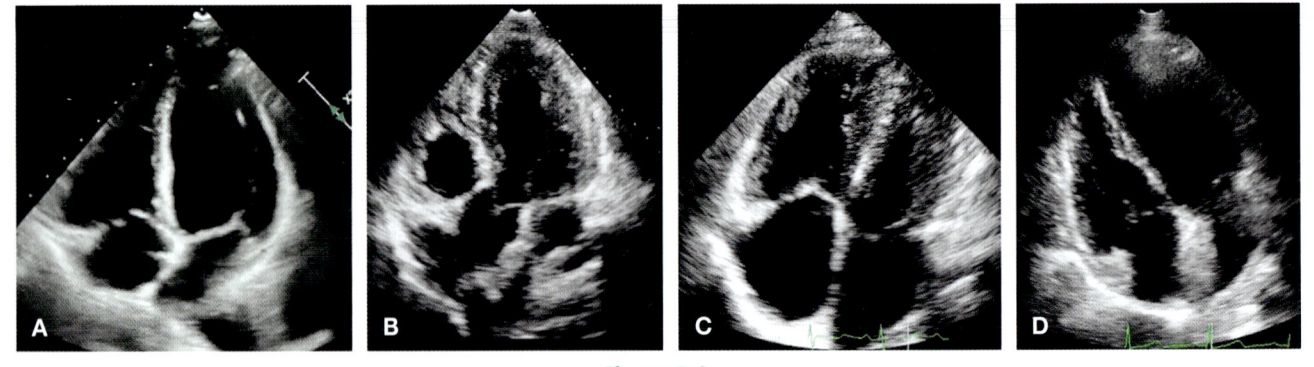

Figure 5.8

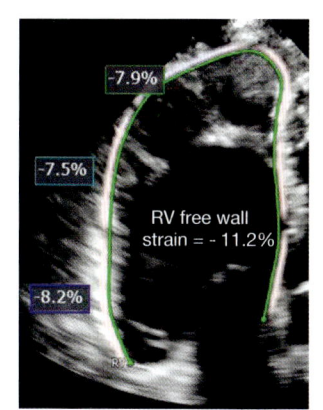

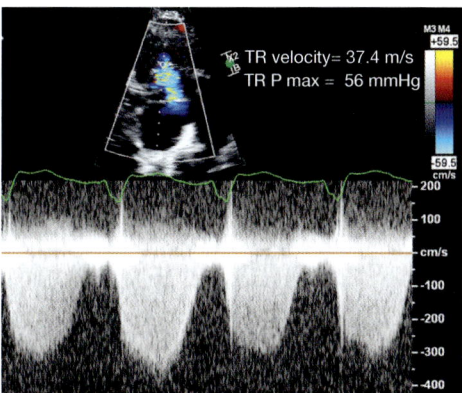

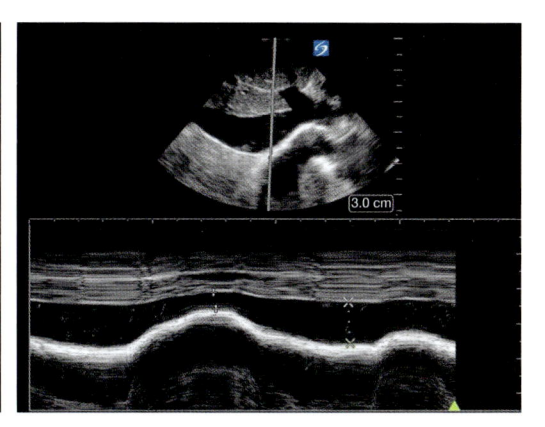

Figure 5.9

41. A 65-year-old man presents to the clinic with shortness of breath and an echocardiogram is performed (**Figure 5.9**).
Which of the following statements is **TRUE** regarding right ventricular function and pulmonary pressures in this 65-year-old man?
A. Normal RV systolic function and pulmonary pressures.
B. Reduced RV systolic function, normal pulmonary pressures.
C. Normal RV systolic function, pulmonary hypertension.
D. Reduced RV systolic function, pulmonary hypertension.

42. In the patient from **Question 41** (**Figure 5.9**), what is the estimated right ventricular systolic pressure?
A. 44 mm Hg.
B. 55 mm Hg.
C. 65 mm Hg.
D. 75 mm Hg.

43. A 35-year-old woman with newly diagnosed pulmonary hypertension is about to start treatment. She has been referred to obtain a baseline assessment of her right ventricular size and systolic function. After assessing the two-dimensional echocardiographic apical 4-chamber view (**Figure 5.10A**), the tissue Doppler image of the lateral tricuspid annulus (**Figure 5.10B**), and the M-mode image through the lateral tricuspid annulus (**Figure 5.10C**), what is her right ventricular size and systolic function?

A. Normal right ventricular size and function.
B. Normal right ventricular size, abnormal systolic function.
C. Abnormal right ventricular size, abnormal systolic function.
D. Abnormal right ventricular size, normal systolic function.

44. A 45-year-old woman with a history of pulmonary embolism is referred for assessment of right ventricular size and systolic function. After evaluating the two-dimensional echocardiographic apical 4-chamber view (**Figure 5.11A**), the tissue Doppler image of the lateral tricuspid annulus (**Figure 5.11B**), and the M-mode image through the lateral tricuspid annulus (**Figure 5.11C**), what is her right ventricular size and systolic function?
A. Normal right ventricular size and function.
B. Normal right ventricular size, abnormal systolic function.
C. Abnormal right ventricular size, abnormal systolic function.
D. Abnormal right ventricular size, normal systolic function.

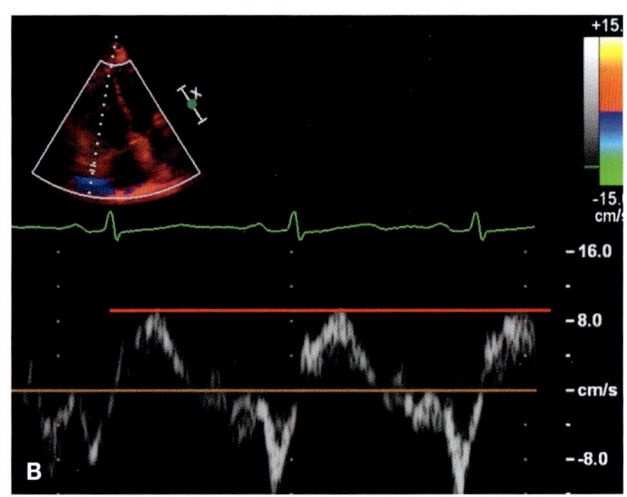

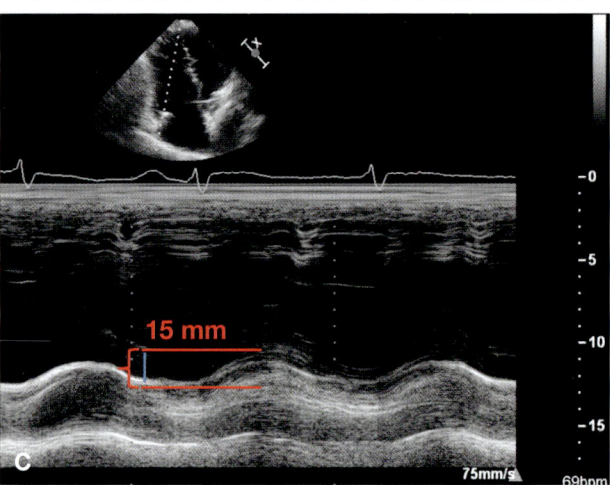

Figure 5.10

45. From the transthoracic echocardiographic study shown in **Figure 5.12**, name the segment indicated by the green arrow in order from 1 to 3.
  A. Basal anterolateral, apical inferior, mid-anteroseptum.
  B. Basal anterior, Apical lateral, mid-anteroseptum.
  C. Basal anterolateral, apical anterior, mid-inferoseptum.
  D. Basal inferoseptum, apical inferior, mid-inferior.

46. Name the coronary artery that typically perfuses the segment indicated by the green arrow in **Figure 5.13**:
  A. LAD or LCX.
  B. LAD.
  C. LCX.
  D. RCA.

47. Match the following conditions with their corresponding strain patterns shown in **Figure 5.14**.
  A. Cardiac amyloidosis (3), pericardial constriction (4), stress cardiomyopathy ("takotsubo") (2), RCA infarction (1).
  B. Cardiac amyloidosis (1), pericardial constriction (2), stress cardiomyopathy ("takotsubo") (3), RCA infarction (4).
  C. Cardiac amyloidosis (2), pericardial constriction (3), stress cardiomyopathy ("takotsubo") (4), RCA infarction (1).
  D. Cardiac amyloidosis (4), pericardial constriction (3), stress cardiomyopathy ("takotsubo") (2), RCA infarction (1).
  E. Cardiac amyloidosis (1), pericardial constriction (4), stress cardiomyopathy ("takotsubo") (2), RCA infarction (3).

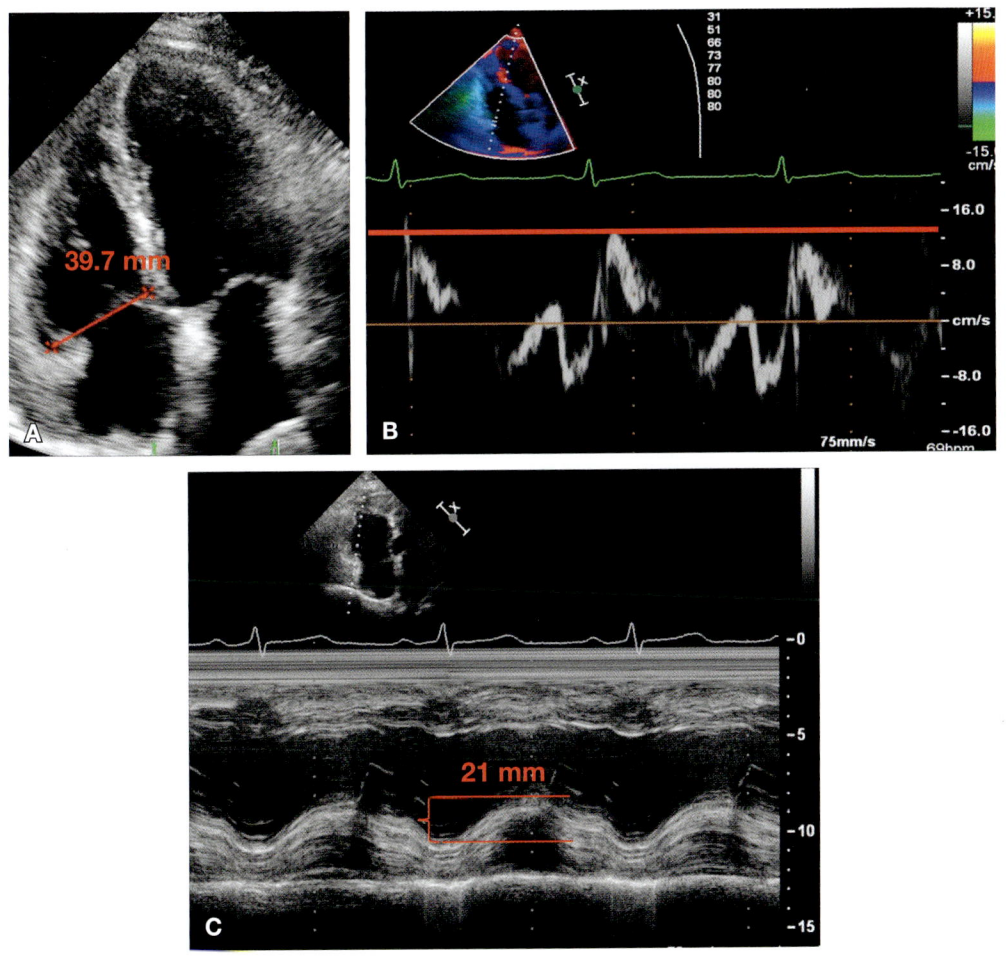

Figure 5.11

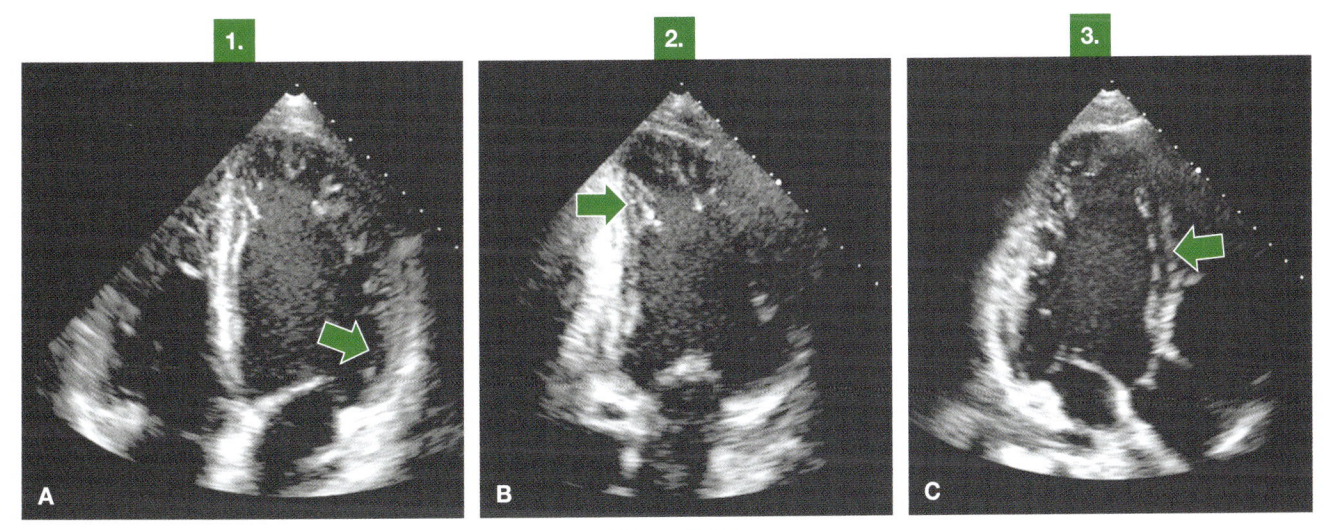

Figure 5.12

48. Which of the following strain patterns shown in **Figure 5.15** would be consistent with hypertrophic cardiomyopathy with fibrosis involving the septum?

A. Figure 5.15A.
B. Figure 5.15B.
C. Figure 5.15C.
D. Figure 5.15D.

90 / Clinical Echocardiography Review

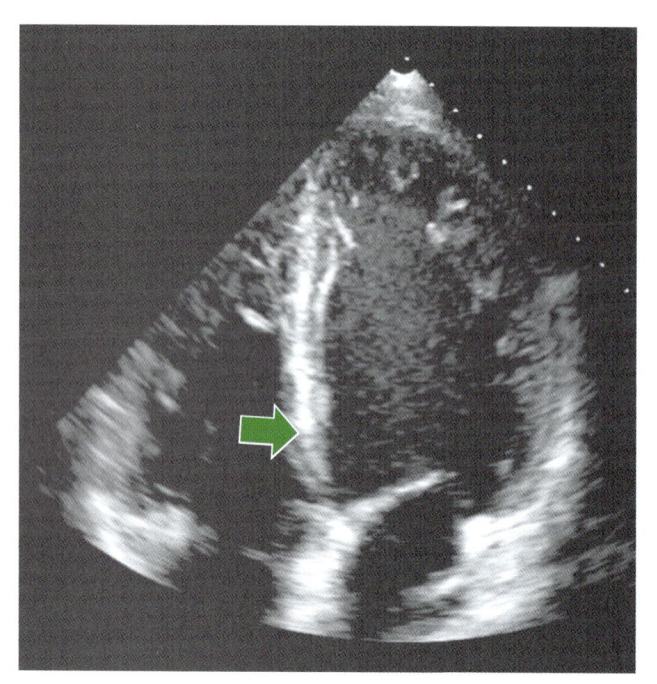

Figure 5.13

49. **Figure 5.16** shows left atrial volume and flow curves for patients of four different ages. Which of the following curves shown in **Figure 5.16** is likely to represent the oldest patient?
A. **Figure 5.16A**.
B. **Figure 5.16B**.
C. **Figure 5.16C**.
D. **Figure 5.16D**.

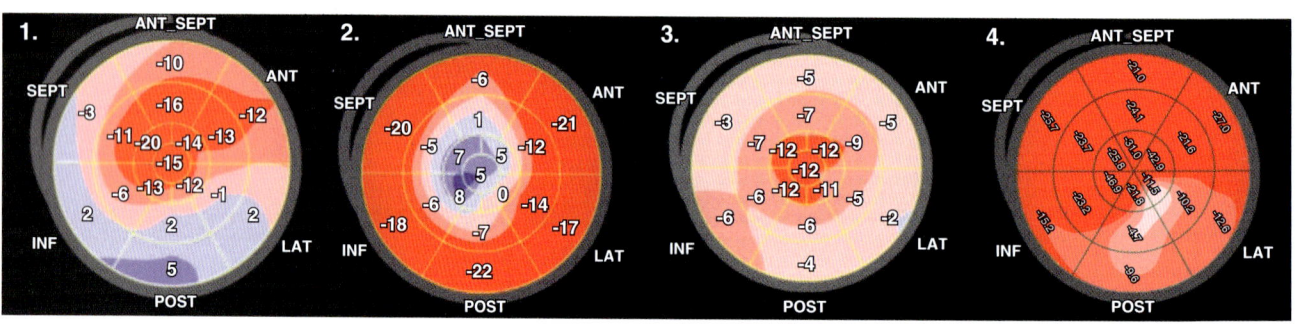

Figure 5.14

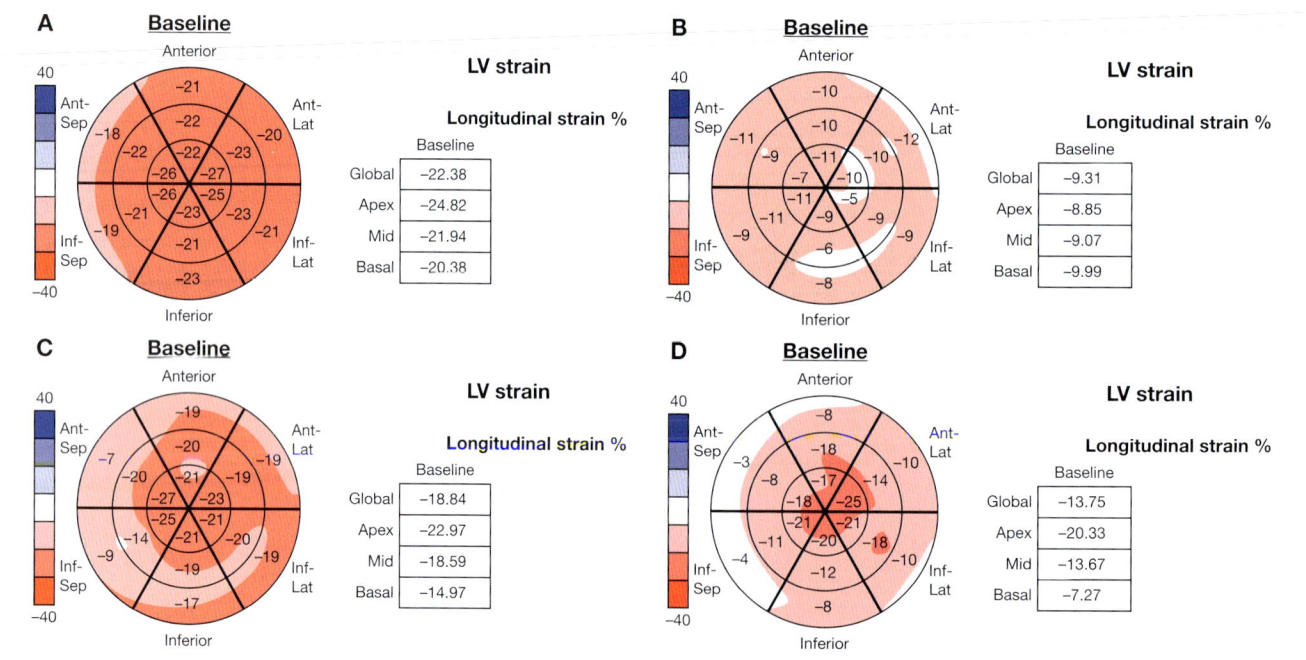

Figure 5.15

Chapter 5 Assessment of Chamber Quantification / 91

Figure 5.16

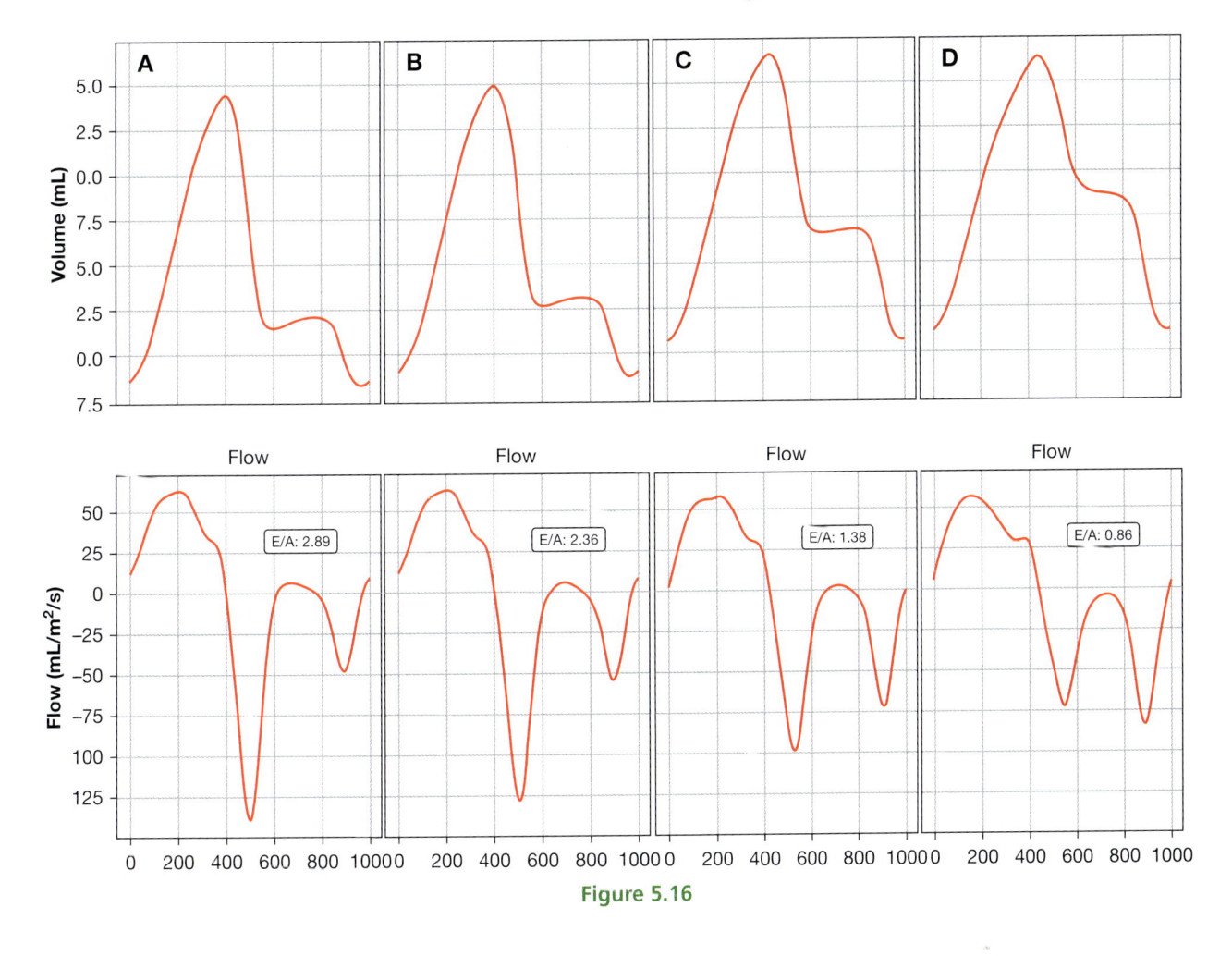

ANSWERS

1. **Answer: C.** The left atrium has three major physiologic roles that affect left ventricular filling and function. The left atrium acts as a (1) contractile pump that delivers 15% to 30% of the entire LV filling, (2) reservoir that collects pulmonary venous return during ventricular systole, and (3) as a conduit for the passage of stored blood from the left atrium to the left ventricle during early ventricular diastole.

2. **Answer: B.** Transthoracic echocardiography is the recommended approach to assess left atrial size. Left atrial size cannot be accurately assessed with TEE because often the entire left atrium cannot fit in the image sector. With respect to the cardiac cycle, the left atrium is largest at the end of left ventricular systole. Accordingly, left atrial size and volumes should be measured at this time in the cardiac cycle rather than during left ventricular diastole. In order to obtain accurate measurements, dedicated left atrial images that avoid foreshortening of the left atrium should be obtained. Measuring the left atrium from standard apical 2- and 4-chamber views acquired to measure left ventricular volumes is inadequate since the longitudinal axis of the left ventricle and left atrium frequently lie in different planes. The base of the left atrium should be at its largest size, indicating that the imaging plane passes through the maximal short-axis area. The left atrial length should also be maximized to ensure alignment along the true long axis of the left atrium. While the left atrial anteroposterior measurement obtained from the parasternal window is often reported because it is highly reproducible, it frequently underestimates left atrial size because this measurement assumes that when the left atrium enlarges, all its dimensions change in the same direction in a similar manner. This is often not the case during LA remodeling, which can be eccentric.

3. **Answer: D.** Left atrial volume is underestimated on two-dimensional echocardiography when compared to computed tomography and cardiac magnetic resonance imaging. This is due to differences in the manner in which the measurement is performed. With computed tomography and cardiac magnetic resonance, imaging slices are taken through the

left atrium. The left atrium is traced on each slice, and knowing the thickness of the slice, the volume of that slice is calculated. The slices are then all added up to obtain the total left atrial volume. With two-dimensional echocardiography, linear measurements of the left atrium from the 4- and 2-chamber views are obtained and then used in formulas to calculate left atrial volume. Left atrial volumes are powerful prognostic variables in disease states such as ischemic heart disease, atrial fibrillation, dilated cardiomyopathy, and diastolic heart failure. Left atrial volumes are also more powerful prognosticators than left atrial anteroposterior diameter. This is because the left atrial anteroposterior diameter frequently underestimates left atrial size because it does not account for eccentric remodeling. Single-plane apical 4-chamber indexed LA volumes are typically 1 to 2 mL/m^2 smaller than apical 2-chamber volumes.

4. **Answer: A.** Left atrial volume can be calculated from three linear measurements using an ellipsoid model. However, this method is not recommended as the relative inaccuracy of the utilized linear measurements limit this method. Instead, the disc summation method is recommended.

   The LA endocardial border is traced, and volume computed by adding the volume of a stack of cylinders of height h and area calculated by orthogonal minor and major transverse axes (D1 and D2) assuming an oval shape: LA volume = π/4 (h) Σ (D1)(D2) (**Figure 5.17A**). Alternatively, a biplane calculation could also be performed using the LA areas and lengths measured from both the apical 4- (A1) and 2-chamber (A2) views. LA volume is calculated as: LA volume = 8 (A1) (A2)/3π L, where L is the shortest distance between the midline of the plane of mitral annulus to the opposite superior side (roof) of the left atrium measured in the 4- and 2-chamber views (**Figure 5.17B**).

   While the area-length method still assumes an ellipsoidal LA shape, it has the advantage of reducing linear dimensions to a single measurement.

5. **Answer: B.** The American Society of Echocardiography guideline recommends that the body surface area–indexed left atrial volume be obtained from the biplane disc summation technique. This is because it is theoretically more accurate than the area-length method because it incorporates fewer geometric assumptions. The upper limit of normality for two-dimensional echocardiography-derived left atrial volume is 34 mL/m^2 for both genders. It is not recommended to report in routine clinical practice apical 4-/2-chamber linear measurements and nonindexed LA area and volume measurements. While left atrial size is dependent on gender, this difference is accounted for when adjusted for body surface area.

6. **Answer: A.** Standardized analysis programs and normative values for three-dimensional echocardiography–derived left atrial volume measurements from ultrasound-enhanced images are not available. Three-dimensional echocardiography–derived left atrial volume measurements are superior to two-dimensional echocardiography–derived measurements as three-dimensional left atrial volumes are typically larger than two-dimensional volumes, which results in better correlation with cardiac computed tomography– and cardiac magnetic resonance imaging–derived left atrial volume measurements. As well, compared to two-dimensional echocardiography, three-dimensional echocardiography–derived left atrial volume is more accurate

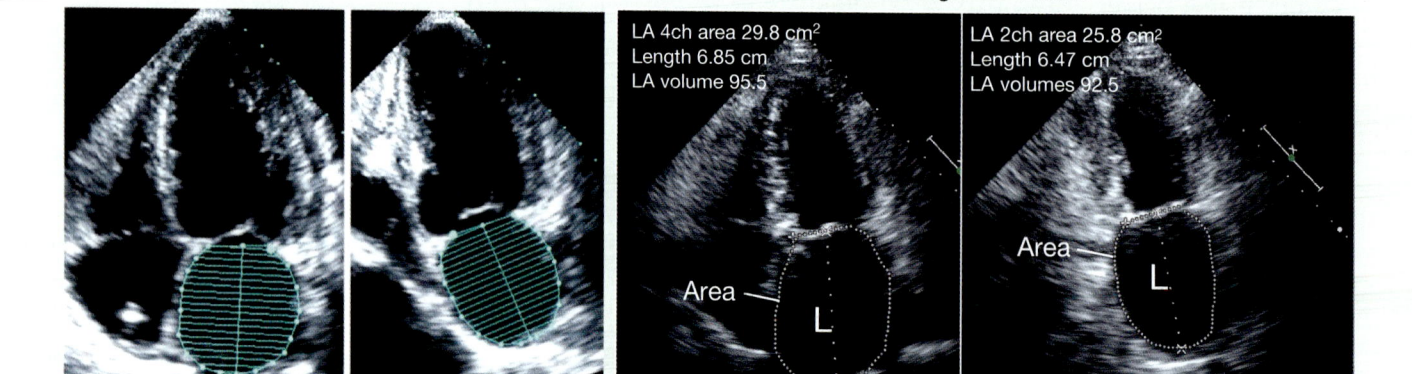

Figure 5.17. Illustration of recommended methods for calculating left atrial volume. **A:** Simpson biplane method in which left atrial (LA) volumes are traced in the 4- and 2-chamber views with volumes calculated by summation of volumes of disks. **B:** Area-length method in which areas rather than volumes are measured using the same standard views with volume calculated using the equation LA volume = (0.85 × area(4ch) × area(2ch))/(shortest atrial length). For either method, tracings should exclude the confluences of the pulmonary veins and the left atrial appendage. The atrio-ventricular interface should be represented by the mitral annulus plane and not by the tip of the mitral leaflets. (**A:** Reprinted from Lang RM, Badano LP, Mor-Avi V, et al. Recommendations for cardiac chamber quantification by echocardiography in adults: an update from the American Society of Echocardiography and the European Association of Cardiovascular Imaging. *J Am Soc Echocardiogr*. 2015;28(1):1-39.e14. Copyright © 2015 Elsevier. With permission.)

when compared to a gold standard and it has a superior prognostic ability.

7. **Answer: C.** Similar to left atrial volume measurements, right atrial volumes are more robust and accurate compared to linear measurements. As well, right atrial volumes are underestimated on two-dimensional echocardiography compared to three-dimensional echocardiography. Unlike left atrial volume measurements, there are no standard orthogonal views to use for apical biplane calculation. Thus, right atrial volume is derived from the apical 4-chamber view using the area-length or disc summation methods. Right atrial volumes are also smaller that left atrial volumes. Finally, right atrial volumes are different between males and females and indexing for body surface area does not account for this difference. The normal range for two-dimensional echocardiography–derived right atrial volumes is 25 ± 7 mL/m^2 in men and 20.5 ± 6 mL/m^2 in women.

8. **Answer: B.** Right atrial strain comprises three components: reservoir, conduit, and booster function (**Figure 5.18**).

    Reservoir function denotes atrial relaxation during atrial filling. Conduit function relates to the passive emptying of the right atrium during ventricular diastole. Finally, booster function represents active emptying, which occurs due to right atrial contraction. In patients with atrial fibrillation, there is loss of sinus rhythm with disorganized atrial activity, resulting in a loss of atrial contraction. Therefore, booster strain function will be absent in these patients.

9. **Answer: D.** Aortic root dilation is associated with aortic valve regurgitation. Aortic regurgitation in the presence of chest pain and a dilated aortic root should raise concerns regarding possible aortic root dissection. Hypertension is associated with enlargement of the distal aortic segments but not the sinuses of Valsalva. Aortic root diameter measurements at the sinuses of Valsalva level are closely related to BSA and age. Therefore, BSA should be used to predict normal aortic root diameter. Aortic root dilatation at the sinuses of Valsalva is defined as an aortic root diameter above the upper limit of the 95% confidence interval of the distribution in a large reference population and can be detected by plotting observed aortic root diameter versus BSA on published nomograms (**Figure 5.19**).

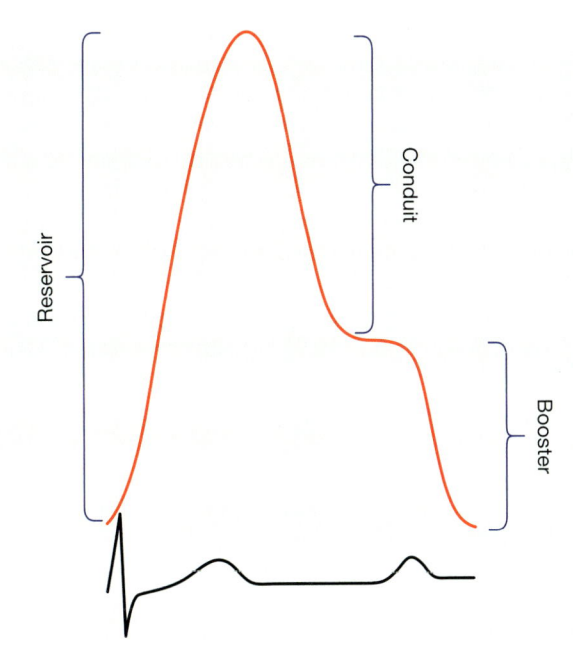

Figure 5.18. Left atrial strain curve (R wave to R wave). Left atrial strain comprises three phases: left atrial relaxation (**reservoir strain**), passive atrial emptying (**conduit strain**), and active atrial contraction (**booster strain**).

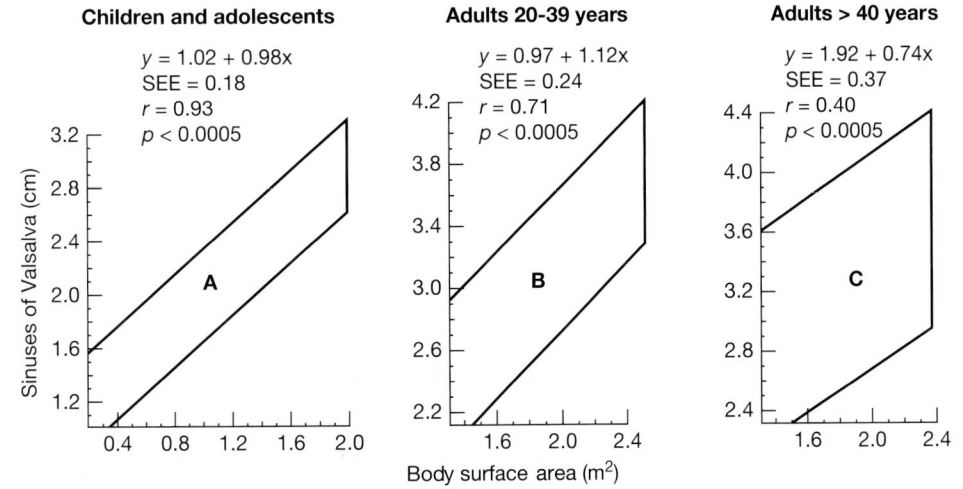

Figure 5.19. Normograms for aortic root dimensions at the level of the sinuses of Valsalva indexed for age and body surface area. (Reprinted from Lang RM, Badano LP, Mor-Avi V, et al. Recommendations for cardiac chamber quantification by echocardiography in adults: an update from the American Society of Echocardiography and the European Association of Cardiovascular Imaging. *J Am Soc Echocardiogr.* 2015;28(1):1-39.e14. Figure 13. Copyright © 2015 Elsevier. With permission.)

10. **Answer: E.** Two-dimensional echocardiography derived aortic diameter measurements are preferable to M-mode measurements, as cardiac motion may result in changes in the position of the M-mode cursor relative to the maximum diameter of the sinuses of Valsalva. This translational motion may result in systematic underestimation (by approximately 2 mm) of the aortic diameter by M-mode in comparison with 2D measurements. While the American Society of Echocardiography/European Association of Cardiovascular Imaging recommends inner edge–to inner edge aortic root measurements to be consistent with other imaging modalities such as cardiac magnetic imaging and computed tomography, previously established echocardiographic normative data were established using leading edge–to–leading edge measurements. The leading edge method results in measurements that are larger on average by about 2 mm compared to the inner edge measurement method. In tricuspid aortic valves, the closure line of the cusps is in the center of the aortic root lumen, and the closed leaflets are seen on the aortic side of a line connecting the hinge points of the two visualized leaflets. An asymmetric closure line, where the tips of the closed leaflets are closer to one of the hinge points, is an indication that the cross section is not encompassing the largest root diameter. Transesophageal echocardiography–derived measurements are typically larger than transthoracic measurements.

11. **Answer: C.** The aortic annular diameter is measured in the parasternal long-axis view, which is not the same plane containing the long-axis of the left ventricle. Calcium is usually considered part of the lumen for the aortic annular diameter measurements and the presence of calcium can affect measurement accuracy. The aortic annular diameter measured in the parasternal long-axis view is typically between the noncoronary cusp and the right coronary cusp. Due to the oval shape of the aortic annulus, 2D-derived linear measurements may systematically underestimate aortic annulus size compared to 3D methods, which does not rely on geometric assumptions.

12. **Answer: A.** Measurement of the aortic annulus should be performed during mid-systole, when the aortic annulus is largest. All other aortic root dimensions (sinus of Valsalva, sinotubular junction ascending aorta) should be performed at end-diastole. No aortic measurements are recommended to be performed during isovolumetric relaxation or contraction.

13. **Answer: C.** Assessment of inferior vena cava size is best performed from the subcostal window and provides valuable information regarding right atrial pressure. However, dilation of the inferior vena cava in athletes is not an indication of elevated right atrial pressures. Studies have demonstrated that trained athletes can have a dilated inferior vena cava with normal collapsibility. Inferior vena cava diameters in mechanically ventilated patients are not reliable in the estimation of right atrial pressure as they may reflect the ventilator settings. An inferior vena cava that measures <1.2 cm with spontaneous collapse is often seen in the presence of intravascular volume depletion.

14. **Answer: D.** In a mechanically ventilated patient, a dilated inferior vena cava (IVC) does not always indicate a high right atrial pressure. As well, an IVC <1.2 cm has a specificity of 100% for a right atrial pressure <10 mm Hg, but sensitivity is not 100% but much lower. IVC diameters have a better correlation with right atrial pressure when measured at end-expiration and end-diastole using M-mode echocardiography.

15. **Answer: E.** Pulmonary artery pressure can be estimated from tricuspid regurgitation (TR) velocity using the following formula:

Systolic pulmonary artery pressure = $4 \times TR^2$ + right atrial pressure,

where right atrial pressure is estimated from the assessment of inferior vena cava diameter (see also **Table 5.1**).

Table 5.1. Estimation of Right Atrial (RA) Pressure From Inferior Vena Cava (IVC) Diameter

IVC Diameter (cm)	IVC Collapsibility	Estimated RA Pressure
<2.1	>50%	3 mm Hg
<2.1	<50%	8 mm Hg
>2.1	>50%	8 mm Hg
>2.1	<50%	15 mm Hg

16. **Answer: E.** The right ventricle is assessed visually integrating multiple views. However, unlike the left ventricle, there are no orthogonal views that allow measurement of a biplane Simpson ejection fraction. This is due to the crescentic shape of the right ventricle (**Figure 5.20**).

Three-dimensional echocardiography allows a true volumetric assessment of the right ventricle, but its use in clinical practice has been limited by lack of integration of three-dimensional echocardiography into clinical practice and the need for off-line analysis and sonographer training. The American Society of Echocardiography guideline recommends that right ventricular function be assessed by at least one or a combination of the following: fractional area change (FAC), tissue Doppler imaging–derived tricuspid lateral annular systolic velocity wave (S′), tricuspid annular plane systolic excursion (TAPSE), and RV index of myocardial performance (RIMP).

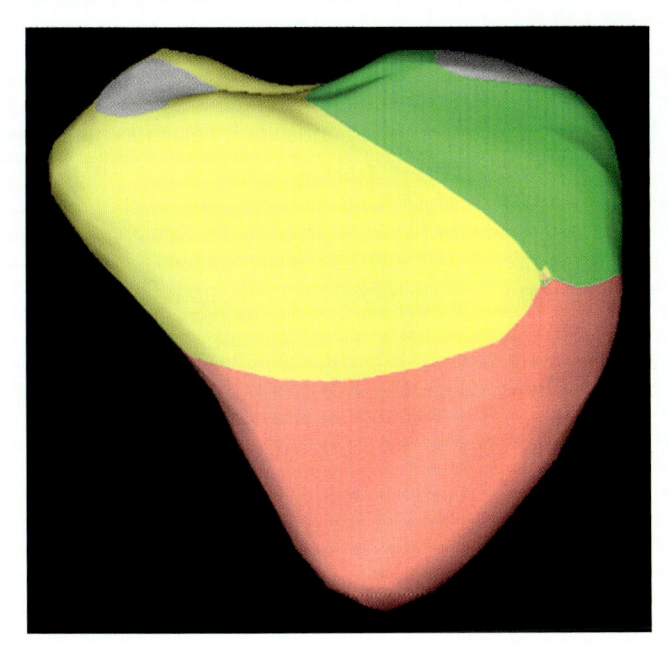

Figure 5.20. Three-dimensional structure of the right ventricle. The right ventricle is crescentic in shape with three distinct regions: an inlet (yellow), body (pink), and outlet (green).

Table 5.2. Abnormal Right Ventricular Function Cutoff Values

Parameter	Abnormal Cutoff
Right ventricular ejection fraction (RVEF)	<45%
Right ventricular fractional area change (RV FAC)	<35%
Tricuspid annular plane systolic excursion (TAPSE)	<17 mm
Tissue Doppler–derived tricuspid lateral annular systolic velocity (S')	<9.5 cm/s
Right ventricular strain	>−20%
Right ventricular index of myocardial performance (RIMP) by pulsed-wave Doppler	>0.43
Right ventricular index of myocardial performance (RIMP) by tissue Doppler imaging	>0.54

Derived from Lang RM, Badano LP, Mor-Avi V, et al. Recommendations for cardiac chamber quantification by echocardiography in adults: an update from the American Society of Echocardiography and the European Association of Cardiovascular Imaging. *J Am Soc Echocardiogr.* 2015;28(1):1-39.e14.

17. **Answer: C.** The proposed right ventricular reference range values in the American Society of Echocardiography guidelines are not indexed to gender, BSA, or height, despite some data suggesting the advantages of indexing. Thus, it is possible that patients at the extreme of height or body surface area may be misclassified as having values outside the reference ranges. This also includes patients with congenital heart disease and endurance athletes where specific reference values are nonexistent. Given these circumstances, physicians should interpret measured values within the context of the clinical scenario when comparing to published reference values. In contrast, right ventricular dimensions are not known to differ in mechanically ventilated patients compared to the general population; therefore, the use of standard, non-indexed values is reasonable.

18. **Answer: D.** Right ventricular ejection fraction is slightly higher in women than in men. This is because they have smaller RV chamber volumes. Thus, when interpreting right ventricular ejection fractions, physicians should consider using gender-specific cutoffs (**Table 5.2**).

    Overall, normal right ventricular ejection fraction is lower than left ventricular ejection fraction. However, because the right ventricular end-diastolic volume is greater than left ventricular end-diastolic volume, both right and left ventricular stroke volumes are similar. For general reference, on two-dimensional echocardiography, a right ventricular end-diastolic volume of 87 mL/m^2 in males and 74 mL/m^2 for females and right ventricular end-systolic volume of 44 mL/m^2 for males and 36 mL/m^2 for females should be used as the upper limits of the corresponding normal ranges.

19. **Answer: D.** A three-dimensional echocardiography–derived right ventricular ejection fraction <45% should be considered abnormal although some laboratories will use age- and gender-specific cutoffs. Three-dimensional echocardiography–derived right ventricular ejection fraction is more accurate and reliable compared to two-dimensional measurements because it accounts for the entire change in the right ventricle rather than a single plane. As well, it is more reliable in patients, such as those imaged postcardiac surgery, where two-dimensional methods (ie, TAPSE, S') are no longer reliable. Three-dimensional echocardiography–derived right ventricular ejection fraction has been extensively validated against cardiac magnetic resonance imaging. In terms of performing the measurement, it is recommended that a volumetric semi-automated border detection approach be used rather than manual tracings. Finally, to ensure that end-systolic frame is not missed, the volume rate of the three-dimensional echocardiographic dataset for analysis should have an acquisition rate of at least 20 volumes per second.

20. **Answer: C.** There are several unique aspects which distinguish the right (RV) from the left ventricle (LV). Due to the lower resistance of the pulmonary vasculature, the right ventricle operates as a low afterload chamber; therefore, **Answer C** is false. The right

ventricle is a thin-walled structure that affords it a high degree of compliance, making **Answer B** true. This low afterload state results in the RV using only 25% of the stroke work of the LV; **Answer E** is therefore true. Unlike the LV which is bullet-shaped, the RV has a complex, crescentic shape; therefore, **Answer A** is true. As the pulmonary and systemic circulation occur in series, LV and RV stroke volumes must be equivalent in the absence of valvular regurgitation or shunt; **Answer D** is therefore true.

21. **Answer: C.** Right ventricular fractional areal change <35% indicates systolic dysfunction. This measurement must be performed on an image that includes the entire right ventricle during systole and diastole in the apical 4-chamber view. As well, it should be measured including the trabeculae in the right ventricular cavity. Right ventricular index of myocardial performance (RIMP) is calculated using the formula: RIMP = (isovolumic contraction time + isovolumic relaxation time)/right ventricular ejection time or RIMP= (tricuspid valve closure-to-opening time − right ventricular ejection time)/right ventricular ejection time. The isovolumic contraction time, the isovolumic relaxation time, and ejection time intervals should be measured from the same heartbeat using either pulsed-wave spectral Doppler or tissue Doppler imaging velocity of the lateral tricuspid annulus (**Figure 5.21**).

    It must be noted that RIMP can be falsely low in conditions associated with elevated right atrial pressures, which will shorten the IVRT. A RIMP >0.43 by PW Doppler and >0.54 by TDI indicate RV dysfunction. Tricuspid annular plane systolic excursion (TAPSE) is measured by M-mode with the cursor aligned in the direction of the tricuspid lateral annulus. Although this index predominantly reflects RV longitudinal function, it has good correlation with parameters estimating global RV systolic function, such radionuclide RV ejection fraction and two-dimensional echocardiography–derived RV fractional area change and ejection fraction. Care should be taken when relying on TAPSE, as the measurements may over- or underestimate RV function due to overall heart motion. While there may be minor variations in TAPSE values according to gender and body surface area, overall a TAPSE < 17 mm is suggestive of right ventricular systolic dysfunction. TDI-derived tricuspid lateral annular systolic velocity (S′) wave should be measured on an image where the basal segment and the annulus are aligned with the Doppler cursor to avoid velocity underestimation. An S′ velocity <9.5 cm/s indicates RV systolic dysfunction.

22. **Answer: B.** Although the right ventricle may be visualized in many transthoracic views, the American Society of Echocardiography recommends that right ventricular measurements be performed in the right ventricular–focused apical 4-chamber view (**Answer B**). This view aligns the probe parallel with the longitudinal axis of the right ventricle, minimizing the risk of underestimation of longitudinal RV functional parameters such as tricuspid annular plane systolic excursion (TAPSE) or Doppler S′. The standard apical 4-chamber (**Answer A**) and modified apical 4-chamber view (**Answer C**) may result in over- or underestimation of right ventricular function. The modified apical 3-chamber view (**Answer D**) is not a recommended view as it is a view that does not exist in the literature (see also Answer 5.40, **Figure 5.23**.).

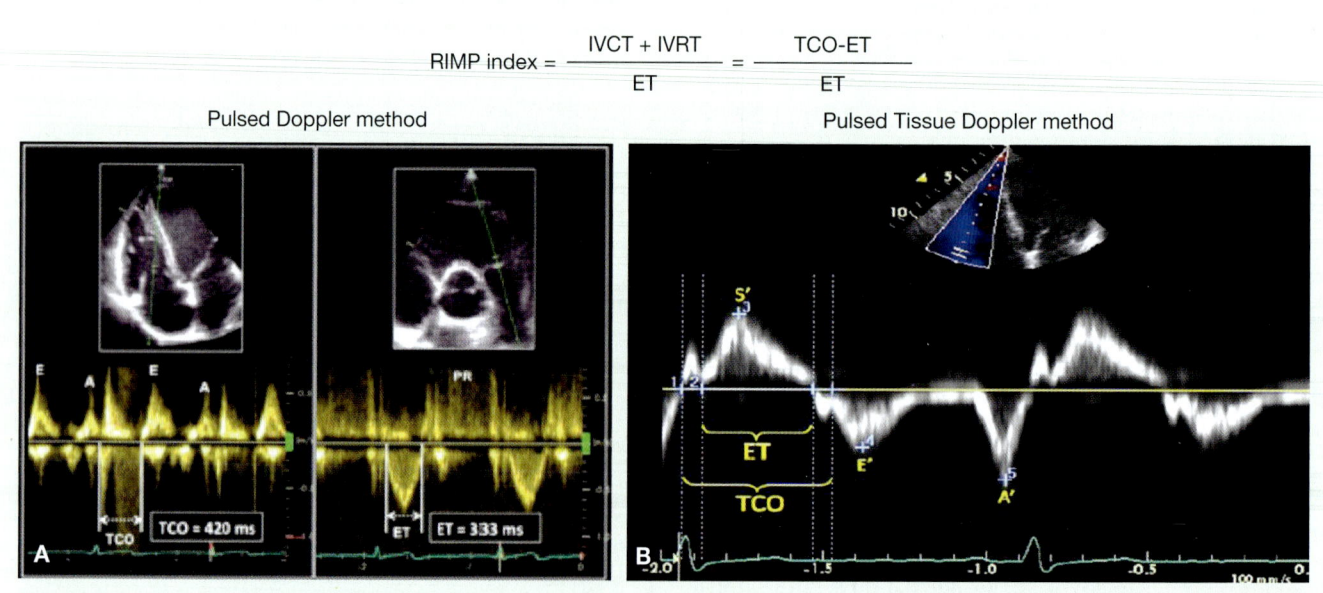

$$\text{RIMP index} = \frac{\text{IVCT} + \text{IVRT}}{\text{ET}} = \frac{\text{TCO-ET}}{\text{ET}}$$

Pulsed Doppler method | Pulsed Tissue Doppler method

Figure 5.21. Right ventricular index of myocardial performance (RIMP). The calculation is performed by adding isovolumic contraction time (IVCT) with isovolumic relaxation time (IVRT) and dividing that total by right ventricular ejection time (ET). Alternatively, subtracting the right ventricular ejection time from tricuspid valve closure-to-opening time (TCO) and dividing that result by the right ventricular ejection time can calculate it. It can be measured using pulsed-wave spectral Doppler **(A)** with a normal cutoff of <0.4 or pulsed tissue Doppler **(B)** with a normal cutoff of <0.55.

23. **Answer: B.** Multiple methods are currently employed to assess right ventricular systolic function. RV TAPSE and S' assess the extent and velocity of tricuspid annular longitudinal excursion during systole, respectively. Although extensively validated, these markers may be less accurate in certain clinical scenarios, such as following sternotomy; in this setting, postoperative changes may result in annular tethering, leading to underestimation of RV function with RV TAPSE and S'. Therefore, **Answer A** is incorrect. As RV TAPSE and S' are 1-dimensional measurements, it is highly dependent on the angle of image acquisition. Care must be taken to align the probe parallel to the direction of tricuspid annular motion; therefore, **Answer C** is incorrect. RV fractional area change relies on changes in RV area in the RV-focused apical 4-chamber view as a surrogate for ejection fraction; similar to 2D volumetric assessment of the LV, RV FAC is prone to error related to image foreshortening. Therefore, **Answer D** is incorrect. Conversely, the assessment of RV systolic function using 3D echocardiography is based on acquisition of the entire 3D RV volume without the need for geometric assumptions or risk of foreshortening; previous studies have shown that RVEF derived from 3D echocardiography more accurately predicts CMR-derived RVEF compared to RV TAPSE, S', and fractional area change.

24. **Answer: E.** The ASE recommends that measurements of RV wall thickness be made below the tricuspid annulus in end diastole. This is typically best obtained from the subcostal view due to the close proximity of the ultrasound probe to the right ventricular free wall. Additionally, the subcostal view is the window in which the right ventricular free wall is oriented most perpendicular to the ultrasound probe. Because axial spatial resolution is substantially better than lateral resolution, measurements of RV wall thickness are more accurate and reproducible in this view. Note that if the subcostal view is unavailable, the right ventricular outflow tract wall thickness in the parasternal long-axis view is considered an acceptable alternative. An RV wall thickness >5 mm is considered abnormal and representative of RV hypertrophy.

25. **Answer: B.** LV volumes may be assessed using either 2D or 3D echocardiography. 2D volumetric assessment rely on the calculation of volumes from the apical 2- and 4-chamber view via the Simpson method. This method relies on the geometric assumption of the heart as a prolate ellipsoid structure. In contrast, 3D echocardiography involves the acquisition of a whole 3D cardiac volume from which endocardial contours can be traced without the need for geometric assumptions. Therefore, **Answer B** is correct. Although 2D geometric assumptions are frequently true, this may not apply in certain cardiac conditions such as regional wall motion abnormalities; therefore, **Answer C** is incorrect. Additionally, 2D volumetric assessment is prone to apical foreshortening, which results in underestimation—not overestimation—of LV volumes; therefore, **Answer A** is incorrect. Both the 2D and 3D assessments of ventricular volumes are highly dependent on image quality. The presence of suboptimal image quality will therefore similarly affect 3D echocardiography, making **Answer D** incorrect.

26. **Answer: B.** Left ventricular volume calculations derived from linear measurements are obsolete and should not be performed. This is because they assume that the left ventricle has a fixed geometric LV shape such as a prolate ellipsoid, which does not apply to patients with cardiac pathology. Thus, Teichholz and Quinones methods for calculating left ventricular volumes are no longer recommended by the American Society of Echocardiography for clinical use. Left ventricular volumes can be measured using two- or three-dimensional echocardiography. On two-dimensional echocardiography, the apical 2- and 4-chamber views should be used for measurements. On three-dimensional echocardiography, either a biplane or a volumetric measurement can be obtained. Contrast agents are indicated to improve endocardial definition when two or more contiguous segments are not well visualized. Measurements obtained with contrast administration result in larger volumes, which are closer to those obtained with cardiac magnetic resonance imaging.

27. **Answer: D.** When acoustic windows are poor on two-dimensional echocardiography, three-dimensional echocardiography will not improve this situation and provide a more accurate measurement. Three-dimensional echocardiographic volume measurements are superior to two-dimensional echocardiographic measurements as the risk of acquiring foreshortened views is decreased since the entire left ventricle is included in the three-dimensional dataset. Also, three-dimensional echocardiography volumetric measurements avoid the geometric assumptions required for biplane calculation on two-dimensional echocardiography. Three-dimensional echocardiography also better accounts for regional abnormalities, which may not be evident in the 2- or 4-chamber view used for the biplane calculation on two-dimensional echocardiography. Overall, if the institution has expertise, the American Society of Echocardiography recommends that three-dimensional volumetric measurements be performed over two-dimensional ones. For two-dimensional echocardiography, the biplane disc summation method should be used and the upper normal limit of left ventricular end-diastolic volume is 74 mL/m^2 for men and 61 mL/m^2 for women. For two-dimensional echocardiographic left ventricular end-systolic volume, it is 31 mL/m^2 for men and 24 mL/m^2 for women. For three-dimensional echocardiography, left ventricular volumes are larger and the upper limits of normal for end-diastole are 79 mL/m^2 for men and 71 mL/m^2 for women.

For three-dimensional echocardiographic measurements of left ventricular end-systolic volume, it is 32 mL/m² for men and 28 mL/m² for women.

28. **Answer: A.** Fractional shortening can be derived from two-dimensional echocardiography–guided M-mode or two-dimensional echocardiographic linear measurements. It is reliable when there are no regional wall motion abnormalities whether these are secondary to conduction abnormalities or coronary disease. The biplane method of discs is also known as the modified Simpson rule and is the currently recommended two-dimensional echocardiographic method for assessing left ventricular ejection fraction. Left ventricular ejection fraction does not differ substantially by gender, age, or body surface area. Global longitudinal strain (GLS) is the most commonly used strain-based measure of left ventricular global systolic function. It is determined using speckle tracking, although tissue Doppler imaging methods may also be used. In two-dimensional echocardiography, peak global longitudinal strain describes the relative length change of the left ventricular myocardium between end-diastole and end-systole: GLS = (MLs – MLd)/MLd, where ML stands for myocardial length at end-diastole (MLd) and end-systole (MLs). This formula results in a global longitudinal strain number that is negative. Thus, the more negative the number, the more normal the strain and the less negative the number, the more abnormal left ventricular function. Overall, a GLS > –18% is considered abnormal, although normal values may vary between measurement packages of different vendors at this time.

29. **Answer: E.** In the 2015 ASE guidelines, the presence of aneurysm is no longer assigned with a separate wall motion score. This is because it is a morphologic entity with a wall motion abnormality that is already described by the other scores. It is a region of focal dilation and thinning secondary to remodeling that is associated with akinetic or dyskinetic myocardial function. The scoring system includes: (1) normal or hyperkinetic, (2) hypokinetic (reduced thickening), (3) akinetic (absent or negligible thickening), and (4) dyskinetic (systolic thinning or stretching).

30. **Answer: D.** Left ventricular mass is an important risk factor for and a strong predictor of cardiovascular events. It can be calculated from M-mode and two- and three-dimensional echocardiographic images acquired at end-diastole. M-mode and two-dimensional echocardiography–derived linear measurements of left ventricular diastolic diameter and wall thickness rely on geometric formulas to calculate the volume of left ventricular myocardium. With two-dimensional echocardiography, either the area-length or truncated ellipsoid techniques are used. In contrast, three-dimensional echocardiography measures left ventricular mass directly. Regardless if M-mode or two- or three-dimensional echocardiography is used, all methods then convert the volume to mass by multiplying the volume of myocardium by the myocardial density (approximately 1.05 g/mL). It must be noted that the left ventricle must be normally shaped for both the M-mode and two-dimensional echocardiography formulas to calculate LV mass reliably. Direct two-dimensional echocardiographic measurements of wall thickness may obtain smaller values than the blind M-mode, which is M-mode obtained without the guidance of the 2D image. If this occurs, then the LV mass calculated using that formula may not be directly comparable. Three-dimensional echocardiography is the only echocardiographic method that directly measures myocardial volume. The upper limits of normal from linear measurements are 95 g/m² in women and 115 g/m² in men. The upper limits of normal from two-dimensional echocardiographic measurements are 88 g/m² in women and 102 g/m² in men. Normal values from three-dimensional echocardiography have not yet been established.

31. **Answer: A.** Left ventricular hypertrophy is defined by the ASE guidelines by the presence of increased left ventricular mass relative to body surface area (BSA). Left ventricular hypertrophy is further categorized by the pattern of left ventricular remodeling based on relative wall thickness (RWT), which is defined as twice the posterior wall thickness divided by left ventricular end-diastolic diameter. This patient has elevation in both LV mass (119 g/m²) and relative wall thickness (0.55) and should be classified as having concentric hypertrophy. Answer C is therefore correct (see **Figure 5.22**).

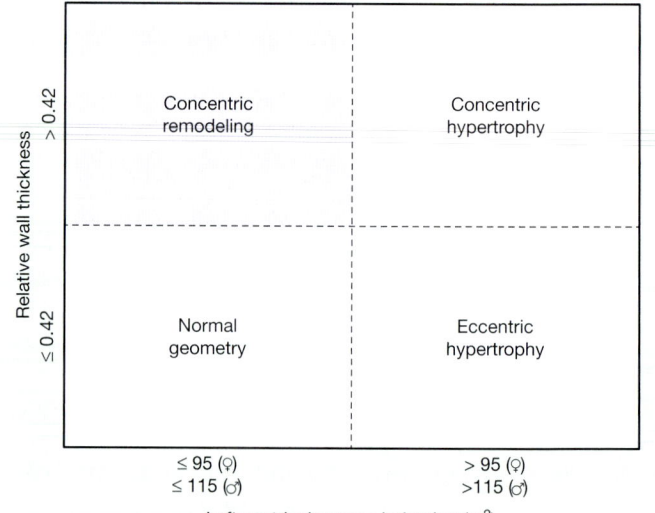

Figure 5.22. Diagram depicting recommended methods for describing left ventricular (LV) chamber hypertrophy patterns. Based on the relative wall thickness and indexed left ventricular mass, the LV may exhibit normal architecture, concentric remodeling, concentric hypertrophy, or eccentric hypertrophy. (Reprinted from Lang RM, Badano LP, Mor-Avi V, et al. Recommendations for cardiac chamber quantification by echocardiography in adults: an update from the American Society of Echocardiography and the European Association of Cardiovascular Imaging. *J Am Soc Echocardiogr*. 2015;28:1-39.e14. Figure 6. Copyright © 2015 Elsevier. With permission.)

Chapter 5 Assessment of Chamber Quantification / 99

32. **Answer: D.** 3D echocardiography relies on the acquisition of whole 3D ventricular volumes; this allows for quantification of the entire LV volume without geometric assumptions. Unlike 2D echocardiography, 3D techniques are not prone to measurement errors related to foreshortening and are therefore more accurate when compared to the gold standard of cardiac magnetic resonance (CMR); therefore, **Answer D** is correct. Linear measurements rely on 2D measurements made in the parasternal long axis, which are highly prone to error due to geometric assumptions; therefore, **Answer A** is incorrect. The use of microbubble contrast agents does improve endocardial delineation. However, this results in increased volumes compared to noncontrast techniques; therefore, **Answer B** is incorrect. Although 3D echocardiography provides the most robust echocardiographic assessment of LV volumes, 3D values systematically underestimate those derived from CMR due to difficulty in differentiating trabeculation from endocardium. Thus, **Answer D** is correct.

33. **Answer: A.** When tracing the borders of the left atrium, the confluences of the pulmonary veins and LA appendage should be excluded. The atrio-ventricular interface should be represented by the mitral annulus plane and not by the tip of the mitral leaflets (see **Answer 5-4, Figure 5.17A**). The left atrium should be traced when it is largest, which is usually during left ventricular end-systole. **Figure 5.1B** is incorrect because it includes part of the ostium of the left upper pulmonary vein. **Figure 5.1C** is incorrect because it includes part of the right lower pulmonary vein. **Figure 5.1D** is incorrect because it is measured during the interval of the cardiac cycle when the left atrium is smallest.

34. **Answer: D.** Left atrial volumes should be measured from the 2- and 4-chamber views with the left atrium optimized at its largest during left ventricular end-systole. The borders should exclude the confluences of the pulmonary veins and the left atrial appendage. The atrio-ventricular interface should be represented by the mitral annulus plane and not by the tip of the mitral leaflets (see **Answer 5-4, Figure 5.17A**). **Figure 5.2A** is incorrect because the left atrium is not optimized to its largest size in both the 2- and 4-chamber views. **Figure 5.2B** is incorrect because a 5-chamber view is used. **Figure 5.2C** is incorrect because a 3-chamber view is used.

35. **Answer: A.** The semilunar attachments of the aortic cusps have the shape of a 3-pronged coronet. The virtual ring (aortic annulus) joins the nadirs (dots) of all three cusps, thereby encircling the cross-sectional area (light gray) of the annulus at the level of the inlet from the left ventricular outflow tract into the aortic root. The upper ring is a true ring of the sinotubular junction. The node of Arantius is the slight thickening at the midpoint of the free edge of the aortic valve cusps.

36. **Answer: B.** The American Society of Echocardiography (ASE) recommends that measurements of the left ventricular outflow tract (LVOT) be made 3 to 10 mm from the valve plane in mid-systole in the parasternal long-axis view, tracing from inner edge to inner edge. This measurement should be made at approximately the same distance from the valve plane as the LVOT pulsed-wave Doppler performed on apical views to provide the most accurate echocardiographic estimation of LV stroke volume. This accurate estimation of LVOT diameter is critical to the assessment of aortic valve area via the continuity equation. Errors in LVOT diameter are the most common source of error in performing the continuity equation and are magnified as the value is squared. Focal calcification of the LVOT—as is seen in this patient—represents a significant challenge, which is frequently encountered in the assessment of aortic stenosis. In these instances, LVOT measurements should again be made 3 to 10 mm from the valve plane, with care taken to exclude the calcium (**Answer B**). Inability to exclude calcification (**Answer A**) will result in erroneous underestimation of LVOT area. In answer choices C and D, the measurement is made too distant from the valve plane. In contrast, aortic annular measurements are made at the base of the valve leaflets. As with LVOT measurement, annular measurements should also be made in mid-systole from inner edge to inner edge. Although typically stroke volume is often estimated from LVOT measurements, it is acknowledged that some experts prefer annular measurements as they may be less error-prone.

37. **Answer: C.** Maximal inferior vena cava diameter should be measured 1 to 2 cm from the inferior vena cava–right atrial junction during expiration using the inferior vena cava long-axis view. Normal inferior vena cava diameter should be less than 2.1 cm. Inferior vena cava diameters may be dilated in ventilated patients, athletes, and patients with congenital heart disease.

38. **Answer: B.** A low estimated right atrial pressure of less 3 mm Hg in a spontaneously breathing patient who is not an athlete or has congenital heart disease is assumed when the inferior vena cava diameter is less than 2.1 cm and has more than 50% collapsibility with sniffing (**Table 5.1**). Patient A (in **Figure 5.6A**) has a normal inferior vena cava dimension at 1.75 cm, but the collapsibility is less than 50% and so has an estimated right atrial pressure of 8 mm Hg. Patient B (in **Figure 5.6B**) has a low estimated right atrial pressure. Their inferior vena cava diameter is 1.66 cm and collapsibility is greater than 50% at 70%. Patient C (in **Figure 5.6C**) has a dilated inferior vena cava at 2.32 cm with collapsibility of 57% and so has an estimated right atrial pressure of 8 mm Hg. Patient D (in **Figure 5.6D**) also has a dilated inferior vena cava

at 3.05 cm with collapsibility of 18% and so has an estimated right atrial pressure of 15 mm Hg.

39. **Answer: C.** As seen in **Figure 5.7A,B**, the inferior vena cava is 1.2 cm, which is within the normal range (<2.1 cm). It also collapses more than 50% with inspiration, indicating that right atrial pressure is normal and therefore estimated to be between 0 and 5 mm Hg. The tricuspid regurgitation velocity is 2.45 m/s (**Figure 5.7C**), which is also within normal limits (<2.8 m/s). Completing the formula: Systolic pulmonary artery pressure = 4 × TR^2 + right atrial pressure = 24 mm Hg+ (0-5 mm Hg) = 24 to 29 mm Hg. This patient does not have an elevated systolic pulmonary artery pressure.

40. **Answer: B.** The apical 4-chamber, right ventricle–focused apical 4-chamber and modified apical 4-chamber, left parasternal long- and short-axis, left parasternal RV inflow, and subcostal views are all recommended by the American Society of Echocardiography to adequately assess the right ventricle. The apical 5-chamber (**Answer B**) view is not a recommended view for assessing the right ventricle. For right ventricular measurements, the RV-focused apical 4-chamber view is the view that should be used (**Answer D**) and is obtained by adjusting the standard apical 4-chamber view slightly to center the right heart on the screen while ensuring that there is no foreshortening. This is achieved by tilting the transducer in the apical 4-chamber view cranially and anteriorly. This is different from the modified right ventricle view where the transducer is tilted laterally and anteriorly (**Answer C**), respectively (see **Figure 5.23**).

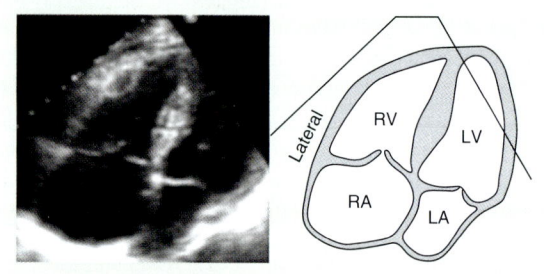

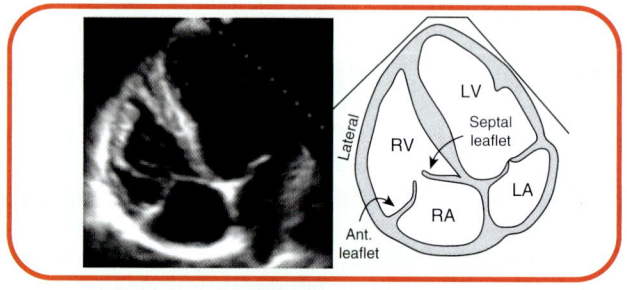

41. **Answer: D.** A variety of parameters are currently used in clinical practice to estimate right ventricular (RV) systolic function including RV tricuspid annular systolic excursion (TAPSE), RV S′, RV fractional area change, and RV free wall strain. Similar to global longitudinal strain, RV free wall strain is quantified using speckle tracking technology with impaired RV systolic function being defined as absolute free wall strain values less than 20%. On echocardiography, pulmonary pressures are estimated noninvasively using the tricuspid regurgitant velocity. This value is proportional to the pressure gradient between the right ventricle and right atrium during systole, which can be added to the estimated central venous pressure to estimate right ventricular systolic pressure (RVSP). TR velocity is markedly elevated in this patient, indicative of pulmonary hypertension. This patient also has impaired RV systolic function and pulmonary hypertension as estimated by RV free wall strain and TR gradient; therefore, Answer D is correct.

42. **Answer: C.** Right ventricular systolic pressure (RVSP) is estimated noninvasively using the tricuspid regurgitation (TR) velocity. This velocity is proportional to the pressure gradient between the right ventricle and right atrium during systole. This pressure gradient is estimated using the simplified Bernoulli equation (P = 4v^2), which in this patient is 4*3.77^2 = 57 mm Hg. This must then be added to the estimated right atrial pressure, which is assessed based on inferior vena cava (IVC) diameter and collapsibility with "sniff" as described in **Table 5.1**. This patient's IVC is dilated but collapsible, indicating an estimated right atrial pressure of 8. The RVSP is therefore 8 + 57 = 65 mm Hg (**Answer C**).

43. **Answer: C.** This patient has an abnormal right ventricular size and systolic function. From the two-dimensional apical 4-chamber view of the right ventricle (Figure A), the dimension of the right ventricle at the base measures 42 mm. This is larger than the normal cutoff of 41 mm at this level, indicating dilation. Alternatively, a dimension >35 mm at the midlevel in the right ventricular–focused view would also indicate right

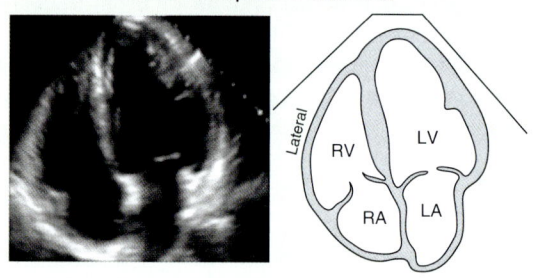

Figure 5.23. Figure depicting the recommended 2-dimensional views for visual assessment of the right ventricle. (Reprinted from Lang RM, Badano LP, Mor-Avi V, et al. Recommendations for cardiac chamber quantification by echocardiography in adults: an update from the American Society of Echocardiography and the European Association of Cardiovascular Imaging. *J Am Soc Echocardiogr*. 2015;28:1-39.e14. Figure 7A. Copyright © 2015 Elsevier. With permission.)

ventricular dilation. With respect to right ventricular function, from the tissue Doppler images of the lateral tricuspid annulus (Figure B), the tissue Doppler–derived tricuspid lateral annular systolic velocity or S' velocity is less than the normal cutoff of 9.5 cm/s (**Table 5.2**), indicating systolic dysfunction. As well, the M-mode image through the lateral tricuspid annulus or TAPSE (Figure C) is also <17 mm, which is consistent with the S' velocity, indicating right ventricular systolic dysfunction. Normal cutoff values for these and other measurements of right ventricular systolic dysfunction are provided in **Table 5.2**.

44. **Answer: A.** This patient has a normal right ventricular size and systolic function. From the two-dimensional apical 4-chamber view of the right ventricle (**Figure 5.11A**), the dimension of the right ventricle at the base measures 39.7 mm. This is smaller than the normal cutoff of 41 mm at this level, indicating normal size. Alternatively, a dimension <35 mm at the midlevel in the right ventricular–focused view would also indicate normal right ventricular size. With respect to right ventricular function, from the tissue Doppler image of the lateral tricuspid annulus (**Figure 5.11B**), the tissue Doppler–derived tricuspid lateral annular systolic velocity or S' velocity is greater than the normal cutoff of 9.5 cm/s (**Table 5.2**), indicating normal systolic function. As well, the M-mode image through the lateral tricuspid annulus or TAPSE (**Figure 5.11C**) is also >17 mm, which is consistent with the S' velocity, indicating normal right ventricular systolic function. Normal cutoff values for these and other measurements of right ventricular systolic dysfunction are provided in **Table 5.2**.

45. **Answer: A.** The standardization of wall segments is paramount to the accurate and reproducible assessment of regional wall motion. The standard method recommended by the ASE for wall segmentation is the 17-segment model. The basal and mid-segments are divided into six segments (anteroseptal, inferoseptal, inferior, inferolateral, anterolateral, anterior). The distal segments, being smaller in size, are divided into four segments (septal, inferior, lateral, anterior), while the apex comprises the final segment. With respect to apical views, the inferoseptum and anterolateral walls are best visualized in the apical 4-chamber view (**Figure 5.12A**). The anterior and inferior walls are best seen in the apical 2-chamber view (**Figure 5.12B**). Finally, the anteroseptal and inferolateral walls are seen in the 3-chamber view (**Figure 5.12C**). Accordingly, the arrowed segments in **Figure 5.12A-C** are the basal anterolateral, apical inferior, and the mid anteroseptal segments, respectively (**Answer A**) (see **Figure 5.24**).

46. **Answer: D.** In addition to the accurate reporting of regional wall motion abnormalities, it is important to localize the coronary artery territories, which are most likely to be affected by ischemia and/or infarction. The LAD territory typically comprises the anteroseptal, anterior, and apical segments (see **Figure 5.25**).

    The RCA typically comprises the inferior segment with or without the inferoseptal and inferolateral segments. The LCX is more variable and may supply areas of the anterolateral and/or inferolateral walls. The regional wall motion abnormality displayed in this question is the basal inferoseptal wall, which corresponds to the RCA territory (**Answer D**) (see **Figure 5.25**).

47. **Answer: A.** Certain patterns of global longitudinal strain (GLS)—as displayed using polar mapping—may be indicative of different diseases. Cardiac amyloidosis is characterized by diffusely reduced GLS with relative sparing of the cardiac apex ("cherry on top") as seen in **Answer Choice 3**. While other conditions can also demonstrate this pattern, typically the ratio of the apex to basal septal GLS is greater than 2.9. and the ratio of GLS to LVEF is greater than 4. Pericardial constriction results in tethering of the lateral portion of the left ventricle, resulting in reduced anterolateral and inferolateral GLS (**Answer Choice 4**). The classical form of stress cardiomyopathy ("takotsubo") results in hyperkinesis of the basal myocardium with akinesis of the distal and apical segments; this also occurs with respect to strain as seen in **Answer Choice 2**. Lastly, ischemia or infarction of the right coronary artery would result in impaired GLS in the inferoseptal and inferior segments corresponding to the typical territory supplied by this vessel (**Answer Choice 1**).

48. **Answer: C.** Panel A demonstrates normal longitudinal strain in all segments and so is normal. Panel B demonstrates a reduction in longitudinal strain in all segments, which would be consistent in a patient with a cardiomyopathy involving all segments. Panel C demonstrates reduced longitudinal strain in the septal segments and preserved strain in the remaining segments and so would be consistent in a patient with hypertrophic cardiomyopathy and fibrosis involving the septum. Panel D demonstrates relative apical sparing with a relative apical sparing ratio (RELAPS)—defined by the ratio of apical longitudinal strain divided by the sum of the basal and mid values—greater than one suggesting cardiac amyloidosis.

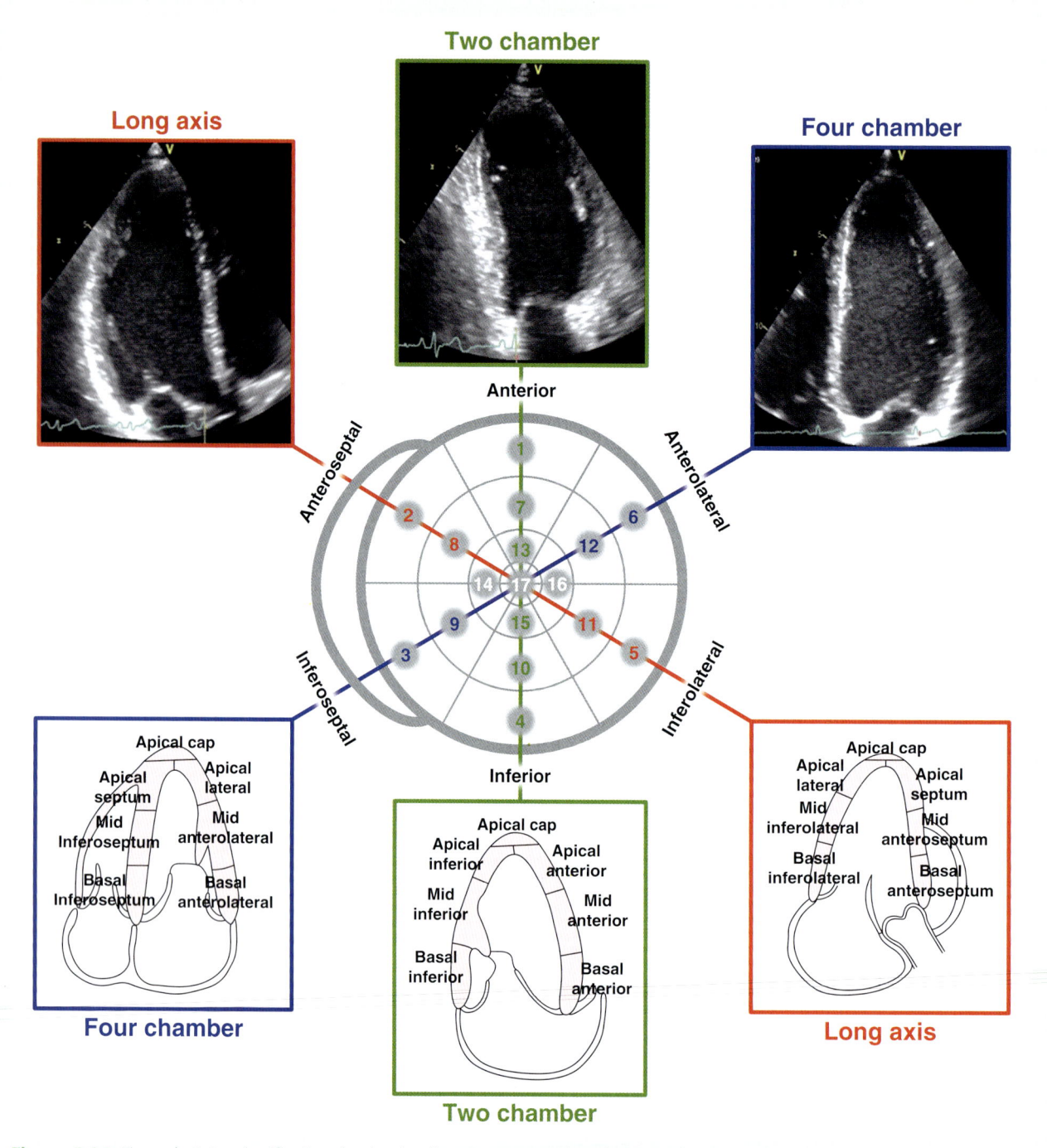

Figure 5.24. Figure depicting classification of regional wall motion segments based on the 17-segment model and the apical views in which these segments are best visualized. (Reprinted from Lang RM, Badano LP, Mor-Avi V, et al. Recommendations for cardiac chamber quantification by echocardiography in adults: an update from the American Society of Echocardiography and the European Association of Cardiovascular Imaging. *J Am Soc Echocardiogr*. 2015;28:1-39.e14. Figure 4. Copyright © 2015 Elsevier. With permission.)

49. **Answer: D.** There are changes in cardiac structure and compliance, which naturally occur because of the aging process. Increases in ventricular stiffness with age lead to decreased passive left atrial emptying in diastole. This results in a greater dependence on left atrial contraction for left ventricular filling. The patient listed in **Answer D** has the least passive atrial emptying and most atrial contractile emptying and is therefore likely to be the oldest.

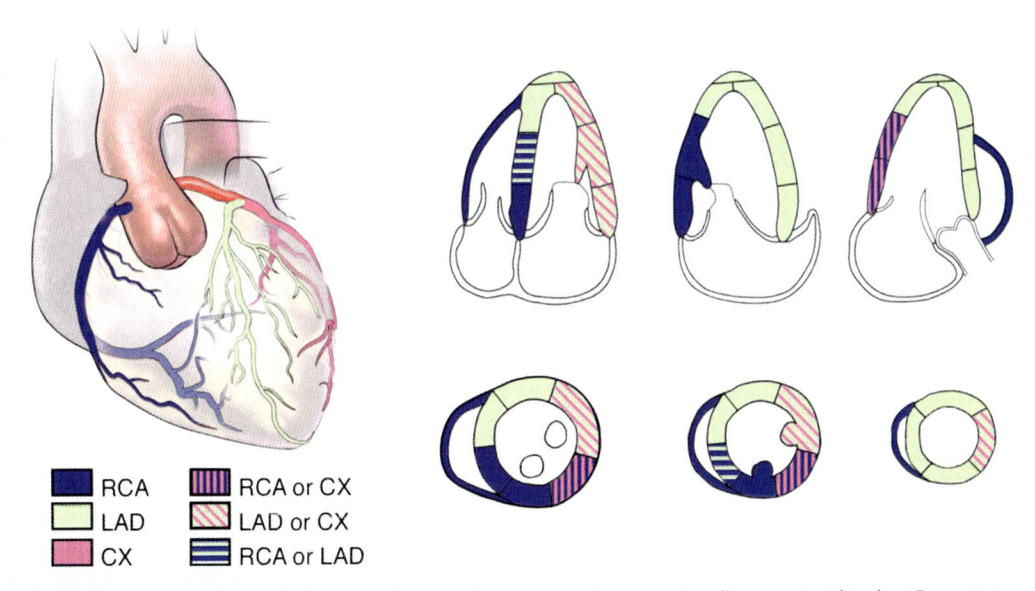

Figure 5.25. Figure displaying the coronary territories corresponding to each wall segment within the 17-segment model. CX, circumflex artery; LAD, left anterior descending artery; RCA, right coronary artery. (Reprinted from Lang RM, Badano LP, Mor-Avi V, et al. Recommendations for cardiac chamber quantification by echocardiography in adults: an update from the American Society of Echocardiography and the European Association of Cardiovascular Imaging. *J Am Soc Echocardiogr.* 2015;28:1-39.e14. Figure 5. Copyright © 2015 Elsevier. With permission.)

SUGGESTED READINGS

Farasat SM, Morrell CH, Scuteri A, et al. Do hypertensive individuals have enlarged aortic root diameters? Insights from studying the various subtypes of hypertension. *Am J Hypertens.* 2008;21(5):558-563.

Galie N, Humbert M, Vachiery JL, et al.. 2015 ESC/ERS guidelines for the diagnosis and treatment of pulmonary hypertension: the Joint Task Force for the Diagnosis and Treatment of pulmonary hypertension of the European Society of Cardiology (ESC) and the European Respiratory Society (ERS)—endorsed by—Association for European Paediatric and congenital Cardiology (AEPC), International Society for Heart and Lung Transplantation (ISHLT). *Eur Heart J.* 2016;37(1):67-119.

Lang RM, Badano LP, Mor-Avi V, et al. Recommendations for cardiac chamber quantification by echocardiography in adults: an update from the American Society of Echocardiography and the European Association of Cardiovascular Imaging. *J Am Soc Echocardiogr.* 2015;16(3):233-270.

Mitchell C, Rahko PS, Blauwet LA, et al. Guidelines for performing a comprehensive transthoracic echocardiographic examination in adults: Recommendations from the American Society of Echocardiography. *J Am Soc Echocardiogr.* 2019;32:1-64.

Pagourelias ED, Mirea O, Duchenne J, et al. Echo parameters for differential diagnosis in cardiac amyloidosis: a head-to-head comparison of deformation and nondeformation parameters. *Circ Cardiovasc Imaging.* 2017;10(3):e005588.

Palmieri V, Bella JN, Arnett DK, et al. Aortic root dilatation at sinuses of valsalva and aortic regurgitation in hypertensive and normotensive subjects: the Hypertension Genetic Epidemiology Network Study. *Hypertension.* 2001;37(5):1229-1235.

Singh A, Carvalho Singulane C, Miyoshi T, et al. Normal values of left atrial size and function and the impact of age: results of the World Alliance Societies of echocardiography study. *J Am Soc Echocardiogr.* 2022;35(2):154-164.e3.

CHAPTER 6

Three-Dimensional Echocardiography

Tiffany Dong and Rhonda Miyasaka

QUESTIONS

1. Which factors affect the quality of 3D reconstructions derived from 2D images?
   A. 2D image quality, motion artifact, and electrocardiogram (ECG) and respiratory gating.
   B. 2D image quality.
   C. Image density.
   D. ECG and respiratory gating.
   E. Image density, gain, persistence, and frame rate.

2. To achieve a higher volume rate (volumes per second or vps), the operator should make which of the following adjustment on the ultrasound system?
   A. Choose a multibeat acquisition.
   B. Decrease the sector size.
   C. Decrease elevation width.
   D. Decrease lateral size.
   E. All of the above.

3. Which of the following is a cause of stitch artifact (**Figure 6.1**)?
   A. Adjusting gain.
   B. Normal sinus rhythm.
   C. Normal respiration.
   D. Narrowing the sector angle.
   E. Zoom imaging.

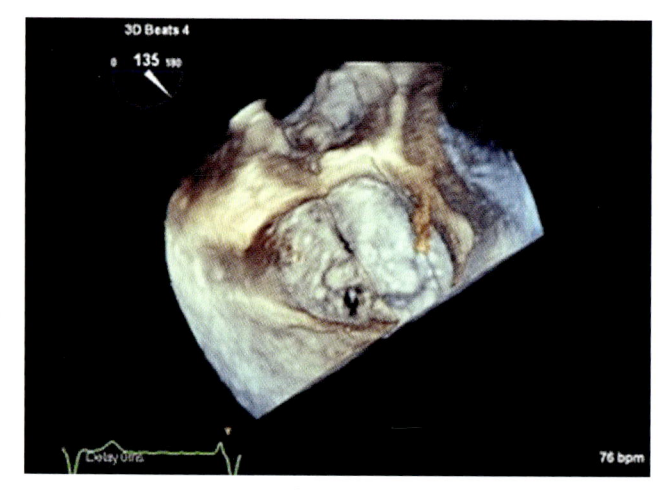

Figure 6.1

4. Which of the following statements is true regarding the accuracy and reproducibility of 2D echocardiography (2DE) versus 3D echocardiography (3DE) in regard to assessment of left ventricular (LV) volumes?
   A. 3DE has superior accuracy and reproducibility compared with 2DE.
   B. 2DE has better accuracy and reproducibility compared with 3DE.
   C. Both 2DE and 3DE have similar accuracy and reproducibility.
   D. Both 2DE and 3DE have similar accuracy but differ in reproducibility.
   E. All of the above are incorrect.

5. Left atrial volume reflects the long-term effects of high left atrial pressure and severity of diastolic dysfunction and is a predictor of mortality and outcome. Which quantitative method has the best test-retest variability?
   A. M-mode echocardiography.
   B. Prolate ellipsoid.
   C. Biplane Simpson.
   D. Area-length method.
   E. 3DE.

6. Which statement pertaining to 3D assessment of the right ventricle (RV) is correct?
   A. Quantitation of RV function by 3DE is an online program using method of discs.
   B. Quantitation of RV volumes is accurate and reproducible using method of discs.
   C. Quantitation of RV volumes is a widespread application since it is accurate and reproducible.
   D. Quantitation of RV volumes involves geometric modeling and mathematical equations easily performed offline.
   E. Quantitation of RV volumes is similar to LV assessment using a bullet-shaped geometric model.

7. Three-dimensional color Doppler imaging with current technology is best described as having:
   A. High temporal resolution but low spatial resolution.
   B. Low temporal resolution but high spatial resolution.
   C. Low temporal resolution and low spatial resolution.
   D. High temporal resolution and high spatial resolution.
   E. None of the above.

8. The mitral valve is correctly displayed from the "surgeon's view" in which panel? See **Figure 6.2**:
   A. Panel A.
   B. Panel B.
   C. Panel C.
   D. Panel D.
   E. None of the above.

CASE 1

*A 34-year-old man presents with shortness of breath and lower extremity edema. He has had fevers, rigors, and poor appetite for several weeks. He has methicillin-sensitive Staphylococcus aureus bacteremia and a history of drug abuse. On examination, he has poor dentition and he has a holosystolic murmur at the apex directed laterally. Transesophageal 2D echocardiogram (***Figure 6.3****, Panels A and B) shows the mitral valve in a 90° angle. Panel C is a transesophageal 3D left atrial orientation of the mitral valve.*

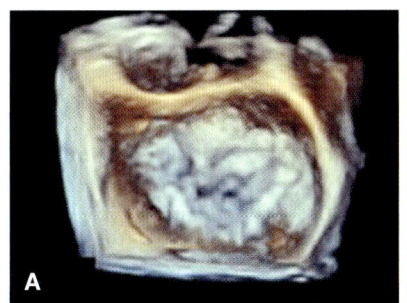

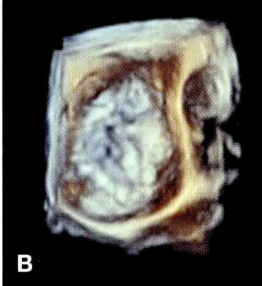

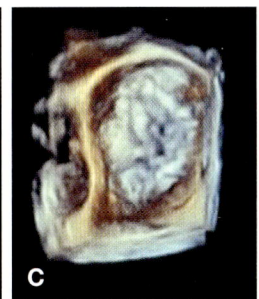

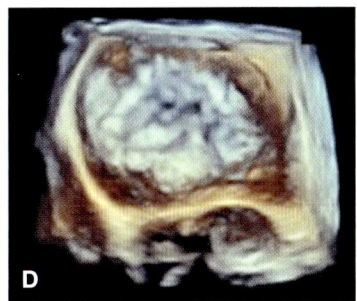

Figure 6.2

106 / Clinical Echocardiography Review

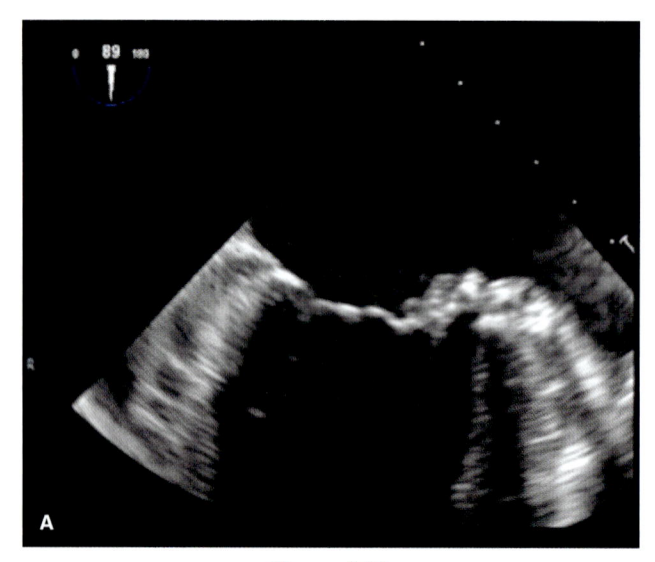

Figure 6.3A

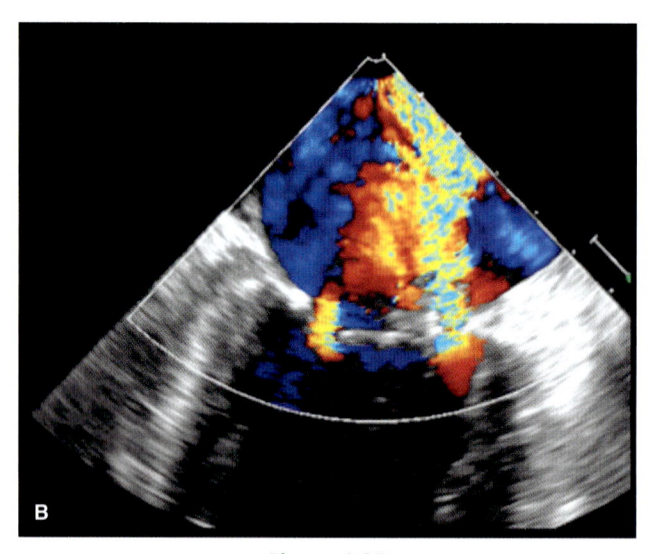

Figure 6.3B

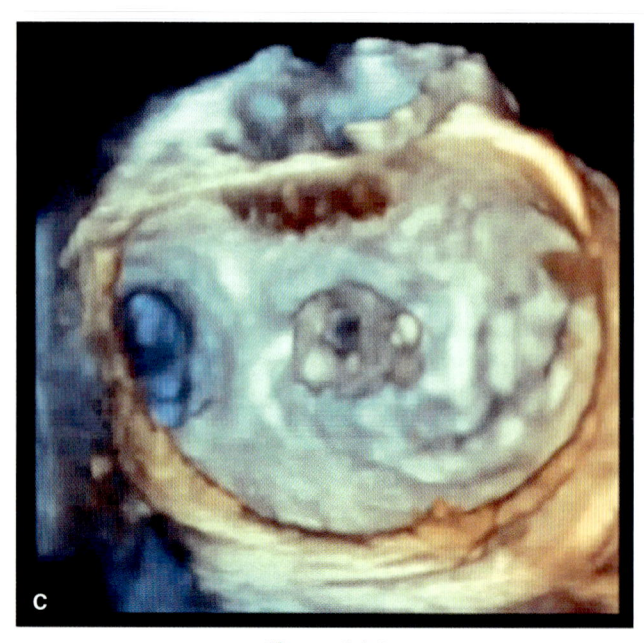

Figure 6.3C

9. Based on the finding in **Case 1**, you conclude that:
   A. There is a posterior leaflet (P1) vegetation with mitral regurgitation.
   B. There is an anterior leaflet (A1) vegetation and perforation with significant mitral regurgitation.
   C. There is a posterior leaflet (P1) vegetation and perforation with significant mitral regurgitation.
   D. There is a ruptured chordae with mitral regurgitation.
   E. There is a flail mitral leaflet with significant regurgitation.

10. After the conclusion made in **Question 9** for the patient in **Case 1**, what would you do next?
    A. Continue with medical management and follow-up with serial echocardiograms.
    B. Continue antibiotic therapy and follow-up with serial transesophageal echocardiograms.
    C. Ask your interventionalist to close this percutaneously.
    D. Ask for a surgical consultation for mitral valve repair.
    E. Discharge to drug rehabilitation, continue medical therapy, and arrange for follow-up in clinic.

CASE 2

A 35-year-old woman from Guatemala has a history of rheumatic fever as a child and balloon valvuloplasty when she was a teenager. She has not had follow-up since her arrival to the United States. She does complain of shortness of breath with housework.

11. The patient's echocardiogram from **Case 2** shows the following (**Figure 6.4**):
    A. Mitral valve prolapse and significant mitral regurgitation.
    B. Normal opening of the mitral valve consistent with successful balloon valvuloplasty.
    C. Decreased opening of the mitral valve leaflets due to low flow.
    D. Decreased mitral valve opening due to restenosis.
    E. Severe mitral stenosis with atrial fibrillation.

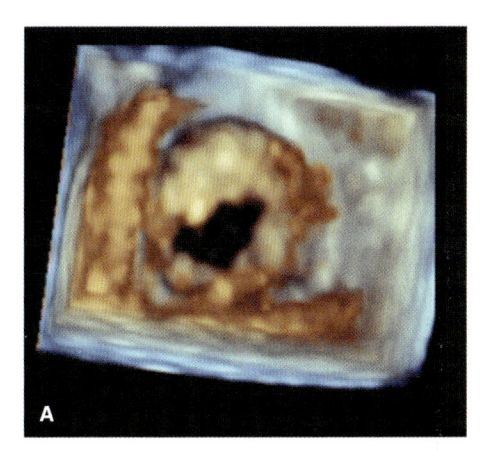

Figure 6.4A

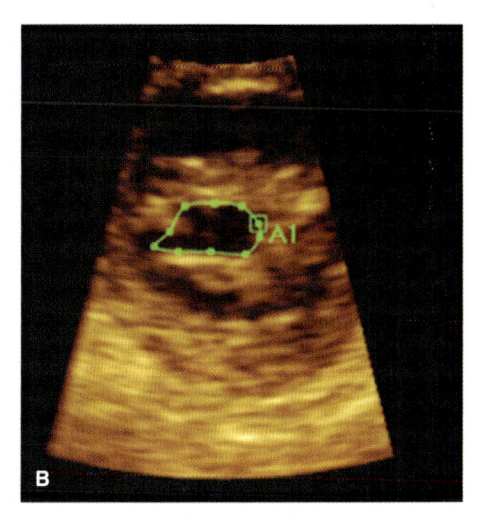

Figure 6.4B

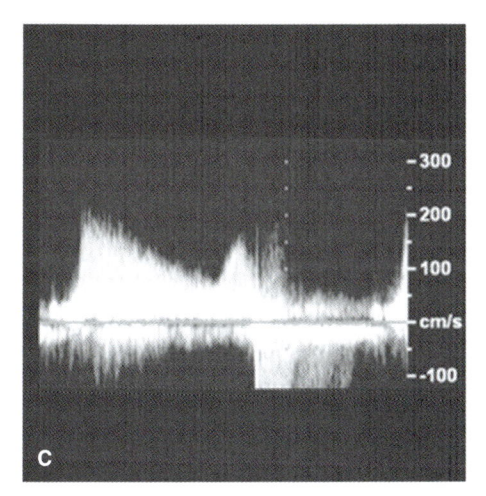

Figure 6.4C

12. The findings from **Case 2** showed that the patient's mitral valve orifice area measured by 3D planimetry demonstrated a mitral valve area of 1.4 cm² with a mean mitral valve gradient of 5 mm Hg. The right ventricular systolic pressure was 45 mm Hg. Since the patient does complain of dyspnea with housework but typically tries not to exert herself, what is your next choice of management?

A. Start amiodarone since she probably has atrial fibrillation as a cause of shortness of breath.
B. Place her on warfarin (Coumadin) since she probably has atrial fibrillation.
C. Inform her that she needs another balloon mitral valvuloplasty.
D. Inform her that she will need a mitral valve repair.
E. Schedule a stress echocardiogram to demonstrate an increase in mitral valve gradient and right ventricular systolic pressure during exercise.

CASE 3

A 60-year-old man with a history of hypertension and hypercholesterolemia has a routine follow-up with a new primary care physician who hears a holosystolic murmur at the apex radiating to the axilla. The patient did not have a history of fever, weight loss, recent trauma to the chest, or rheumatologic illness. He noted difficulty working in his garden because of fatigue. At the end of the visit, he remembered that on a previous health physical examination for the Army he was told that he had a murmur. A transthoracic echocardiogram revealed severe mitral regurgitation but was unable to elucidate the mechanism of mitral regurgitation. After being referred to a cardiologist, a 2D and 3D transesophageal echocardiogram (TEE) was performed. **Figure 6.5** *is a view from a left atrial perspective demonstrating the mitral valve from a surgeon's view.*

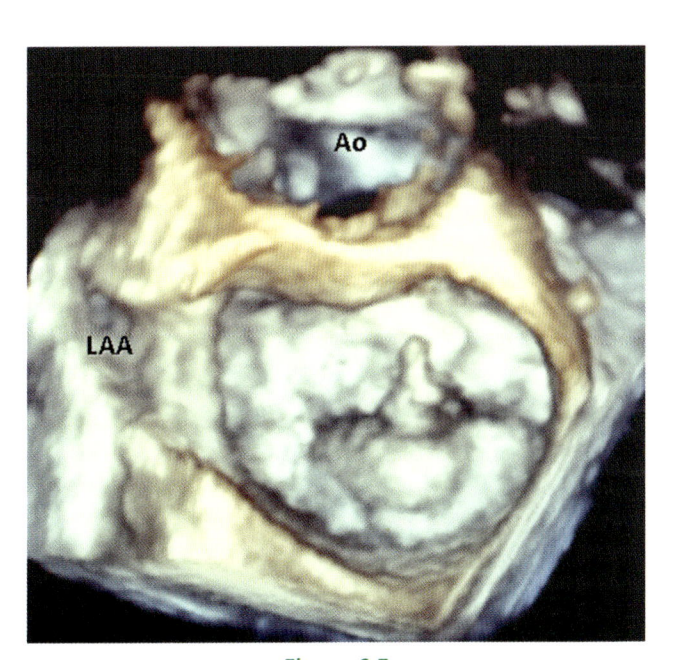

Figure 6.5

13. Based on **Case 3** and **Figure 6.5,** which segment of the mitral valve is the cause of the mitral regurgitation?
    A. A1.
    B. A2.
    C. P1.
    D. P2.
    E. P3.

14. What is the mechanism of mitral regurgitation in the patient from **Case 3**?
    A. Bacterial endocarditis with a vegetation on the P2 scallop.
    B. Barlow disease.
    C. Rheumatic heart disease.
    D. Systemic lupus erythematosus (SLE) with P2 Libman-Sacks lesion.
    E. Flail P2 scallop.

CASE 4

A 75-year-old woman with a history of a mitral valve replacement, hypertension, and hypercholesterolemia presents with progressive shortness of breath, lower extremity edema, and palpitations. She has been faithfully taking all her medications including warfarin. Her blood pressure is 180/100 mm Hg, and heart rate is 100 beats/min, and on auscultation, she has loud mechanical heart sounds and a 2/4 diastolic and 2/6 systolic murmur at the apex.

15. From the TTE demonstrated in **Figure 6.6**, what type of mechanical valve does the patient from **Case 4** have?
    A. Bioprosthetic valve.
    B. Homograft.
    C. Ball-cage valve.
    D. Single tilting disc valve.
    E. Bileaflet tilting disc valve.

16. After giving the patient in **Case 4** furosemide, a beta-blocker, and angiotensin-converting enzyme inhibitor, her blood pressure is 120/80 mm Hg and heart rate is 65 beats/min. She still has lower extremity edema and feels breathless vacuuming. Reviewing her echocardiogram again, she has a mean mitral valve gradient of 4 mm Hg and mitral regurgitation. She undergoes a transesophageal echocardiogram for further evaluation (**Figure 6.7**). What do you decide to do next?

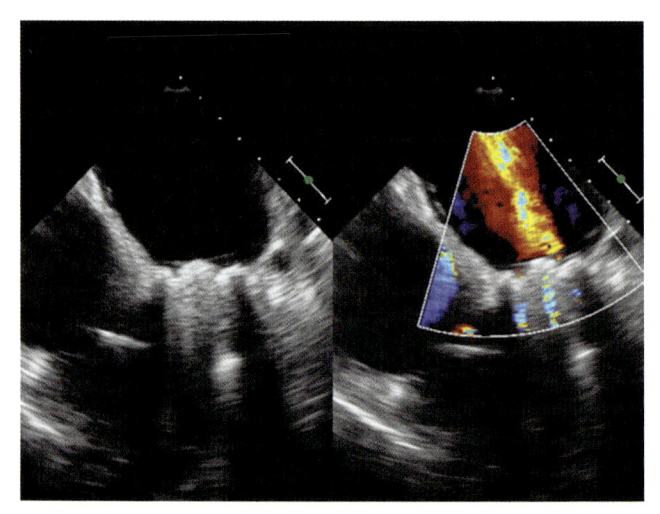

Figure 6.7

A. Increase her doses of diuretics and beta-blocker.
B. Increase anticoagulation and consider heparin therapy.
C. Add high-dose statin therapy.
D. Thrombolytics.
E. Mitral valve replacement.

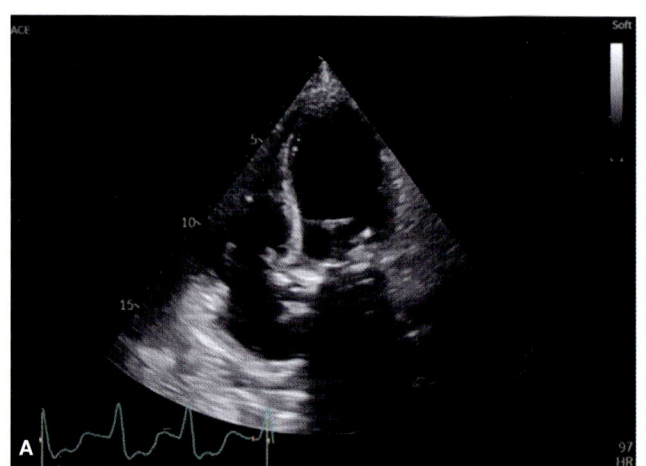

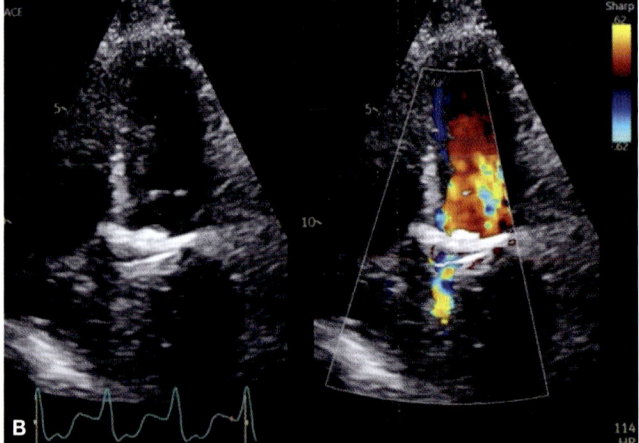

Figure 6.6

CASE 5

A 60-year-old man has a history of mitral valve prolapse and severe mitral regurgitation. He does not admit to having symptoms and tells you that his wife told him to go to the physician's office. She notices that he is more sedentary and does not walk as fast as he used to. On auscultation, he has a 3/6 murmur at the apex radiating to his axilla and back with an absent S1 and loud P2 component. He has severe mitral regurgitation by transthoracic echocardiogram (TTE). Because of poor acoustic windows on the TTE study, he agrees to a TEE. A 3D image of the mitral valve as visualized from a left atrial perspective is shown in **Figure 6.8**.

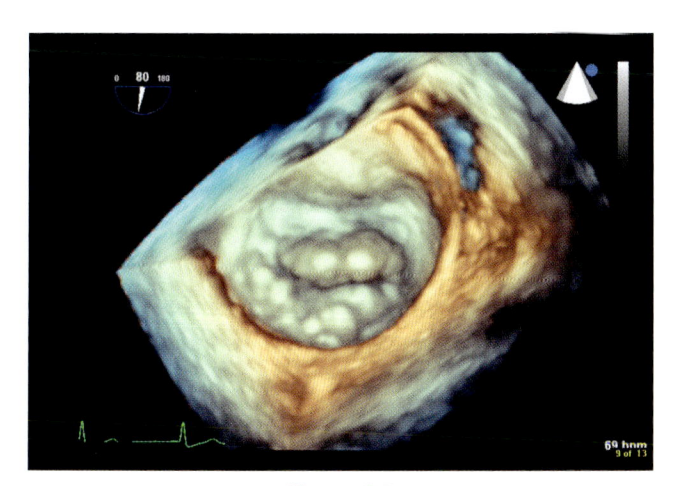

Figure 6.8

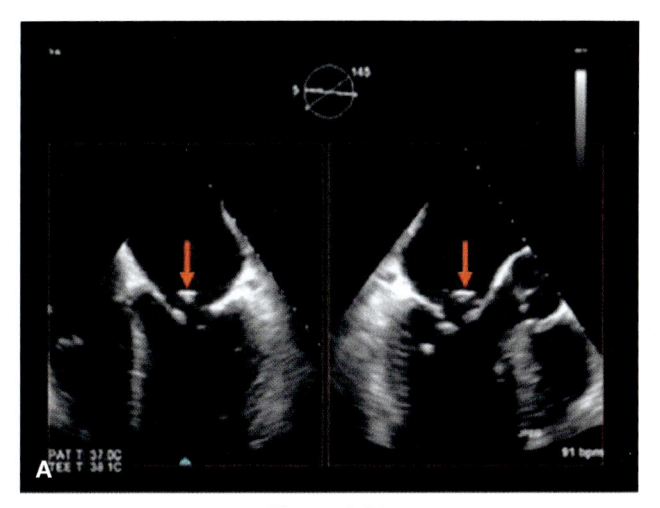

Figure 6.9A

17. After reviewing **Case 5** and **Figure 6.8,** what are your findings?
    A. There is mitral stenosis.
    B. There is a P2 scallop flail.
    C. There is A2 and P2 prolapse.
    D. There is multiscallop prolapse including A2, A3, P1, P2, P3, and the medial commissure.
    E. There is multiscallop prolapse including A1, A2, P2, P1, and the lateral commissure.

CASE 6

A 70-year-old man with a history of dilated cardiomyopathy and severe mitral regurgitation underwent mitral valve repair. A 29-mm Carpentier-Edwards ring was placed in the mitral position. After 6 months, the patient returned complaining of shortness of breath and lower extremity edema. A holosystolic murmur was heard at the apex and pulmonary edema was seen on chest x-ray film. A TEE was performed to reevaluate the mitral regurgitation with findings best described as follows (see **Figure 6.9**): **Figure 6.9** *shows 2D TEE (Panel A) and a 3D left atrial view of the mitral valve (Panel B).*

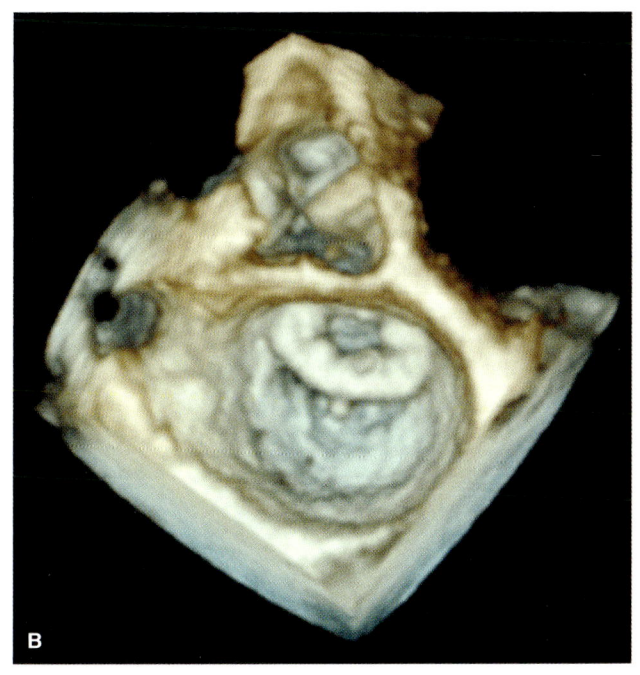

Figure 6.9B

18. What is the arrow pointing to in **Figure 6.9A** from **Case 6**?
    A. A bright echodensity on 2DE at the level of the mitral annulus that corresponds to the mitral valve ring dehiscence on 3DE.
    B. A bright echodensity on 2DE at the level of the mitral annulus that corresponds to the normal mitral valve ring seen from the left atrium on 3DE.
    C. A bright echodensity on 2DE that is probably calcification and corresponds to calcification seen on the posterior mitral annulus on 3DE.
    D. A bright echodensity on 2DE that is probably vegetation and corresponds to the likely mobile echodensity attached to the mitral ring on 3DE.
    E. None of the above.

110 / Clinical Echocardiography Review

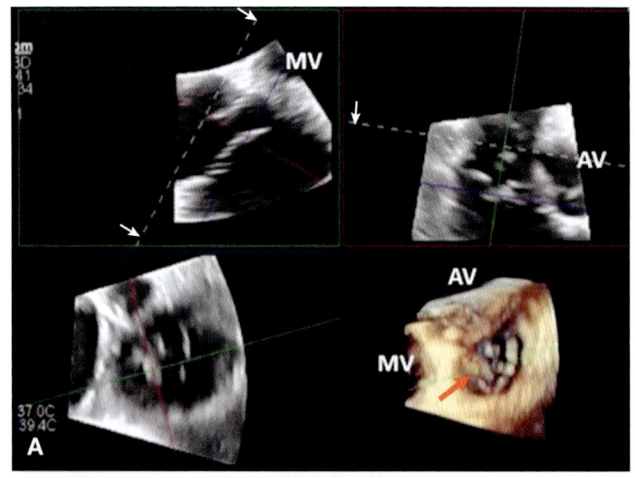

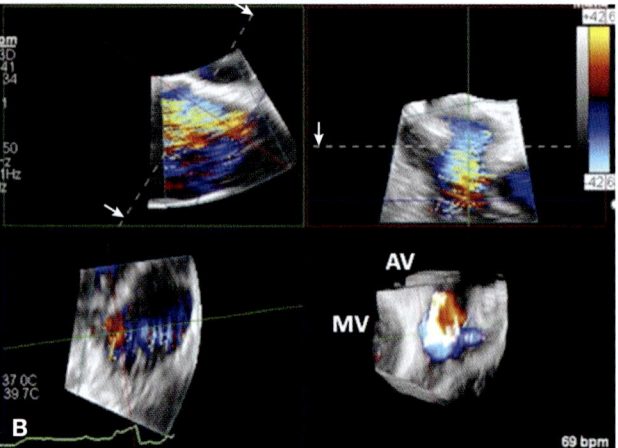

Figure 6.10. AV, aortic valve; MV, mitral valve.

CASE 7

A 65-year-old woman presents with lower extremity edema and abdominal fullness for the past year. She underwent heart transplant 10 years ago for end-stage hypertrophic cardiomyopathy.

19. What is the tricuspid valve pathology on TEE (**Figure 6.10**, *arrow*) obtained from patient in **Case 7**?
    A. Annular dilatation.
    B. Anterior leaflet flail.
    C. Septal leaflet flail.
    D. Posterior leaflet flail.

20. Please label the structures seen in **Figure 6.11** on the interatrial septal view as visualized from the left atrial perspective.
    A. A, mitral valve; B, aortic valve; C, superior vena cava; D, coronary sinus.
    B. A, aortic valve; B, mitral valve; C, superior vena cava; D, fossa ovalis.
    C. A, pulmonic valve; B, inferior vena cava; C, tricuspid valve; D, coronary sinus.
    D. A, aortic valve; B, mitral valve; C, right upper pulmonary vein; D, inferior vena cava.
    E. None of the above.

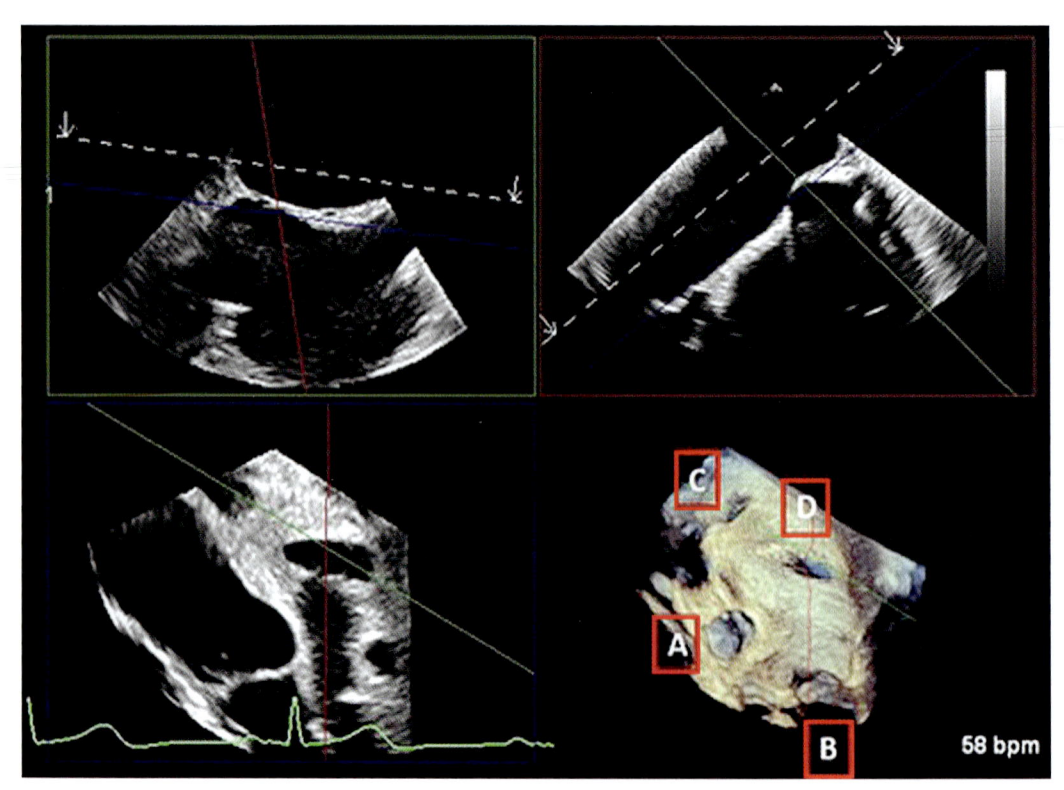

Figure 6.11

CASE 8

An 80-year-old man with paroxysmal atrial fibrillation undergoes Watchman placement for recurrent diverticular bleeds.

21. On 45-day TEE assessment of the Watchman (**Figure 6.12**), where is the peridevice leak in the patient from **Case 8**?
    A. Anterior.
    B. Posterior.
    C. Superior.
    D. Inferior.
    E. None of the above.

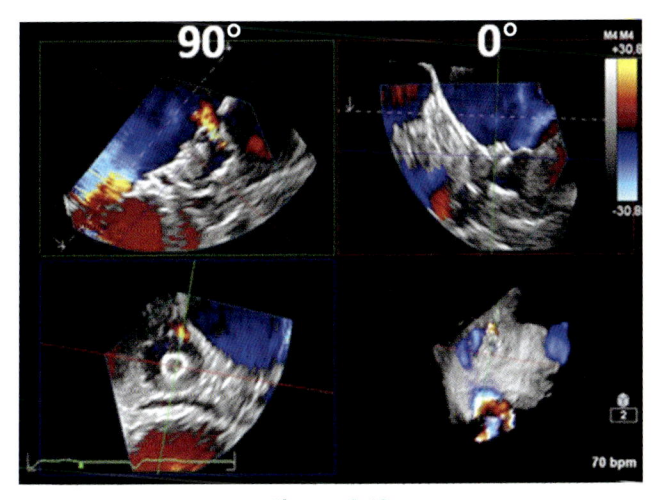

Figure 6.12

22. Where is the pacemaker lead relative to the tricuspid valve in **Figure 6.13** (*arrow*)?
    A. Center of the tricuspid valve.
    B. Anterior-septal commissure.
    C. Posterior-septal commissure.
    D. Anterior-posterior commissure.
    E. None of the above.

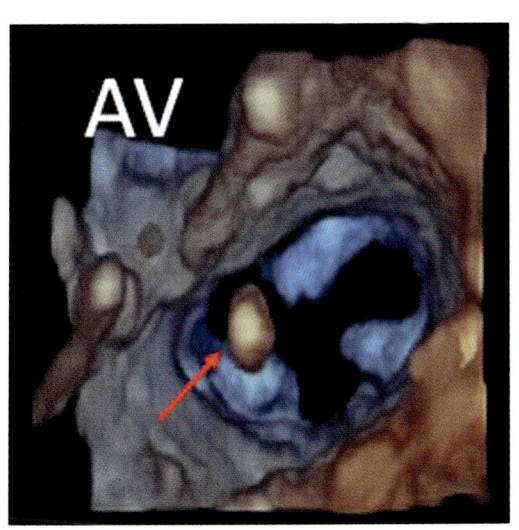

Figure 6.13. AV, aortic valve.

CASE 9

A 58-year-old woman underwent bioprosthetic mitral valve replacement 4 years ago for native mitral valve endocarditis caused by Staphylococcus aureus. She presents to clinic with dyspnea on exertion and evidence of hemolysis on labs (see ▶ Video 6.1 and Figure 6.14).

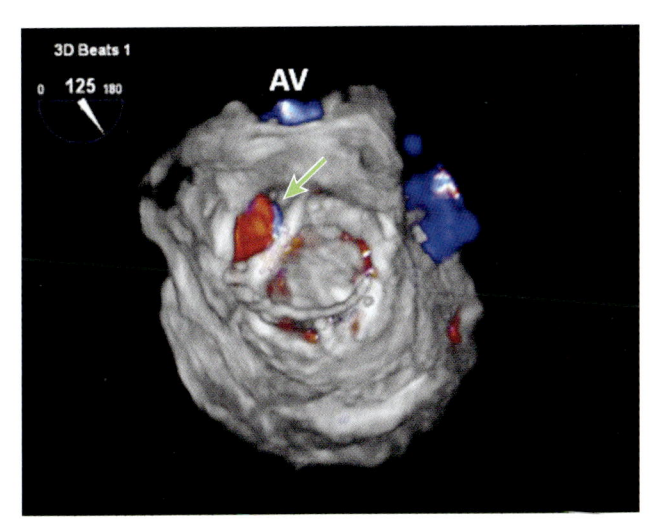

Figure 6.14. AV, aortic valve.

23. Based on the findings in **Case 9**, localize the paravalvular leak on this bioprosthetic mitral valve as indicated by the *green arrow*.
    A. Anteromedial.
    B. Posterolateral.
    C. Posteromedial.
    D. Anterolateral.
    E. None of the above.

112 / Clinical Echocardiography Review

24. Viewed from the left ventricle (▶ Video 6.2 and Figure 6.15), where is the jet of mitral regurgitation located?
   A. Anterior.
   B. Posterior.
   C. Medial.
   D. Lateral.
   E. None of the above.

25. Which image (Figure 6.16) would most accurately measure the mitral valve area?
   A. A
   B. B
   C. C
   D. D
   E. None of the above.

CASE 10

A 29-year-old woman experienced transient loss of vision. She has not had any fevers or palpitations. On TEE, a mobile echodensity is noted.

26. Based on **Case 10**, the finding on this 3D image (▶ Video 6.3) is probably a:
   A. Myxoma.
   B. Fibroelastoma.
   C. Calcification.
   D. Lambl excrescence.
   E. Vegetation.

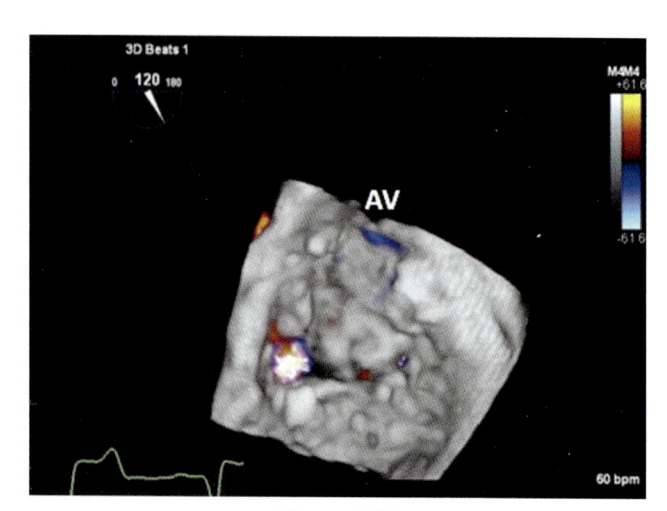

Figure 6.15

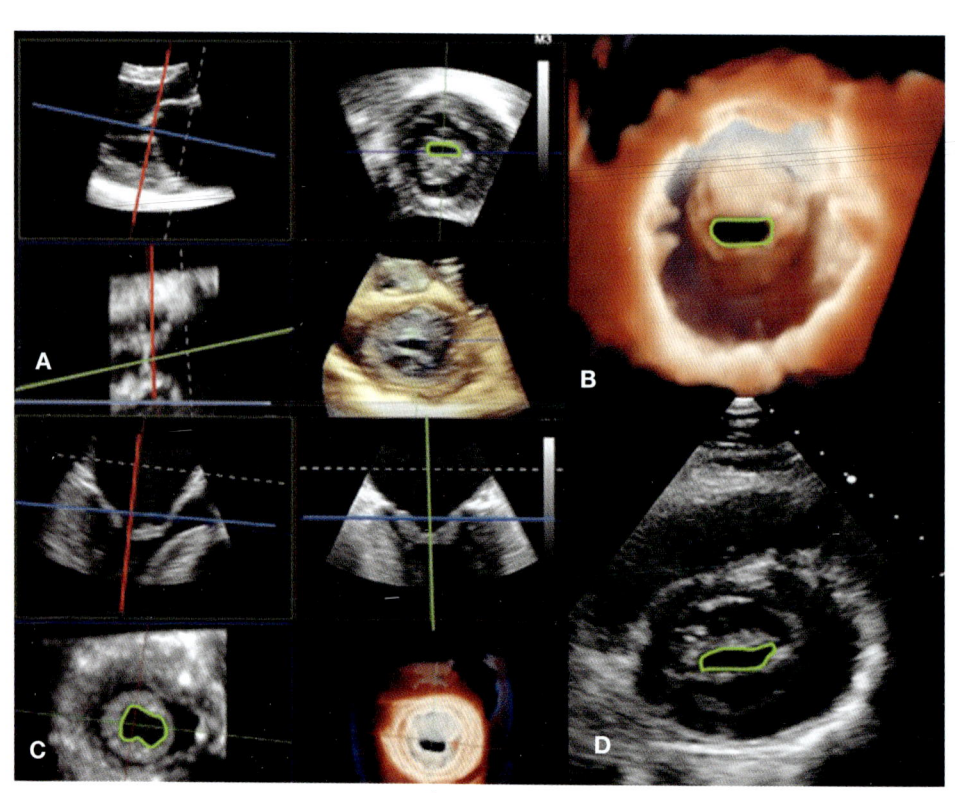

Figure 6.16

CASE 11

A 63-year-old man with a history of a mitral valve replacement presented with chest discomfort. On physical examination, an audible click is heard with a diastolic murmur. He was evaluated with a cardiac catheterization and was found to have no significant coronary obstruction. On further investigation, he admits that he has not been taking warfarin regularly over many months but has not noticed a change in his physical activity. A TEE was performed revealing the 3D image in diastole from a left atrial perspective (**Figure 6.17**); please review ▶ **Video 6.4A,B**.

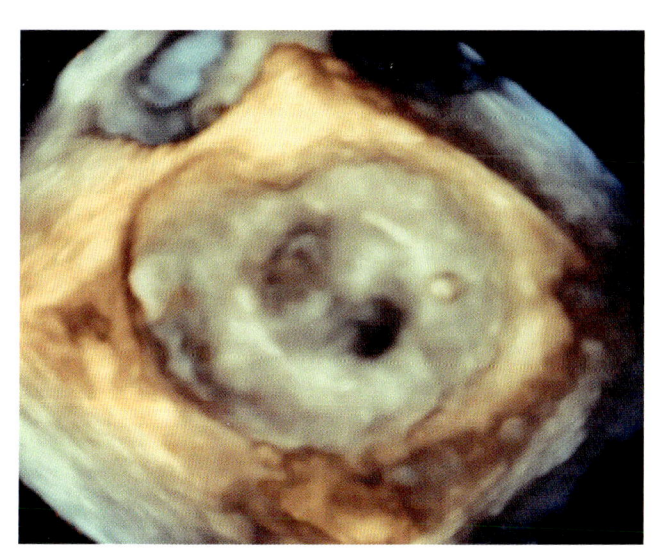

Figure 6.17

27. What are the findings shown in **Figure 6.17** and ▶ **Video 6.4A** from the patient in **Case 11**?
    A. This is a normal bileaflet mechanical mitral valve.
    B. This is a single tilting disc valve.
    C. There is a valve vegetation.
    D. There is a valvular dehiscence and an immobile mitral valve disc.
    E. There is a thrombosed mitral valve leaflet.

CASE 12

A 66-year-old man is referred to you because his primary physician noted a murmur during his first office visit. He tells you that he has known about the murmur since he was a teenager but has never gone to a physician for follow-up. He still works taking care of school maintenance. He walks on the treadmill for exercise at 4 mph and a 10% incline on occasion for half an hour 4 days a week. He fervently denies shortness of breath with this activity. On TTE, you find severe mitral regurgitation based on flow convergence calculation (effective regurgitant orifice = 0.4 cm^2) with normal LV function (EF = 65%). Since the mechanism of regurgitation was difficult to discern on TTE, a TEE was performed revealing the abnormality as shown in **Figure 6.18**.

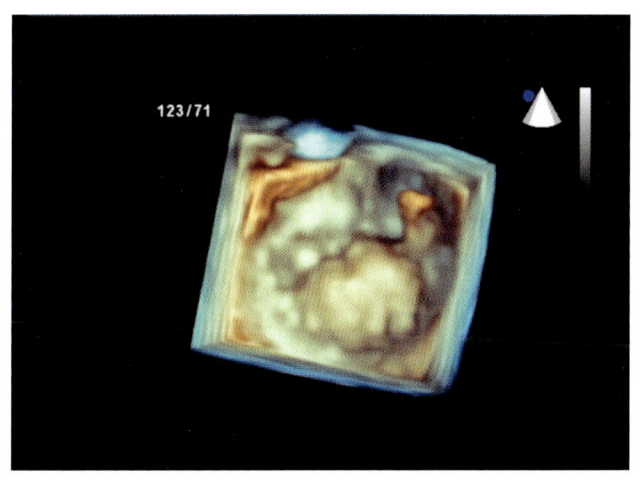

Figure 6.18

28. What is the mechanism of mitral regurgitation shown in **Figure 6.18** and ▶ **Video 6.5** from the patient in **Case 12**?
    A. P1 flail.
    B. P2 flail.
    C. P3 prolapse.
    D. Severe prolapse of P2 and P3 flail.
    E. Severe prolapse of P2 to P3.

CASE 13

A 45-year-old Hispanic woman has a history of rheumatic fever as a child and had balloon mitral valvuloplasty as a young adult. She now feels fatigued doing housework such as vacuuming her living room and has been unable to walk up a hill to get to the market. She is currently on a beta-blocker with a heart rate of 55 beats/min. On TTE, she has a mean mitral valve gradient of 5 mm Hg, moderate mitral regurgitation, and moderate aortic stenosis. On TEE, 3D imaging of the mitral valve, a 3D mitral valve area planimetry demonstrates an orifice area of 0.6 cm^2, as shown in **Figure 6.19A**. The mitral valve anatomy is shown from a left atrial (**Figure 6.19B**) and LV (**Figure 6.19C**) perspective (see also ▶ **Video 6.6**).

114 / Clinical Echocardiography Review

29. What findings are shown in **Figure 6.19B,C** from the patient in **Case 13**?
   A. There is asymmetric fusion of the medial commissure with severe subvalvular fibrosis.
   B. There is asymmetric fusion of the lateral commissure with severe subvalvular fibrosis.
   C. There is asymmetric fusion of the medial commissure with mild subvalvular fibrosis.
   D. There is mild mitral stenosis with equal fusion of medial and lateral commissures.
   E. None of the above.

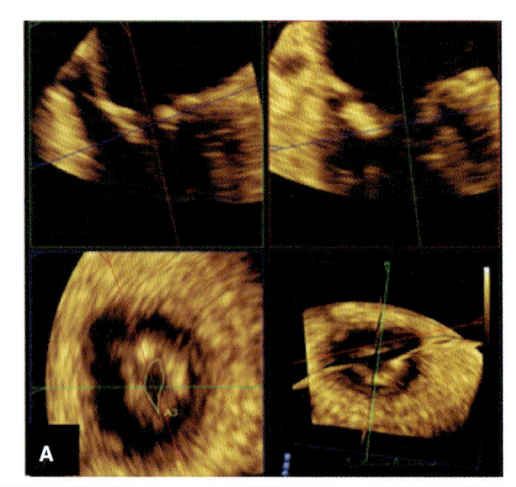

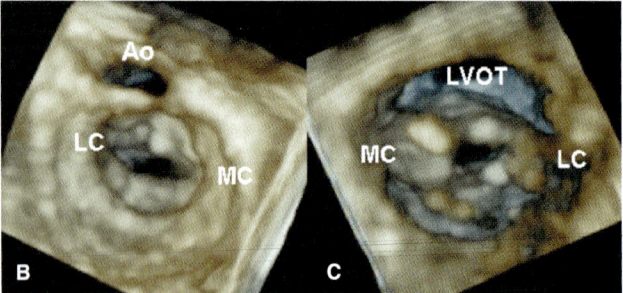

Figure 6.19. In Panel A: a 3D multiplanar reconstruction images of the mitral valve are displayed. The short axis of the mitral valve is seen in the bottom left of the quad image. A view of the mitral valve from the left atrial view (Panel B) and a left ventricular view of the mitral valve (Panel C). Ao, aorta; LC, left commissure; LVOT, left ventricular outflow tract; MC, medial commissure.

30. With these findings from **Case 13**, what would you recommend?
   A. Increasing beta-blockers to achieve a heart rate in the 40s.
   B. Perform a bicycle stress test to measure an increase in right ventricular (RV) systolic pressure.
   C. Warfarin for stroke prevention.
   D. Balloon mitral valvuloplasty.
   E. Mitral valve replacement and aortic valve replacement.

CASE 14

*A 67-year-old woman with a history of a bioprosthetic valve replacement for rheumatic mitral valve disease 7 years prior to presentation was brought to the hospital by her son because of failure to thrive, decreased exercise capacity, shortness of breath, and occasional fevers. A loud systolic ejection murmur and diastolic rumble are heard at the lower left sternal border and apex. On TTE, the mitral valve mean gradient was 11 mm Hg and a TEE was performed (**Figure 6.20**). Please view ▶ Video 6.7A,B.*

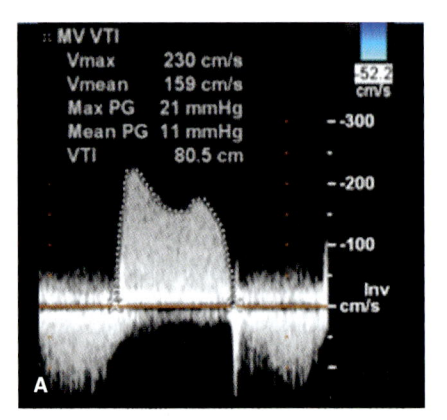

Figure 6.20A

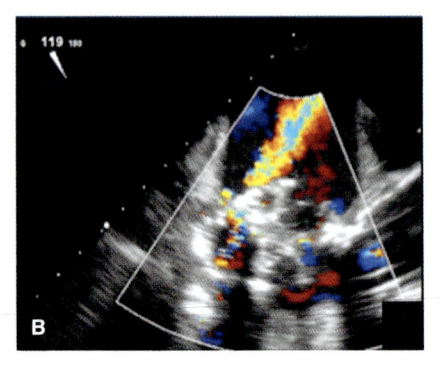

Figure 6.20B

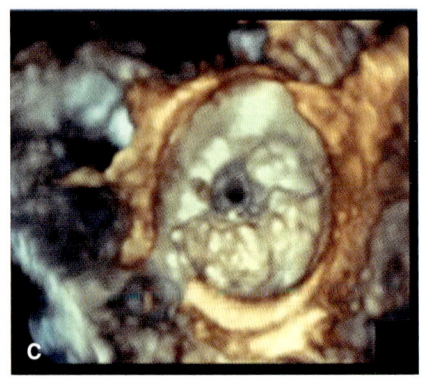

Figure 6.20C

31. What are the findings for **Case 14** based on the 2D and 3D TEE (**Figure 6.20** and ▶ Video 6.7)?
    A. Severe valvular mitral regurgitation.
    B. Severe mitral stenosis.
    C. Combination of severe paravalvular regurgitation and mitral stenosis due to the vegetation causing obstruction.
    D. Combination of severe valvular regurgitation and mitral stenosis due to the vegetation causing obstruction and malcoaptation.
    E. None of the above.

CASE 14 CONTINUED

A mechanical mitral valve replacement was performed. Though her symptoms were alleviated initially, she has recently experienced progressive dyspnea on exertion a month after her surgery. A TEE was performed with the findings shown in **Figure 6.21** *and* ▶ Video 6.8A,B.

32. Based on **Figure 6.21** and ▶ Video 6.8A,B which of the following is most likely causing the patient's symptoms from **Case 14**?
    A. Prosthetic valve thrombosis.
    B. Failed occlusion of prosthetic paravalvular regurgitation.
    C. Hemolytic anemia.
    D. Vegetations on the prosthetic valve ring.
    E. Pannus overgrowth with prosthetic stenosis.

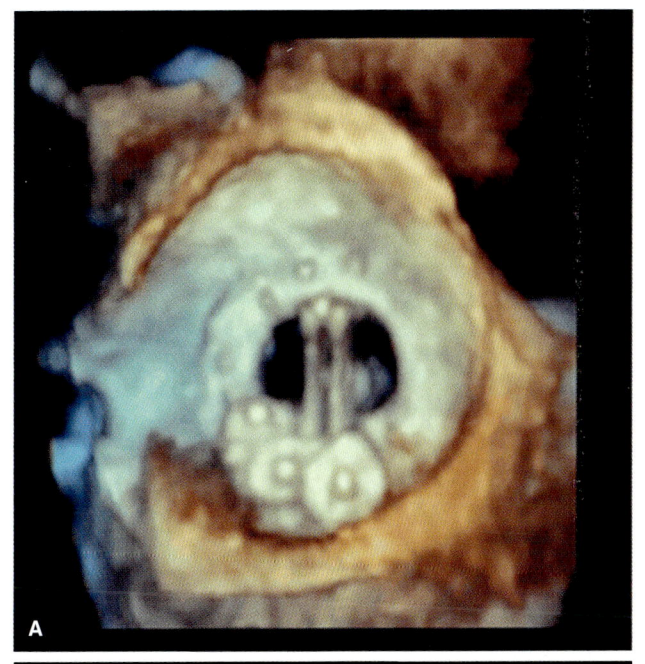

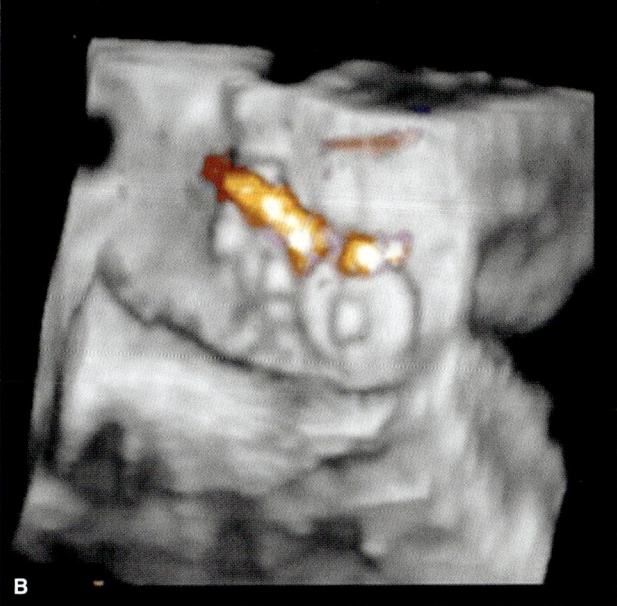

Figure 6.21. A 3D transesophageal echocardiogram is displayed from a left atrial view (Panel A) and with color flow Doppler (Panel B).

ANSWERS

1. **Answer: A.** The quality of a 3D reconstruction using multiple 2D images depends on the quality of the 2D images and the ability to avoid motion during acquisition by either the operator or the patient. ECG and respiratory gating were also essential in ensuring the location in time and space. Hence, patients with atrial fibrillation or irregular heartbeats were usually excluded in studies. The data integrity in such patients could not be ensured. However, if patients are not extremely tachycardic, 3D images can be obtained in patients with atrial fibrillation with the understanding that the severity of valvulopathies may vary across 3D datasets.

2. **Answer: E.** A multibeat acquisition enables the user to achieve better temporal resolution compared with a single beat acquisition, while maintaining high spatial resolution. In addition, decreasing the imaging depth, decreasing sector width (elevation and lateral), and using a zoom mode of imaging will also increase the volume rate. Magnification does not change spatial or temporal resolution.

3. **Answer: C.** Stitch artifact (**Figure 6.22**) occurs during a multibeat acquisition where several subvolumes are sequentially obtained over two to seven cardiac cycles. Operator or patient movement, respiratory motion, arrhythmias, or even esophageal motility can cause misalignment of these subvolumes.

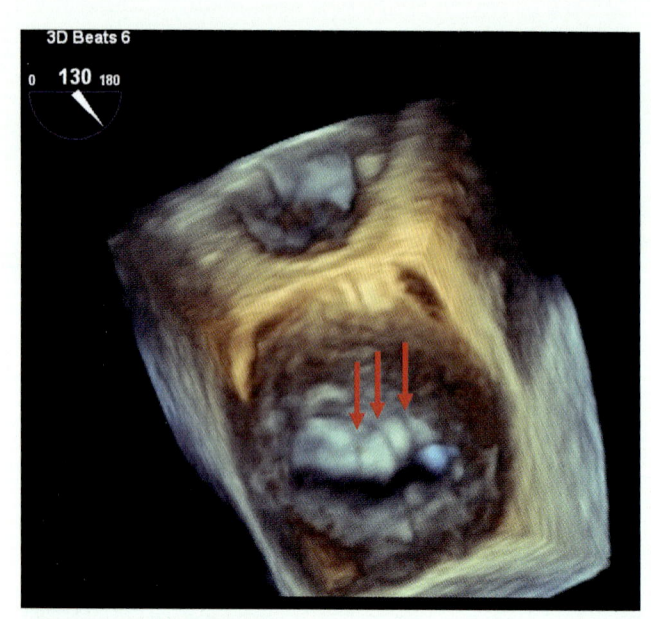

Figure 6.22. Stitch artifact (shown by the red arrows), which is a malignment of adjacent volumes during acquisition.

4. **Answer: A.** Three-dimensional echocardiography has repeatedly been shown to be superior to 2DE when compared with cardiac magnetic resonance imaging (MRI) as a gold standard. Specifically, real-time 3DE studies have demonstrated less variability in repeated measurements (intra- and interobserver variability), which is explained by the ease of obtaining a common long axis in 3D volume data. Image alignment is pivotal in the accuracy of 2D quantitation of LV volumes. Although both 2DE and 3DE underestimate LV volumes, underestimation occurs mostly when using 2DE methods for quantitation (biplane Simpson method or method of discs).
5. **Answer: E.** Three-dimensional echocardiography has the lowest test-retest variability compared with other methods, making it the best modality to use for serial follow-up of patients long term.
6. **Answer: B.** The RV has been described as a crescent-shaped ventricle not easily conforming to any geometric shape. Therefore, its quantitative assessment is very difficult. Current techniques to measure the RV using 3D include the method of disks, a rotational approach, and a semiautomatic border detection approach.
7. **Answer: C.** Although we are able to perform 3D color Doppler imaging, the current limitations of this technology are low temporal and spatial resolution. Better temporal resolution can be obtained using multibeat acquisitions over seven cardiac cycles, but this creates a high risk of stitch artifacts. Using a smaller sector size can also aid in increasing temporal resolution, but this decreases the available spatial and anatomic information.
8. **Answer: A.** The standard display orientation of the mitral valve is shown with labels in **Figure 6.23**. The aortic valve is usually rotated to the 11 to 12 o'clock position and the left atrial appendage is at approximately 9 o'clock. The posterior mitral valve leaflet is centered at 6 o'clock (specifically the P2 scallop) and the interatrial septum is between 2 and 3 o'clock. This display is described as the "surgeon's view," which is the orientation of the mitral valve when visualized from the left atrium by a surgeon standing on the patient's right side.
9. **Answer: B.** This patient has an A1 scallop vegetation

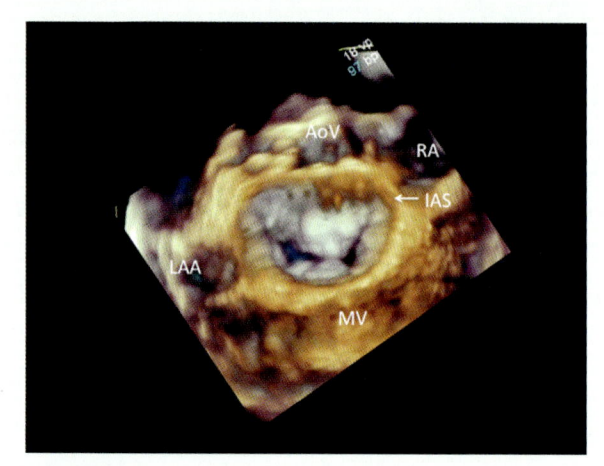

Figure 6.23. "Surgeon's view" of the mitral valve from a left atrial orientation. AoV, aortic valve; IAS, interatrial septum; LAA, left atrial appendage; MV, mitral valve; RA, right atrium.

and perforation with significant mitral regurgitation. At 90° on a 2D transesophageal echocardiogram, the leaflet scallops coapting in this view are P3 and A3. There is an echodensity on the anterior leaflet adjacent to the left atrial appendage, which is usually the A1 scallop. When color flow Doppler is applied, the jet penetrates through the leaflet. From a left atrial perspective, this vegetation and perforation can be visualized easily on 3D echocardiography.

See **Figure 6.24**. Two-dimensional transesophageal echocardiography (Panels A and B) demonstrates a vegetation (red arrow) at the A1 scallop in 90° with mitral regurgitation going through the A1 scallop indicative of a perforation. On 3D transesophageal echocardiography, there is a vegetation (red arrow) with a visible hole through the A1 scallop seen from a left atrial orientation.

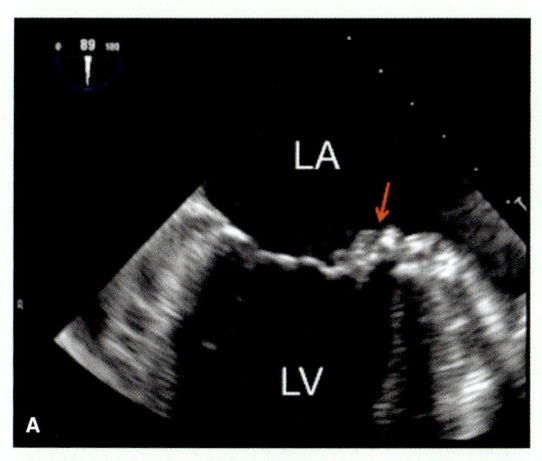

Figure 6.24A

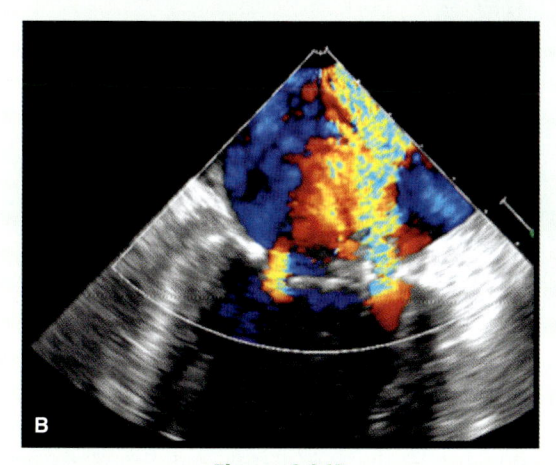

Figure 6.24B

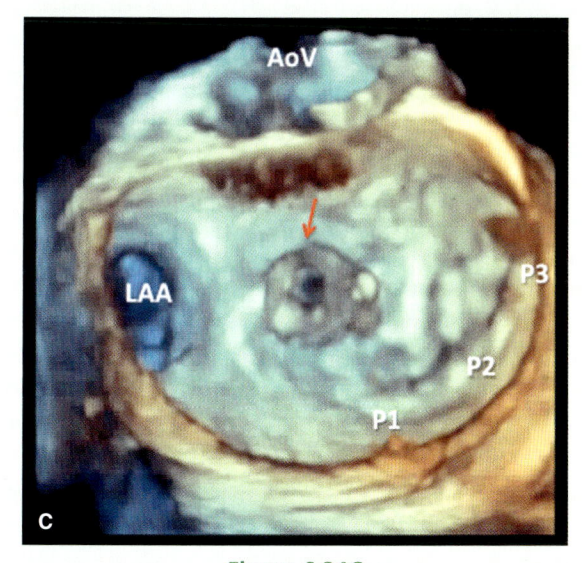

Figure 6.24C

10. **Answer: D.** The class I indications for mitral valve surgery in the setting of endocarditis include severe mitral regurgitation resulting in heart failure, fungal or highly resistant organisms causing endocarditis, or those complicated by heart block, abscess, or destructive lesions (eg, mitral leaflet perforation; or infection of the mitral-aortic intervalvular fibrosa). Severe mitral regurgitation with heart failure and a perforated leaflet were indications for surgery in this patient. Three-dimensional echocardiographic findings were confirmed with intraoperative surgical pathology.

11. **Answer: D.** This patient has severe mitral stenosis with a moderate transmitral gradient. **Figure 6.4** is a view of the mitral valve from a LV perspective. There is doming of the anterior mitral leaflet with medial and lateral commissural fusion. Using multiplanar reconstruction, a 2D cut plane can be placed at the tips of the mitral leaflet en face to the valve opening to derive a mitral valve area as shown in **Figure 6.25**. In this case, the mitral valve orifice area was 1.4 cm^2.

12. **Answer: E.** This patient with mitral stenosis has a valve area of ≤1.5 cm^2 with a gradient of 5 mm Hg and mild pulmonary hypertension. For this patient with symptomatic severe mitral stenosis, there is an indication to perform stress echocardiography to evaluate a rise in mean mitral valve gradients of >15 mm Hg with exercise. If patients have valve morphology amenable to valvuloplasty and meet these criteria, then there is an indication for percutaneous balloon mitral valvuloplasty.

13. **Answer: D.** The abnormal scallop in this case is the P2 scallop. The P2 scallop is most frequently affected and is typically across from the aorta (**Figure 6.26**) (Ao, aorta; LAA, left atrial appendage).

14. **Answer: E.** This is a P2 scallop that is flail (**Figure 6.27A,B**). The tip of the ruptured chordae can be seen from this left atrial perspective, noted by the arrows.

15. **Answer: C.** This is a ball-cage valve (**Figure 6.28**). In Panel A, a three-dimensional transthoracic image displayed from an anterior perspective demonstrates the ball and cage during a systolic phase. A 2D transthoracic echocardiogram from an apical window shows the ball and cage valve during diastole (Panel B) and with color flow Doppler (Panel C).

16. **Answer: E.** Since the patient's symptoms persist even with maximum medical therapy, mitral valve replacement is advised. The patient takes warfarin regularly with a therapeutic international normalized ratio (INR) and her symptoms are progressive, which indicates that this is probably not an acute event such as valve thrombosis. The most likely problem since she has had this valve for many years is pannus. On transesophageal echocardiogram, she has mitral regurgitation that is significant. Typically, there is only a small amount of physiologic mitral regurgitation with a ball-cage valve due to the movement of the ball upward toward the left atrium.

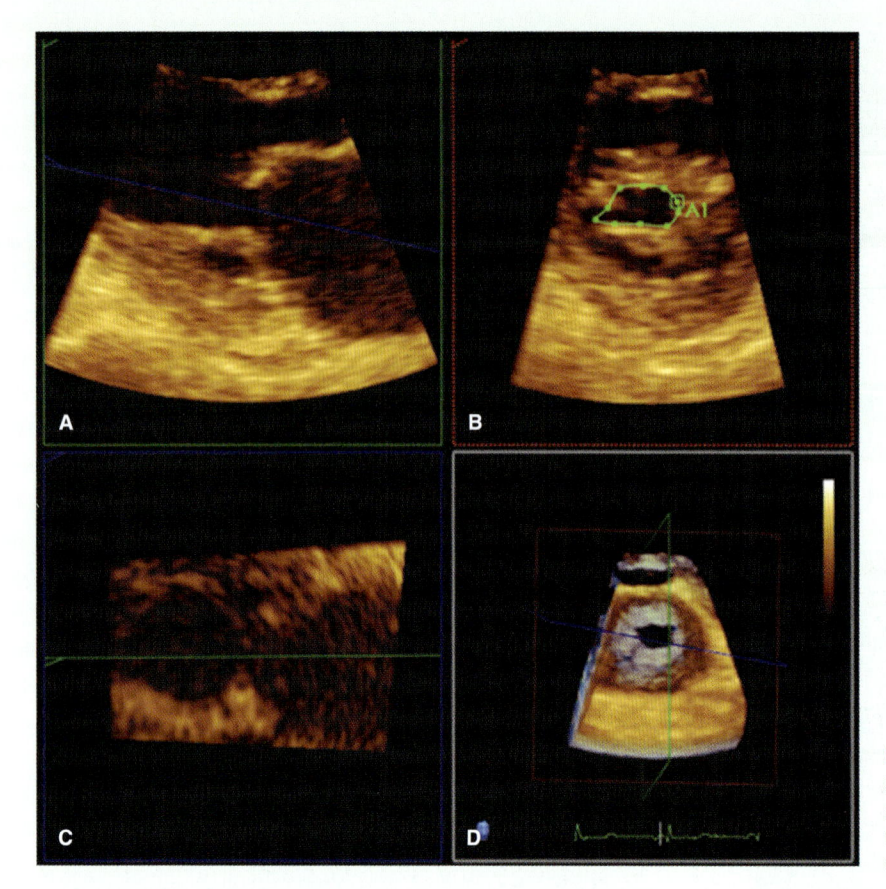

Figure 6.25. Multiplanar reconstruction of a zoom mode acquisition in this patient with mitral stenosis. On the short-axis cross section of the mitral valve, a mitral valve area planimetry was obtained.

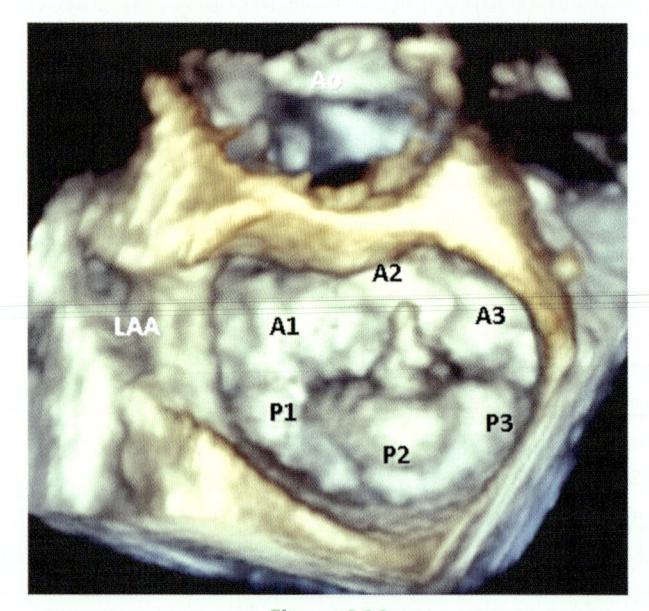

Figure 6.26

17. **Answer: D.** Besides the multisegmental prolapse and the medial commissural involvement, there is calcification over the P2 scallop noted by the arrow (**Figure 6.29**) (AV, aortic valve; C, commissure).
18. **Answer: A.** On 2DE, there is a bright echodensity at the level of the mitral valve seen in the biplane image with 4-chamber and long-axis views. The mitral leaflets appear too close below the mitral annulus. The cause of the holosystolic murmur is annular dilatation. A normal mitral ring should be seen adjacent to the anterior and posterior aspects of the annulus. On the 3DE image of the mitral valve in **Figure 6.30** (displayed from the left atrial orientation), the aortic valve is seen at 12 o'clock, left atrial appendage at 9 o'clock, and posterior mitral annulus at 6 o'clock. The bright echodensity corresponds to the dehisced mitral ring that remains mostly sutured anteriorly from trigone to trigone. The entire posterior aspect of this mitral ring is dehisced.
19. **Answer: C.** There is flail of the tricuspid septal leaflet. The TR jet is visualized in the green plane on the 3D image with color. The green plane cuts through the tricuspid valve in a septal to lateral orientation, in this case, through the septal and anterior leaflets as visualized on the 3D image. The leaflet closest to the MV, that is, the septal leaflet, is seen to be flail. Patients with heart transplants are at higher risk for tricuspid valve injury usually causing flail or perforation from serial endomyocardial biopsies.
20. **Answer: B.** In this view of the interatrial septum as viewed from the left atrium, A is the aortic valve best seen on the blue plane running oblique to the septum. The green plane cuts through the superior vena cava labeled C. The image is centered on the fossa ovalis labeled D with the mitral valve inferiorly, as seen in the red plane labeled B. This view can be

Chapter 6 Three-Dimensional Echocardiography / 119

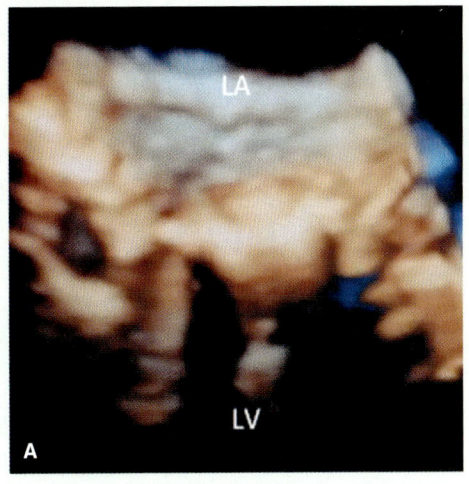

Figure 6.28A

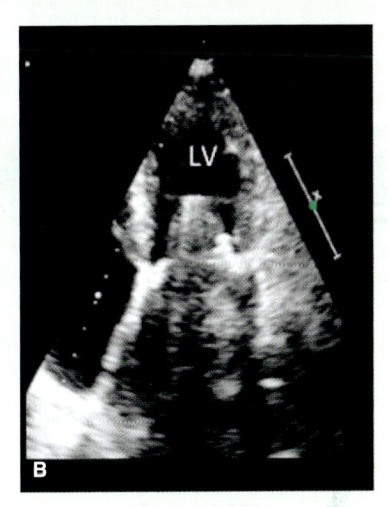

Figure 6.28B

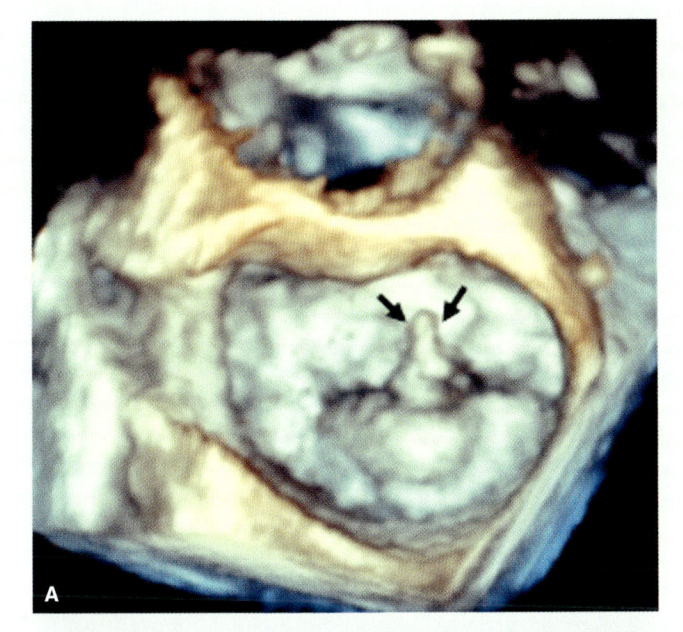

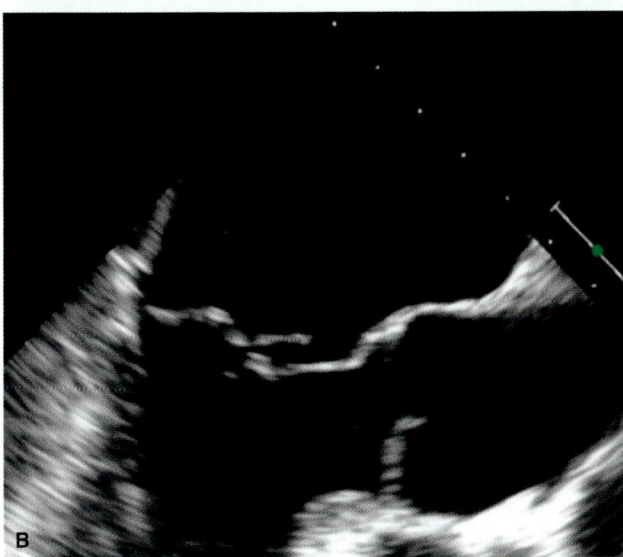

Figure 6.27

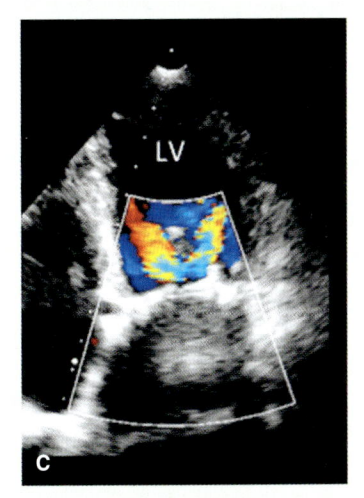

Figure 6.28C

particularly helpful in measuring transseptal puncture height relative to the mitral valve.

21. **Answer: C.** The peridevice leak is superior. The TEE image at 90° shows a small peridevice leak confirmed on the 3D image. The 90° view typically establishes the superior to inferior axis with the mitral valve located inferiorly to the Watchman device. This may vary on individual patient anatomy. The 0° view offers an anterior to posterior axis of the left atrial appendage.

22. **Answer: B.** The pacemaker lead is in the anteroseptal commissure, with the aortic valve establishing the anterior orientation and the interatrial septum adjacent to the septal leaflet.

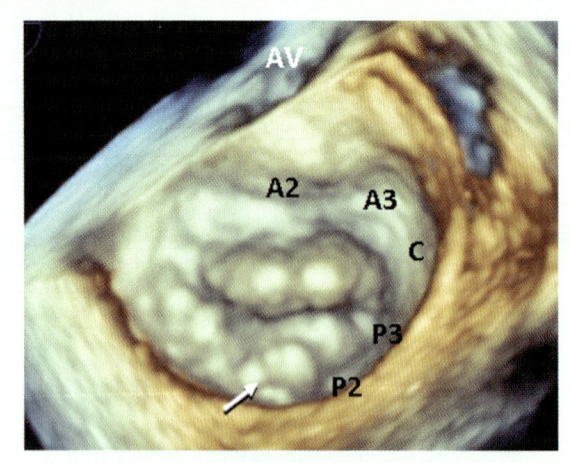

Figure 6.29. Three-dimensional echocardiogram of the mitral valve from a left atrial view.

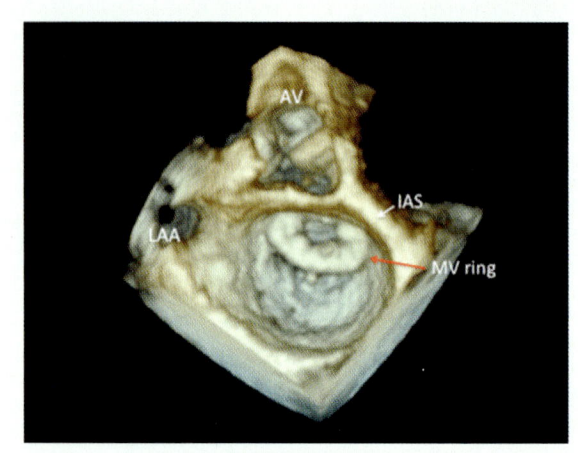

Figure 6.30. Three-dimensional transesophageal echocardiogram of the mitral valve displayed from a left atrial orientation shows the dehisced mitral ring from the posterior aspect of the mitral valve annulus. AV, aortic valve; IAS, interatrial septum; LAA, left atrial appendage; MV, mitral valve.

23. **Answer: D.** The paravalvular leak is anterolateral to the mitral valve replacement adjacent to the left atrial appendage.
24. **Answer: C.** The mitral regurgitation is located on the medial aspect of the mitral valve. In 3D, when the valve is viewed from the ventricular side, the medial and lateral aspects are mirrored relative to when viewing from the atrial side. It can be helpful to assess mitral regurgitation jets from the ventricular side to localize origin and size of the jets.
25. **Answer: A.** Answer choice A shows the correct way to measure the mitral valve area with multiplanar reconstruction, confirming the tracing is at the level of the leaflet tips. Answer choice C is a multiplanar reconstruction of the mitral valve. However, the blue plane is not at the mitral leaflet tips, so the MVA is overestimated. Answer choices B and D are incorrect because it is unclear if the image is on the axis or at the mitral valve tips. In general, measurements should not be made on the 3D image itself.

26. **Answer: B.** On the left side of the video (▶ **Video 6.3**) is an aortic view and on the right is a 5-chamber view from the midesophageal level. The echodensity is located on the aortic side, appears round, and has a stalk. This is most likely a pedunculated fibroelastoma that appears attached to the commissure of the right and noncoronary cusps.

KEY POINTS
- 3DE aids in identifying the etiology of aortic valve echodensities by characterizing the shape, mobility, and attachment point.

27. **Answer: D.** From this left atrial view of the mitral valve in diastole, only one leaflet appears to open (**Figure 6.31**). The opened leaflet (black arrow) reveals a darker background since the ventricle is segmented during a zoom acquisition, whereas the thrombosed leaflet is the same appearance as the surrounding structure. This can be better appreciated in ▶ **Video 6.4A**. Two-dimensional TEE images in ▶ **Video 6.4B** (a 4-chamber and long-axis view) are shown. In the midesophageal 4-chamber view, there is an immobile mitral valve leaflet also confirmed in a long-axis view. With color flow Doppler imaging, there is a laterally directed eccentric jet and color flow through the mitral valve leaflet that is not thrombosed. Three-dimensional color Doppler imaging reconfirms this finding, demonstrating flow through the mobile leaflet and also the area of dehiscence (indicated by the double white arrows)—please review ▶ **Video 6.4C**. Hence, there is a thrombosed leaflet and a paravalvular leak due to dehiscence.

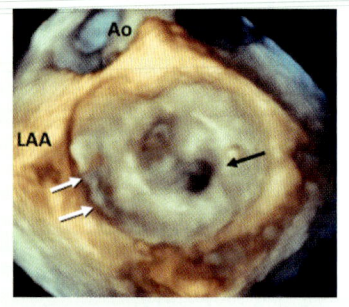

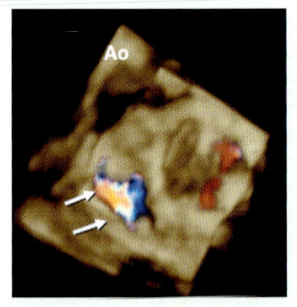

Figure 6.31. Three-dimensional echocardiogram from a left atrial orientation shows a mechanical prosthetic valve with one leaflet opening. With color flow Doppler, there is a large area of flow at 9 o'clock, which is an area of dehiscence (double arrows). (Ao, aorta; LAA, left atrial appendage).

KEY POINTS

- 3DE may aid in demonstrating a thrombosed mechanical leaflet.
- 3DE is able to demonstrate the exact site of valvular dehiscence for paravalvular regurgitation allowing for precise presurgical planning.

28. **Answer: D.** In this systolic phase, the mitral valve is seen from a left atrial orientation. Most of the P2 leaflet appears myxomatous, prolapsing into the left atrium. The P3 scallop tip is flail since the tip of the leaflet is directed superiorly to the left atrium.

    Figure 6.32 shows a 3D echocardiogram showing the mitral valve from a left atrial view. The arrow shows the flail P3 scallop.

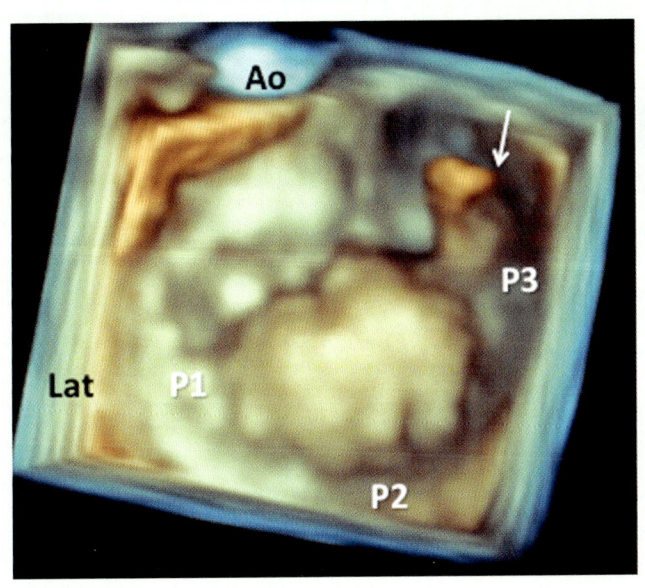

Figure 6.32

KEY POINTS

- 3DE is able to determine the involved mitral valve scallop and the presence of prolapse or flail.

29. **Answer: A.** Figure 6.19A shows a multiplanar reconstruction from a zoomed acquisition of the mitral valve. There are two orthogonal views on the top panels and in the bottom left panel, there is a short-axis plane that is placed at the tips of the mitral leaflets. This ability to place this plane at the tips of the mitral leaflets allows better accuracy and reproducibility of the mitral valve orifice area. From a left atrial perspective (**Figure 6.19B**), the posterior leaflet appears smooth and short. There is a calcific nodule on the A2 scallop. The lateral and medial commissures are sometimes seen from this left atrial view. Typically, the LV orientation (**Figure 6.19C**) demonstrates the nature of the commissures best. Here the medial commissure appears thickened with significant fusion compared with the lateral commissure, which has less thickening.

30. **Answer: E.** This patient who is symptomatic with severe mitral stenosis, moderate mitral regurgitation, and moderate aortic stenosis does not need further stress testing. This patient has maximum medical therapy with beta blockers and so further AV nodal blocking is not warranted. There is no mention of whether this patient had atrial fibrillation, a previous embolic event, or evidence of left atrial thrombus that are all class I indications for warfarin therapy. Since she has moderate mitral regurgitation, there are no indications for balloon mitral valvuloplasty and the patient should have a mitral valve and aortic valve replacement due to the concomitant aortic stenosis. A left atrial thrombus is usually an absolute contraindication, while a Wilkins score >8 may be a relative contraindication to mitral valvuloplasty.

KEY POINTS

- Mitral valve area determined by 3DE allows for improved accuracy and reproducibility due to confirmation of assessment done at the tips of the leaflets.

31. **Answer: C.** There is a combination of severe paravalvular regurgitation and mitral stenosis due to a vegetation that is obstructing flow through the bioprosthetic mitral valve. This increased gradient is reflected by the gradient using continuous-wave Doppler. There is a regurgitant jet originating outside the bioprosthetic valve and on 3DE, there is a bulky vegetation that spans from 9 o'clock till 12 o'clock. There is also a rocking of the mitral valve

prosthesis on 2D echocardiography, which is indicative of prosthetic valve dehiscence.

Figure 6.33 shows bioprosthetic valve vegetation with increased mitral valve mean gradient by continuous-wave Doppler (Panel A), paravalvular prosthetic regurgitation (Panel B), and 3DE of the mitral prosthesis and vegetation from a left atrial orientation (Panel C, white arrow).

32. **Answer: C.** The videos show three Amplatzer occluder devices adjacent to the posterior aspect of the prosthetic ring. These were implanted during the attempts at percutaneous paravalvular leak occlusion. While there is residual regurgitation between the occluder devices and prosthetic ring, it appears at most moderate in severity and was likely present immediately after the procedure. The regurgitant jet does demonstrate high velocities with aliasing, increasing the likelihood of significant hemolysis over time. The patient's blood hemoglobin concentration was found to be reduced to 5.7 g/dL. There is no evidence of stenosis as both mechanical valve leaflets appear to move freely. There does not appear to be any thrombus, vegetation, or pannus present.

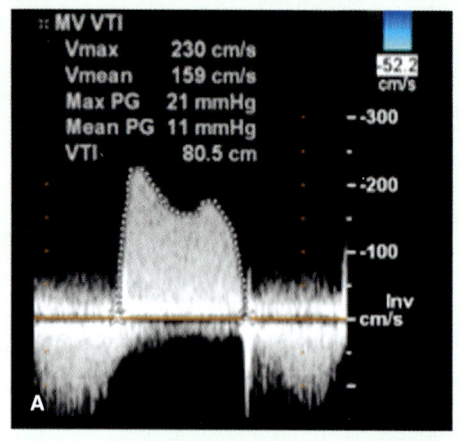

Figure 6.33A

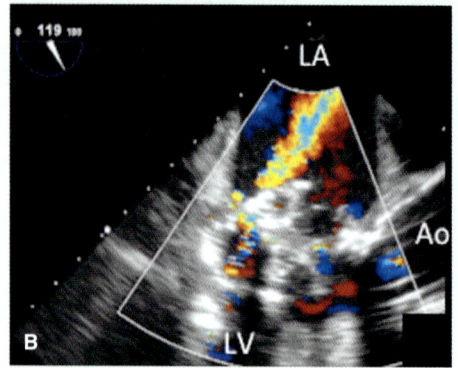

Figure 6.33B

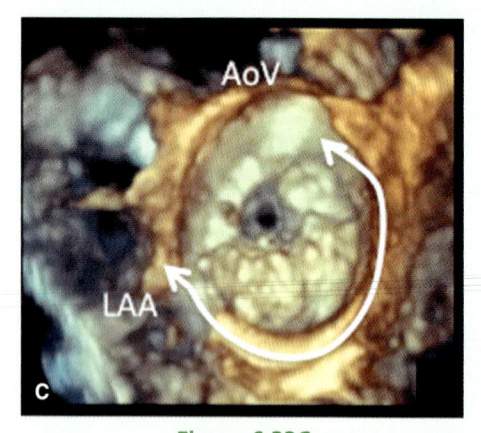

Figure 6.33C

> **KEY POINTS**
> - 3DE is valuable in determining the mechanism of prosthetic valve regurgitation and associated complications.

SUGGESTED READINGS

Altszuler D, Vainrib AF, Bamira DG, et al. Left atrial occlusion device implantation: the role of the echocardiographer. *Curr Cardiol Rep*. 2019;21(7):66.

Bruun NE, Habib G, Thuny F, Sogaard P. Cardiac imaging in infectious endocarditis. *Eur Heart J*. 2014;35(10):624-632.

Faletra FF, Saric M, Saw J, Lempereur M, Hanke T, Vannan MA. Imaging for patient's selection and guidance of LAA and ASD percutaneous and surgical closure. *JACC Cardiovasc Imaging*. 2021;14(1):3-21.

Gheorghe LL, Mobasseri S, Agricola E, et al. Imaging for native mitral valve surgical and transcatheter interventions. *JACC Cardiovasc Imaging*. 2021;14(1):112-127.

Hahn RT, Saric M, Faletra FF, et al. Recommended standards for the performance of transesophageal echocardiographic screening for structural heart intervention: from the American Society of echocardiography. *J Am Soc Echocardiogr*. 2022;35(1):1-76.

Hahn RT. State-of-the-art review of echocardiographic imaging in the evaluation and treatment of functional tricuspid regurgitation. *Circ Cardiovasc Imaging.* 2016;9(12):e005332.

Hung J, Lang R, Flachskampf F, et al. 3D echocardiography: a review of the current status and future directions. *J Am Soc Echocardiogr.* 2007;20(3):213-233.

Lang RM, Bierig M, Devereux RB, et al. Recommendations for chamber quantification: a report from the American Society of Echocardiography's guidelines and standards committee and the Chamber Quantification Writing Group, developed in conjunction with the European Association of Echocardiography, a branch of the European Society of Cardiology. *J Am Soc Echocardiogr.* 2005;18(12):1440-1463.

Lang RM, Tsang W, Weinert L, Mor-Avi V, Chandra S. Valvular heart disease. The value of 3-dimensional echocardiography. *J Am Coll Cardiol.* 2011;58(19):1933-1944.

Little SH, Rigolin VH, Garcia-Sayan E, et al. Recommendations for special competency in echocardiographic guidance of structural heart disease interventions: from the American Society of Echocardiography. *J Am Soc Echocardiogr.* 2023;36(4):350-365.

Mor-Avi V, Sugeng L, Lang RM. Real-time 3-dimensional echocardiography: an integral component of the routine echocardiographic examination in adult patients? *Circulation.* 2009;119(2):314-329.

Otto CM, Nishimura RA, Bonow RO, et al. 2020 ACC/AHA guideline for the management of patients with valvular heart disease: executive summary—a report of the American College of Cardiology/American Heart Association Joint committee on clinical practice guidelines. *Circulation.* 2021;143(5):e35-e71.

Perk G, Kronzon I. Interventional echocardiography in structural heart disease. *Curr Cardiol Rep.* 2013;15(3):338.

Skolnick A, Vavas E, Kronzon I. Optimization of ASD assessment using real time three-dimensional transesophageal echocardiography. *Echocardiography.* 2009;26(2):233-235.

Vaidyanathan B, Simpson JM, Kumar RK. Transesophageal echocardiography for device closure of atrial septal defects: case selection, planning, and procedural guidance. *JACC Cardiovasc Imag.* 2009;2(10):1238-1242.

Vainrib AF, Harb SC, Jaber W, et al. Left atrial appendage occlusion/exclusion: procedural image guidance with transesophageal echocardiography. *J Am Soc Echocardiogr.* 2018;31(4):454-474.

Zoghbi WA, Asch FM, Bruce C, et al. Guidelines for the evaluation of valvular regurgitation after percutaneous valve repair or replacement: a report from the American Society of Echocardiography developed in collaboration with the Society for Cardiovascular Angiography and Interventions, Japanese Society of Echocardiography, and Society for Cardiovascular Magnetic Resonance. *J Am Soc Echocardiogr.* 2019;32(4):431-475.

CHAPTER 7

Transesophageal Echocardiography and Intraoperative Echocardiography

Ben Alencherry, Nakul S. Kumar, and L. Leonardo Rodriguez

QUESTIONS

1. In the midesophageal transesophageal echocardiography (TEE) short-axis view of the aortic valve:
   A. The noncoronary cusp is the most anterior cusp.
   B. The left coronary cusp is the most anterior cusp.
   C. The right coronary cusp is adjacent to the interatrial septum.
   D. The noncoronary cusp is adjacent to the interatrial septum.

2. During TEE guidance of a transseptal puncture, the two-dimensional view to best direct the needle anteriorly or posteriorly is:
   A. Midesophageal 4-chamber view.
   B. Bicaval view.
   C. Short-axis view at the level of the aortic valve.
   D. Midesophageal 5-chamber view.

3. Which of the following statements is **CORRECT** regarding TEE findings in patients with atrial fibrillation?
   A. Cardioversion can be safely performed without anticoagulation if the TEE is negative for thrombus.
   B. Spontaneous echo contrast is common and does not offer independent prognostic value.
   C. Spontaneous echo contrast is highly associated with previous stroke or peripheral embolism in patients with atrial fibrillation.
   D. Surgical ligation (by all techniques) excludes flow into the left atrial appendage (LAA) in >90% of the cases.

4. Which is a **TRUE** statement regarding TEE complications?
   A. The mortality is 0.1% to 0.2%.
   B. Esophageal perforation occurs in 0.4% to 0.9%.
   C. Major bleeding occurs in <0.01%.
   D. Heart failure occurs in 0.5%.

5. Which of the following statements is **CORRECT** regarding methemoglobinemia occurring after benzocaine topical anesthetic for TEE?
   A. Oxygen saturation is low, arterial Po_2 is normal, and there is no cyanosis.
   B. There is no cyanosis, low oxygen saturation, and low arterial Po_2.
   C. Higher levels (methemoglobin level >70%) may result in dysrhythmias, circulatory failure, neurologic depression, and death.
   D. Treatment of choice is 100% oxygen.

6. Which of the following is an absolute contraindication for TEE?
   A. History of radiation to the neck and mediastinum.
   B. History of gastrointestinal surgery.
   C. Barrett esophagus.
   D. Esophageal diverticulum.

7. The pulmonary valve can be best visualized from which of the following standard transesophageal views?
   A. Midesophageal short-axis.
   B. Midesophageal bicaval.
   C. Transgastric right ventricular inflow.
   D. Transgastric long-axis.

8. Intraoperative air embolization to a coronary artery is more often associated with wall motion abnormalities in which coronary territory?
   A. Right coronary artery.
   B. Left anterior descending artery.
   C. Left circumflex artery.
   D. Global regions.

9. In a patient with a known severe esophageal stricture with dysphagia, what should be done regarding intraoperative echocardiography?
   A. Passage of the TEE probe can proceed as usual, because the risk of perforation is low.
   B. Use of a pediatric probe is the only way to do a TEE.
   C. Epicardial echo is an alternative imaging modality.
   D. A standard TEE probe can be used, but it should not be passed beyond the gastroesophageal junction.
   E. Intraoperative echocardiography is not recommended.

10. Intraoperative TEE during implantation of a left ventricular assist device (LVAD) is useful for:
    A. Exclusion of mitral regurgitation (MR), which makes the LVAD ineffective.
    B. Deciding on the location of the inflow cannula into the left ventricle.
    C. Exclusion of significant aortic regurgitation, which reduces LVAD effectiveness.
    D. Quantitation of tricuspid regurgitation (TR).

11. Immediately after implantation of a stented bioprosthesis, the most common transient abnormality is:
    A. Minimal amounts of periprosthetic regurgitation.
    B. Immobility of valve prosthetic leaflets.
    C. Moderate central prosthetic regurgitation.
    D. LV outflow tract obstruction by mitral prosthetic stents.

12. What are the high-risk findings for recurrent aortic regurgitation after aortic valve repair?
    A. Level of cusp coaptation <9 mm and cusp coaptation height <4 mm.
    B. Level of cusp coaptation >9 mm and cusp coaptation height >4 mm.
    C. Aortic annulus <25 mm and cusp coaptation height >4 mm.
    D. Aortic annulus <25 mm and level of cusp coaptation >9 mm.

13. A 70-year-old man presents with chest and back pain and a computed tomographic scan discovers a localized dissection of the distal ascending aorta. On arrival for the intraoperative TEE, you find aortic dilation but no dissection. What is the cause of the "blind spot" for TEE imaging?
    A. The esophagus is between the aorta and the right mainstem bronchus.
    B. The esophagus is between the aorta and trachea.
    C. The trachea is between the aorta and the esophagus.
    D. The left mainstem bronchus is between the aorta and the esophagus.

14. Which of the following TEE views best guide transseptal puncture performed during a MitraClip procedure?
    A. Midesophageal (ME) bicaval view, ME short-axis view, ME 4-chamber view.
    B. ME bicaval view, ME long-axis view, ME 4-chamber view.
    C. ME short-axis view, ME bicaval view, deep transgastric view.
    D. ME bicommissural view, ME bicaval view, ME SAX view.

126 / Clinical Echocardiography Review

15. When encountering resistance to insertion of the TEE probe in the midesophagus, which of the following maneuvers is recommended?
    A. Withdraw the probe to the mouth and reinsert.
    B. Withdraw the probe slightly, anteflex, and try again to advance the probe forward.
    C. Withdraw the probe slightly, retroflex, and try again to advance the probe forward.
    D. Withdraw the probe and recommend an endoscopy.

16. A TEE is performed for source of stroke in a young otherwise healthy male. The TEE does not identify any definite source of stroke. By color Doppler and agitated saline, no patent foramen ovale (PFO) is seen. Which of the following statements is **CORRECT**? See **Figure 7.1**.
    A. No source of embolism is seen.
    B. A potential source of embolism is seen.
    C. A definite source of embolism is seen.

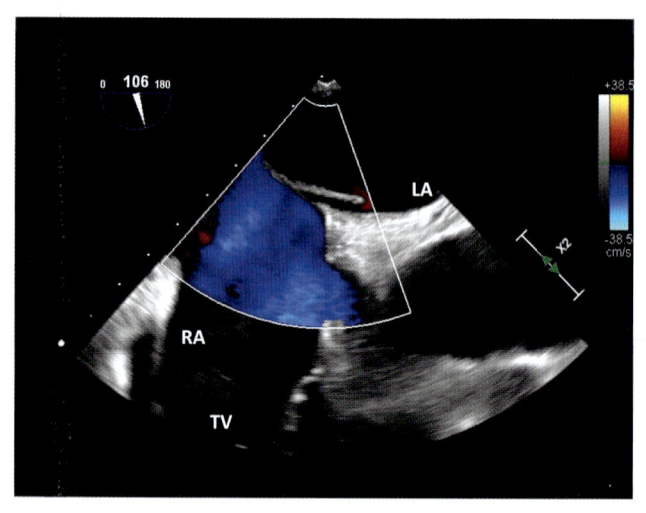

Figure 7.1

17. A TEE is performed prior to cardioversion of recent onset atrial fibrillation. A 4-chamber midesophageal view with retroflexion and mild probe advancement is obtained. The *arrow* points to what finding (see **Figure 7.2**)?
    A. Thrombus.
    B. Vegetation.
    C. Eustachian valve.
    D. Thebesian valve.

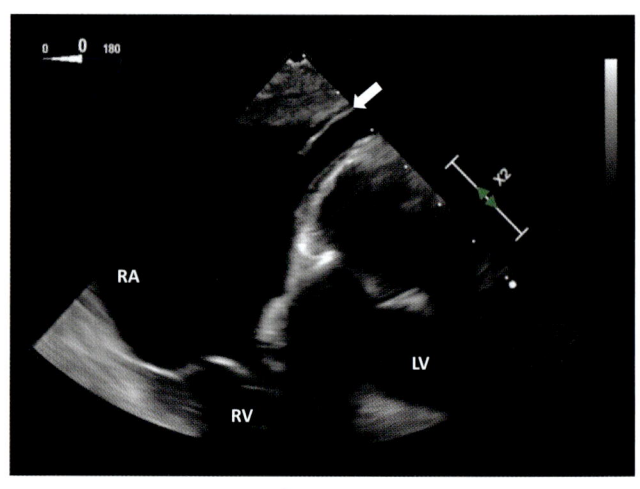

Figure 7.2

18. This color Doppler image (**Figure 7.3**) of the pulmonary vein bifurcation (midesophageal, 110° view) most likely represents:
    A. The left pulmonary veins.
    B. The right pulmonary veins.
    C. The right and left upper pulmonary veins.
    D. The right lower and left lower pulmonary veins.

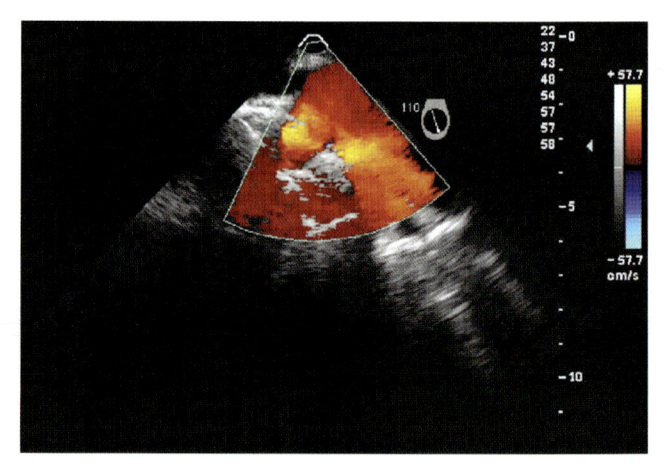

Figure 7.3

19. Which of the following structures is visualized in **Figure 7.4**?
    A. Right coronary artery.
    B. Periaortic abscess.
    C. Anomalous origin of the left main coronary artery.
    D. Normal left main trunk.

Figure 7.4

20. The abnormality of the aortic valve seen in **Figure 7.5** is consistent with:
  A. Rheumatic aortic valve disease.
  B. Normal bioprosthetic valve.
  C. Bicuspid aortic valve.
  D. Unicuspid aortic valve.

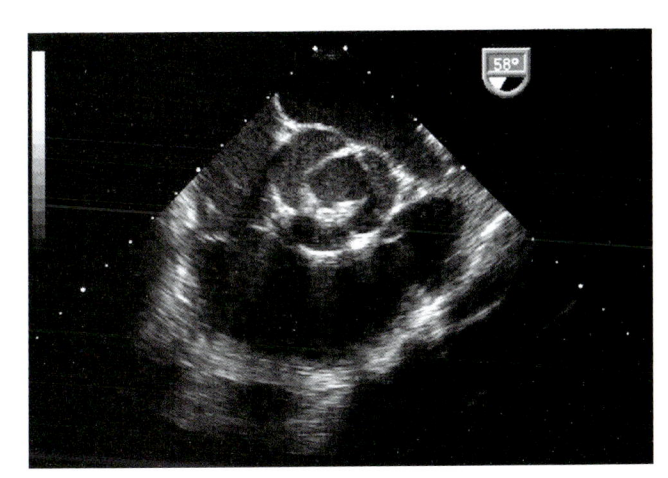

Figure 7.5

21. **Figure 7.6A, B** were acquired minutes apart. What is the most likely explanation for the difference between **Figure 7.6A** and **Figure 7.6B**?
  A. Phenylephrine infusion.
  B. Change in equipment settings.
  C. Failed mitral valve repair.
  D. Systolic anterior motion of the mitral valve.

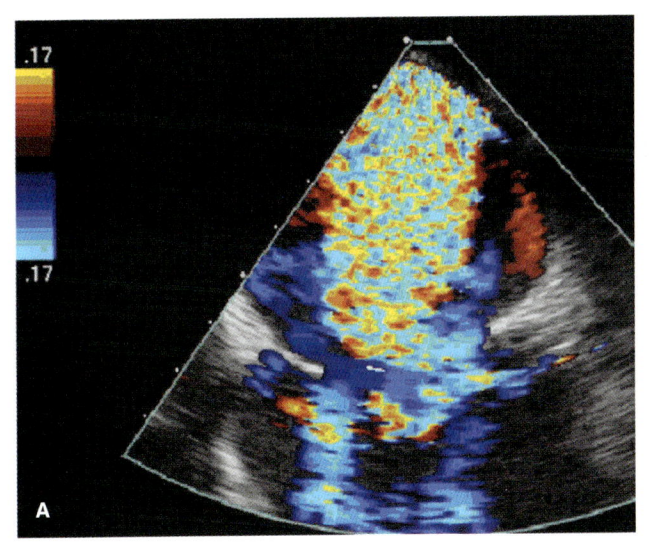

Figure 7.6A

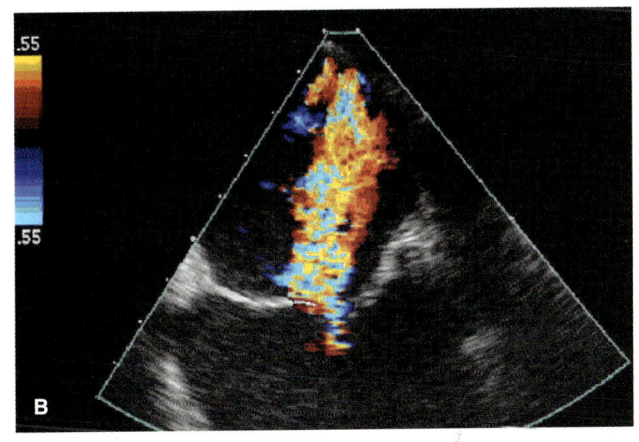

Figure 7.6B

22. A 67-year-old man undergoes echocardiographic assessment after aortic valvular replacement. Which type of valve replacement is seen in **Figure 7.7**?
  A. Aortic homograft.
  B. Stented bioprosthetic valve.
  C. Mechanical On-X valve.
  D. Mechanical Bentall.

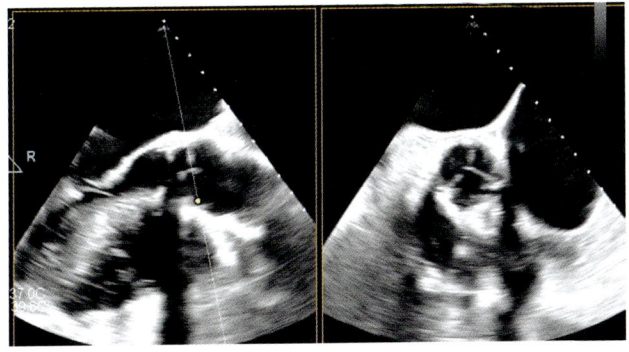

Figure 7.7

128 / Clinical Echocardiography Review

23. Which of the following measurements is a predictor for the pathology shown in the following images, **Figure 7.8A,B**?

A. Anterior-to-posterior leaflet height ratio of 2:1.
B. Coaptation (C)-septal distance of 2.4 cm.
C. Posterior leaflet height of 1.2 cm.
D. LV end-diastolic diameter of 5 cm.

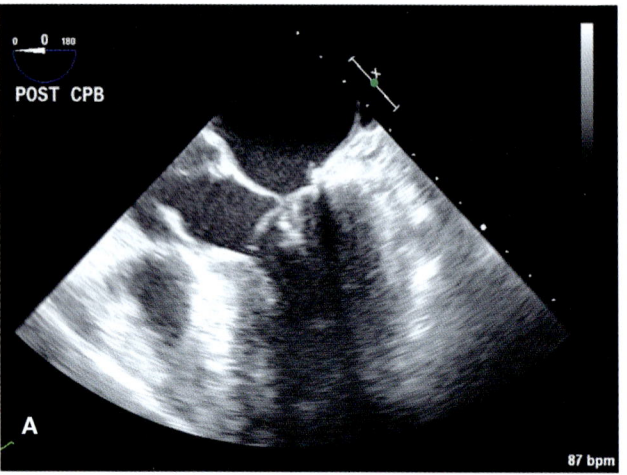

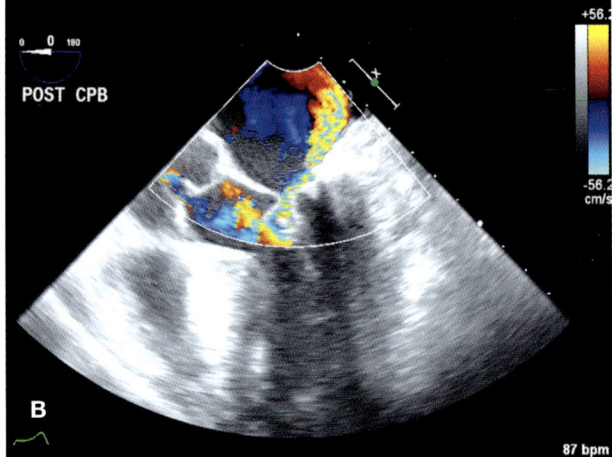

Figure 7.8

24. Which of the following measurements best represents the recommendation for depth of an Impella 5.5 insertion shown in **Figure 7.9**?
A. 2.0 cm.
B. 3.5 cm.
C. 5.0 cm.
D. 6.5 cm.

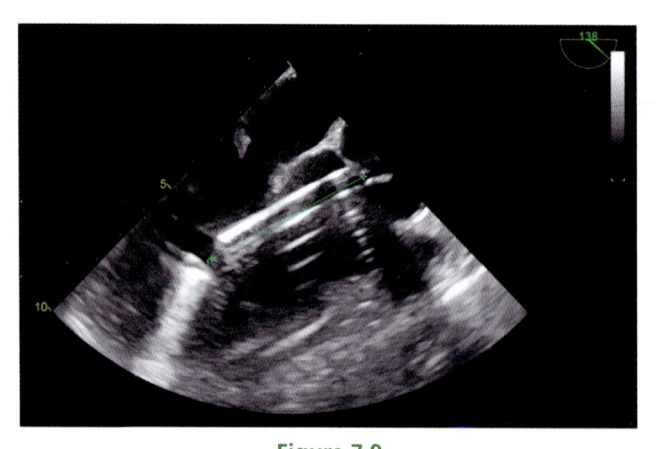

Figure 7.9

25. A 70-year-old woman with previous aortic and tricuspid valve replacements presents with leg edema and ascites, with clear lung fields. The frames in **Figure 7.10A, B** are recorded from a midesophageal TEE transverse 4-chamber view at a multiplane angle of 0°, rotated to the right to view the right atrium and right ventricle.
From where is the high-velocity flow originating?
A. Pulmonary artery.
B. Aorta.
C. Right ventricle.
D. Coronary sinus.

Chapter 7 Transesophageal Echocardiography and Intraoperative Echocardiography / 129

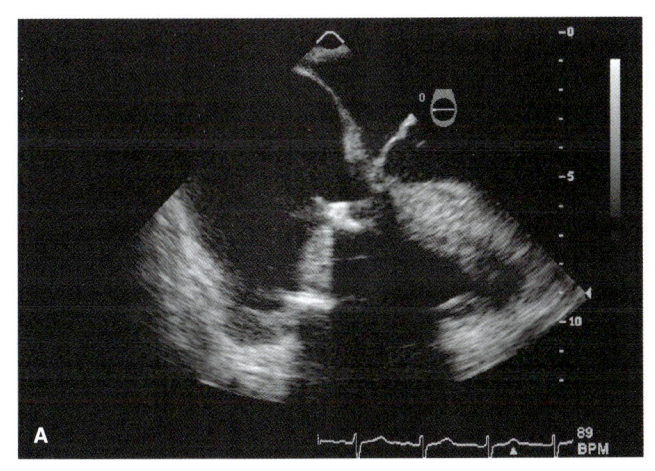

Figure 7.10A

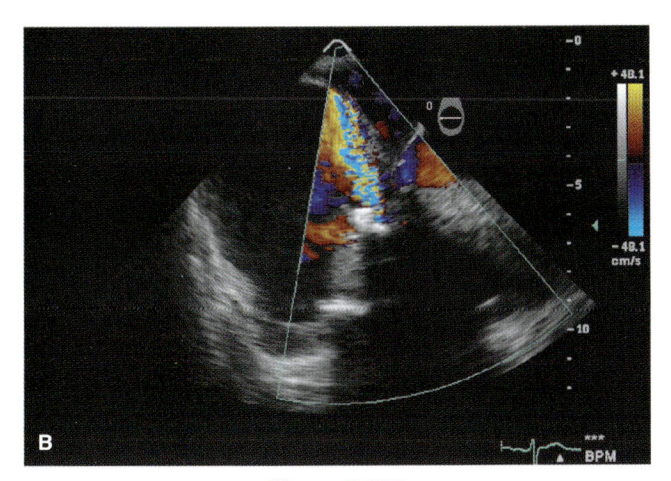

Figure 7.10B

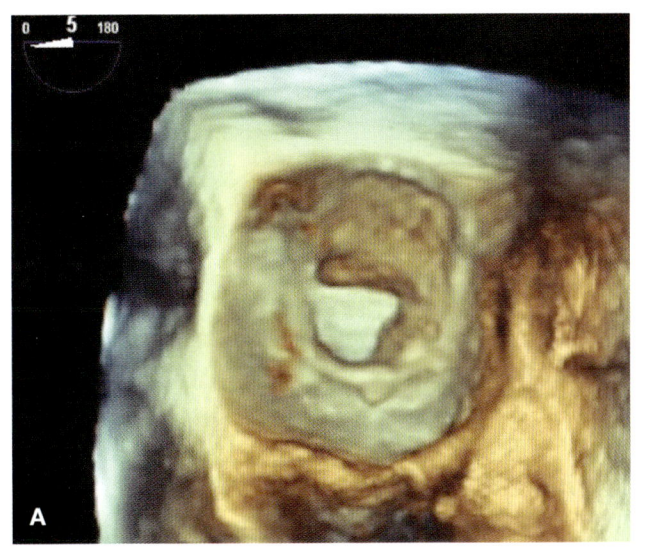

Figure 7.11A

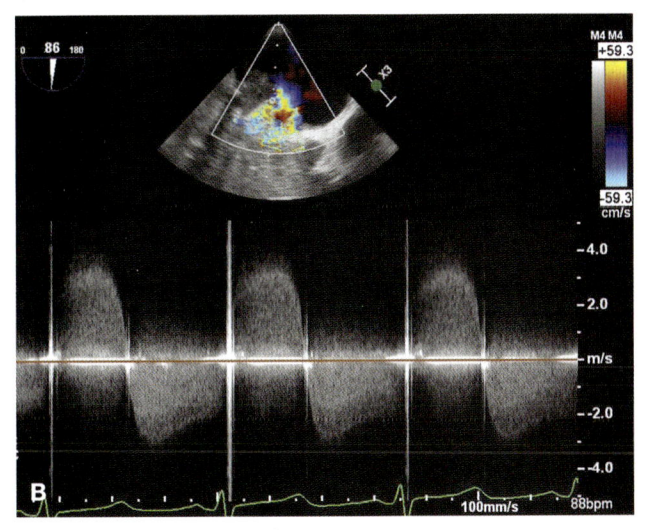

Figure 7.11B

26. A 55-year-old man with a previous St. Jude bileaflet mechanical mitral prosthesis stopped his warfarin and presented to the hospital with pulmonary edema and hypotension. He was taken directly to the operating room. A three-dimensional intraoperative transesophageal echo of the mitral valve from the left atrial perspective is shown in **Figure 7.11A**. A continuous-wave Doppler through the prosthesis is shown in **Figure 7.11B**.
What has occurred?
   A. A mitral prosthetic disc has embolized, leaving severe regurgitation and secondarily a high antegrade velocity.
   B. A tumor has overlapped the mitral prosthesis, likely an atrial myxoma.
   C. A clot has formed on the valve causing moderate stenosis.
   D. A clot has formed on the valve with severe mitral stenosis and some mitral regurgitation.

27. A 55-year-old woman was studied with a prepump TEE prior to tricuspid and mitral valve surgery. **Figure 7.12A,B** was recorded from a long-axis view of the atrial septum after intravenous injection of agitated saline.
What can be said about the presence of shunting?
   A. There is a right-to-left shunt.
   B. There is a left-to-right shunt.
   C. There is no shunt.
   D. There is a bidirectional shunt.

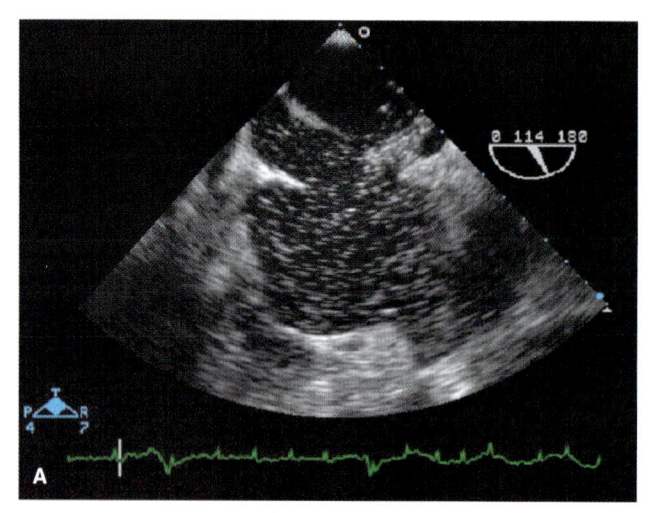

Figure 7.12A

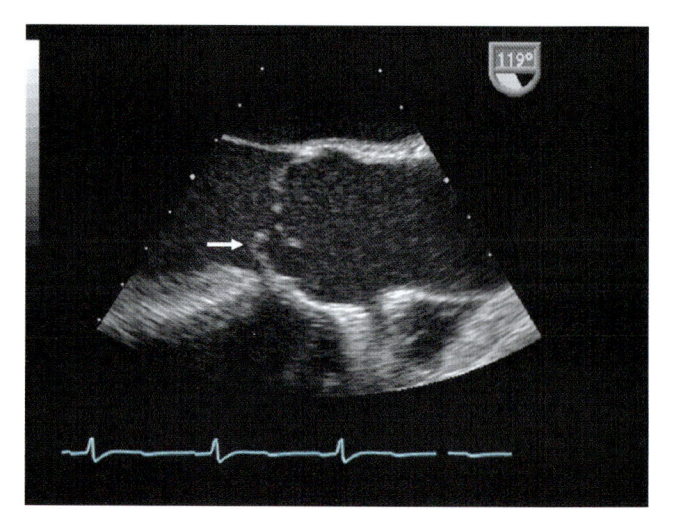

Figure 7.13

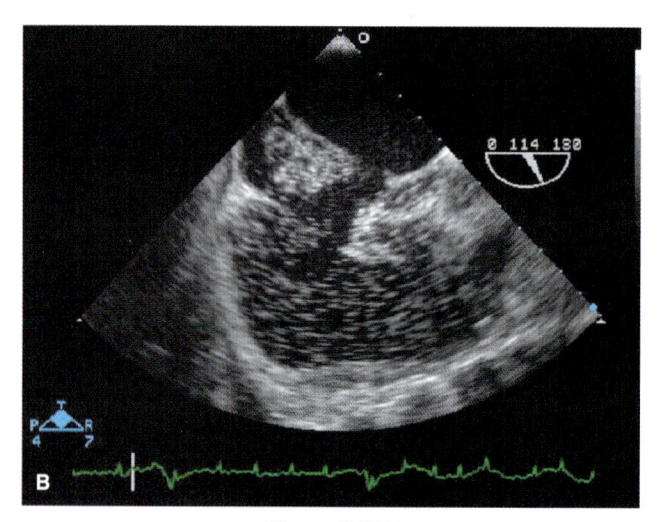

Figure 7.12B

28. The use of intraoperative TEE in patients during CABG:
    A. Lacks benefits when performed routinely.
    B. Decreases morbidity but not mortality.
    C. Decreases mortality particularly in high-risk patients.
    D. Decreases mortality only in patients with associated tricuspid regurgitation.

29. A 32-year-old man is undergoing valve surgery and has a TEE with this midesophageal long-axis view of the aortic valve (**Figure 7.13**). What is the structure to which the small *arrow* points in **Figure 7.13**?
    A. An aortic valve vegetation.
    B. A prolapsing noncoronary cusp.
    C. A fibroelastoma.
    D. A portion of the patient's bicuspid aortic valve.

30. ▶ Video 7.1 and **Figure 7.14** show the ascending aorta on the prepump intraoperative TEE. As indicated, the diameter of the tubular ascending aorta is 4.0 cm. What is the echo-free space posterior to the ascending aorta highlighted by the *arrow* in **Figure 7.14**?
    A. A double lumen consistent with a small localized aortic dissection.
    B. A pericardial cyst.
    C. A reflection of the pericardium with small amount of normal pericardial fluid.
    D. The transverse portion of the hemiazygos vein.

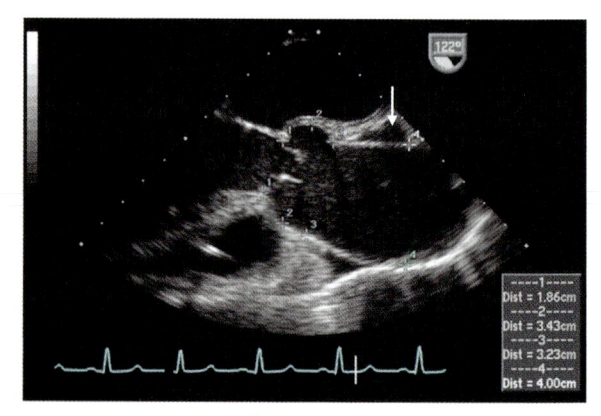

Figure 7.14

CASE 1

A 50-year-old woman is evaluated for right ventricular dilatation (see ▶ Video 7.2A,B).

31. The finding shown in **Figure 7.15** of the patient from **Case 1** is frequently associated with:
    A. Cleft anterior mitral valve.
    B. Normal variant.
    C. Anomalous pulmonary drainage.
    D. Continuous murmur.

Chapter 7 Transesophageal Echocardiography and Intraoperative Echocardiography / 131

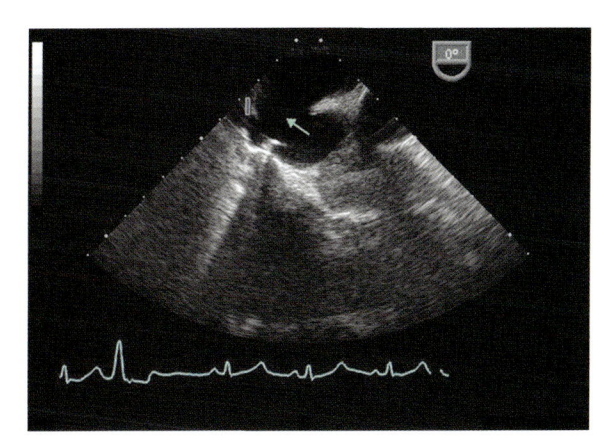

Figure 7.15

32. The pathology from **Question 31** for the patient in **Case 1** often requires:
A. Medical management.
B. Surgical closure.
C. Percutaneous closure.
D. No treatment.

CASE 2

A 65-year-old patient with atrial fibrillation underwent a TEE prior to cardioversion.

33. What does the structure incidentally found and marked with the *arrow* in **Figure 7.16** represent for the patient in **Case 2** (See also ▶ **Video 7.3**.)?
A. Descending aorta.
B. Aneurysm of the circumflex artery.
C. Left lower pulmonary vein.
D. Dilated coronary sinus.

34. The best way to corroborate the diagnosis for the patient in **Case 2** is:
A. Coronary angiogram.
B. Agitated saline injected through the left arm.
C. Transthoracic echocardiogram with microbubbles (contrast).
D. Posterior rotation of the probe and longitudinal view of the aorta.

CASE 3

A 46-year-old patient with a history of prior aortic valve replacement (AVR) and coronary artery bypass grafting (CABG) has developed severe mitral regurgitation.

35. For the patient in **Case 3**, the midesophageal long-axis view in **Figure 7.17A** and 3D echocardiography view in **Figure 7.17B** shows:
A. Commissural mitral regurgitation.
B. A small atrial septal defect (ASD).
C. Mitral stenosis.
D. Anterior mitral leaflet perforation.

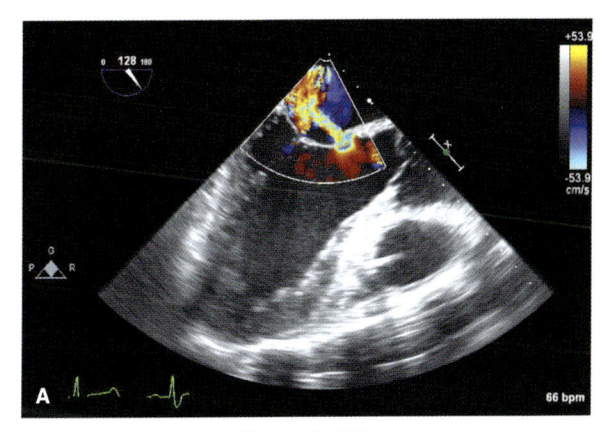

Figure 7.17A

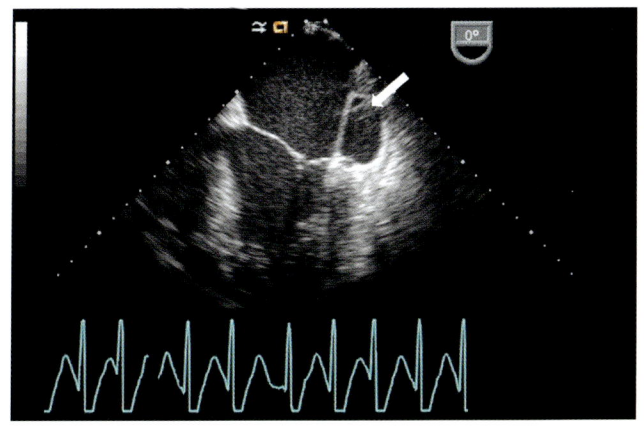

Figure 7.16

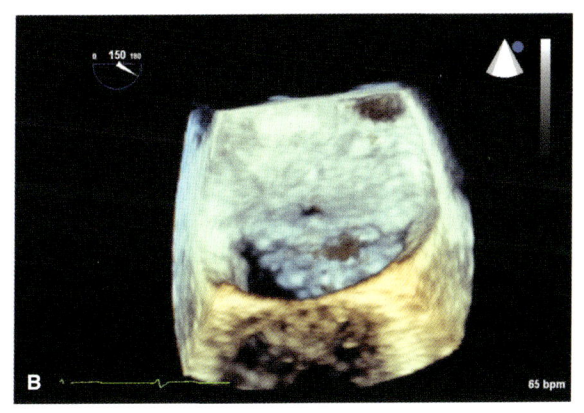

Figure 7.17B

CASE 4

An asymptomatic patient underwent a TEE because of an abnormality suspected on a prior TTE.

36. For the patient in **Case 4**, a midesophageal view of the aortic valve in **Figure 7.18A,B** (and ▶ **Video 7.4**) shows:
    A. Sinus of Valsalva aneurysm of the right coronary sinus.
    B. Quadricuspid aortic valve.
    C. Periaortic abscess.
    D. Ruptured noncoronary sinus into the right atrium.

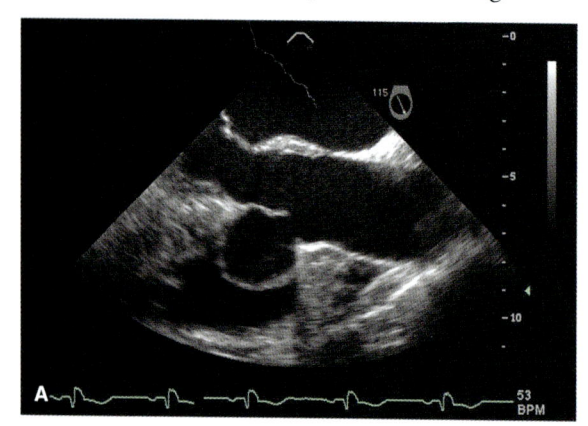

Figure 7.18A

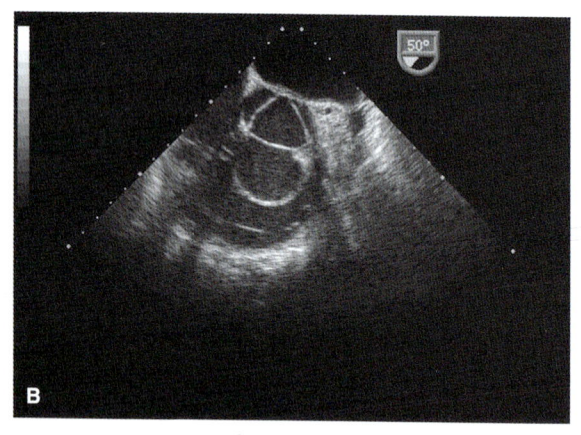

Figure 7.18B

CASE 5

▶ **Video 7.5A-J** *pertains to a 71-year-old man who presents with progressive weakness, associated with fever of 1-week duration. He also gives a 2-month history of progressive abdominal swelling and leg edema. Four years ago, he underwent a tissue aortic valve replacement and mitral valve repair for aortic stenosis and posterior mitral prolapse. Physical examination on admission revealed BP of 162/88 mm Hg, temperature of 39°, severe jugular venous distention with "V" waves in the jugular pulse contour, a pulsatile liver, a moderate diastolic murmur, Roth spots, and Janeway lesions. He was taken to the operating room several days later, and this TEE was recorded.*

37. ▶ **Video 7.5A,B** from the patient in **Case 5** shows two views from a prepump intraoperative TEE in the midesophageal 4-chamber view. What is the severity of the TR at the time of this study?
    A. No TR.
    B. Mild TR.
    C. Moderate TR.
    D. Severe TR.

38. For the patient in **Case 5**, presuming that he had significant tricuspid regurgitation (TR) prior to surgery, evidenced by the "V" waves in his jugular vein pressure waveform, the leg edema, and the pulsatile liver, what has changed, as of the intraoperative echo?
    A. He has become volume overloaded and hypertensive.
    B. He has become volume overloaded and hypotensive.
    C. He has become volume depleted and hypertensive.
    D. He has become volume depleted and hypotensive.

39. For the patient in **Case 5**, the three-dimensional echocardiographic structural image in ▶ **Video 7.5E** shows that the echo lucent space is posterior to the aortic prosthesis. Where and what is this space?
    A. Periprosthetic pseudoaneurysm within the posterior mitral annulus.
    B. Periprosthetic abscess within the intervalvular fibrosa.
    C. Periprosthetic abscess within the posterior mitral annulus.
    D. Periprosthetic abscess within the coronary sinus.
    E. An aneurysm of the coronary artery.

40. The patient in **Case 5** underwent AVR with a homograft (a cryopreserved human cadaver valve), tricuspid valve repair with an annuloplasty, and mitral valve repair with an annuloplasty (▶ **Video 7.5I,J**). The hinging side of the anterior mitral valve was sutured to the homograft tissue and reinforced by suturing to it a new mitral annuloplasty band. Besides providing tissue for the intervalvular fibrosa for the mitral valve attachments, what other advantages, compared to a stented bioprosthesis, does the AVR homograft have in this case?
    A. Reduction in postoperative infection.
    B. Higher gradient.
    C. Less regurgitation.
    D. Easier implantation.
    E. More available.

ANSWERS

1. **Answer: D.** The noncoronary cusp is adjacent to the interatrial septum. The midesophageal TEE short-axis view allows detailed visualization of the aortic valve anatomy. In typical trileaflet aortic valves, the right coronary cusp is the most anterior cusp (farthest from the transducer).

2. **Answer: C.** Guidance of percutaneous interventions in structural heart disease is an expanding indication for TEE. Some of these procedures require a transseptal puncture (eg, mitral valve procedures and left atrial appendage closure). Correct placement of the needle for transseptal puncture is paramount for the safety of the procedure. To avoid aortic puncture, the needle has to be manipulated posteriorly. The best two-dimensional view for guidance in the anterior-posterior direction is the short-axis view at the level of the aortic valve. See **Figure 7.19** showing optimal sites for transseptal puncture for intracardiac interventions.

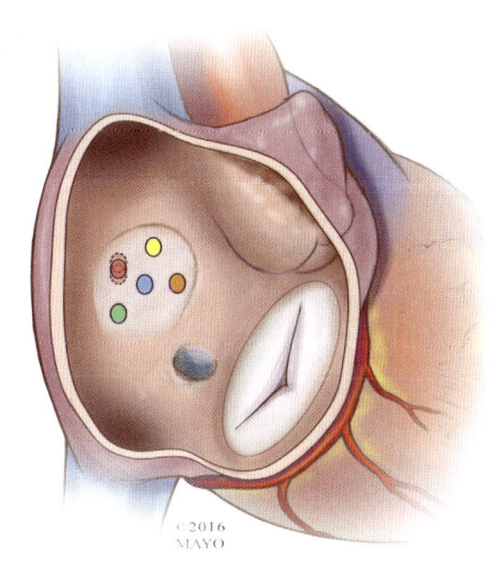

Figure 7.19. Red: MitraClip, paravalvular leak closure (a higher crossing site is recommended for medial leaks, and a lower crossing site is recommended for lateral leaks; dashed red circles). Yellow: transseptal patent foramen ovale closure. Blue: percutaneous left ventricular assist device placement, hemodynamic studies. Green: left atrial appendage closure. Orange: pulmonary vein interventions. (Site-Specific Transseptal Puncture for Various Intracardiac Interventions. From Alkhouli M, Rihal CS, Holmes DR Jr. Transseptal techniques for emerging structural heart interventions. *JACC Cardiovasc Interv*. 2016;9(24):2465-2480. Used with permission of Mayo Foundation for Medical Education and Research. All rights reserved.)

3. **Answer: C.** In patients with atrial fibrillation, the presence of severe spontaneous contrast or smoke is a marker of increased risk of thromboembolic events. Electrical cardioversion causes left atrial appendage stunning with increased severity of echo contrast immediately after the procedure. There have been published case series of embolic stroke after cardioversion in patients with a negative TEE for left atrial thrombus who are not anticoagulated. For that reason, patients should have therapeutic levels of anticoagulation before proceeding with cardioversion. Depending on the surgical technique of left atrial appendage closure, there can be varying rates of residual flow between the left atrium (LA) and LAA, ranging from 10% to 55% in older series of suture exclusion of the appendage. However, recent occlusion devices with a LAA clip have found >90% success rate.

4. **Answer: C.** TEE is a safe technique in the proper setting and in experienced hands. The overall incidence of complications is very low (0.18%-2.8%). The highest complication rates (>10%) are hoarseness and lip injury. Overall mortality is <0.02%. These incidences are roughly similar between diagnostic TEE and intraoperative TEE (**Table 7.1**).

Table 7.1. Diagnostic TEE and Intraoperative TEE Mortality

Complication	Diagnostic TEE	Intraoperative TEE
Overall complication rate	0.18%-2.8%	0.2%
Mortality	<0.01%-0.02%	0%
Major morbidity	0.2%	0%-1.2%
Major bleeding	<0.01%	0.03%-0.8%
Esophageal perforation	<0.01%	0%-0.3%
Tracheal intubation	0.02%	
Heart failure	0.05%	
Hoarseness	12%	
Dental injury	0.1%	0.03%

TEE, transesophageal echocardiography
Adapted from Hahn RT, Abraham T, Adams MS, et al. Guidelines for performing a comprehensive transesophageal echocardiographic examination: recommendations from the American Society of Echocardiography and the Society of Cardiovascular Anesthesiologists. *J Am Soc Echocardiogr*. 2013;26(9):921-964. Copyright © 2013 by the American Society of Echocardiography. With permission.

5. **Answer: C.** Methemoglobinemia related to benzocaine topical anesthetic given during TEE is a rare reaction occurring in 0.07% to 0.12% of patients. Methemoglobin levels are elevated due to conversion of iron from a reduced to oxidized form of hemoglobin, which results in poor oxygen-carrying capacity. This results in cyanosis, low oxygen saturation levels, and normal arterial Po_2 levels. Patients with methemoglobin levels >70% may develop circulatory collapse, neurologic depression, and death. The treatment of choice is intravenous methylene blue 1% solution (10 mg/mL) 1 to 2 mg/kg administered intravenously slowly for more than 5 minutes, followed by intravenous flush with normal saline.

6. Answer: D. There are a few absolute contraindications to TEE, including esophageal or pharyngeal obstruction, esophageal diverticulum, active gastrointestinal bleeding from an unknown source, and perforated viscus. The list of relative contraindications is extensive, including esophageal varices, history of radiation to the neck, Barrett esophagus, and coagulopathy. When these arise in an individual patient case, it is important to balance the strength of indication with the relative risks of the procedure. Furthermore, there are ways to modify the procedure to still add clinical value, for example, avoiding transgastric views in those patients with small or medium nonbleeding esophageal varices (**Table 7.2**).

Table 7.2. TEE Contraindications

Pathology	Absolute Contraindication
Upper GI bleed—gastric	<1 mo duration; for transgastric views, consider GI consult
Esophageal stricture or dysphagia	Significant esophageal dysphagia, unable to tolerate secretions, requiring G tube for feeding
Esophagitis/peptic ulcer disease	Grade C-D esophagitis, acute, symptomatic
Neck/mediastinum radiation	Dysphagia, active esophagitis, radiation <4 wk
Esophageal surgery	Dysphagia and surgery <6 mo. With esophagectomy, consider GI or thoracic surgery clearance
Esophageal stent	Contraindicated
S/p fundoplication	Surgery <6 wk; needs surgical clearance
S/p bariatric or gastric surgery	Surgery <6 wk; needs surgical clearance
Perforated esophagus or stomach	Unrepaired or <6 wk from repair
Esophageal tumor	Requires gastroenterologist or thoracic surgeon consult
Unrepaired esophageal diverticulum	Requires imaging or consultation
Neck immobility	Uncleared or unstable C-spine

GI, gastrointestinal, s/p, status post; TEE, transesophageal echocardiography.
Adapted from Mishra KL, Baker MT, Siegrist KK. Multidisciplinary approach to improving safety in transesophageal echocardiography in patients with relative contraindications. *J Am Soc Echocardiogr*. 2022;35:1195. Copyright © 2022 by the American Society of Echocardiography. With permission.

7. Answer: A. The pulmonary valve is anterior, and thus, far-field structure for TEE. This can make it more challenging to visualize because of interference from other structures such as the bronchus. The midesophageal short-axis view is one of the most common views for imaging the pulmonary valve. **Figure 7.20** shows the midesophageal short-axis view and other common TEE views that are used to visualize the pulmonary valve. These views are commonly utilized during pulmonary valve transcatheter interventions and to rule out pulmonary valve endocarditis.

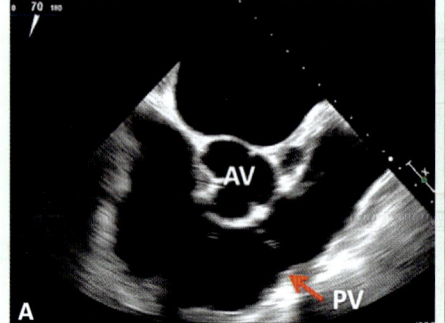

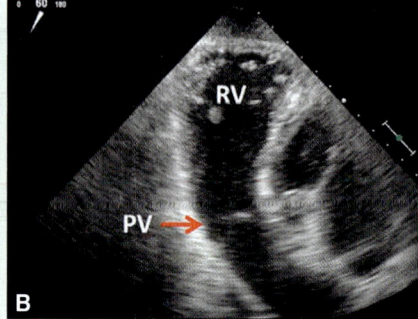

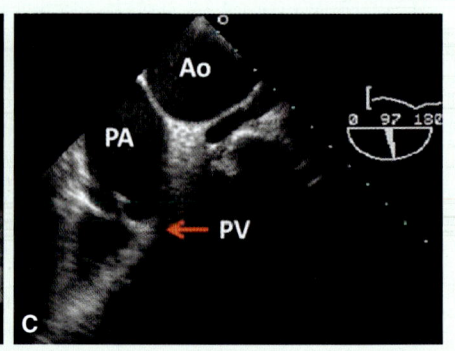

Figure 7.20. Pulmonary valve imaging from the midesophageal right ventricular (RV) inflow-outflow view (A, red arrow), transgastric basal RV view (B, red arrow), and upper esophageal aortic arch short-axis view (C, red arrow). (Reprinted from Hahn RT, Abraham T, Adams MS, et al. Guidelines for performing a comprehensive transesophageal echocardiographic examination: recommendations from the American Society of Echocardiography and the Society of Cardiovascular Anesthesiologists. *J Am Soc Echocardiogr*. 2013;26(9):921-964. Copyright © 2013 by the American Society of Echocardiography. With permission.)

8. **Answer: A.** The right coronary artery is located anteriorly within the sinuses of Valsalva, which is the highest portion of the aorta (farthest off the ground) with the patient in the supine position for a midsternal thoracotomy. Therefore, air that enters the heart during open-heart surgery is pushed by pressure into this coronary preferentially. This occurs more commonly in mitral repair than in other types of heart surgery, because of insufflation of the left ventricle (filling it with fluid under pressure) done to examine leaflet coaptation. Most cases of coronary air embolization can be treated conservatively. Sometimes, it is necessary to put the patient back on cardiopulmonary bypass (CPB) or to treat ventricular arrhythmias pharmacologically.

9. **Answer: C.** The need for intraoperative echo still exists for those who have a contraindication to blind TEE passage, and these can readily be accomplished by epicardial echo. A standard transthoracic echo transducer is placed within a sterile sleeve with ultrasound gel inside the sleeve for elimination of air. It has been suggested that those with esophageal stricture and no dysphagia represent a relative contraindication to TEE, and it would be reasonable to proceed cautiously with TEE in those situations.

10. **Answer: C.** Intraoperative TEE is an important monitoring tool for patients undergoing implantation of an LVAD. The presence of aortic regurgitation (AR) makes an LVAD ineffective because the AR would return blood back to the left ventricular (LV) cannula without providing systemic arterial perfusion. The presence of LV enlargement and mitral regurgitation (MR) is irrelevant to the placement of the device. Placement of the inflow LVAD cannula into the left ventricle does not require TEE guidance. The presence and severity of tricuspid regurgitation (TR) are less important objectives of TEE.

11. **Answer: A.** It is common to see one or more small color jets of periprosthetic regurgitation early after cessation of cardiopulmonary bypass. When small, these resolve progressively after protamine administration or within a few hours.

12. **Answer: A.** There are several factors after aortic valve repair that help predict success of repair. In the midesophageal long-axis view, a distance from the aortic annulus to the leaflet tips greater than 9 mm has a high probability of near normal aortic valve function. In the same view, cusp coaptation height ≥4 mm predicts a minimal likelihood of moderate or severe AR at long-term follow-up. Finally, a large aortic annulus ≥25 mm has been associated with a high failure rate. See **Figure 7.21**.

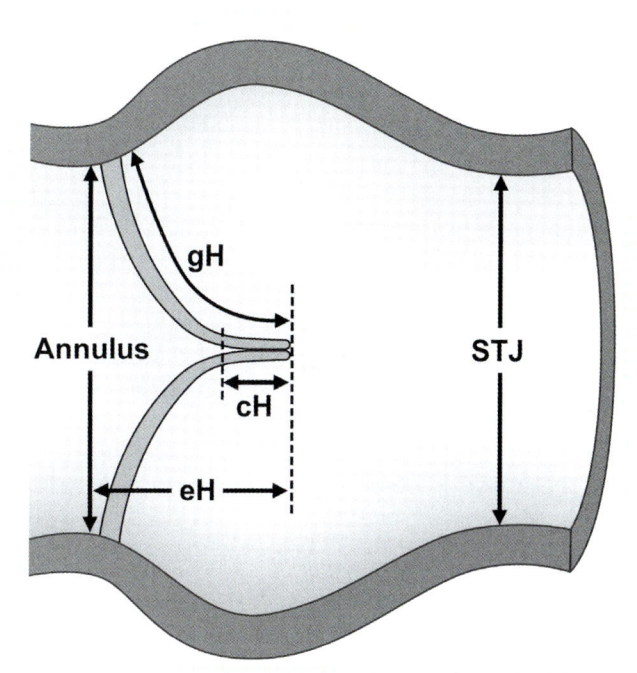

Figure 7.21. Echocardiographic measurements of the aortic root performed in the preprocedure assessment for aortic valve repair. *cH*, coaptation height; *eH*, effective height; *gH*, geometric height of the aortic valve cusps; *STJ*, sinotubular junction. (From Nicoara A, Skubas N, Ad N, et al. Guidelines for the use of transesophageal echocardiography to assist with surgical decision-making in the operating room: a surgery-based approach: from the American Society of Echocardiography in Collaboration with the Society of Cardiovascular Anesthesiologists and the Society of Thoracic Surgeons. *J Am Soc Echocardiogr.* 2020;33(6):692-734. Figure 4. Redrawn with permission of Nancy International Ltd. from Berrebi A, Monin JL, Lansac E. Systematic echocardiographic assessment of aortic regurgitation-what should the surgeon know for aortic valve repair?. *Ann Cardiothorac Surg.* 2019;8(3):331-341; permission conveyed through Copyright Clearance Center, Inc.)

13. **Answer: C.** The trachea, and sometimes bronchus, is between the aorta and the esophagus. Because air provides a poor propagation of ultrasound, the trachea or bronchus does not transmit the reflected images from the mid-ascending aorta.

14. **Answer: A.** TEE guidance for transseptal puncture during MitraClip procedures requires multiple imaging planes to best determine a 3-dimensional position that allows an optimal approach toward the mitral valve. It begins initially with a midesophageal (ME) bicaval view as the needle and sheath approach the interatrial septum from the IVC and begin tenting the fossa. Once the superior-inferior plane has been established, the probe is rotated to the ME aortic valve short-axis view, which allows positioning in the anterior-posterior direction. For a MitraClip procedure, puncture should be performed in a more posterior location, away from the aortic valve. Finally, the probe is rotated toward the ME 4-chamber

view to measure tenting/puncture height to the mitral valve, where a >4-cm distance is targeted, depending on the etiology of mitral regurgitation and anticipated clip placement.

15. **Answer: C.** Sometimes the TEE probe will become coiled in the esophagus with the tip pointed toward the mouth. Often, this can be remedied by withdrawing the probe to a slight extent, retroflexing the probe, and then attempting to advance the probe forward. However, it is always true that if simple maneuvers such as this do not work, then the TEE should not be continued and an endoscopy should be performed to rule out a stricture or obstructing lesion.

16. **Answer: B.** A potential source of embolism is seen. The image is obtained at 106°, beyond a typical midesophageal bicaval view. It demonstrates the interatrial septum with color Doppler showing no apparent patent foramen ovale and the question confirms no shunt is seen with agitated saline. However, a septal pouch (SP), an embryologic variant, is shown with the pouch formed on the left atrial side of the septum due to incomplete fusion of the septum primum and the septum secundum, and without interatrial shunting or flow to prevent stasis in this region. Although controversial, some studies have suggested that in this space, thrombotic material can collect and lead to a stroke or embolic event.

17. **Answer: D.** The structure seen is a prominent Thebesian valve. The Thebesian valve is the valve of the coronary sinus (CS), which is seen in the image entering the right atrium (RA). This view is obtained with retroflexion and advancement of the TEE probe from a standard 4-chamber view. The Thebesian valve is a membranous, fibromuscular, embryologic remnant structure that originates and covers a portion of the ostium of the CS. It prevents back flow into the CS during atrial contraction. It may be confused with vegetations or thrombus and may interfere with CS cannulation. The Eustachian valve is the valve at the junction of the IVC and RA.

18. **Answer: A.** Visualization of the pulmonary veins is important in a variety of situations: after pulmonary vein ablation, in patients with sinus venosus ASD, and in the assessment of mitral regurgitation. The easiest vein to visualize is the left upper pulmonary vein that runs next to the left atrial appendage. However, it is possible to visualize the bifurcation of the left and right pulmonary veins. The left pulmonary veins are typically seen from 110° to 140° with counterclockwise rotation. In the example, the bifurcation can be easily seen with a transducer position at 110°. **Figure 7.22A** corresponds to the left upper and lower pulmonary veins and **Figure 7.22B** corresponds to the right upper and lower pulmonary veins. The right pulmonary veins are usually visualized from 45° to 60° transducer position with clockwise rotation.

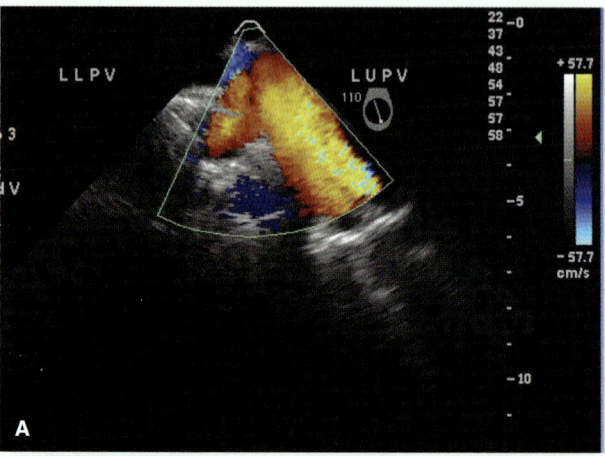

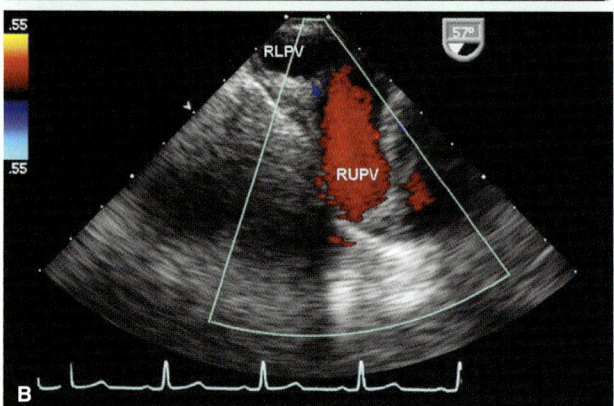

Figure 7.22. LLPV, left lower pulmonary vein; LUPV, left upper pulmonary vein; RLPV, right lower pulmonary vein; RUPV, right upper pulmonary vein.

19. **Answer: D.** The proximal coronary arteries can be visualized using TEE. In patients with normal coronary origins, the left main can present as in the example. The right coronary artery can be more challenging due to its anterior origin and can be masked by aortic calcification.

20. **Answer: D.** This is an example of a unicuspid aortic valve, a rare entity accounting for less than 5% of the adult population with aortic stenosis requiring surgery. Unicuspid valves can be unicommissural (most common) or acommissural.

21. **Answer: B.** The answer is a change in equipment settings, in particular, the Nyquist limit. This is a frequent mistake in evaluating regurgitant lesions. The appearance of a jet by color Doppler depends on jet

momentum (flow × velocity). In addition, changes in gain, pulse repetition frequency, and Nyquist limit may markedly change the size of the jet. The standard Nyquist limit to evaluate a regurgitant lesion is around 45 to 60 cm/s. In this example, the Nyquist limit was lowered to interrogate the interatrial septum (low-velocity patent foramen ovale [PFO] flow) and then was not changed back to assess the degree of mitral regurgitation.

22. **Answer: A.** Among the different types of prostheses, aortic homografts have the appearance closest to a native aortic valve due to their human cadaveric origin. They are stentless grafts with a tricuspid leaflet shape as noted by a lack of struts at annular points; therefore, they require some native aortic tissue for stability with different surgical techniques based on pathology and surgeon experience. These stentless bioprosthetic valves can also be designed with ascending aortic conduits that extend distally beyond the aortic root and can be used for ascending aorta replacement. They are most used in cases of infective endocarditis as they are more resilient against reinfection and where aortic root replacement may also be required. It can be difficult to distinguish between stentless bioprosthesis such as a homografts or xenografts due to a similar appearance on echocardiography. The main echocardiographic characteristic of an aortic homograft is an increased thickness of the annulus and root/ascending aortic tissue. Of the available answer choices, only the aortic homograft fits the criteria presented for the bioprosthetic aortic valve replacement shown in the image (eliminating Choices C and D) along with ascending aortic replacement (eliminating Choice B).

23. **Answer: B.** Systolic anterior motion (SAM) after mitral valve repair is a known complication that may require intraoperative return to cardiopulmonary bypass. There are a multitude of intraoperative transesophageal echocardiographic parameters that predict the risk of SAM following repair such as: (1) anterior to posterior leaflet height ratio of ≤1.3, (2) bileaflet prolapse and anterior displacement of papillary muscle, (3) coaptation-septal distance of <2.5 cm, (4) posterior leaflet height >1.5 cm, (5) LV end-diastolic diameter of <4.5 cm, (6) LV end-systolic diameter of <2.5 cm, (7) aortomitral angle of <120°, (8) basal septal hypertrophy ≥1.5 cm, and (9) hyperdynamic ventricle. The aortomitral angle and coaptation-septal distance, described as the end-systolic distance from the coaptation point perpendicular to the interventricular septum, are shown in **Figure 7.23**.

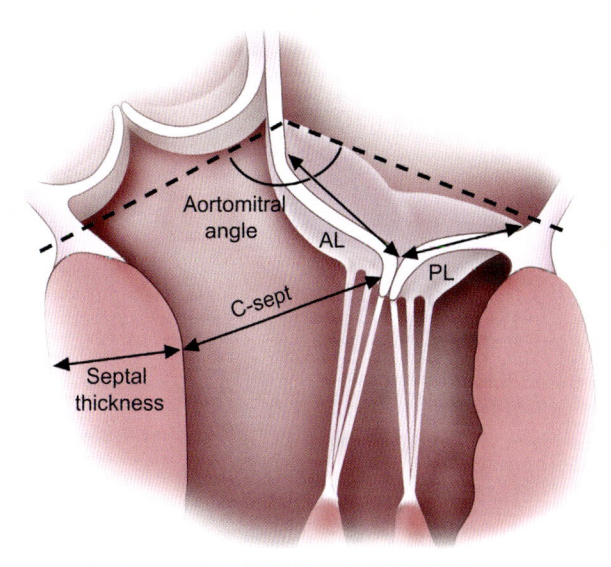

Figure 7.23. Echocardiographic measurements for predicting the risk of systolic anterior motion after mitral valve repair. *AL*, anterior leaflet height measured from the aortic annulus to the coaptation point; *C-sept*, distance from the coaptation point to the interventricular septum measured at end-systole perpendicular to the septum; *PL*, posterior leaflet height measured from the aortic annulus to the coaptation point. (Reprinted from Nicoara A, Skubas N, Ad N, et al. Guidelines for the use of transesophageal echocardiography to assist with surgical decision-making in the operating room: a surgery-based approach—from the American Society of Echocardiography in Collaboration with the Society of Cardiovascular Anesthesiologists and the Society of Thoracic Surgeons. *J Am Soc Echocardiogr*. 2020;33(6):692-734. Copyright © 2020 by the American Society of Echocardiography. With permission.)

24. **Answer: C.** TEE guidance for Impella 5.5 (Abiomed, Danvers, MA) temporary left ventricular assist device is important to ensure appropriate positioning within the LV cavity, assess both left and right ventricular function, and evaluate any interference with valve function. Unlike the Impella 5.0, which consisted of a short pigtail catheter extending distally from the inlet of the device, this pigtail catheter is no longer present on the Impella 5.5, allowing a slightly deeper position in the LV cavity. According to manufacturer guidance, the aortic valve annulus to mid-inlet distance should be approximately 5 cm and the cannula bend should be seated at the aortic valve. Avoiding further depth of insertion should allow for the cannula outlet to be safely above the aortic valve. The midesophageal long-axis view provides the best visualization of cannula insertion depth for this procedure.

25. **Answer: C.** The patient has a partially dehisced tricuspid prosthesis, with a periprosthetic leak of TR, located medial to the valve. The key in this case is to understand the imaging plane, which is stated in the question given. Note that the right atrium is very large and that the interatrial septum bows

toward the left atrium due to right atrial hypertension. The anterior mitral leaflet is shown in the image, while the aortic prosthesis is not shown.

26. **Answer: D. Figure 7.11A** shows a 3D echo image of a mass, likely a thrombus, that obliterates the entire upper half of the atrial side of the prosthesis. **Figure 7.11B** shows high velocity, diastolic antegrade mitral flow, with a long pressure half-time, indicating severe prosthetic stenosis. There is also a systolic flow, shown above the baseline, with a moderate signal density consistent with moderate mitral regurgitation. The upper color Doppler portion of **Figure 7.11B** shows antegrade mitral flow only in the rightward portion of the prosthetic ring with an immobile posterior leaflet due to thrombotic obstruction. A mass like this, presenting acutely after stopping warfarin, is more likely thrombus than tumor or vegetation.

27. **Answer: D. Figure 7.12A** shows a positive contrast effect with bubbles in the left atrium that have passed from the right atrium. **Figure 7.12B** shows a negative contrast effect with a streak of blood without bubbles that has passed into the right atrium from the left atrium. Hence, there is a bidirectional shunt.

28. **Answer: C.** In a retrospective review, intraoperative TEE has been associated with lower operative mortality, especially in those with the highest predicted operative risk. Furthermore, the use of TEE is also associated with increased likelihood of a valve procedure at the time of coronary artery bypass graft (CABG), likely due to a comprehensive assessment of valvular pathology at the time of surgery.

29. **Answer: D.** This is a patient without fever or any signs of infection. He has a congenital bicuspid aortic valve of the horizontal type, with fusion of what would have been the right and left coronary cusps. In patients like this, the conjoined cusp has a longer length of its free edge, causing it to prolapse (*small arrow,* **Figure 7.13**) back into the outflow tract, resulting in aortic regurgitation.

30. **Answer: C.** The images (anechoic space indicated by the arrow) show a reflection of the normal pericardium posterior to the aorta in the transverse sinus, with a small amount of physiologic pericardial fluid.

31. **Answer: C.** Atrial septal defects can occur in multiple locations of the interatrial septum. This case shows a superior sinus venosus defect, which is commonly associated with anomalous drainage of the right pulmonary veins and frequently requires surgical treatment. The diagnosis can be missed unless there is a high index of suspicion (**Figure 7.24**). This figure shows a 0° view at the level of the great vessels with slight counterclockwise rotation. The objective of this view is to visualize the superior vena cava that normally appears as a closed circle.

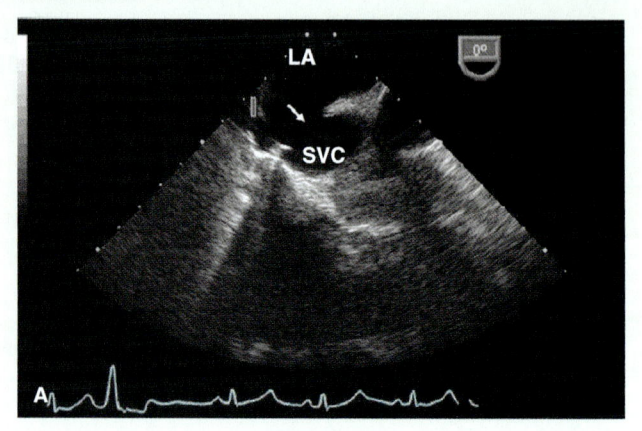

Figure 7.24A

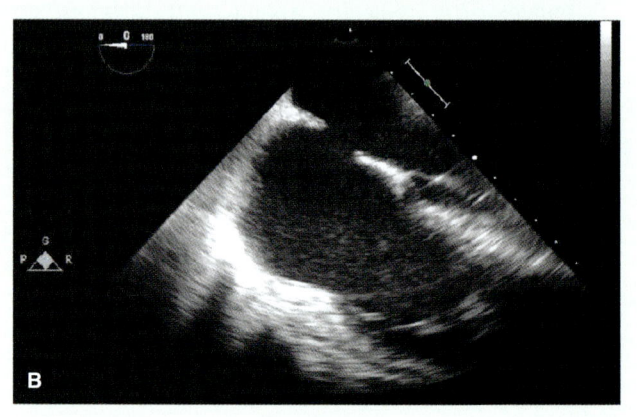

Figure 7.24B

In the case of a sinus venosus ASD, a defect in the superior vena cava (SVC) can be seen in **Figure 7.24A** (seen also in ▶ **Video 7.6A**). This should be confirmed in a bicaval view (90°-120°) (see ▶ **Video 7.6B**). Careful interrogation of all pulmonary veins is mandatory. The most common ASD is the ostium secundum type as shown in **Figure 7.24B**. This defect is located in the fossa ovalis. Another type of interatrial septal defect is ostium primum (a type of endocardial cushion defect) that is usually accompanied by a cleft mitral leaflet.

32. **Answer: B.** A sinus venosus defect is not amenable to percutaneous closure.

KEY POINTS

- Sinus venosus defects are associated with right ventricular enlargement and anomalous drainage of the right pulmonary veins.
- Detection of a sinus venosus defect requires that appropriate views are obtained to visualize the superior vena cava.
- Sinus venosus-type atrial septal defects require surgical closure.

33. **Answer: D.** This structure represents a severely dilated coronary sinus (CS). The most common cause of CS dilatation is right atrial hypertension due to right-sided heart failure, tricuspid regurgitation, or pulmonary hypertension. However, the degree of dilatation as seen in this example is usually caused by a persistent left superior vena cava draining into the CS. Another rarer cause of significant dilatation of the CS is anomalous pulmonary vein drainage. Additional imaging at 0° by advancing the probe deeper will also show the CS draining into the right atrium (RA) (**Figure 7.25A**). A persistent left SVC is a benign variant and usually does not require other diagnostic tests. Incidentally, the case shown had anomalous right pulmonary vein drainage in the right SVC (small white arrows) found on a CT scan (**Figure 7.25B**). (L-SVC, persistent left superior vena cava; PA, pulmonary artery; SVC, superior vena cava.)

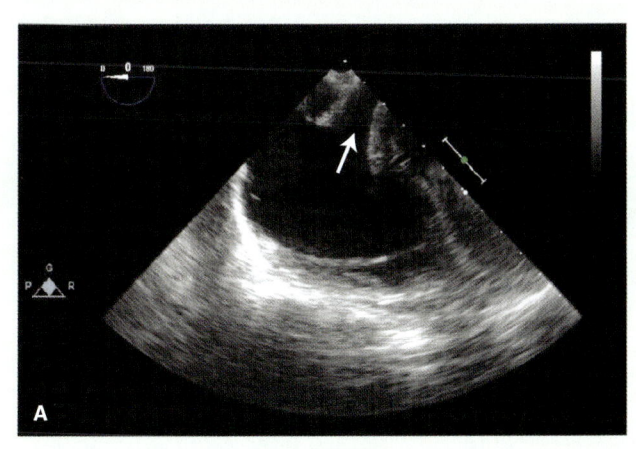

Figure 7.25A

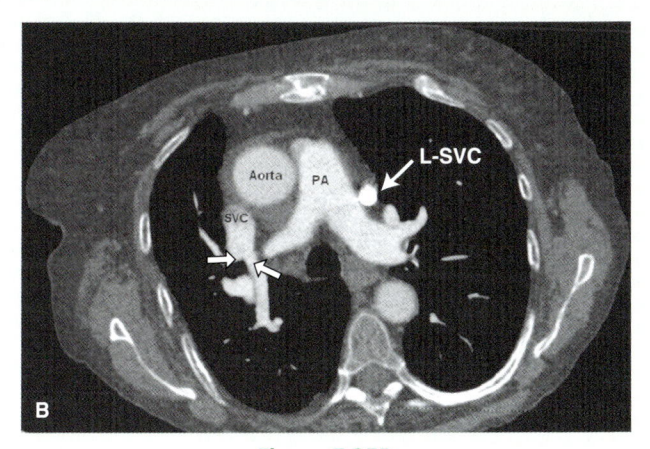

Figure 7.25B

34. **Answer: B.** Confirmation of the suspected persistent left SVC is done by injecting agitated saline into the left arm and showing early appearance of the bubbles in the coronary sinus before the right atrium (▶ **Video 7.7**).

KEY POINTS
- A dilated CS is most often due to right atrial hypertension but other causes include a fistula to the CS, anomalous pulmonary vein drainage to the CS, or a left SVC to the CS.
- A left SVC is almost always a benign anatomic variant.
- Confirmation of a left SVC to CS connection can be obtained by demonstrating bubbles injected into the left arm vein appearing in the CS prior to the right atrium.

35. **Answer: D.** This is a typical perforation at the base of the anterior mitral valve leaflet. In most cases, this is the result of endocarditis involving the aortic valve with aortic regurgitation. The aortic valve infection seeds the anterior leaflet at the site where the aortic regurgitation jet hits the anterior mitral leaflet. Secondary mitral valve involvement in cases of aortic valve endocarditis can appear as "windsock" lesions (**Figure 7.26A,B**) or frank perforations. In this patient, the perforation was a rare, late presentation of an iatrogenic complication after aortic valve replacement.

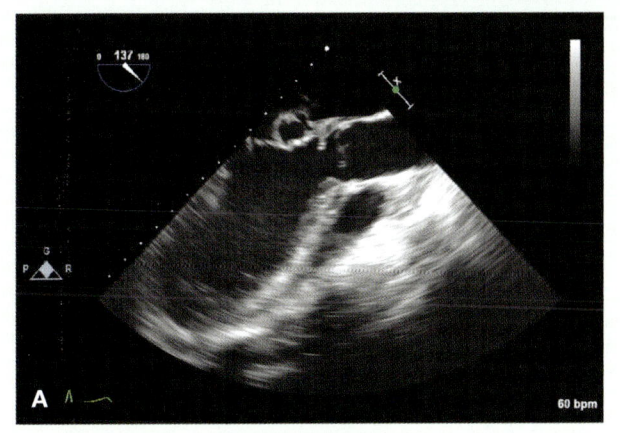

Figure 7.26A

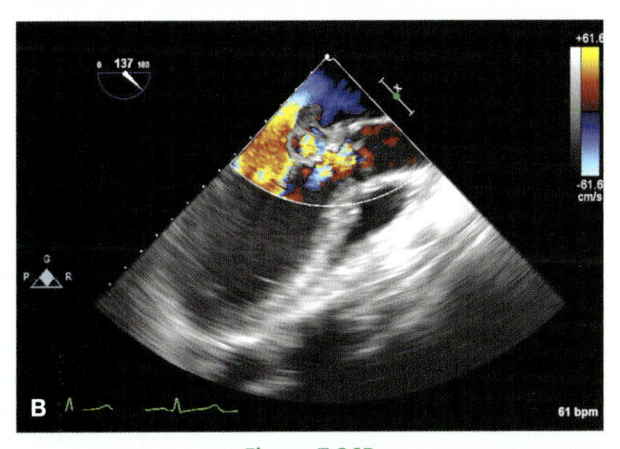

Figure 7.26B

> **KEY POINTS**
> - Perforation of the base of the anterior mitral leaflet is most often due to endocarditis as a result of a jet lesion from aortic valve endocarditis associated with aortic regurgitation.
> - Iatrogenic perforation of the mitral leaflet at the time of heart surgery is rare but another etiology of mitral regurgitation.

36. **Answer: A.** Aneurysm of the sinus of Valsalva of the right coronary cusp is a rare anomaly, usually congenital, although it can also be traumatic. Nonruptured aneurysm of the sinus of Valsalva is not associated with symptoms, although it may result in aortic regurgitation. In cases of intracardiac rupture into the right atrium or right ventricle, acute heart failure and physical findings consistent with severe aortic regurgitation may develop. Once ruptured, the morphology of the aneurysm may change and appears more like a fistulous tract and can be confused with tricuspid valve vegetation and severe tricuspid regurgitation. The continuous timing of the spectral Doppler helps make the diagnosis of aorta to right atrial communication.

> **KEY POINTS**
> - Sinus of Valsalva aneurysm is usually a congenital anomaly but may also result from trauma.
> - Nonruptured sinus of Valsalva aneurysms may be associated with aortic regurgitation.
> - Ruptured sinus of Valsalva aneurysms can result in acute heart failure, severe aortic regurgitation, and hypotension.
> - Spectral Doppler continuous flow may be helpful to distinguish a ruptured aneurysm from other pathologies.

37. **Answer: B.** Video 7.5A,B shows mild TR, based on spatial mapping. Not shown here is that the mitral repair looks good with only trivial MR. No vegetations were noted.

38. **Answer: D.** He has become volume depleted and hypotensive. All valve lesions are load-dependent, especially TR and MR. TR is the most load-dependent of all of them. Many ambulatory patients have excess sympathetic tone during heart failure with activation of the renin-angiotensin system and the sympathetic nervous system. This patient was hypertensive at the time of admission. In the next few days, he was probably diuresed and put on various vasodilators. In the operating room, he may have been volume depleted relative to his hemodynamics when he initially was admitted. In addition, anesthesia reduces sympathetic tone, often resulting in a drop in systemic and pulmonary arteriolar resistance; therefore, regurgitant valve lesions may decrease in severity. This accounts for the reduction in the severity of TR. The severity of the valve dysfunction seen under "street conditions" is a better handle to decide long-term plans like valve surgery.

39. **Answer: B.** There is a periprosthetic abscess within the intervalvular fibrosa. Three-dimensional echo allows postexamination exploration of different imaging planes. The images show that the abscess extends almost 180° around the prosthesis and extends superiorly along the area of the sinuses of Valsalva posteriorly. This is why it extended up into the interatrial septum as shown previously in Video 7.5C,D.

40. **Answer: A.** The AVR homograft has an advantage in patients with active endocarditis of lower rates of persistent infection compared to a stented bioprosthesis, likely due to less foreign material. Video 7.5I,J shows the results of surgery on the postpump TEE, with no TR or AR, and only mild MR. Note that the normal homograft has a unique appearance, which is different than stented aortic prostheses. Note the double density at the walls of the homograft tissue. This results from its implantation as an "inclusion cylinder," which includes the walls of the aortic sinuses from the donor. Actually, the homograft is less available, the systolic gradient from a homograft is lower, and the homograft is more difficult to implant, compared to a standard stented bioprosthesis. There is often trivial regurgitation of either a homograft or a stented bioprosthesis. The band of soft tissue between the double densities should be relatively uniform in thickness and free of any flow in that space demonstrable by color Doppler.

> **KEY POINTS**
> - This case shows severe perivalvular regurgitation and an abscess that started around the aortic prosthesis, destroyed part of the intervalvular fibrosa, and extended into the atrial septum. It was fixed by extensive debridement of infected tissue and placement of an aortic homograft, with its posterior tissue accessible for attaching the patient's normal mitral valve.
> - Abscesses of the heart most commonly occur adjacent to an infected prosthesis.
> - The patient also had severe functional TR when the patient was volume overloaded at the time of admission, though the TR diminished to mild on the prepump intraoperative TEE, likely due to diuresis and reduction of sympathetic tone by the anesthesia. The risk of postoperative TR warranted tricuspid annuloplasty, despite the prepump TEE.

SUGGESTED READINGS

Alkhouli M, Rihal CS, Holmes DR. Transseptal techniques for emerging structural heart interventions. *J Am Coll Cardiol.* 2016;9(24):2465-2480.

Hahn RT, Abraham T, Adams MS, et al. Guidelines for performing a comprehensive transesophageal echocardiographic examination: recommendations from the American Society of Echocardiography and the Society of Cardiovascular Anesthesiologists. *J Am Soc Echocardiogr.* 2013;26(9): 921-964.

Mishra KL, Baker MT, Siegrist KK, et al. Multidisciplinary approach to improving safety in transesophageal echocardiography in patients with relative contraindications. *J Am Soc Echocardiogr.* 2022;35(11):1195-1197.

Nicoara A, Skubas N, Ad N, et al. Guidelines for the use of transesophageal echocardiography to assist with surgical decision making in the operating room: a surgery-based approach. From the American Society of Echocardiography in collaboration with the Society of Cardiovascular Anesthesiologists and the Society of Thoracic Surgeons. *J Am Soc Echocardiogr.* 2020;33(6):692-734.

Novaro GM, Aronow HD, Militello MA, Garcia MJ, Sabik EM. Benzocaine-induced methemoglobinemia: experience from a high-volume transesophageal echocardiography laboratory. *J Am Soc Echocardiogr.* 2003;16(2):170-175.

Tugcu A, Okajima K, Jin Z, et al. Septal pouch in the left atrium and risk of ischemic stroke. *JACC Cardiovasc Imaging.* 2010;3(12):1276-1283.

CHAPTER 8

Doppler and Hemodynamics

Daniel Bamira and Muhamed Saric

QUESTIONS

1. A 72-year-old man had undergone surgical aortic valve replacement using a 19-mm bioprosthesis a year ago. One month after surgery his echocardiogram demonstrated normal LV ejection fraction. Aortic valve (AV) and left ventricular outflow tract (LVOT) values from that study are listed in **Table 8.1** in the TTE #1 column. Recently, he presented with a gastrointestinal bleed and severe shortness of breath. TTE is repeated and corresponding values are listed in the TTE #2 column. Which one of the following best describes the change in echocardiographic parameters of the aortic bioprosthesis seen in TTE #2 compared to TTE #1?
   A. Patient has now developed severe bioprosthetic stenosis.
   B. Aortic valve area remains unchanged.
   C. LVOT stroke volume has now decreased.
   D. Aortic valve area has now increased.
   E. None of the above

2. A 32-year-old woman is referred for the evaluation of rheumatic mitral valve stenosis. No mitral regurgitation was noted. The following values were obtained using Doppler echocardiography:

E wave deceleration time	910 ms
Mean diastolic mitral gradient	17 mm Hg
Diastolic mitral inflow velocity-time integral	66 cm
Heart rate	85 bpm

   The following statements are **TRUE**:
   A. Mitral valve area can be calculated by dividing 220 into deceleration time.
   B. Stroke volume across the mitral valve is 72 mL/beat.
   C. Pressure half-time is 355 ms.
   D. Mitral valve area is 0.8 cm^2.
   E. During exertion, her mean gradient is expected to decrease.

Table 8.1. AV and LVOT Values

	Units	TTE #1	TTE #2
AV Vmax	m/s	3.1	4.2
AV VTI	cm	65	87
LVOT Vmax	m/s	0.90	1.2
LVOT VTI	cm	18	24
LVOT Diameter	cm	2.0	2.0

AV, aortic valve; AV Vmax, aortic valve maximum velocity; LVOT Vmax, left ventricular outflow tract maximum velocity; LVOT VTI, left ventricular outflow tract velocity-time integral.

3. A 21-year-old man presented with dyspnea on exertion and enlarged pulmonary artery on chest X-ray underwent transthoracic echocardiography. The study revealed patent ductus arteriosus and the following:

Left ventricular outflow tract (LVOT) diameter	2.0 cm
LVOT velocity-time integral	31 cm
Right ventricular outflow tract (RVOT) diameter	2.5 cm
RVOT velocity-time integral	12 cm
Heart rate	80 bpm

The following statement is **TRUE**:
A. Systemic blood flow (Qs) is 7.8 L/min.
B. The ratio of pulmonic to systemic blood flow (Qp:Qs) is less than one.
C. Stroke volume entering the lungs is 38 mL/beat.
D. Patient is cyanotic in the lower parts of the body.
E. The ratio of stroke volume through the LVOT and the stroke volume through the RVOT are equal to Qp:Qs ratio in this patient.

4. A 39-year-old woman was admitted for severe shortness of breath on exertion. On transthoracic echocardiogram, there was mild pulmonic regurgitation. Continuous wave spectral Doppler tracings of the pulmonic regurgitant jet reveal the following:

Early diastolic peak velocity	3.0 m/s
End-diastolic velocity	2.0 m/s

Examination of the inferior vena cava by M-mode echocardiography demonstrated the following:

IVC diameter during expiration	2.6 cm
IVC diameter during inspiration	2.6 cm

The following statement is **TRUE**:
A. Right atrial pressure is estimated at 6 mm Hg.
B. Pulmonary artery diastolic pressure is approximately 31 mm Hg.
C. Pulmonary artery diastolic pressure is 36 mm Hg minus the right atrial pressure.
D. Pulmonary artery diastolic pressure cannot be assessed if the pulmonic regurgitation is only mild.
E. Pulmonary artery diastolic pressure is normal.

5. A 42-year-old man was admitted to the hospital after a 1-month history of intermittent fever and progressive shortness of breath. Blood cultures grew *Streptococcus viridans*. On transesophageal echocardiogram, perforation of the anterior mitral leaflet and mitral regurgitation was seen. On color Doppler imaging, a well-formed flow convergence (PISA) shell was visualized on the ventricular side of the mitral valve in systole. In addition, the following was noted:

Maximal mitral regurgitation PISA radius	1.0 cm
Aliasing velocity at which PISA radius was measured	45 cm/s
Peak velocity of mitral regurgitation jet	500 cm/s
Velocity-time integral of mitral regurgitation	140 cm

The following statement is **TRUE**:
A. Vena contracta of the mitral regurgitant flow is expected to be less than 0.3 cm.
B. Effective regurgitant orifice area of mitral regurgitation is approximately 0.6 cm^2.
C. Instantaneous flow rate across the mitral valve using the PISA method is 70 mL/s.
D. Mitral regurgitation is moderate (2+).
E. Regurgitant volume is 40 mL/beat.

6. An 84-year-old obese woman with history of hypertension and chronic renal insufficiency experienced shortness of breath at a rehabilitation facility 2 weeks after elective hip replacement. Transthoracic echocardiogram revealed normal left ventricular systolic function, no mitral or aortic valve disease, and the following:

Peak velocity of the mitral E wave	125 cm/s
Flow propagation velocity of mitral inflow on color M mode	31 cm/s
Peak velocity of tricuspid regurgitant jet	4 m/s
Estimated right atrial pressure	15 mm Hg

The following statement is **TRUE**:
A. Mean pulmonary artery wedge pressure is markedly elevated.
B. On mitral inflow, E to A ratio is expected to be less than 1.
C. Pulmonary artery systolic pressure is 64 mm Hg.
D. The ratio of peak E wave velocity to the peak medial mitral annular tissue Doppler velocity is expected to be less than 8.
E. Flow propagation velocity of mitral inflow on color M mode is normal for her age.

7. A 44-year-old man with trileaflet aortic valve and dilated aortic root measuring 5.5 cm at the level of sinuses of Valsalva is being evaluated for aortic regurgitation. The following statement is **TRUE**:
A. When the regurgitant fraction is 65%, it would indicate that the aortic regurgitation is severe.
B. Like the size of flow convergence (PISA) radius, the size of vena contracta is strongly influenced by Nyquist limit setting.
C. Vena contracta of at least 0.2 cm would indicate that the aortic regurgitation is severe.
D. Regurgitant volume of 30 mL per beat is consistent with severe aortic regurgitation.
E. Vena contracta obtained using two-dimensional echocardiography can be used to calculate regurgitant volume.

8. A 62-year-old man with history of treated hypertension, chronic atrial fibrillation, and bicuspid aortic valve had a transthoracic echocardiogram done. The study showed the following:

Peak velocity of mitral regurgitant jet	6.0 m/s
dP/dt of mitral regurgitant jet	1900 mm Hg/s
Ratio of peak mitral E wave to average peak velocity of medial and lateral mitral annulus (E/e')	16
Vena contracta of mitral regurgitation	0.2 cm

Systemic blood pressure at the time of study was 120/70 mm Hg.
The following statement is **TRUE**:
A. Peak-to-peak aortic gradient is 90 mm Hg.
B. Patient is in cardiogenic shock due to left ventricular systolic dysfunction.
C. Mean left atrial pressure is approximately 20 mm Hg.
D. The size of vena contracta is diagnostic of severe mitral regurgitation.
E. Left atrial pressure cannot be estimated by E/e' method in patients with atrial fibrillation.

9. A 67-year-old man with aortic regurgitation underwent transthoracic echocardiographic examination. There was no mitral stenosis or regurgitation. The following values were obtained:

Peak diastolic velocity of aortic regurgitant jet	5.0 m/s
End-diastolic velocity of aortic regurgitant jet	3.7 m/s
Pressure half-time of aortic regurgitant jet	656 ms
Peak aortic antegrade flow velocity	2.2 m/s
Blood pressure	130/65 mm Hg

Based on the data, one can conclude:
A. Pressure half-time is consistent with severe aortic regurgitation.
B. Aortic valve area can be estimated as 220 divided by pressure half-time.
C. Peak left ventricular systolic pressure is lower than the systolic blood pressure.
D. Left ventricular end-diastolic pressure is estimated at 10 mm Hg.
E. Aortic valve area cannot be calculated using a continuity equation because there is aortic regurgitation.

10. A 25-year-old woman is being evaluated for percutaneous closure of her secundum atrial septal defect (ASD). Transthoracic echocardiography demonstrated mild tricuspid regurgitation, no pulmonic stenosis, and the following:

Pulmonary artery systolic pressure	55 mm Hg
Pulmonary artery diastolic pressure	25 mm Hg
Left atrial pressure	10 mm Hg
Right ventricular outflow tract (RVOT) diameter	2.6 cm
RVOT velocity-time integral	30 cm
Left ventricular outflow tract (LVOT) diameter	2.0 cm
LVOT velocity-time integral	20 cm
Heart rate	75 bpm

Based on the data, one can conclude:
A. Patient should be advised against ASD closure because pulmonary hypertension is present.
B. Pulmonary vascular resistance is approximately 16 Wood units.
C. The ratio of pulmonary to systemic blood flow (Qp:Qs) is approximately 2.5 to 1.
D. Shunt flow is larger than the pulmonic flow (Qp).
E. Patient is cyanotic.

11. A 35-year-old woman was noted on clinical exam to have a systolic murmur and was referred for transthoracic echocardiography. The exam revealed perimembranous ventricular septal defect (VSD), mild tricuspid regurgitation, pulmonic stenosis, intact aortic valve and the following:

Blood pressure	120/80 mm Hg
Peak systolic velocity across the VSD	3.0 m/s
End-diastolic velocity across the VSD	1.0 m/s
Estimated right atrial pressure	10 mm Hg
Peak systolic gradient across the pulmonic valve	55 mm Hg
Left ventricular end-diastolic pressure	12 mm Hg

The following statement is **TRUE**:
A. Right ventricular systolic pressure is 46 mm Hg.
B. Pulmonary artery systolic pressure is 29 mm Hg.
C. Right ventricular systolic pressure is 84 mm Hg above the right atrial pressure.
D. Pulmonary artery systolic pressure is 45 mm Hg higher than the right ventricular systolic pressure.
E. Right ventricular end-diastolic pressure is 28 mm Hg.

12. A 21-year-old college student is noted to have fixed splitting of the second heart sound and right bundle branch block. Real-time three-dimensional transesophageal echocardiogram revealed a 1.2-cm secundum atrial septal defect (ASD) that was circular in shape. On color Doppler, a well-formed hemispheric flow convergence (PISA) shell is seen on the left atrial side of the ASD. The following data were also obtained:

Blood pressure	120/80 mm Hg
Heart rate	100 bpm
PISA radius	0.7 cm
Velocity-time integral of left-to-right flow across ASD	80 cm
Left ventricular outflow tract (LVOT) diameter	2.0 cm
LVOT velocity-time integral	19 cm

The following statement is **TRUE**:
A. Ratio of pulmonic to systemic flow (Qp:Qs) is 1.8 to 1.0.
B. Shunt flow across the ASD is approximately 9.0 L/min.
C. The difference between the pulmonic and systemic stroke volume is 180 mL.
D. Systemic stroke volume is 150 mL.
E. Pulmonic blood flow (Qp) is approximately 7.0 L/min.

13. A 35-year-old woman presents with sudden onset of dyspnea and pulmonary edema. She underwent bedside transthoracic echocardiography which revealed hyperdynamic left ventricular systolic function, normal aortic valve, and mitral regurgitation. The following data were obtained using transthoracic echocardiogram:

Blood pressure	95/50 mm Hg
Heart rate	120 bpm
Peak velocity of mitral regurgitant jet	4.0 m/s
Time interval from onset of mitral regurgitation to jet velocity of 1 m/s	5 ms
Time interval from onset of mitral regurgitation to jet velocity of 3 m/s	25 ms
Vena contracta of mitral regurgitation	0.8 cm

The following statement is **TRUE**:
A. Peak velocity of the mitral inflow E wave is expected to be low.
B. Left atrial pressure is low.
C. Pulmonary venous flow velocity pattern on spectral Doppler is likely to reveal flow reversal during early diastole.
D. Rate of pressure rise (dP/dt) in the left ventricle is 1600 mm Hg/s.
E. Left ventricular systolic function is markedly diminished.

14. A 29-year-old Bangladeshi woman with rheumatic mitral stenosis is referred to the cardiac catheterization laboratory for percutaneous mitral balloon valvuloplasty. Upon placement of the pigtail catheter in the left ventricle, the following values were obtained:

Left ventricular peak systolic pressure	124 mm Hg
Early left ventricular diastolic pressure	7 mm Hg
Left ventricular end-diastolic pressure	10 mm Hg

Transesophageal echocardiogram prior to valvuloplasty revealed the absence of both mitral and aortic regurgitation as well as the following:

Heart rate	104 bpm
Time-velocity integral of diastolic mitral flow	65 cm
Mean mitral valve gradient in diastole	21 mm Hg
Mitral pressure half-time	270 ms

The following statement is **TRUE**:
A. Mean left atrial pressure is expected to be lower than the mean left ventricular diastolic pressure.
B. Peak velocity of the mitral inflow E wave is expected to be low.
C. Pressure half-time may be unreliable in patients prior to valvuloplasty.
D. Mitral valve area is 0.6 cm^2.
E. Mean left atrial pressure is approximately 28 mm Hg.

15. An 81-year-old woman with systolic heart murmur was referred for an echocardiogram. A heavily calcified aortic valve and normal mitral valve were noted on two-dimensional echocardiographic imaging. Doppler echocardiography of the aortic valve revealed:

Left ventricular outflow tract (LVOT) diameter	1.9 cm
Peak velocity across the aortic valve	5.0 m/s
Peak LVOT velocity	1.0 m/s
LVOT velocity-time integral (VTI)	20 cm

The following statement is **TRUE**:
A. Aortic valve area cannot be calculated because aortic valve velocity-time integral is not stated.
B. Aortic valve stenosis is subvalvular.
C. Aortic valve area is likely to be less than 1 cm^2.
D. Left ventricular stroke volume is 80 mL/beat.
E. Systolic blood pressure is approximately 100 mg Hg above the left ventricular systolic pressure.

16. A 52-year-old woman presents for the evaluation of mitral regurgitation. **Figure 8.1** demonstrate continuous wave Doppler tracing obtained using transthoracic echocardiography. Which one of the following most likely represents the type of mitral regurgitation recorded in this patient?
A. Moderate chronic mitral regurgitation.
B. Severe acute mitral regurgitation.
C. Partly diastolic mitral regurgitation.
D. Mitral regurgitation due to mitral valve prolapse.
E. None of the above.

17. A 41-year-old man is admitted to the intensive care unit with severe hypoxic respiratory failure in the setting of severe mitral regurgitation. Transesophageal echocardiography is performed and spectral Doppler tracings from a pulmonary vein are obtained. Which one of the following 4 panels in **Figure 8.2** is most consistent with the diagnosis of severe mitral regurgitation?
A. Panel A.
B. Panel B.
C. Panel C.
D. Panel D.
E. None of the above.

18. A 65-year-old woman undergoes transesophageal echocardiography in the intensive care unit. Mitral valve spectral Doppler recordings are obtained at baseline and post intervention and shown in **Figure 8.3**. Which one of the following interventions is most likely to explain the change in the mitral inflow pattern?
A. Fluid resuscitation with 1 liter of normal saline.
B. Direct current cardioversion.
C. Transcatheter mitral valve repair.
D. Development of severe aortic regurgitation post balloon valvuloplasty.
E. None of the above.

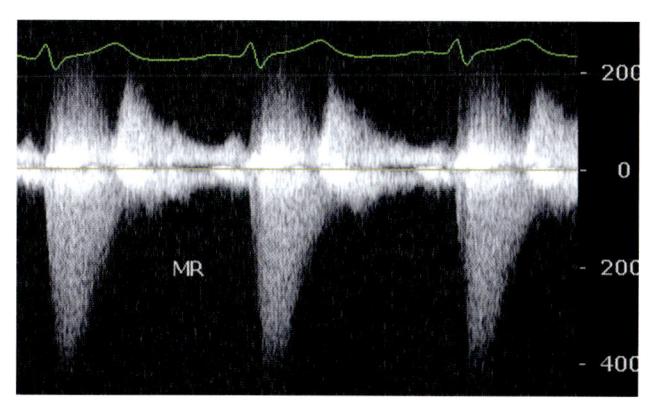

Figure 8.1

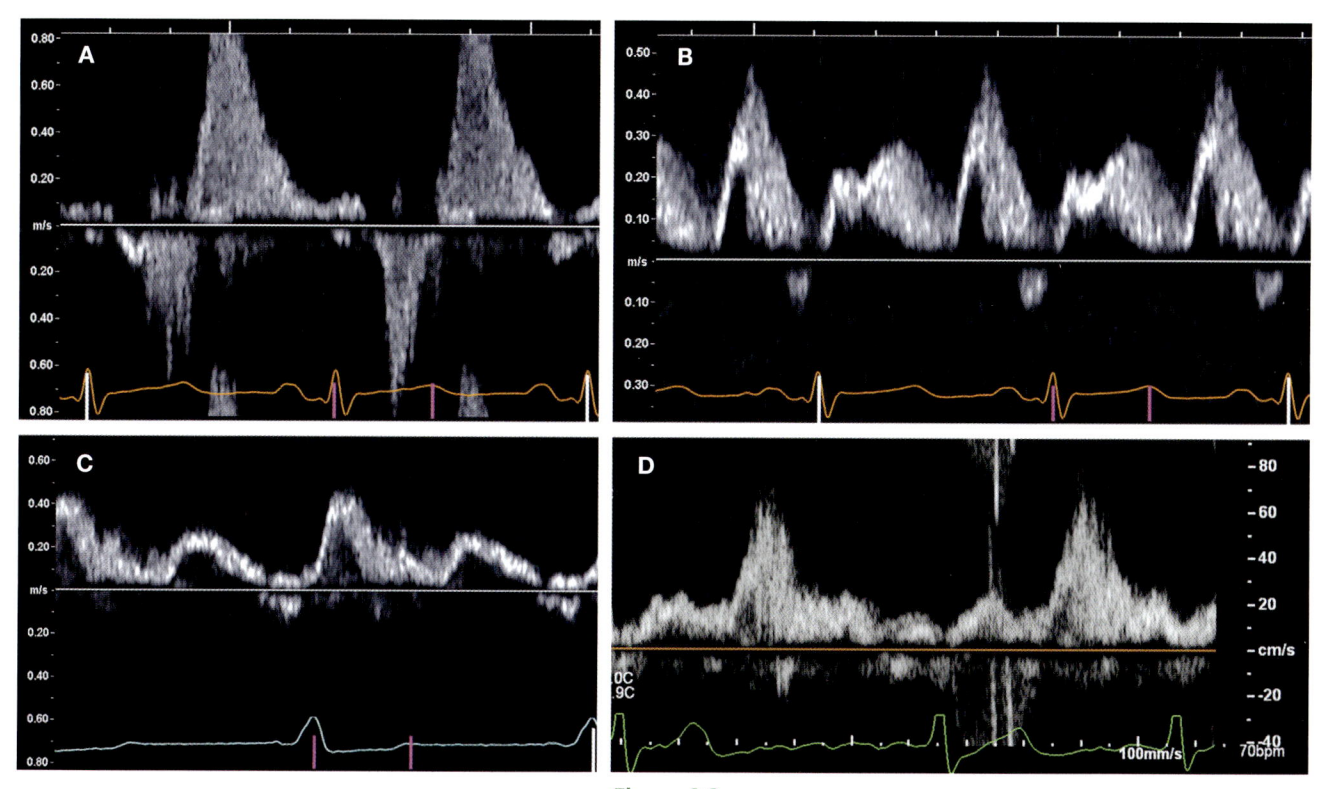

Figure 8.2

148 / Clinical Echocardiography Review

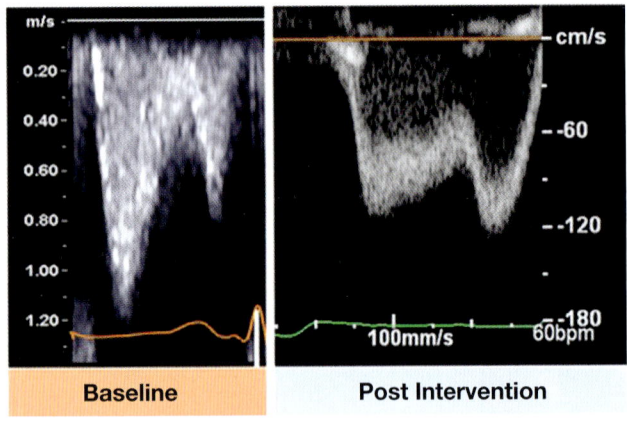

Figure 8.3

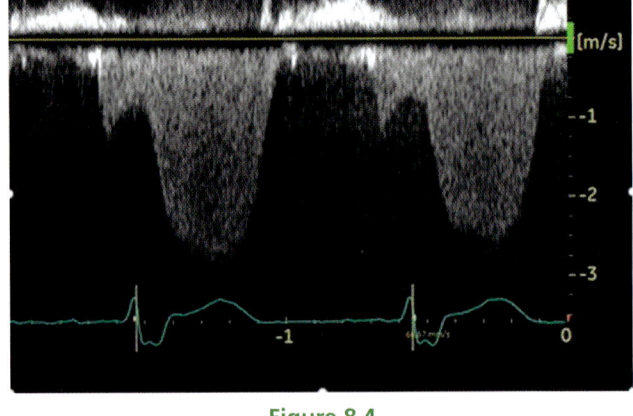

Figure 8.4

19. An 88-year-old man is referred for the evaluation of syncope. Transthoracic echocardiography is performed and a continuous wave spectral Doppler recording across the tricuspid valve is obtained and shown in **Figure 8.4**. Which of the following is the most likely explanation for the tricuspid spectral Doppler flow velocity pattern in this patient?
A. First degree atrioventricular block.
B. Atrial fibrillation.
C. Severe acute tricuspid regurgitation.
D. Ebstein anomaly.
E. None of the above.

20. A 32-year-old man undergoes transcatheter intervention for a congenital heart defect. Continuous wave spectral Doppler recordings are obtained at baseline and post intervention and shown in **Figure 8.5**. Which one of the following is the intervention most likely performed in this patient?
A. Patent ductus arteriosus closure.
B. Aortic balloon valvuloplasty.
C. Stenting of aortic coarctation.
D. Atrial septal defect closure.
E. None of the above.

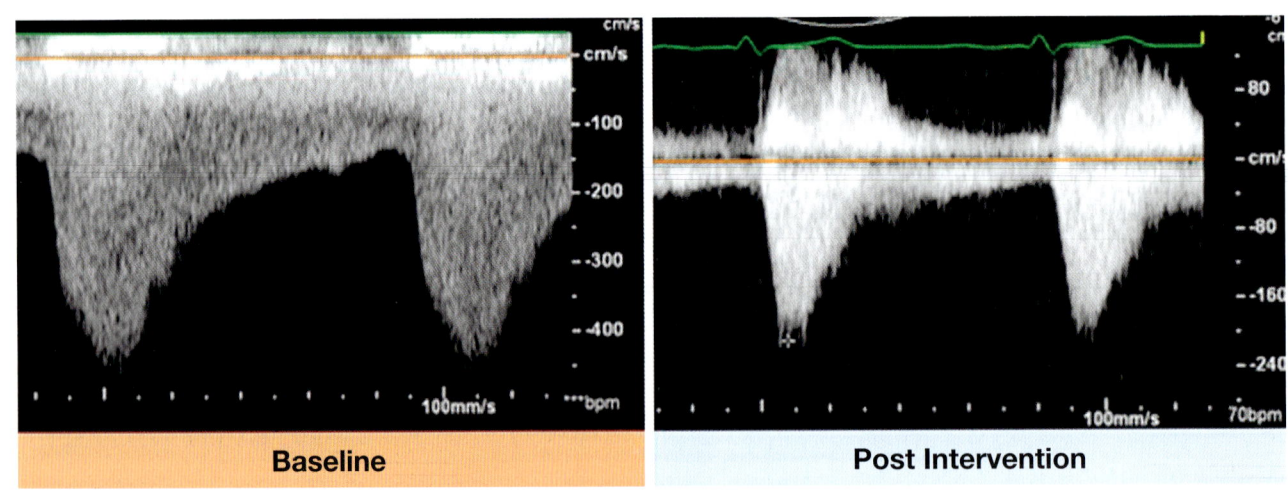

Figure 8.5

21. A 43-year-old woman presents with severe shortness of breath, anorexia, and lower extremity edema. TTE was performed and spectral pulsed-wave Doppler recording at the level of the mitral valve with simultaneous respirometry was obtained and shown in **Figure 8.6**. The upstroke of respirometry tracings represents inspiration and the downstroke represents expiration. Which one of the following conditions is most consistent with the recordings shown?
    A. Restrictive cardiomyopathy.
    B. Constrictive pericarditis.
    C. Pericardial tamponade.
    D. Acute pericarditis.
    E. None of the above.

22. A 37-year-old woman with scleroderma and severe pulmonary hypertension underwent transthoracic echocardiography for the evaluation of worsening dyspnea. Which one of the spectral Doppler recordings at the level of the pulmonic valve in **Figure 8.7** is most consistent with her diagnosis of severe systolic pulmonary hypertension?
    A. Panel A.
    B. Panel B.
    C. Panel C.
    D. Panel D.
    E. None of the above.

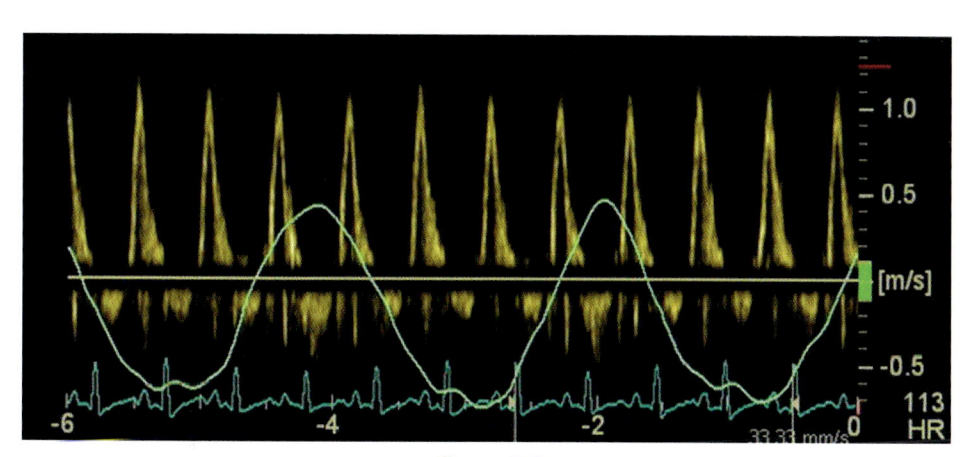

Figure 8.6

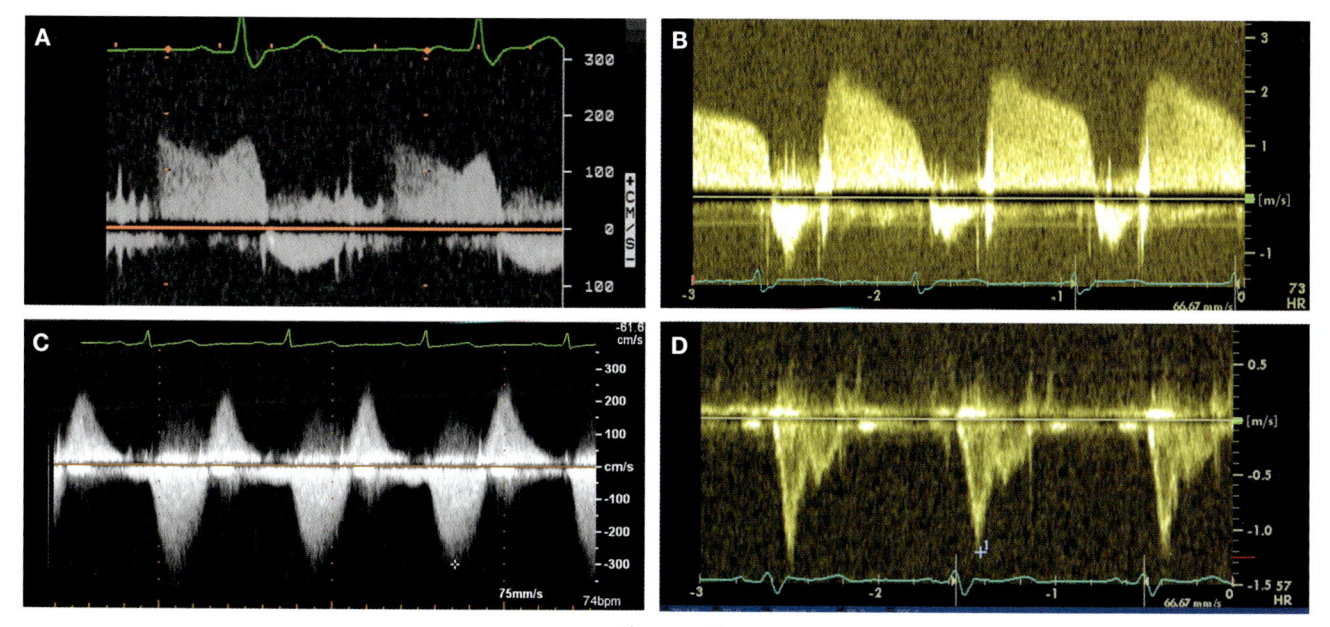

Figure 8.7

23. **Figure 8.8** shows continuous wave spectral Doppler tracing of the tricuspid regurgitant jet from an 18-year-old woman with pulmonic valve stenosis. The peak pulmonic valve gradient is 24 mm Hg. Right atrial pressure is estimated at 10 mm Hg. The following is **TRUE** about this patient:
    A. Peak pulmonary artery systolic pressure is higher than the right ventricular peak systolic pressure.
    B. Right ventricular peak systolic pressure is 64 mm Hg above the pulmonary artery peak systolic pressure.
    C. Pulmonary artery peak systolic pressure is 50 mm Hg.
    D. Right ventricular peak systolic pressure is 24 mm Hg less than the peak pulmonary artery systolic pressure.
    E. Right ventricular peak systolic pressure is 108 mm Hg.

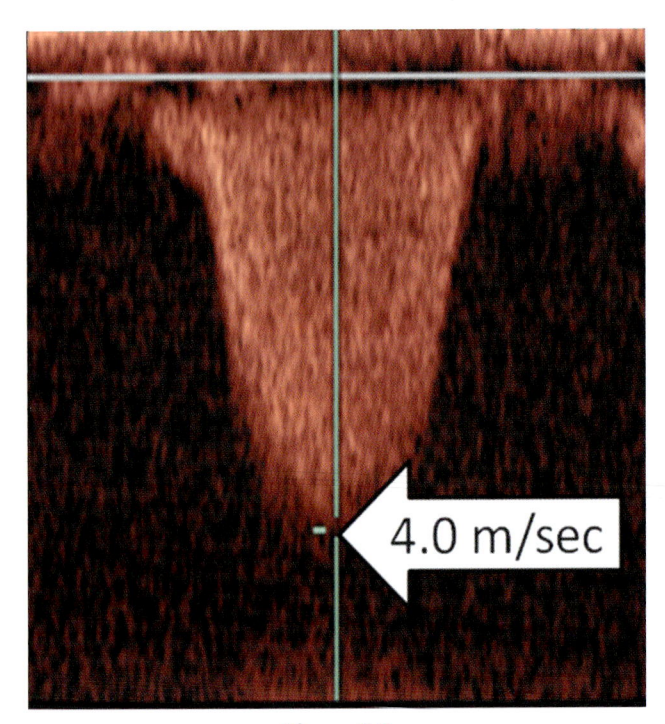

Figure 8.8

24. An 82-year-old man was referred for the evaluation of a systolic ejection murmur. On parasternal long-axis view, the left ventricular outflow tract diameter was measured at 2.0 cm. The spectral Doppler tracings in **Figure 8.9** were obtained in or through the left ventricular outflow tract in the apical 5-chamber view. The following statement is **TRUE**:
    A. Increased cardiac output alone may explain the elevated gradient across the aortic valve.
    B. Marked difference between the subvalvular and valvular velocities in this patient may also be seen in severe aortic regurgitation.
    C. Patient has a very severe aortic valve stenosis with a mean gradient of approximately 60 mm Hg.
    D. Aortic valve area is greater than 1.0 cm².
    E. Patient has hypertrophic obstructive cardiomyopathy (HOCM).

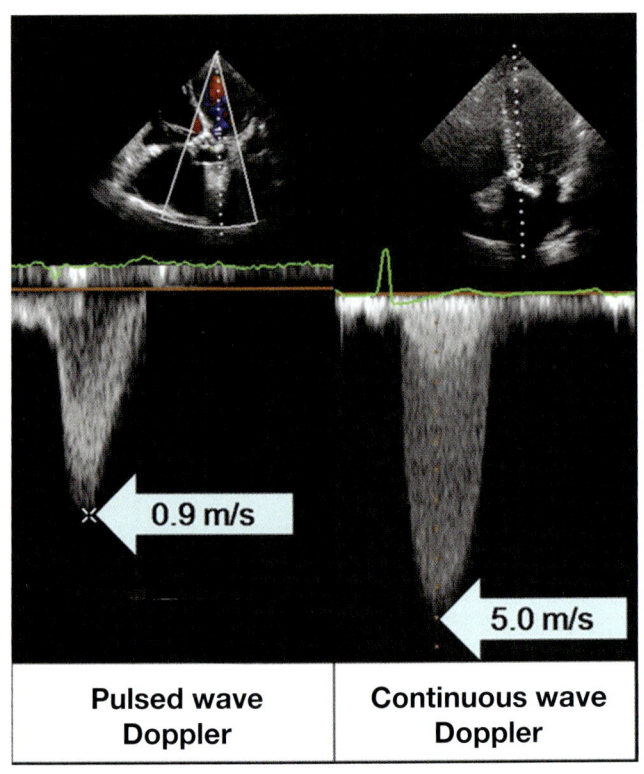

Figure 8.9

25. **Figure 8.10** shows a continuous wave spectral Doppler tracing from a 21-year-old woman that represents the flow velocity profile in the main pulmonary artery. Based on **Figure 8.10**, the following is **TRUE** about this patient:
    A. End-diastolic gradient across the pulmonic valve is high.
    B. There is severe pulmonic valve stenosis.
    C. Pulmonary artery systolic pressure is 9 mm Hg above the right ventricular pressure.
    D. Pulmonic valve regurgitation is severe.
    E. The velocity profile is diagnostic of patent ductus arteriosus.

Figure 8.10

26. The tracings in **Figure 8.11** were obtained from an 82-year-old woman with a normal left ventricular ejection fraction of 65%. The LEFT panel represents blood flow velocity pattern obtained by placing a pulsed-wave Doppler sample volume at the mitral leaflet tips. The RIGHT panel represents tissue Doppler of the lateral mitral annulus. Based on these two tracings, the following is **TRUE**:

A. The patient has excellent exercise capacity.
B. Abnormal left ventricular relaxation alone explains the mitral inflow pattern.
C. Left atrial pressure is elevated.
D. Patient has normal left ventricular diastolic function.
E. Mitral E wave velocity is expected to increase following the Valsalva maneuver.

27. The two panels in **Figure 8.12** were obtained from the same patient at the same heart rate. The following statement is **TRUE**:

A. Mitral inflow pattern is diagnostic of restrictive filling.
B. Left ventricular end-diastolic pressure is elevated.
C. The higher the peak velocity of the atrial reversal wave in pulmonary veins, the lower the left ventricular pressure.
D. The absence of atrial reversal wave in pulmonary vein tracings indicates pulmonary hypertension due to left ventricular dysfunction.
E. Ratio of peak systolic to peak diastolic velocity in pulmonary veins of more than one is indicative of elevated left atrial pressure.

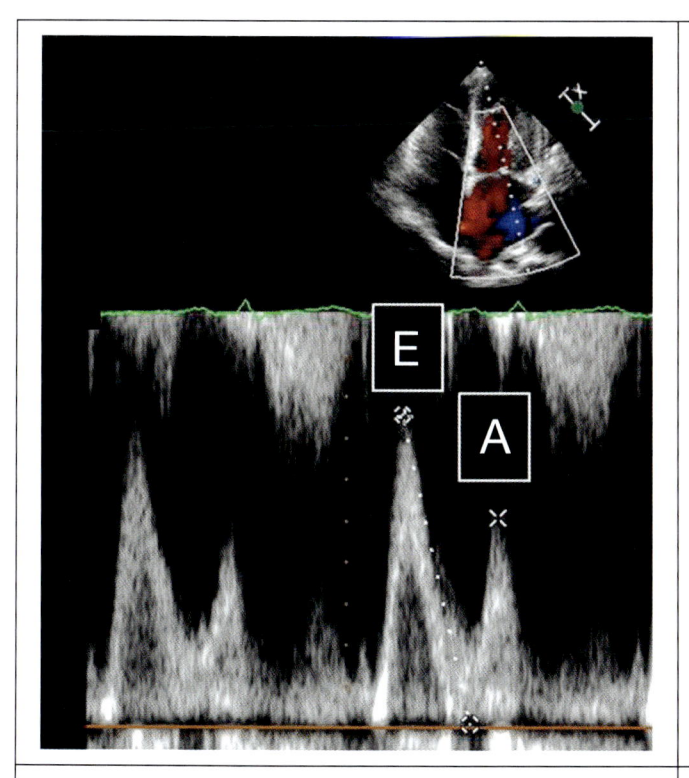

MITRAL INFLOW
Peak E wave velocity = 142 cm/s
E wave deceleration time = 148 ms

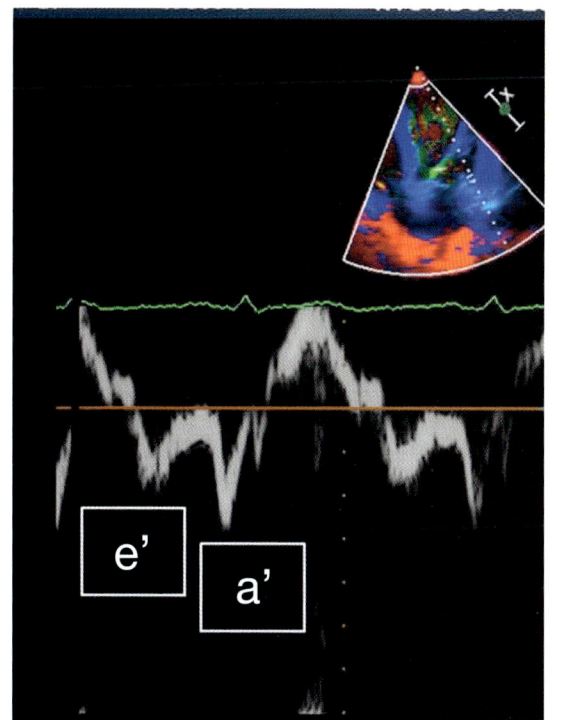

LATERAL MITRAL ANNULUS
Peak e' velocity = 8 cm/s
Peak a' velocity = 10 cm/s

Figure 8.11

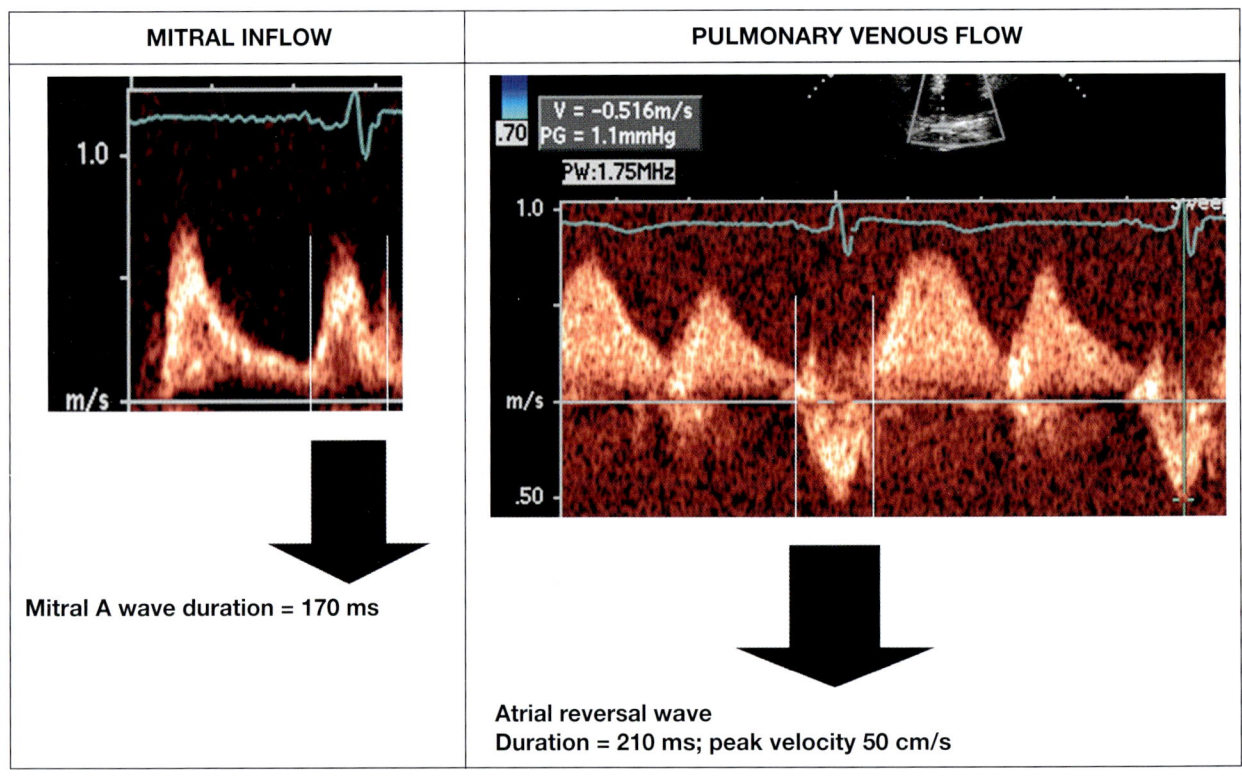

Figure 8.12

MITRAL INFLOW	PULMONARY VENOUS FLOW
Mitral A wave duration = 170 ms	Atrial reversal wave Duration = 210 ms; peak velocity 50 cm/s

28. Upward deflection in respirometry recordings from **Figure 8.13** indicate inspiration while the downward deflection indicates expiration. The following statement is **TRUE**:
    A. There is no ventricular interdependence.
    B. Expiratory increase in diastolic flow reversal in hepatic veins suggests constriction.
    C. Abnormal interventricular septal motion is due to right ventricular volume overload.
    D. Inspiratory increase in antegrade hepatic vein flow velocities is abnormal.
    E. Above M-mode recordings are diagnostic of a large pericardial effusion and tamponade.

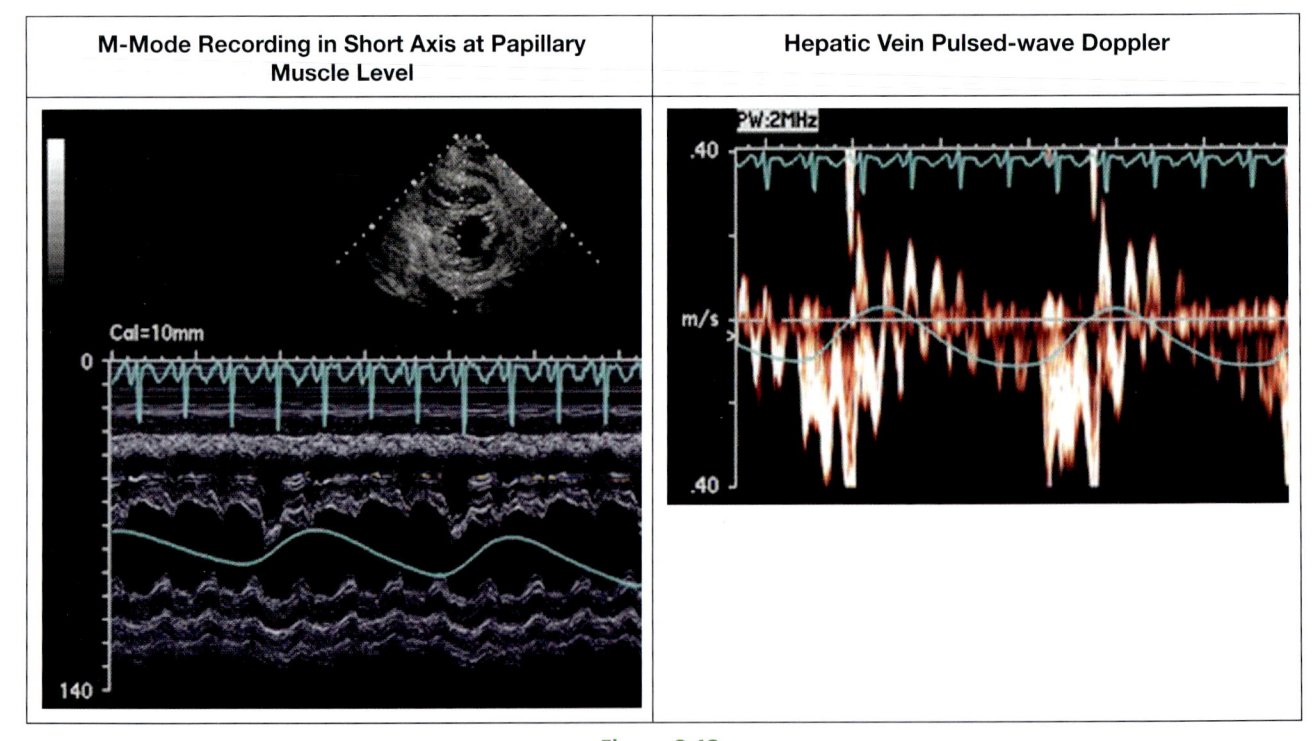

Figure 8.13

M-Mode Recording in Short Axis at Papillary Muscle Level	Hepatic Vein Pulsed-wave Doppler

29. A 33-year-old man has had a murmur since childhood. The transthoracic spectral Doppler tracings in **Figure 8.14** are obtained from the suprasternal view. Which of the following statements is **TRUE**:
    A. The pattern of diastolic flow is indicative of severe aortic regurgitation.
    B. The tracings are diagnostic of aortic coarctation.
    C. Quadricuspid aortic valve is the most common cause of aortic stenosis associated with the above flow velocity pattern.
    D. The recordings are obtained from the ascending aorta and represent severe aortic stenosis.
    E. Patient's blood pressure in the legs is markedly higher than in the arms.

30. A 91-year-old woman presents with severe shortness of breath. The two spectral Doppler recordings in **Figure 8.15** were obtained from two different valves. The vertical line in each tracing marks the onset of QRS. The following statement is **TRUE**:
    A. Panel B represents tricuspid regurgitant jet and the patient has severely elevated right ventricular systolic pressure.
    B. Panel A represents severe aortic stenosis because the jet starts during isovolumic contraction period.
    C. The jet with the shorter duration represents aortic stenosis.
    D. Peak velocity of 5.0 m/s in Panel B is not compatible with a tricuspid regurgitant jet.
    E. Systolic function of both ventricles is severely diminished.

Peak systolic velocity	3.77 m/s
End-diastolic velocity	1.0 ms

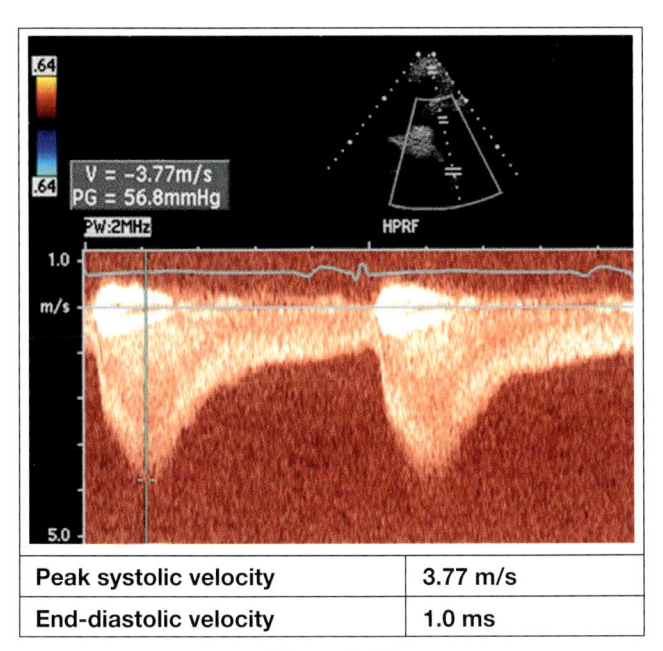

Figure 8.14

Peak velocity = 4.5 m/s
Jet duration = 515 ms

Peak velocity = 5.0 m/s
Jet duration = 345 ms

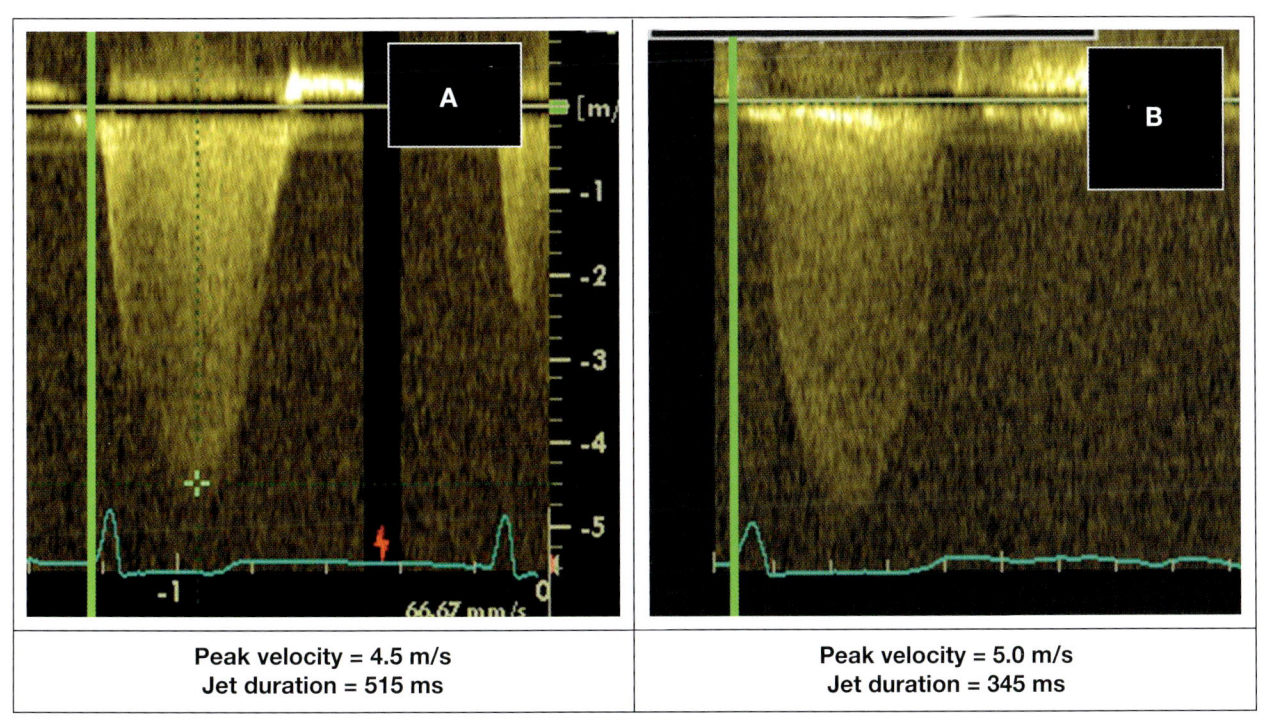

Figure 8.15

31. A 55-year-old man with hypertension treated with a beta-blocker and advanced gastric carcinoma presents with sudden onset of severe shortness of breath. The spectral pulsed-wave Doppler recordings were obtained at the mitral leaflet tips as shown in **Figure 8.16**. Upward deflection in respirometry recordings above indicates inspiration, while the downward deflection indicates expiration. The following statement is **TRUE**:
   A. Respiratory variations in peak velocity of late diastolic flow (A wave) of more than 25% favor constriction over tamponade.
   B. Marked decrease in peak E wave velocity seen at the onset of inspiration is consistent with the diagnosis of tamponade.
   C. Findings are characteristic of restrictive cardiomyopathy.
   D. The ratio of early to late diastolic peak mitral velocity (E/A ratio) of less than one favors the diagnosis of constrictive pericarditis.
   E. Treatment with diuretics would markedly improve patient's shortness of breath.

32. A 28-year-old man with liver disease presents with jugular venous distension. (See **Figure 8.17**.) The following statement is **TRUE**:
   A. Right atrial pressure rises progressively toward the end of ventricular systole.
   B. Right ventricular systolic function is markedly diminished.
   C. Peak velocity of 2.2 m/s excludes the diagnosis of pulmonary hypertension.
   D. Tricuspid regurgitation is likely mild.
   E. There is a right ventricular midcavitary gradient during systole.

Peak velocity of tricuspid regurgitant jet = 2.2 m/sec

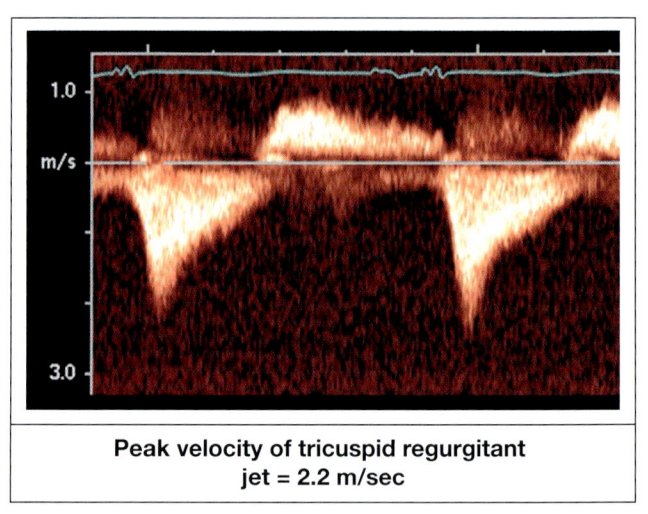

Figure 8.17

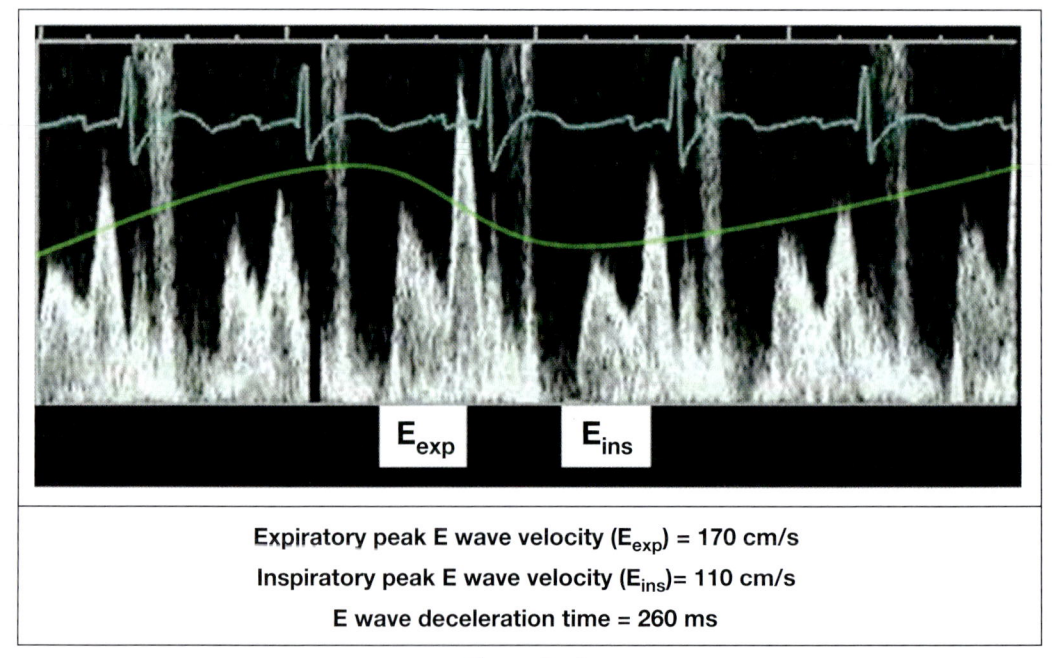

Expiratory peak E wave velocity (E$_{exp}$) = 170 cm/s
Inspiratory peak E wave velocity (E$_{ins}$) = 110 cm/s
E wave deceleration time = 260 ms

Figure 8.16

33. A 59-year-old man was diagnosed with perimembranous ventricular septal defect (VSD) by transthoracic echocardiography.

His blood pressure was 90/45 mm Hg and his end-diastolic right atrial pressure was estimated at 10 mm Hg. There was no aortic or tricuspid valve stenosis. The continuous wave spectral Doppler shown in **Figure 8.18** was obtained across his VSD. What is this patient's left ventricular end-diastolic pressure (LVEDP)?
A. 39 mm Hg.
B. 6 mm Hg.
C. 19 mm Hg.
D. 26 mm Hg.
E. 35 mm Hg.

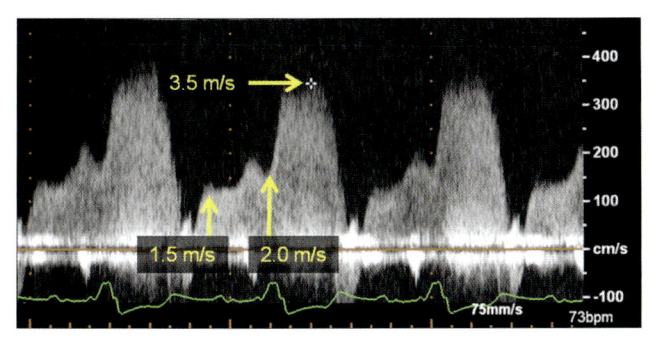

Figure 8.18

34. A 55-year-old Vietnamese woman presents with progressive dyspnea on exertion, increased abdominal girth and bilateral pitting edema over the past several months. The mitral annular tissue Doppler tracings in **Figure 8.19** were obtained. These tissue Doppler recordings are most consistent with the following diagnosis:

A. Carcinoid heart disease.
B. Amyloidosis.
C. Constrictive pericarditis.
D. Mitral annular calcifications.
E. Flail posterior mitral leaflet.

35. A 29-year-old woman on transesophageal echocardiography in preparation to have a secundum atrial septal defect (ASD) closure was found to have a left-to-right shunt with a continuous wave Doppler flow pattern. Her right atrial pressure was estimated at 8 mm Hg. Based on **Figure 8.20**, what is the peak left atrial pressure in this patient?
A. 1 mm Hg.
B. 17 mm Hg.
C. 21 mm Hg.
D. 36 mm Hg.
E. 52 mm Hg.

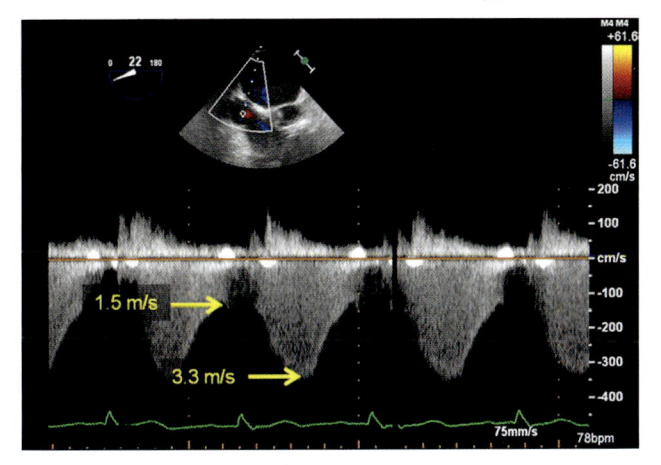

Figure 8.20

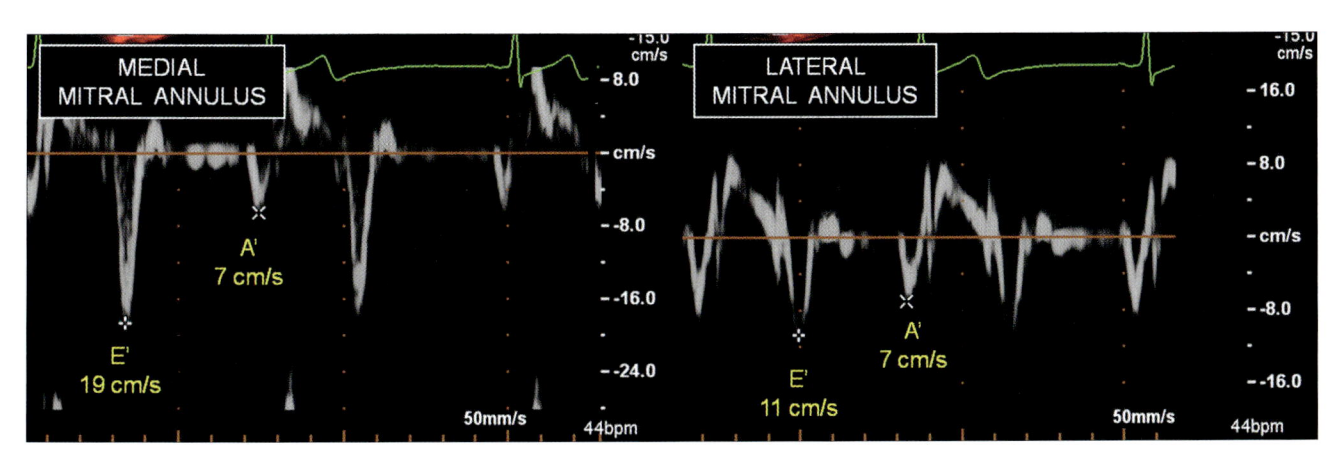

Figure 8.19

36. A 49-year-old man was referred for transthoracic echocardiogram for the evaluation of a murmur. The continuous wave Doppler tracing across the mitral valve was obtained from the apical 4-chamber view (**Figure 8.21**). In addition, the effective regurgitant orifice area (EROA) of mitral regurgitation is calculated at 0.48 cm², left atrial pressure is estimated at 10 mm Hg and no aortic stenosis is present. Regarding this patient, which of the following statements is **CORRECT**?
    A. Mitral regurgitation occurs only in early systole.
    B. EROA accurately reflects the severity of mitral regurgitation in this patient.
    C. Patient is hypotensive at the time of the study.
    D. Regurgitant fraction of mitral regurgitation is 60%.
    E. Regurgitant volume of this patient is indicative of moderate (2+) mitral regurgitation.

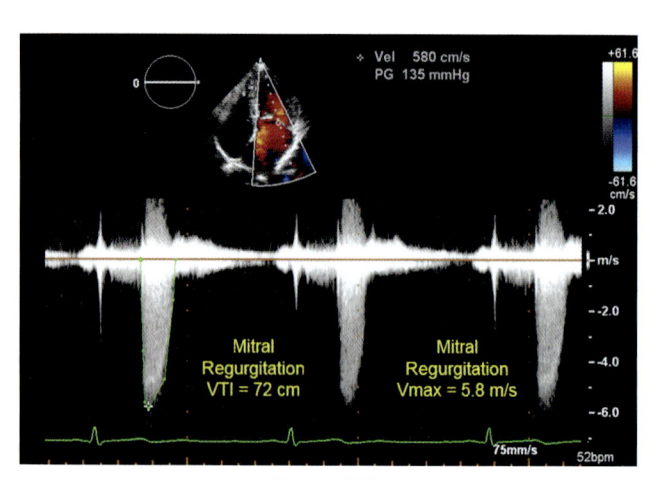

Figure 8.21

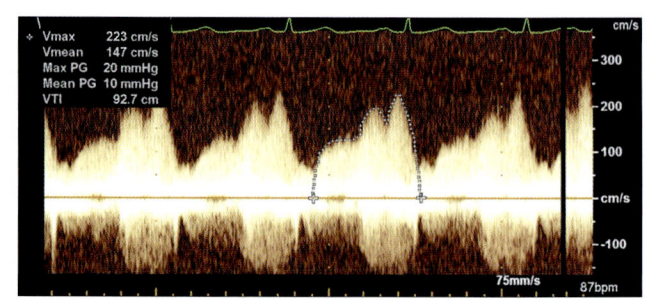

Figure 8.22

37. A 35-year-old man who grew up in Venezuela reports a history of rheumatic fever in his childhood. He was referred for transthoracic echocardiogram for the evaluation of a murmur. The continuous wave spectral Doppler tracing across the mitral valve was obtained in the apical 4-chamber view (**Figure 8.22**). Based on **Figure 8.22**, which is the **CORRECT** diagnosis?
    A. Mitral stenosis due to supravalvular ring.
    B. Shone complex.
    C. Rheumatic mitral stenosis.
    D. Cor triatriatum.
    E. Subvalvular mitral stenosis.

CASE 1

A 78-year-old obese woman with history of hypertension and poorly controlled diabetes mellitus developed progressive chest pain and shortness of breath for the past 2 days. She had no prior history of coronary revascularization or heart surgery. Her son brought her to the emergency department where she was noted to be diaphoretic and tachypneic.

Electrocardiogram in the emergency department revealed normal sinus rhythm, right bundle branch block, and nonspecific ST/T wave changes.

Blood pressure 90/50 mm Hg; heart rate 100 beats/min; and oral temperature 98.7°. On auscultation of the lungs, rales were noted bilaterally throughout the lung fields. The heart exam revealed prominent S3 and no murmur. Serum troponin was elevated at 40 ng/mL (normal <5 ng/mL). There was marked pulmonary edema on chest X-ray.

Transthoracic echocardiogram at the time of presentation revealed hypokinesis of six left ventricular segments supplied by the left anterior descending artery; ejection fraction was estimated at 40%. There was mild regurgitation of a structurally normal native mitral valve.

38. The patient in **Case 1** was transferred to the intensive care unit where a Swan–Ganz catheter was placed. Pulmonary artery wedge pressure was 38 mm Hg. Tissue Doppler of the medial mitral annulus and pulsed-wave Doppler recordings with the sample volume at the tips of the mitral valve leaflets were obtained at that time. Patient was in normal sinus rhythm. Peak velocity of the early annular tissue Doppler wave (e′) was 5 cm/s. Which of the following mitral flow velocity patterns shown in **Figure 8.23** is most likely at this time?

A Peak E wave velocity = 45 cm/s

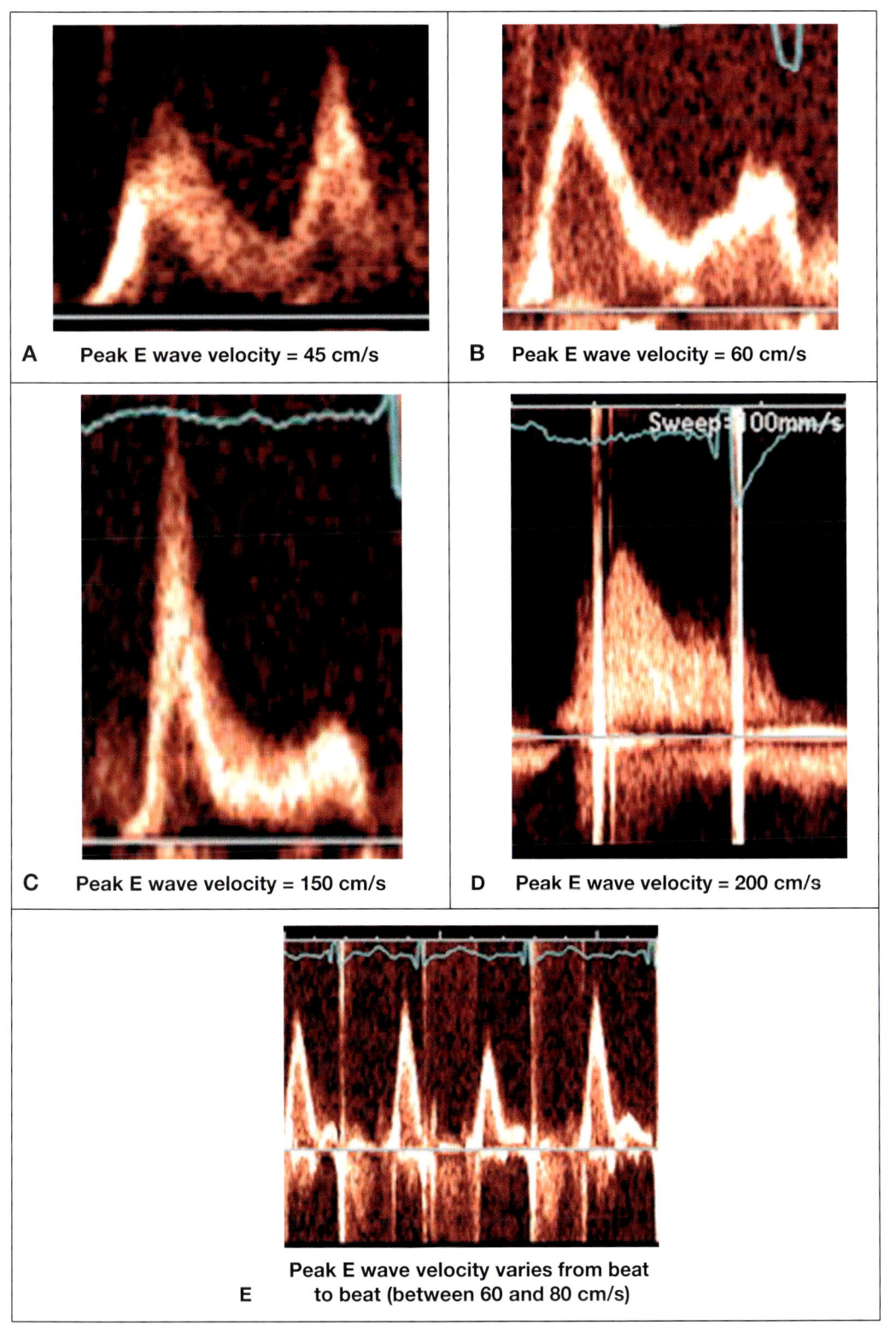

B Peak E wave velocity = 60 cm/s

C Peak E wave velocity = 150 cm/s

D Peak E wave velocity = 200 cm/s

E Peak E wave velocity varies from beat to beat (between 60 and 80 cm/s)

Figure 8.23

158 / Clinical Echocardiography Review

39. From the emergency department, the patient in **Case 1** was taken for coronary angiogram which revealed total occlusion of the proximal left anterior descending artery and diffuse atherosclerosis in the left circumflex artery. Percutaneous coronary intervention was attempted but the stent could not be deployed in the left anterior descending artery. She was then transferred to the intensive care unit. After appropriate medical therapy, she was discharged home free of symptoms on hospital day 5.

Three days later, she collapsed. Emergency services were activated and the patient was intubated in the field for severe hypoxemia. On admission, she was afebrile. Laboratory data revealed normal white blood cell count. Chest X-ray in the emergency department demonstrated massive bilateral pulmonary edema. Transesophageal echocardiography was performed and ▶ **Video 8.1** was obtained. In addition, the following data were obtained in **Figure 8.24**. The degree of mitral regurgitation is:

A. Trivial.
B. Mild (1+).
C. Moderate (2+).
D. Moderate to severe (3+).
E. Severe (4+).

40. The most likely etiology of mitral regurgitation in the patient in **Case 1** is:
A. Papillary muscle rupture.
B. Bacterial endocarditis.
C. Mitral annular dilatation.
D. Rheumatic heart disease.
E. Mitral valve prolapse.

CASE 2

A 56-year-old man, a recent immigrant from Argentina has been an avid soccer player since childhood. He reports that over the past year or so, he no longer can run around the soccer field as he used to because of exertional dyspnea. He initially saw a pulmonary specialist who ruled out exercise-induced asthma.

On examination, his blood pressure was 170/70 mm Hg; heart rate was 72 beats/min with a regular rhythm; room air oxygen saturation by pulse oxymetry was 98%. He has no central or peripheral cyanosis. His lungs are clear. First heart sound (S_1) is normal while the second heart sound (S_2) is obscured by the continuous, machinery-type murmur best heard in the left upper chest. There is no peripheral edema.

Echocardiography revealed patent ductus arteriosus, normal left ventricular systolic function, no valvular disease, and no hypertrophic cardiomyopathy. Right atrial pressure was estimated at 10 mm Hg.

Color Doppler demonstrating PISA on the left ventricular side of the mitral valve; radius is 0.9 cm	PISA r = 0.9 cm
Peak systolic velocity of mitral regurgitant jet	4.2 m/s

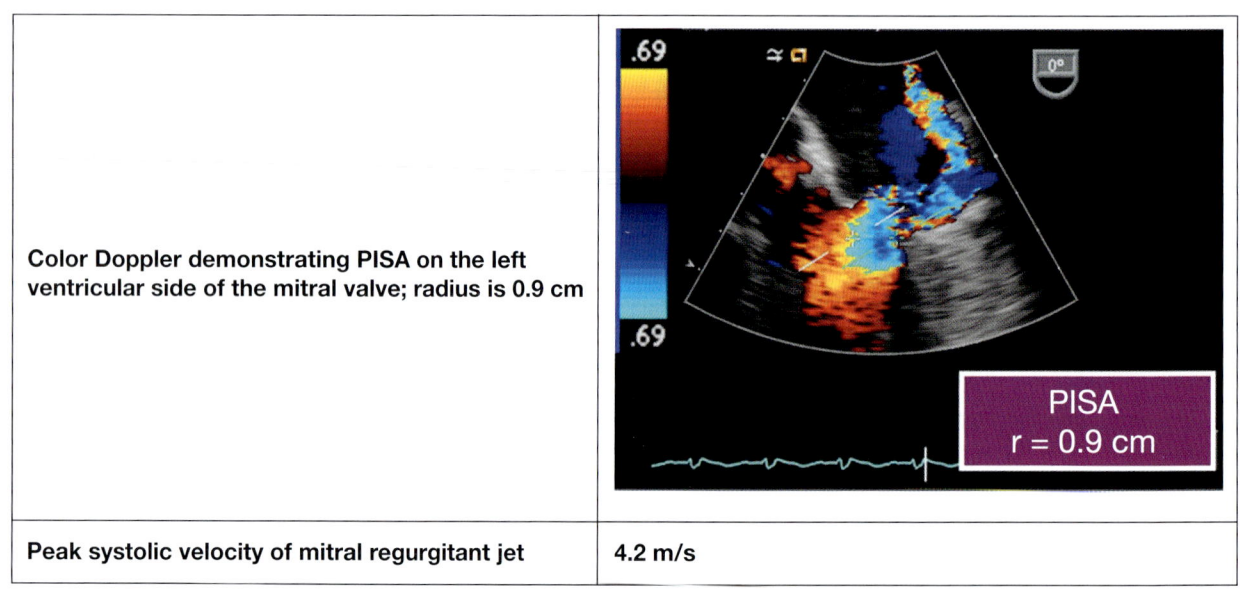

Figure 8.24

41. For the patient in **Case 2**, the spectral Doppler tracing shown in **Figure 8.25** represents flow across the patent ductus arteriosus obtained by transthoracic echocardiography. The following statement is **TRUE**:
   A. Pulmonary artery diastolic pressure is 21 mm Hg above the right atrial pressure.
   B. The tracing was obtained by pulsed-wave Doppler technique.
   C. Pulmonary artery pressure is estimated at 26/12 mm Hg.
   D. Pulmonary artery systolic pressure is 110 mm Hg.
   E. Patent ductus arteriosus is very large because the flow occurs throughout the cardiac cycle.

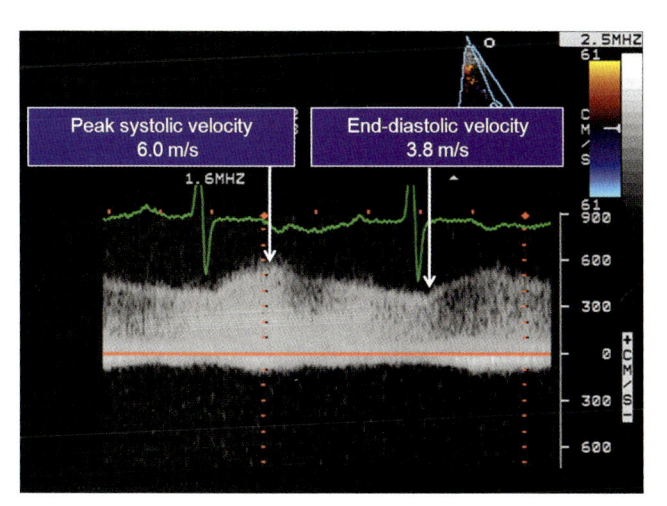

Figure 8.25

42. For the patient in **Case 2**, the transthoracic echocardiographic color Doppler image (**Figure 8.26**) in the parasternal short-axis view at the level of the patent ductus arteriosus comes from the same study as the spectral tracing in **Question 8.41**. Using the PISA method, the cross-sectional area of the patent ductus arteriosus at its aortic end during maximum flow is:
   A. 0.01 cm².
   B. 0.11 cm².
   C. 0.22 cm².
   D. 1.3 cm².
   E. 2.2 cm².

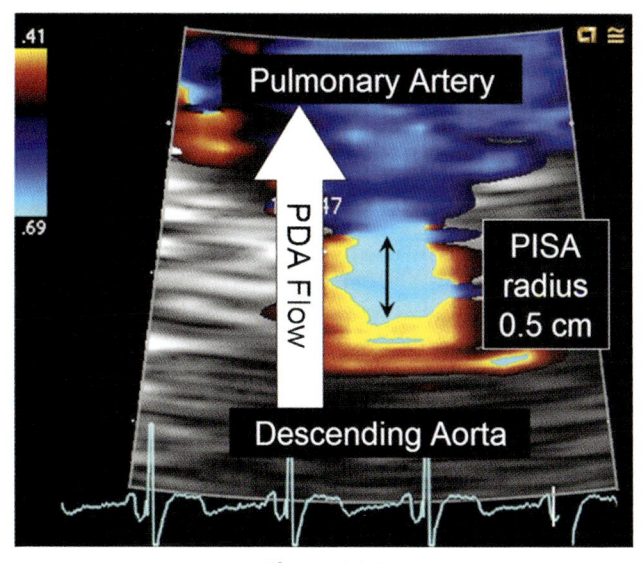

Figure 8.26

CASE 3

A 24-year-old college athlete collapsed on the basketball court. The coach promptly used the automatic external defibrillator which delivered an appropriate shock and revived the patient. The patient was then brought to the emergency department.

On physical examination, he was lying comfortably in bed, fully awake, alert and oriented. Blood pressure 144/72 mm Hg; heart rate 64 beats/min. Lungs were clear on auscultation. Cardiac exam revealed a crescendo–decrescendo systolic ejection murmur along the left sternal border which increased with Valsalva maneuver. The carotid upstroke was brisk and there was a bisferiens pulse.

43. For the patient in **Case 3**, transthoracic echocardiogram performed in the emergency department demonstrated hypertrophic cardiomyopathy with asymmetric septal hypertrophy, systolic anterior motion, and normal left ventricular systolic function. Aortic valve was normal. Left atrial pressure was estimated at 10 mm Hg. There was eccentric mitral regurgitation; the spectral Doppler of the mitral regurgitant jet is depicted in **Figure 8.27**. The following statement is **TRUE**:
   A. Envelope of the mitral regurgitant jet is not fully recorded because the early systolic portion of the jet is missing.
   B. Left ventricular systolic pressure is low.
   C. Maximal instantaneous left ventricular outflow gradient is 122 mm Hg.
   D. Mitral regurgitation is partly diastolic.
   E. Peak left ventricular systolic pressure is 246 mm Hg.

Peak velocity of mitral regurgitant jet = 8 m/s

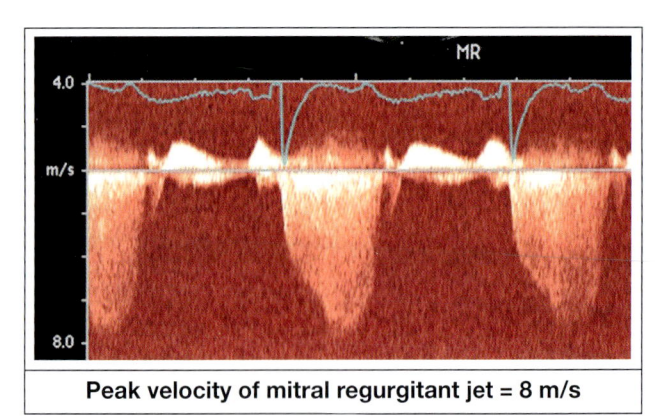

Figure 8.27

44. The patient in **Case 3** was started on oral disopyramide. Repeat echocardiogram was done and spectral tracing was obtained (**Figure 8.28**). Left atrial pressure was again estimated at 10 mm Hg. Otherwise, there were no significant changes in his echocardiogram. The following statement is **TRUE**:
    A. The shape of the mitral regurgitant jet is now suggestive of mitral valve prolapse with click and systolic murmur.
    B. Flow velocity pattern of jet #2 is typical of valvular aortic stenosis.
    C. Left ventricular outflow gradient has dropped by about 50% compared to the initial echocardiogram.
    D. The patient has developed intracavitary gradient as demonstrated by jet #1.
    E. Peak left ventricular systolic pressure is now 159 mm Hg minus the left atrial pressure.

CASE 4

A 66-year-old man with a long-standing history of ethanol abuse complains of orthopnea, paroxysmal nocturnal dyspnea, and lower extremity edema.

He is tachypneic and tachycardic. Blood pressure 90/50 mm Hg, heart rate 110 bpm; weight 80 kg; height 175 cm; and body surface area 2.1 m². Auscultation of the lungs reveals bibasilar rales. Cardiac exam demonstrates an S_3 gallop and no murmur. There is bilateral lower extremity pitting edema pretibially.

Transthoracic echocardiogram revealed global left ventricular hypokinesis with an estimated ejection fraction of 25%.

45. To calculate the left atrial volume for the patient in **Case 4**, the data in **Figure 8.29** were obtained. The left atrial volume index is approximately:
    A. 20 mL/m².
    B. 30 mL/m².
    C. 40 mL/m².
    D. 50 mL/m².
    E. 60 mL/m².

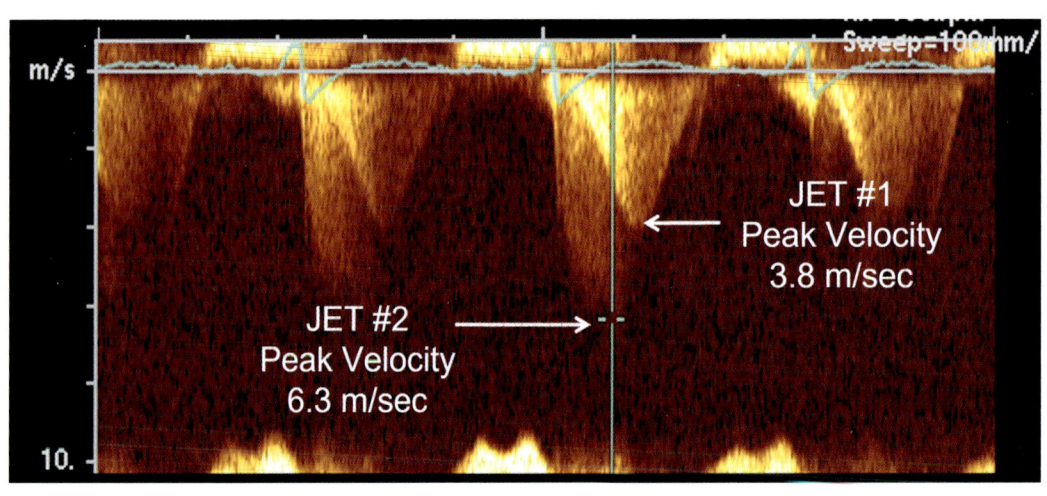

JET #1 Peak Velocity 3.8 m/sec

JET #2 Peak Velocity 6.3 m/sec

Figure 8.28

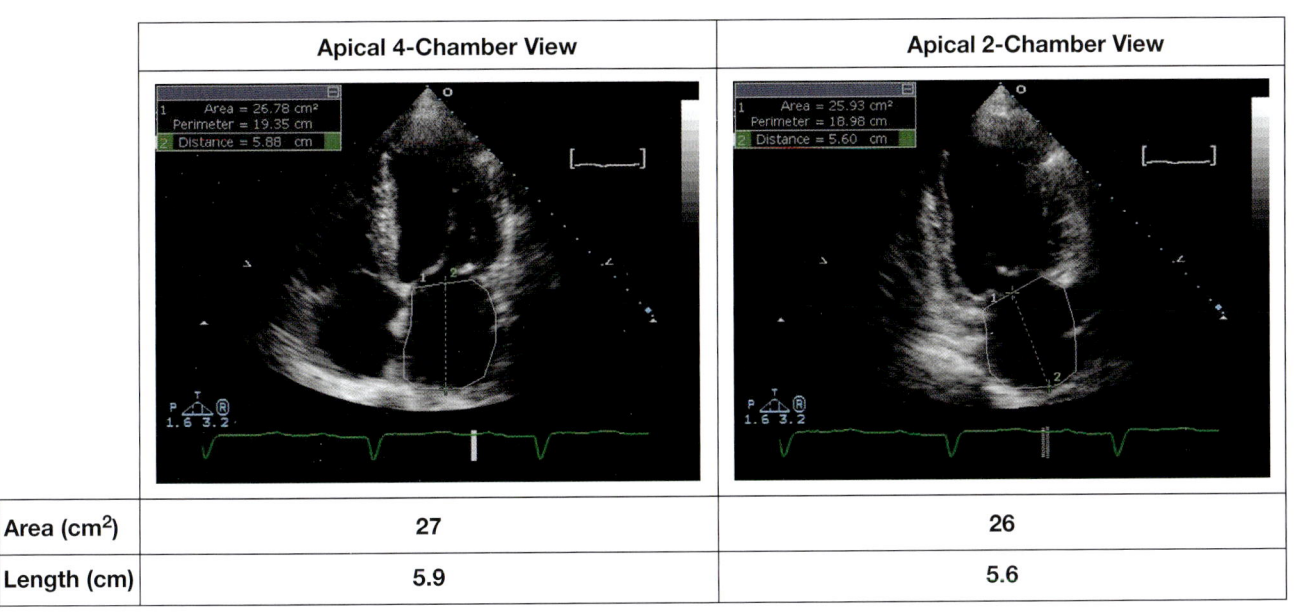

	Apical 4-Chamber View	Apical 2-Chamber View
Area (cm²)	27	26
Length (cm)	5.9	5.6

Figure 8.29

46. For the patient in **Case 4**, mitral inflow and pulmonary venous flow velocity spectral Doppler tracings (**Figure 8.30**) were obtained on admission and after 5 days of appropriate medical therapy, including intravenous diuretics. The following was the result of what medical therapy?
  A. Left ventricular preload has increased.
  B. Left atrial pressure has decreased.
  C. Normal mitral filling pattern was replaced with the pattern of abnormal relaxation.
  D. Patient has developed atrial flutter.
  E. The change in mitral filling pattern seen in this patient portends grave long-term prognosis.

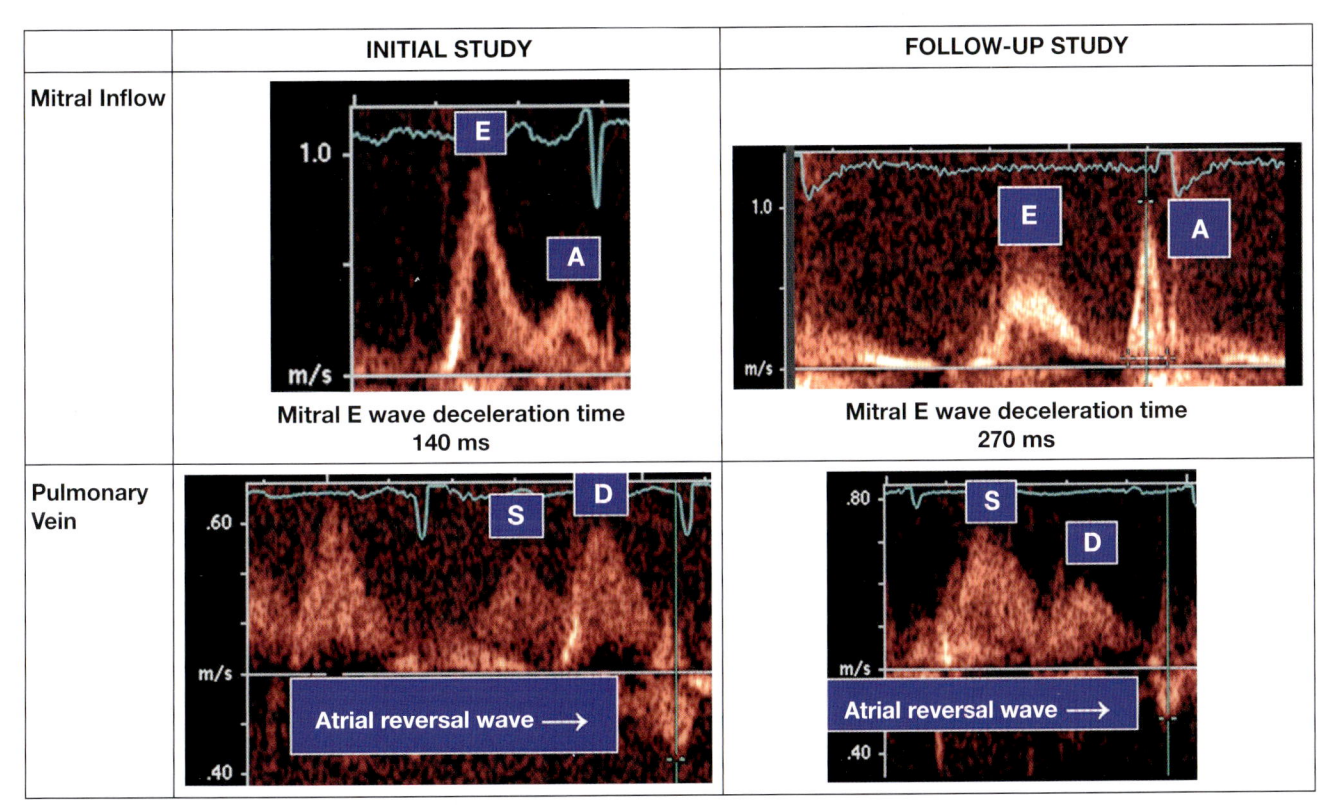

	INITIAL STUDY	FOLLOW-UP STUDY
Mitral Inflow	Mitral E wave deceleration time 140 ms	Mitral E wave deceleration time 270 ms
Pulmonary Vein	Atrial reversal wave →	Atrial reversal wave →

Figure 8.30

CASE 5

A 23-year-old college student came back to the United States from an extended trip to rural areas of the Indian subcontinent complaining of dyspnea on exertion and chest pain on deep inspiration.

*On initial outpatient examination, he was afebrile. His lungs were clear on auscultation. There was a friction rub throughout the precordium. Electrocardiogram was suggestive of pericarditis (**Figure 8.31**).*

He was prescribed an oral course of a nonsteroidal anti-inflammatory agent (NSAID) and sent home.

Despite taking the NSAID for 2 weeks, his chest pain worsened. Computed tomography of the chest revealed a large pericardial and left pleural effusion with clinical and echocardiographic signs of tamponade. Skin test for tuberculosis (PPD) was positive. Pericardial effusion was drained percutaneously and the patient was started on appropriate anti-tuberculosis medical therapy.

His chest pain resolved completely. However, his shortness of breath persisted and he started developing bilateral ankle edema. Transthoracic echocardiogram was ordered.

47. For the patient in **Case 5**, **Figure 8.32** was also obtained on the echocardiogram. In **Figure 8.32**, the upstroke of the respirometer curve denotes inspiration, and the downstroke indicates expiration. The following is **TRUE**:
    A. Restrictive cardiomyopathy of the left ventricle is present.
    B. Right atrial pressure is low.
    C. Left ventricular flow propagation velocity (Vp) is abnormal.
    D. Patient has constrictive pericarditis.
    E. Degree of respiratory variations in the mitral inflow is normal.

48. ▶ **Video 8.2**, from the patient in **Case 5**, obtained in the apical 4-chamber view, demonstrates abnormal septal motion which is due to:

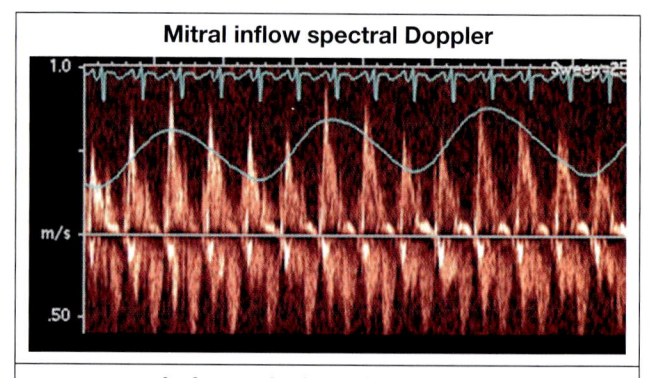

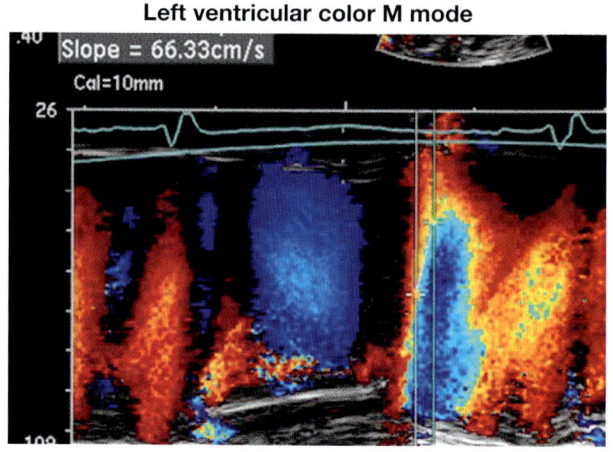

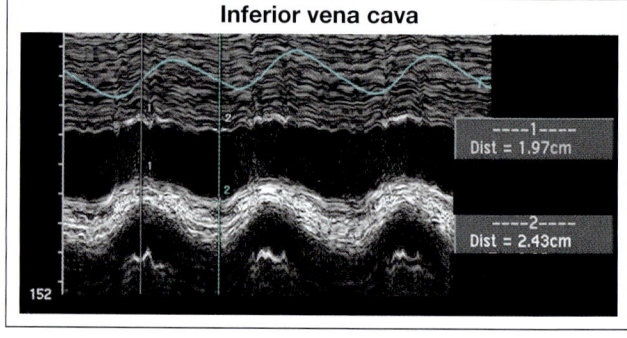

Figure 8.32

A. Right ventricular pressure overload.
B. Right ventricular volume overload.
C. Left bundle branch block.
D. Ventricular interdependence.
E. Cardiac surgery.

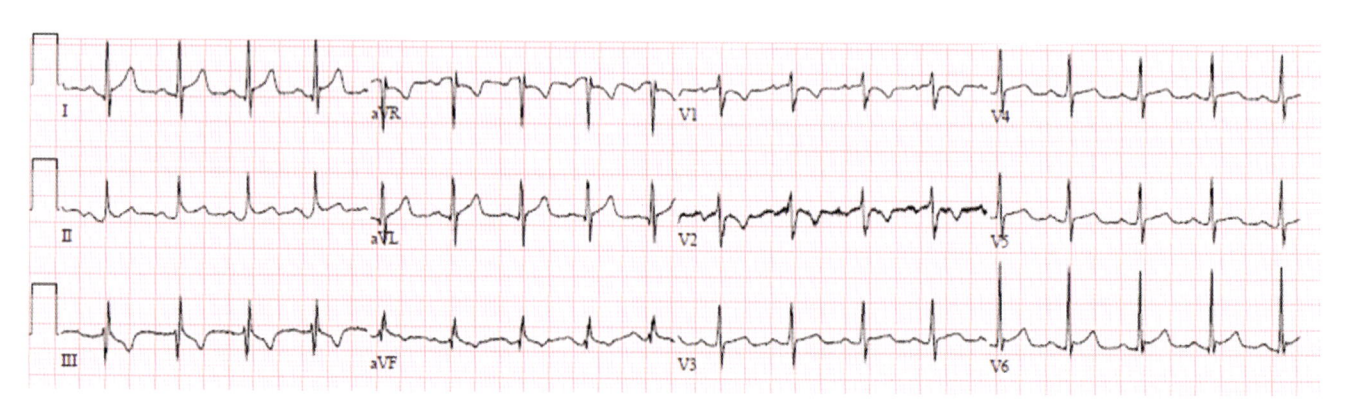

Figure 8.31

ANSWERS

1. **Answer: B.** By the continuity equation, AVA can be calculated as follows:

$$AVA = LVOT\ area * \frac{LVOT\ VTI}{AV\ VTI}$$

AVA on TTE #1

$$AVA = 3.14 * \frac{18}{65} = 0.87\ cm^2$$

AVA on TTE #2

$$AVA = 3.14 * \frac{24}{87} = 0.87\ cm^2$$

Thus, there was no significant change in the AVA between the two studies.

Answer A is incorrect because there was no significant change in the dimensionless velocity index (DVI) between the two studies despite the significant change in aortic valve velocities as shown in **Table 8.2**. DVI is defined as the ratio of LVOT to aortic valve Vmax.

Answer C is incorrect because the LVOT stroke volume has actually increased on TTE #2 compared to TTE #1, as shown in **Table 8.3**.

LVOT stroke volume is calculated as the product of LVOT area.

Table 8.2

	Units	TTE #1	TTE #2
AV Vmax	m/s	3.1	4.2
LVOT Vmax	m/s	0.90	1.2
DVI		0.29	0.29

AV Vmax, aortic valve maximum velocity; DVI, dimensionless velocity index; LVOT Vmax, left ventricular outflow tract maximum velocity.

Table 8.3

	Units	TTE #1	TTE #2
LVOT VTI	cm	18	24
LVOT Diameter	cm	2.0	2.0
LVOT Area	cm^3	3.14	3.14
SV	mL	57	75

LVOT VTI, left ventricular outflow tract velocity-time integral; SV, stroke volume.

LVOT area on both TTE #1 and TTE #2:

$$LVOT\ area = \pi * \left(\frac{1}{2} * LVOT\ diameter\right)^2$$

$$LVOT\ area = 3.14 * \left(\frac{1}{2} * 2.0\ cm\right)^2$$

$$LVOT\ area = 3.14\ cm^2$$

LVOT stroke volume on TTE #1

LVOT stroke volume = LVOT area * LVOT VTI
LVOT stroke volume = 3.14 cm^2 * 18 cm
LVOT stroke volume = 57 cm^3 = 57 mL

LVOT stroke volume on TTE #2

LVOT stroke volume = LVOT area * LVOT VTI
LVOT stroke volume = 3.14 cm^2 * 24 cm
LVOT stroke volume = 75 cm^3 = 75 mL

The increase in the LVOT stroke volume from 57 mL on TTE #1 to 75 mL on TTE #2 in this patient may be due to a hyperdynamic circulatory state in the setting of GI bleed.

Answer D is incorrect because the calculated aortic valve area (AVA) has not substantially changed between the two TTEs.

By the continuity equation, AVA can be calculated as follows:

$$AVA = LVOT\ area * \frac{LVOT\ VTI}{AV\ VTI}$$

AVA on TTE #1

$$AVA = 3.14 * \frac{18}{65} = 0.87\ cm^2$$

AVA on TTE #2

$$AVA = 3.14 * \frac{24}{87} = 0.87\ cm^2$$

2. **Answer: D.**
Mitral valve area (MVA) can be calculated using the pressure half-time (PHT) method:

$$MVA = \frac{220}{PHT} \qquad (8.1)$$

In this question, PHT was not given. However, PHT can be calculated from the stated mitral deceleration time (DT) using the following formula:

$$PHT = 0.29 * DT \qquad (8.2)$$

164 / Clinical Echocardiography Review

Thus, in our patient:

PHT = 0.29 * DT = 0.29 * 910 = 264 ms

MVA = 220/PHT = 220/264 = 0.8 cm².

Alternatively, Equations (8.1) and (8.2) can be combined into the following one:

$$MVA = \frac{759}{DT} \quad (8.3)$$

In our patient then:

MVA = 759/DT = 759/910 = 0.8 cm².

Therefore, answer D is correct.

Answer A is incorrect because the MVA is calculated by dividing 220 into PHT (Equation 8.1) and not DT.

Answer B is incorrect because the stroke volume (SV) across the mitral valve in this patient is 53 mL/beat. Once the MVA is calculated, SV and cardiac output (CO) can be derived using the following formulas:

SV = MVA * VTI

CO = SV * HR

where VTI is the mitral velocity-time integral during diastole, and HR is the heart rate.

In our patient, mitral VTI during diastole was 66 cm and the heart rate was 85 bpm:

SV = 0.8 cm² * 66 cm = 53 mL:

CO = 53 mL * 85 bpm = 4.5 L/min.

Answer C is incorrect because as shown above, PHT in this patient was 264 ms and not 355 ms.

Answer E is incorrect because the resting gradient of mitral stenosis is expected to increase with the augmentation of cardiac output such as during exercise, fever, or pregnancy.

3. **Answer: E.** The patient has patent ductus arteriosus (PDA) which is an extracardiac shunt resulting from a communication between the descending thoracic aorta (DTA) and the proximal left pulmonary artery.

In utero, the blood that reaches the pulmonary artery from the right ventricle cannot enter the collapsed lungs; instead, it is diverted across the ductus arteriosus into the DTA. Soon after birth, the pressure in the pulmonary artery falls below the pressure in DTA and the blood flow in the ductus arteriosus reverses its direction. It now flows from the DTA into the pulmonary artery. High oxygen content of the ductal blood triggers the closure of ductus arteriosus in most newborns. In rare instances, the communication persists in the post-neonatal period giving rise to PDA.

In individuals with PDA, the systemic blood flow (Qs) reaches the right heart through systemic veins and continues through the right ventricular outflow tract (RVOT) into the main pulmonary artery. At that level, Qs is joined by the shunt flow (SF) entering the pulmonary artery through the PDA. The sum of Qs and SF represents the amount of blood flow that enters the pulmonary circulation (Qp).

After passing through the lungs, Qp enters the left heart through the pulmonary veins and exits through the left ventricular outflow tract (LVOT) into the aorta. At the level of the descending aorta, Qp divides into SF which enters the PDA, and Qs which continues into the peripheral systemic circulation to ultimately reach the right heart through systemic veins.

Note that in individuals with PDA, the flow across the RVOT represents Qs and the flow across the LVOT represents Qp. Therefore, the answer E is correct.

This is in contrast to atrial and ventricular septal defects where LVOT flow represents Qs and the RVOT flow represents Qp. Since in most individuals with PDA, Qp > Qs, it is the left heart and not the right heart that dilates to accommodate the excess blood flow.

The general echocardiographic formula to calculate volumetric flow (Q) is:

$$Q = CSA * VTI * HR \quad (8.4)$$

where CSA is the cross-sectional area, VTI is velocity-time integral, and HR is the heart rate.

One can use right and left ventricular outflow tracts to calculate volumetric flow. Since both tracts are assumed to be circular in shape, the CSA can be expressed in the above equations as:

$$CSA = \left(\frac{1}{2} * D\right)^2 * \pi \quad (8.5)$$

where D is the diameter of the outflow tract. Equation (8.4) after expressing CSA in terms of Equation (8.5) becomes:

$$Q = \left(\frac{1}{2} * D\right)^2 * \pi * VTI * HR$$

Calculations for our patient are summarized in **Table 8.4**:

Answer A is incorrect because the flow rate of 7.8 L/min across the LVOT represents Qp and not Qs in patients with PDA.

Answer B is incorrect because Qp:Qs in this patient is greater than 1 (it is 1.7:1).

Answer C is incorrect because the stroke volume that enters the lungs (97 mL/beat) is the sum

Table 8.4

	LVOT	RVOT	Shunt Across PDA
Diameter (cm)	2.0	2.5	
Area (cm²)	3.1	4.9	
VTI (cm)	31	12	
Stroke Volume (mL)	97	59	97 − 59 = 38
HR	80	80	
	Qp	Qs	
Flow (L/min)	7.8	4.7	
Qp:Qs	1.7	1	

HR, heart rate; LVOT, left ventricular outflow tract; PDA, patent ductus arteriosus; Qp, pulmonic flow; Qs, systemic flow; RVOT, right ventricular outflow tract; VTI, velocity-time integral.

of the systemic stroke volume (59 mL/beat) that entered the main pulmonary artery through the RVOT and the shunt flow (38 mL/beat) that came into the pulmonary artery through the PDA.

Answer D is incorrect because Qp is much greater than Qs, the shunt flow is in the left-to-right direction and the patient is unlikely to be cyanotic. In patients with PDA who develop Eisenmenger physiology, there is a right-to-left shunt. Such patients are cyanotic in the lower parts of the body because the deoxygenated blood from the pulmonary artery crosses the PDA and enters the descending thoracic aorta past the origins of the aortic arch vessels, which supply fully oxygenated blood to the head and the arms.

4. **Answer: B.** (Pulmonary artery diastolic pressure is 31 mm Hg).

This patient with severe shortness of breath has elevated pulmonary artery diastolic pressure (PADP). Using the end-diastolic velocity (V) of the pulmonic regurgitant jet and the $4V^2$ formula, one can calculate the pressure gradient (ΔP) between the PADP and the end-diastolic right ventricular pressure (RVDP).

$$\Delta P = PADP - RVDP = 4 * V^2 \quad (8.6)$$

In the absence of tricuspid stenosis, RVDP is the same as the right atrial pressure (RAP). Thus the pressure gradient can also be expressed as:

$$\Delta P = PADP - RAP = 4 * V^2 \quad (8.7)$$

Rearranging Equation (8.7), PADP can be calculated in the following manner:

$$PADP = 4 * V^2 + RAP \quad (8.8)$$

where V is the end-diastolic velocity of the pulmonic regurgitant jet, and RAP is right atrial pressure.

RAP can be estimated from the expiratory size of the inferior vena cava (IVC) and the percent decrease in diameter change with inspiration as recommended by the 2015 chamber quantification guidelines by the American Society of Echocardiography and the European Association of Cardiovascular Imaging. In our patient, the IVC is dilated (>2.1 cm) and the IVC diameter does not change with inspiration. The estimated RAP is thus approximately 15 mm Hg ((range, 10-20 mm Hg).

Once RAP is known, we can then calculate PADP:

$$PADP = 4 * (2 \text{ m/s})^2 + 15 = 16 + 15 = 31 \text{ mm Hg}.$$

Therefore, answer B is correct.

Answer A is incorrect because RAP in this patient is >15 mm Hg as demonstrated in the previous section.

Answer C is incorrect for two reasons: (1) Pressure gradient between PADP and RVDP is 16 mm Hg and not 36 mm Hg; and (2) PADP is calculated by adding RAP to the gradient between PADP and RVDP and not subtracting from it.

Answer D is incorrect because even in mild pulmonic regurgitation appropriate spectral Doppler tracings of the regurgitant jet can be obtained.

Answer E is incorrect because normal PADP range is typically between 5 to 16 mm Hg.

5. **Answer: B.** (Effective regurgitant orifice area of mitral regurgitation is approximately 0.6 cm²).

Severe mitral regurgitation (grades 3+ and 4+) is defined by the following criteria:

	Severe MR
Regurgitant orifice (cm²)	≥0.4
Regurgitant fraction	≥50%
Regurgitant volume (mL)	≥60
Vena contracta (cm)	≥0.7

Regurgitant orifice area (ROA) can be calculated using the following formula:

$$ROA_{MR} = 2 * \pi * r^2 * \frac{V_{alias}}{V_{max}} \quad (8.9)$$

where r is the PISA radius, Valias is the aliasing velocity at which PISA radius is measured, and Vmax is the maximum velocity of the mitral regurgitant jet on spectral Doppler.

In Equation (8.9), the expression $2 * \pi * r^2 * V_{alias}$ represents instantaneous flow rate (IFR):

$$IFR = 2 * \pi * r^2 * V_{alias} \quad (8.10)$$

Now Equation (8.9) can be expressed as:

$$ROA_{MR} = \frac{IFR}{V_{max}} \quad (8.11)$$

In our patient, IFR is calculated as:

IFR = 2 * 3.14 *(1.0 cm)² * 45 cm/s = 283 mL/s

And ROA as:

$$ROA_{MR} = 283/500 \text{ cm/s} = 0.6 \text{ cm}^2.$$

Therefore, answer B is correct.

Answer A is incorrect because the vena contracta in severe mitral regurgitation is ≥0.7 cm.

Answer C is incorrect because the instantaneous flow rate (IFR) of the mitral regurgitant jet in this patient is 283 mL/s as calculated as above.

Answer D is incorrect because mitral regurgitation is severe since ROA ≥ 0.4 cm² (it is 0.6 cm²).

Answer E is incorrect because the regurgitant volume (RegV) in this patient is 79 mL/beat. RV can be calculated as:

$$RegV = ROA_{MR} * VTI_{MR} \quad (8.12)$$

where VTI_{MR} is the velocity-time integral of the mitral regurgitant jet.

In our patient, RV equals 0.6 cm² * 140 cm, or 79 mL/beat. This is again consistent with severe mitral regurgitation (RV ≥ 60 mL/beat).

6. **Answer: A.** (Mean pulmonary artery wedge pressure is markedly elevated).

The patient presents with shortness of breath due to elevated pulmonary artery wedge pressure (PAWP). In most instances, PAWP elevation is the result of high left atrial pressure (LAP) elevation.

PAWP can be estimated from the following formula:

$$PAWP = 4.6 + 5.27 * \frac{E}{Vp}$$

where E is the peak blood flow velocity of the mitral inflow in cm/s, and Vp is the flow propagation velocity of the mitral inflow (in cm/s) obtained by color M-mode. Vp recording of this patient is demonstrated in **Figure 8.33**.

Vp measures the rate at which red blood cells reach the LV apex from the mitral valve level during early diastole. The rate of blood flow from the mitral valve to the LV apex is determined by the rate of LV relaxation during early diastole. Therefore, Vp is an indirect measure of the rate of LV relaxation; the lower the Vp, the slower the LV relaxation and higher the left ventricular diastolic pressure (LVDP).

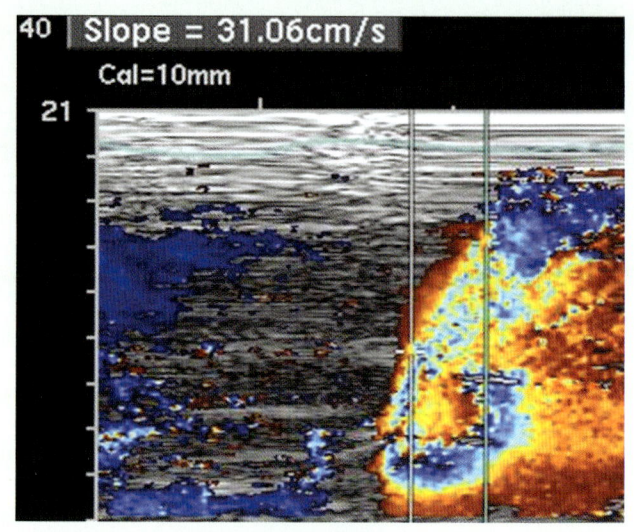

Figure 8.33

In our patient:

$$PAWP = 4.6 + 5.27 * \frac{125}{31} = 26$$

With the value of 26 mm Hg, PAWP is elevated; normal PAWP is ≤12 mm Hg. Therefore, answer A is correct.

Answer B is incorrect because in patients with markedly elevated LAP and PAWP, the peak velocity of the mitral E wave is typically higher than that of the mitral A wave. The patients have either the pseudonormal filling pattern (E/A is between 1.0 and 2.0; E wave deceleration time ≥160 ms) or the restrictive filling pattern (E/A > 2 and E wave deceleration time <160 ms).

Answer C is incorrect because the pulmonary artery systolic pressure (PASP) is 64 mm Hg plus the right atrial pressure, or 64 + 15 = 79 mm Hg. In the absence of pulmonic stenosis, PASP is the same as the right ventricular systolic pressure (RVSP). Peak velocity (V) of the tricuspid regurgitant flow can be used to estimate the RV-to-RA pressure gradient (ΔP) at peak systole:

$$\Delta P = 4 * V^2 = (4 \text{ m/s})^2 = 64 \text{ mm Hg}.$$

By adding right atrial pressure (RAP) to ΔP, RVSP (and, by extension, PASP) can be calculated:

RVSP = PASP = ΔP + RAP = 64 + 15 = 79 mm Hg.

Answer D is incorrect because the ratio of mitral E wave to mitral annular tissue Doppler e' wave is expected to be greater than 15 in patients with markedly elevated LAP and PAWP.

Answer E is incorrect because the normal Vp velocity >55 cm/s in young individuals and >45 cm/s in middle-aged and elderly individuals.

7. **Answer: A.** (Regurgitant fraction of 65% would indicate that the aortic regurgitation is severe).

Severe aortic regurgitation (grades 3+ and 4+) is defined by the following criteria:

	Severe AR
Regurgitant orifice (cm²)	≥0.3
Regurgitant fraction	≥50%
Regurgitant volume (mL)	≥60
Vena contracta (cm)	>0.6

Therefore, answer A is correct; the regurgitant fraction of 65% indicates a severe aortic regurgitation.

Answer B is incorrect because vena contracta is not strongly influenced by Nyquist limit color Doppler settings. This is in contrast to PISA radius. By changing the color Doppler Nyquist limit, one also automatically changes the velocity filter. The role of the velocity filter is to prevent color encoding of low velocities. By lowering the color Doppler Nyquist limit, one lowers the velocity filter allowing for the inclusion of lower velocities and an increase in the color area. Because vena contracta contains predominantly high velocities, altering the Nyquist limit will not significantly change the size of vena contracta diameter. This is in contrast to PISA radius, which becomes progressively larger with lower Nyquist limits.

The impact of changes in color Doppler Nyquist limit on vena contracta is demonstrated in **Figure 8.34**:

Answer C is incorrect because in severe aortic regurgitation vena contracta is >0.6 cm.

Answer D is incorrect because in severe aortic regurgitation, regurgitant volume is ≥60 mL/beat.

Answer E is incorrect because the diameter of vena contracta obtained by two-dimensional echocardiography should not be used to calculate the regurgitant volume. Instead, the two-dimensional diameter of vena contracta should be used for semi-quantitative assessment of the degree of aortic regurgitation.

8. **Answer: C.** (Mean left atrial pressure is approximately 20 mm Hg).

The E/e' ratio is directly proportional to left atrial pressure (LAP). The peak velocity of the mitral annular tissue Doppler e' wave is directly proportional to the rate of LV relaxation during early diastole. The slower the LV relaxation, the higher the left ventricular diastolic pressure (LVDP). Once LVDP rises, there is a concomitant rise in the LAP and PAWP rise to allow for better filling of a stiff LV. The higher the LAP, the taller the mitral E wave. In summary, as the LV diastolic dysfunction worsens, the peak velocity of the annular tissue e' wave gets smaller, the mitral E wave gets higher, and the E/e' ratio becomes progressively larger reflecting the rising LAP and PAWP.

The E/e' ratio can be used to estimate LAP in two ways. One approach is to use it semi-quantitatively; when an E/e' ratio using an average of medial and lateral e' peak velocities is greater than 14, this is suggestive of elevated LAP pressure.

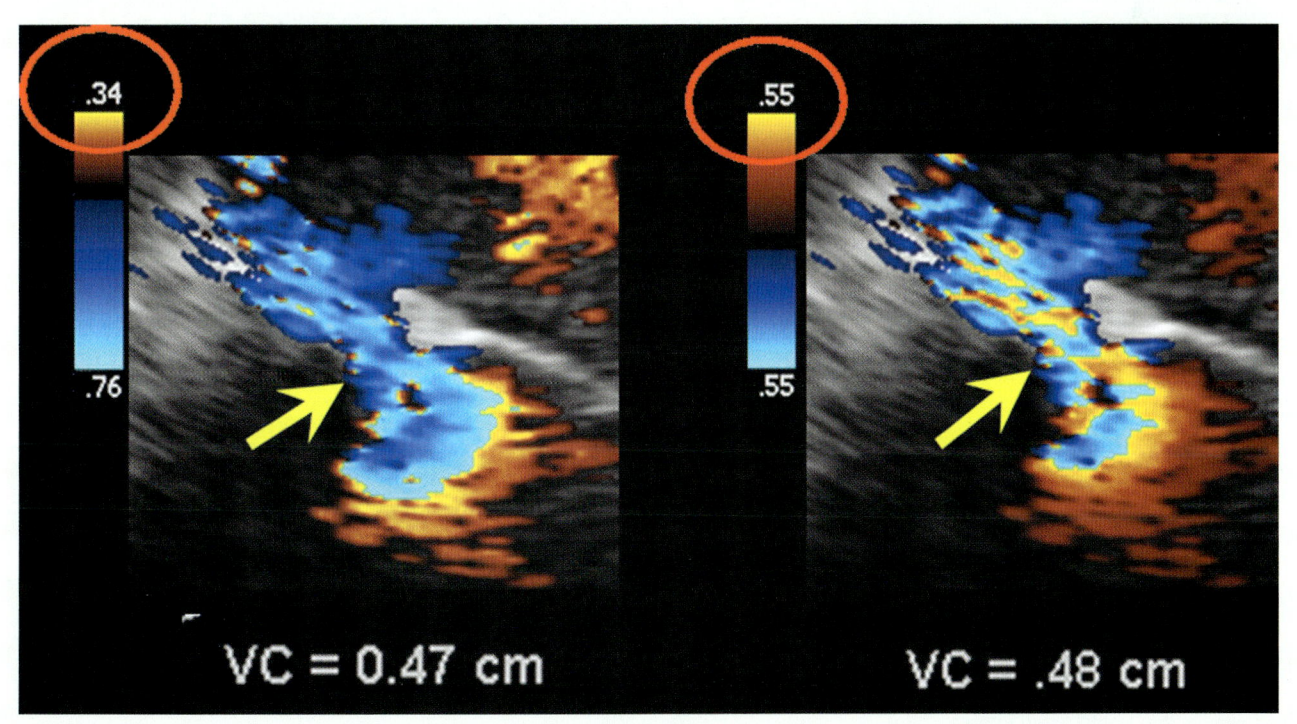

Figure 8.34

168 / Clinical Echocardiography Review

Thus, by E/e' ratio of 16 alone, an elevated LAP is likely in this patient. The other approach is to estimate LAP numerically using the following equation:

$$LAP = 1.9 + 1.24 * \frac{E}{e'} \quad (8.13)$$

In our patient:

$$LAP = 1.9 + 1.24 * 16 = 22$$

An LAP of 22 mm Hg is significantly elevated; normal LAP is <12 mm Hg.

A simplified form of Equation (8.13) is:

$$LAP = 4 + \frac{E}{e'} \quad (8.14)$$

In our patient, LAP can be estimated using Equation (8.14) as 4 + 16, or 20 mm Hg.

Therefore, answer C is correct.

Answer A is incorrect because the peak-to-peak gradient of aortic stenosis in this patient is 44 mm Hg.

To calculate the peak-to-peak gradient of aortic stenosis, we first need to calculate the peak left ventricular systolic pressure (LVSP) using the following formula:

$$LVSP = \Delta P_{MR} + LAP \quad (8.15)$$

where ΔP_{MR} is the peak systolic gradient of the mitral regurgitant jet, and LAP is the left atrial pressure. After expressing ΔP_{MR} in terms of the peak velocity (V) of the mitral regurgitant jet, Equation (8.15) becomes:

$$LVSP = 4 * V^2 + LAP \quad (8.16)$$

In our patient:

$$LVSP = 4*(6.0 \text{ m/s})^2 + 20 = 164 \text{ mm Hg}.$$

Once LVSP is known, the peak-to-peak aortic gradient (P2P) can be calculated as:

$$P2P = LVSP - SBP \quad (8.17)$$

where SBP is the systolic blood pressure.
In our patient:

$$P2P = 164 - 120 = 44 \text{ mm Hg}.$$

It is important to emphasize that this pressure gradient, which is commonly measured on cardiac catheterization, is not a physiologic one because it represents a pressure difference at separate points in time as demonstrated in **Figure 8.35**. P2P is lower than the peak instantaneous gradient (PIG) obtained by continuous wave Doppler across the aortic valve.

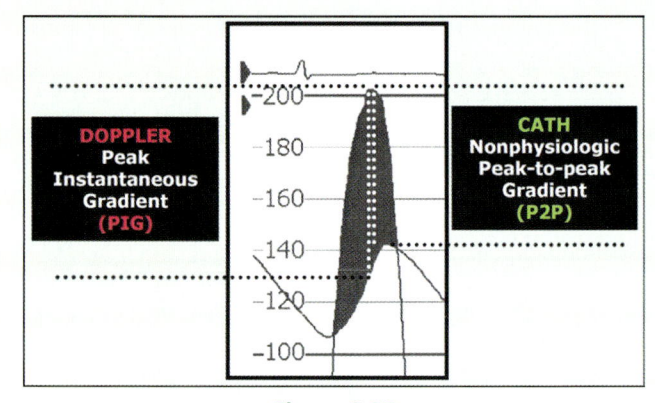

Figure 8.35

Answer B is incorrect because left ventricular dP/dt is normal. Patients with cardiogenic shock have low dP/dt values. Normal dP/dt = 1661 + 323 mm Hg/sec.

Answer D is incorrect because in severe mitral regurgitation vena contracta of ≥0.7 cm.

Answer E is incorrect because either Equation (8.13) or Equation (8.14) is applicable irrespective of the atrial rhythm (normal sinus rhythm, atrial fibrillation, etc).

9. **Answer: D.** (Left ventricular end-diastolic pressure is estimated at 10 mm Hg).

Figure 8.36 shows continuous wave spectral Doppler tracings of our patient:

Using the end-diastolic velocity (V) of the aortic regurgitant jet, one can calculate the pressure gradient (ΔP) between diastolic blood pressure (DBP) and left ventricular end-diastolic pressure (LVEDP).

$$\Delta P = DBP - LVEDP = 4 * V^2 \quad (8.18)$$

Rearranging Equation (8.18), LVEDP can be calculated in the following manner if the DBP is known:

$$LVEDP = DBP - 4 * V^2 \quad (8.19)$$

In our patient:

$$LVEDP = 65 \text{ mm Hg} - 4*(3.7 \text{ m/sec})^2 = 10 \text{ mm Hg}.$$

Therefore, answer D is correct.

Answer A is incorrect because in severe aortic regurgitation pressure half-time is <200 ms.

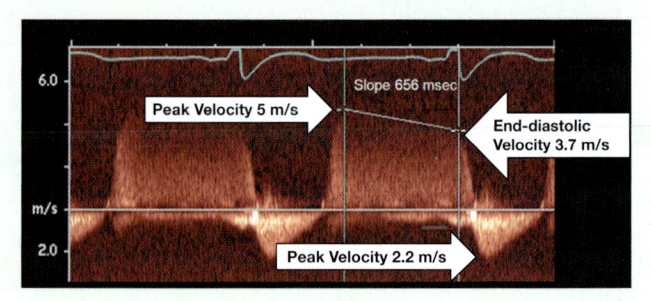

Figure 8.36

Answer B is incorrect because the aortic valve area cannot be calculated by 220 into pressure half-time; that is the formula for calculating the mitral valve area.

Answer C is incorrect because the peak left ventricular systolic pressure (LVSP) is always higher than systolic blood pressure in patients with aortic stenosis. LVSP becomes progressively higher than SBP as aortic stenosis becomes more severe. The LVSP-to-SBP pressure gradient is referred to as the peak-to-peak aortic gradient as discussed in answer to **Question 8**.

Answer E is incorrect because the continuity equation can be used to calculate the aortic valve area in patients with or without aortic regurgitation. The continuity principle states that the stroke volume across the left ventricular outflow tract (LVOT) is the same as the stroke volume across the aortic valve (AV):

LVOT Stroke Volume = AV Stroke Volume

(8.20)

Since stroke volume can be expressed as the product of the cross sectional area (CSA) and the flow velocity integral (VTI), Equation (8.20) becomes:

$$CSA_{LVOT} * VTI_{LVOT} = CSA_{AV} * VTI_{AV} \quad (8.21)$$

In patients with aortic regurgitation, there is an increase in antegrade flow from the left ventricle into the aorta due to augmentation of the true left ventricular stroke volume by the aortic regurgitant volume. However, this increase equally affects the flow through the left ventricular outflow tract and the aortic valve in systole. In Equation (8.21), this will be reflected in a proportional increase in VTI_{LVOT} and VTI_{AV}.

By continuity equation, aortic valve area (CSA_{AV}) can be calculated as follows:

$$CSA_{AV} = CSA_{LVOT} * \frac{VTI_{LVOT}}{VTI_{AV}} \quad (8.22)$$

In aortic regurgitation, there is augmentation of VTI_{LVOT} and VTI_{AV}. However, the ratio of the two VTIs remains the same, and therefore the calculated value of CSA_{AV} is not affected by the presence of aortic regurgitation.

10. **Answer: C.** (The ratio of pulmonary to systemic blood flow (Qp:Qs) is approximately 2.5-1).

The patient has an atrial septal defect (ASD) with a left-to-right shunt. ASD is an intracardiac shunt at the atrial level. Systemic blood flow (Qs) reaches the right atrium through systemic veins. At the level of the right atrium, it is joined by the shunt flow which enters the right atrium from the left atrium across the ASD. The sum of Qs and the shunt flow then passes through the right ventricular outflow tract (RVOT) into pulmonary circulation. Therefore, the sum of Qs and the shunt flow represents the pulmonary blood flow (Qp). This Qp reaches the left atrium through the pulmonary veins. At the left atrial level, Qp divides into shunt flow (which traverses ASD to reach the right atrium), and Qs which enters the left ventricle. Qs then passes through the left ventricular outflow tract (LVOT) into the aorta and eventually reaches the right atrium through systemic veins.

Table 8.5. Shunt Calculations for Patient With ASD

	RVOT	LVOT	Comment
Diameter (cm)	2.6	2.0	
Area (cm²)	5.3	3.1	Calculated using formula Area = (0.5 * Diameter)² * π
VTI (cm)	30	20	
Stroke Volume (mL)	159	63	Calculated using formula Stroke Volume = Area * VTI
Heart Rate (beats per minute)	75	75	Calculated using formula Flow = Stroke Volume * Heart Rate
Flow (L/min)	11.9	4.7	Shunt flow is the difference between Qp and Qs, or 7.2 L/min.
	Pulmonic Flow (Qp)	Systemic Flow (Qs)	
Qp: Qs	2.5:1		

Because Qp:Qs = 2.5:1, the answer C is correct.
LVOT, left ventricular outflow tract; RVOT, right ventricular outflow tract; VTI, velocity-time integral.

170 / Clinical Echocardiography Review

In summary, flow through LVOT represents Qs, while the flow through RVOT represents Qp in patients with ASD.

Shunt calculations for this patient are summarized in **Table 8.5**:

Answer A is incorrect because the presence of pulmonary hypertension per se does not preclude ASD closure. It is the degree of pulmonary vascular resistance (PVR) that determines whether a patient is a candidate for ASD closure or not, as discussed below.

Answer B is incorrect because the patient's PVR is essentially normal. Using the Ohm's law, PVR can be calculated as:

$$PVR = \frac{\Delta P}{Qp} \quad (8.23)$$

where Qp is the pulmonary blood flow (in L/min), and ΔP is the pressure gradient across pulmonary circulation. ΔP is the difference between the mean pulmonary artery pressure (MPP) and the mean left atrial pressure (LAP). Equation (8.23) then becomes:

$$PVR = \frac{MPP - LAP}{Qp} \quad (8.24)$$

MPP can be calculated from pulmonary artery systolic pressure (PASP) and the pulmonary artery diastolic pressure (PADP) using the following equation:

$$MPP = PADP + \frac{1}{2} * (PASP - PADP) \quad (8.25)$$

In this patient:

$$MPP = 25 + \frac{1}{2} * (55 - 25) = 40 \text{ mm Hg}$$

Once MPP is known, we can use Equation (8.24) to calculate PVR:

$$PVR = \frac{40 - 10}{11.9} = \frac{30}{11.9} = 2.5 \text{ Wood units}$$

Normal PVR is 1-2 Wood units (80-160 dyne*sec*cm^{-5}). In this patient, PVR is only modestly elevated. In principle, ASD closure should not be performed if PVR is 2/3 or more of the systemic vascular resistance (SVR). Since normal SVR is approximately 13 Wood units (range 11-16 Wood units, or 900-1300 dyne*sec*cm^{-5}), PVR ≥ 9 Wood units usually precludes ASD closure.

Answer D is incorrect because the shunt flow in this patient is 7.2 L/min. Shunt flow is the difference between Qp and Qs. In this patient:

$$SF = Qp - Qs = 11.9 - 4.7 = 7.2 \text{ L/min.}$$

Answer E is incorrect because Qp is much larger than Qs, the shunt flow is in the left to right direction and thus the patient is not expected to be cyanotic.

11. **Answer: B.** (Pulmonary artery systolic pressure is 29 mm Hg).

The presence of ventricular septal defect (VSD) allows for calculation of the right ventricular systolic pressure (RVSP) and, by extension, the pulmonary artery systolic pressure (PASP) if the systolic blood pressure (SBP) is known.

RVSP in a patient with VSD and no left ventricular outflow obstruction can be calculated as:

RSVP = SBP − Peak systolic VSD gradient

$$(8.26)$$

Using the peak systolic velocity (V) across the VSD, the peak systolic VSD gradient can be calculated as:

Peak systolic VSD gradient = 4 * V^2 (8.27)

By combining Equations (8.26) and (8.27), RVSP is then calculated as:

RVSP = SBP − 4 * V^2 (8.28)

Thus, in this patient, RVSP = 120 − 4 * (3.0 m/s)^2 = 84 mm Hg.

When there is no pulmonic stenosis, PASP = RVSP. However, this patient has pulmonic stenosis with a peak systolic gradient of 55 mm Hg across the pulmonic valve. In the presence of pulmonic stenosis (PS), the relationship between RVSP and PASP is as follows:

PASP = RVSP − Peak PS Gradient (8.29)

In our patient, PASP = 84 − 55 = 29 mm Hg. Therefore, the answer B is correct.

Answer A is incorrect because RVSP in this patient is 84 mm Hg.

Answer C is incorrect because the right atrial pressure is not required for RVSP estimation using the VSD method.

Answer D is incorrect because PASP is lower than RVSP due to the presence of pulmonic stenosis. RVSP exceeds PASP by 55 mm Hg, which is the peak gradient across the stenosed pulmonic valve.

Answer E is incorrect because the right ventricular end-diastolic pressure (RVEDP) in this patient is, if the left ventricular end-diastolic pressure is known (LVEDP), the RVEDP can be calculated as:

RVEDP = LVEDP − End-diastolic VSD gradient

$$(8.30)$$

Using the end-diastolic velocity (V) across the VSD, the end-diastolic VSD gradient can be calculated as:

End-diastolic VSD gradient = 4 * V²   (8.31)

By combining Equations (8.30) and (8.31), RVEDP is then calculated as:

RVEDP = LVEDP − 4 * V²   (8.32)

where V is the end-diastolic velocity across the VSD. In our patient:

$RVEDP = 12 - 4*(1\,m/s)^2 = 12 - 4 = 8\,mm\,Hg.$

12. **Answer: B.** (Shunt flow across the ASD is approximately 9.0 L/min).

The pulmonic flow (Qp) in patients with atrial septal defect (ASD) is the sum of the shunt flow (SF) across the ASD and the systemic flow (Qs). SF can be calculated either directly or as the difference between Qp and Qs.

One method for direct calculation of SF is the standard echocardiographic formula for determining flow rate through an orifice:

Flow = CSA * VTI * HR

where CSA is the cross-sectional area of the orifice, VTI is the velocity-time integral at the level of the orifice, and HR is the heart rate.

In the first step, we will calculate the CSA of the atrial septal defect whose diameter is 1.2 cm. Since the ASD is circular in shape, then ASD area can be calculated as:

$$CSA_{ASD} = \left(\frac{1}{2} * ASD\,diameter\right)^2 * \pi$$

In our patient:

$CSA_{ASD} = \left(\frac{1}{2} * 1.2\,cm\right)^2 * 3.14 = 0.36 * 3.14 = 1.13\,cm^2.$

Next, we can calculate the stroke volume across the ASD as:

ASD shunt stroke volume = CSA$_{ASD}$ * VTI$_{ASD}$

In our patient:

ASD shunt stroke volume = 1.13 cm² * 80 cm
= 90 mL per beat.

In the final step, by multiplying the ASD shunt stroke volume by the heart rate, one can calculate the shunt flow across the ASD. In our patient:

ASD shunt flow = 90 mL * 100 bpm = 9.0 L/min.

Therefore, the answer B is correct.

Answer A is incorrect because the Qp:Qs in this patient is 2.5:1. In this patient, Qs is calculated at the level of the left ventricular outflow tract (LVOT) using the formula:

Qs = CSA$_{LVOT}$ * VTI$_{LVOT}$ * HR

Where CSA$_{LVOT}$ is the cross-sectional area of LVOT, VTI$_{LVOT}$ is the velocity-time integral at LVOT level, and HR is the heart rate. In our patient:

$Qs = \left(\frac{1}{2} * 2.0\,cm\right)2 * \pi * 19\,cm * 100\,bpm$
$= 60\,mL * 100\,bpm = 6.0\,L/min$

In the next step, we can calculate Qp as:

Qp = Qs + ASD shunt flow

In our patient:

Qp = 6.0 L/min + 9.0 L/min = 15.0 L/min

Once Qp and Qs are known, we can calculate Qp:Qs ratio:

Qp:Qs = 15.0 L/min : 6.0 L/min = 2.5:1

Answer C is incorrect because the difference between the pulmonic and systemic stroke volumes in this patient is 90 mL/beat. This value represents the ASD shunt stroke volume calculated above.

Answer D is incorrect because the systemic stroke volume in this patient is 60 mL/beat as calculated above.

Answer E is incorrect because the Qp in this patient is 15.0 L/min as calculated above.

Calculations related to this question are summarized in **Table 8.6**.

13. **Answer: D.** Continuous Doppler spectral tracing of the mitral regurgitant jet can be used to estimate the rate of pressure rise (dP) in the left ventricle over time (dt), a measure of left ventricular systolic function, using the following formula:

$$dP/dt = \frac{\Delta P}{RTI}$$ (8.33)

where RTI is the relative time interval, measured in seconds, between mitral regurgitant jet velocities of 1 m/s (V$_1$) and 3 m/s (V$_2$). ΔP represents the pressure difference between the left ventricular to left atrial pressure gradients at V$_2$ and V$_1$ (**Figure 8.37**).

This pressure difference can be calculated as:

$\Delta P = \left(4V_2^2 - 4V_1^2\right)$
$\Delta P = 4 * (3\,m/s)^2 - 4 * (1\,m/s)^2 = 4*9 - 4*1 = 36 - 4$
$\Delta P = 32\,mm\,Hg$

172 / Clinical Echocardiography Review

Table 8.6

	LVOT	ASD	RVOT	Comments
Diameter (cm)	2.0	1.2		
Area (cm²)	3.10	1.13		
VTI (cm)	19	80		
Stroke Volume (mL)	60	90	150	RVOT stroke volume is the sum of LVOT and ASD stroke volumes.
Heart Rate (beats/min)	100	100		
Flow (L/min)	6.0	9.0	15.0	Qp is the sum of Qs and ASD shunt flow.
	Systemic Flow (Qs)	Shunt Flow	Pulmonic Flow (Qp)	Qp:Qs = 2.5

ASD, atrial septal defect; LVOT, left ventricular outflow tract; RVOT, right ventricular outflow tract.

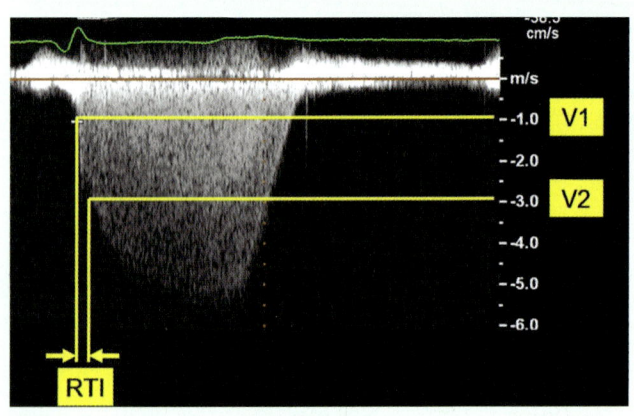

Figure 8.37

Now, Equation (8.33) can be expressed as:

$$dP/dt = \frac{32}{RTI} \quad (8.34)$$

In the next step, we will calculate RTI in our patient:

$$RTI = \text{Time at } V_2 - \text{Time at } V_1$$
$$= 25 \text{ msec} - 5 \text{ msec} = 20 \text{ msec}$$

Because in Equation (8.34) RTI is expressed in seconds, we have to convert our patient RTI from milliseconds to seconds:

$$RTI = 20 \text{ ms} = 0.02 \text{ seconds.}$$

Once RTI is known, we can calculate dP/dt in our patient:

$$dP/dt = \text{to } 32/0.02 = 1600 \text{ mm Hg/s.}$$

Therefore, answer D is correct.

Answer A is incorrect because the peak velocity of mitral E wave in severe mitral regurgitation is expected to be high. Peak velocity across an orifice is directly related to flow across that orifice. Since the flow is the product of stroke volume and heart rate, peak velocity is then a direct function (f) of stroke volume:

$$\text{E wave velocity} = f(SV) \quad (8.35)$$

In mitral regurgitation, SV that crosses the mitral valve in diastole is the sum of the systemic stroke volume (SV_{LVOT}) and the regurgitant volume (RegV). Thus, Equation (8.35) can be expressed as:

$$\text{E wave velocity} = f(SV_{LVOT} + RegV) \quad (8.36)$$

The more severe the mitral regurgitation, the larger the RegV, and therefore, the higher the peak velocity of the mitral inflow E wave. When native mitral regurgitation is severe (as is the case in this patient as judged by the vena contracta ≥0.7 cm), peak E velocity is expected to be >1.5 m/s. In severe prosthetic mitral regurgitation, the peak E velocity is usually >2.0 m/s.

Answer B is incorrect because LAP in this patient is elevated. The patient presents with severe mitral regurgitation (vena contracta ≥0.7 cm) and pulmonary edema due to elevated left atrial pressure (LAP).

Using the peak velocity (Vmax) of the mitral regurgitant jet, one can calculate the pressure gradient (ΔP) between the peak left ventricular systolic pressure (LVSP) and the LAP:

$$\Delta P = 4 * V\max^2 \quad (8.37)$$

In our patient:

$$\Delta P = 4 * (4.0 \text{ m/sec})^2 = 4 * 16 = 64 \text{ mm Hg}$$

The sum of this pressure gradient and LAP during systole represents the peak left ventricular systolic pressure (LVSP):

$$LVSP = \Delta P + LAP \quad (8.38)$$

By rearranging Equation (8.38), we can solve the LAP:

$$LAP = LVSP - \Delta P \quad (8.39)$$

The LAP calculated by this method represents a value on the CV wave portion of the left atrial pressure tracing.

LVSP is not given in the question. In this patient who does not have aortic stenosis or left ventricular outflow obstruction, LVSP is equal to systolic blood pressure (SBP). Thus we can express Equation (8.39) as:

$$LAP = SBP - \Delta P \quad (8.40)$$

In our patient, whose SBP was 95 mm Hg and whose ΔP was calculated above at 64 mm Hg, LAP is then calculated as:

$$LAP = 95 \text{ mm Hg} - 64 \text{ mm Hg} = 31 \text{ mm Hg}$$

This LAP of 31 mm Hg is highly elevated (normal LAP is ≤12 mm Hg).

Answer C is incorrect because in severe mitral regurgitation there may be flow reversal in systolic (S) but not diastolic (D) wave on pulmonary venous flow velocity tracings. An example of S wave reversal due to severe mitral regurgitation is shown in **Figure 8.38**.

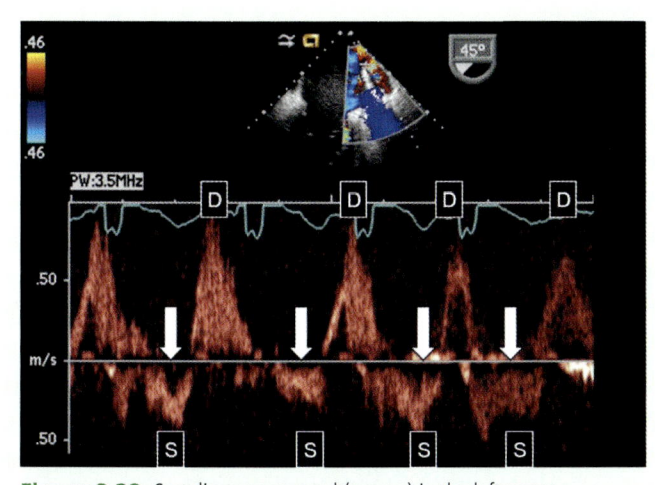

Figure 8.38. Systolic wave reversal (arrows) in the left upper pulmonary vein due to severe mitral regurgitation is seen in spectral Doppler recordings on a transesophageal echocardiography. S, systolic wave; D, diastolic wave.

Answer E is incorrect because dP/dt in this patient is estimated at 1600 mm Hg/s, which is normal. (Normal dP/dt = 1661 ± 323 mm Hg/s). The value of 800 mm Hg/s would indicate a markedly diminished LV systolic function as seen in cardiogenic shock, for example.

14. **Answer: E.** In mitral stenosis, there is a pressure gradient between the left atrium and the left ventricle during diastole. In this patient, the mean diastolic pressure gradient is markedly elevated (21 mm Hg). Mean diastolic pressure gradient of >10 mm Hg is typically consistent with very severe mitral stenosis as shown in **Table 8.7** which is based on the 2020 ACC/AHA guidelines on valvular heart disease.

It is important to emphasize that the transmitral gradient alone should not be used to judge the severity of mitral stenosis due to the variability of the mean pressure gradient with heart rate and forward flow; the gradient is therefore only an ancillary criterion in judging the severity of mitral stenosis.

In this young patient, left ventricular diastolic pressures are normal. Mean left atrial pressure (LAP) can be calculated as:

LAP = Mean mitral gradient in diastole + Early LV diastolic pressure

In our patient:

LAP is 21 mm Hg + 7 mm Hg = 28 mm Hg.

Therefore, the answer E is correct.

Answer A is incorrect because in mitral stenosis there is an antegrade flow driven by a pressure gradient between the left atrium and the left ventricle in diastole. Therefore, the mean left atrial pressure is higher than the mean left ventricular diastolic pressure.

Answer B is incorrect because in mitral stenosis the peak velocity of the mitral E wave is expected to be high. Velocity (V) across an orifice is inversely related to the cross-sectional area (CSA) of the orifice:

$$V \approx \frac{1}{CSA} \quad (8.41)$$

Table 8.7

	Severe MS	Very Severe MS
Mitral Valve Area (cm^2)	<1.5	<1.0
Typical Mean Diastolic Gradient (mm Hg)	5 - 10	>10

MS, mitral stenosis.

For mitral stenosis, CSA equals to the mitral valve area (MVA) and Equation (8.41) becomes:

$$V \approx \frac{1}{MVA} \quad (8.42)$$

Therefore, the smaller the mitral valve area (ie, the more severe the mitral stenosis), the higher the peak velocity of the mitral E wave.

Answer C is incorrect because the pressure-half time method may be unreliable immediately <u>after</u> but not before mitral valvuloplasty. Pressure-half time method assumes that the left ventricular pressure and compliance are normal, and therefore, the deceleration slope of the mitral E wave on spectral Doppler tracings in diastole is the function of the mitral valve area alone.

Immediately after valvuloplasty, there is a sudden increase in the mitral orifice area leading to an increase in the stroke volume delivered to the left ventricle in early diastole. Because the left ventricle compliance cannot change acutely, the left ventricular diastolic pressure increases. With the rise in left ventricular diastolic pressure, the diastolic gradient between the left atrium and the left ventricle decreases and the mitral pressure half-time shortens above and beyond what would be expected by an increase in the mitral valve area alone after valvuloplasty. Therefore, the pressure-half time method may lead to the calculation of an erroneously large mitral valve area.

Answer D is incorrect because the mitral valve area (MVA) by pressure-half time (PHT) method in this patient is 0.8 cm²:

$$MVA = \frac{220}{PHT} = \frac{220}{270} = 0.8 \quad (8.43)$$

15. **Answer: C.** (Aortic valve area is likely to be less than 1 cm²).

When velocity-time integrals are not available, aortic valve area (AVA) can be calculated using the following modified continuity equation:

$$AVA = CSA_{LVOT} * \frac{V_{LVOT}}{V_{AV}} \quad (8.44)$$

where CSA_{LVOT} is the cross-sectional area of the left ventricular outflow tract (LVOT), V_{LVOT} is the peak systolic LVOT velocity, and V_{AV} is the peak systolic aortic valve (AV) velocity.

The V_{LVOT}/V_{AV} ratio of the two velocities is referred to as the dimensionless index (DI). Thus Eq. can be expressed as:

$$AVA = CSA_{LVOT} * DI \quad (8.45)$$

After expressing the LVOT area in term of LVOT diameter (D), Equation (8.45) becomes:

$$AVA = \left(\frac{1}{2}*D\right)^2 * DI \quad (8.46)$$

In our patient:

$$AVA = \left(\frac{1}{2}*[1.9\ cm]^2\right)*(1\ m\ per\ s/5\ m\ per\ s)$$
$$AVA = 2.84\ cm^2 * 0.2$$
$$AVA = 0.6\ cm^2$$

Therefore, answer C is correct.

Incorrect Answers

Answer A is incorrect because the modified continuity equation using the dimensionless index, as explained above, can be used to calculate the aortic valve area when velocity-time integrals are unavailable.

Answer B is incorrect because the subvalvular (LVOT) velocity is normal (1.0 m/s).

Answer D is incorrect because the left ventricular stroke volume in this patient is 57 mL/beat. Left ventricular stroke volume (SV) can be calculated as follows:

$$SV = \frac{1}{2}*(LVOT\ diameter)^2 * VTI_{LVOT}$$
$$SV = \frac{1}{2}*(1.9\ cm)^2 * 20\ cm$$
$$SV = 57\ mL/beat$$

Answer E is incorrect because in aortic stenosis left ventricular peak systolic pressure exceeds the systolic blood pressure. The magnitude of this pressure difference (peak-to-peak gradient) is proportional to the severity of aortic stenosis.

16. **Answer: B.** Correct answer is B because (1) mitral regurgitation Vmax is relatively low (around 3.5 m/s); and (2) there is a triangular, early peaking flow velocity pattern of mitral regurgitant flow on continuous wave spectral Doppler imaging.

Low Vmax and the rapidly decelerating triangular jet in severe acute mitral regurgitation may result from a combination of low systolic blood pressure in the setting of acute shock and high left atrial pressures in a noncompliant left atrium. This results in rapid equalization of the LV to LA systolic gradient giving rise to a relatively low MR Vmax and the triangular MR jet shape.

Answer A is incorrect because chronic mitral regurgitation tends to have (1) parabolic shape of continuous wave spectral Doppler tracing of the mitral regurgitant flow; and (2) higher peak mitral regurgitation velocity (typically in the range of 5.0 m/s but depending on the systolic blood pressure), as **Figure 8.39**.

Answer C is incorrect because in this patient the mitral regurgitant flow occurs only during systole. For comparison, **Figure 8.40** is an example of a partly diastolic mitral regurgitation tracing on spectral Doppler.

Chapter 8 Doppler and Hemodynamics / 175

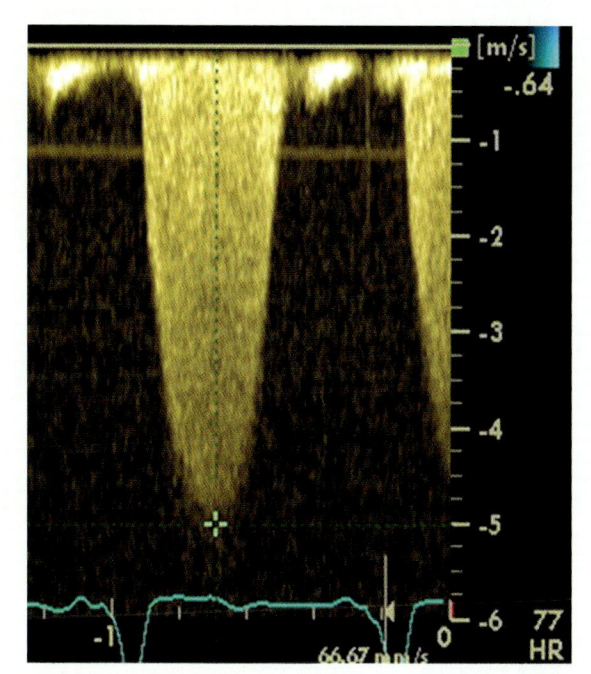

Figure 8.39

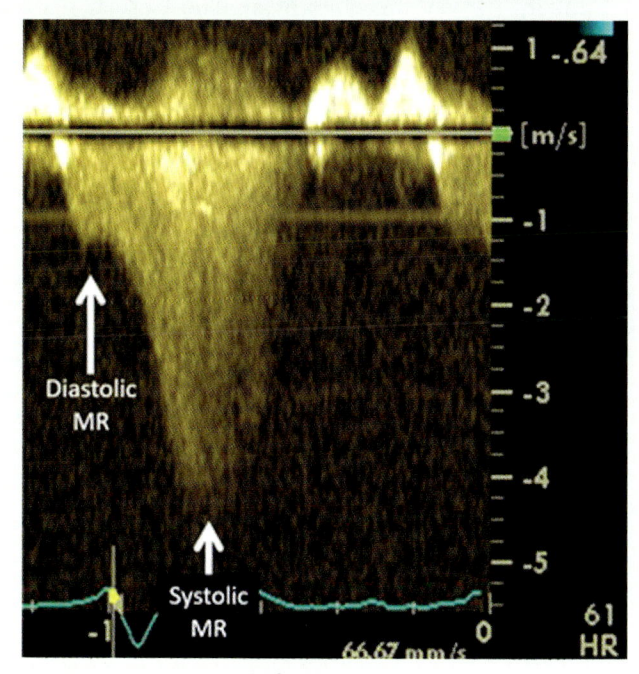

Figure 8.40

left atrial pressure and may be consistent with mitral regurgitation. However, another panel is more consistent with severe mitral regurgitation than this one (**Figure 8.43**).

Answer C is incorrect because it demonstrates systolic (S) wave dominance, which is typically

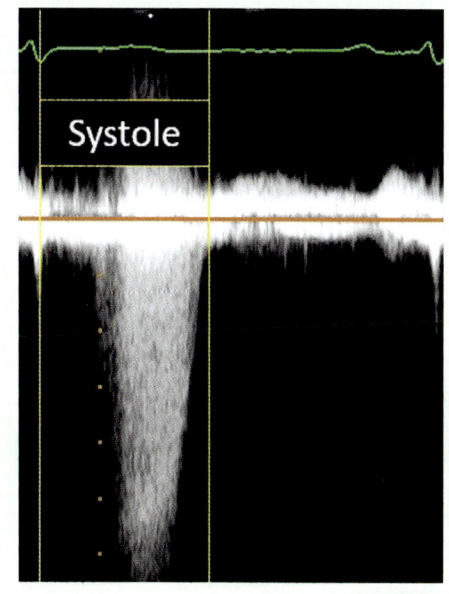

Figure 8.41

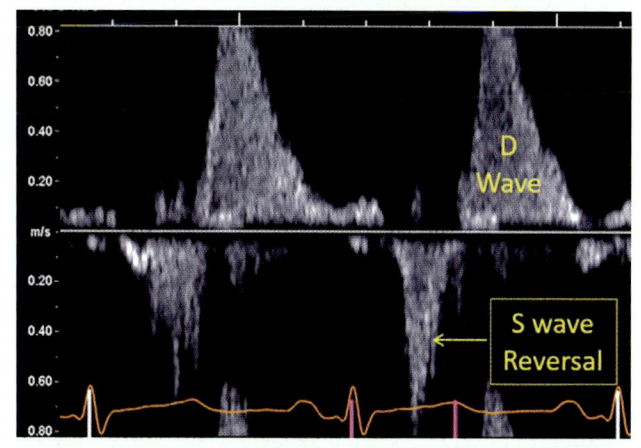

Figure 8.42

Answer D is incorrect because in mitral valve prolapse, mitral regurgitation tends to occur in late systole as shown in **Figure 8.41**. In contrast, mitral regurgitation shown in the question begins in early systole.

17. **Answer: A.** **Figure 8.2**, Panel A demonstrates systolic (S) wave reversal in a pulsed-wave spectral Doppler tracing from a pulmonary vein. Of all the choices, this finding is most consistent with the diagnosis of severe mitral regurgitation (**Figure 8.42**).

Answer B is incorrect. It demonstrates systolic (S) wave blunting, which is indicative of an elevated

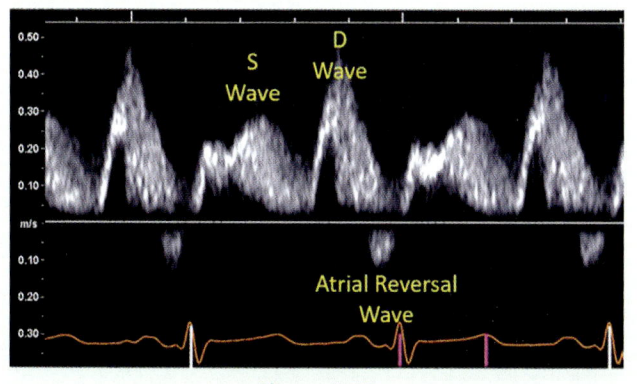

Figure 8.43

associated with normal LA pressure and thus inconsistent with severe acute mitral regurgitation (**Figure 8.44**).

Answer D is incorrect. It demonstrates pulmonary venous flow velocity pattern seen in atrial fibrillation with systolic (S) wave blunting and no definite atrial reversal wave. This finding is not specific for severe mitral regurgitation (**Figure 8.45**).

18. **Answer: C.** At baseline, there is E wave predominance with rapid E wave velocity deceleration in the pulsed-wave spectral Doppler recording of the mitral valve. Post mitral valve repair, there is A wave predominance and prolonged E wave velocity deceleration. This sequence of findings is indicative of interval decrease in left atrial pressure and of all the choices given; transcatheter mitral valve repair is the most appropriate choice.

Answer A is incorrect because the administration of 1 L of normal saline would typically lead to an interval increase in the E wave peak velocity. In contrast, here we see an interval decrease in the peak velocity of the E wave and a decrease in the E/A ratio.

Answer B is incorrect as the patient is in sinus rhythm in both recordings and there would have been no need for direct current cardioversion.

Answer D is incorrect because a development of severe aortic regurgitation would have likely resulted in elevated left pressures. In this case, one observes an interval decrease in LA pressures as demonstrated by the interval decrease in both the peak E wave velocity and the E/A ratio.

19. **Answer: A.** The continuous wave spectral Doppler recording of the tricuspid valve demonstrates a combination of diastolic (pre-systolic) and systolic tricuspid regurgitation. This finding is observed in various forms of atrioventricular blocks (first, second, and third degree) (**Figure 8.46**).

Answer B is incorrect as the patient is in sinus rhythm with 1st degree AV block (**Figure 8.47**).

Answer C is incorrect because the flow velocity pattern of tricuspid regurgitation is mostly parabolic in shape. In contrast, in severe acute tricuspid regurgitation one would expect a triangular shape indicative of rapid equalization of RV to RA systolic pressure gradient. In severe acute tricuspid regurgitation, one would also likely see a low peak velocity of the TR jet (**Figure 8.48**).

Answer D is incorrect because while Ebstein anomaly leads to tricuspid regurgitation, the spectral Doppler finding is not specific for Ebstein anomaly.

20. **Answer: C.** At baseline, the continuous wave spectral Doppler tracing from the aortic arch region demonstrates typical findings of severe aortic coarctation, namely the abnormally high systolic velocities as well as the abnormal antegrade diastolic flow. Post coarctation stenting, the peak systolic velocity becomes markedly lower and there is no longer very prominent antegrade diastolic flow.

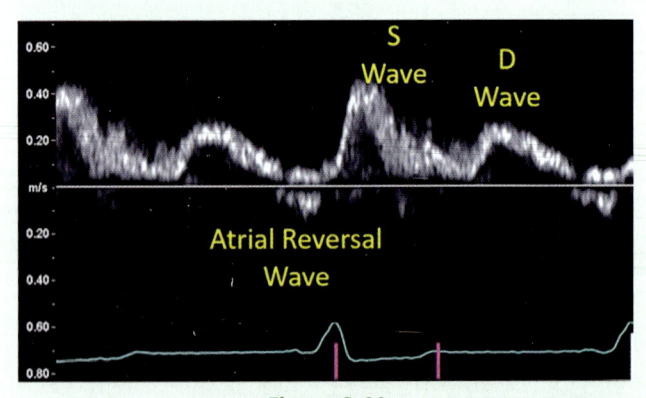

Figure 8.44

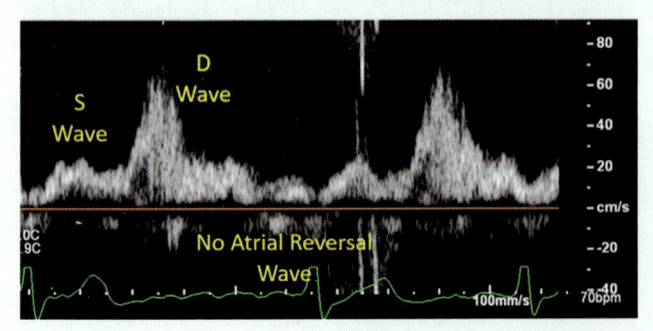

Figure 8.45

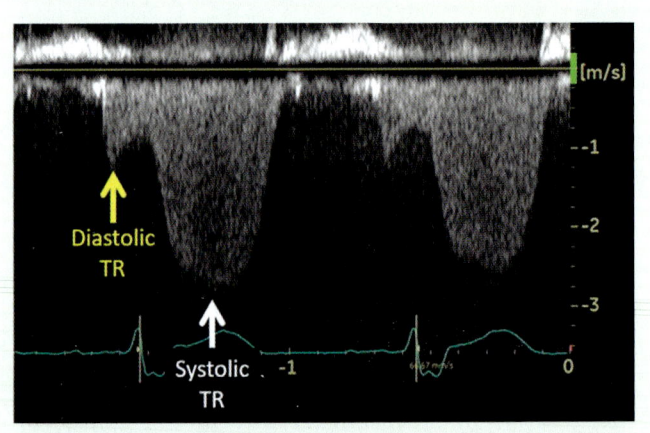

Figure 8.46

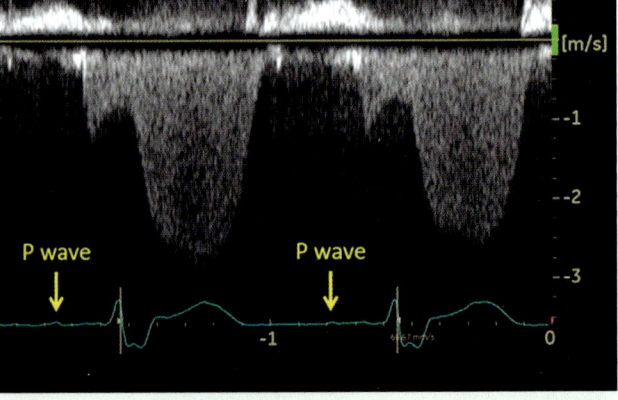

Figure 8.47

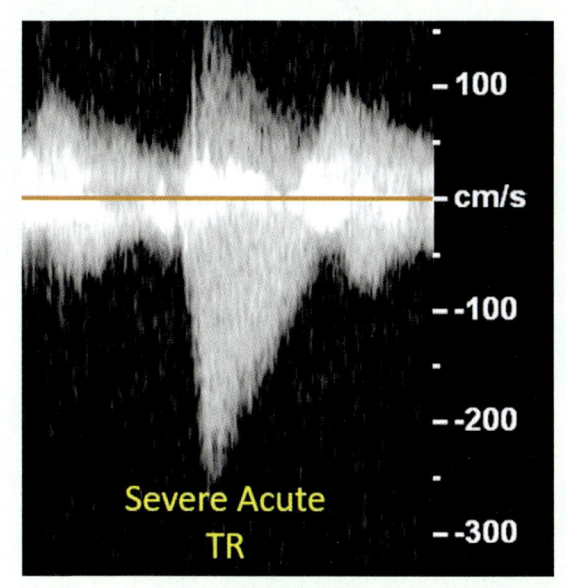

Figure 8.48

Answer A is incorrect because the baseline recording is not consistent with a typical patent ductus arteriosus flow velocity pattern. Typically, PDA flow demonstrates higher peak diastolic velocities than those shown in the question's recording. Typical continuous wave spectral Doppler recordings from an uncomplicated PDA are shown in **Figure 8.49**.

Answer B is incorrect because the baseline tracing is not consistent with severe aortic stenosis. In severe aortic stenosis, the antegrade transvalvular gradient is elevated during systole but not during diastole (**Figure 8.50**).

Answer D is incorrect because the flow velocity pattern of an atrial septal defect is unlikely to demonstrate such high systolic and diastolic velocities at baseline. In ASD, there is typically continuous low-velocity antegrade flow pattern, as shown in **Figure 8.51**. Initially, the flow peaks in late systole with an additional increase in flow across the ASD after atrial contraction (atrial kick). Moreover, after ASD closure, typically there would have been no residual flow across the ASD.

21. **Answer: A.** The pulsed-wave spectral Doppler recordings of the mitral inflow with simultaneous respirometry tracings demonstrated no significant respiratory variations in the peak E wave velocity. Moreover, there is marked E wave predominance with no discernible A wave despite the patient being in sinus rhythm. The E wave deceleration is very rapid. These findings are consistent with a restrictive mitral inflow pattern. In the absence of significant respiratory variations, the findings are most consistent with restrictive cardiomyopathy.

Answer B is incorrect as in constrictive pericarditis one would typically expect significant respiratory variations in the peak E wave velocities, as shown below. However, it is important to emphasize that in a small percentage of patients with constriction, respiratory variations may be absent (**Figure 8.52**).

Answer C is incorrect because as in tamponade one would typically expect significant respiratory variations in the peak E wave velocities and the E/A ration tends to be less than 1, as shown in **Figure 8.53**. Because the pericardial fluid is incompressible, LV filling is impaired in early diastole which is responsible for an E/A ratio <1. In contrast, with constriction, the LV filling is primarily impaired in late diastole which then results in a restrictive mitral filling pattern characterized by E/A much greater than 1.

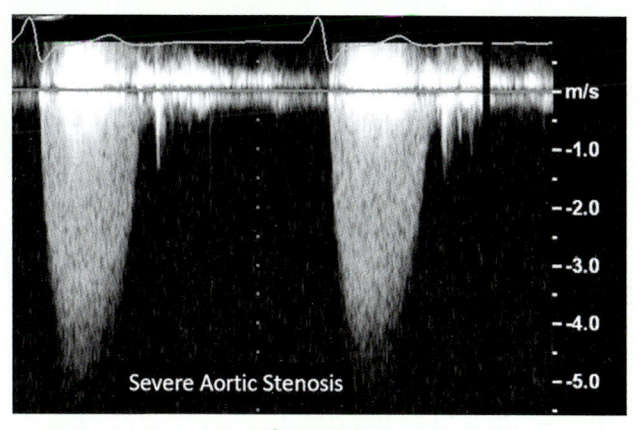

Figure 8.50

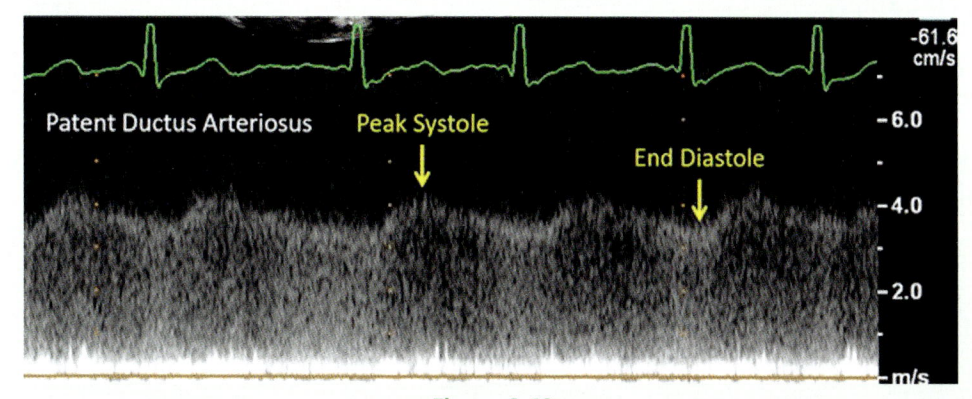

Figure 8.49

178 / Clinical Echocardiography Review

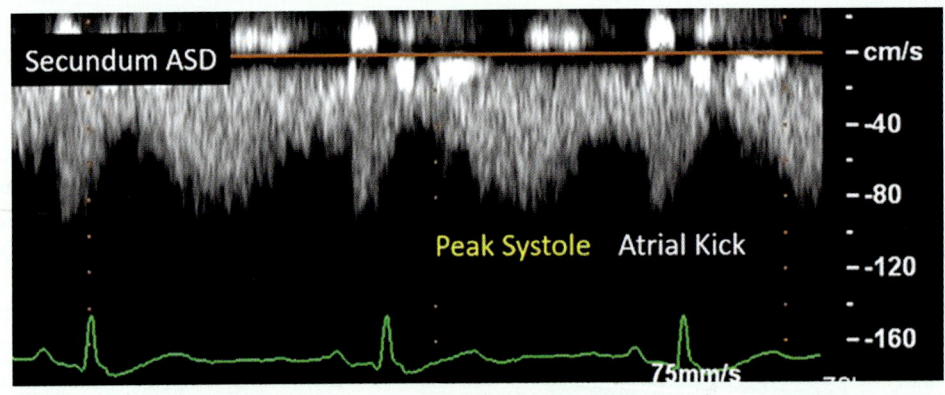

Figure 8.51

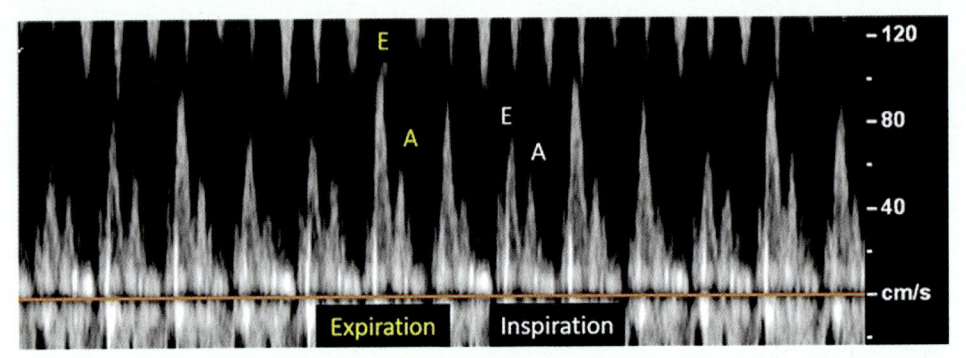

Figure 8.52

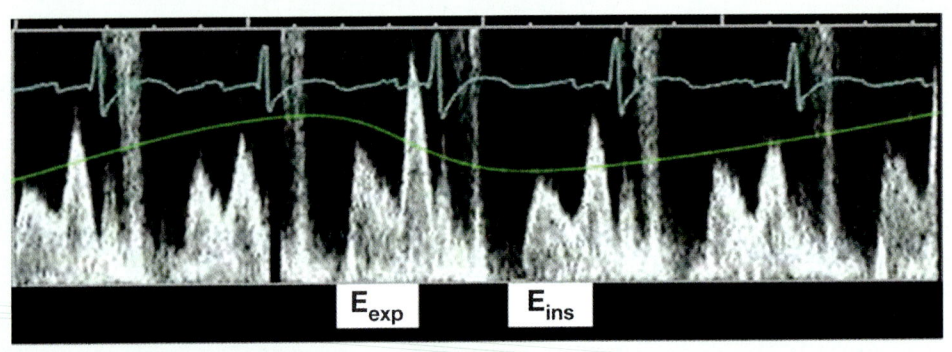

Figure 8.53

Answer D is incorrect because there are no spectral Doppler findings that are specific for acute pericarditis.

22. **Answer: D. Figure 8.7**, Panel D is correct because it demonstrates midsystolic notching of the pulmonic flow velocity pattern. This is the spectral Doppler equivalent of the flying W sign observed in M mode recording from the pulmonic valve (**Figure 8.54**).

It should be noted that the above pattern of midsystolic notching with secondary flow acceleration post notching may not be the only pattern seen in patients with pulmonary hypertension. In some patients with pulmonary hypertension, the acceleration time is short but there is no notching. Yet in other patients with pulmonary hypertension there is rectilinear mid-systolic deceleration with an inflection point and no post-notching acceleration flow.[1]

Answer A is incorrect because Panel A spectral Doppler tracing is not specific for pulmonary arterial hypertension. It rather demonstrates normal antegrade systolic flow pattern. During diastole, there is pulmonic regurgitation flow with characteristic notching after atrial contraction and a transient increase in RV diastolic pressure which transiently decreases PA to RV diastolic gradient (**Figure 8.55**).

[1] For further details please see Takahama H, McCully RB, Frantz RP, Kane GC. Unraveling the RV ejection doppler envelope: insight into pulmonary artery hemodynamics and disease severity. *JACC Cardiovasc Imaging*. 2017;10(10 pt B):1268-1277.

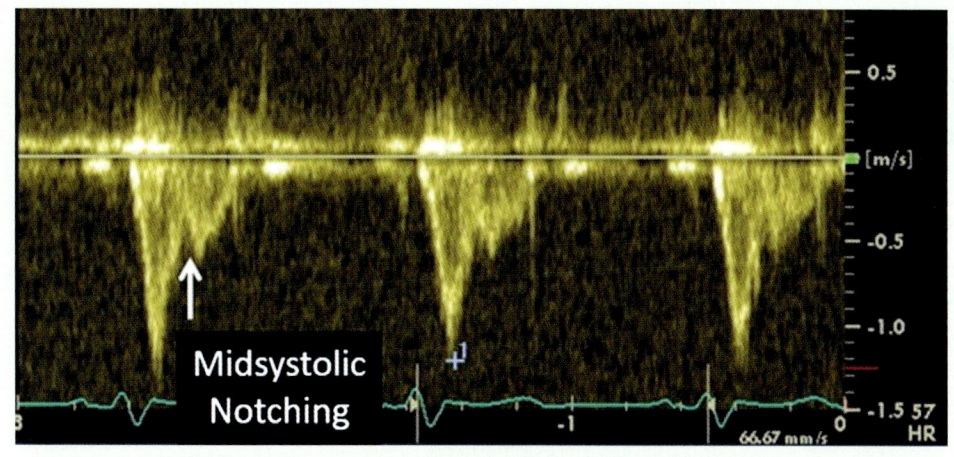

Figure 8.54

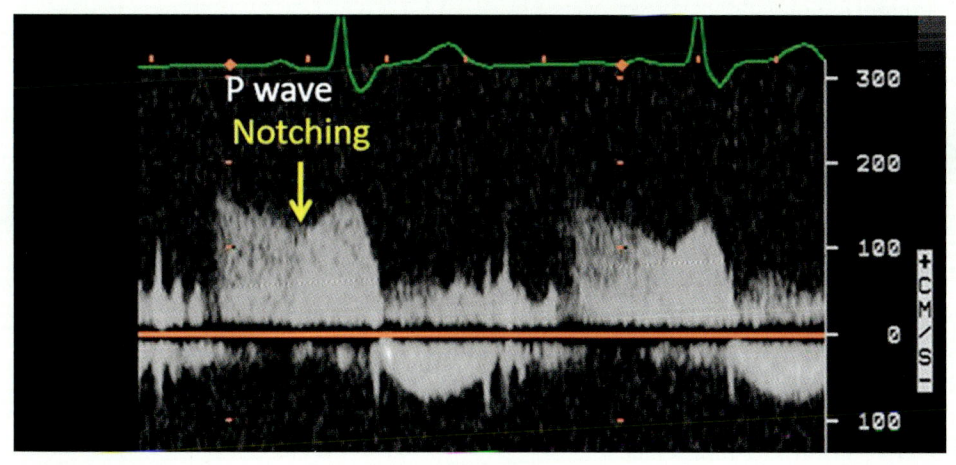

Figure 8.55

Answer B is incorrect because the finding is not specific for severe systolic pulmonary hypertension. It merely demonstrates pulmonic regurgitant flow in a patient with atrial fibrillation and variability in end-diastolic velocities.

Answer C is incorrect because it demonstrates severe pulmonic regurgitation with a rapidly decelerating and prematurely terminating pulmonic regurgitation flow, as shown in Figure 8.56. There is also an increase in the peak systolic velocity, which may be consistent with severe pulmonic regurgitation alone or due to a combination of pulmonic stenosis and regurgitation.

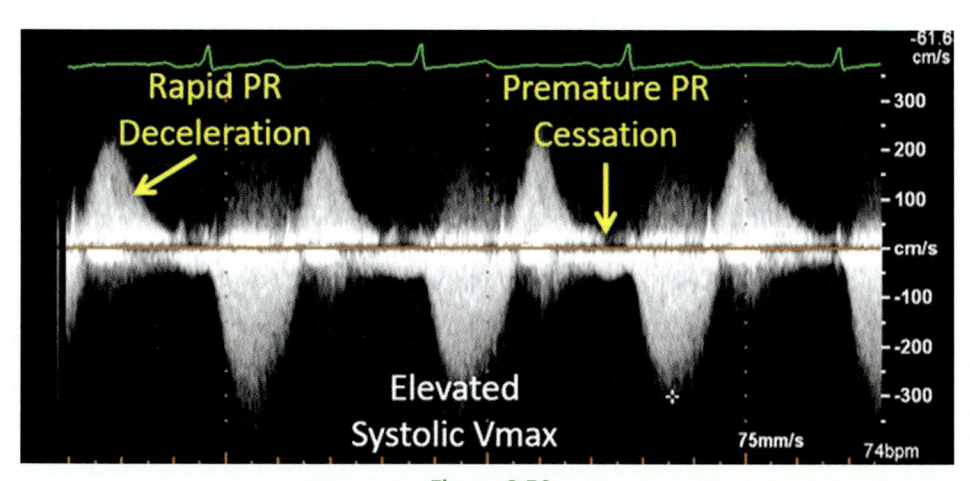

Figure 8.56

180 / Clinical Echocardiography Review

23. Answer: C. Peak right ventricular systolic pressure (RVSP) in a patient with or without pulmonic stenosis can be calculated as:

$$\text{RVSP} = \text{Peak RV-to-RA systolic gradient} + \text{RAP} \quad (8.47)$$

where RAP is the right atrial pressure. Since RV-to-RA systolic gradient can be estimated from the peak systolic velocity of the tricuspid regurgitant (V), Equation (8.47) can be expressed as:

$$\text{RVSP} = 4 * V^2 + \text{RAP} \quad (8.48)$$

In the absence of pulmonic stenosis, RVSP is equal to pulmonary artery systolic pressure (PASP). In pulmonic stenosis, however, peak RVSP exceeds PASP. The difference between the two pressures represents the peak gradient of pulmonic stenosis (PS). Therefore, in patients with PS, PASP is estimated as:

$$\text{PASP} = \text{RVSP} - \text{PS Gradient} \quad (8.49)$$

In our patient:

$$\text{RVSP} = 4 * (4.0 \text{ m/s})^2 + 10 = 74 \text{ mm Hg}$$
$$\text{PASP} = 74 - 24 = 50 \text{ mm Hg}.$$

Therefore, answer C is correct.

All calculations are graphically summarized in **Figure 8.57**; RVP, right ventricular pressure; RAP, right atrial pressure; PAP, pulmonary artery pressure.

Answer A is incorrect because in the presence of pulmonic valve stenosis, RVSP exceeds PASP as shown in **Figure 8.57**.

Answer B is incorrect because RVSP exceeds PASP by 24 mm Hg, the value of the peak systolic gradient across the pulmonic valve.

Answer D is incorrect because RVSP is 24 mm Hg more than PASP.

Answer E is incorrect because RVSP is 74 mm Hg as calculated above.

24. Answer: C. Peak gradient (ΔPmax) of aortic stenosis can be calculated from the peak systolic velocity (V) across the aortic valve obtained by continuous wave Doppler using the modified Bernoulli equation:

$$\Delta P\text{max} = 4 * V^2 \quad (8.50)$$

The mean aortic valve gradient (ΔPmean) is approximately 60% of the peak gradient (ΔPmax):

$$\Delta P\text{mean} = 0.6 * \Delta P\text{max} \quad (8.51)$$

In our patient:

$$\Delta P\text{max} = 4 * (5.0 \text{ m/s})^2 = 100 \text{ mm Hg}$$
$$\Delta P\text{mean} = 0.6 * 100 \text{ mm Hg} = 60 \text{ mm Hg}$$

Therefore, answer C is correct.

Answer A is incorrect because increased cardiac output (as during pregnancy, for instance) leads to a proportional increase in both LVOT and aortic velocities. In this patient, there is a marked difference between the peak systolic LVOT velocity (0.9 m/s) and the peak systolic aortic velocity (5.0 m/s) indicative of aortic stenosis.

Answer B is incorrect because in aortic regurgitation there is a proportional increase in both LVOT and aortic velocities in systole due augmentation of the left ventricular stroke volume by the recirculating regurgitant volume. A wide discrepancy in the peak LVOT and aortic velocities in systole is not expected in severe aortic regurgitation.

Answer D is incorrect because the aortic valve area in this patient is less than 1.0 cm².

Aortic valve area (AVA) in this patient can be estimated using the modified continuity equation:

$$\text{AVA} = \text{CSA}_{\text{LVOT}} * \frac{V_{\text{LVOT}}}{V_{\text{AV}}} \quad (8.52)$$

After expressing the LVOT area in terms of LVOT diameter (D), Equation (8.52) becomes:

$$\text{AVA} = \left(\frac{1}{2} * D\right)^2 * \frac{V_{\text{LVOT}}}{V_{\text{AV}}} \quad (8.53)$$

where CSA_{LVOT} is the cross-sectional area of the LVOT, V_{LVOT} is the LVOT peak systolic velocity, and V_{AV} is the peak aortic velocity in systole.

In this patient:

$$\text{AVA} = \left(\frac{1}{2} * 2.0\right)^2 * \frac{0.9}{5.0} = 0.57 \text{ cm}^2$$

Answer E is incorrect because the subvalvular (LVOT) velocity of 0.9 m/s is normal.

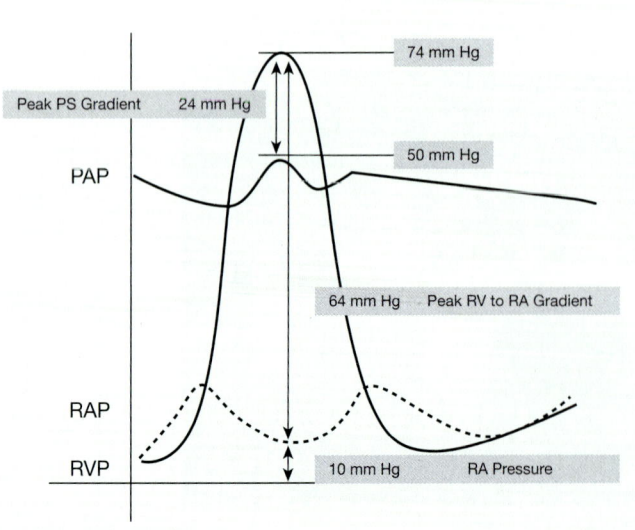

Figure 8.57

25. **Answer: D.** (Pulmonic valve regurgitation is severe).

The patient has severe pulmonic valve regurgitation, a common long-term complication of tetralogy of Fallot repair.

Because of a large regurgitant orifice, the pressure gradient between pulmonary artery and the right ventricle equalizes rapidly. Equalization is achieved by mid diastole and there is no measurable end-diastolic gradient as demonstrated in **Figure 8.58**.

This rapid deceleration and premature cessation of the pulmonic regurgitant jet is a characteristic finding of severe pulmonic regurgitation. Therefore, answer D is correct.

Answer A is incorrect because the end-diastolic gradient in severe pulmonic regurgitation is approaching zero.

Answer B is incorrect because the peak antegrade velocity across the pulmonic valve in systole is only elevated to about 1.5 m/s (peak systolic gradient = 4 * 1.5^2 = 9 mm Hg). This is consistent with pulmonic regurgitation alone. During systole, stroke volume is augmented by the recirculating regurgitant volume. This flow augmentation leads to higher systolic velocities across the pulmonic valve based on the fundamental equation of fluid dynamics:

$$V = \frac{Q}{PVA} = \frac{SV * HR}{PVA}$$

Where V is the antegrade velocity across the pulmonic valve, Q is the volumetric flow across the pulmonic valve in systole, SV is the stroke volume, HR is the heart rate, and PVA is the pulmonic valve area. Thus, when the PVA remains constant, any increase in stroke volume leads to elevation in the transvalvular velocity.

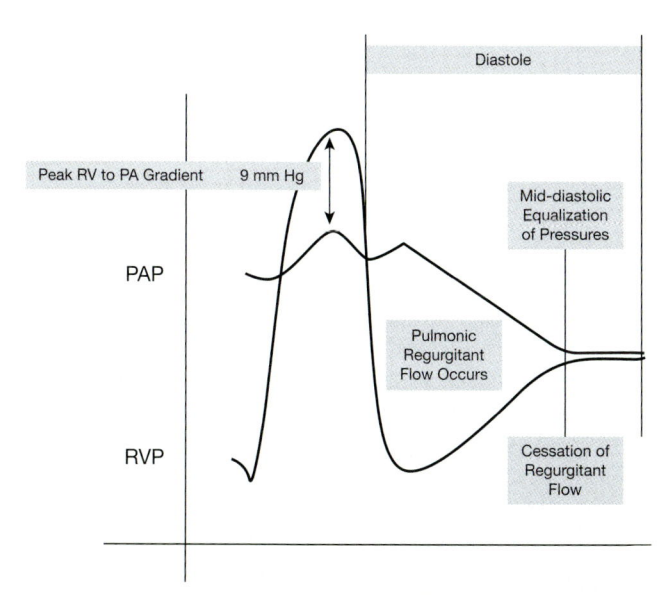

Figure 8.58

Answer C is incorrect, the right ventricular systolic pressure exceeds pulmonary artery by 9 mm Hg (see **Figure 8.58**).

Answer E is incorrect because in uncomplicated patent ductus arteriosus, antegrade flow occurs during both systole and diastole. In the patient's tracing, there is antegrade flow in systole and retrograde flow in diastole.

26. **Answer: C.** The tracings were obtained from an elderly woman presenting with acutely decompensated heart failure.

The E/e' ratio can be used to estimate LAP in two ways. One approach is to use it semi-quantitatively; when an E/e' ratio using an average of medial and lateral e' peak velocities is greater than 14, this is suggestive of elevated LAP pressure.

In our patient, the average peak e' velocity is (10 + 6)/2 = 8 cm/s. Thus, E/e' is 142/8, or 18. This ratio is consistent with elevated left atrial pressure. Therefore, answer C is correct.

Answer A is incorrect because the patient is likely to have poor exercise capacity with exertional dyspnea given the elevation of left atrial pressure even at rest. With exertion, left atrial pressure is expected to rise even further.

Answer B is incorrect because the patient's mitral inflow pattern is a combination of abnormal left ventricular relaxation and elevated left atrial pressure. The mitral E/A ratio that is greater than two in conjunction with a rapid E wave deceleration time (<160 ms) indicates a restrictive filling pattern. The features of different filling patterns in individuals older than 60 years are summarized in **Table 8.8**.

Answer D is incorrect because the patient has a restrictive filling pattern. This is an abnormal finding and consistent with severe left ventricular diastolic dysfunction.

Answer E is incorrect because with a Valsalva maneuver the peak velocity of the mitral E wave is expected to decrease. Valsalva maneuver decreases preload and leads to a lower early diastolic pressure gradient between the left atrium and left ventricle. This leads to a lower peak velocity of the mitral E wave, and a lower mitral E/A ratio.

27. **Answer: B.** In sinus rhythm, the left atrium contracts following the P wave on EKG and the blood is propelled both forward into the left ventricle across the mitral valve, as well as backwards into the pulmonary veins, which lacks valves. The velocity profile of the forward flow is responsible for the mitral inflow A wave, while the retrograde flow into the pulmonary veins is responsible for the atrial reversal (AR) wave.

When the left ventricular diastolic pressure is elevated at the time of atrial contraction, both the peak velocity and the duration of the AR wave are

Table 8.8. Filling Patterns in Patients 60 and Older

Diastolic Dysfunction	Filling Pattern	Mitral Inflow E/A	E wave Deceleration Time (ms)	Pulmonary Vein S/D	Mitral Annular e' (cm/s)
None	Normal	0.6-1.3	≤258	>1	>8
Grade I (Mild)	Abnormal Relaxation	<0.8	>258		<8
Grade II (Moderate)	Pseudonormal	0.8-2	160-258	<1	
Grade III (Severe)	Restrictive Filling	>2	<160		

increased. A peak AR velocity of ≥35 cm/s is indicative of elevated LV end-diastolic pressure.

Elevation of LV end-diastolic pressure can also be inferred when the duration of the AR wave is ≥30 ms more than the duration of the mitral inflow A wave. In our patient, peak velocity of AR was 50 cm/s, and AR outlasted mitral A wave by 40 ms (210-170 ms); both are indicative of an elevated LV diastolic pressure. Therefore, answer B is correct.[2]

Answer A is incorrect because a restrictive filling pattern is characterized by a mitral inflow E/A ratio greater than 2; in this patient, peak E wave velocity is barely higher than the peak A wave velocity.

Answer C is incorrect because the higher the peak velocity of the atrial reversal wave in the pulmonary vein spectral tracing, the higher the left ventricular diastolic pressure.

Answer D is incorrect because with left ventricular dysfunction, there is an increase in the left ventricular diastolic pressure leading to secondary pulmonary hypertension. Because of LV diastolic pressure elevation, the pulmonary vein atrial reversal wave is likely to be prominent (as explained above) rather than absent. Atrial reversal wave is absent in atrial arrhythmias such as atrial fibrillation.

Answer E is incorrect because when left atrial pressure is elevated in older patients, the peak velocity of the systolic wave (S wave) in the pulmonary vein tracings is generally lower than the peak velocity of the diastolic wave (D wave). The higher the left atrial pressure, the lower the S/D ratio is.

28. **Answer: B.** In constrictive pericarditis, ventricular filling is constrained by an inelastic pericardial sac, which envelopes the entire heart except for the cranial portion of the left atrium and the pulmonary veins. This results in (1) ventricular interdependence, and (2) a differential impact of negative intrathoracic pressure that develops during inspiration on pulmonary veins and the heart.

Ventricular interdependence refers to diastolic filling of one ventricle at the expense of the other depending on the respiratory phase. In inspiration, the pressure in the intrathoracic systemic vein decreases. This leads to a larger pressure gradient between extra- and intrathoracic systemic veins, which result in improved RV filling. At the same time, the drop in the intrathoracic pressure with inspiration decreases the pulmonary venous pressure. Because of the thickened rigid pericardium, the drop in the intrathoracic pressure cannot be transmitted to the heart; this results in a decreased pressure gradient between pulmonary veins and the left atrium, and decreased LV filling in the diastole.

The net effect of inspiration is such that the right ventricle fills at the expense of the left ventricle, and the interventricular septum moves toward the left ventricle. The opposite occurs in expiration. This is illustrated in the M-mode recordings of our patient. The recordings also demonstrate no pericardial effusion.

With inspiration, the drop in intrathoracic pressure enhances forward flow in the hepatic veins in normal individuals; in constrictive pericarditis, there is an exaggeration of this inspiratory forward flow enhancement. During expiration, the rightward shift of the interventricular septum impedes RV filling; the rise in the RV diastolic pressure then leads to an expiratory increase in hepatic vein flow reversal. Therefore, answer B is correct.

Answer A is incorrect because of the presence of marked reciprocal changes in the right and left ventricular filling that are phasic with respiration and indicative of ventricular interdependence.

Answer C is incorrect because the abnormal septal motion due to right ventricular overload (as in atrial septal defect or severe tricuspid regurgitation) is characterized by flattening of the interventricular septum with each diastole rather than being phasic with respiration.

---

[2]For further explanation, the reader is referred to Recommendations for the evaluation of left ventricular diastolic function by echocardiography: an update from the American Society of Echocardiography and the European Association of Cardiovascular Imaging. *J Am Soc Echocardiogr.* 2016;29:277-314.

Answer D is incorrect because inspiratory increase in antegrade velocities is a normal finding. During inspiration, the drop in intrathoracic pressures enhances systemic venous return. This increased flow into the right heart elevates antegrade velocities in the hepatic veins.

Answer E is incorrect because the M-mode reveals no echo lucency posterior to the left ventricle that would be diagnostic of a large pericardial effusion. Instead, it shows pericardial thickening. It is important to emphasize, however, that the abnormal interventricular septal motion phasic with respiration is encountered in both tamponade and constrictive pericarditis.

29. **Answer: B.** In a normal descending aorta, antegrade flow occurs only in systole, and there is a small flow reversal in early diastole as depicted in the following pulsed-wave Doppler tracing in **Figure 8.59**.

    The pulsed-wave Doppler tracings in **Question 8.29** is abnormal as it demonstrates that antegrade flow is throughout the cardiac cycle. In addition, there is a large peak systolic gradient across the coarctation of almost 60 mm Hg. The presence of a holodiastolic antegrade flow in conjunction with a large systolic gradient is indicative of severe aortic coarctation. Therefore, answer B is correct.

    Answer A is incorrect because in severe aortic regurgitation, there is a retrograde flow throughout diastole (holodiastolic flow reversal) as demonstrated in **Figure 8.60**.

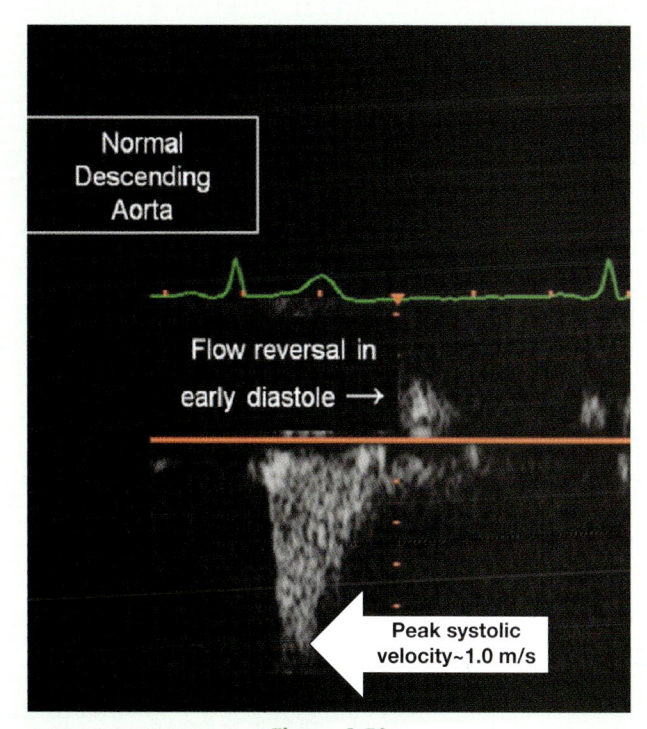

Figure 8.59

Answer C is incorrect because it is the bicuspid and not quadricuspid aortic valve that is typically associated with aortic coarctation. It is estimated that at least 50% of all individuals with coarctation have bicuspid aortic valve.

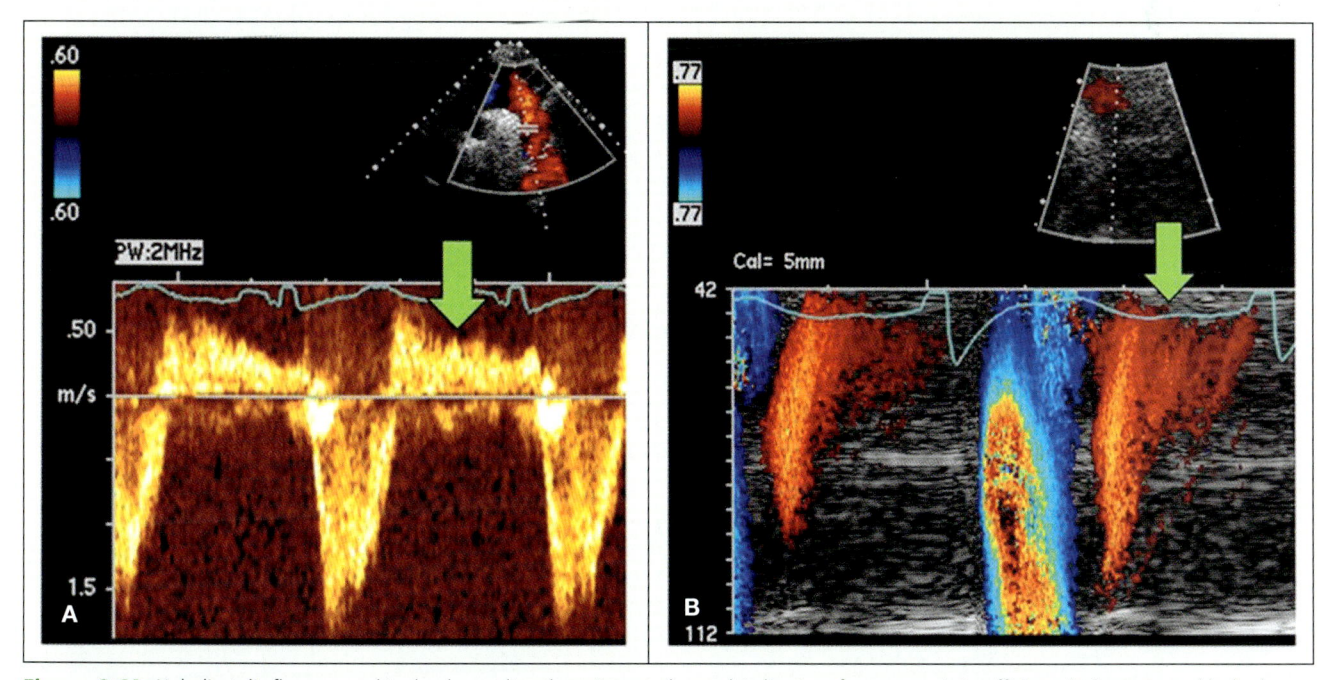

Figure 8.60. Holodiastolic flow reversal in the descending thoracic aorta (arrows) indicative of severe aortic insufficiency is demonstrated by both spectral Doppler (**A**, left panel) and color M-mode recordings (**B**, right panel).

Answer D is incorrect for two reasons. First, if this were a recording from the ascending aorta, forward velocities would have been recorded above the baseline and not below it. Second, aortic stenosis is not characterized by an antegrade diastolic gradient across the aortic valve.

Answer E is incorrect because coarctation usually occurs distal to the origin of the neck arteries, and the blood pressure in the arms is higher than in the legs.

30. **Answer: C.** Normal systole consists of isovolumic contraction time and ejection period. Flow across the aortic valve, whether the valve is normal or stenotic, occurs only during the ejection period of systole. In contrast, tricuspid regurgitant jet extends throughout the systole. Thus, on the spectral Doppler tracing, the aortic stenosis jet is of shorter duration and has a later onset compared to the tricuspid regurgitant as demonstrated in **Figure 8.61**. Therefore, answer C is correct.

    Answer A is incorrect because the panel on the right represents the flow velocity pattern across the aortic valve. Note the short time interval (isovolumic contraction time) between the QRS and the onset of flow in the right panel. In contrast, the onset of tricuspid regurgitant jet on the left panel coincides with the QRS on EKG.

    Answer B is incorrect because the aortic jet starts after the isovolumic contraction period.

    Answer D is incorrect because a peak velocity of 5 m/s does not exclude a tricuspid regurgitant jet; such a tricuspid jet velocity can be recorded in a patient with very severe pulmonary hypertension (pulmonary systolic pressure >100 mm Hg).

    Answer E is incorrect because the systolic function of both ventricles appears normal given the rapid rise in velocities from their baseline to their peak values. This rapid flow acceleration is consistent with a normal dP/dt, a measure of systolic function.

31. **Answer: B.** In both tamponade and constrictive pericarditis, there is impairment in ventricular filling during diastole. In tamponade, the impediment is caused by the pericardial fluid around the heart, while in constrictive pericarditis, the impediment is caused by a thickened rigid and sometimes calcified pericardium.

    In tamponade, the left ventricular filling is impaired from the onset of diastole. On spectral Doppler tracings of mitral inflow, this is manifested by the pattern of abnormal relaxation (peak velocity of the mitral E wave is lower than that of the A wave, and the deceleration time of the E wave is prolonged) (**Figure 8.62**).

    In contrast, in constrictive pericarditis, early diastolic filling is rapid then abruptly decreases in late diastole when the expanding myocardium reaches the rigid pericardium. This can be demonstrated using either cardiac catheterization or Doppler echocardiography. On cardiac catheterization, there is a rapid y descent in right atrial pressure tracings, and a dip-and-plateau pattern on right ventricular pressure tracings. On spectral Doppler recordings of mitral inflow, there is a restrictive filling pattern (the

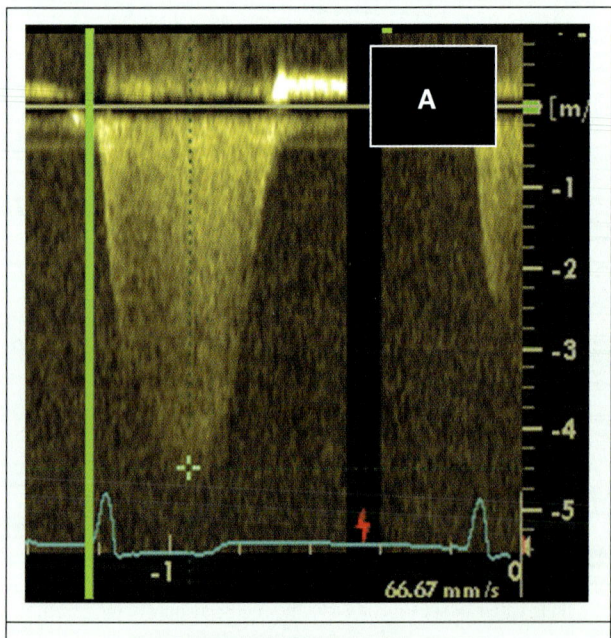

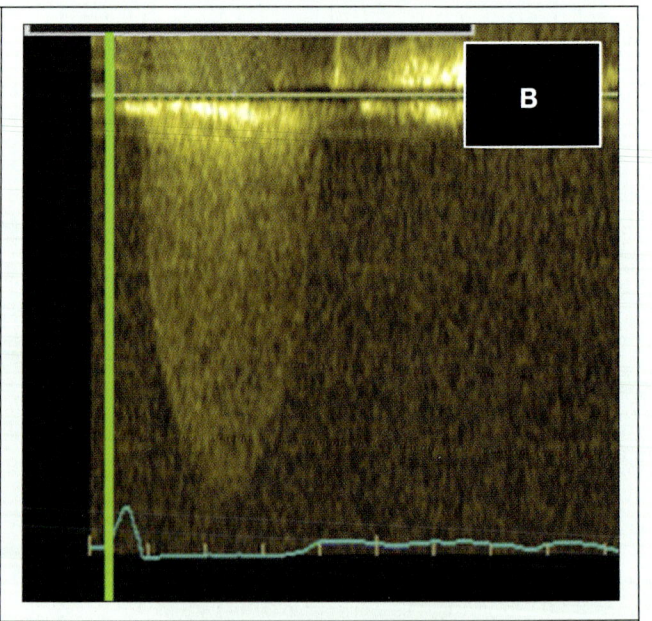

TRICUSPID REGURGITANT JET	AORTIC STENOSIS JET
Peak velocity = 4.5 m/s	Peak velocity = 5.0 m/s
Jet duration = 515 ms	Jet duration = 345 ms

Figure 8.61

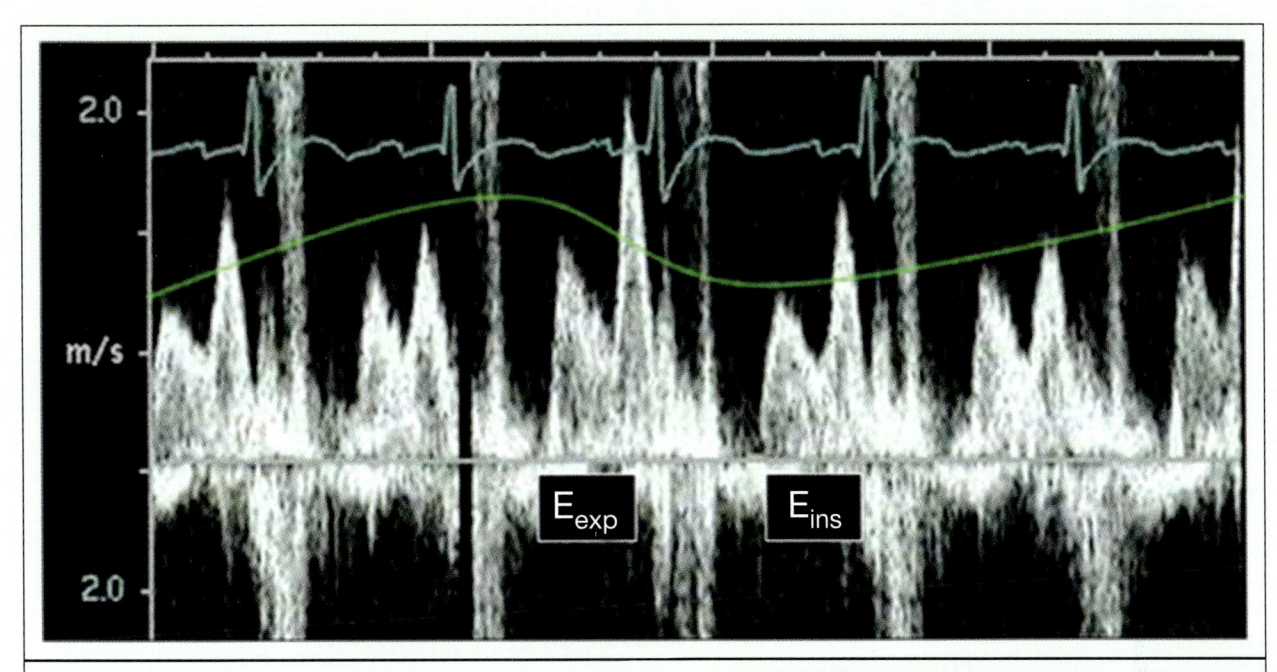

Expiratory peak E wave velocity (E$_{exp}$) = 170 cm/sec
Inspiratory peak E wave velocity (E$_{ins}$) = 110 cm/sec

Figure 8.62

ratio of peak E wave to peak A wave velocity >2; deceleration time of E wave <160 ms).

Both in tamponade and constrictive pericarditis, there is ventricular interdependence. Because of ventricular interdependence, there is marked decrease in left ventricular filling during inspiration. The magnitude of inspiratory drop in early diastolic filling (as measured by peak velocity of mitral E wave) is directly proportional to the severity of either tamponade or constrictive pericarditis.

In normal individuals, inspiratory drop in peak E wave velocity with inspiration is small; in tamponade and constrictive pericarditis, the inspiratory drop is ≥30% and ≥25%, respectively. One uses the following formula to calculate percent respiratory variation in the peak velocity of mitral E wave (ΔE):

$$\Delta E = \frac{E_{Expiration} - E_{Inspiration}}{E_{Expiration}}$$

Bear in mind that marked respiratory variations are not unique to tamponade and constrictive pericarditis; they also occur with labored breathing, asthma, chronic obstructive lung disease, pulmonary embolism, and obesity.

In our patient:

$$\Delta E = \frac{170 - 110}{170} = \frac{60}{170} = 35\%$$

In summary, the combination of the abnormal relaxation mitral inflow pattern and the marked respiratory variations in the peak velocity of the mitral inflow E wave are consistent with the diagnosis of cardiac tamponade. Therefore, answer E is correct.

Answer A is incorrect because in both tamponade and constrictive pericarditis, the respiratory variations are measured in the peak velocity of the E wave, not the A wave.

Answer C is incorrect for two reasons. First, the mitral inflow filling pattern in this patient demonstrates abnormal relaxation (E/A < 1) rather than restrictive filling (E/A > 2 and E wave deceleration time <160 ms). Second, there are no significant respiratory variations in mitral inflow in patients with restrictive cardiomyopathy. An additional distinction between restrictive cardiomyopathy and constrictive pericarditis is the peak velocity of the mitral annular tissue Doppler early diastolic e' wave. The e' velocity is normal in constrictive pericarditis and diminished in restrictive cardiomyopathy.

Answer D is incorrect because an E/A < 1 favors tamponade over constrictive pericarditis as discussed above.

Answer E is incorrect because diuretics should not be administered to patients with tamponade physiology since the decrease in preload caused by diuretics would further impair ventricular filling.

186 / Clinical Echocardiography Review

32. Answer: A. (Right atrial pressure rises progressively toward the end of ventricular systole).

The spectral recordings were obtained from a patient with very severe tricuspid regurgitation. When the tricuspid regurgitant orifice is large, there is ventricularization of the right atrial pressures (RAP) which results in a very rapid pressure equilibration between right ventricular pressure (RVP) and the RAP as demonstrated in pressure tracings in **Figure 8.63**.

The rapid rise in the right atrial pressure results in a rapid deceleration slope of the tricuspid regurgitant jet (*arrow* in the continuous Doppler tracing [**Figure 8.64**] of the tricuspid regurgitant jet). Therefore, answer A is correct.

Clinically, a patient with this type of tricuspid regurgitation typically has a pulsatile liver. An echocardiographic correlate of pulsatile liver is the systolic wave reversal in hepatic vein spectral Doppler tracings shown in **Figure 8.65**.

Answer B is incorrect because the acceleration rate in tricuspid regurgitant jet velocities from baseline to the peak velocity is fast indicative of a normal dP/dt and a normal RV systolic function.

Answer C is incorrect because the peak velocity of the tricuspid regurgitant jet is often low even in the presence of significant pulmonary hypertension.

Answer D is incorrect because the flow velocity profile of this patient's tricuspid regurgitant jet is typical of severe tricuspid regurgitation (low peak velocity; rapid deceleration slope due to rapid pressure equilibration between RV and RA.

Answer E is incorrect because the spectral Doppler tracing of a midcavitary right ventricular gradient has its peak in late systole. In this patient, the jet peaks in early systole.

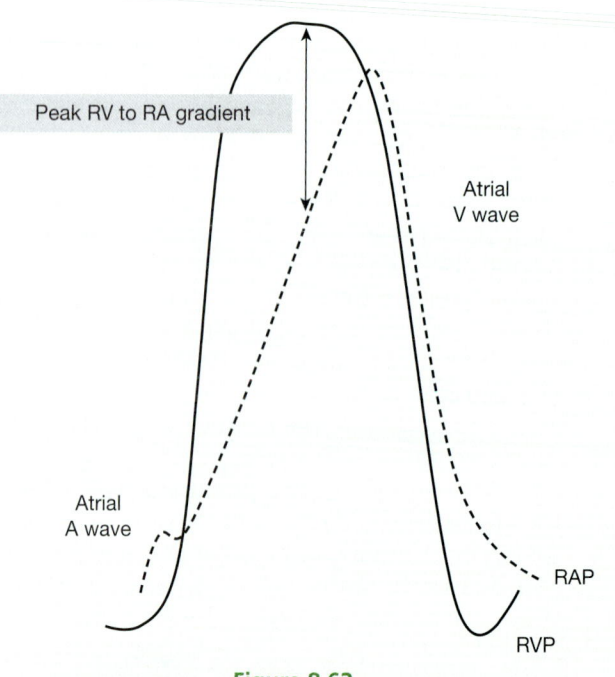

Figure 8.63

33. Answer: D. In patients with uncomplicated VSD, there is antegrade flow from the left ventricle to the right ventricle during both systole and diastole.

Using the $4 * V^2$ formula to calculate the peak systolic and end-diastolic pressure gradients from VSD spectral Doppler recordings, one can estimate right ventricular peak systolic pressure (RVSP) and left ventricular end-diastolic pressure (LVEDP), respectively (**Figure 8.66**).

As shown in the figure given above, this patient's peak systolic and end-diastolic pressure gradients are as follows:

$$\text{VSD Peak systolic gradient} = 4 * (3.5 \text{ m/s})^2$$
$$= 4 * 12.25 \text{ mm Hg}$$
$$= 49 \text{ mm Hg}$$
$$\text{VSD End-diastolic gradient} = 4 * (2.0 \text{ m/s})^2$$
$$= 4 * 4 \text{ mm Hg}$$
$$= 16 \text{ mm Hg}$$

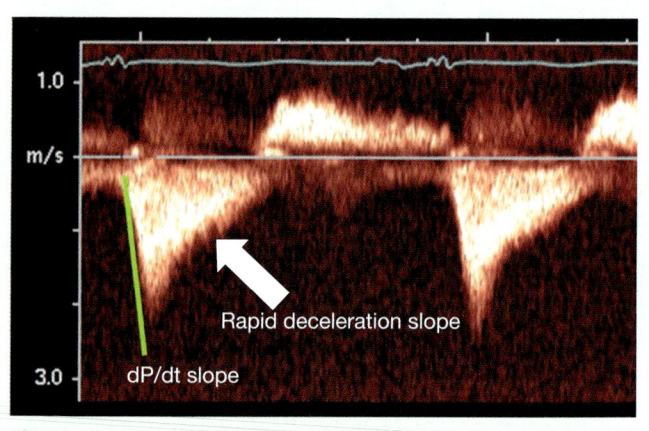

Figure 8.64. Continuous spectral Doppler of tricuspid regurgitant jet.

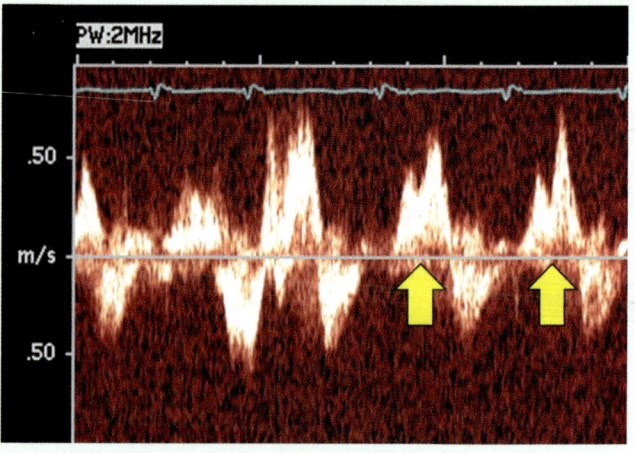

Figure 8.65. Systolic wave reversal in hepatic vein spectral Doppler tracing indicative of severe tricuspid regurgitation.

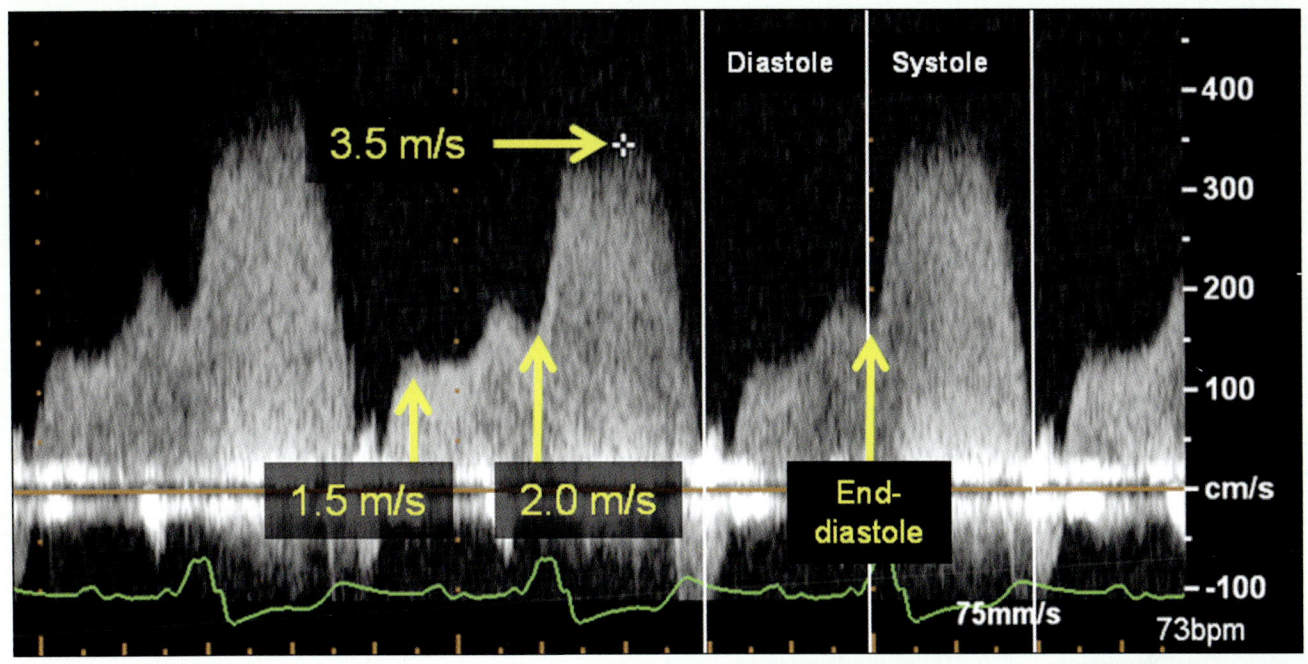

Figure 8.66

To calculate the LVEDP, we need to add the estimate of the RV end-diastolic pressure to the VSD end-diastolic gradient. In the absence of tricuspid stenosis, RV end-diastolic pressure equals the end-diastolic RA pressure (which is given in the question as 10 mm Hg). Thus:

LVEDP = VSD End-diastolic gradient
+ RA end-diastolic pressure.

LVEDP = 16 + 10 = 26 mm Hg.

Additionally, we can calculate the RV peak-systolic pressure in this patient as well by subtracting the VSD Peak systolic gradient from the patient's systolic blood pressure (SBP):

RV peak systolic pressure = SBP − VSD Peak-systolic gradient
RV peak systolic pressure = 90 − 49 mm Hg = 41 mm Hg.

34. **Answer: C.** Normal mitral annular tissue Doppler recordings demonstrate the following:
- Peak velocity of the early diastolic (E') wave of at least 10 cm/s at either medial or lateral mitral annulus.
- Peak E' velocity is normally higher in the lateral compared to the medial annulus. In other words, E' lateral/E' medial >1.
- E' velocity is typically higher than the peak velocity of the late diastolic (A') wave

In this patient, overall peak E' velocities are within normal range. However, the medial E' velocity is much higher than the lateral E' velocity.

Therefore, in this patient, E' lateral/E' medial <1. This phenomenon when E' lateral/E' medial is reversed from what is normally observed is referred to as *annulus reversus*.

The finding of annulus reversus on mitral annular tissue Doppler is consistent with the diagnosis of constrictive pericarditis. The lateral E' velocity diminishes relative to the medial E' velocity because fibrosis and calcifications of the surrounding pericardium restrict the motion of the lateral annulus. The medial E' velocity is typically not affected in constrictive pericarditis as the septal annulus is not surrounded by the pericardium.

Answer A is incorrect as the left heart valves (mitral and aortic valve) are not typically affected by carcinoid heart disease. Carcinoid disease typically affects the right heart valves rendering the leaflets of the tricuspid and pulmonic valve immobile; this results in both stenosis and regurgitation of the tricuspid and pulmonic valve.

Answer B is incorrect as both medial and lateral annular tissue Doppler velocities are diminished in patients with amyloidosis but the ratio of E' lateral to E' medial of >1 is maintained as in normal individuals.

Answer D is incorrect because mitral annular calcification leads to a decrease of both medial and lateral annular tissue Doppler velocities but the ratio of E' lateral to E' medial of >1 is maintained as in normal individuals.

Answer E is incorrect as patients with mitral regurgitation due to a flail leaflet typically have lateral E' velocities higher than medial E' velocities.

35. Answer: E. (Peak left atrial pressure is 52 mm Hg).

Normally, the peak gradient across an uncomplicated ASD is small and measures only a few mm Hg as the LA pressure is only slightly higher than the RA pressure.

However, in patients with left ventricular dysfunction and/or severe mitral valve disease, the LA pressure may rise to high levels and lead to pulmonary edema. If such a patient has an ASD with a left-to-right shunt, the peak LA pressure can be calculated as the sum of the peak trans-ASD gradient and the RA pressure estimate. In this patient:

Peak trans-ASD gradient = 4 * 3.3^2 m/s = 4 * 11 = 44 mm Hg

Since the RA pressure is given as 8 mm Hg, then:

Peak LA pressure = Peak trans-ASD gradient + RA pressure
Peak LA pressure = 44 + 8 = 52 mm Hg.

36. Answer: E. Typically, mitral regurgitation is holosystolic and both EROA and regurgitant volume are accurate measures of mitral regurgitation severity as shown in **Table 8.9**

However, when mitral regurgitation is only late systolic (as is in many cases of mitral valve prolapse), there is discordance between the EROA and the regurgitant volume.

This patient's EROA of 0.48 cm^2 would suggest severe mitral regurgitation. However, since the MR jet is only late systolic, its velocity-time integral (VTI) is relatively small and consequently the calculated regurgitant volume is not consistent with severe mitral regurgitation.

In general, regurgitant volume is a product of EROA and the regurgitant jet VTI:

Regurgitant volume = EROA * VTI

In this patient:

Regurgitant volume = 0.48 cm^2 * 72 cm = 35 mL

Thus, the regurgitant volume of 35 mL in this patient is indicative of moderate mitral regurgitation.

In summary, in patients with mitral valve prolapse and late systolic regurgitant jet, EROA overestimates the severity of mitral regurgitation. In such instances, regurgitant volume and fraction are better measures of mitral regurgitation severity compared to EROA.

In contrast, in patients with holosystolic mitral regurgitation, EROA and regurgitant volume are concordant as illustrated in the right panel of **Figure 8.67**.

In the above patient with annular dilatation, let us assume that EROA is also 0.48 cm^2 as in the patient with mitral valve prolapse. Note, however, that the VTI in the patient with annular dilatation is much higher than in the patient with mitral valve prolapse (141 vs 72 cm).

The regurgitant volume in the patient with annular dilatation and holosystolic mitral regurgitation can be calculated as follows:

Regurgitant volume = EROA * VTI

Regurgitant volume = 0.48 cm^2 * 141 cm = 68 mL

A regurgitant volume of 68 mL is consistent with severe mitral regurgitation.

Answer A is incorrect because mitral regurgitation in this patient is late systolic and not early systolic.

Answer B is incorrect because EROA overestimates the severity of mitral regurgitation in patients with mitral valve prolapse and late systolic mitral regurgitation as discussed above.

Answer C is incorrect because the peak systolic LV to LA gradient based on the mitral regurgitant jet is 135 mm Hg:

Peak LV to LA gradient = 4 * $(5.8 \text{ m/s})^2$ = 135 mm Hg

Table 8.9. Grading of Mitral Regurgitation Severity

	Mild (1+)	Moderate (2+)	Moderate-Severe (3+)	Severe (4+)
EROA (cm^2)	<0.2	0.20-0.29	0.30-0.39	≥0.4
Regurgitant Fraction	<30%	30%-39%	40%-49%	≥50%
Regurgitant Volume (mL)	30	30-44	45-59	≥60
Vena contracta (cm)	≤0.3	0.4-0.6		≥0.7

EROA, effective regurgitant orifice area.

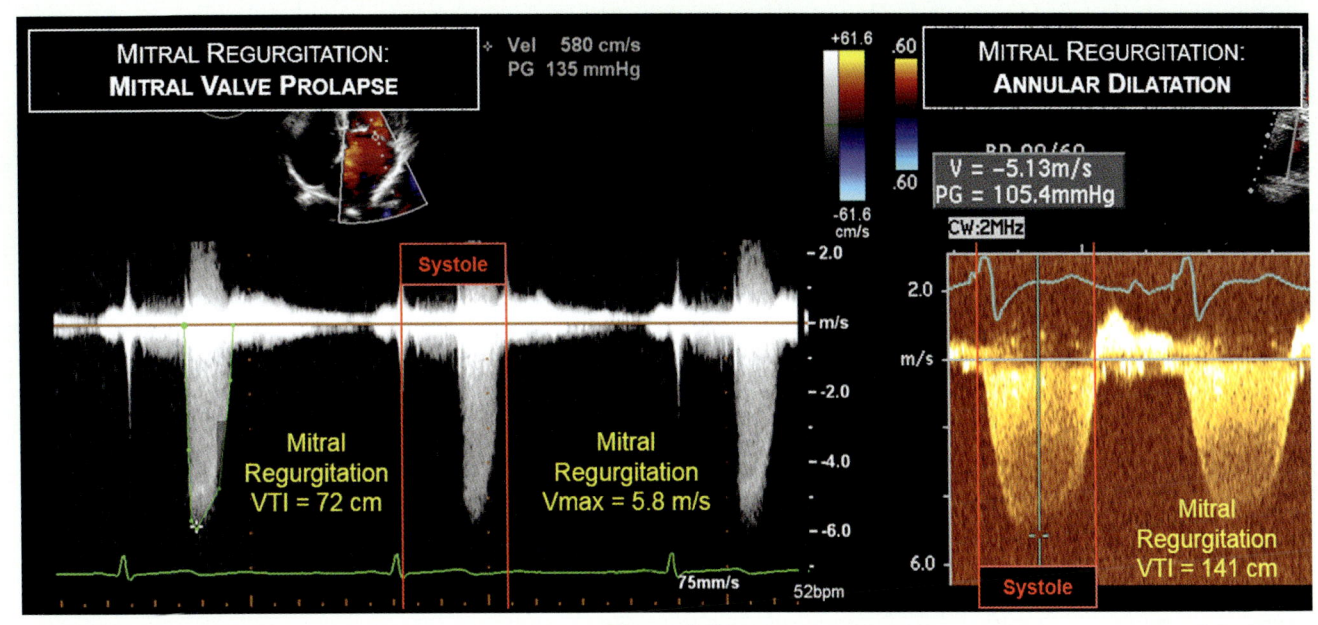

Figure 8.67

Peak LV systolic pressure can be calculated as follows:

Peak LV systolic pressure = Peak LV to LA gradient + LA pressure

In this patient:

Peak LV systolic pressure = 135 + 10 = 145 mm Hg

Systolic blood pressure = Peak LV systolic pressure

In the absence of aortic stenosis:

Systolic blood pressure = Peak LV systolic pressure

Thus this patient's systolic blood pressure is approximately 145 mm Hg and the patient is hypertensive rather than hypotensive.

Answer D is incorrect as the regurgitant fraction cannot be calculated from the provided data as the forward stroke volume across a nonregurgitant orifice (such as the LV outflow tract in the absence of aortic regurgitation) is not provided for this patient.

In general:

Regurgitant fraction = Regurgitant volume/ (Regurgitant volume + Forward stroke volume).

37. Answer: D. The spectral Doppler tracing demonstrates antegrade flow in both systole and diastole. Since the patient is in normal sinus rhythm, the flow is triphasic and consists of a systolic (S) wave and two diastolic waves: early diastolic (E) wave and late diastolic (A) wave. The mean gradient of 10 mm Hg in this patient is indicative of significant stenosis.

This triphasic flow is characteristic of cor triatriatum (literally, a heart with three atria). In this congenital malformation, a perforated membrane divides the left atrium into two chambers: the posterior left atrium which receives the pulmonary veins, and the anterior left atrium which is connected to the left atrial appendage and is bound by the mitral valve.

Clinical presentation of cor triatriatum is similar to that of mitral stenosis. However, mitral stenosis (whether supravalvular, valvular, or subvalvular) is characterized by an elevated transmitral pressure gradient that is present only during diastole. In contrast, the elevated gradient of cor triatriatum is present in both systole and diastole. This is illustrated in **Figure 8.68**.

Answers A, C, and E refer to various forms of mitral stenosis (supravalvular mitral stenosis due to supravalvular ring, valvular rheumatic mitral stenosis, subvalvular stenosis). All three answers are incorrect as systolic antegrade flow across the mitral valve is absent in all of them.

Shone complex is a congenital syndrome of sequential obstructions in the left heart and the aorta. Patients with Shone complex may be present with one or more of the following: supravalvular mitral ring, parachute mitral valve (single papillary muscle with maldeveloped chordae resulting in subvalvular mitral stenosis), subaortic membrane and coarctation of the aorta. Cor triatriatum is not a manifestation of Shone complex.

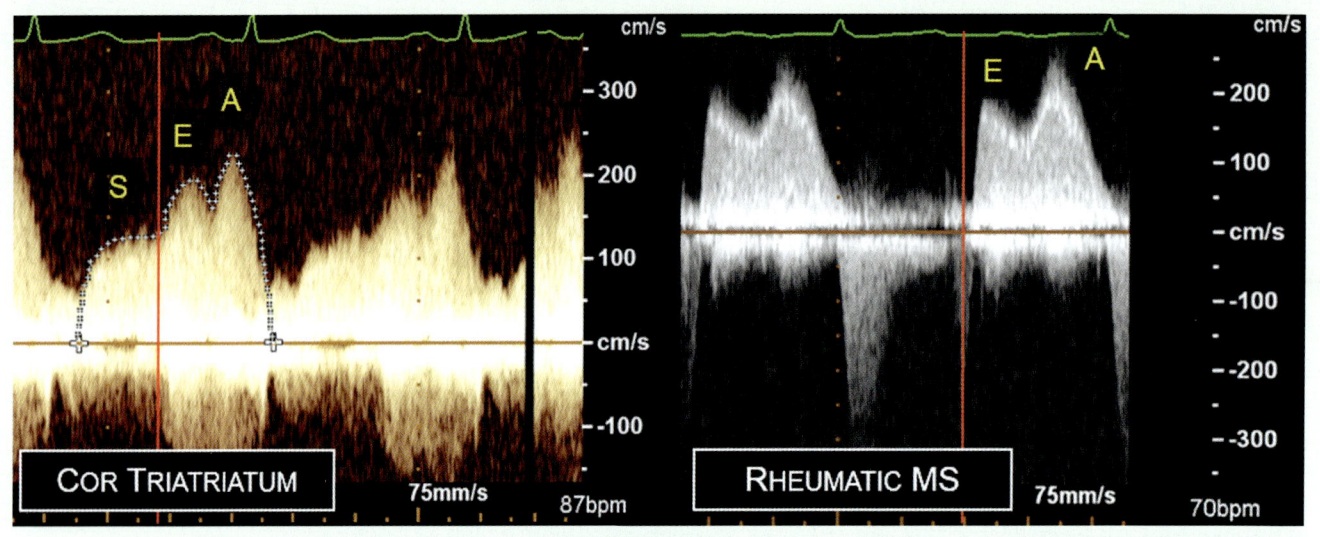

Figure 8.68

38. Answer: C. The patient initially presents with acutely decompensated heart failure due to acute coronary syndrome (non-ST elevation myocardial infarction) in the distribution of the left anterior descending coronary artery.

The five mitral inflow patterns presented in **Question 8.38** were as follows:

A	Abnormal relaxation pattern (Grade I diastolic dysfunction)
B	Pseudonormal pattern (Grade II diastolic dysfunction)
C	Restrictive filling pattern (Grade III diastolic dysfunction)
D	Mitral inflow in a patient with mechanical mitral valve (note the vertical line artifact due to opening and closing of the prosthetic leaflets).
E	Mitral inflow in a patient with atrial fibrillation.

Since the patient has a normal native mitral valve and was in normal sinus rhythm at the time of study, patterns D and E do not belong to this patient.

Using the E/e' ratio concept (discussed in answer to **Question 8.8**) we can estimate the mean pulmonary artery wedge pressure (PAWP) for the remaining three patterns:

Pattern	Peak E Velocity (cm/s)	Peak e' Velocity (cm/s)	PAWP = 1.9 + 1.24*(E/e') (mm Hg)	PAWP = 4 + E/e' (mm Hg)
Image A (Grade I)	45	5	13	13
Image B (Grade II)	60	5	17	16
Image C (Grade III)	150	5	39	34

Of the three remaining patterns, only the restrictive filling (pattern C) predicts a PAWP that is in general agreement with the 38 mm Hg value obtained invasively by Swan–Ganz catheter. Therefore, answer C is correct.

39. Answer: E. (Severe 4+)

The severity of mitral regurgitation can be assessed using the PISA method to calculate the effective regurgitant orifice area (EROA):

$$EROA = 2 * \pi * r^2 * \frac{Valias}{Vmax}$$

In our patient, radius was 0.9 cm, Valias was 69 cm/s, and Vmax was 420 cm/s:

$$EROA = 2 * 3.14 * (0.9)^2 * (69/420) = 0.8 \text{ cm}^2$$

This EROA is very large (see **Table 8.9**) and indicative of severe mitral regurgitation. Therefore, answer E is correct.

40. Answer: A. Patient presented with severe acute mitral regurgitation 8 days after myocardial infarction in the territory of the left anterior descending artery that resulted in the rupture of the anterolateral papillary muscle. The course of events is consistent with the timeframe in which papillary muscle rupture, a mechanical complication of myocardial infarction, typically occurs.

Rupture of the anterolateral papillary muscle is less common than the rupture of the posteromedial one. Anterolateral papillary muscle usually has dual blood supply from both left anterior descending and left circumflex arteries. In contrast, posteromedial papillary muscle has solitary blood supply from either right coronary or left circumflex artery. Our patient had total proximal occlusion of the left anterior descending artery and diffuse disease in the left circumflex artery.

Answer B is incorrect because the clinical findings are inconsistent with bacteremia: the patient is afebrile and has a normal white blood count. In addition, a vegetation would appear as a shaggy, independently mobile echo density attached typically to the atrial side of the mitral valve. The mass seen in this patient is attached to the mitral chordae and represents a severed head of the anterolateral papillary muscle.

Answer C is incorrect because mitral annular dilatation typically leads to mitral regurgitation with a central jet. In this patient, the jet is highly eccentric which is consistent with papillary muscle rupture.

Answer D is incorrect because rheumatic mitral valve disease is a chronic disorder that typically begins in childhood and progresses over many years. In our patient, the mitral valve was normal on initial admission and became severely regurgitant only days later. In addition, TEE imaging of the mitral valve in this patient lacks typical findings of rheumatic valve disease such as leaflet thickening and calcification, chordal fusion, and shortening.

Answer E is incorrect because mitral valve prolapse due to myxomatous degeneration is a chronic valvulopathy that would have been recognized on the initial echocardiogram at the time of first hospitalization. Mitral valve prolapse is characterized by floppy mitral leaflets that protrude into the left atrium above the mitral annular plane in systole due to leaflet and chordal elongation. Papillary muscle rupture is not a typical complication of mitral valve prolapse.

KEY POINTS
Case 1
- In normal elderly patients, the typical mitral inflow filling pattern is A dominant (E < A). Increase in LA pressure leads to progressive increase in E wave velocity.
- In a patient with recent myocardial infarction and elevated LA pressures, mechanical complications of myocardial infarction, including acute severe mitral regurgitation due to papillary muscle rupture should be considered

41. Answer: C. (Pulmonary artery pressure is estimated at 26/12 mm Hg).

This patient has a patent ductus arteriosus (PDA) with a left-to-right shunt from the descending thoracic aorta to the left pulmonary artery throughout the cardiac cycle.

Using the spectral Doppler tracings of the PDA flow, one can calculate the peak systolic gradient (PSG) and end-diastolic gradient (EDG) across the PDA.

$$PSG = 4 * PSV^2$$
$$EDG = 4 * EDV^2$$

Where PSV is the peak systolic velocity and EDV is the end-diastolic velocity across the PDA.

In our patient:

$$PSG = 4 * (6.0 \text{ m/s})^2 = 4 * 36 = 144 \text{ mm Hg}$$
$$EDG = 4 * (3.8 \text{ m/s})^2 = 4 * 14.4 = 58 \text{ mm Hg}$$

By subtracting PSG and EDG from systolic and diastolic blood pressure, respectively, one can estimate pulmonary artery systolic blood pressure (SBP) and diastolic blood pressure (DBP).

$$PASP = SBP - PSG$$
$$PADP = DBP - EDG$$

In our patient:

$$PASP = 170 - 144 = 26 \text{ mm Hg}$$
$$PADP = 70 - 58 = 12 \text{ mm Hg}$$

Therefore, answer B is correct. This patient's calculations are summarized as follows:

	Velocity (m/sec)	PDA Gradient (mm Hg)	Blood Pressure (mm Hg)	Estimated Pulmonary Artery Pressure (mm Hg)
Systole	6.0	144	170	26
Diastole	3.8	58	70	12

Answer A is incorrect because the right atrial pressure is not needed to calculate PADP in a patient with PDA when DBP and EDG are known.

Answer B is incorrect because a pulsed-wave Doppler technique would not have been able to record such high velocities (including a peak velocity of 6 m/sec) without aliasing in an adult.

Answer D is incorrect because PASP in this patient is 26 mm Hg as calculated above.

Answer E is incorrect because flow across an uncomplicated PDA occurs throughout the cardiac cycle irrespective of a PDA size. This is because in uncomplicated PDA, the pressures in the descending aorta are higher than the pressures in the pulmonary artery throughout the cardiac cycle.

42. Answer: B. 0.11 cm².

PISA method can be used to estimate the effective orifice area (EOA) of the PDA at its aortic end:

$$EOA = 2 * \pi * r^2 * \frac{V_{alias}}{V_{max}}$$

where r is the PISA radius, Valias is the PISA aliasing velocity, and Vmax is the peak systolic velocity across the PDA.

In our patient:

$$EOA = 2*3.14*(0.5 \text{ cm})^2 * 41/600 = 0.11 \text{ cm}^2.$$

Note that the color bar baseline was shifted upward. Of the two Nyquist limits (41 cm/s for antegrade flow and 69 cm/s for retrograde flow), one should use the one in the direction of PDA flow, which is 41 cm/s.

Assuming a circular shape, the PDA orifice in this patient would then have a diameter of approximately 4 mm. The area (A) of a circle is calculated as:

$$A = \left(\frac{d}{2}\right)^2 * \pi$$

where d is the PDA diameter. In our patient:

$$0.11 = \left(\frac{d}{2}\right)^2 * 3.14 = \frac{0.11}{3.14} = \left(\frac{d}{2}\right)^2$$

Solving for diameter (d):

$$d = 2*\sqrt{\frac{0.11}{3.14}} = 0.37 \text{ cm} = 3.7 \text{ mm}$$

The diameter of a PDA usually ranges between 0.9 and 11.2 mm (median 2.6 mm).

KEY POINTS
Case 2
- In patients with a patent ductus arteriosus, one can calculate PA systolic and diastolic pressures by subtracting the peak systolic and end-diastolic trans-PDA gradients from systolic and diastolic blood pressure, respectively. It is important to emphasize that RA pressure estimate is not needed for these calculations.
- PISA method can be used to estimate the size of the PDA orifice

43. **Answer: C.** This patient has hypertrophic obstructive cardiomyopathy (HOCM) with asymmetric septal hypertrophy. Systolic anterior motion of the mitral leaflets in HOCM leads to (1) dynamic left ventricular outflow tract (LVOT) obstruction, and (2) mitral regurgitation. Both the gradient across the LVOT and the gradient across the mitral valve peak late in systole.

One can calculate the peak systolic LVOT gradient from the following three parameters: peak gradient of mitral regurgitant jet, left atrial pressure, and systolic blood pressure.

Step 1: Calculate the peak systolic LV-to-LA gradient

Using the peak velocity of the mitral regurgitant jet, one can calculate the peak systolic pressure gradient (ΔP_{MR}) between the left ventricle (LV) and the left atrium (LA):

$$\Delta P_{MR} = 4 V^2$$

where V is the peak velocity of the mitral regurgitant jet.

In our patient:

$$\Delta P_{MR} = 4*(8 \text{ m/s})^2 = 4*64 = 256 \text{ mm Hg}$$

Step 2: Calculate the peak LV systolic pressure (LVSP)

By definition, ΔP_{MR} is the difference between the peak LVSP and the LA pressure (LAP):

$$\Delta P_{MR} = LVSP - LAP$$

Solving for LVSP:

$$LVSP = \Delta PMR + LAP$$

In our patient:

$$LVSP = 256 \text{ mm Hg} + 10 \text{ mm Hg} = 266 \text{ mm Hg}$$

Step 3: Calculate maximal instantaneous left ventricular outflow gradient ($\Delta PLVOT$)

ΔP_{LVOT} is the pressure difference between the LVSP and the systolic blood pressure (SBP):

$$\Delta P_{LVOT} = LVSP - SBP$$

In our patient:

$$\Delta P_{LVOT} = 266 \text{ mm Hg} - 144 \text{ mm Hg} = 122 \text{ mm Hg}$$

Therefore, answer C is correct. All these calculations are summarized **Figure 8.69**:

Answer A is incorrect because in HOCM, mitral regurgitation increases progressively toward mid to

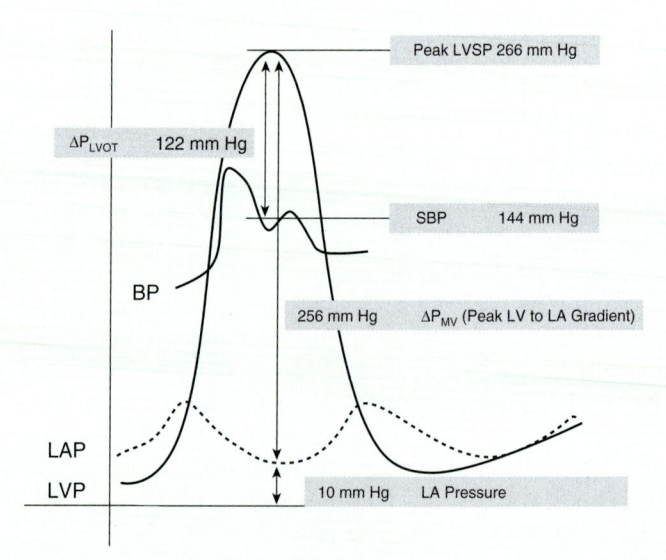

Figure 8.69

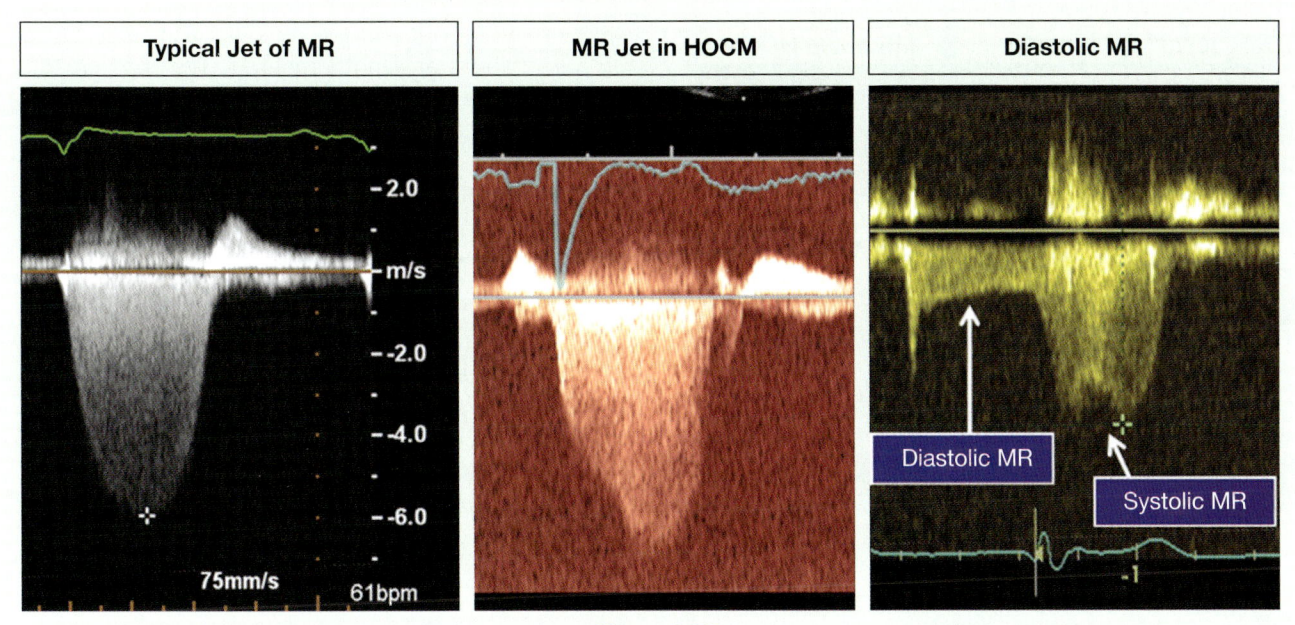

Figure 8.70

| Typical Jet of MR | MR Jet in HOCM | Diastolic MR |

late systole. MR in HOCM is the result of systolic anterior motion (SAM); the anterior leaflet moves progressively toward the interventricular septum and away from the coaptation line with the posterior leaflet. This results in an MR velocity profile that peaks late in systole. Therefore, in our patient, the initial portion of the mitral regurgitant jet is not missing from the Doppler tracing; the Doppler velocity profile is typical for HOCM-related MR.

Answer B is incorrect because LVSP is very high. It is calculated above at 266 mm Hg. Normal LVSP is the same as the normal SBP, which is around 120 mm Hg.

Answer D is incorrect because there is no diastolic MR in this patient. Typically, MR is a systolic phenomenon. In rare instances, MR can start in late diastole (diastolic MR) and continue into systole. Diastolic MR may occur in severe LV systolic dysfunction or with complete heart block.

Different MR velocity profiles are summarized in **Figure 8.70**.

Answer E is incorrect because the peak LV systolic pressure in this patient is 266 mm Hg.

44. **Answer: C.** In this patient with hypertrophic obstructive cardiomyopathy (HOCM), jet #1 represents the systolic flow velocity pattern across the left ventricular outflow tract (LVOT), and jet #2 represents the flow velocity pattern of the mitral regurgitant (MR) jet.

Jet #1 has a saw tooth appearance because the gradient characteristically peaks late in systole. The systolic anterior motion of the mitral valve in HOCM progressively narrows the LVOT toward the end of systole. This in turn results in ever-increasing systolic blood velocities through the LVOT and the late peaking velocity profile typical of HOCM.

Using the $\Delta P = 4V^2$ formula, we can calculate peak systolic instantaneous gradient (ΔP_{LVOT}) across the LVOT where V represents the peak velocity of jet #1.

$$\Delta P_{LVOT} = 4*(3.8 \text{ m/s})^2 = 4*14.4 = 58 \text{ mm Hg}$$

Since the pre-treatment ΔP_{LVOT} was 122 mm Hg, there was an approximately 50% drop in the gradient on the repeat echocardiogram:

Percent drop in ΔP_{LVOT} = (122 − 58)/122 = 64/122 ≈ 50%

Therefore, answer C is correct.

Answer A is incorrect because in mitral valve prolapse with click and systolic murmur, mitral regurgitation characteristically does not occur in early systole. The prolapse usually does not create a regurgitant orifice until mid-systole. Once the regurgitant orifice is created, mitral regurgitation continues until the end of systole. The difference in the shape of the mitral regurgitant spectral jet between mitral valve prolapse and HOCM is depicted in **Figure 8.71**.

Answer B is incorrect because jet #2 starts immediately after the QRS complex on the EKG. Therefore, the jet encompasses the isovolumic contraction time. Aortic stenosis flow does not occur in that early portion of systole.

Answer D is incorrect because an intracavitary left ventricular gradient tapers off and peaks even later in systole than the LVOT gradient as shown in **Figure 8.72**.

Answer E is incorrect because the peak left ventricular systolic pressure (LVSP) is calculated as:

$$LVSP = \Delta P_{MR} + LAP \qquad (8.54)$$

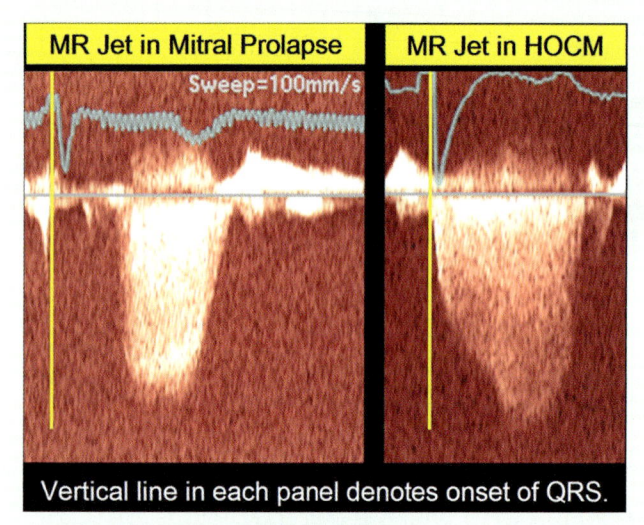

194 / Clinical Echocardiography Review

Figure 8.71 — MR Jet in Mitral Prolapse | MR Jet in HOCM. Sweep=100mm/s. Vertical line in each panel denotes onset of QRS.

where ΔP_{MR} is the peak systolic gradient of the mitral regurgitant jet, and LAP is the left atrial pressure. After expressing ΔP_{MR} in terms of the peak systolic velocity (V) of the mitral regurgitant jet, Equation (8.54) becomes:

$$LVSP = 4*V^2 + LAP \qquad (8.55)$$

In our patient:

$$LVSP = 4*(6.3 \text{ m/s})^2 + 10$$
$$LVSP = 159 + 10 = 169 \text{ mm Hg}.$$

KEY POINTS
Case 3
- In patients with obstructive hypertrophic cardiomyopathy, it is important to differentiate spectral Doppler patterns of LVOT obstruction from mitral regurgitation
- Spectral Doppler of mitral regurgitant flow in patients with obstructive hypertrophic cardiomyopathy typically has high peak velocity and the velocity peaks late in systole.

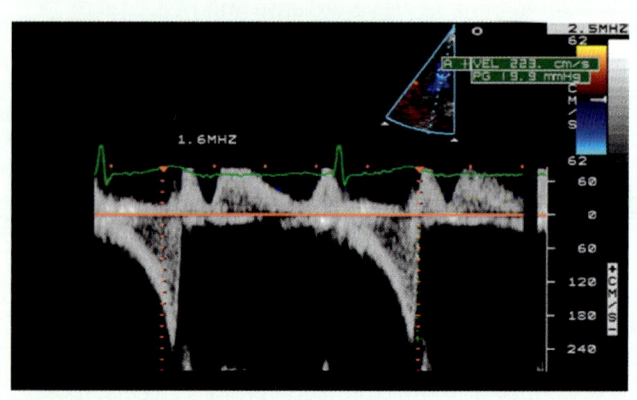

Figure 8.72. Pulsed-wave spectral Doppler tracing of a left ventricular intracavitary gradient.

---

45. **Answer: D.** Left atrial volume (LAV) can be calculated using the area–length method. The mathematical formula requires three parameters: left atrial area in the apical 4-chamber view (A1), left atrial area in the apical 2-chamber view (A2), and the shorter of the two atrial lengths (L) either in the apical 4- or apical 2-chamber view.

$$LAV = \frac{8*A1*A2}{3*\pi*L}$$

The formula can be simplified by calculating the $8/3\pi$ ratio as 0.85:

$$LAV = 0.85 * \frac{A1*A2}{L}$$

In our patient:

$$LAV = 0.85 * \frac{27*26}{5.6} = 107 \text{ mL}$$

LAV index (LAVI) is calculating by dividing LAV into the body surface area(BSA):

$$LAVI = \frac{LAV}{BSA}$$

In our patient:

LAVI = 107 mL / 2.1 m² ≈ 50 mL/m²

Therefore, answer D is correct. This is a severely elevated LAVI as shown in the data that follows:

	LA Volume Index (mL/m²)
Normal	≤34
Mild dilatation	35–41
Moderate dilatation	42–48
Severe dilatation	>48

46. **Answer: B.** The initial echocardiogram, which was obtained at the time of acutely decompensated heart failure, demonstrates a restrictive filling pattern. Because of the high left atrial pressure, the early diastolic gradient across the mitral valve is high. This results in a tall mitral E wave and the ratio of peak mitral E to peak mitral A wave that is usually >2. In addition, the mitral E wave has rapid deceleration (deceleration time <160 ms). In the pulmonary venous spectral Doppler tracings, the peak of the systolic (S) wave is lower than the peak of the diastolic (D) wave. The height of the S wave is inversely related to the left atrial pressure. All these findings in mitral and pulmonary vein pulsed-wave Doppler tracings are consistent with the restrictive filling pattern.

With appropriate medical treatment, including diuretics, left atrial pressure decreases and the mitral inflow reverts to the pattern of abnormal relaxation common in the patient's age group. The pattern is characterized by an E < A pattern in the mitral inflow and a prolonged deceleration time of the mitral E wave. In the pulmonary veins, the peak velocity of the S wave now exceeds the peak velocity of the D wave (S > D), reflective of lower left atrial pressures.

Therefore, answer B is correct.

Different mitral and pulmonary vein filling patterns as well as their relationship to mean left atrial pressure is summarized in **Figure 8.73**.

Answer A is incorrect because the preload has decreased from the initial to the subsequent study as judged by the decrease in the mean left atrial pressure.

Answer C is incorrect because the initial filling pattern was not normal; it was restrictive. A normal pattern cannot be distinguished from a pseudonormal pattern by mitral and pulmonary flow patterns alone. Ancillary data such as the peak velocity of the mitral annular tissue Doppler e' prime wave is required to distinguish normal (e' > 8 cm/s) from pseudonormal pattern (e' < 8 cm/s).

Answer D is incorrect because the presence of a prominent and normally timed A wave in mitral inflow and the S wave in the pulmonary vein argue against atrial arrhythmias such as atrial flutter or atrial fibrillation. In these atrial arrhythmias, the peak velocities of the mitral A wave and the pulmonary vein S wave are greatly diminished.

Answer E is incorrect because it is the persistence of the restrictive pattern despite appropriate medical therapy that portends a grave prognosis, the prognosis is grave with a 2-year mortality estimated at 50% in patients with left ventricular ejection fraction of <40%. In this patient, the change from restrictive filling to the abnormal relaxation pattern actually portends a better prognosis.

> **KEY POINTS**
> **Case 4**
> - LA volume index can be calculated using either the area-length method or the biplane method of discs.
> - The magnitude of E wave velocity depends on the preload. Following successful diuresis therapy, E wave Vmax and E/A ratio are expected to decrease compared to pre-diuresis. A failure to decrease E wave Vmax and E/A ratio with diuresis may imply an irreversible restrictive filling pattern (Grade IV diastolic dysfunction), which carries a grave prognosis.

47. **Answer: D.** The three recordings from this patient are consistent with the diagnosis of constrictive pericarditis.

Filling Pattern	Mitral Inflow	Pulmonary Vein	Typical Mean LA Pressure
Abnormal Relaxation	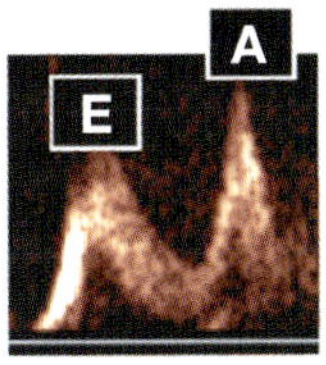	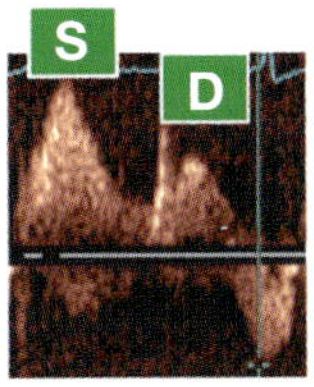	8 – 14 mm Hg
Pseudonormalization	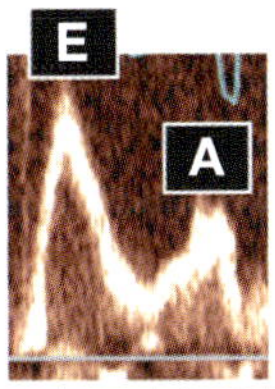	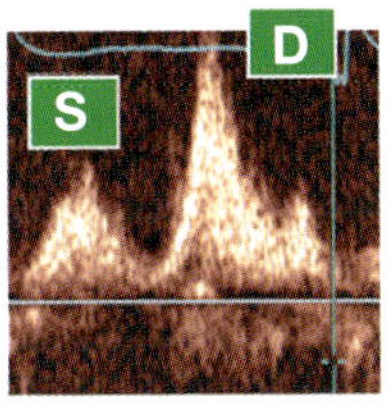	15 – 22 mm Hg
Restrictive Filling	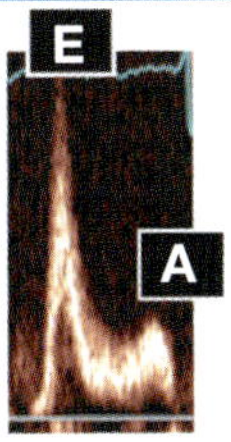	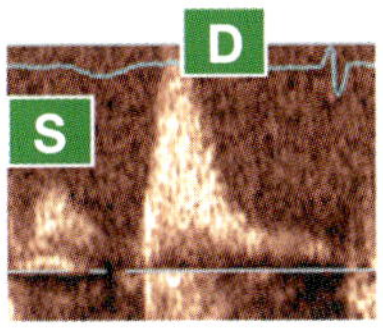	> 22 mm Hg

Figure 8.73

1. MITRAL INFLOW—The mitral inflow spectral Doppler tracings demonstrate marked respiratory variations in the mitral E wave velocities. Such a finding would be consistent with either constrictive pericarditis or tamponade, as well as obesity, labored breathing, asthma, chronic obstructive lung disease, etc. However, in each cardiac cycle, the peak velocity of the mitral E wave is larger than that of the mitral A wave (E > A). This indicates that there is no impediment to early mitral filling which would be consistent with constrictive pericarditis. In contrast, tamponade is characterized by an impediment in early diastolic filling and an E < A.

2. COLOR M-MODE - The flow propagation velocity (Vp) of the early diastolic mitral flow is normal (66 cm/s). Normal Vp values are age-dependent as shown in the data that follows:

	Normal Vp (cm/sec)
Young	>55
Elderly	>45

Vp measures the rate of left ventricular myocardial relaxation. The faster the rate of myocardial relaxation, the higher the Vp. Typically, there is no significant myocardial involvement in constrictive pericarditis, Vp is normal. This is in contrast to restrictive cardiomyopathy which is a myocardial disorder characterized by impaired relaxation and compliance. In restrictive cardiomyopathy, Vp is low.

3. INFERIOR VENA CAVA—In constrictive pericarditis, there is plethora of the inferior vena cava (IVC) as demonstrated by M-mode recordings of the IVC in this patient. The IVC is dilated (2.43 cm in expiration), and collapses less than 50% with inspiration (inspiratory diameter of IVC = 1.97 cm). The finding is indicative of an elevated right atrial pressure (RAP; 15 mm Hg). Such a finding is consistent with the diagnosis with constrictive pericarditis.

However, IVC plethora is also found in other conditions of elevated right atrial pressure such as tricuspid stenosis, severe tricuspid regurgitation, right ventricular infarct, etc.

Therefore, answer D is correct.

Answer A is incorrect because in restrictive cardiomyopathy, there are no marked respiratory variations in the mitral E wave velocities. In addition, Vp is low in restrictive cardiomyopathy.

Answer B is incorrect because the IVC plethora is indicative of an elevated right atrial pressure.

Answer C is incorrect because Vp in this patient is normal (>55 cm/s).

Answer E is incorrect because there is marked respiratory variations (>30%) in the peak velocity of the mitral E wave.

48. **Answer: D.** The patient has constrictive pericarditis. With each inspiration, the filling of the right ventricle increases, and the filling of the left ventricle decreases.

The characteristic movement of the interventricular septum that is phasic with respiration occurs in both tamponade and constrictive pericarditis. The absence of pericardial effusion on the apical 4-chamber view argues against the diagnosis of tamponade.

The abnormal septal motions stated in the remaining four answers are not phasic with respiration. Their characteristics are summarized in **Table 8.10**.

> **KEY POINTS**
> **Case 5**
> - Pericardial constriction may be preceded by effusive-constrictive pericarditis
> - Worldwide, tuberculosis remains the leading cause of effusive-constrictive pericarditis and pericardial constriction
> - Ventricular interdependence is a key finding of pericardial constriction (as well as tamponade).

Table 8.10. Abnormal Interventricular Septal Motions

Right ventricular pressure overload	Interventricular septum flattens in systole and diastole. In the short-axis, left ventricular contour becomes D-shaped rather than circular in both systole and diastole.
Right ventricular volume overload	Interventricular septum flattens in diastole. In the short-axis, left ventricular contour becomes D-shaped rather than circular during diastole.
Left bundle branch block	Interventricular septum moves posteriorly in the pre-ejection period, and then moves anteriorly (away from the posterior left ventricular wall) during ejection phase of systole.
Cardiac surgery	Movement of the interventricular septum toward the right ventricle rather than the left ventricle in systole, with normal thickening.

SUGGESTED READINGS

Baumgartner H, Hung J, Bermejo J, et al. Recommendations on the echocardiographic assessment of aortic valve stenosis: a focused update from the European association of cardiovascular imaging and the American Society of echocardiography. *J Am Soc Echocardiogr.* 2017;30(4):372-392.

Klein AL, Abbara S, Agler DA, et al. American Society of echocardiography clinical recommendations for multimodality cardiovascular imaging of patients with pericardial disease: endorsed by the Society for Cardiovascular Magnetic Resonance and Society of Cardiovascular Computed tomography. *J Am Soc Echocardiogr.* 2013;26(9):965-1012.e15.

Lang RM, Goldstein SA, Kronzon I, et al., eds. *ASE's Comprehensive Echocardiography.* 3rd ed. Elsevier; 2021.

Nagueh SF, Smiseth OA, Appleton CP, et al. Recommendations for the evaluation of left ventricular diastolic function by echocardiography: an update from the American Society of echocardiography and the European association of cardiovascular imaging. *J Am Soc Echocardiogr.* 2016;29(4):277-314.

Otto CM, Nishimura RA, Bonow RO, et al. 2020 ACC/AHA guideline for the management of patients with valvular heart disease: executive summary—a report of the American College of Cardiology/American Heart Association Joint Committee on clinical practice guidelines. *Circulation.* 2021;143(5):e35-e71. Erratum in: *Circulation.* 2021;143(5):e228. Erratum in: *Circulation.* 2021;143(10):e784.

Stout KK, Daniels CJ, Aboulhosn JA, et al. 2018 AHA/ACC guideline for the management of adults with congenital heart disease: a report of the American College of Cardiology/American Heart Association task force on clinical practice guidelines. *Circulation.* 2019;139(14):e698-e800. Erratum in: *Circulation.* 2019;139(14):e833-e834.

Zoghbi WA, Jone PN, Chamsi-Pasha MA et al; American Society of Echocardiography's Guidelines and Standards Committee Task Force on Prosthetic Valves. *J Am Soc Echocardiogr.* 2024;37:2-63.

Zoghbi WA, Adams D, Bonow RO, et al. Recommendations for noninvasive evaluation of native valvular regurgitation: a report from the American Society of Echocardiography developed in collaboration with the society for cardiovascular magnetic resonance. *J Am Soc Echocardiogr.* 2017;30(4):303-371.

CHAPTER 9

Tissue Doppler and Strain

Juan Carlos Plana and Srikanth Koneru

QUESTIONS

1. When compared with standard Doppler, tissue Doppler uses:
   A. The lesser reflectivity of tissue.
   B. The faster motion of tissue.
   C. Filters to exclude highly reflective tissue.
   D. Filters to exclude higher velocities.

2. Strain rate for tissue Doppler is defined as:
   A. Measured tissue velocity × time.
   B. Absolute difference in velocities.
   C. The change in velocity between two points divided by their distance.
   D. It cannot be measured with tissue Doppler.

3. When compared with two-dimensional strain, the biggest disadvantage of tissue Doppler imaging (TDI)–based strain is:
   A. Only strain rate can be calculated, not strain.
   B. Angle dependency.
   C. Susceptibility to tethering.
   D. Low sensitivity to signal noise.

4. If two-dimensional strain imaging is used to evaluate pathologic processes involving the subendocardium, the preferred modality should be:
   A. Radial strain.
   B. Longitudinal strain.
   C. Circumferential strain.
   D. Torsion.

5. Which of the following hemodynamic parameters best correlates with a combination of mitral E-wave velocity and early diastolic longitudinal velocities of the myocardium (e′)?
   A. Superior vena cava pressure.
   B. Right atrial pressure.
   C. Right ventricular systolic pressure.
   D. Mean left atrial pressure.

6. When reporting global longitudinal strain (GLS), it is important to bear in mind the impact of:
   A. Country of origin.
   B. Gender.
   C. Age.
   D. All of the above.

7. Which of the following radial strain rates obtained at the mid-inferior wall during systole of a patient with ischemic cardiomyopathy is consistent with dyskinesis?
   A. 0.
   B. 1.
   C. −1.
   D. 10.

8. In left ventricular (LV) torsion:
   A. During ejection, the basal segments of the LV myocardium rotate counterclockwise.
   B. During ejection, the apical segments rotate counterclockwise.
   C. During diastole, the basal segments of the LV myocardium rotate counterclockwise.
   D. Basal twisting is the main component of LV systolic torsion.

9. Which of the following is a **TRUE** statement about TDI?
   A. It is more preload dependent than traditional Doppler imaging.
   B. A normal velocity and pattern of mitral annular velocities do not always indicate normal diastolic function.
   C. It is unable to discriminate passive motion from active motion.
   D. M-mode color TDI has lower spatial resolution than pulsed TDI.

10. Based on the expert consensus for the multimodality imaging of the adult patient during and after cancer therapy, subclinical LV dysfunction is defined as:
    A. GLS <−16%.
    B. GLS <−18%.
    C. 15% reduction in GLS when compared to reference values from the JUSTICE study.
    D. 15% reduction in GLS when compared to baseline value.

11. In asymmetric septal hypertrophic cardiomyopathy, tissue Doppler e′:
    A. Is abnormal in the lateral wall.
    B. Is normal in the septum.
    C. Has an inverse relationship with septal thickness.
    D. Has a direct relationship with septal thickness.

12. In diabetic patients, which of the following statements is **CORRECT**?
    A. HgbA$_{1C}$ correlates with E/e′.
    B. Diabetic patients have a higher Doppler e′.
    C. Asymptomatic diabetic patients do not demonstrate an abnormal E/e′.
    D. The mechanism for any diastolic dysfunction is thought to be related to concomitant renal dysfunction.

13. The polar map for LV strain pattern shown in **Figure 9.1** is most consistent with:
    A. Cardiac amyloidosis.
    B. Variant of hypertrophic cardiomyopathy.
    C. Cardiac sarcoidosis.
    D. Nonischemic cardiomyopathy.

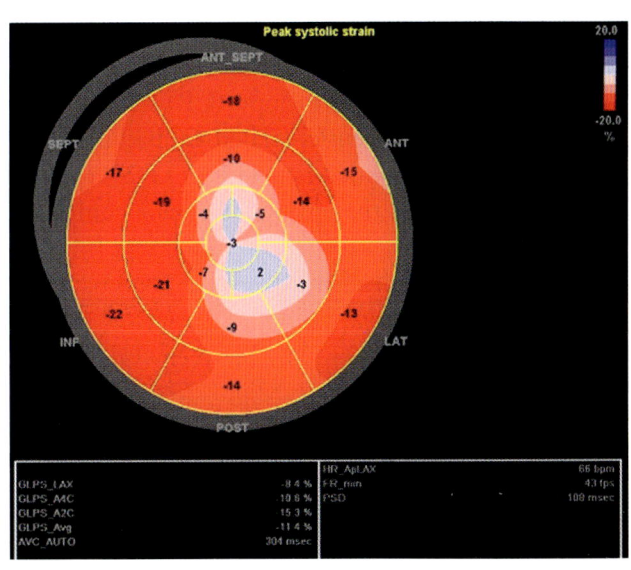

Figure 9.1

14. Which of the following tissue Doppler indices has been shown to carry the most prognostic value after myocardial infarction (MI)?
    A. Mitral E-wave velocity.
    B. Mitral annular e′ velocity.
    C. E/e′ ratio.
    D. Systolic annular velocity.

15. Cardiac function/performance is assessed by various methods, which of the following parameters is independent on changes in loading conditions?
    A. Left ventricular ejection fraction (LVEF).
    B. Global longitudinal strain (GLS).
    C. Myocardial work.
    D. None of the above.

16. Which of the following cardiac conditions is associated with a normal or high e′?
    A. Friedreich ataxia.
    B. Fabry disease.
    C. Hypertrophic cardiomyopathy.
    D. Cardiac amyloidosis.
    E. Myocardial hypertrophy in athletic hearts.

17. Which of the following is observed when initiating cardioprotective therapy (CPT) in patients with cancer therapeutics-related cardiac dysfunction (CTRCD) guided by LVEF or GLS?
    A. LVEF-guided therapy was superior compared to GLS.
    B. GLS-guided therapy was superior compared to LVEF.
    C. No difference in EF between GLS- and EF-guided CPT.
    D. There is no evidence of improving LVEF by initiating CPT.

18. The following clinical conditions have abnormal or reduced left ventricular twist mechanics, **EXCEPT** for:
    A. Heart failure with reduced EF.
    B. Heart failure with preserved EF.
    C. Transplanted hearts.
    D. Constrictive pericarditis.

19. The radial strain map in **Figure 9.2** obtained from a patient with chest pain demonstrates:
    A. Normal LV function.
    B. Segmental dyskinesis.
    C. Anterolateral hypokinesis.
    D. Anteroseptal akinesis.

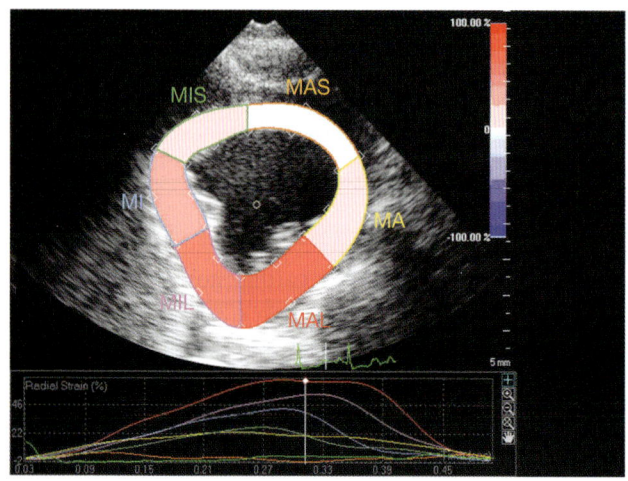

Figure 9.2. MA, mid anterior; . MAL, mid anterolateral; MAS, mid anteroseptal; MI, mid inferior; MIL, mid inferolateral; MIS, mid inferoseptal.

20. The strain rate pattern in **Figure 9.3** is consistent with:
    A. Anteroseptal infarct.
    B. Anterolateral infarct.
    C. Extensive apical infarct.
    D. Normal LV function.

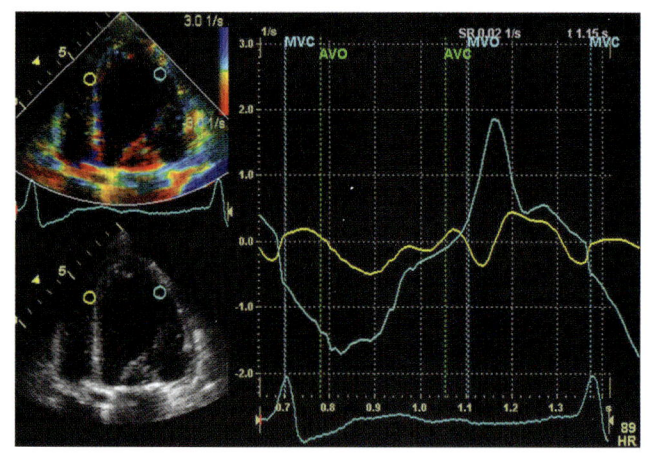

Figure 9.3

21. A 70-year-old woman with ischemic heart disease and chronic obstructive pulmonary disease (COPD) presents for evaluation of dyspnea. What would you recommend on the basis of the echo Doppler findings in **Figure 9.4A,B**?
    A. Evaluation for pulmonary embolism.
    B. Intravenous diuresis and evaluation for ischemia.
    C. Initiation of therapy for COPD exacerbation.
    D. Right heart catheterization.

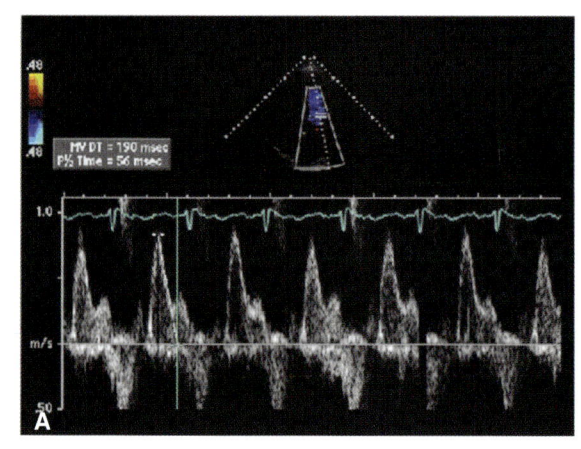

Figure 9.4A

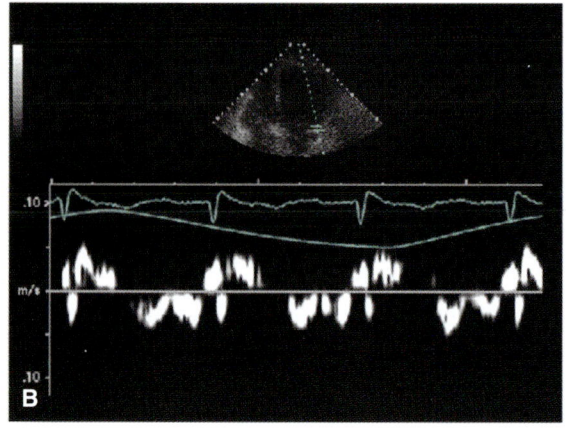

Figure 9.4B

22. Two days after successful medical treatment in the previous case, symptoms of dyspnea have resolved. An echocardiogram is repeated, and the Doppler images are shown in **Figure 9.5A,B**. What can you conclude?

   A. The patient requires more aggressive diuresis.
   B. The patient has abnormal diastolic function.
   C. The patient has a restrictive filling pattern.
   D. The patient requires Doppler pulsed-wave interrogation of the pulmonary veins to assess diastolic function.

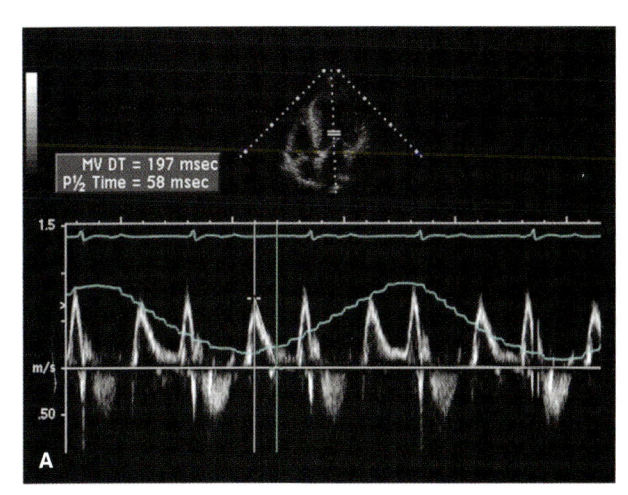

Figure 9.5. **A:** Mitral inflow. **B:** Medial tissue Doppler annular velocities.

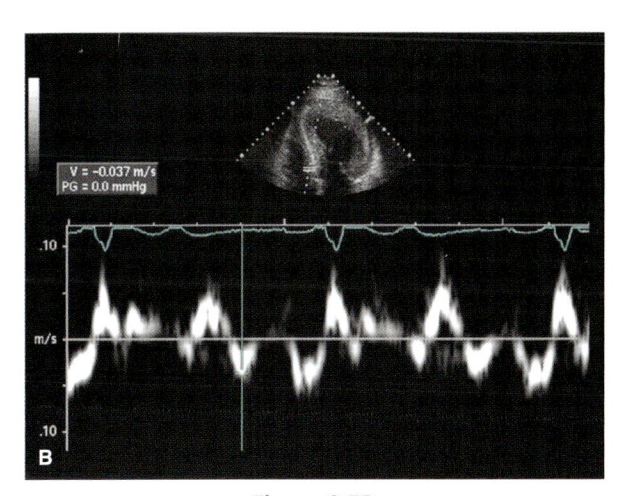

Figure 9.5B

23. A 46-year-old woman with previous history of breast cancer treated with mastectomy, chemotherapy, and radiation therapy presents for evaluation of symptoms of fatigue. On examination, she has a heart rate (HR) of 100 beats/min, BP of 85/60 mm Hg, elevated jugular venous pressure (JVP), decreased breath sounds at the lung bases, ascites, and 3+ peripheral edema. Transesophageal and transthoracic echocardiographic Doppler images are shown in **Figure 9.6A-C**. The most likely diagnosis is:

   A. Hypertrophic cardiomyopathy.
   B. Constrictive pericarditis.
   C. Cardiac amyloidosis.
   D. Restrictive cardiomyopathy post radiation.

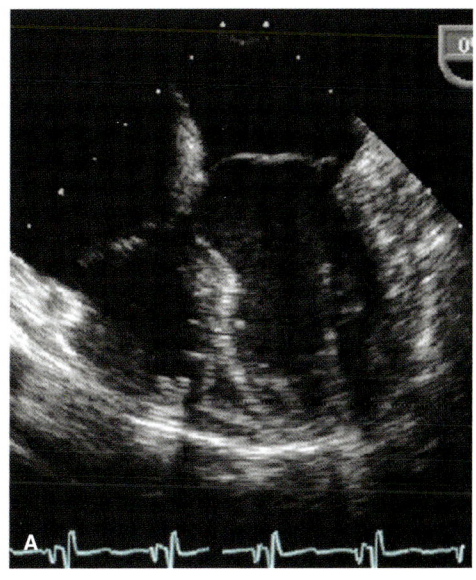

Figure 9.6. **A:** Transesophageal echocardiography mid-esophageal four-chamber view. **B:** Transthoracic echocardiography mitral inflow. **C:** Transthoracic echocardiography medial tissue Doppler annular velocity.

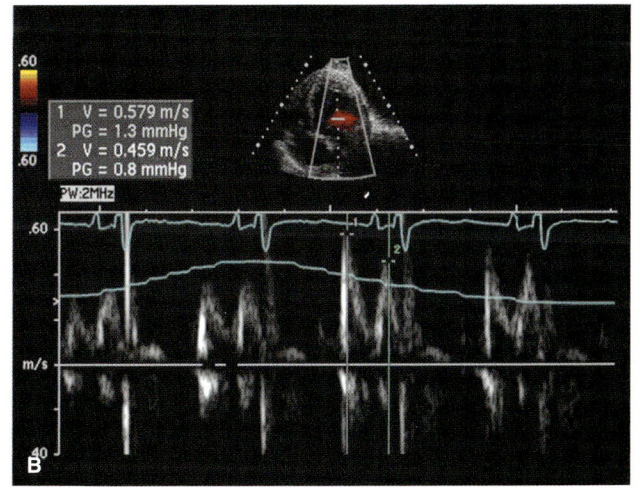

Figure 9.6B

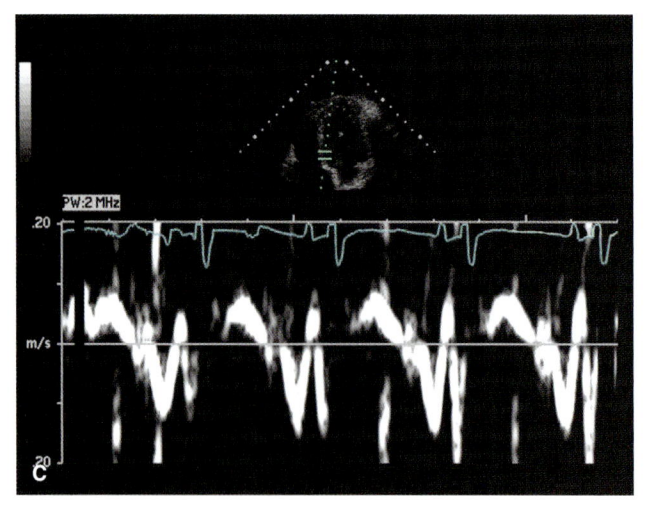

Figure 9.6C

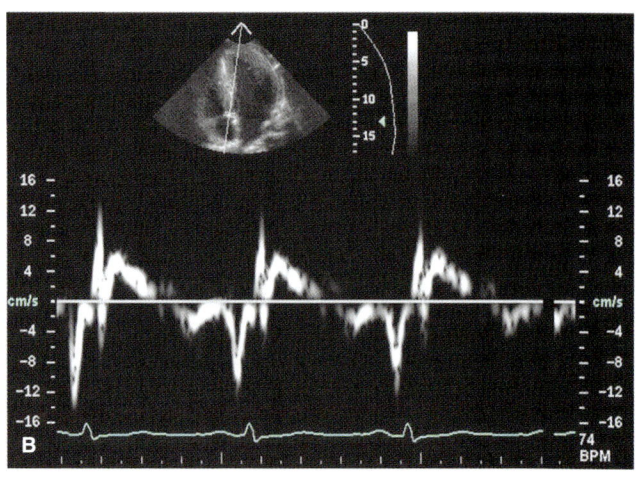

Figure 9.7B

24. In this patient, you would be concerned about the presence of:
   A. Annulus reversus.
   B. Annulus paradoxus.
   C. Annulus reversus and paradoxus.
   D. Increased global circumferential strain (GCS).

25. A 68-year-old woman presents for evaluation of dyspnea on exertion. Tissue Doppler images are shown in **Figure 9.7A,B**. The most likely diagnosis is:
   A. Asymmetric septal hypertrophic cardiomyopathy.
   B. Anterolateral infarction.
   C. Cardiac amyloidosis.
   D. Constrictive pericarditis.

26. A 40-year-old asymptomatic man presents with a diagnosis of severe aortic regurgitation. LVEF is 51%. On the basis of his global longitudinal strain (GLS) (**Figure 9.8**), you would state:
   A. At a GLS worse than approximately −19%, there is a progressive increase in mortality.
   B. LV GLS improves reclassification of risk for longer term mortality.
   C. LV GLS worse than approximately −19%, provides incremental prognostic value.
   D. All of the above statements are correct.

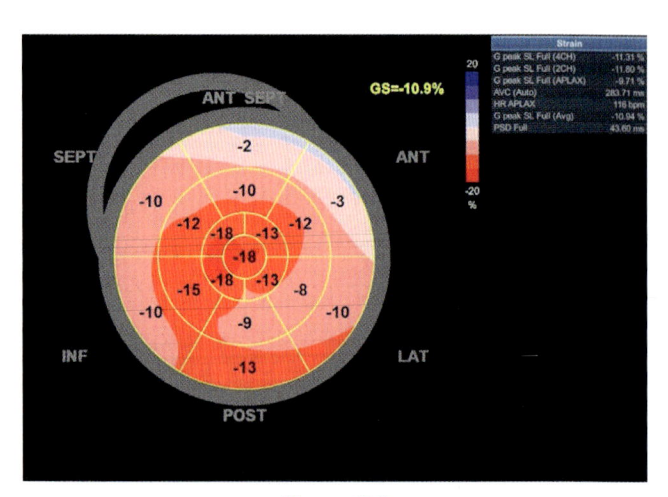

Figure 9.8

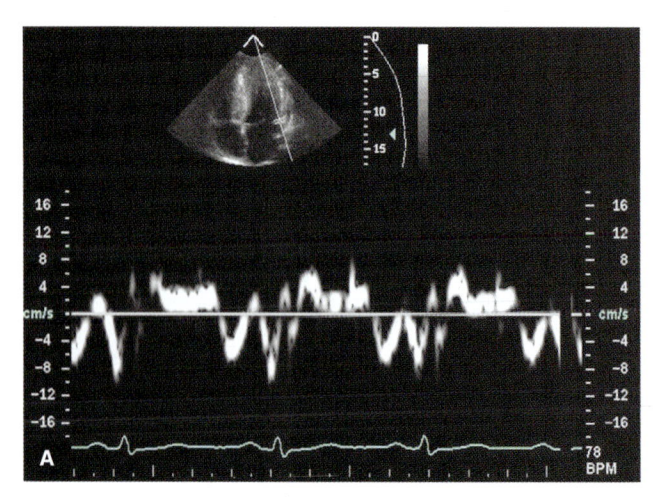

Figure 9.7A

27. A 64-year-old diabetic woman is referred for evaluation of heart failure symptoms. The two-dimensional echocardiographic (**Figure 9.9A**), color tissue Doppler (**Figure 9.9B**) images and strain (**Figure 9.9C**) data obtained from the apical four-chamber view are consistent with:
    A. Dilated cardiomyopathy.
    B. Ischemic heart disease.
    C. Restrictive cardiomyopathy.
    D. Hypertrophic cardiomyopathy.

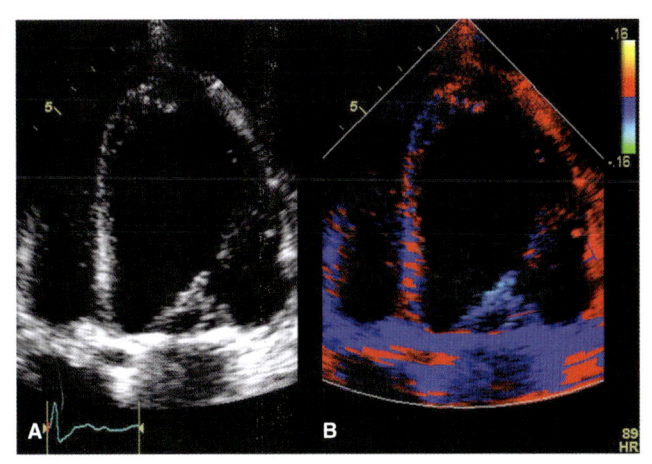

Figure 9.9A, B

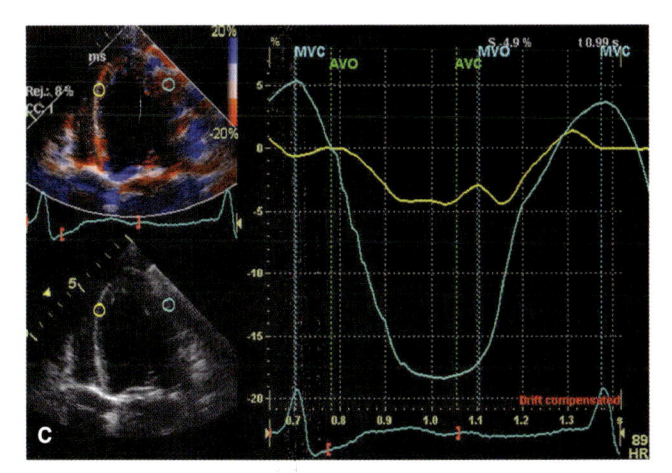

Figure 9.9C

28. A 52-year-old man is sent to you after receiving 550 mg/m^2 of doxorubicin (Adriamycin) for the treatment of a tibial sarcoma. His ultrasensitive troponin I was 20 pg/mL. After reviewing **Figure 9.10**, you would recommend to his oncologist:
    A. To interrupt therapy as there is concern for subclinical LV dysfunction.
    B. To continue therapy as the GLS and the biomarkers are normal.
    C. To repeat the global longitudinal strain (GLS) in 3 weeks and then discuss.
    D. To obtain a cardiac magnetic resonance (CMR) study, as the risk of congestive heart failure is too high, and echocardiography may be unreliable to identify small differences in ejection fraction.

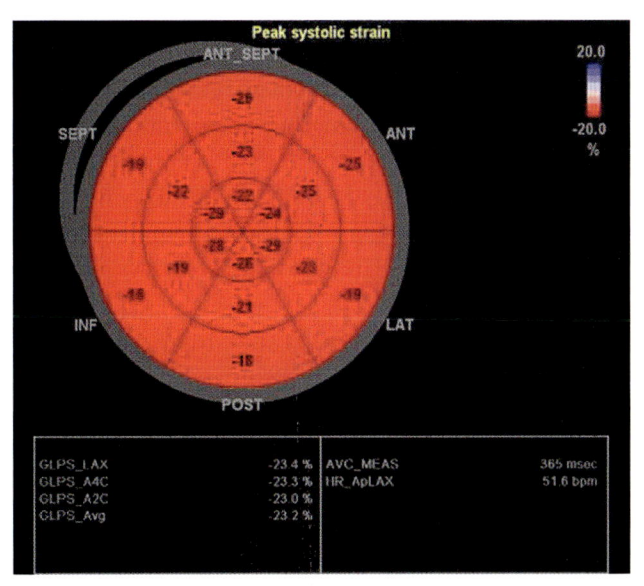

Figure 9.10

29. A 62-year-old man with a history of rheumatic heart disease and previous mitral valve repair undergoes echocardiographic examination for evaluation of a heart murmur. The color M-mode tissue Doppler (**Figure 9.11**) parasternal long-axis images are consistent with:
    A. Anteroseptal MI.
    B. Inferolateral MI.
    C. LV dyssynchrony.
    D. Normal postoperative findings.

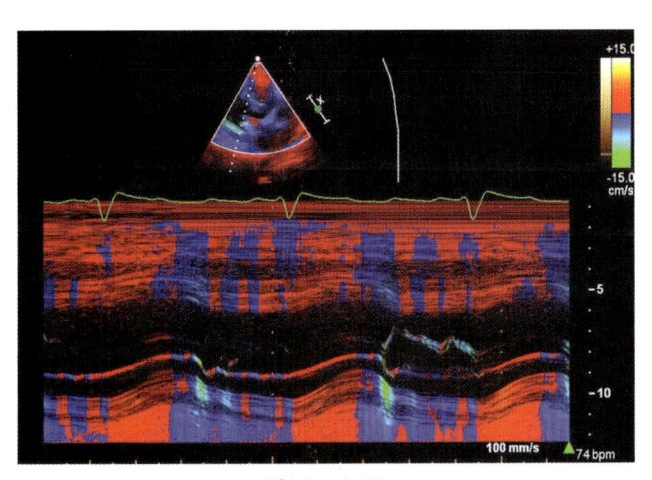

Figure 9.11

30. A 78-year-old woman with a history of congestive heart failure and COPD presents to the emergency department with worsening symptoms of dyspnea. On physical examination, BP is 160/90 mm Hg, HR is 60 beats/min, and respiratory rate (RR) is 28/min. On auscultation, a II/VI ejection systolic murmur is detected at the left upper sternal border (LUSB). Breath sounds have both bibasilar rales and expiratory wheezing. Oxygen saturation is 90%. Blood work demonstrates hemoglobin count = 10 mg/dL, BUN = 50 mg/dL, and serum creatinine level = 2.0 mg/dL. An echocardiogram is obtained immediately at the bedside while the patient has labored breathing. Apical four-chamber images obtained at end diastole (**Figure 9.12A**) and end systole (**Figure 9.12B**) as well as pulsed Doppler LV filling (**Figure 9.12C**) and basal septal tissue Doppler (**Figure 9.12D**) images are shown. In addition to oxygen, you should initially recommend:

A. Intravenous furosemide.
B. Intravenous beta-blockers.
C. Inhaled bronchodilators.
D. Blood transfusion.

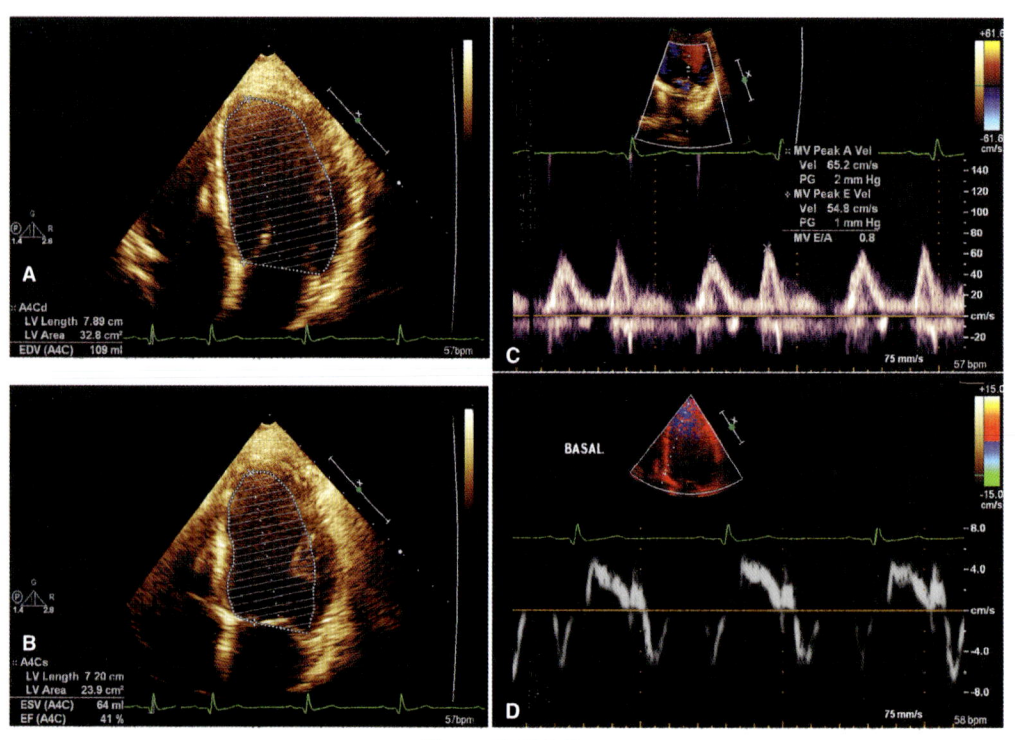

Figure 9.12A-D

ANSWERS

1. **Answer: D.** Standard Doppler measures blood flow velocities using the Doppler effect. The change in frequency between transmitted sound and reflected sound is termed "Doppler shift" and is used to calculate the velocity of the moving red blood cells. When using standard Doppler, filters are used to exclude low-velocity objects, like the myocardium. Conversely, since tissue moves at a slower velocity, Doppler tissue imaging employs filters, which exclude high velocities.
2. **Answer: C.** *Strain rate* (SR) may be derived from the velocity data using the equation: SR = $(V_1 - V_2)/L$, where V_1 = velocity at point 1, V_2 = velocity at point 2, and L = length usually set at 10 mm.
3. **Answer: B.** Doppler tissue imaging–derived strain, like all Doppler techniques, is sensitive to alignment. The instantaneous gradient of velocity, along a sample length, may be quantified by performing a regression calculation between the velocity data from adjacent sites along the scan line, and this instantaneous data may then be combined to generate a SR curve. Integration of this curve provides instantaneous data on deformation (strain). The comparison of adjacent velocities is extremely sensitive to signal noise. TDI is not susceptible to tethering to adjacent tissue, as the myocardial motion is measured relative to the adjacent myocardium and not relative to the transducer.
4. **Answer: B.** Several studies have explored the deformation of the ventricle, describing myocyte arrangements as a continuum of two helical fiber geometries. In the subendocardium, the fibers are roughly longitudinally oriented, with an angle of 80° with respect to the circumferential direction of the fibers located in the mid-aspect of the thickness of the myocardium. As a result, global longitudinal strain (evaluating the longitudinal fibers) should be the modality of choice when evaluating pathology involving the subendocardium. See **Figure 9.13** demonstrating different forms of strain.
5. **Answer: D.** The early diastolic velocity of the longitudinal motion of the myocardium (e′) reflects the rate of myocardial relaxation. Decreased e′ is one of the earliest signs of diastolic dysfunction and is present in all stages of diastolic dysfunction. Because e′ velocity is reduced and mitral E velocity increases with higher filling pressures, the ratio between E and e′ correlates well with LV filling pressures. This combination of early mitral E velocity and early diastolic longitudinal velocities of the myocardium has a linear relationship to the pulmonary capillary wedge pressure or mean left atrial pressure.
6. **Answer: D.** The WASE Normal Values Study is a multicenter international, observational, prospective, cross-sectional study of healthy adult individuals. Participants recruited in each country were evenly distributed among six predetermined subgroups according to age and gender. Two thousand eight subjects were enrolled in 15 countries. Global WASE normal ranges for LV dimensions and volumes were larger in male subjects, while LVEF and GLS were higher in female subjects. Significant intercountry variation was identified for all LV parameters reflecting LV size (dimensions, mass, and volumes) even after indexing to body surface area, with LV end-diastolic and end-systolic volumes having the highest variation. The largest volumes were noted in Australia, while the smallest were measured in India for both genders. This finding suggests that in addition to gender and body surface area, specific country should be considered when evaluating LV volumes. Intercountry variation for LVEF and GLS was smaller but still statistically significant ($P < .05$ for all).
7. **Answer: C.** Strain rate (SR) imaging simultaneously measures the velocities in two adjacent points as well as the relative distance between these two points. Expressed as SR = $(V_1 - V_2)/L$. Positive radial

ε_r : Radial strain
ε_c : Circumferential strain
ε_l : Longitudinal strain
ε_t : Torsional strain

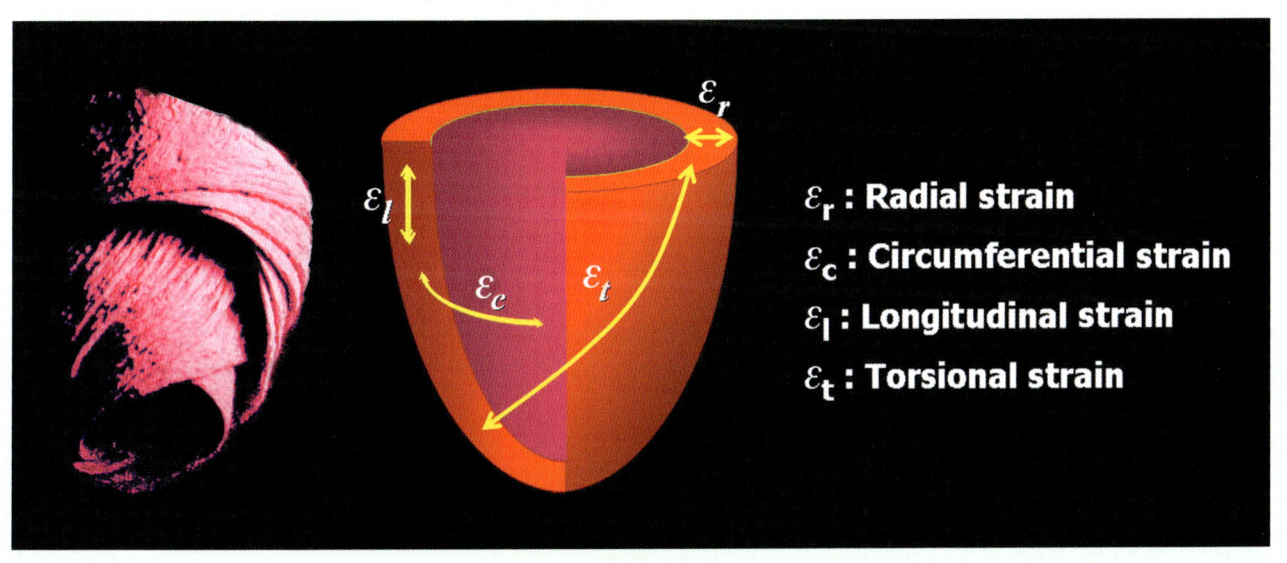

Figure 9.13

SR represents active contraction. Negative values for radial strain represent either relaxation (if measured during diastole) or dyskinesis (if measured during systole).

8. **Answer: B.** The LV myocardium has a spiral architecture with myocardial fibers that vary in orientation depending on where in the myocardium they are located. Fiber direction is predominantly longitudinal in the endocardial region, transitioning into a circumferential direction in the mid wall and becoming longitudinal again over the epicardial surface. In addition to radial and longitudinal deformation, there is torsional deformation of the LV during the cardiac cycle due to the helical orientation of the myocardial fibers. During isovolumic contraction (phase 1), the apex shows a brief clockwise rotation and the base a short counterclockwise rotation. During ejection (phase 2), the direction of the rotation changes to counterclockwise at the LV apex and clockwise at the LV base, respectively (**Table 9.1**).

9. **Answer: C.** Standard Doppler measurement of mitral inflow velocities can be used to assess diastolic function by measuring the early rapid filling wave (E) and the late filling wave due to atrial contraction (A). The velocities and ratios of E/A are used to determine diastolic function, but as they are reflective of the pressure gradient between the left atrium and the left ventricle, they are directly related to preload and inversely related to ventricular relaxation. Doppler tissue myocardial diastolic velocities are less load dependent. In adults, an early diastolic longitudinal (e′) velocity of the lateral aspect of the mitral valve annulus >0.10 m/s is associated with normal LV diastolic function. TDI measures only vector motion that is parallel to the ultrasound beam and is not able to differentiate between active motion (like myocardial contraction) and passive motion (like tethering). M-mode color TDI is acquired by color-coding images of tissue motion during an M-mode image acquisition. Different colors specify direction of motion and allow images to have both high temporal and spatial resolution.

10. **Answer: D.** In a systematic review and meta-analysis of 21 prognostic studies, worse absolute GLS during chemotherapy and a greater relative deterioration compared with baseline were associated with a higher risk of CTRCD (Oikonomou EK et al). Currently, a relative GLS decrease of >15% compared with baseline is the recommended threshold as it reflects the 95% upper limit in the meta-analysis of GLS to predict future significant LVEF reduction. Using the 15% threshold will maximize specificity and minimize overdiagnosis of CTRCD and guide cardioprotective therapy (2022 ESC Guidelines on cardio-oncology) (**Figure 9.14**).

Table 9.1. Definitions and Parameters Used to Assess LV Twist Mechanics

Parameters	Definition
Systolic	
Apical rotation (°)	Peak counterclockwise systolic rotation of the LV apical short-axis cross section as viewed from the apex
Basal rotation (°)	Peak clockwise systolic rotation of the LV basal short-axis cross section level as viewed from the apex
LV twist (°)	Peak difference in systolic rotations of LV apex and base as viewed from the apex
LV torsion (°/cm)	Normalized twist: Twist angle divided by the distance between the measured locations of base and apex
LV twist rate (°/s)	Peak velocity of LVT
Diastolic	
Apical reverse rotation (°)	Peak clockwise diastolic reverse rotation of the LV apical short-axis cross section as viewed from the apex
Basal reverse rotation (°)	Peak counterclockwise diastolic reverse rotation of the LV basal short-axis cross section as viewed from the apex
LV untwist (°)	Difference in diastolic reverse rotations of LV apex and base as viewed from the apex, measured as percentage of untwist from aortic valve closure to mitral valve opening (% UT in IVR)
Untwist rate (°/s)	Peak velocity of UT

IVR, isovolumic relaxation; LV, left ventricle; LVT, LV twist; and UT, untwist.
Reprinted with permission from Omar AM, Vallabhajosyula S, Sengupta PP. Left ventricular twist and torsion: research observations and clinical applications. *Circ Cardiovasc Imaging*. 2015;8(6):e003029. Table 1. Copyright © 2015 American Heart Association, Inc.

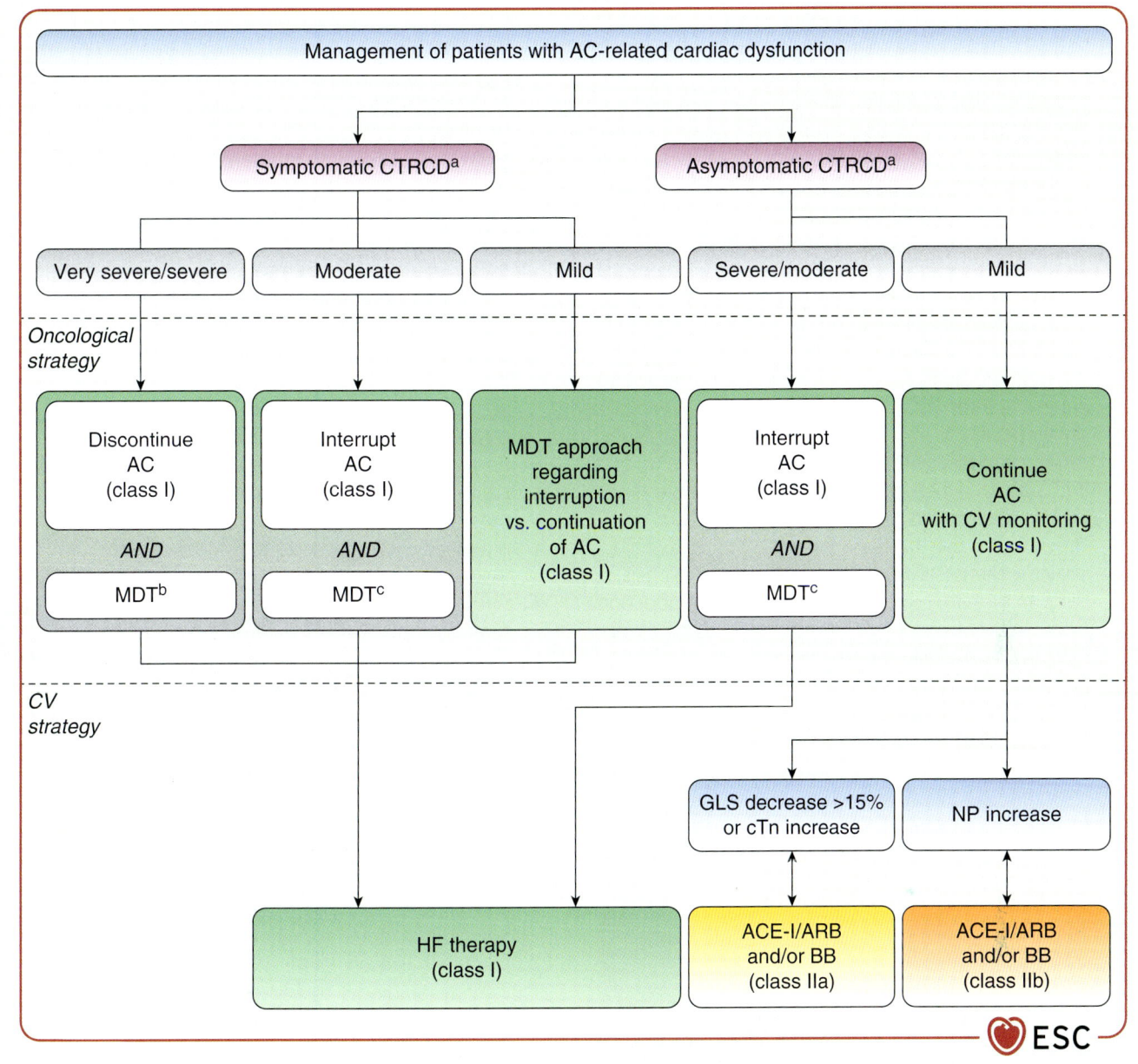

Figure 9.14. Management of anthracycline chemotherapy–related cardiac dysfunction. AC, anthracycline chemotherapy; ACE-I, angiotensin-converting enzyme inhibitors; ARB, angiotensin receptor blockers; BB, beta-blockers; cTn, cardiac troponin; CTRCD, cancer therapy–related cardiac dysfunction; CV, cardiovascular; GLS, global longitudinal strain; HF, heart failure; MDT, multidisciplinary team; NP, natriuretic peptides. [a]Symptomatic CTRCD: symptomatic confirmed HF syndrome; asymptomatic severe CTRCD: LVEF 50%. [b]In rare exceptions, anthracycline chemotherapy may be restarted after recovery of LV function with optimal HF therapy. [c]An MDT discussion is recommended before restarting anthracycline chemotherapy after recovery of LV function. (From Lyon AR, López-Fernández T, Couch LS, et al. 2022 ESC Guidelines on cardio-oncology developed in collaboration with the European Hematology Association (EHA), the European Society for Therapeutic Radiology and Oncology (ESTRO) and the International Cardio-Oncology Society (IC-OS). *Eur Heart J*. 2022;43(41):4229-4361. Reproduced by permission of The European Society of Cardiology.)

11. **Answer: C.** Tissue Doppler can also identify abnormal regional function in areas of localized hypertrophy. In fact, it appears that the greater the extent of segmental wall thickness, the greater is the reduction in myocardial velocities. These abnormalities can often be found in asymptomatic carriers of hypertrophic cardiomyopathy genetic mutations, even in the absence of phenotypic expression.

12. **Answer: A.** Glycemic control in diabetic patients has been associated with microvascular complications. Microvascular disease may lead to ischemia and subsequent impaired LV relaxation and increased myocardial stiffness. Advanced glycation end products have been associated with microvascular complications of type 1 diabetes mellitus and may be a pathophysiologic mechanism for diastolic

dysfunction in these patients. Type 1 diabetic patients have worse diastolic function with lower tissue Doppler e'. Furthermore, HgbA$_{1c}$ is correlated with E/e'. These results demonstrate that asymptomatic diastolic dysfunction is common in patients with type 1 diabetes mellitus and that its severity is correlated with glycemic control. Furthermore, asymptomatic diabetic patients have increased LV filling pressure as measured by E/e' and a larger left atrial size.

13. **Answer: B.** The pattern of segmental LV strain seen on polar map is typical for apical variant hypertrophic cardiomyopathy, which correlated with myocardial disarray and apically predominant scar pattern. This pattern is often referred to as "blueberry-on-top". A similar pattern is also seen in patients with takotsubo cardiomyopathy with hypokinesis of apical segments and normal/hyperkinetic basal to midsegments. In cardiac amyloidosis, an apical sparing pattern of LV strain (bull's eye pattern) is seen with reduced LV strain in the basal to midsegments. In sarcoidosis, a pattern of patchy nonspecific segmental reduction in LV strain is observed. Non-ischemic cardiomyopathy has a globally reduced LV strain pattern with no significant segmental variation, on contrary to ischemic heart disease showing an LV strain pattern corresponding to coronary arterial territory involved (see **Figure 9.15** and ▶ **Video 9.1**).

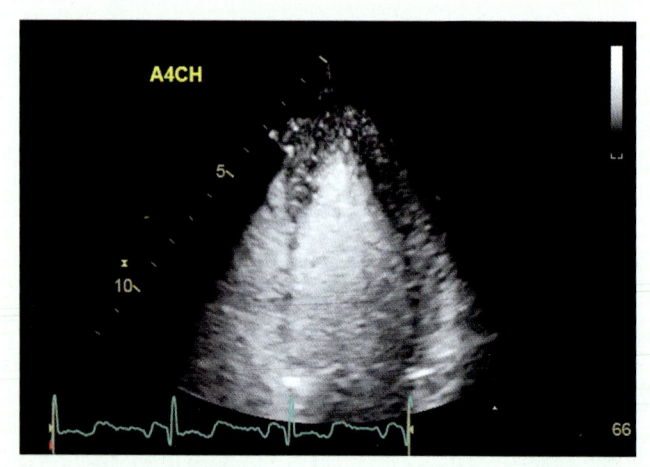

Figure 9.15. Apical four-chamber view with contrast showing apical hypertrophic cardiomyopathy.

14. **Answer: C.** After an MI, E/e' has been shown to be associated with an increased risk of death or need for heart transplantation. Patients with an E/e' ratio >17 had a mortality rate of approximately 40% at 36 months compared with 5% in those with an E/e' ratio <17. In a study that included 250 nonselected patients who had an echocardiogram 1.6 days after an MI followed up for a median of 13 months, the most powerful predictor of survival was an E/e' ratio >15. E/e' was a stronger predictor than other Doppler echocardiographic indices, including the LV filling pulsed Doppler deceleration time. Increased E/e' has also correlated with increased LV end-diastolic volume post-MI and has been attributed to a relationship to LV remodeling and progressive LV dilation.

15. **Answer: C.** LVEF has inherent limitations and load dependency, which compromise its reliability and usefulness as a comprehensive assessment of cardiac function. Two-dimensional (2D) global longitudinal strain (GLS) has been shown to detect early deterioration in myocardial function. Although GLS exhibits lower load dependency compared with LVEF, it is still vulnerable to changes in load. Pressure-strain loop (PSL) analysis is an innovative echocardiographic method used to quantify myocardial work (MW), which involves the combination of information derived from speckle tracking strain imaging and noninvasive estimate of the LV pressure (LVP). By incorporating the LV loading condition, PSL analysis offers a superior approach for assessing myocardial performance.

16. **Answer: E.** Tissue Doppler velocities may help differentiate myocardial hypertrophy seen in athletes from hypertrophic cardiomyopathy, where these velocities are abnormally decreased. Similar findings have been reported in Fabry disease, a cardiomyopathy secondary to α-galactosidase A deficiency. Patients with mutation-positive Fabry disease have significant reduction of e' and higher E/e' compared with normal control subjects, even before the development of LV hypertrophy. Tissue Doppler has been used to study myocardial performance in patients with Friedreich ataxia. Asymptomatic patients who are homozygous for the GAA expansion in the Friedreich ataxia gene have reduced myocardial velocity gradients during systole and in early diastole. Patients with a restrictive cardiomyopathy from an infiltrative disease process like cardiac amyloidosis will have impaired relaxation and therefore reduced e' velocities.

17. **Answer: C.** Cardio protection using strain-guided management of potentially cardiotoxic cancer therapy (SUCCOUR trial) is an international multicenter prospective randomized controlled trial, initiating CPT either by GLS-guided (>12% relative reduction) or EF-guided (>10% absolute reduction of EF < 55%) therapy. Patients were followed up by serial LVEF from baseline to 3 years, preferentially measured using 3D EF. Among patients taking potentially cardiotoxic chemotherapy for cancer, the 3-year data showed improvement of LV dysfunction compared with 1 year, with no difference in EF between GLS- and EF-guided CPT.

18. **Answer: B.** The presence of macroscopic structural abnormalities, from longstanding cardiovascular risk factors, can lead to LV dysfunction at the subendocardial level and the resultant subendocardial

dysfunction will reduce LV mechanics in the longitudinal direction; however, the LV twist remains preserved or even increased because of unopposed contraction of subepicardial fibers. This increased LV twist might serve as compensatory mechanism to preserve LV systolic function. However, the reduction in LVEF in association with LV twist signifies more advanced stage of myocardial dysfunction (**Table 9.2**). On the contrary, in patients with constrictive pericarditis, there is marked epicardial dysfunction leading to impairment of circumferential shortening and twist mechanics, whereas the subendocardial longitudinal mechanics are relatively spared. Finally, in patients with heart transplant, there is baseline reduced LV twist mechanics, which worsens with evidence of rejection (**Table 9.2**).

Table 9.2. Comparison of Myocardial Mechanics in HFPEF and HFREF

	HFPEF	HFREF
Longitudinal strain	Markedly decreased	Markedly decreased
Circumferential strain	Preserved/mild decrease	Markedly decreased
Radial strain	Preserved/mild decrease	Markedly decreased
Twist	Preserved	Markedly decreased
Untwist	Delayed/may decrease	Delayed and decreased
Global EF	Preserved	Markedly decreased

EF, ejection fraction; HFPEF, heart failure patients with preserved ejection fraction; and HFREF, heart failure patients with reduced ejection fraction.
Reprinted with permission from Omar AM, Vallabhajosyula S, Sengupta PP. Left ventricular twist and torsion: research observations and clinical applications. *Circ Cardiovasc Imaging*. *Circ Cardiovasc Imaging*. 2015;8(6):e003029. Table 3. Copyright © 2015 American Heart Association, Inc.

19. **Answer: D.** As the ventricle contracts, muscle fibers shorten in the longitudinal and circumferential directions and thicken or lengthen in the radial direction. Strain represents the change in segment length throughout a cardiac cycle. Strain rate or strain velocity is the local rate of myocardial deformation and can be derived from TDI velocities. TDI-derived strain rate is a strong index of LV contractility. In **Figure 9.2**, a parasternal short-axis image of the mid-left ventricle is shown. The myocardium has been color coded by segment and by its percent strain value with a scale of 100% (red) and −100% (blue). The time plot at the bottom of the imaging graphs the percent radial strain of each color-coded segment. The color of the plot corresponds to the outlined color of the segment selected. **Figure 9.2** shows that the best motion is seen in the mid-anterolateral wall, which has the darkest red coloring and is also plotted on the graph as the red line with a marked positive percent strain during systole. The mid-anteroseptal wall, colored white and outlined in orange, shows akinesis based upon the white color coding and the flat plot of the orange curve. Radial strain can provide quantitative data to assist in the interpretation of segmental wall motion and can be of particular use in the interpretation of stress echocardiograms.

20. **Answer: A. Figure 9.3** shows strain rate imaging with regions of interest selected in the septum (yellow circle and corresponding plot) and lateral wall (blue circle and corresponding plot) in the apical four-chamber views (AVC, aortic valve closure; AVO, aortic valve opening; MVC, mitral valve closure; MVO, mitral valve opening). A strain rate of zero indicates akinesis. A strain rate of >0 indicates expansion, and a strain rate of <0 indicates compression. The strain rate of the selected area of the septum (yellow) shows that it maintains a strain rate of approximately zero throughout systole and diastole. This finding is consistent with akinesis and scar formation. The strain rate of the selected area of the lateral wall (blue), however, demonstrates a negative strain rate in systole (from MVC to AVC), signifying appropriate myocardial compression, and a positive strain rate in diastole (from AVC to MVC), signifying appropriate myocardial expansion.

21. **Answer: B.** The common clinical presentation of dyspnea in an elderly patient with a history of heart disease with concurrent pulmonary pathology is a diagnostic dilemma that can be greatly clarified with echo tissue Doppler use. Specifically, Doppler and TDI can provide information regarding LV preload and relaxation. This information, in conjunction with standard information about biventricular size and function as well as assessment of right ventricular systolic pressure, can provide a wealth of actionable information. **Figure 9.4A** shows an elevated E wave and elevated E/A ratio of 3 from standard Doppler interrogation of mitral inflow. **Figure 9.4B** shows decreased TDI velocities obtained from the lateral mitral annulus. The E/e′ ratio in this example is 18. E/e′ ratios of >14 have been correlated with pulmonary capillary pressures greater than 18 to 20 mm Hg. An elevated E/e′ ratio has also been related to poor prognosis in both ischemic and nonischemic LV dysfunction.

22. **Answer: B.** Compared with the prior images, the mitral inflow E wave shows a markedly reduced velocity in early diastole after the patient was

successfully treated with intravenous diuretics. This finding, in combination with symptomatic improvement, indicates that her mean left atrial pressure or preload has been reduced. This is further confirmed by a reduction in the E/e' ratio. Despite normal preload conditions after diuresis, both the early to late diastolic filling waves in the standard Doppler, as well as the tissue Doppler findings, suggest that the patient has underlying diastolic dysfunction. As the deceleration time is >160 ms, this pattern is not consistent with a restrictive filling pattern. Although pulmonary venous filling patterns may give additional information about LV filling patterns, the current information about mitral inflow velocity and tissue Doppler allows for the diagnosis of diastolic function.

23. **Answer: B.** Diastolic dysfunction in constrictive pericarditis results from increased pericardial constraint on the LV that is related to the thickness and rigidity of the pericardium. Patients present with signs and symptoms of right-sided heart failure, which are similar to those found in restrictive cardiomyopathy. Two-dimensional echocardiography may not demonstrate increased pericardial thickness and the typical interventricular septal bounce. Right and left ventricular Doppler filling patterns may demonstrate respiratory variability. However, these findings are not always present and are not specific. Acute respiratory illnesses can increase intrathoracic pressure swings, and respiratory flow variability may also increase. Excessive preload may attenuate the effect of intrathoracic pressure swings and decrease respiratory variability, whereas low preload can decrease the constraining effect of the pericardium also masking the characteristic Doppler signs of constriction. Tissue Doppler myocardial velocities are useful in differentiating restrictive cardiomyopathy from constrictive pericarditis. In restrictive cardiomyopathy patients, both relaxation and stiffness are abnormal. On the contrary, relaxation is preserved in pure constrictive pericarditis, in the absence of other myocardial disease. Patients with constrictive pericarditis and normal systolic function have normal or elevated e' velocities (>8 cm/s), reflecting their preserved ventricular relaxation. In this example, the mitral inflow demonstrates some respiratory variation, and its morphology is suggestive of a restrictive filling pattern; however, Doppler tissue at the mitral annulus demonstrates preservation of relaxation, making a cardiomyopathy such as cardiac amyloidosis and hypertrophic cardiomyopathy unlikely. The E/e' ratio is approximately 4, which does not correspond to an elevated left ventricular end-diastolic pressure.

24. **Answer: C.** The concept of annulus paradoxus was introduced in 2001. Paradoxical to the positive correlation between E/e' and pulmonary capillary wedge pressure (PCWP) in patients with myocardial disease, an inverse relationship in patients with constrictive pericarditis was found. Subsequently, the use of mitral "annulus reversus" to diagnose constrictive pericarditis was also introduced. In patients with constrictive pericarditis, the average lateral e' velocity is 2% lower than the medial e' velocity, while in controls, the lateral e' velocity was 25% higher than the medial e' velocity. After pericardiectomy, all annular velocities decreased significantly. The reduction in medial e' velocity was greater than that of mitral lateral e' velocity, and the mitral lateral/medial e' ratio normalized.

25. **Answer: A. Figure 9.7** shows tissue Doppler in the lateral wall and in the septal wall. The key finding is reduction in e' velocity that is much more pronounced in the septum consistent with hypertrophic cardiomyopathy. The most common form of hypertrophic cardiomyopathy is characterized by a prominent increase in global or segmental LV wall thickness and histologically by myocardial fiber disarray. Diastolic function is characterized by increased LV chamber stiffness and decreased relaxation of variable severity due to the asynchronous deactivation of the muscle fibers. This asynchronous deactivation is manifested in Doppler tissue as a decreased velocity seen in hypertrophic segments (septum in this example) in early diastole when compared with segments that do not demonstrate hypertrophy (lateral wall in this example).

26. **Answer: D. Figure 9.8** shows an abnormal GLS of −10.9%. The study by Alashi et al concludes that in asymptomatic patients with ≥3+ chronic aortic regurgitation and preserved LVEF, worsening LV GLS was associated with longer term mortality, providing incremental prognostic value and improved reclassification.

27. **Answer: B.** The two-dimensional image in **Figure 9.9** demonstrates a dilated LV cavity, consistent with either dilated or ischemic cardiomyopathy. The tissue Doppler image shows a different color velocity pattern in the septum and the lateral wall, and strain imaging shows reduced deformation in the apical septum (yellow curve) compared with the apical lateral wall (red curve); these findings are consistent with a septal MI.

28. **Answer: B. Figure 9.10** shows the bull's eye plot reporting a normal GLS for vendor, gender, and age of this patient. The ultrasensitive troponin I is also normal (<30 pg/mL). Using the data from Sawaya et al., a GLS < 19% or troponin I > 30 pg/mL predicted subsequent cardiotoxicity. As such, it would be appropriate to reassure the referring oncologist and to have them continue with the prescribed treatment.

29. Answer: D. The color M-mode tissue Doppler in **Figure 9.11** indicates paradoxical anterior systolic motion of the interventricular septum, a common finding after pericardiotomy. The red coloration of the septum shows movement toward the transducer, paradoxical to normal motion.

30. Answer: C. In this patient, the E/e' ratio is 8, the E/A ratio is 0.9, and the E deceleration time is normal. All findings are consistent with normal LV filling pressures. Therefore, the most likely cause of the patient's symptoms is decompensated COPD.

SUGGESTED READINGS

Alashi A, Mentias A, Abdalla A et al. Incremental prognostic utility of left ventricular global longitudinal strain in asymptomatic patients with significant chronic aortic regurgitation and preserved left ventricular ejection fraction. *JACC Cardiovasc Imaging*. 2018;11:673-682.

Ha JW, Oh JK, Ling LH, et al. Annulus paradoxus: transmitral flow velocity to mitral annular velocity is inversely proportional to pulmonary capillary wedge pressure in patients with constrictive pericarditis. *Circulation*. 2001;104:976-978.

Lyon AR, López-Fernández T, Couch LS, et al. 2022 ESC Guidelines on cardio-oncology developed in collaboration with the European Hematology association (EHA), the European Society for Therapeutic Radiology and Oncology (ESTRO) and the International Cardio-Oncology Society (IC-OS). *Eur Heart J Cardiovasc Imaging*. 2022;23(10):e333-e465. Erratum in: *Eur Heart J Cardiovasc Imaging*. 2023;24(6):e98.

Marwick TH, Abraham TP. *American Society of Echocardiography Comprehensive Strain Imaging*, 1st ed. Elsevier; 2021.

Negishi K, Negishi T, Hare JL, et al. Independent and incremental value of deformation indices for the prediction of trastuzumab-induced cardiotoxicity. *J Am Soc Echocardiogr*. 2013;26:493-498.

Oikonomou EK, Kokkinidis DG, Kampaktsis PN, et al. Assessment of prognostic value of left ventricular global longitudinal strain for early prediction of chemotherapy-induced cardiotoxicity: a systematic review and meta-analysis. *JAMA Cardiol*. 2019;4(10):1007-1018.

Omar AM, Vallabhajosyula S, Sengupta PP. Left ventricular twist and torsion: research observations and clinical applications. *Circ Cardiovasc Imaging*. 2015;8(6):e003029. Erratum in: *Circ Cardiovasc Imaging*. 2015;8(8).

Sengupta PP, Tajik AJ, Chandrasekaran K, et al. Twist mechanics of the left ventricle: principles and application. *JACC Cardiovasc Imaging*. 2008;1:366-376.

CHAPTER 10

Contrast-Enhanced Ultrasound Imaging

Thomas R. Porter and Feng Xie

QUESTIONS

1. Which of the following conditions are contraindications to ultrasound enhancing agent (UEA) use?
   A. Intracardiac shunts.
   B. Pulmonary hypertension.
   C. Severe aortic stenosis.
   D. Allergy to perflutren.

2. Which FDA-approved UEA contains the lowest molecular weight gas?
   A. Lumason.
   B. Optison.
   C. Sonazoid.
   D. Definity.

3. The very-low–mechanical index fundamental frequency nonlinear imaging techniques available on most ultrasound systems have been shown to improve all of the following aspects of enhancing imaging **EXCEPT**:
   A. Myocardial perfusion imaging.
   B. Endocardial border resolution.
   C. Basal segment delincation.
   D. Spatial resolution.

4. A 69-year-old obese man is getting an echocardiogram because of shortness of breath and hypotension. An ultrasound enhancing bolus injection is given. You are using a 1.7 MHz harmonic transducer at a 0.3 mechanical index. You see acoustic shadowing from the mid-left ventricular cavity preventing delineation of the basal myocardial segments. All of the following can be utilized to improve basal segment delineation **EXCEPT**:
   A. Further reduce the mechanical index to <0.2.
   B. Switch to a 1.8 MHz fundamental nonlinear imaging modality.
   C. Give a brief high–mechanical index impulse and return to 0.3 mechanical index.
   D. Waiting 10 seconds.

5. You are asked to define the mechanical index to a group of cardiology fellows. **TRUE** statements about the mechanical index are all of the following **EXCEPT**:
   A. Higher values of the mechanical index indicate higher potential for cavitation.
   B. It is inversely proportional to the transmit frequency.
   C. It is directly proportional to the peak negative pressure.
   D. It is directly proportional to transmit gain.

6. Clinical trials of myocardial perfusion imaging with ultrasound enhancing agents during stress echocardiography have demonstrated all of the following **EXCEPT**:
   A. Improved sensitivity of myocardial contrast echo over radionuclide imaging to detect angiographically significant coronary artery disease.
   B. Reduced specificity of myocardial contrast echo over radionuclide imaging to detect angiographically significant coronary artery disease.
   C. Improved sensitivity of perfusion imaging over wall motion analysis in detecting coronary artery disease during dobutamine stress echocardiography.
   D. No difference between wall motion analysis alone versus wall motion analysis with myocardial perfusion in predicting patient outcome following stress echocardiography.

7. Myocardial perfusion imaging with contrast echocardiography using real-time techniques has not been shown clinically useful in predicting the outcomes of patients in which of the following clinical scenarios?
   A. Dobutamine stress echocardiography.
   B. Dipyridamole stress echocardiography.
   C. Emergency room chest pain evaluation.
   D. Post-myocardial infarction echocardiography.
   E. Stress cardiomyopathy.

8. A 74-year-old man with a history of hyperlipidemia and hypertension undergoes a dobutamine stress echocardiogram with a continuous infusion of an ultrasound enhancing agent to evaluate both myocardial perfusion and wall motion. At 20 u/kg/min dobutamine infusion rate at a heart rate of 90 bpm, a delay in contrast replenishment following a high–mechanical index impulse is observed in the mid anteroseptal, distal septal, and apical segments. Basal segment replenishment appeared normal. Wall thickening remained normal in all segments. The most likely explanation for these findings is:
   A. True positive findings for left anterior descending ischemia.
   B. False positive findings because wall thickening is still normal.
   C. These are attenuation artifacts.
   D. Wall thickening will remain normal even at >85% predicted maximum heart rate.

9. One of the impediments to using ultrasound contrast has been obtaining intravenous access. Which statement is **TRUE** regarding qualifications for starting an intravenous (IV) line?
   A. It should only be performed by certified phlebotomy technicians.
   B. It requires a nurse in all US hospitals.
   C. It is not routinely required for other imaging techniques such as radionuclide or magnetic resonance imaging.
   D. It can be performed by sonographers.

10. Which of the following is **NOT** an advantage of a continuous infusion of ultrasound contrast when compared to a bolus injection?
    A. Improved left ventricular opacification.
    B. Reduced left ventricular cavity acoustic shadowing.
    C. It allows quantification of myocardial perfusion.
    D. Reduced far-field attenuation.

11. Studies examining the risk versus benefit of ultrasound enhancing agents in acute critical care settings have demonstrated:
    A. Using IV ultrasound enhancing agents is associated with a slight increase in all-cause early mortality.
    B. An increased risk for anaphylactic reactions when compared to an outpatient setting.
    C. A significant reduction in all-cause mortality when an ultrasound enhancing agent is utilized.
    D. Less beneficial effects but no difference in risk when compared to an outpatient setting.

12. A 72-year-old woman with a history of hypertension, type 2 diabetes, and obstructive sleep apnea presents to the emergency department with chest pain, relieved by sublingual nitroglycerin. An EKG is obtained, which demonstrates nonspecific ST depression (<0.1 mV) in V5 and V6. High-sensitivity troponin level is 10 ng/liter. A perfusion echocardiogram is ordered. Which of the following findings has been associated with the **WORST** prognosis?
  A. Resting myocardial perfusion abnormality, with normal wall thickening.
  B. Resting myocardial perfusion abnormality, with abnormal wall thickening.
  C. Basal inferior segment perfusion abnormality with normal wall thickening.
  D. Resting normal myocardial perfusion, with abnormal wall thickening.

13. You are giving an ultrasound enhancing agent (Definity) to a patient and she experiences back pain. Which of the following statements is **FALSE**?
  A. You could switch to Optison if she needed additional contrast.
  B. This is considered a precursor to a severe anaphylactic reaction.
  C. This is most likely related to the lipid shell of the microbubble.
  D. The back pain usually resolves with discontinuation of the contrast agent use.

14. In which of the following clinical scenarios has fundamental nonlinear imaging with an ultrasound enhancing agent not been the preferred imaging modality to detect a left ventricular apical abnormality?
  A. Detecting an apical left ventricular pseudoaneurysm.
  B. Detecting left ventricular noncompaction.
  C. Detecting a distal septal and apical perfusion defect.
  D. Detecting a left ventricular apical thrombus.

15. In the absence of a resting flow-limiting stenosis, animal studies have confirmed that the regulation of coronary blood flow during any form of hyperemic stress (adenosine, dobutamine, exercise) is mediated by:

  A. Capillaries.
  B. Large arterioles.
  C. Small arterioles.
  D. Postcapillary venules.

16. A 77-year-old man with a history of hypertension, chronic kidney disease, congestive heart failure with preserved LVEF, and remote history of liposarcoma had an echocardiogram ordered with a continuous infusion of an ultrasound enhancing agent to assess for chemotherapy-induced cardiotoxicity. An apical short axis image at the plateau intensity is displayed in **Figure 10.1**. The left ventricular apical mass is most likely:
  A. A prominent false tendon.
  B. Apical variant hypertrophic cardiomyopathy.
  C. Metastases.
  D. A fibroma.

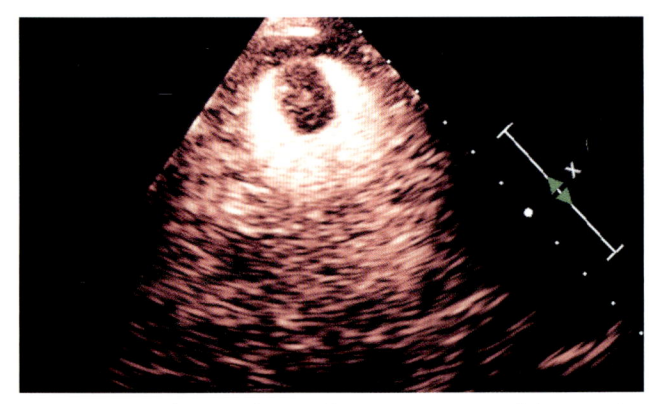

Figure 10.1. Left ventricular apical mass in a patient with hypertension and heart failure receiving chemotherapy.

17. Figure 10.2 was obtained from a patient undergoing an evaluation for a nonischemic cardiomyopathy.
The images on the left are during a continuous infusion of an ultrasound enhancing agent during very-low–mechanical index fundamental nonlinear imaging, and the images on the right are obtained with a low–mechanical index (0.3) and harmonic imaging. The underlying diagnosis is **BEST** detected with:
  A. The very-low–mechanical index imaging pulse sequence scheme.
  B. An alternative imaging modality such as radionuclide SPECT.
  C. An alternative imaging modality such as transesophageal echocardiography.
  D. The low–mechanical index harmonic imaging.

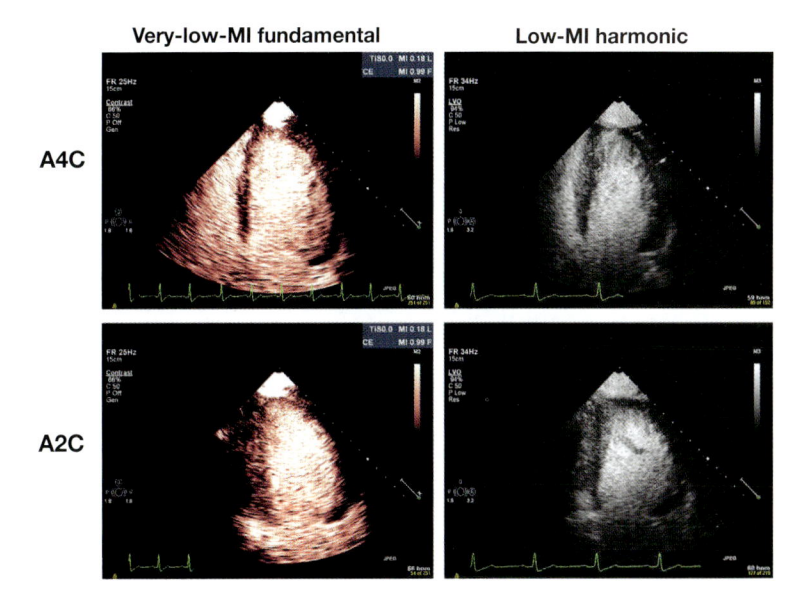

Chapter 10 Contrast-Enhanced Ultrasound Imaging / 215

Figure 10.2. A patient being evaluated for heart failure with depressed systolic function. MI, mechanical index.

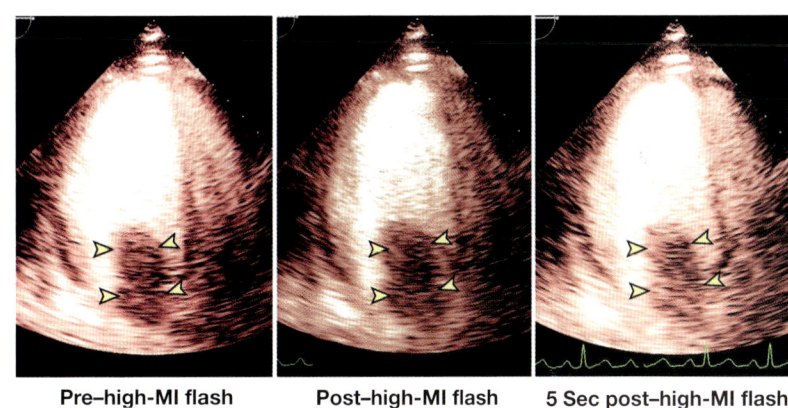

Figure 10.3. Apical three-chamber imaging with very-low–mechanical index nonlinear imaging in a patient with a stroke.

18. A 65-year-old woman with no prior cardiac history presented with a stroke. She had no prior history of hypertension or atrial fibrillation, but did have some recent fevers. Carotid Doppler exam was normal. An echocardiogram was ordered to evaluate for a source of embolus. An apical three-chamber contrast-enhanced image at different points before and after a high–mechanical index impulse is displayed (**Figure 10.3**).
This intracardiac mass (yellow arrows) is most likely:
   A. A thrombus.
   B. A metastasis.
   C. A myxoma.
   D. An atrial septal aneurysm.

19. A 56-year-old man with nonobstructive coronary artery disease is referred back to cardiology for persistent shortness of breath on exertion and episodes of near-syncope. The contrast-enhanced apical four chamber is shown in **Figure 10.4**. Which of the following statements is **NOT TRUE** regarding this patient's findings?

   A. There is probably no subaortic obstruction.
   B. The patient probably needs a defibrillator.
   C. An intracavitary Doppler gradient is probably present.
   D. The EKG probably demonstrates no resting ST- or T-wave abnormalities.

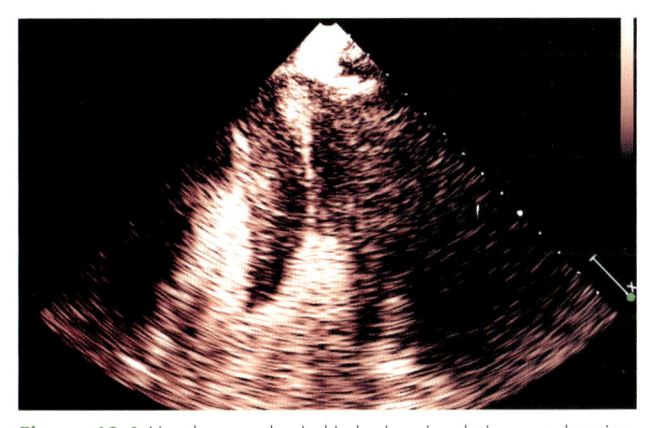

Figure 10.4. Very-low–mechanical index imaging during an enhancing agent infusion in the apical four-chamber view in a patient with an abnormal electrocardiograph and shortness of breath.

216 / Clinical Echocardiography Review

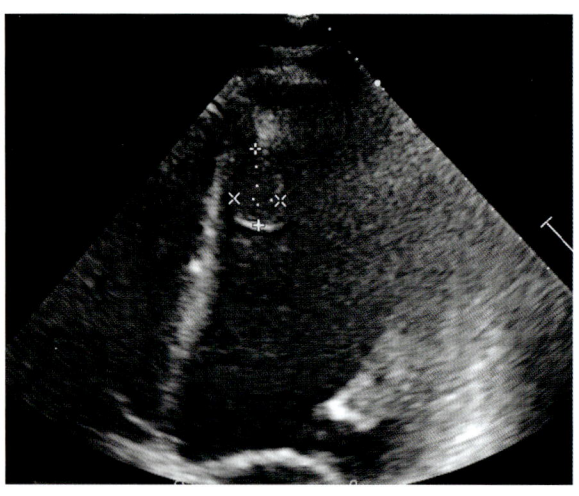

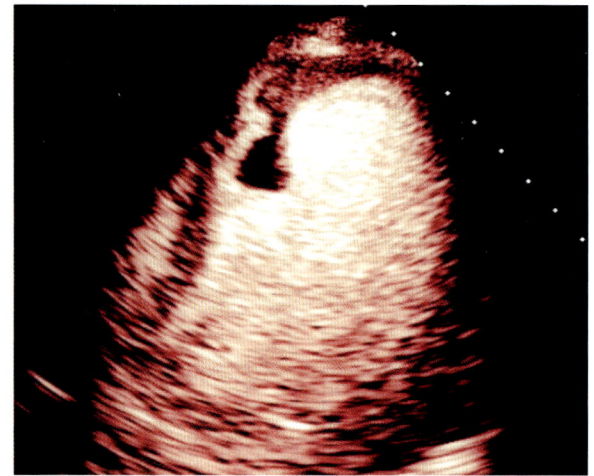

Figure 10.5. Unenhanced and enhanced images in the apical four-chamber view.

20. The series of images in **Figure 10.5** was obtained from a patient who had a prior history of coronary artery disease and myocardial infarction. The unenhanced image is demonstrated on the left. The contrast-enhanced image is displayed on the right. The **CORRECT** diagnosis is:
    A. Apical aneurysm.
    B. Apical thrombus.
    C. False tendon.
    D. Apical pseudoaneurysm.

21. A 65-year-old man was admitted for congestive heart failure. He had a history of hypertension and methamphetamine use. He was diuresed and had an echocardiogram performed. Contrast enhancement was utilized to better delineate left ventricular borders. An end-diastolic off-axis reverse apical four-chamber view is displayed below at the plateau intensity prior to a high–mechanical index impulse (**Figure 10.6**).
    The most remarkable finding is:

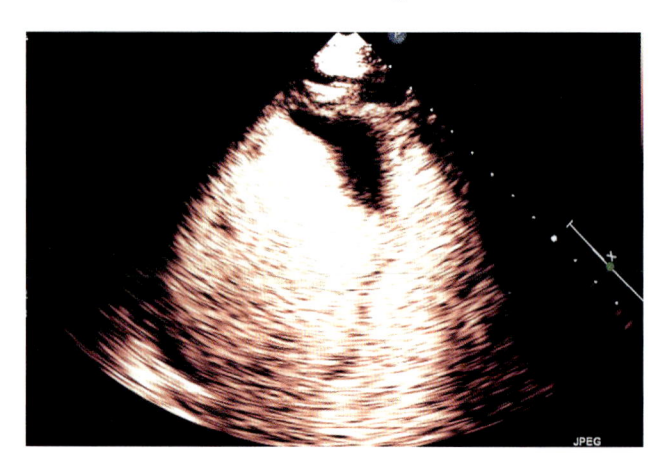

Figure 10.6. Contrast-enhanced apical three-chamber view.

   A. Apical thrombus.
   B. Findings consistent with a left anterior descending occlusion.
   C. Apical hypertrophic cardiomyopathy.
   D. Isolated noncompaction of the left ventricle.

22. A 67-year-old woman with known coronary artery disease, previous history of proximal left circumflex stenting, had acute ST changes noted during an intraoperative procedure. This was associated with chest pain. She was taken directly to the cardiac catheterization laboratory where the coronary angiogram demonstrated acute left circumflex occlusion at the previous site of the stent. She had successful restenting of the left circumflex vessel (**Figure 10.7A**, **prestenting**; **Figure 10.7B**, **poststenting**). A subsequent echocardiogram was ordered and end-systolic contrast-enhanced myocardial perfusion images are displayed in the apical four-chamber view (**Figure 10.7C**). The patient was symptom-free at the time of the echocardiogram.
    The most likely explanation for the perfusion findings are:
    A. Recurrent left circumflex ischemia.
    B. Microvascular obstruction.
    C. Severe residual stenosis in the left anterior descending artery segment.
    D. Artifact from contrast attenuation.

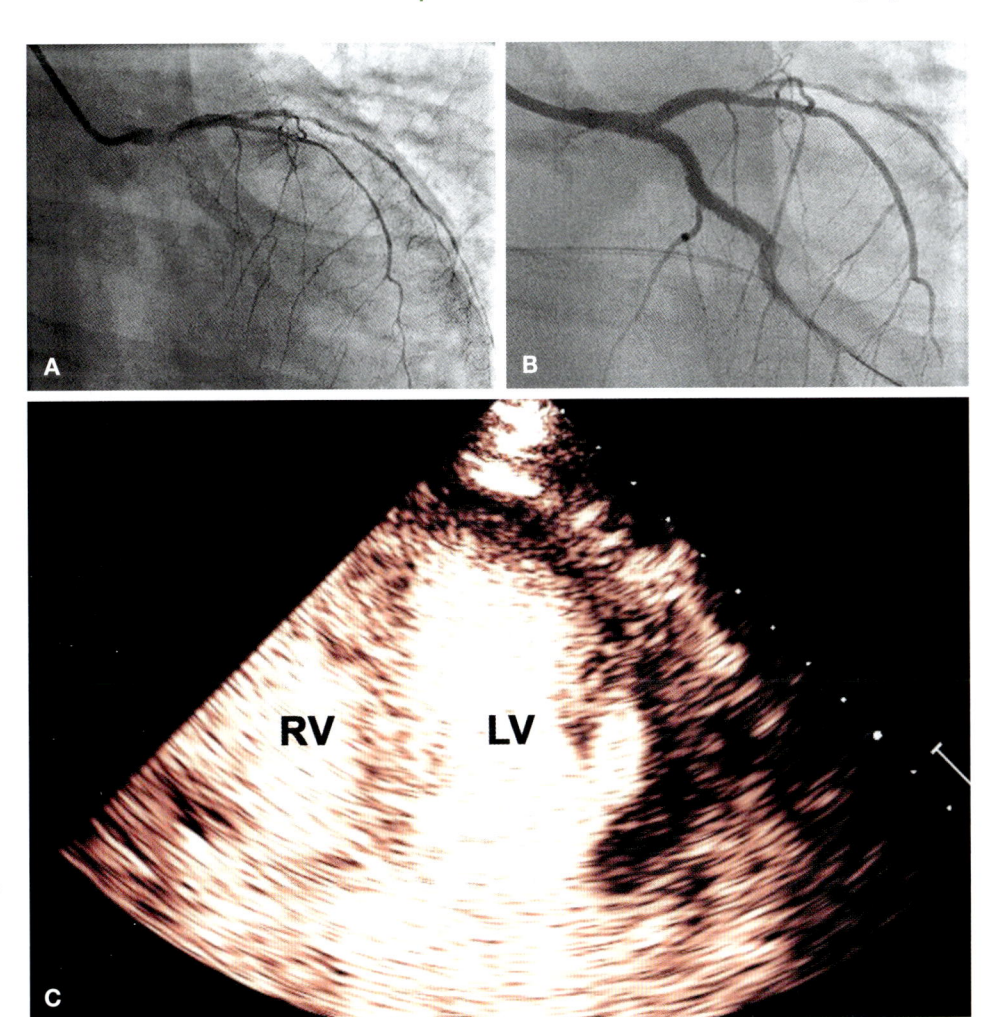

Figure 10.7. **A** and **B:** Coronary angiogram of a patient with an acute ST segment elevation myocardial infarction involving the left circumflex artery before and after successful emergent percutaneous coronary intervention. **C:** Contrast-enhanced images during the plateau intensity. LV, left ventricle; RV, ventricle.

23. A 70-year-old obese man is admitted with hypoxic respiratory failure and has an elevation in serum troponin. ▶ Video 10.1A-C displays the unenhanced apical four-chamber (▶ Video 10.1A) and very-low-mechanical index imaging using a fundamental nonlinear imaging technique (▶ Video 10.1B) and harmonic enhancing imaging (▶ Video10.1C). Which of the following statements in **INCORRECT**?
    A. The end-diastolic and end-systolic volumes with fundamental nonlinear imaging will be higher.
    B. The harmonic enhanced imaging has basal segment attenuation.
    C. The endocardium is not visualized on the unenhanced images.
    D. The harmonic enhanced images should have the mechanical index turned down further to improve image quality.

24. A 65-year-old woman is admitted with left arm discomfort that radiates to her jaw. The symptoms have recently started bothering her at rest, which brought her into the emergency department. Initial EKG demonstrated normal sinus rhythm at 86 bpm without ST- or T-wave abnormalities. Initial high-sensitivity troponin was elevated slightly and increased slightly at 2 hours. The resting unenhanced apical two-chamber video (▶ Video 10.2) is displayed on the left. The resting plateau intensity images on the right using fundamental nonlinear imaging are displayed on the right. **Figure 10.8** displays the end-systolic images pre–high-MI flash impulse and at 1, 2, and 3 seconds post–high-MI impulse. Which of the following statements about these images is **TRUE**?
    A. There is basal segment attenuation.
    B. Acoustic shadowing in the left ventricular cavity is prohibiting detection of inferior segments.
    C. There is mid to distal anterior hypokinesis with a resting perfusion defect.
    D. There is basal inferior hypokinesis with a resting perfusion defect.

Figure 10.8. Apical 2-chamber view.

25. A 48-year-old man with a prior history of a myocardial infarction is being seen for recurrent resting chest pain that is sharp and transient in nature. No associated diaphoresis or SOB. He does not experience the pain with exertion. EKG demonstrates normal sinus rhythm with Q waves in V4 and V5 with 0.1 mV ST elevation. Initial and 2-hour high-sensitivity troponin values were normal. A resting echocardiogram was obtained with small boluses of intravenous ultrasound enhancing agent added using fundamental non-linear imaging at a 0.18 mechanical index in the apical two-chamber (▶ **Video 10.3A**) and apical three-chamber (▶ **Video 10.3B**) windows. The most likely explanation for the findings in the apical two- and three-chamber views with and without contrast is:
   A. An apical aneurysm.
   B. Acute left anterior descending ischemia.
   C. Near-field contrast destruction.
   D. Takotsubo cardiomyopathy.

CASE 1

*A 58-year-old woman with a 30-pack-year history of smoking cigarettes, known coronary artery disease with prior left circumflex stenting, was seen in the emergency department for left precordial discomfort that awakened her from sleep. She had relief with nitroglycerin. She is currently symptom free. EKG was normal. Initial high-sensitivity troponin was normal. A dobutamine stress echo was ordered. A diluted ultrasound enhancing agent was infused during very-low–mechanical index imaging. Rest and stress apical three-chamber images during replenishment are shown (▶ **Video 10.4**; **Figure 10.9**).*

26. Based on **Case 1** (▶ **Video 10.4, Figure 10.9**), which of the following statements about the stress and rest images is **TRUE**?
   A. There is an inferolateral wall perfusion defect during stress only.
   B. Resting myocardial perfusion is abnormal.
   C. Stress wall thickening appears abnormal.
   D. There is a distal lateral segment attenuation artifact.

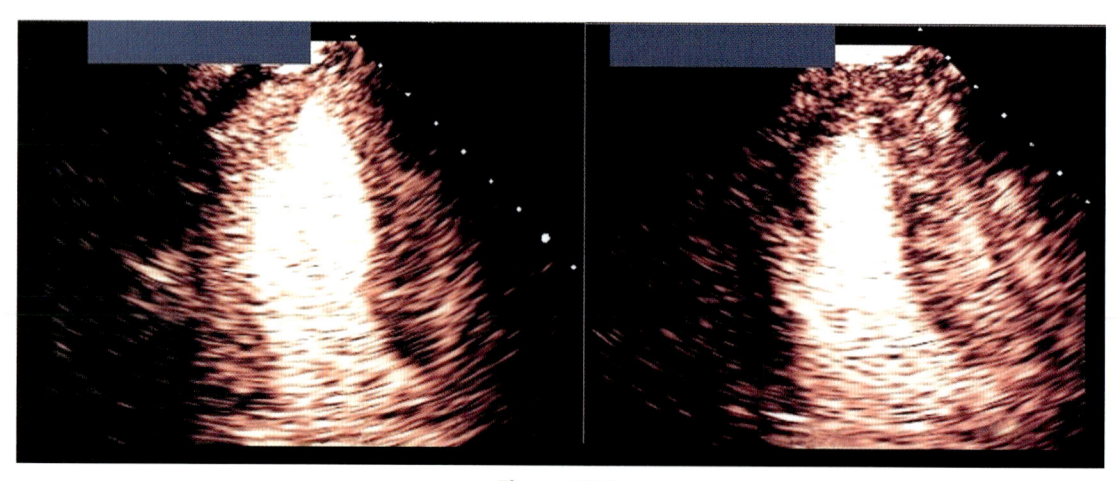

Figure 10.9

CASE 2

A 55-year-old woman with a history of hypertension and hyperlipidemia was admitted for acute onset of nausea, vomiting, and fever. An EKG was obtained in the emergency department, which exhibited T-wave inversions in the anterior precordial leads. High-sensitivity troponin was elevated slightly. The echo images without contrast and with very-low-MI imaging are demonstrated in ▶ **Video 10.5A** *and* ▶ **Video 10.5B**. *The patient was placed on intravenous heparin, dual antiplatelet therapy, high-intensity statin, and a beta blocker. Coronary angiography demonstrated nonobstructive coronary artery disease. The follow-up apical four-chamber contrast perfusion image obtained 3 days later is shown in* ▶ **Video 10.5C**.

27. The findings in **Case 2** and ▶ **Video 10.5** demonstrate:
    A. Resting normal perfusion but wall motion abnormality in one coronary artery territory.
    B. Resting abnormal perfusion and wall motion in more than one coronary artery territory.
    C. Resting normal perfusion but abnormal wall motion in more than one coronary artery territory.
    D. Abnormal perfusion in the segments exhibiting normal wall motion.

CASE 3

A 45-year-old woman with steatohepatitis and exertional shortness of breath had a dobutamine stress echocardiogram performed for a liver transplant evaluation. Very-low-MI imaging was performed during a continuous infusion of ultrasound contrast (3% Definity at 4 mL/min during rest, 2 mL/min during stress). The apical four-chamber rest (left) and stress (right) images are displayed in ▶ **Video 10.6**

28. Based on **Case 3** and the view displayed in ▶ **Video 10.6**, the **BEST** interpretation of the results of the stress echo should be?
    A. Inducible distal septal, mid anterolateral to distal anterolateral, and apical perfusion defect with wall motion abnormality.
    B. Inducible basal inferoseptal ischemia (wall motion and perfusion; 1 segment).
    C. A prior distal septal, distal lateral, and apical infarction, with inducible mid anterolateral perfusion defect.
    D. Normal microvascular perfusion but abnormal wall thickening in the left anterior descending and left circumflex territory.

CASE 4

A 56-year-old man with a history of methamphetamine and cigarette use was seen in the emergency department for chest pain along with elevated resting high-sensitivity troponin assay. EKG demonstrated no acute ST changes. However, resting high-sensitivity troponin was elevated. ▶ **Video 10.7A** *demonstrates unenhanced apical four- and two-chamber windows. Despite what appeared to be adequate windows, a diluted ultrasound enhancing agent infusion was administered and the apical four- and two-chamber views repeated before and following a high–mechanical index impulse followed by contrast replenishment (* ▶ **Video 10.7B**).

29. Unlike the unenhanced images, the contrast-enhanced images in **Case 4** (▶ **Videos 10.7A,B**) display:
    A. Normal regional wall motion.
    B. Resting wall motion abnormality in the anterolateral segments.
    C. Resting wall motion abnormality in the distal septum and apex.
    D. Inadequate border resolution to determine resting regional wall motion.

220 / Clinical Echocardiography Review

CASE 5

A 61-year-old man with morbid obesity, hypertension, and systolic murmur is referred for echocardiography. His body mass index is >40 kg/m². He is referred for an echocardiogram. The windows are difficult, and the left ventricular outflow tract and aortic valve continuous wave Doppler signal is displayed in **Figure 10.10**.

30. Ultrasound enhancing agents would be useful in the patient in **Case 5** for all the following indications **EXCEPT**:
    A. Doppler enhancement.
    B. Left ventricular volumes.
    C. Left ventricular ejection fraction.
    D. Left atrial volumes.

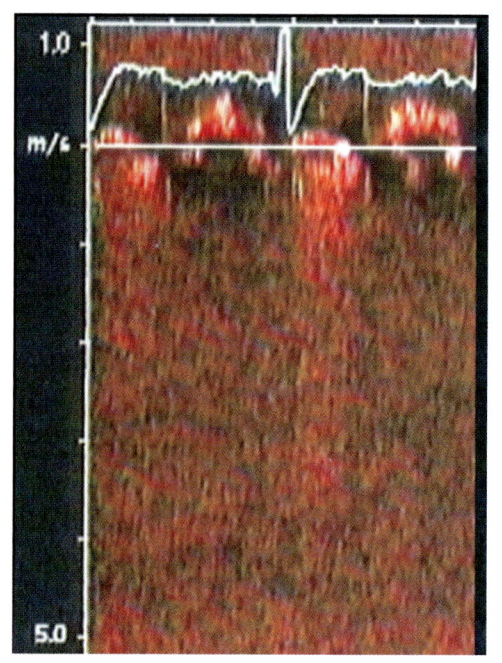

Figure 10.10. Apical continuous wave Doppler of the aortic valve without ultrasound enhancing agent.

ANSWERS

1. **Answer: D.** According the current package insert, the only remaining contraindication is an allergy or hypersensitivity to perflutren. The intracardiac shunt contraindication has been removed for all three commercially available agents. The ultrasound enhancing agents have also been given safely in patients with pulmonary hypertension. The composition and dosage recommendations for the three approved ultrasound enhancing agents are listed in **Table 10.1**.

Table 10.1. Currently Available Ultrasound Enhancing Agents

	Definity/Luminity	Optison	Lumason/SonoVue
Shell	Phospholipids	Human albumin	Phospholipids
Gas	Octafluoropropane (C_3F_8)	Octafluoropropane (C_3F_8)	Sulfur hexafluoride (SF_6)
Size	1.1-3.3 μm	3.0-4.5 μm	1.5-2.5 μm
Concentration (microbubbles/mL)	1.2×10^{10}	$5-8 \times 10^8$	$1.5-5.6 \times 10^8$
Volume	2.0 mL	3.0 mL	4.5 mL
Preparation	Activate by Vialmix for 45 s	Ready for use after resuspension	Shake with saline for 20 s
Storage	2-8°C	2-8°C	15-30°C
Administration Continuous infusion	3%	7.5%	12%
Administration Bolus injection	0.1 mL	0.2 mL	0.5 mL

2. **Answer: A.** The change from room air encapsulated gas to higher molecular weight (MW) gases has led to longer persistence of microbubbles (due to reduced diffusivity and solubility) and consistent left ventricular opacification following venous injection or infusion. Lumason microbubbles contain sulfur hexafluoride (MW: 146 g/mole), Optison and Definity contain perfluoropropane (MW: 188 g/mole), and Sonazoid contains decafluorobutane (MW: 238 g/mole).
3. **Answer: D.** Very-low–mechanical index (MI) imaging techniques are available on most commercially available systems (**Table 10.2**). These permit the enhancement of microbubble nonlinear behavior at these very low MIs at the fundamental frequency while simultaneously reducing background tissue signals (which do not exhibit nonlinear behavior at very low MIs). Very-low-MI imaging is the term given to this fundamental nonlinear imaging technique. This has been utilized not only to provide improved endocardial border delineation but also to detect myocardial perfusion and perfusion of intracardiac masses. Spatial resolution is improved with increased transmit frequency but not with ultrasound enhancing agents. **Table 10.2** depicts the recommended instrumentation settings for very-low-MI imaging.
4. **Answer: A.** One of the limitations of harmonic imaging for detection of ultrasound contrast is the higher frequency returning signals attenuate in the far field. This far-field attenuation can be made worse by either reducing the mechanical index further or by giving too high a concentration of microbubbles, which occurs more commonly with bolus intravenous injections. Methods to overcome this problem would be to use a fundamental nonlinear cancellation technique that results in enhanced signal from microbubbles at a lower mechanical index and less far-field attenuation because of the lower frequency used for imaging. A brief high–mechanical index impulse (which destroys microbubbles) will reduce left ventricular cavity microbubble concentration and allow better delineation of basal segments. Conversely, simply waiting for a brief period of time to allow the bolus injection to pass through the left ventricular cavity, you also see a decrease in cavity microbubble concentration.
5. **Answer: D.** The mechanical index is equal to the peak negative pressure divided by the square root of the transmit frequency (in Megahertz). The higher the mechanical index, the greater the potential for cavitation. Microbubbles (ultrasound enhancing agents) lower the threshold for cavitation. The transmit gain only alters incoming signals and does not affect the potential for cavitation.

Table 10.2. Recommended System Settings

System Setting	Philips EPIQ	GE E95[a]
Depth	140-160 mm	160 mm
Transducer	X5 or S5	-
XRES	on	N/A
Flash Power	1.0-1.2 MI	1.0 MI
Flash Frames	5-15, adjust as needed to clear myocardium and not cavity	15
Mechanical Index (MI) for imaging	0.12-0.16 MI	0.12-0.2 MI
Frame rate	20-30 Hz	25-30 Hz
Color Map	Chroma Map 7 (Heated Object)	yes
Gray	Map 2	N/A
Loop	Type: Time (10)	yes
Focus	Mitral Valve Level	Mitral Valve Level
Gain	72%-75%, but 65%-68% for IE33	0 dB
TGC and LGC	Set potentiometers in midline; adjust near-field potentiometers to reduce near field-gain	Near-field attenuation

LGC, lateral gain compensation; TGC, time gain compensation.
[a]GE system settings are provided by Dr. Tian Gang Zhu.

6. **Answer: D.** A multicenter European study comparing real-time myocardial contrast echocardiography (RTMCE) with radionuclide SPECT during dipyridamole stress testing found that RTMCE had higher sensitivity but lower specificity for the detection of angiographically significant coronary artery disease (Senior R et al. *J Am Coll Cardiol*. 2013;62:1353-1361). This translated into no differences in test accuracy between the two perfusion imaging techniques. During dobutamine stress echocardiography, the addition of perfusion imaging performed at experienced centers has improved not only the detection of significant coronary artery stenoses but also the predictive value of the test for hard events, such as death or nonfatal myocardial infarction. (Porter et al *2018 American Society of Echocardiography Guidelines Update*)

7. **Answer: E.** Myocardial contrast echocardiography has provided perfusion imaging information that has added incremental value over wall motion and clinical variables during stress echocardiography, in the evaluation of chest pain with a nondiagnostic EKG in the emergency department, and in the post-myocardial infarction setting. Although contrast improves the delineation of the apex and detects myocardial perfusion in patients with stress cardiomyopathy, there are no data published on its ability to predict recovery or regional wall motion in these patients (see Abdelmoneim SS et al. *J Am Soc Echocardiogr*. 2009;11:1249-1255).

8. **Answer: A.** Preclinical and clinical data have demonstrated during demand ischemia that myocardial perfusion abnormalities precede the development of wall thickening abnormalities, which is what was occurring in this patient example. Attenuation would be much less likely since this typically involves basal segments in the apical windows, and these were exhibiting normal replenishment following a high-MI impulse. Wall thickening will not typically become abnormal until a higher degree of demand stress has been achieved.

9. **Answer: D.** Several hospitals throughout the United States now allow sonographers to start their own intravenous (IV) lines and administer an ultrasound enhancing agent. Both the 2014 and 2018 American Society of Echocardiography guidelines recommend sonographers be trained in both IV starting using sterile technique and in ultrasound enhancing agent administration. Several hospitals now include training for sonographers to be qualified for starting of the IV line and administration of contrast. With radionuclide imaging and CT imaging, IV lines are routinely required for contrast or tracer administration.

10. **Answer: A.** Continuous infusions of ultrasound enhancing agents permits quantification of myocardial perfusion using destruction replenishment curves. Since the concentration of contrast is constant, the 1-exponential function can be utilized to examine contrast replenishment following destructive impulses. This cannot be done following a bolus injection, because of the varying contrast concentration. The bolus of contrast also can produce temporary acoustic shadowing and far-field attenuation that is seen to a lesser degree with continuous infusions.

11. **Answer: C.** Large propensity-matched clinical outcomes data from the Premier database have demonstrated that patients receiving contrast-enhanced echocardiograms have an actual reduction in mortality when compared to patients receiving noncontrast echocardiograms. The mechanism as to how early use of UEAs reduces mortality is not clear, but earlier detection of left ventricular regional and globally systolic function abnormalities may play a role. The study by Kurt et al demonstrated that additional diagnostic procedures were avoided in over 30% of patients and drug management was altered in over 10 % of patients when ultrasound contrast was utilized in critical care settings.

12. **Answer: B.** In the evaluation of a patient with chest discomfort and a nondiagnostic EKG, regional wall motion and myocardial perfusion provide additive information in detecting a high-risk patient with an acute coronary syndrome. The combination of both a resting regional wall motion abnormality and resting myocardial perfusion defect has been associated with the highest risk for in-hospital and short-term mortality.

13. **Answer: B.** Back pain is an infrequent complication that has been seen almost exclusively with intravenous Definity use. It has not been reported with Optison and rarely is reported with Lumason. It is not an anaphylactic reaction and is most likely related to complement-mediated retention of microbubbles within the renal cortex. Although the exact cause for back pain is unknown, it is most likely related to the lipid shell composition since it is not seen with albumin-shelled agents.

14. **Answer: B.** Very-low–mechanical index imaging with fundamental nonlinear imaging pulse sequence schemes has been shown to improve the delineation of apical abnormalities because it does not destroy contrast in the near field, but enhances the signal intensity produced by the enhancing agent. Because it does not destroy the microbubbles, fundamental nonlinear imaging has the limitation of not being able to distinguish the noncompacted myocardial layer and the intertrabecular recesses of contrast. To optimize detection of the noncompacted layer, a mechanical index which destroys the microbubbles in the noncompacted myocardium but not the higher flowing intertrabecular recesses is needed.

15. **Answer: A.** Carefully controlled canine studies performed in the late 1990s using models of nonflow limiting coronary stenoses demonstrated that all the way up to an 85% stenosis, the arterioles are the main mediator of resting coronary blood flow, while the capillaries become the major regulator of coronary blood flow during hyperemic stress. The myocardial contrast defects observed during hyperemic stress with fundamental nonlinear imaging are due to capillary derecruitment and form the basis for ischemia detection during stress testing.

16. **Answer: C.** In this patient, there is a left ventricular apical mass noted that has evidence of perfusion prior to the high–mechanical index impulse. The degree of enhancement is similar to the myocardial contrast enhancement and therefore is most consistent with a metastases. Thrombus would exhibit virtually no myocardial contrast enhancement, and benign tumors would exhibit a small amount of contrast enhancement but less than the surrounding myocardium.

17. **Answer: D.** The very-low-MI images on the left exhibit increased contrast signal when compared to the low-MI harmonic image (right panel) and clearly allow visualization of the apex. Although the 0.3 MI harmonic image is considered "low MI," it still results in apical myocardial contrast destruction and normally is not preferred except in this case where it is detecting noncompacted myocardium (right panel). The very-low-MI nonlinear fundamental imaging does not destroy myocardial or cavity contrast and therefore the noncompacted myocardium cannot be distinguished from the intertrabecular cavity contrast. The low-MI imaging destroys the noncompacted myocardial contrast and allows for better delineation of the noncompacted myocardial thickness. Transesophageal echocardiography has difficulty seeing apical images due to far-field attenuation and foreshortening of apical windows. The reduced spatial resolution of radionuclide SPECT would not be able to detect the noncompacted myocardium.

18. **Answer: C.** This patient has a contrast enhancing mass that is heterogenous and lower in intensity when compared to the adjacent myocardium. This is consistent with a benign tumor, in this case a myxoma. Note that the presentation in this case was embolic, but certainly could also have presented as syncope in view of the large mobile mass obstructing mitral valve flow. It also could have presented as a mitral stenosis–like picture in view of its diastolic obstruction of left ventricular inflow. Intracardiac metastases are typically more vascular and have greater degrees of contrast enhancement. Intracardiac thrombi exhibit virtually no enhancement. Atrial septal aneurysms are thin mobile structures within the fossa ovalis.

19. **Answer: D.** The contrast-enhanced images here with very-low–mechanical index imaging are detecting the midcavity variant of hypertrophic cardiomyopathy. This is characterized by marked end-diastolic thickening of the mid to distal left ventricular segments and apical segment. There is typically cavity obliteration in systole with these variants but no dynamic subaortic obstruction. Although this end-systolic image demonstrates apical akinesis, there is no evidence of apical aneurysm formation. The presence of any size apical aneurysm is now an indication for a defibrillator. These patients also have diastolic dysfunction that causes shortness of breath and characteristic electrocardiographic abnormalities consisting of deep T-wave inversions in the precordial leads.

20. **Answer: D.** The contrast enhancement in the left ventricular cavity and myocardium, when used with very-low-MI imaging, can be utilized to pick up subtle abnormalities in the left ventricular apex. In this particular case, the unenhanced images in **Figure 10.5** appear to indicate a thrombus in the distal septum and apex. However, the ultrasound enhancing agent detects a pseudoaneurysm forming in this region with a narrow neck (*arrow* in **Figure 10.11**; ▶ **Video 10.8**). Pseudoaneurysms are contained ruptures of the left ventricular cavity, which complicate 0.2% to 0.3% of infarctions. Ultrasound enhancing agents have been very beneficial in detecting these surgical emergencies.

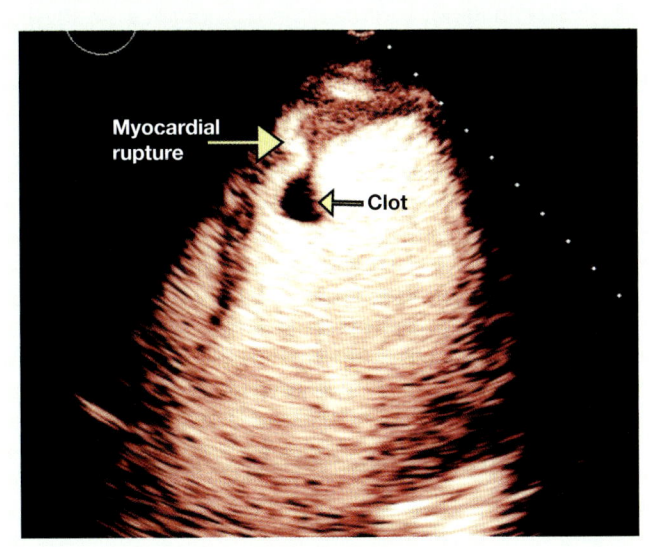

Figure 10.11

21. **Answer: A.** Patients with methamphetamine-related cardiomyopathies are at high risk for intracavitary thrombus. In this particular case, the thrombus was easily visualized with an ultrasound enhancing agent using very-low–mechanical index imaging. Often off-axis views are needed to delineate the perfusion within the mass and better delineate the extent of the mass. Although myocardial perfusion appeared normal, there was no contrast evident in the mid anteroseptal, distal septal, and apical intracavity mass, consistent with thrombus (which is avascular). The very-low–mechanical index fundamental nonlinear imaging mode enhances the signal from contrast and is much less destructive, permitting a clear delineation of the thrombus.

22. **Answer: B.** There is resting microvascular perfusion defect in the lateral segments on this apical four-chamber view. Since the patient is asymptomatic, it is unlikely due to recurrent left circumflex ischemia but rather microvascular obstruction. Microvascular obstruction occurs in over 40% of successfully treated myocardial infarctions, even if normal epicardial flow has been achieved in the infarct vessel. The microvascular perfusion in the inferoseptal, distal septal, and apical segments appear normal, and therefore the resting left anterior descending and right coronary artery segments appear normal. Attenuation primarily affects basal segments and is not apparent on these images.

23. **Answer: D.** Intravenous ultrasound enhancing agents are indicated in this patient's case because of poor endocardial definition. According to the 2018 American Society of Echocardiography contrast guidelines, the preferred imaging modality to detect contrast in this setting would be fundamental nonlinear imaging. The fundamental nonlinear imaging technique detects nonlinear nondestructive contrast enhancement at very low (<0.2) mechanical indices (unlike harmonic imaging which requires a higher mechanical index to get a contrast response that results in near-field destruction). Because it transmits and receives at a low frequency and is less destructive, there is less far-field attenuation and better delineation of both basal and apical segments with fundamental very-low–mechanical index nonlinear imaging when compared to harmonic imaging.

24. **Answer: D.** This is another example where fundamental nonlinear imaging with a very low mechanical index was utilized to detect a resting basal inferior wall motion abnormality and perfusion defect that was not evident on unenhanced images. Since a continuous infusion of a diluted ultrasound enhancing agent was utilized, there was also less likelihood of left ventricular cavity shadowing. The combination of both a resting perfusion defect and wall thickening abnormality in this setting increases the likelihood of significant cardiovascular events, including death and nonfatal myocardial infarction.

25. **Answer: A.** The unenhanced apical two- and three-chamber views could not visualize the apical segments. With very-low–mechanical index fundamental nonlinear imaging and small bolus intravenous injections of an ultrasound enhancing agent with a slow intravenous flush, the apex is visualized without microbubble destruction, permitting the delineation of a persistent apical thinning deformity in systole and diastole consistent with aneurysm. There was no clinical evidence to suggest myocardial ischemia was occurring, so this was unlikely. Takotsubo cardiomyopathy typically involves a larger segmental distribution and troponin elevations.

26. **Answer: A.** During demand stress imaging (eg, dobutamine, exercise), perfusion abnormalities precede the development of wall thickening abnormalities. This was true in this case where an inducible inferolateral and distal lateral perfusion defect was evident despite relatively normal wall thickening in these same segments. Attenuation artifacts typically only involve basal segments and this defect extended into the distal segments.

> **KEY POINTS**
> - Contrast attenuation typically only affects the basal segment of any particular view and does not extend into the mid and apical segments, as was the case here.
> - Delays in replenishment (beyond 3 seconds during stress imaging) should be considered abnormal and can be confined to just the subendocardial layers.

27. **Answer: C.** The contrast echocardiogram findings in this particular case, and the demographic profile, is consistent with takotsubo cardiomyopathy. The patient is perimenopausal and has an acute concomitant illness, which is the typical clinical scenario. The extent of the wall motion abnormality goes beyond any coronary artery distribution and resting microvascular perfusion remains normal. As could be seen on the follow-up echo in just 2 days, there was already recovery of systolic function on beta blockers (▶ **Video 10.5C**).

KEY POINTS
- The apical form of takotsubo cardiomyopathy typically displays an extensive regional wall motion abnormality that extends beyond any one coronary artery territory.
- Resting microvascular perfusion with very-low–mechanical index real-time perfusion imaging is helpful in that it usually depicts normal perfusion in the segments with abnormal wall motion.
- Real-time very-low–mechanical index imaging also depicts the hyperkinetic basal segments often seen with apical takotsubo cardiomyopathy.
- When there is resting myocardial ischemia due to coronary artery plaque rupture, a microvascular perfusion defect and wall motion abnormality often coexist and are confined to the one affected vascular territory.

28. **Answer: A.** The real-time myocardial contrast echocardiogram in the apical four-chamber window in this patient demonstrates normal resting myocardial perfusion and wall motion. However, during dobutamine stress imaging, there are inducible perfusion defects and wall thickening abnormalities in several segments including the mid anterolateral, distal septal, distal lateral, and apical segments. This is a pattern typical of multivessel coronary artery disease, which was confirmed at subsequent coronary angiography. This would be inconsistent with a prior infarction in this territory since resting wall motion and perfusion were normal in these segments. Similarly, the basal to mid inferoseptal segments exhibit replenishment within 2 seconds during stress, indicative of normal stress perfusion when using a two-dimensional transducer, and thus choices B and D would not be correct. The peak stress images indicate a delay in contrast replenishment in the mid anterolateral, distal lateral, distal septal, and apical segments *with wall motion abnormalities*.

KEY POINTS
- Perfusion defects occur prior to the onset of wall thickening abnormalities during demand stress. The presence of both an inducible perfusion and wall thickening abnormality during dobutamine stress identifies a higher risk of complications.
- When using a two-dimensional imaging transducer with a typical elevation plane of 4 to 5 mm (since normal resting capillary blood velocity is approximately 1 mm/s), normal myocardial contrast replenishment should be within 4 to 5 seconds under resting conditions, and within 2 seconds during stress imaging (since capillary blood velocity increases over twofold during hyperemic stress).
- Perfusion defects with real-time myocardial contrast imaging typically appear as subendocardial defects that assist in detecting subendocardial wall thickening abnormalities.

29. **Answer: B.** This patient had what appeared to be adequate windows on the apical four- and two-chamber windows without ultrasound enhancing agent. However, visualization of the compacted border is difficult in the anterolateral and apical segments. The very-low–mechanical index perfusion imaging permits better delineation of the compacted myocardium. He was subsequently found to have a >90% large diagonal lesion coming off the left anterior descending artery.

KEY POINTS
- Very-low-MI imaging (<0.2), when combined with pulse sequences schemes that elicit nonlinear responses from microbubbles, can produce myocardial contrast that detects myocardial perfusion abnormalities in real time.
- Very-low-MI imaging techniques can be used to improve regional wall motion analysis and should be considered in high-risk chest pain situations even when initial wall motion analysis appeared normal with unenhanced imaging.
- In the acute setting, the combination of both a resting myocardial perfusion defect and wall thickening abnormality identifies a high-risk patient for death or nonfatal myocardial infarction.

30. **Answer: D.** One of the key additional indications for ultrasound enhancing agents is enhancing Doppler signals. In this particular case, the use of ultrasound enhancing agents permitted the detection of the aortic peak velocity and time velocity integral for measurements of aortic stenosis severity (**Figure 10.12**). The infusion rate required to

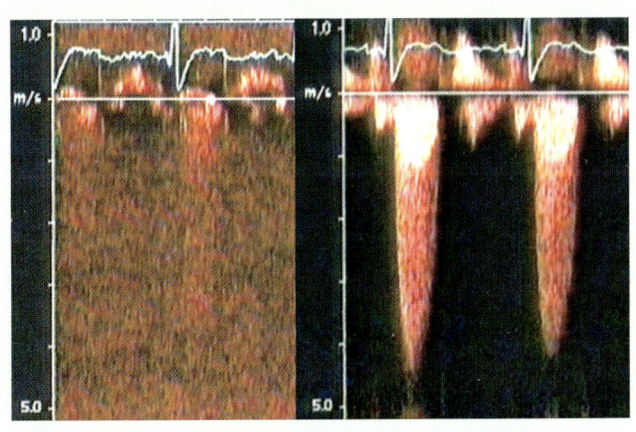

Figure 10.12. Continuous wave Doppler of the aortic valve.

enhance Doppler signals is less than that required for left ventricular endocardial border definition, and the Doppler gain settings required to detect this enhanced spectral profile are lower (30% or less). Left ventricular volumes and ejection fraction determinations have been improved with the use of ultrasound enhancing agents, but unfortunately left atrial volumes are in the far field and their enhancement with contrast agents has not been demonstrated.

SUGGESTED READINGS

Abdelmoneim SS, Bernier M, Scott CG, et al. Safety of contrast agent use during stress echocardiography in patients with elevated right ventricular systolic pressure: a Cohort Study. *Circ Cardiovasc Imaging*. 2010;3(3):240-248.

Abdelmoneim SS, Mankad SV, Bernier M, et al. Microvascular function in Takotsubo cardiomyopathy with contrast echocardiography: prospective evaluation and review of literature. *J Am Soc Echocardiogr*. 2009;22(11):1249-1255.

Aggarwal S, Xie F, Porter TR. Masking and unmasking of isolated noncompaction of the left ventricle with real-time contrast echocardiography. *Circ Cardiovasc Imaging*. 2017;10(11):e006999.

Gaibazzi N, Reverberi C, Lorenzoni V, Molinaro S, Porter TR. Prognostic value of high-dose dipyridamole stress myocardial contrast perfusion echocardiography. *Circulation*. 2012;126(10):1217-1224.

Hoffman R, von Bardeleben S, Kasprzak JD, et al. Analysis of regional left ventricular function by cineventriculography, cardiac magnetic resonance imaging, unenhanced and contrast-enhanced echocardiography: a multicenter comparison of methods. *J Am Coll Cardiol*. 2006;47:121-128.

Kurt M, Shaikh KA, Peterson L, et al. Impact of contrast echocardiography on evaluation of ventricular function and clinical management in a large prospective cohort. *J Am Coll Cardiol*. 2009;53(9):802-810.

Kutty S, Bisselou Moukagna KS, Craft M, Shostrom V, Xie F, Porter TR. Clinical outcome of patients with inducible capillary blood flow abnormalities during demand stress in the presence or absence of angiographic coronary disease. *Circ Cardiovasc Imaging*. 2018;11(10):e007483.

Leong-Poi H, Le E, Rim S-J, Sakuma T, Kaul S, Wei K. Quantification of myocardial perfusion and determination of coronary stenosis severity during hyperemia using real-time myocardial contrast echocardiography. *J Am Soc Echocardiogr*. 2001;14(12):1173-1182.

Porter TR, Abdelmoneim S, Belcik T, et al. Guidelines for the cardiac sonographer in the performance of contrast echocardiography: a focused update from the American Society of Echocardiography. *J Am Soc Echocardiogr*. 2014;27(8):797-810.

Porter TR, Mulvagh SL, (Co-Chair), Abdelmoneim SS, et al. Clinical applications of ultrasonic enhancing agents in echocardiography: 2018 American Society of Echocardiography Guidelines Update. *J Am Soc Echocardiogr*. 2018;31(3):241-274.

Senior R, Moreo A, Gaibazzi N, et al. Comparison of sulfur hexafluoride microbubble (SonoVue)-enhanced myocardial contrast echocardiography with gated single-photon emission computed tomography for detection of significant coronary artery disease: a large European multicenter study. *J Am Coll Cardiol*. 2013;62(15):1353-1361.

Wei KJ. Utility contrast echocardiography in the emergency department. *Am Coll Cardiol Imaging*. 2010;3:197-203.

Xie F, Qian L, Goldsweig A, Xu D, Porter TR. Event-free survival following successful percutaneous intervention in acute myocardial infarction depends on microvascular perfusion. *Circ Cardiovasc Imaging*. 2020;13(6):e010091.

CHAPTER 11

Systolic Function Assessment

Thomas H. Marwick

QUESTIONS

1. The change in left ventricular (LV) function attributable to therapy is sought in a postinfarct patient. Which of the following echocardiographic measures is the most feasible and closest analog of systolic elastance as a marker of myocardial contractility?
   A. Ejection fraction.
   B. Systolic strain rate.
   C. Myocardial performance ("Tei") index.
   D. Systolic strain.
   E. dp/dt measured from the mitral regurgitant jet.

2. A patient after inferior infarction is thought on clinical grounds to have right ventricular (RV) infarction. Which parameters give a reliable assessment of RV function?
   A. Two-dimensional (2D) echocardiography RV ejection fraction (EF).
   B. RV-free wall strain.
   C. Tricuspid annular plane displacement (TAPSE).
   D. RV S'.
   E. Three-dimensional (3D) echocardiography RV ejection fraction (EF).

3. The development of end-systolic cavity obliteration during stress echocardiography reduces the development of ischemia, likely because of reduced wall stress. Wall stress is:
   A. Proportionate to transmural pressure and chamber size.
   B. Inversely proportionate to transmural pressure and chamber size.
   C. Proportionate to wall thickness.
   D. The same as systolic strain.
   E. Readily measured on a regional basis.

4. Visual assessment of ejection fraction is sometimes required (eg, in an emergency). What are the potential limitations of visual EF?
   A. Inability to interrogate multiple imaging planes simultaneously.
   B. Image quality.
   C. Extremes of heart rate.
   D. Experience of the reviewer.
   E. All of the above.

5. A patient presenting with chest pain undergoes an echocardiogram during pain. The presence of a wall motion abnormality is:
   A. A marker of abnormal myocardium.
   B. Indicative of a high likelihood of myocardial ischemia.
   C. Identified with thickening of <50% or excursion <5 mm.
   D. Uninterpretable in the setting of left bundle branch block (LBBB).
   E. Useful in a diagnostic sense but not prognostically.

6. After implantation of a biventricular pacing device, a 55-year-old patient with dilated cardiomyopathy continues to complain of functional class III symptoms and there is no reduction of LV volumes. What factors are important in considering device optimization?
   A. There is no evidence to support the value of optimization.
   B. The role of mechanical dyssynchrony is in question since publication of the PROSPECT results.
   C. The iterative technique for AV optimization is based on observation of the LV filling curve at various pacing settings.
   D. The site of previous infarction.
   E. The site of the LV lead.

7. Following anterior myocardial infarction, a 70-year-old man has an ejection fraction of 40% with an end-systolic volume of 95 mL (50 mL/m^2). In what range is his 5-year mortality?
   A. 10%.
   B. 15%.
   C. 20%.
   D. 30%.
   E. 50%.

8. In the course of auditing the activity of your echocardiography laboratory, you find that 18% of studies have had a previous study. On investigating the matter further, you find that many are being performed for the follow-up of heart failure (HF). Which of the following are **TRUE** regarding repeat echocardiograms?
   A. A repeat echocardiogram for HF is a class 1 indication from the ACC/AHA guidelines only in symptomatic patients.
   B. 95% confidence intervals for EF are ±11%.
   C. 95% confidence intervals for LV mass are ±60 g.
   D. All of the above.
   E. None of the above.

9. LV strain has been proposed as a simple quantitative tool for assessing LV function. Which of the following is associated with reduced strain, irrespective of myocardial status?
   A. Decreased afterload.
   B. Decreased preload.
   C. Decreased heart rate.
   D. All of the above.
   E. None of the above.

10. Accurate measures of LV volumes are needed in the course of follow-up of patients with asymptomatic mitral regurgitation (MR). Which is the most accurate option for LV volume measurement?
    A. 2D echocardiography.
    B. 2D echocardiography with contrast.
    C. M-mode.
    D. 3D echocardiography.
    E. Transesophageal echocardiography.

11. Given its high workload and distance from nutrient supply, the subendocardium is an important site of pathology. Which techniques could be used to assess subendocardial function?
    A. Longitudinal and circumferential strain.
    B. Radial strain.
    C. Myocardial contrast echocardiography with high mechanical index (MI).
    D. None of the above.
    E. All of the above.

12. Which of the statements regarding the application of new echo technologies is **TRUE**?
    A. Systolic velocity is a reliable marker of regional systolic function.
    B. 3D measurements are useful for assessment of diastolic function.
    C. Deformation analysis is useful for assessment of myocardial viability.
    D. None of the above.
    E. All of the above.

13. Which of the following statements is true regarding the application of new technologies to the different stages of heart failure?
    A. Myocardial deformation is of value in the detection of stage B heart failure.
    B. 3D volume measurements are of most value in stages C and D.
    C. Tissue velocity is of use in all stages.
    D. None of the above.
    E. All of the above.

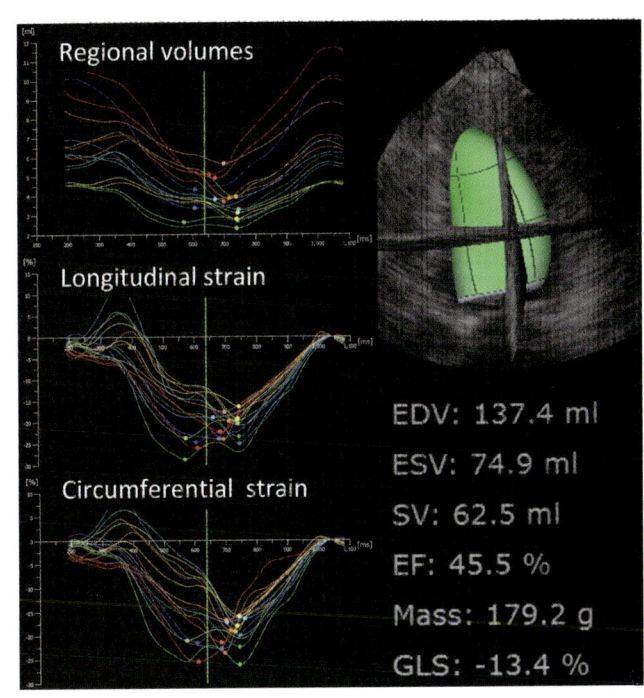

Figure 11.1

14. A 58-year-old woman (height 165 cm, weight 66 kg, BSA 1.74 kg/m²) with controlled hypertension has septal and posterior wall thickness of 12 and 13 mm, respectively, with an end-diastolic dimension of 52 mm (LV mass index 151 g/m²). How would you characterize these LV dimensions?
A. Normal LV geometry.
B. Concentric remodeling.
C. Concentric hypertrophy.
D. Eccentric hypertrophy.
E. None of the above.

15. An echocardiogram taken after an acute coronary syndrome shows a mild apical wall motion abnormality with mild LV impairment (EF = 45%) and normal LV volumes. However, global longitudinal strain is decreased (GLS = −13%), while global circumferential strain is preserved (**Figure 11.1**). What are the potential explanations for these findings?
A. Type 2 diabetes mellitus.
B. Obesity.
C. Previous hypertensive heart disease.
D. Extensive coronary artery disease.
E. All of the above.

16. A 67-year-old man with hypertrophic obstructive cardiomyopathy (HOCM) is seen in the clinic for follow-up. He is treated with high-dose beta-blockers. Prior to a subsequent treatment, he was NYHA class 3 with exertional dyspnea and chest pain, with a left ventricular outflow tract gradient (LVOT) at rest of 70 mm Hg, and 3+ posteriorly directed mitral regurgitation due to systolic anterior motion (SAM) of the mitral valve. Since treatment, he is now NYHA class 2 with less symptoms. Based on **Figure 11.2**, **Panel A** (before treatment) and **Figure 11.2**, **Panel B** (after treatment), what is the most likely intervention that occurred?
A. Myectomy.
B. Alcohol septal ablation.
C. Medical therapy.
D. Transcatheter edge-edge repair.
E. No intervention.

Figure 11.2A

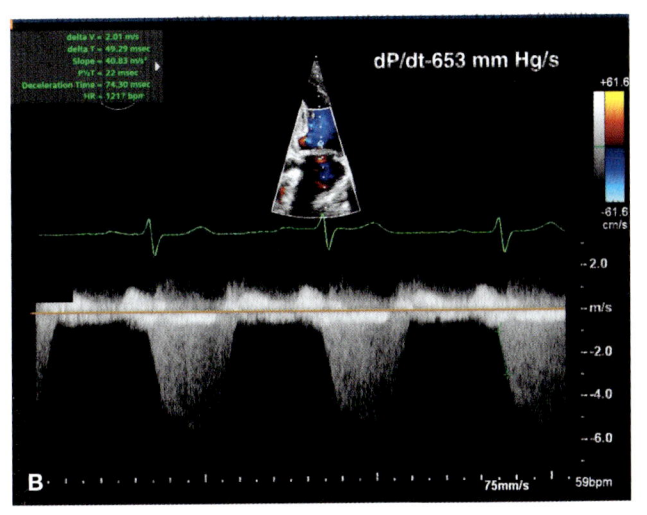

Figure 11.2B

230 / Clinical Echocardiography Review

17. A 70-year-old man is seen in the emergency room for dyspnea. He is morbidly obese with a BMI of 45 kg/m². The fellow on call does a bedside echocardiogram. 2D images of the left ventricle are very poor and the LVEF cannot be determined, even with the use of an ultrasound-enhancing agent. Doppler images are obtainable and the following profiles of the mitral valve are seen in **Figure 11.3, Panel A** (pulsed-wave Doppler), and **Figure 11.3, Panel B** (continuous-wave Doppler). What is the most likely explanation for the patient's dyspnea?

A. Heart failure with reduced ejection fraction (HFrEF).
B. Heart failure with preserved ejection fraction (HFpEF).
C. Cannot be determined.
D. Noncardiac etiology.
E. Severe mitral regurgitation.

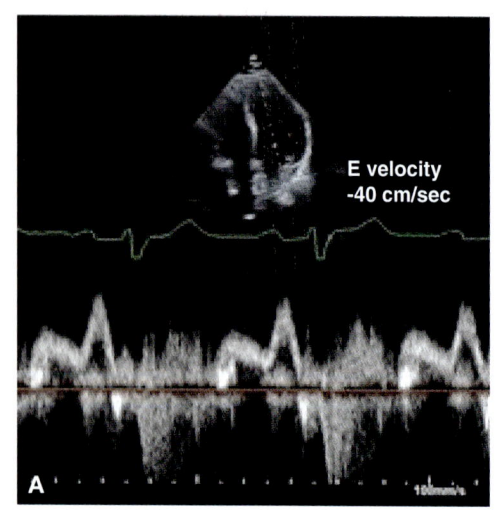

Figure 11.3A

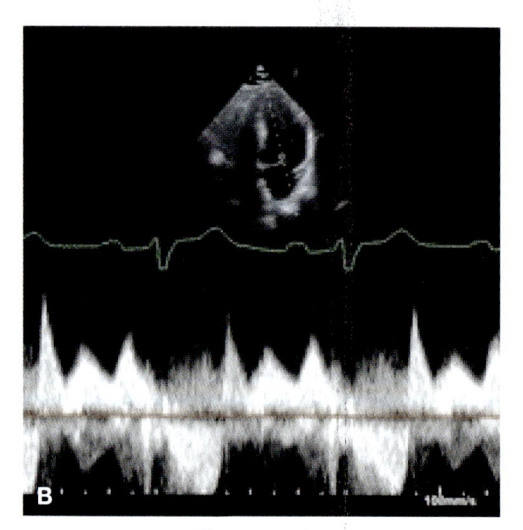

Figure 11.3B

18. A 50-year-old man undergoes a routine echocardiogram for palpitations. He has no cardiac history and his EKG is normal. Which of the following best describes the images seen in the apical 4-chamber view of the left ventricle in **Figure 11.4, Panel A** (diastole), and **Figure 11.4, Panel B** (systole), obtained with an ultrasound enhancing agent, and ▶ **Video 11.1**?

A. An apical aneurysm.
B. An apical pseudoaneurysm.
C. A congenital abnormality.
D. A healed ventricular septal defect.
E. A myocardial cleft.

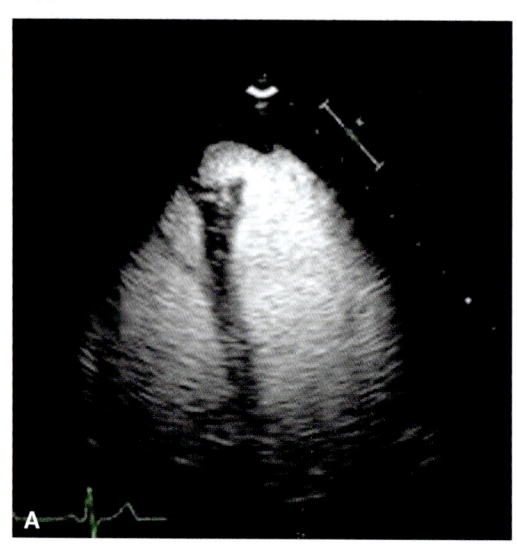

Figure 11.4A

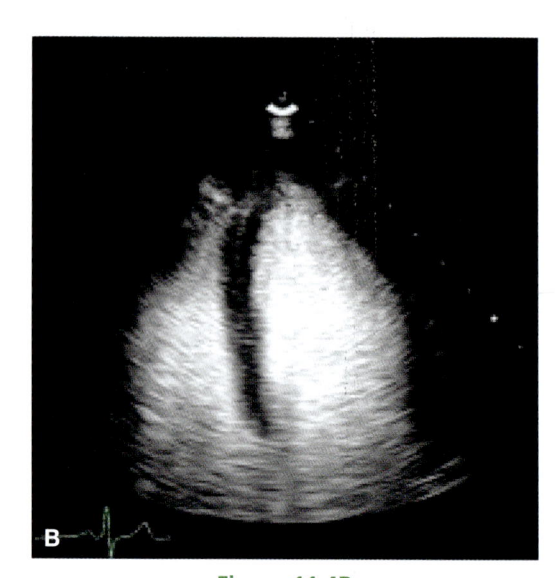

Figure 11.4B

19. A 48-year-old man with renal impairment has presented late after a myocardial infarction. On ECG, there are no Q waves and there is preservation of R waves. On echocardiography, there is an apical wall motion abnormality. Coronary angiography has been withheld because of concerns regarding possible nephrotoxicity, so a myocardial contrast perfusion study is performed with a destruction-replenishment protocol. The findings (**Figure 11.5A-C** and ▶ **Video 11.2A,B**) suggest:

A. Left circumflex artery territory scar.
B. Medical management is appropriate.
C. Right coronary artery territory scar.
D. Stunned myocardium in the left anterior descending artery territory.
E. Left anterior descending artery territory scar.

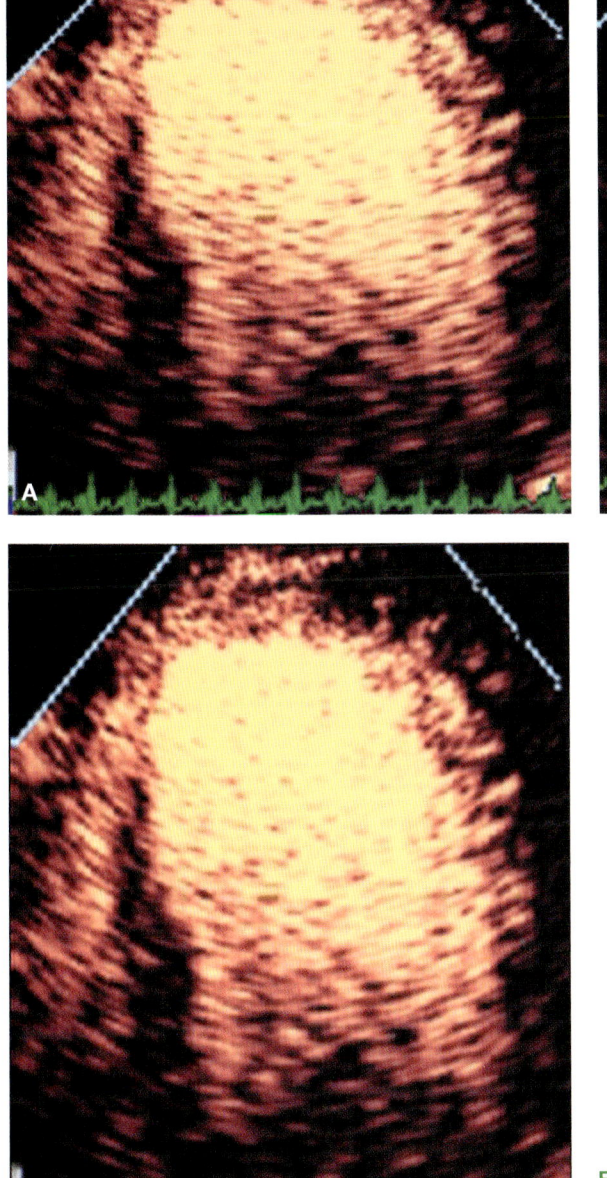

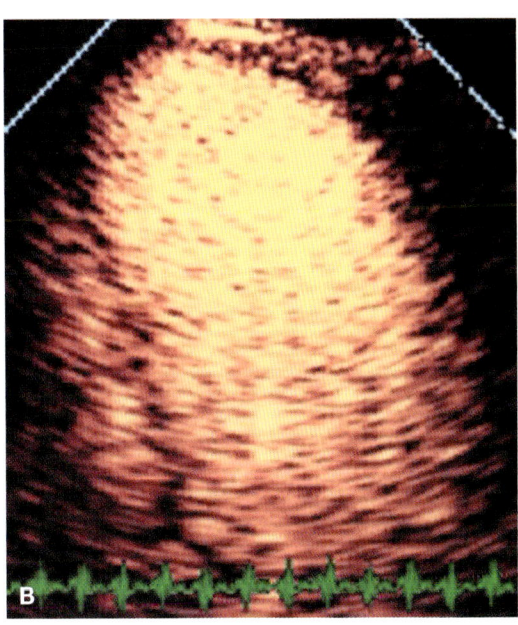

Figure 11.5. Apical 4-chamber view pre-flash (upper left), apical 4-chamber view 5 beats post-flash (lower left), apical 2-chamber view (upper right).

20. A tissue Doppler image of the lateral annulus (**Figure 11.6**) was obtained in a 34-year-old woman with bileaflet mitral valve prolapse with moderate midsystolic mitral regurgitation and a history of palpitations associated with non-sustained ventricular tachycardia and syncope. **Figure 11.6** is significant for what reason?
   A. It demonstrates a high-velocity S′ wave, which suggests there is hyperdynamic left ventricular systolic function.
   B. It demonstrates a normal e′ velocity, which suggests there is hyperdynamic left ventricular systolic function.
   C. There is no significance to mitral annular tissue Doppler in patients with mitral valve prolapse and mitral regurgitation.
   D. It demonstrates a high-velocity S′ wave, which suggests enhanced systolic tethering of the mitral annulus.

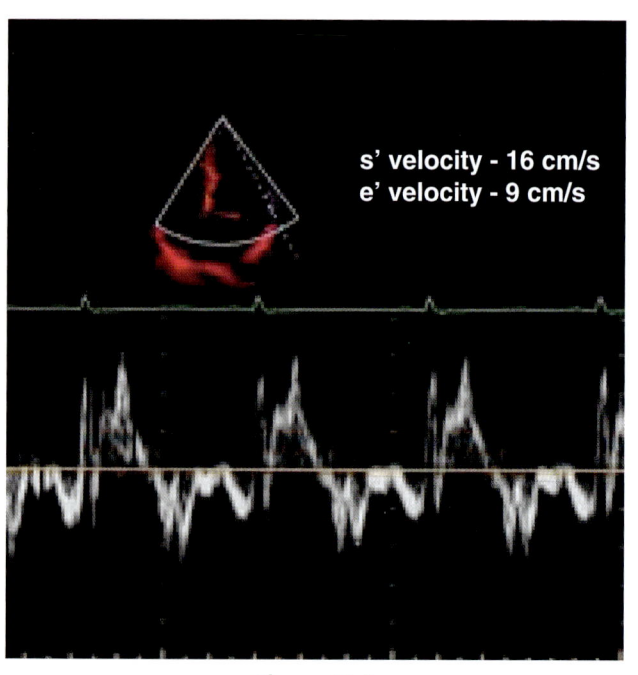

Figure 11.6

21. A 77-year-old man with congestive heart failure undergoes a transthoracic echocardiogram. Findings include severe increased left ventricular (LV) wall thickness with preserved LV systolic function. Tissue Doppler image of the lateral mitral annulus is shown with corresponding values for s′, e′, and a′ in **Figure 11.7**.
Which of the following diagnoses is most likely?
   A. Hypertrophic cardiomyopathy.
   B. Hypertensive heart disease.
   C. Fabry disease.
   D. Amyloidosis.
   E. Sarcoidosis.

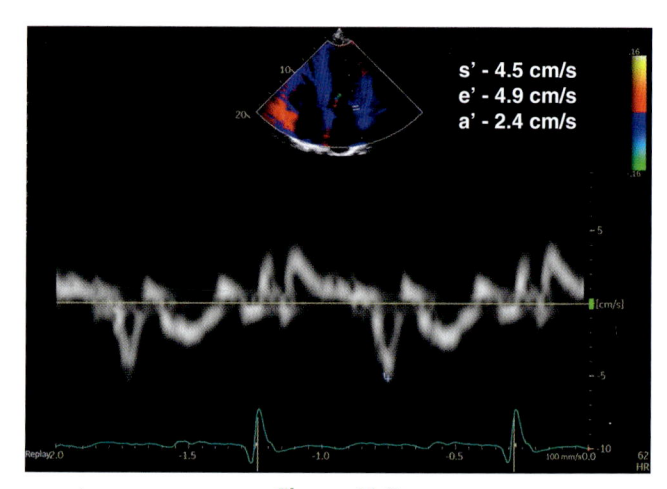

Figure 11.7

22. A 58-year-old man presents for follow-up of aortic regurgitation. He is asymptomatic with average functional capacity. Echocardiogram shows an LVEF = 55%, LVIDd = 6.2 cm, LVIDs = 4.2 cm, and ROA = 0.35 cm^2 with flow reversal in the abdominal aorta. Additional GLS imaging is performed and shown in **Figure 11.8**.
Which of the following statements is most appropriate?
   A. There is no ACC/AHA guideline indication for surgery and prognosis is very good.
   B. Surgery is indicated based on ACC/AHA guidelines.
   C. There is no ACC/AHA guideline indication for surgery, but patient will likely have a poorer long-term survival.
   D. Surgery is indicated based on ACC/AHA guidelines but prognosis is poor.

Chapter 11 Systolic Function Assessment / 233

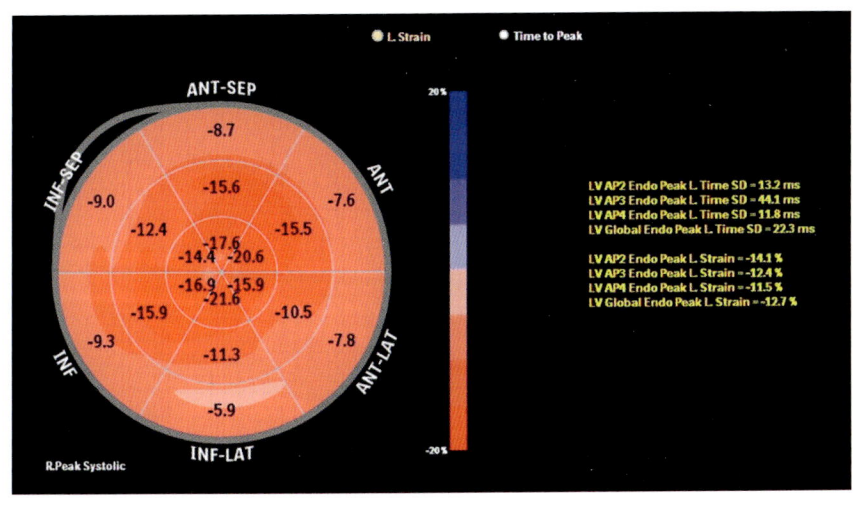

Figure 11.8

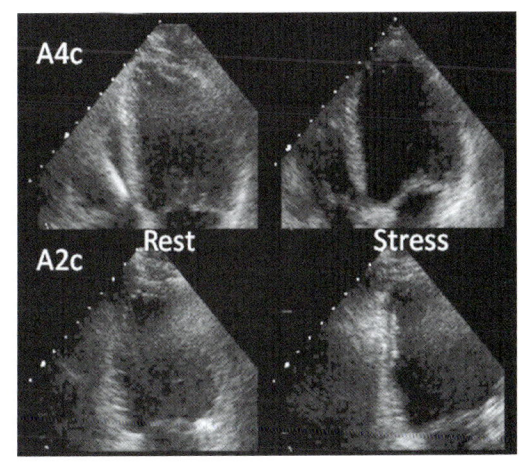

Figure 11.9

23. An asymptomatic patient with normal LV function but severe MR has bileaflet prolapse. She is uncertain as to whether to proceed to mitral repair and undergoes an exercise echocardiogram. The apical 4- and 2-chamber views (**Figure 11.9** and ▶ **Video 11.3**) before and after exercise suggest:

A. Normal LV response to stress.
B. Left anterior descending artery territory scar.
C. Loss of contractile reserve.
D. Right coronary artery territory scar.
E. Left circumflex artery territory scar.

CASE 1

A 72-year-old woman undergoes an echocardiogram because of heart failure symptoms.

24. The resting wall motion abnormalities suggest infarctions in (**Figures 11.10** and **11.11**; ▶ **Video 11.4**):

A. No discrete territory (nonischemic cardiomyopathy).
B. Left anterior descending territory.
C. Right coronary artery territory.
D. Left circumflex artery territory.
E. Multiple vessels.

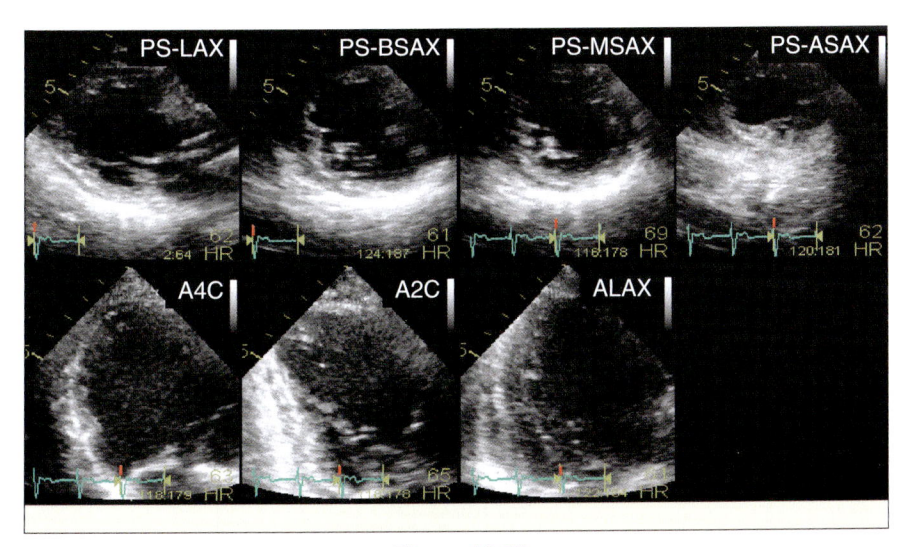

Figure 11.10

234 / Clinical Echocardiography Review

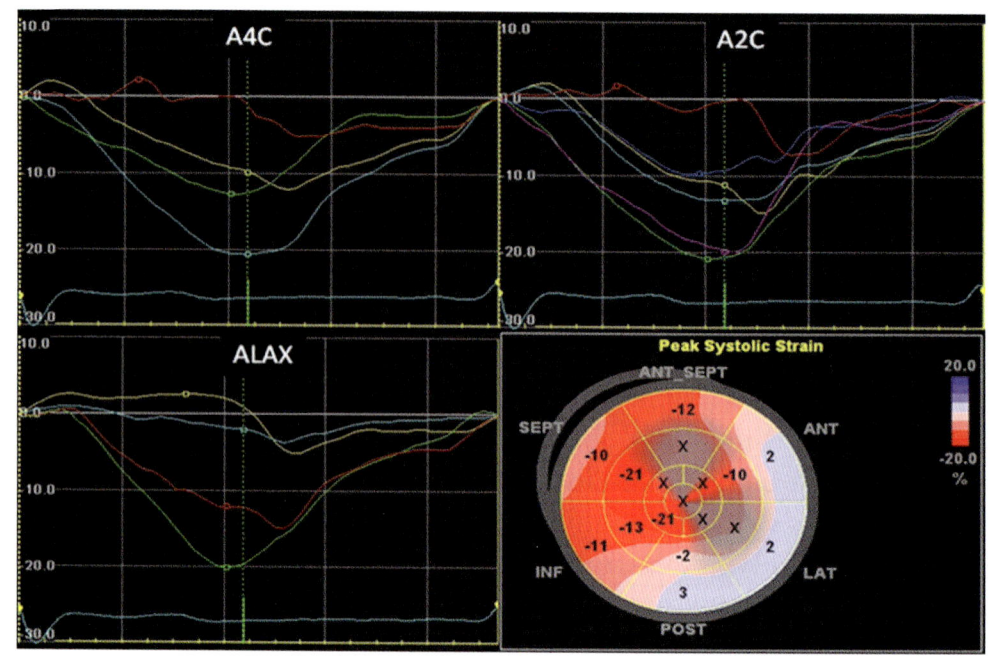

Figure 11.11

25. The strain pattern in the posterior wall of **Figure 11.12** suggests:
    A. No discrete abnormality.
    B. Loss of longitudinal function in the base but not the apex.
    C. Loss of longitudinal function in the apex but not the base.
    D. Loss of longitudinal function in both the apex and the base.
    E. Loss of thickening in the whole posterior wall.

CASE 2

A 63-year-old man undergoes an echocardiography prior to stress echocardiography. The biplane Simpson EF is 37% (end-diastolic volume 172 mL, end-systolic volume 108 mL).

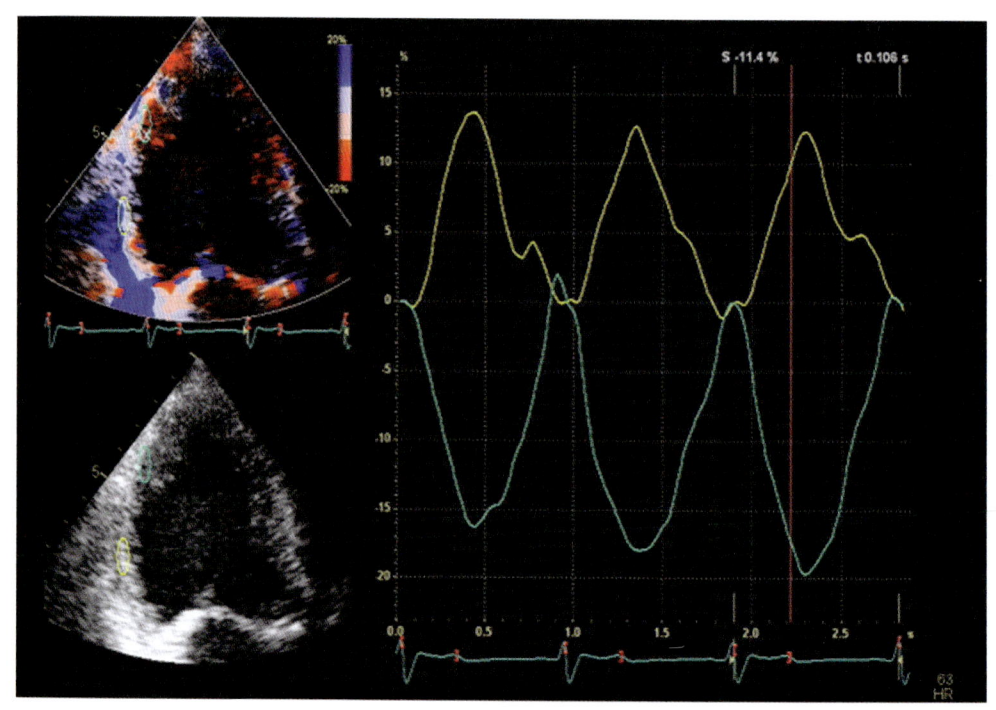

Figure 11.12

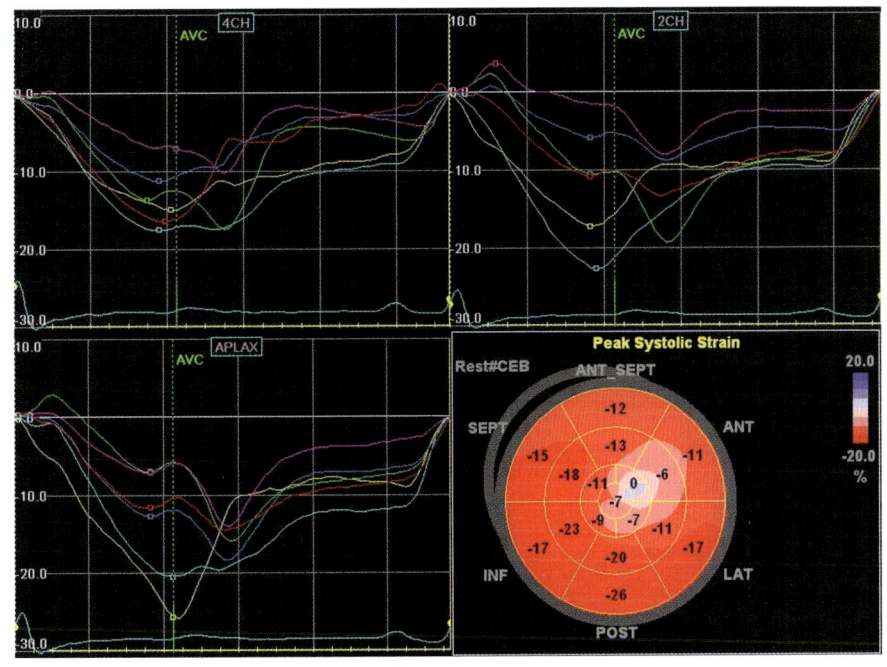

Figure 11.13

26. In the presence of a mean global strain of 14% and segmental waveforms as shown in **Figure 11.13** and ▶ **Video 11.5**, the findings:
    A. Are concordant in showing mildly reduced LV function.
    B. Show a discrepancy between radial and longitudinal function.
    C. Underestimate the severity of LV dysfunction.
    D. Show extensive late contraction (which may identify viability).
    E. The problem appears to be nonischemic.

27. The resting wall motion abnormalities suggest infarctions in (**Figure 11.14** and ▶ **Video 11.6**):
    A. No discrete territory (nonischemic cardiomyopathy).
    B. Left anterior descending artery territory.
    C. Right coronary artery territory.
    D. Left circumflex artery territory.
    E. Multiple vessels.

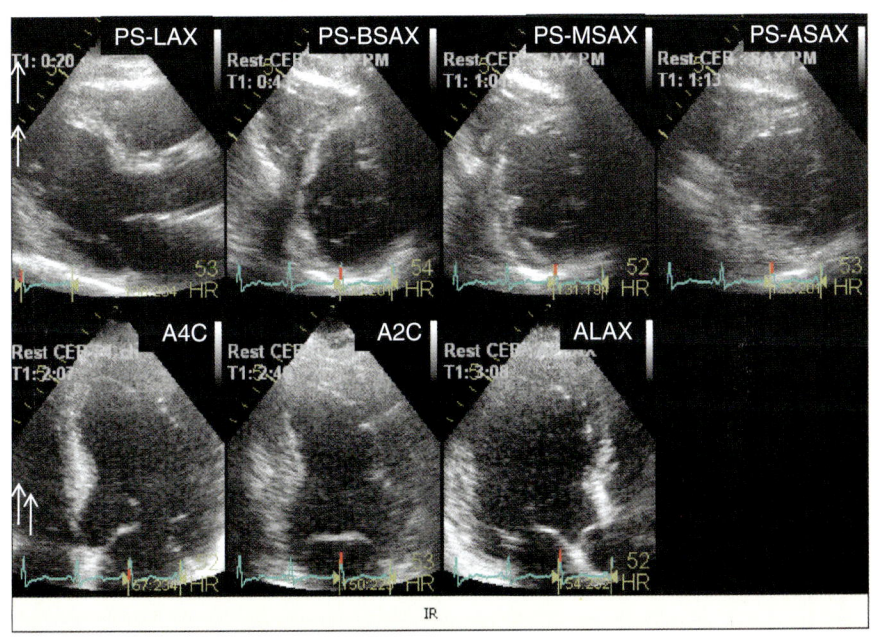

Figure 11.14

CASE 3

After an inferior myocardial infarction, this 68-year-old woman developed heart failure, and a new systolic murmur was noted.

28. The baseline echocardiogram (**Figure 11.15** and ▶ **Video 11.7A-C**) demonstrates severe, posteriorly directed MR due to:
    A. Papillary muscle rupture.
    B. Anterior mitral valve prolapse.
    C. Severe LV dysfunction.
    D. Mitral annular enlargement.
    E. Posterior mitral leaflet restriction.

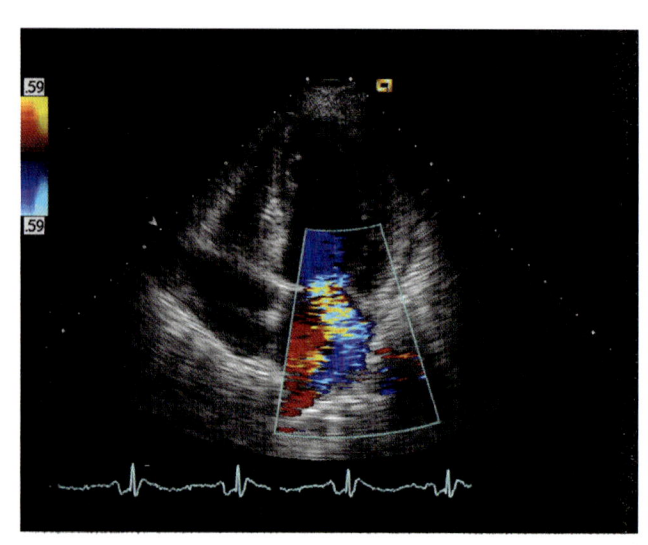

Figure 11.15

CASE 4

*A 63-year-old woman presents to the hospital after reversing her vehicle into another car at a shopping center. She had developed chest pain after an altercation with the other driver, followed by increasing dyspnea. She has anterior ST segment elevation and an echocardiogram is performed because of pulmonary congestion. You are unable to view movie images remotely, so the fellow uses the strain software to send deformation traces of the apical views (**Figure 11.16**).*

29. These findings are consistent with:
    A. Cardiac contusion.
    B. Large anteroseptal myocardial infarction.
    C. Stress (takotsubo) cardiomyopathy.
    D. Multivessel ischemia.
    E. None of the above.

30. What other potential explanations for dyspnea and pulmonary congestion associated with stress cardiomyopathy may be present?
    A. Left ventricular (LV) outflow tract obstruction.
    B. Increased LV diastolic pressure.
    C. Mitral regurgitation.
    D. All of the above.
    E. None of the above.

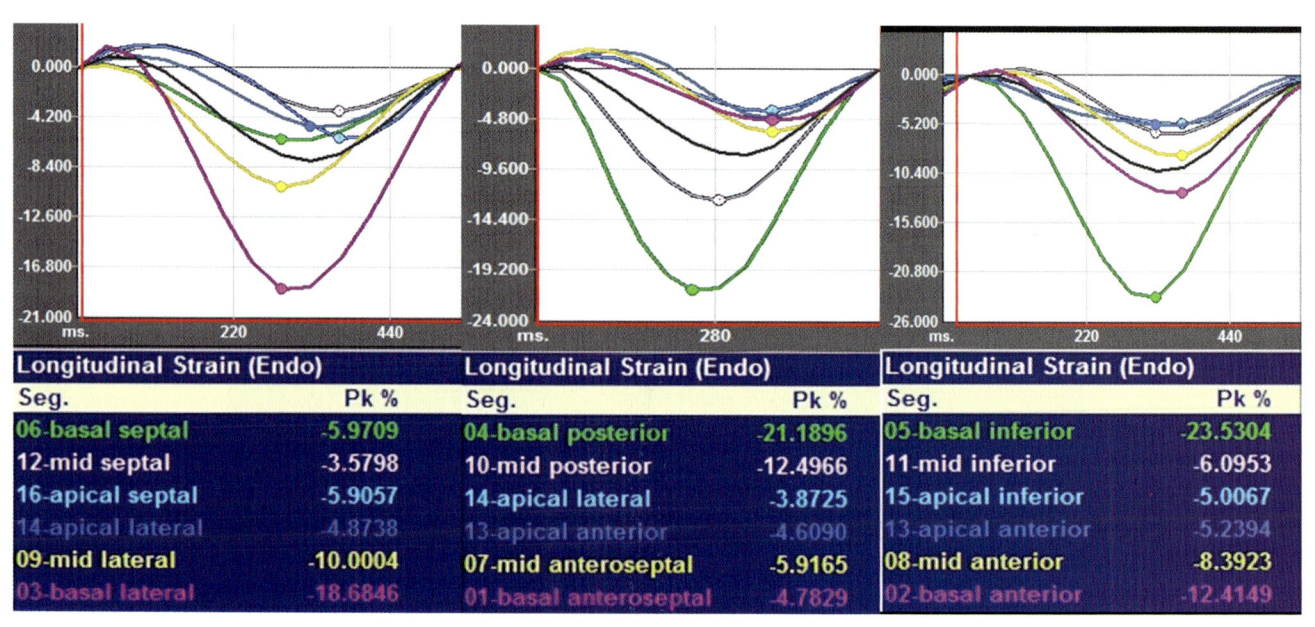

Longitudinal Strain (Endo)	
Seg.	Pk %
06-basal septal	-5.9709
12-mid septal	-3.5798
16-apical septal	-5.9057
14-apical lateral	-4.8738
09-mid lateral	-10.0004
03-basal lateral	-18.6846

Longitudinal Strain (Endo)	
Seg.	Pk %
04-basal posterior	-21.1896
10-mid posterior	-12.4966
14-apical lateral	-3.8725
13-apical anterior	-4.6090
07-mid anteroseptal	-5.9165
01-basal anteroseptal	-4.7829

Longitudinal Strain (Endo)	
Seg.	Pk %
05-basal inferior	-23.5304
11-mid inferior	-6.0953
15-apical inferior	-5.0067
13-apical anterior	-5.2394
08-mid anterior	-8.3923
02-basal anterior	-12.4149

Figure 11.16

CASE 5

A 39-year-old man presents with heart failure.

31. The LV findings are consistent with (**Figure 11.17A,B** and ▶ **Video 11.8A-D**):

A. Apical hypertrophic cardiomyopathy.
B. Laminated apical thrombus.
C. LV noncompaction.
D. Hemangioma of the LV.
E. None of the above.

32. The LV filling pattern in the same patient (**Figure 11.18**) identifies:
A. Restrictive filling pattern.
B. Grade 2 diastolic dysfunction.
C. Atrial fibrillation.
D. Mitral regurgitation

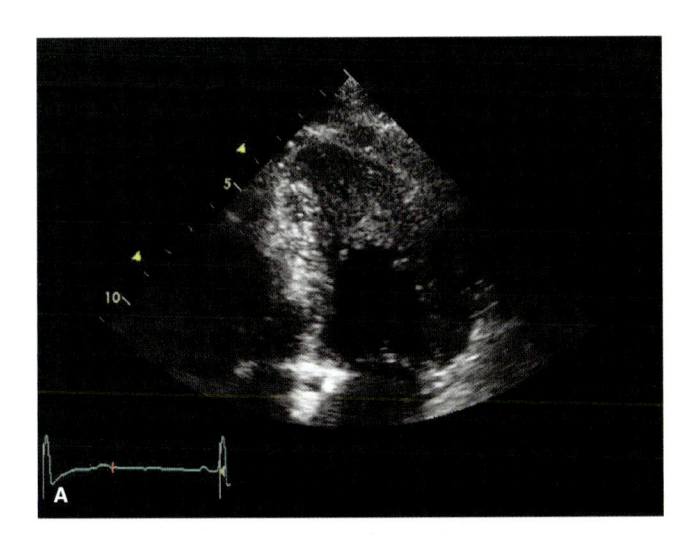

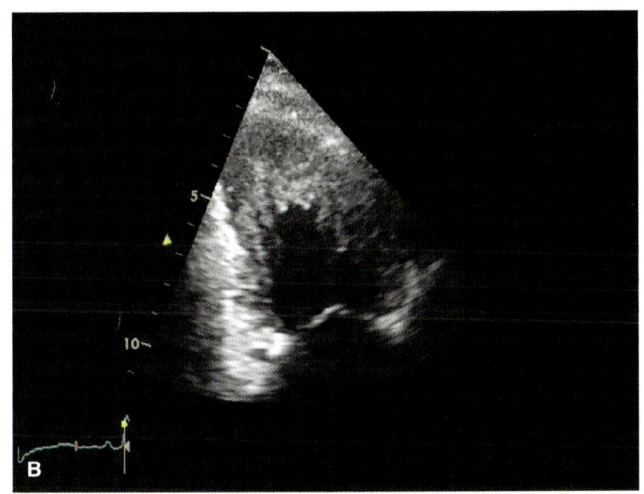

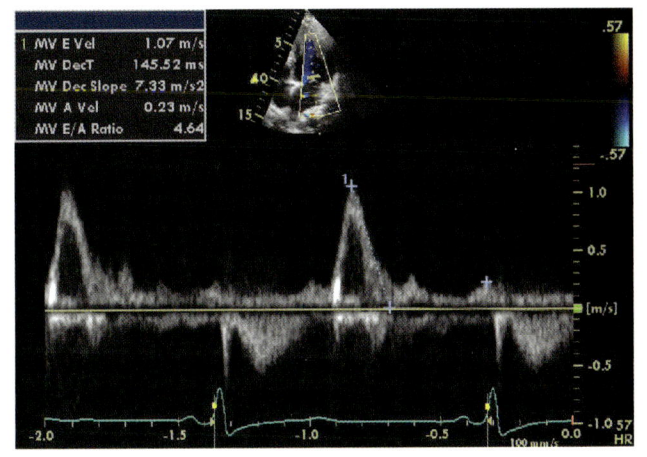

Figure 11.18

Figure 11.17. **A:** Apical 4-chamber view. **B:** Apical 2-chamber view.

ANSWERS

1. **Answer: B.** Contractility is a term that is often misused to describe systolic function. In fact, this parameter describes systolic function independent of loading. Changes in cardiac function can be attributed to alterations in contractility if heart rate, conduction velocity, preload, and afterload are held constant. Strain rate corresponds to the contractility marker, dp/dt. In contrast, ejection fraction and the Tei index are load-dependent. Strain has been described in some reviews as load-independent, but this is mistaken. The assessment of myocardial work is a relatively new technique that takes account of blood pressure by creating a hypothetical pressure-strain loop (**Figure 11.19**), effectively superimposing the product of pressure and strain on the end-systolic and end-diastolic points of the strain curve. The global work index (GWI) is the average work calculated from the area of the pressure-strain loop. The software calculates constructive work (CW, positive work during systole and negative work during isovolumic relaxation), wasted work (WW, negative work during systole and positive work during isovolumic relaxation), and work efficiency (CW/[CW + WW]). Normal ranges,

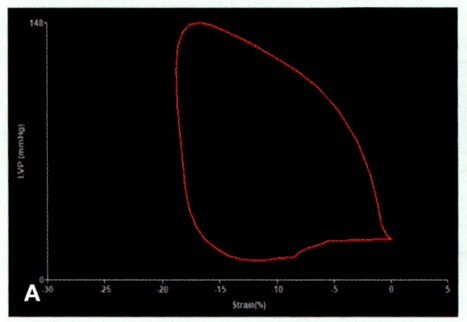

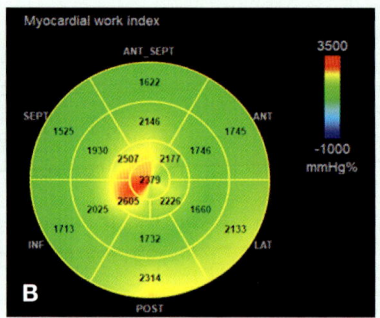

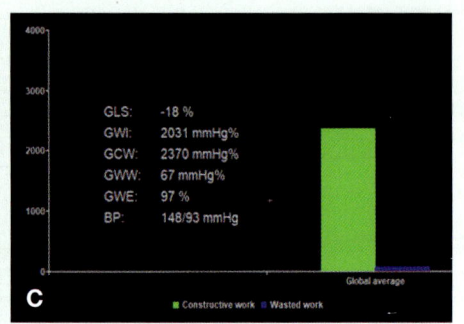

Figure 11.19. Assessment of myocardial work in a patient with hypertension but a normal heart. **A:** The first step is integration of BP (estimated left ventricular pressure, y-axis) and strain (x-axis). **B:** The resulting work index (area within the curve) can be expressed globally and regionally. **C:** Assessment of work during various intervals (see text) allows calculation of constructive and wasted work and work efficiency.

developed in the EACVI's NORRE study, show substantial variance (**Table 11.1**). The other problems are that it is only available from one manufacturer and averages work throughout systole, so it might be considered a marker of "average contractility." Although LV dp/dt can be measured from the MR jet, this is restricted to when an MR signal is available and may be compromised in severe MR, as the calculation assumes that LA pressure is zero.

Table 11.1. Normal Ranges From EACVI's NORRE Study

Parameter	Normal—Males	Normal—Females
GWI (mm Hg%)	1270-2428	1310-2538
GCW (mm Hg%)	1650-2807	1543-2924
GWW (mm Hg%)	238 ± 33	239 ± 39
GWE (%)	90 ± 1.6	91 ± 1

EACVI, European Association of Cardiovascular Imaging.

2. Answer: E. The diagnosis of RV infarction should be suspected with hemodynamic changes in a patient after inferior MI, and echocardiography is confirmatory in a qualitative sense. The problem relates to quantitation—the RV is a nongeometric chamber and 2D volumes are often underestimated because images are frequently off-axis. Depending on whether end-systolic and end-diastolic volumes are underestimated to the same degree (they may not be), 2D EF (or fractional area change) may even vary according to view. TAPSE, RV S', and strain reflect longitudinal displacement. Although they offer a means of overcoming the geometric limitations of EF calculation in global RV dysfunction, they are regional measures that may be influenced by the site of MI. Potentially, they might be averaged over multiple segments (this necessitates an RV view orthogonal to the standard 4-chamber view). The Tei index is also a reasonable choice, as it is independent of RV geometry but is not purely a measure of systolic function. RV systolic function is notoriously difficult to quantify! 3D echocardiography (3DE) can overcome the complexities that derive from its crescentic and irregular shape, and a variety of software approaches have become available to facilitate this measurement. RV evaluation has become an important indication for 3DE.

3. Answer: A. Wall stress appears to be a determinant of local remodeling and the development of cell therapies will eventually mandate an approach to the measurement of this entity. Wall stress is proportionate to transmural pressure and chamber size and inversely related to wall thickness. However, accurate quantification of wall stress using the law of Laplace without cognizance of material properties (or time in systole) is an oversimplification. Moreover, although global equations for stress are described, regional stress varies in accordance with regional curvature. The measurement of wall stress is one of the Holy Grails of hemodynamic assessment and should be matched to systolic strain—although there are sufficient ranges of error with the measurement of both as to make this correlation difficult with current technologies.

4. Answer: E. Visual EF should not be considered the "standard of care"; current guidelines propose the biplane Simpson method as the methodology of choice for volume and EF measurement and support the use of 3D echocardiography when possible. Accuracy and reproducibility are especially important when echo measurements of EF may be a component of major decisions, such as suitability for implantable defibrillator or cardiac resynchronization devices. However, although quantitation is accepted as the preferred method, this may not be achievable under all circumstances. As in other qualitative assessments in echocardiography, an expert eye has been shown to be analogous to the trackball for EF measurements, and it is dependent on image quality. Extremes of heart rate can make the assessment challenging and tomographic approach to the postinfarct ventricle is important.

Although quantitation is accepted as the preferred method, potential problems with respect to spatial and temporal resolution need to be considered.

Concerns about spatial resolution can be addressed by appropriate depth and zoom; LV opacification should be considered if two or more myocardial segments are inadequately visualized. Temporal resolution is an issue to the extent that the time course of contraction is neglected by assessment of only end-diastolic and end-systolic images, and global strain and strain rate may help address this.

5. **Answer: C.** Wall motion abnormalities are usually identified with thickening of <50% or excursion <5 mm. They are not necessarily a marker of abnormal myocardium (normal inferior and posterior walls in particular may be hypokinetic) and do not necessarily indicate ischemia (they may be preexisting). Wall thickening (rather than motion or timing) is interpretable with a LBBB. The extent and severity of wall motion abnormality have similar prognostic values to ejection fraction.

6. **Answer: C.** The benefit of AV optimization is supported by its performance in the landmark CRT studies and smaller trials. The most feasible is the iterative technique for AV optimization. This involves pulsed Doppler mitral inflow estimation, with shortening and lengthening of AV delay, and observation of the morphology of the transmitral filling wave. If AV delay is too short, ventricular activation will occur before completion of the mitral A wave. If AV delay is too long, ventricular systole will encroach on diastolic filling time. At the optimal setting of paced AV delay, the time-velocity integral of transmitral flow will be optimized, with no truncation of the mitral A wave (see **Figure 11.20**).

Patient selection for CRT is based on clinical, ECG, and ejection fraction criteria. Despite the best efforts for appropriate selection, 30% of implanted subjects fail to demonstrate a symptomatic or physiologic response to CRT. However, while enthusiasm for using measures of mechanical synchrony (tissue Doppler and strain) has abated since the report of the PROSPECT trial, newer work has pointed toward the value of septal "flash" (an early systolic inward motion of the septum, before the delayed lateral wall contracts) and apical rocking (seen in the 4-chamber view as movement toward the septum as this shortens in early systole, and then toward the lateral as delayed lateral contraction occurs in late systole) as markers of mechanical dyssynchrony (**Figure 11.21** and ▶ **Video 11.9**). Nonetheless,

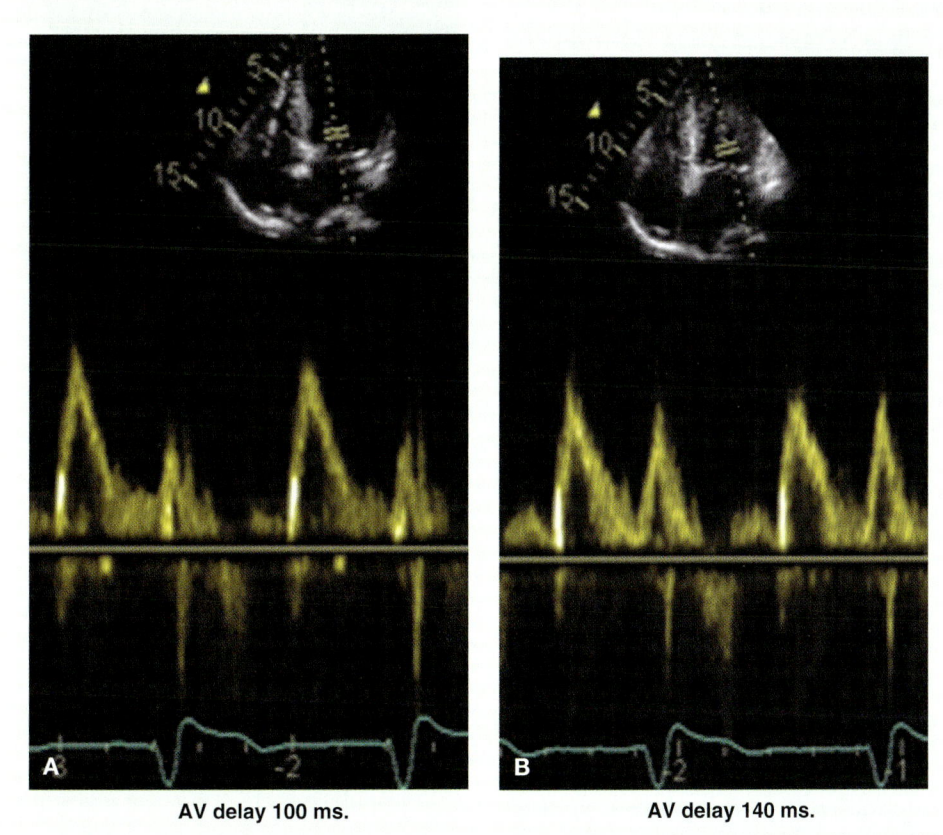

Figure 11.20. A: AV delay 100 ms. **B:** AV delay 140 ms. The iterative method for optimization of atrioventricular delay using pulsed-wave Doppler of mitral inflow. The initial AV delay setting of 100 ms shows truncation of the mitral A wave. Optimization at 140 ms avoids truncation of the mitral A wave and maintains an optimal time-velocity integral. Further lengthening of AV delay would be at the cost of delayed systole encroaching on passive filling.

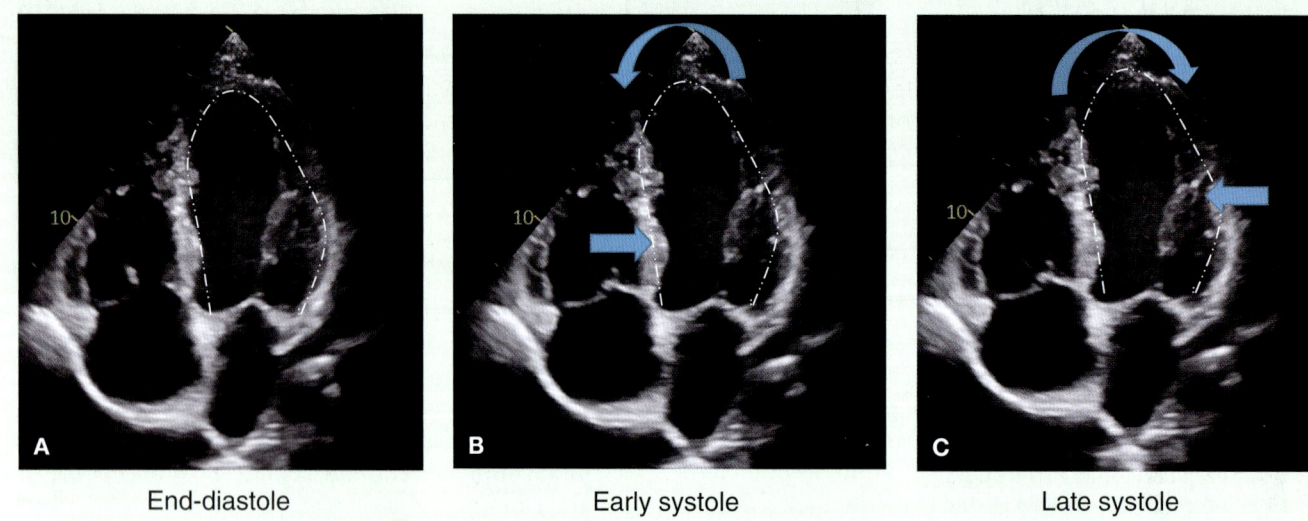

Figure 11.21. View in association with ▶ **Video 11.9**. Evidence of mechanical dyssynchrony by 2D echocardiography. Compared to end diastole, early systole shows septal motion ("septal flash") and motion of the apex toward the septum. Late systole shows delayed movement of the lateral wall, and apical movement toward the lateral wall ("apical rocking").

these considerations are relevant to selection rather than optimization.

The adverse effects of extensive scarring and lead malposition on CRT response have been shown by studies showing response to be predicted by concordance between pacing site and strain magnitude and/or time to maximal delay. However, the site of previous infarction and position of the LV lead offer limited opportunities for optimization.

7. **Answer: D.** The assessment of LV volumes carries incremental prognostic information to ejection fraction alone. Angiographic data have shown that in patients with mild LV dysfunction, end-systolic volume (ESV) <95 mL is associated with a 5-year mortality of 10%, but more dilated ventricles are associated with a much worse outcome (30%), and similar findings have been described with echocardiography. Because of avoidance of geometric assumptions, 3D echocardiography may be especially useful for assessment of volumes (see **Figure 11.22**). The evidence of incremental information on the basis of LV volumes is an argument for more accurate LV volume calculations (eg, with 3D echocardiography). Importantly, these studies have assessed systolic volume rather than diastolic volume, which may be increased in the setting of mitral regurgitation.

8. **Answer: D.** Repeat 2D echocardiography—although often performed for the reassessment of LV function—is not a sensitive or reliable tool for this purpose. The reliability of a measurement is often expressed as 95% confidence intervals (95% CI). Applied to EF, the 95% CI is ±11%, meaning that 95% of estimations are within an absolute difference of 11% from the actual EF, or only 2.5% of measurements are less than the actual one. What this means in real life is that an EF of 40% is highly likely to be abnormal, whereas an EF of 46% is not. For LV

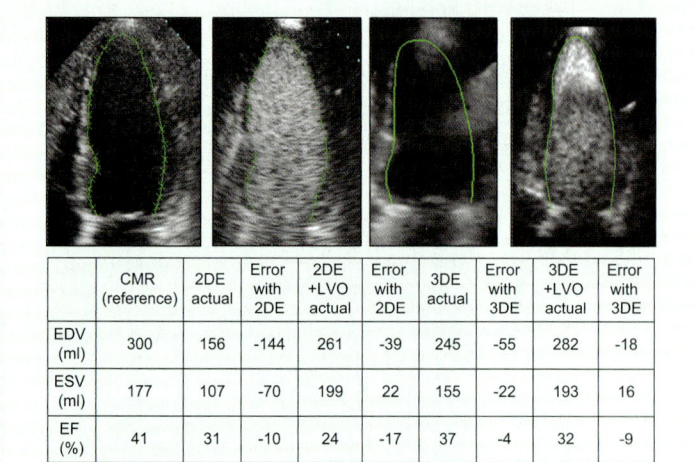

	CMR (reference)	2DE actual	Error with 2DE	2DE +LVO actual	Error with 2DE	3DE actual	Error with 3DE	3DE +LVO actual	Error with 3DE
EDV (ml)	300	156	-144	261	-39	245	-55	282	-18
ESV (ml)	177	107	-70	199	22	155	-22	193	16
EF (%)	41	31	-10	24	-17	37	-4	32	-9

Figure 11.22. Comparison of LVEDV measurements with 2D and 3D echocardiography with and without contrast, with measurements compared with MRI EDV of 300 mL. The above illustration and table shows the degree of underestimation (difference in volume) between 4 echo techniques (2D and 3D, with and without contrast) and MRI. The underestimation by 2D echocardiography is substantially reversed by the use of 3D echocardiography or contrast and minimized by the combination of both. EF, ejection fraction; ESV, end-systolic volume; LVEDV, left ventricular end-diastolic volume; LVO, left ventricular outflow.

mass, the 95% CI is ±60 g. Both are large changes in biologic terms, meaning that minor changes (such as may occur from year to year in the progression of heart failure—maybe 5%—or in response to antihypertensive therapy over a year or two—maybe 20 g) are well under the limits of variability of the measurement. The resulting changes are more meaningful in populations than they are in individuals.

Sources of variability include not only intra- and interobserver variation but also acquisition issues (equipment and sonographers), regression to mean, and biologic variation. As some of this variation arises from differences in imaging axis between studies, it is potentially reducible using 3D imaging techniques, and there is some evidence to support this.

9. **Answer: B.** Strain can be considered as an analog of regional ejection, as it reflects shortening from the beginning to the end of systole. Reduced preload—which is associated with reduced LV cavity size—will reduce strain, reflecting the lower position of the ventricle on the Frank-Starling curve as well as the lower deformation of an already empty LV cavity. Conversely, reduction of afterload is associated with increased strain, reflecting the lower impedance to LV ejection. Higher heart rate is associated with a reduction of LV filling and reduced strain. These observations are important in understanding the strain and strain rate response to dobutamine stress. Strain rate (which is time dependent) shows a linear increment with dobutamine, whereas strain increases initially but decreases toward peak dose, as the stroke volume falls at higher heart rates.

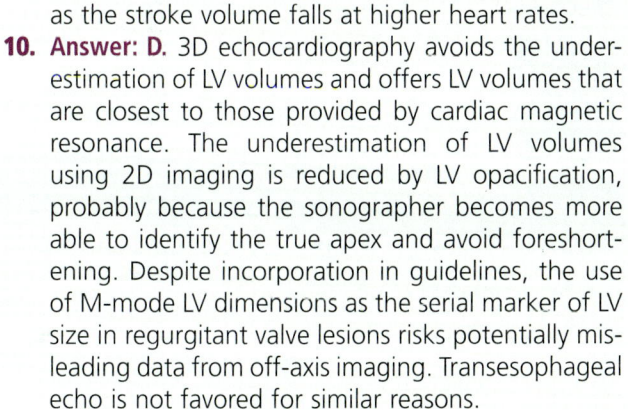

10. **Answer: D.** 3D echocardiography avoids the underestimation of LV volumes and offers LV volumes that are closest to those provided by cardiac magnetic resonance. The underestimation of LV volumes using 2D imaging is reduced by LV opacification, probably because the sonographer becomes more able to identify the true apex and avoid foreshortening. Despite incorporation in guidelines, the use of M-mode LV dimensions as the serial marker of LV size in regurgitant valve lesions risks potentially misleading data from off-axis imaging. Transesophageal echo is not favored for similar reasons.

11. **Answer: A.** The ability to derive strain from 2D images (rather than tissue Doppler, which is directional) has enabled strain assessment in not only the longitudinal but also the circumferential plane. Subendocardial dysfunction causes a reduction of longitudinal function (as subendocardial fibers have a longitudinal orientation). Infarctions of relatively limited extent may cause a reduction in longitudinal strain, and the susceptibility of this to worsening strain in proportion to the infarct extent is not completely clear. However, the degree of reduction of circumferential strain is related to the transmural extent of subendocardial dysfunction (see **Figure 11.23**).

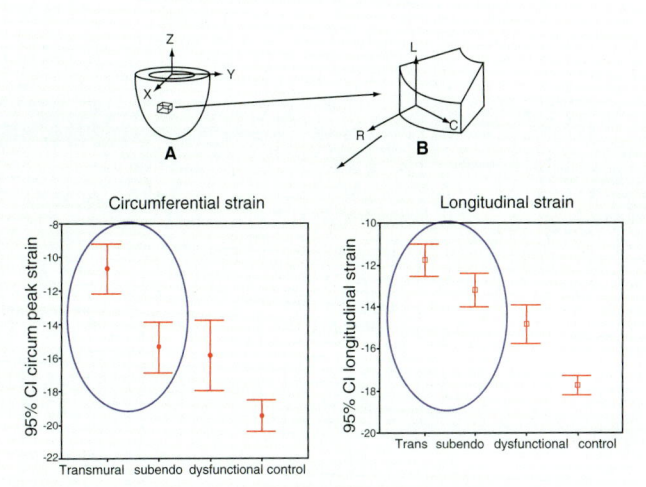

Figure 11.23. Derivation of longitudinal, circumferential, and transverse strain as the association of these with scar extent, defined by contrast-enhanced magnetic resonance imaging.

Radial (or transverse) strain is not a reliable clinical marker, probably because the numbers of speckles are insufficient for accurate measurement.

Real-time perfusion imaging has been used to delineate the extent of subendocardial scar, as flow and function can be appreciated in the same sequence (triggered imaging provides perfusion data alone).

12. **Answer: C.** There has been a prolific expansion of new technologies, and it has been difficult to keep track of which modality can help with which clinical question. Generally, tissue velocity has been useful for timing (eg, synchrony) and measurement of global phenomena (eg, e' velocity), but it is subject to tethering by adjacent segments, so it is not a good marker of segmental function. Accurate volumetric measurements are possible with 3D, but at a low temporal resolution. It seems unlikely this modality will be useful for the assessment of diastolic function, where the time for volume changes is critical. Deformation analysis with speckle strain can provide information on the transmural distribution of scar, and the response to low-dose dobutamine has been quantified with both tissue velocity and speckle strain (see **Table 11.2**).

Table 11.2. Contributions of New Technologies to Particular Diagnostic Questions

	Tissue Doppler	Deformation[a] (TVI and 2D)	3D Volumes
Systolic dysfunction	+	++	++
Viability	–	++	–
Ischemia	–	++	–
Diastolic dysfunction	++	–	–
LV synchrony	++	–	+
Myocardial characterization	++	++	–

[a]Strain imaging can be used for assessing viability, and the morphology of the wave form may be informative in assessing ischemia. The initial (and most robust) ischemia data were obtained with strain rate (SR), but time-velocity integral (TVI)-based SR is technically challenging and the temporal resolution of current speckle strain is too low. The feasibility of speckle SR may improve as high frame rate acquisitions become available.

Table 11.3. Combinations of HF Risk Factors, Cardiac Function and Structure Disturbances and Clinical Features

	HF History	HF Signs	Abnormal Structure/Function	Risk Factors for HF
Normal	No	No	No	No
Stage A	No	No	No	Yes
Stage B	No	No	Yes	Yes
Stage C1	No	Yes	Yes	Yes
Stage C2	Yes	No	Yes	Yes
Stage D	Yes	Yes	Yes	Yes

13. **Answer: E.** The ongoing adverse outcomes associated with heart failure have spurred an increasing interest in recognition of the earlier stages of heart failure and attempts to prevent progression. The main contribution of tissue velocity has been for the assessment of tissue e', which is a sensitive marker of myocardial impairment that may be reduced even in the presence of risk factors, and in the estimation of LV filling pressure, which may support the diagnosis of later-stage heart failure. Myocardial strain may be a sign of preclinical dysfunction in early-stage disease, although its ability to quantify scar may also make it helpful in later disease. The main contributions of LV volume calculation are of most value in late-stage disease, where the LV cavity is dilated and EF reduced (see **Table 11.3**).

14. **Answer: C.**

    Relative wall thickness (RWT) = 2 × PWd/LVd

    = 2 × 13/52 = 0.5.

    Both LV mass and LV geometry are important determinants of outcome. In this patient, both LV mass and relative wall thickness are increased, indicating concentric LVH. Concentric remodeling (wall thickening without increased mass) is also associated with adverse outcome (**Figure 11.24**). Eccentric hypertrophy relates to increased mass that is driven by LV enlargement—indeed the walls may not be particularly thick. This too is associated with adverse outcome.

    The question is often raised as to whether it is acceptable to add IVS + PW (rather than 2PW) to determine RWT. The problem with doing this is that the parameter has been defined based on PW, and hence the prognostic evidence pertains to this. The use of PW also avoids the potential for overestimation due to the basal septal bulge—which is problematic in the very patients with hypertensive heart disease in whom remodeling would be desirable to measure.

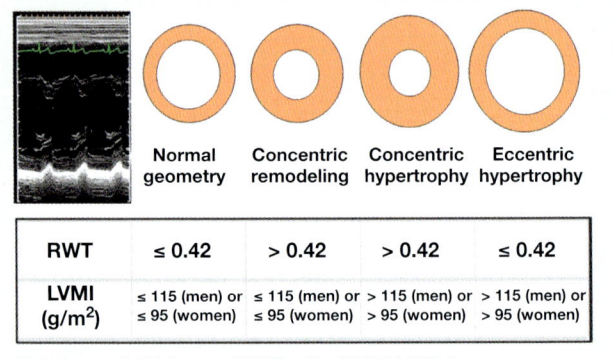

	Normal geometry	Concentric remodeling	Concentric hypertrophy	Eccentric hypertrophy
RWT	≤ 0.42	> 0.42	> 0.42	≤ 0.42
LVMI (g/m²)	≤ 115 (men) or ≤ 95 (women)	≤ 115 (men) or ≤ 95 (women)	> 115 (men) or > 95 (women)	> 115 (men) or > 95 (women)

Relative wall thickness (RWT) = 2 × PWd / LVDd.
LV mass index (LVMI) = 1.04 ((LVDd+IVSd+PWd)^3-LVDd^3)-13.6

Figure 11.24

15. **Answer: E.** All of the above. Generally, an EF of ~35% corresponds to a strain of ~12%, so this case exemplifies a situation in which the degree of GLS impairment exceeds what might be expected from a relatively minor regional wall motion abnormality. GLS may be impaired by a variety of causes of subclinical LV dysfunction (impairment in asymptomatic individuals with normal ejection fraction), which may have preceded the ACS. Importantly, strain is an independent determinant of outcome, especially in the normal or near-normal LV.

16. **Answer: C.** The patient was initiated on mavacamten, a myosin inhibitor that reduces the number of myosin-actin cross-bridges and effectively reduces the hypercontractile state of hypertrophic cardiomyopathy (HCM). Attenuation of hypercontractility with HCM has been shown to reduce LVOT obstruction, improve symptoms and functional class, and reduce eligibility for septal reduction therapy. **Figure 11.2**, Panel A and B, shows continuous-wave Doppler tracings of mitral regurgitation (MR). Using the MR jet, dp/dt can be calculated, which is a surrogate measure of left ventricular contractility. Briefly, the time it takes for the pressure to go from 1 m/s to 3 ms/s is calculated (a pressure change of 32 mm

Hg), and divided by the time difference in seconds (not milliseconds). See Chapter 8: Doppler and Hemodynamics for a detailed discussion of dp/dt. For **Figure 11.2**, Panel A, before treatment the dp/dt is 1143 mm Hg/s. For **Figure 11.2**, Panel B, after treatment the dp/dt is 653 mmHg/sec. Generally, a normal dp/dt is in the range of 1300 to 1600 mm Hg/s, though this patient was also on high dose beta-blockers. None of the other choices would generally be expected to reduce the contractile state.

17. **Answer: D.** The most likely explanation is that dyspnea in this patient is not cardiac in etiology. In **Figure 11.3**, Panel A, pulsed-wave Doppler mitral inflow is notable for a low velocity e wave velocity of 40 cm/s that would typically not be associated with an elevated left atrial pressure. In **Figure 11.3**, Panel B, continuous-wave Doppler through the mitral inflow shows three waves (first wave—exaggerated flow during isovolumic relaxation period; second wave—early filling, e wave; third wave—atrial contraction, a wave). Exaggerated flow during isovolumic relaxation period (IVRP) results due to a hyperdynamic contractile function and often cavity obliteration. This results in early left ventricular relaxation and enhanced diastolic inflow from base to apex. Note that exaggerated IVRP flow is not seen by pulsed-wave Doppler at the mitral leaflet tips since the flow occurs within the cavity. The other choices HFrEF, HFpEF, and severe MR would likely have a tall mitral e wave and absent exaggerated IVRP flow due to less vigorous contraction.

18. **Answer: C.** A congenital abnormality is present, which is a left ventricular apical diverticulum. This is most evident because with systole, the apical outpouching disappears since it is contracting muscle. This is best seen in ▶ **Video 11.1**. In addition, it is very localized, not thinned, and the adjacent myocardium appears normal thickness and with normal contractility. A left ventricular diverticulum is rare and generally benign, but must be differentiated from a true aneurysm, which is a focal dilatation that is thinned, and either akinetic or dyskinetic. However, a pseudoaneurysm is a contained rupture, which usually has a narrow neck with to-and-fro low-velocity flow, stasis and surrounding hematoma, effusion, and pericardium. Both aneurysms and pseudoaneurysm are seen in the context of a sizable area of infarction. Healed muscular ventricular septal defects and clefts cause more limited discrete myocardial abnormalities.

19. **Answer: D.** Despite the apical wall motion abnormality, bubbles return to this area after the flash (arrows) (**Figure 11.25**), indicating an intact microcirculation. Although there is contrast attenuation in the right coronary artery (RCA) and left circumflex

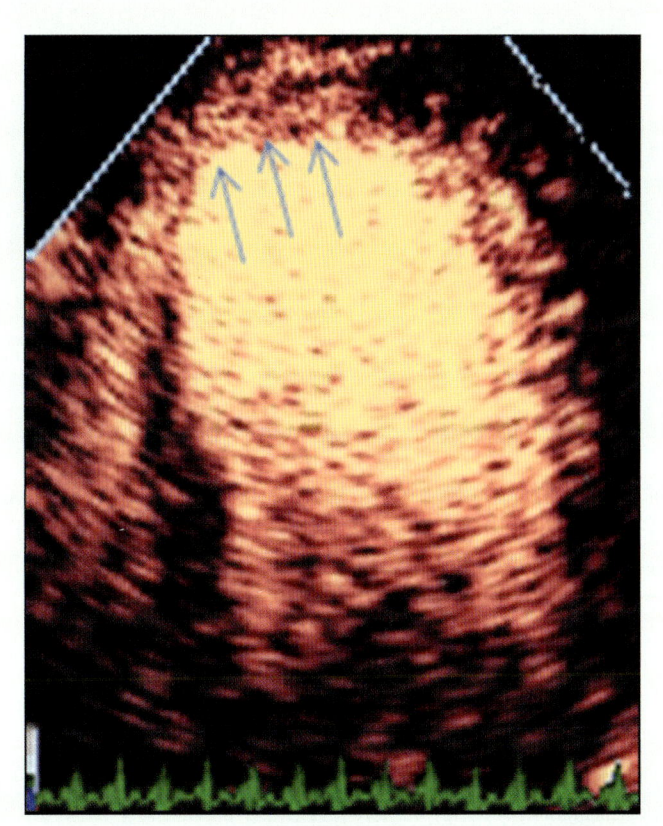

Figure 11.25

coronary artery (LCX) segments, these are still thickening. Myocardial contrast echocardiography has been used to define the transmural extent of infarction and to differentiate stunned from necrotic myocardium. Its accuracy in the prediction of functional recovery is comparable to dobutamine stress echocardiography, perfusion scintigraphy, and cardiac magnetic resonance imaging.

20. **Answer: D.** The tissue Doppler profile of the lateral mitral annulus shows a characteristic finding of malignant mitral valve prolapse (MVP), called the Pickelhaube sign. The Pickelhaube sign is so named due to the systolic tissue Doppler spiked, high peaked (high-velocity) appearance, which is similar to a German war helmet. It is thought due to the mid-systolic traction from the posterior medial papillary muscle tugging at the prolapsing leaflet and pulling the posterior basal wall rapidly toward the left ventricular apex in systole. It has been associated with various other echocardiographic features (mitral annular dysjunction, posterior left ventricular basal fibrosis, bileaflet prolapse with myxomatous leaflets) and clinical and electrocardiographic features including ventricular tachycardia and possibly sudden cardiac death.

21. **Answer: D.** Cardiac amyloidosis is the most likely diagnosis given severe increased left ventricular wall thickness and low mitral annular tissue Doppler velocities. Although not diagnostic for cardiac

244 / Clinical Echocardiography Review

amyloidosis, three 5s sign (s', e', and a' velocities <5 cm/s) should heighten suspicion. Other forms of hypertrophy like hypertrophic cardiomyopathy or hypertensive heart disease and infiltrative or storage disorders less likely have preserved LV function with severe reduction in s' (representing impaired contractile function), e' (representing impaired relaxation), and a' (representing impaired atrial contractile function).

22. **Answer: C.** There is no ACC/AHA guideline indication for surgery, but patient will likely have a poorer long-term survival. Current 2020 ACC/AHA Valvular Heart Disease Guidelines recommend surgery (2a indications) for severe aortic regurgitation (AR) in asymptomatic patients when LVEF < 55% (class 1 indication) or LVIDs > 50 mm or 25 mm/m² (class 2a indication). However, these recommendations are based on older data, and linear dimensions on echocardiography. Due to the high preload, high afterload, and high wall stress associated with severe AR, subclinical LV dysfunction may occur prior to symptoms or a decrease in LVEF < 55%. Several newer indicators for timing of surgery for severe AR include an LVIDd > 20 mm/m2 and LV GLS < −19%, which has been associated with an increased risk of mortality in patients with preserved LV function.

23. **Answer: C.** Traces of the resting dimensions have been superimposed on the postexercise image to show LV enlargement and LV dysfunction postexercise (**Figure 11.26**). Subclinical LV dysfunction may be identified on the basis of a reduced EF response or LV dilatation with exercise. No regional changes are detected.

Although technical advances have reduced the risk of failed mitral repair, the prospect of surgery may be confronting for asymptomatic patients. In this situation, the assessment of contractile reserve (CR) may permit the detection of subclinical myocyte contractile abnormalities. This may be assessed with LV volumes and EF, and also with GLS. A simpler approach may be the performance of myocardial strain imaging at rest to identify subclinical dysfunction in this setting.

24. **Answer: E.** There is thinning of the posterior wall, akinesis of the inferior and basal septal walls, and lateral hypokinesis. The apical function appears reduced in the apical 4- and 3-chamber views. This combination is most commonly seen with multivessel disease.

The accompanying strain displays show low strains in these regions, and the distribution of reduced function is summarized in the polar map display. GLS adds incremental prognostic value to both LV hypertrophy and wall motion assessment, but segmental strain remains subject to noise, and is technically difficult.

25. **Answer: B.** The behavior of the basal-mid posterior and apical walls is different. The longitudinal deformation in the basal-mid wall shows lengthening (the curve is above the baseline). In the apex, the strain curve varies between −16% and 20%, indicating normal shortening. Note that this assessment of endocardial (longitudinal) function may not correspond to the visual assessment of regional function (mainly radial). The proviso regarding the limitations of regional strain remains pertinent—strain in this setting is an adjunct rather than a replacement to visual assessment.

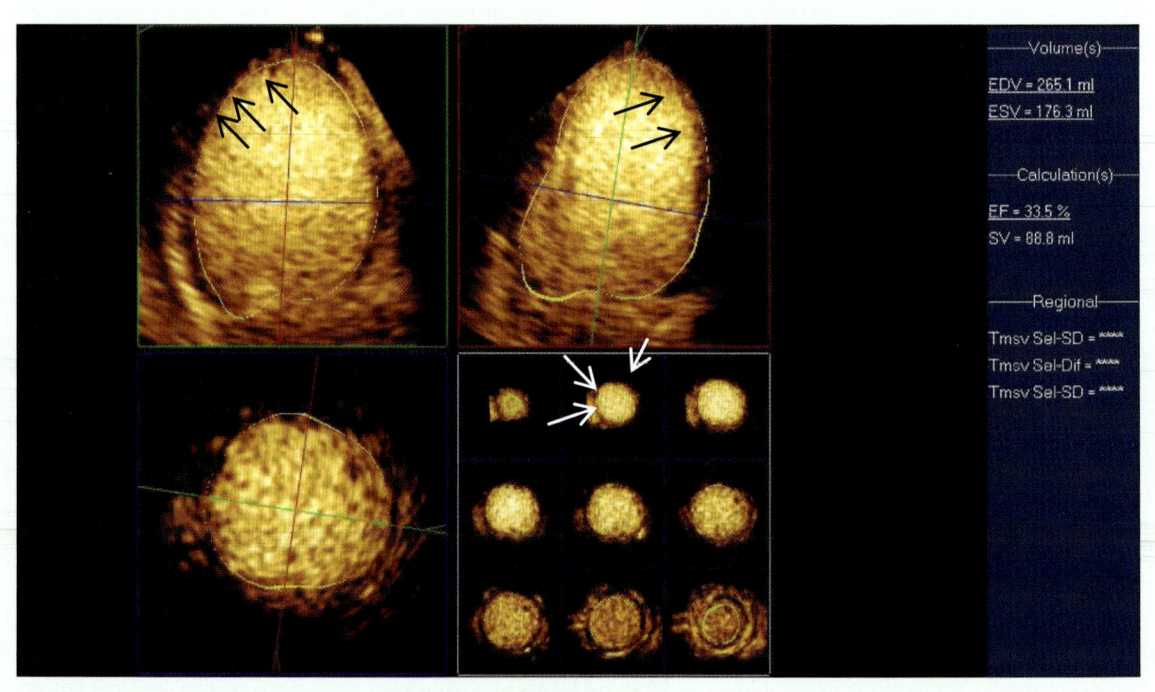

Figure 11.26

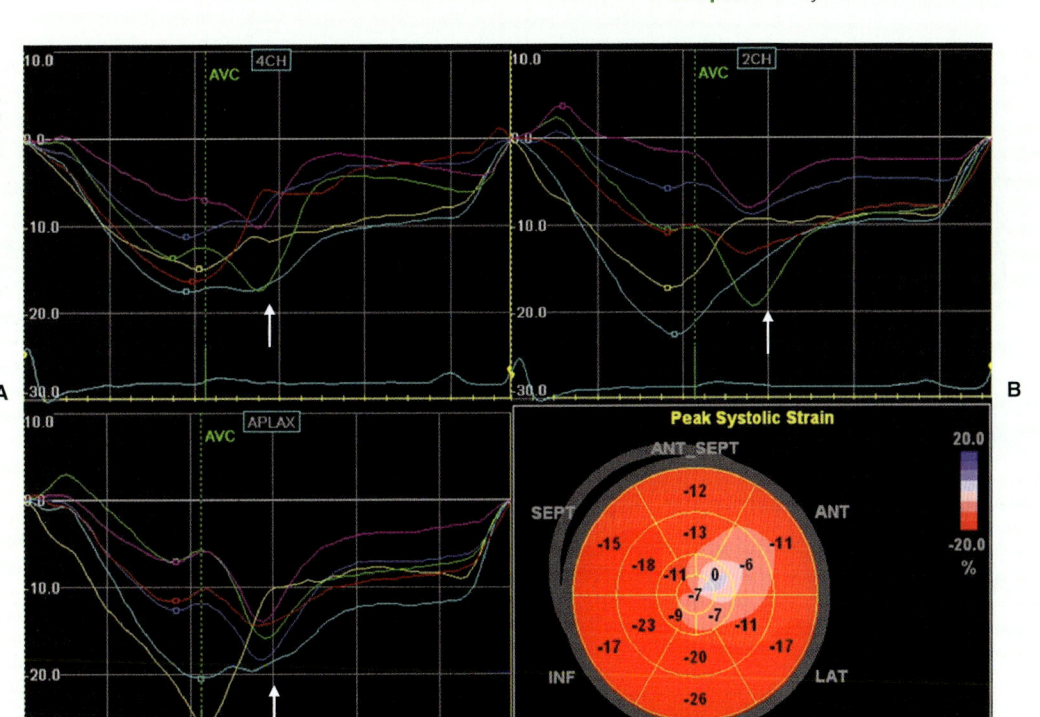

Figure 11.27

KEY POINTS

- LV wall thinning is an important clue that should not be neglected in wall motion analysis.
- Strain quantification may be readily applied to resting images and stress response and can be obtained in the longitudinal and circumferential directions. Radial strain is unreliable and should not be used.
- GLS data provide incremental prognostic information to standard analysis.

26. **Answer: D.** The strain curves in each view all include a marker for aortic valve closure (AVC). Curves relating to the left anterior descending artery territory show postsystolic contraction (ie, arrows point to peak strain following AVC). This phenomenon of postsystolic contraction can be seen in normal myocardium, but in that case is mild. It may, on occasion, be a passive phenomenon (eg, in the setting of dyskinesis), but in this case is due to the delayed development of shortening, which reflects reduction of myocardial force generation.

The other alternatives are incorrect. Findings of 37% EF and global strain of −14% both attest to moderate LV dysfunction and seem analogous (A, C). Radial strain is unreliable, and not measured in this case, although 2D imaging provides information on radial function and both radial and longitudinal functions seem impaired (B). The delayed contraction suggests that this is most likely ischemic (e).
See **Figure 11.27**.

27. **Answer: B.** The shape of the LV apex is altered and thickening is reduced. Function in the other territories appears preserved.

KEY POINTS

- The allocation of segments into coronary territories caries a risk of erroneous allocation to a coronary artery simply because of variations in coronary anatomy. Despite this risk, recognition of patterns corresponding to standard coronary artery distributions is a very useful guide to wall motion analysis. Failure of motion to coincide with standard coronary distributions implies the possibility of false-positive interpretation or the presence of a noncoronary cause for regional dysfunction.
- The timing of contraction is a component that is often neglected in regional wall motion analysis. It would be highly unusual for an ischemic segment to demonstrate synchronous contraction. Identification of hypokinesis without delay should cause reconsideration about whether the hypokinesis is truly present. Subtle changes cannot be seen visually and require freezing and stepping through the images or quantitation of the strain curve with comparison of the morphology of curves in different segments.

28. **Answer: E.** The findings are consistent with ischemic mitral regurgitation due to posterior leaflet restriction caused by inferoposterior infarction. The resulting anterior leaflet "override" leads to posteriorly directed mitral regurgitation. Ischemic MR is a disease caused by changes of LV structure and function and contrasts with acute MR, which is an infarct complication related to rupture or stretching of the papillary muscle. Ischemic MR is identified in 50% of post-MI patients, of whom 12% are moderate or severe. Moderate or severe ischemic MR is associated with a 3-fold increase in heart failure risk and a 1.6-fold increased risk of death at 5 years.

There are two major mechanisms—displacement of the posterior papillary muscle (causing anterior leaflet "override" and posteriorly directed MR) and LV enlargement, tethering both leaflets and a more central jet.

KEY POINTS

- Ischemic MR is a common finding after MI, and the clues to its recognition are based on the morphology of the mitral valve, the presence of leaflet restriction, and the pattern of the jet direction.
- Although this problem is manifested as MR, it is nonetheless an LV process, and consideration should be given to myocardial ischemia and viability, particularly posterior wall.
- Quantitation of ischemic MR may be difficult, as the process is governed by LV geometry, which changes during systole. It is typical for the amount of regurgitation to be greater during early than mid-systole, as the ventricle empties and the valve is pushed back into the annulus. These features need to be considered when judging regurgitation severity.

29. **Answer: C.** The history of chest pain onset following emotional stress is the classical presentation of stress cardiomyopathy (takotsubo cardiomyopathy [TTC]). TTC mimics acute STEMI with normal epicardial coronary arteries, and spontaneously resolves with a favorable prognosis. The most common trigger is severe emotional stress, and women are more often involved than men. The distribution is atypical for coronary territories—although the wall motion abnormalities involve the apex, they are usually symmetrical, and involvement of the entire mid-apical LV would be an improbable ischemic pattern in the absence of multivessel CAD. Nonetheless, TTC is heterogeneous, with apical, mid- and basal patterns, and even localized involvement. While it has been reported that a strain pattern of lengthening may be seen in TTC, an infarct-related aneurysm can certainly show the same pattern.

30. **Answer: D.** In most cases, stress cardiomyopathy is a benign and self-limiting disease. However, in some instances, the distortion of the LV anatomy provoked by the apical wall motion abnormality, together with hyperkinesis of the basal segments, leads to narrowing of the LV outflow tract and resulting obstruction. The same process may provoke mitral regurgitation. Large wall motion abnormalities are common, with resulting effects on stroke volume and filling pressure.

KEY POINTS

- Stress cardiomyopathy results in a noncoronary artery territory distribution of regional abnormalities, usually with apical akinesis and basal hyperkinesis. Strain analysis may provide complementary information to visual wall motion analysis.
- Left ventricular outflow tract (LVOT) obstruction with systolic anterior motion of the mitral valve, MR, reduced stroke volume, and high LV filling pressures may be associated findings with stress cardiomyopathy.

31. **Answer: C.** LV noncompaction is a developmental abnormality that shows a wide phenotypic spectrum—patients with the most extensive disturbances may develop heart failure, systemic thromboembolism, and arrhythmias. Although apical soft-tissue thickening is seen with all of the above, the characteristic color flow mapping profile showing flow into recesses is typical of noncompaction (**Figures 11.28A-C**). While hopes were held for myocardial torsion as a means of characterizing this entity, the reproducibility and robustness of this parameter make it challenging for clinical use. Patients with noncompaction and preserved EF have a larger mass and relative wall thickness, LA remodeling, pulmonary hypertension and reduced GLS. Excessive trabeculation is a nonspecific feature, detected in normal people, pregnancy, and athletes, as well as in pathologic settings. Indeed, it does not appear that the trabeculation carries risk, which is instead attributable to impaired function and tissue properties. Thus, there is an emerging consensus that diagnosis based on the presence and severity of trabeculation is probably insufficiently exact (see Petersen et al in Suggested Readings below). While the existing criteria regarding compacted-to-noncompacted ratio seem inescapable at present, the presence and degree of LV enlargement and dysfunction can inform prognostic discussions and frequency of follow-up.

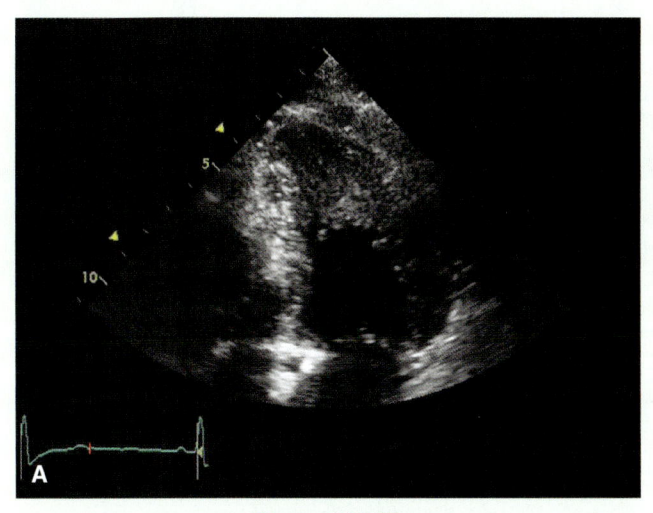

Figure 11.28A

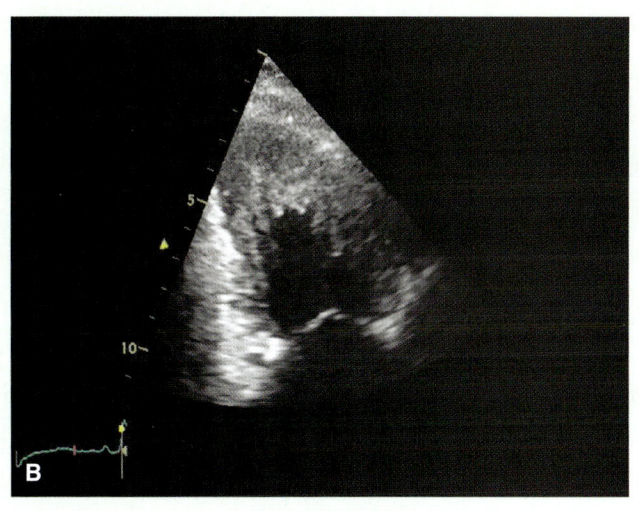

Figure 11.28B

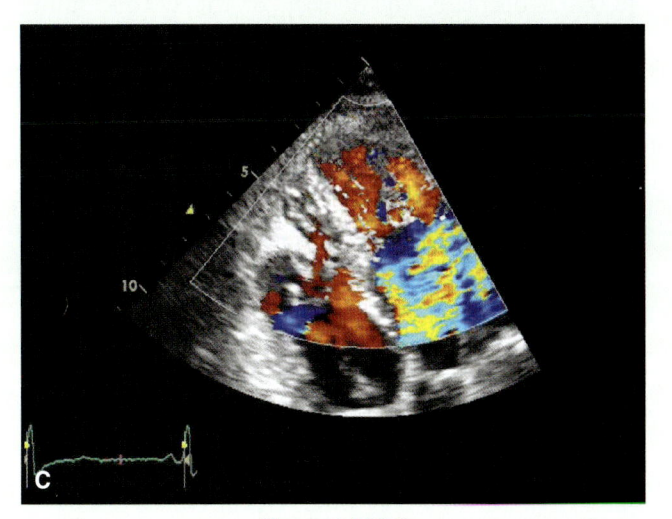

Figure 11.28C

32. **Answer: A.** Noncompaction behaves like a cardiomyopathic process. In this case, the anatomic changes and impaired systolic function are associated with a restrictive filling pattern. (grade 3 diastolic function)

SUGGESTED READINGS

Kittleson MM, Maurer MS, Ambardekar AV, et al. Cardiac amyloidosis: evolving diagnosis and management—a Scientific statement from the American heart association. *Circulation*. 2020;142(1):e7-e22.

Lancellotti P, Pellikka PA, Budts W, et al. The clinical use of stress echocardiography in non-ischaemic heart disease: recommendations from the European Association of Cardiovascular Imaging and the American Society of Echocardiography. *J Am Soc Echocardiogr*. 2017;30(2):101-138.

Lang RM, Badano LP, Mor-Avi V, et al. Recommendations for cardiac chamber quantification by echocardiography in adults: an update from the American Society of Echocardiography and the European Association of Cardiovascular Imaging. *J Am Soc Echocardiogr*. 2015;28:1-39.e14.

Mor-Avi V, Lang RM, Badano LP, et al. Current and evolving echocardiographic techniques for the quantitative evaluation of cardiac mechanics: ASE/EAE consensus statement on methodology and indications endorsed by the Japanese Society of Echocardiography. *J Am Soc Echocardiogr*. 2011;24(3):277-313.

Pellikka PA, Arruda-Olson A, Chaudhry FA, et al. Guidelines for performance, interpretation, and application of stress echocardiography in ischemic heart disease: from the American Society of Echocardiography. *J Am Soc Echocardiogr*. 2020;33:1-41.e8.

Petersen S, Jensen B, Aung N, et al. Excessive trabeculation of the left ventricle: JACC—cardiovascular imaging expert panel paper. *J Am Coll Cardiol Img*. 2023;16(3):408-425.

Porter TR, Mulvagh SL, Abdelmoneim SS, et al. Clinical applications of ultrasonic enhancing agents in echocardiography: 2018 American Society of Echocardiography guidelines update. *J Am Soc Echocardiogr*. 2018;31(3):241-274.

Potter E, Marwick TH. Assessment of left ventricular function by echocardiography: the case for routinely adding global longitudinal strain to ejection fraction. *JACC Cardiovasc Imaging*. 2018;11(2 pt 1):260-274.

Zaidi A, Knight DS, Augustine DX, et al. Echocardiographic assessment of the right heart in adults: a practical guideline from the British Society of Echocardiography. *Echo Res Pract*. 2020;7(1):G19-G41.

Zoghbi WA, Adams D, Bonow RO, et al. Recommendations for noninvasive evaluation of native valvular regurgitation: a report from the American Society of Echocardiography developed in collaboration with the Society for cardiovascular magnetic resonance. *J Am Soc Echocardiogr*. 2017;30(4):303-371.

CHAPTER 12

Diastology

Tahir S. Kafil, Patrick H. Collier, Tom Kai Ming Wang, and Allan L. Klein

QUESTIONS

1. The best two-dimensional (2D) and Doppler echocardiographic finding to differentiate restrictive cardiomyopathy from constrictive pericarditis would be to evaluate:
   A. Mitral inflow pattern.
   B. Pulmonary venous flow pattern.
   C. Atrial size.
   D. Inferior vena cava dilatation.
   E. Early diastolic mitral annular velocity.

2. Comorbidities that do not typically confound assessment of diastolic function include:
   A. Tachycardia, atrial fibrillation, recent MAZE procedure, or pulmonary vein isolation.
   B. Hypertension, aortic stenosis, or pulmonary hypertension.
   C. Severe mitral annular calcification, mitral stenosis, or mitral valve surgery.
   D. Significant aortic or mitral regurgitation (MR).
   E. Ventricular pacing, left ventricular assist device (LVAD) insertion, or cardiac transplantation.

3. How will the pulmonary venous Doppler flow pattern immediately change in the case of left atrial stunning (eg, after cardioversion for persistent atrial fibrillation)? *S1: first velocity of systolic pulmonary venous flow; S2: second velocity of systolic pulmonary venous flow; D: diastolic velocity of pulmonary venous flow; AR: atrial reversal of pulmonary venous flow:*
   A. The systolic filling fraction (S1) will increase.
   B. The systolic filling fraction (S2) will increase.
   C. A decrease will be seen of the diastolic filling fraction (D).
   D. A decrease will be seen of the systolic filling fraction, particularly S1.
   E. An increase in the AR velocity will be seen.

4. Which of the following statements are **TRUE** about the pulmonary venous flow pattern?
   A. Peak atrial reversal (AR) >35 cm/s suggests elevated left ventricular (LV) end-diastolic filling pressures.
   B. The pulmonary vein S1 wave is related to LV relaxation.
   C. The S/D ratio provides an accurate estimation of LV filling pressures in patients with preserved and reduced systolic function.
   D. Pulmonary venous AR duration < mitral inflow A duration indicates an increased LV end-diastolic pressure (LVEDP).
   E. Pulmonary venous flow AR can be obtained in only 50% of patients.

5. In patients with atrial fibrillation, LV filling pressures could be best estimated using which of the following statements?
   A. E/é ≥ 11 correlates well with elevated pulmonary capillary wedge pressure (PCWP).
   B. A short deceleration time in patients with a normal ejection fraction (EF) correlates with elevated PCWP.
   C. Higher left atrial size (>34 mL/m^2) will reflect chronically elevated filling pressures.
   D. Peak velocity of the diastolic pulmonary venous flow will reflect atrial pressure.
   E. It is impossible to estimate PCWP since there is no A wave and the variability in cycle length precludes any accurate estimation.

6. A 61-year-old male patient with a history of hypertension complains of exercise intolerance. His lung function tests are normal and has no obstructive coronary artery disease. His heart rate (HR) at rest is 60 beats/min. He has a normal ejection fraction, mild LV hypertrophy, and no valvular pathology. Doppler echocardiography data are included in **Table 12.1**.
Based on this information:
   A. The cause of his symptoms is unlikely cardiac. Refer him to internal medicine.
   B. Consider a cardiac magnetic resonance imaging study.
   C. We can conclude that the patient has elevated filling pressures and should be given a diuretic.
   D. Consider a diastolic stress test.
   E. Brain natriuretic peptide (BNP) is 500 pg/mL.

Table 12.1

E-wave velocity	48 cm/s
A-wave velocity	60 cm/s
E/A ratio	0.8
Deceleration time	300 ms
e′ velocity	8 cm/s
Tricuspid regurgitation jet velocity	2.5 m/s
E/e′	6

7. The patient in Question 6 above undergoes stress testing with a supine bike protocol. Doppler echocardiography is performed 2 minutes after peak exercise (HR = 136 beats/min, ~85% maximum predicted heart rate [MPHR]). Findings are included in **Table 12.2**.
Which statement is **TRUE**?
   A. This patient has grade I diastolic dysfunction with exercise.
   B. These findings raise concern for pulmonary embolism.
   C. More information is needed to make any definite statement concerning the patient's diastolic function.
   D. These are normal values for this patient's age and gender, given the fact that he just underwent stress testing and his HR is increased.
   E. The patient has elevated LV filling pressures with exercise.

Table 12.2

E-wave velocity	130 cm/s
A-wave velocity	70 cm/s
E/A ratio	1.9
Deceleration time	160 ms
e′ velocity	8 cm/s
Tricuspid regurgitation jet velocity	3.7 m/s
E/e′	16

8. A dialysis patient undergoes cardiac catheterization. His ventricular angiogram shows normal systolic function. The pulmonary capillary wedge tracing shows significant V waves. However, the ventriculogram and a carefully performed echocardiogram do not show significant MR. What is the most likely explanation?
   A. MR can be very dynamic. In addition, there could be a very eccentric jet.
   B. Grade 3 diastolic dysfunction due to LV hypertrophy and volume overload.
   C. Atrial rhythm disturbance.
   D. Loss of left atrial reservoir function.
   E. Congenital anomaly.

9. When performing pulsed-wave Doppler imaging in the apical 4-chamber view to acquire mitral annular velocities, which of the following is true?
   A. The sample volume should be positioned at or 1 cm within the septal and lateral insertion sites of the mitral leaflets.
   B. The sample volume should be small enough (usually 2-3 mm) to evaluate the longitudinal excursion of the mitral annulus in both systole and diastole.
   C. In general, the velocity scale should be set at ~30 cm/s above and below the zero-velocity baseline.
   D. Angulation up to 40° between the ultrasound beam and the plane of cardiac motion is acceptable.
   E. Spectral recordings are ideally obtained during inspiration and measurements should reflect the average of three consecutive cardiac cycles.

10. Which statement is **FALSE**? First-degree AV block:
  A. May have the same effect on the mitral inflow pattern as sinus tachycardia.
  B. May prolong isovolumetric contraction time.
  C. May cause E-A fusion and hamper evaluation of LV diastolic function when only pulsed Doppler interrogation of the mitral inflow is performed.
  D. May lead to diastolic MR in the presence of restrictive filling.
  E. Will decrease the LV diastolic filling period. Therefore, it may have an adverse effect on filling pressures and cardiac output in patients with severe systolic dysfunction.

11. Color Doppler M-mode (CMM) echocardiography provides information on flow propagation (Vp), which is unique in that it is relatively independent of which of the following?
  A. Cardiac output.
  B. LV compliance.
  C. Left atrial size.
  D. Loading conditions.
  E. HR.

12. What is the strongest determinant of mitral deceleration time?
  A. Left atrial mechanical function.
  B. LV operating stiffness.
  C. Left ventricular end-diastolic pressure (LVEDP).
  D. Ejection fraction.
  E. Left atrial reservoir function.

13. In patients with dilated cardiomyopathy, pulsed-wave Doppler mitral flow velocity variables and filling patterns correlate with which of the following?
  A. Cardiac filling pressures and functional class, but not prognosis.
  B. Prognosis, but not filling pressures or functional class.
  C. Cardiac filling pressures, functional class, and prognosis, but less so than does LV ejection fraction.
  D. Cardiac filling pressures, functional class, and prognosis better than does LV ejection fraction.
  E. Cardiac filling pressures, functional class, and prognosis, but to a lesser degree than in patients with LV ejection fraction >50%.

14. Which statement is most correct with respect to the application of the Valsalva maneuver in the assessment of diastolic function?
  A. The lack of reversibility in E/A ratio with Valsalva in patients with advanced diastolic dysfunction indicates irreversible restrictive physiology and implies a very poor prognosis.
  B. The Valsalva maneuver is a sensitive and specific way to differentiate normal from grade I diastolic function.
  C. The Valsalva maneuver should be used in every patient when assessing diastolic function.
  D. In cardiac patients, a decrease of ≥50% in E/A ratio is highly specific for increased LV filling pressures.

15. Figure 12.1 represents three different pulsed-wave Doppler recordings of mitral inflow velocity in a 63-year-old man with a diagnosis of cardiac amyloidosis.
The Doppler recordings were acquired at different grades in the progression of his disease. Atrial fibrillation is a common complication in these patients. At what grade in his disease would sudden onset of atrial fibrillation most likely cause a marked increase in symptoms?
  A. Around the time of the Doppler recording represented in **Figure 12.1A**.
  B. Around the time of the Doppler recording represented in **Figure 12.1B**.
  C. Around the time of the Doppler recording represented in **Figure 12.1C**.
  D. No matter how advanced the diastolic dysfunction, atrial fibrillation is always highly symptomatic in cardiac amyloidosis.
  E. More information is needed to answer this question.

Mitral inflow

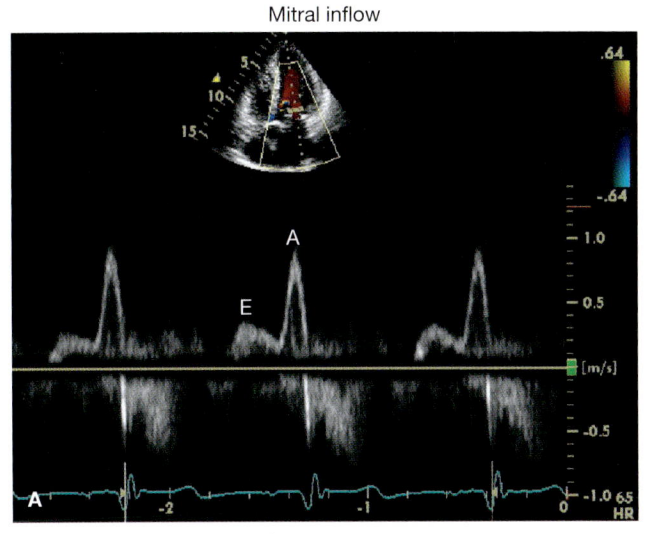

Figure 12.1A

Mitral inflow

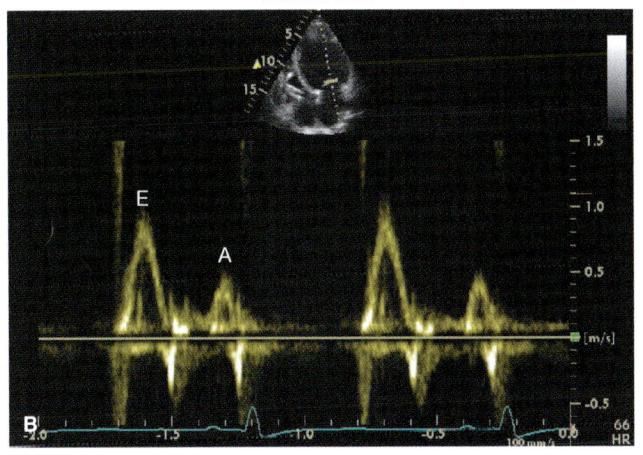

Figure 12.1B

Mitral inflow

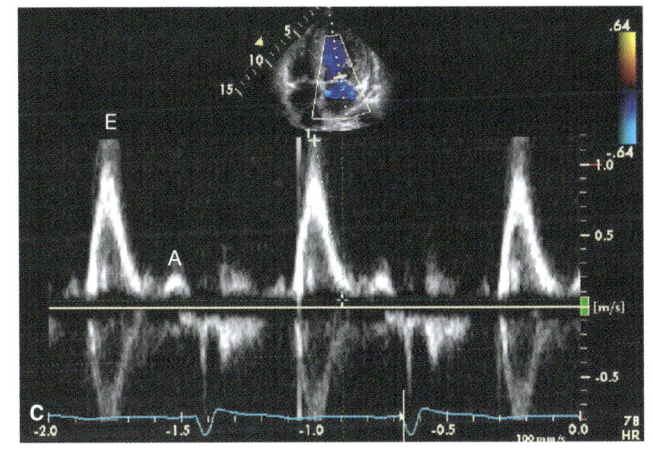

Figure 12.1C

16. Based on **Figure 12.2**, what could you say about the underlying diastolic function in this patient?
    A. The transmitral gradient suddenly increases in mid-diastole because of a decrease in LV compliance and normal relaxation.

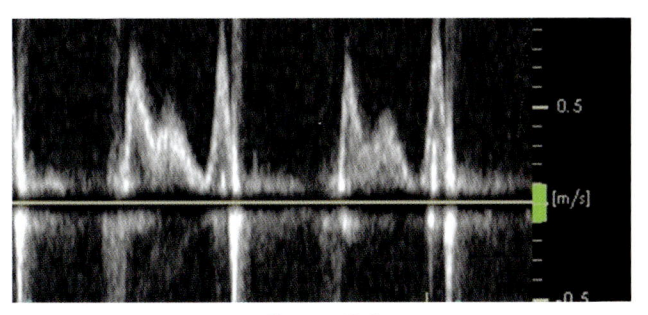

Figure 12.2

B. This type of inflow pattern is consistent with constrictive physiology.
C. This finding represents a very early grade of diastolic dysfunction.
D. This patient has markedly prolonged relaxation and evidence of pseudonormalization. Preload reduction will reveal grade I diastolic dysfunction.
E. The Doppler tracing is suggestive of atrial mechanical dysfunction, possibly due to a recent episode of atrial tachyarrhythmia.

17. A 35-year-old male athlete complains of exercise intolerance. An echocardiogram shows a normal left ventricular (LV) systolic function (ejection fraction = 60%) and no valvular dysfunction. Based on the Doppler recording of his mitral inflow pattern in **Figure 12.3**, which additional echocardiographic parameter is most helpful in confirming whether his symptoms should be attributed to elevated filling pressure?
    A. Left atrial volume index of 34 mL/m^2.
    B. The presence of mild concentric LV hypertrophy.
    C. Tissue Doppler early diastolic velocity of the mitral annulus of 6 cm/s.
    D. Prolonged diastolic filling time.
    E. Indexed LV end-diastolic volume of 80 mL/m^2.

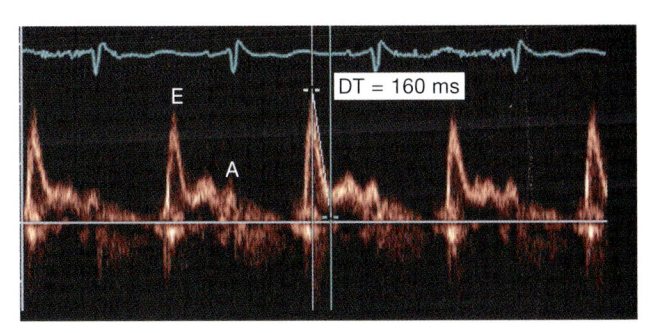

DT = deceleration time

Figure 12.3

252 / Clinical Echocardiography Review

18. A patient with severe LV dysfunction due to long-standing untreated hypertension is referred for initiation of medical therapy. Based on the Doppler findings in **Figure 12.4A,B**, one should be extra cautious when starting what medical therapy?
   A. Diuretics.
   B. Nitrates.
   C. Angiotensin-converting enzyme (ACE) inhibitors.
   D. Beta-blocking agents.
   E. Hydralazine.

19. Figure 12.5 represents the continuous Doppler trace of aortic regurgitation flow in a patient with shortness of breath. The BP is 154/78 mm Hg. What is the most likely cause of his shortness of breath?
   A. LVEDP is in the normal range—consider an alternative etiology.
   B. LVEDP is low indicative of an underfilled LV and possible anemia.
   C. LVEDP is elevated consistent with severe aortic regurgitation.
   D. LVEDP is elevated consistent with significant diastolic dysfunction.
   E. Assessment of LVEDP is unreliable because of the presence of significant aortic regurgitation.

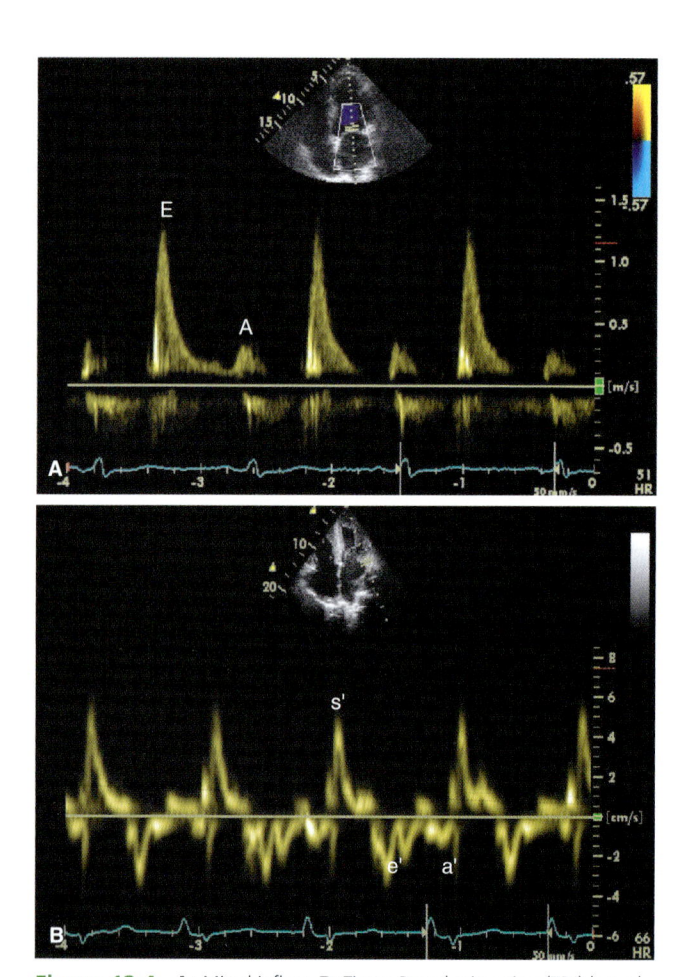

Figure 12.4. **A:** Mitral inflow. **B:** Tissue Doppler imaging (TDI) lateral annulus.

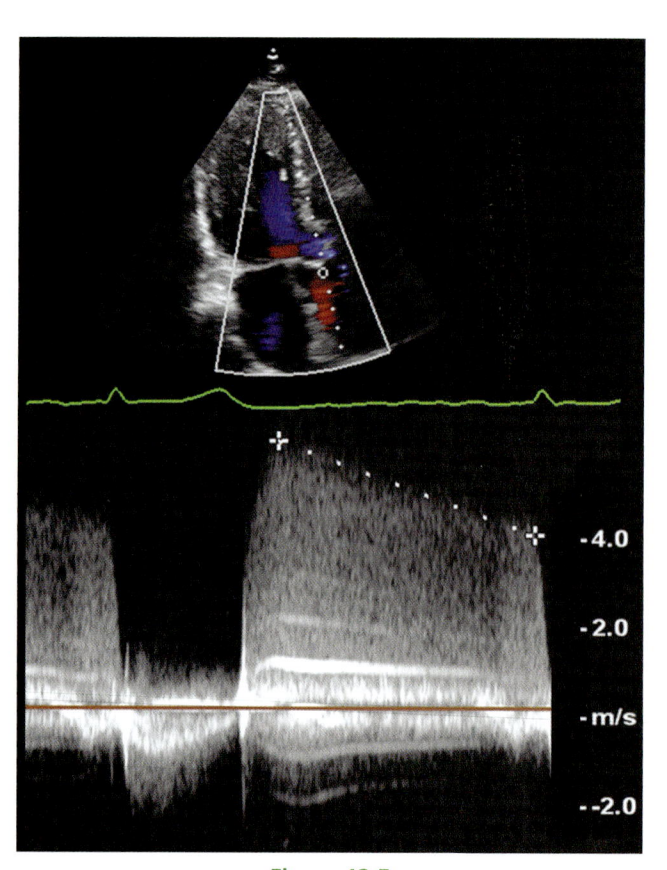

Figure 12.5

20. The Doppler findings in **Figure 12.6A,B** are most likely to be found in which clinical scenario?
    A. A 35-year-old male athlete.
    B. A 50-year-old woman with 3+ MR.
    C. A 60-year-old man with advanced hypertensive heart disease.
    D. A 40-year-old man with asymptomatic newly diagnosed hypertrophic cardiomyopathy.
    E. A 50-year-old woman with atrial fibrillation.

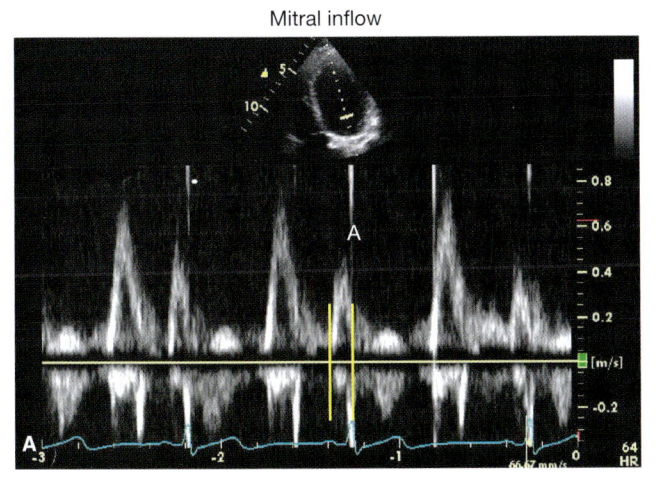

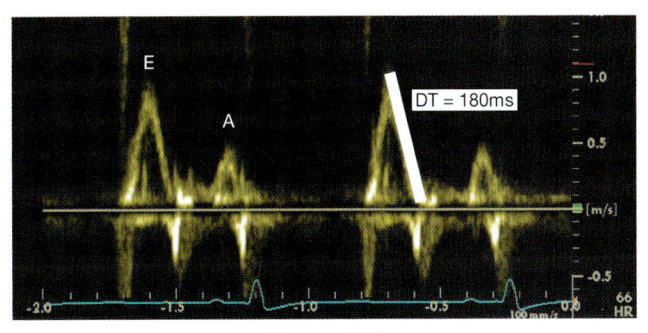

Figure 12.7

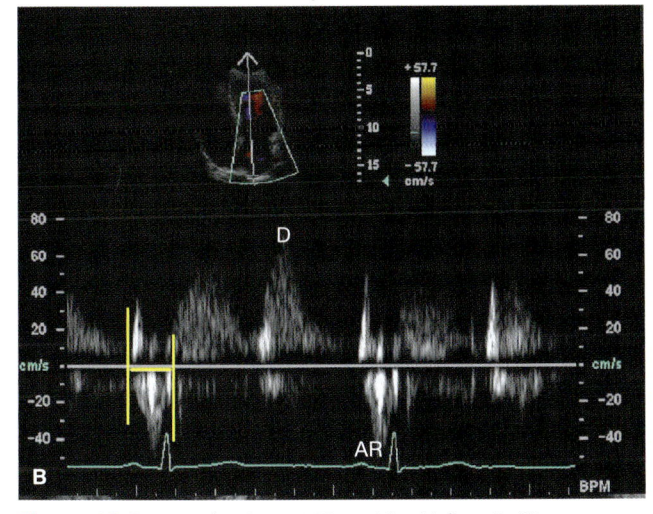

Figure 12.6. A: A duration = 100 ms. Mitral inflow. **B:** AR duration = 180 ms. Pulmonary venous flow.

21. The mitral inflow pattern shown in **Figure 12.7** is by itself suggestive of elevated filling pressures if:
    A. The patient has an ejection fraction of 25%.
    B. The patient has an ejection fraction of 60%.
    C. The patient has a dilated left atrium and a prior history of paroxysmal atrial fibrillation.
    D. The patient has mitral valve prolapse and moderately severe MR.
    E. The maximal jet velocity of the tricuspid regurgitant jet is 3.5 m/s.

22. A 56-year-old patient was referred to you because of increasing shortness of breath. Pulsed-wave Doppler echocardiography in the hepatic veins reveals the tracing in **Figure 12.8**.
    What is the most appropriate statement?
    A. There is evidence for an increased right ventricular end-diastolic pressure (RVEDP).
    B. There must be severe tricuspid regurgitation.
    C. This pattern can be seen in patients with constrictive pericarditis.
    D. There is a right ventricular relaxation abnormality.
    E. Chronic obstructive pulmonary disease can be the cause of this finding.

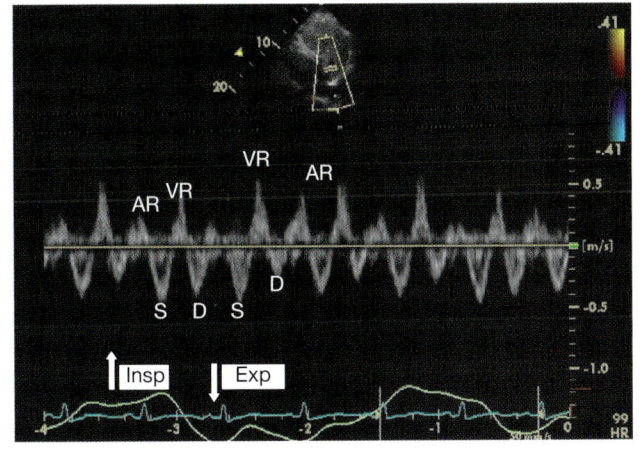

Figure 12.8. AR, atrial reversal; D, diastolic; Exp, expiratory reversal; Insp, inspriration; S, systolic; VR, venous reversal.

23. A 70-year-old male patient with ischemic heart disease and normal left ventricular function (LVEF) is being assessed for diastolic function. His septal e′ velocity is 5 cm/s, E/e′ is 12, TR velocity is 2.0 m/s, and LA volume index is 27 mL/m². What is the diastolic function?
    A. Normal diastolic function.
    B. Indeterminate.
    C. Cannot determine LAP and diastolic dysfunction grade.
    D. Further information such as E/A is needed.
    E. Grade I diastolic dysfunction.

CASE 1

A 91-year-old man with a history of hypertension, bilateral carpal tunnel syndrome, and medication intolerance presents to your clinic for evaluation. He complains of bilateral neuropathy and has had to be weaned off his blood pressure medications due to low blood pressures. He complains of dyspnea on exertion. ECG is notable for low voltages and atrial fibrillation.

Physical examination reveals blood pressure of 92/45 mm Hg and HR of 90 beats/min. He appears frail. Cardiovascular examination is noted for an irregularly irregular pulse and 2/6 holosystolic murmur at the apex. Echocardiographic findings are shown in **Figure 12.9A-D**.

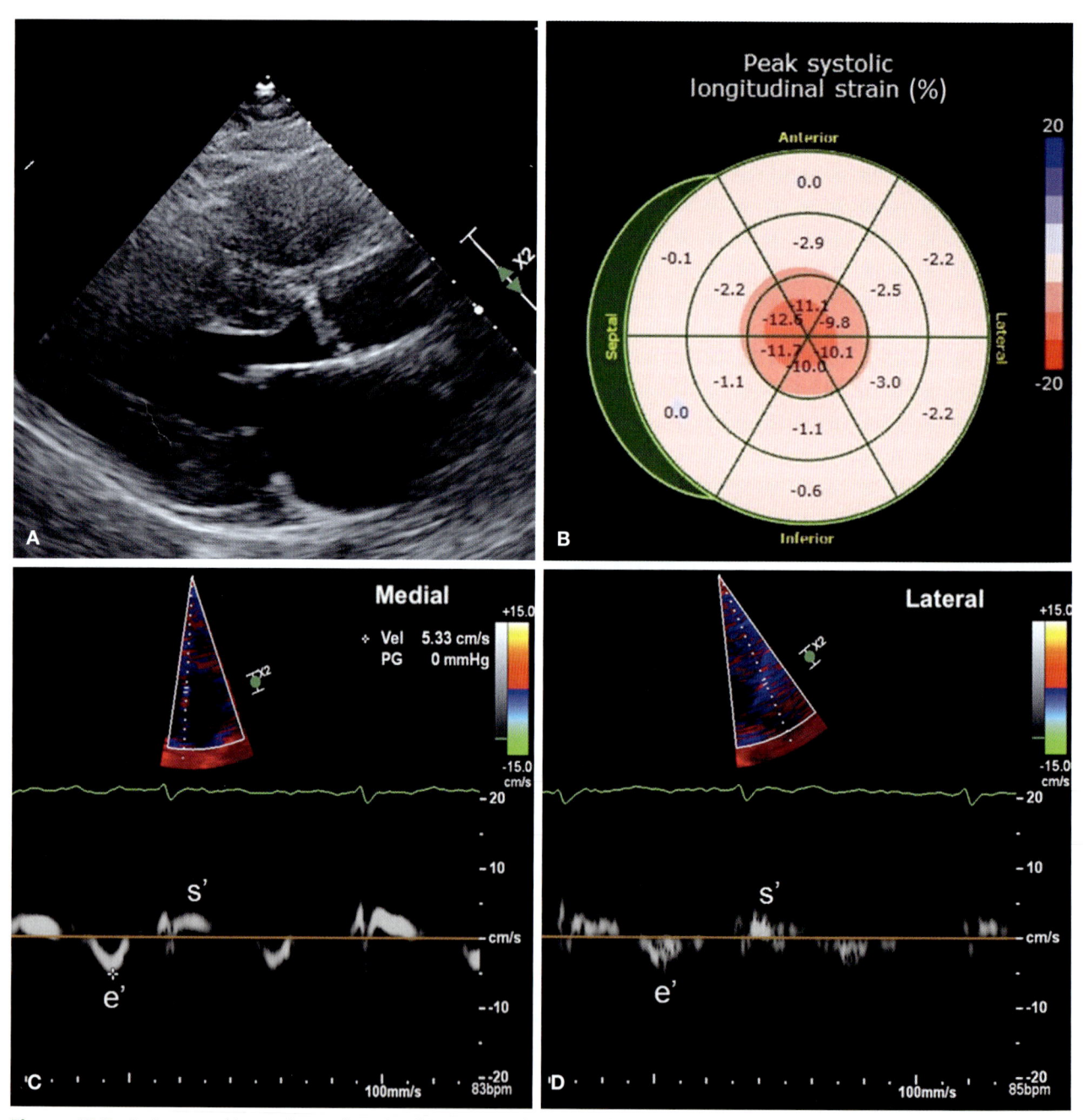

Figure 12.9. **A:** Parasternal long-axis two-dimensional image. **B:** Peak systolic left ventricular longitudinal strain polar plot. **C:** Medial tissue Doppler imaging (TDI) annulus. **D:** Lateral TDI annulus.

24. In **Case 1**, what are the septal and lateral e' velocities (3-4 cm/s) and polar plot of LV longitudinal strain demonstrating?
    A. Diastolic dysfunction with the apical region being most affected.
    B. Constrictive pericarditis.
    C. Restrictive cardiomyopathy with apical sparing.
    D. This finding is nonspecific.
    E. Left ventricular systolic dysfunction.

25. The findings in **Case 1** are found in which clinical scenario?
    A. TTR Cardiac amyloidosis.
    B. Cardiac sarcoidosis.
    C. Hypertrophic cardiomyopathy.
    D. Fabry disease.
    E. Loeffler endocarditis.

CASE 2

A 48-year-old male commercial real estate developer presents to the hospital with increasing shortness of breath, abdominal swelling, and lower extremity edema developing over the past 6 months. For the last 2 years, he has been seen in the clinic for evaluation of multiple episodes of syncope and atrial fibrillation has been documented on Holter monitoring. ECG is notable for sinus tachycardia and low voltage.

Physical examination is remarkable for blood pressure = 100/74 mm Hg, HR = 100 beats/min, and oral temperature = 37.9 °C. Cardiovascular examination is notable for elevated neck veins at 8 cm and a normal S1 and S2 with a soft S4. In addition, he has a nondisplaced point of maximal impulse. Lungs are clear on auscultation. Abdomen does not demonstrate organomegaly. His extremities are cool, with mild pitting edema extending up to the mid-tibia bilaterally.

Echocardiographic findings are shown in **Figure 12.10A,B** *and in* ▶ **Video 12.1**.

26. What finding in **Case 2** and ▶ **Video 12.1** could explain his symptoms?
    A. Pericardial effusion, suggesting imminent tamponade.
    B. Abnormal systolic function.
    C. Septal bounce, suggesting constrictive pericarditis.
    D. Restrictive cardiomyopathy.

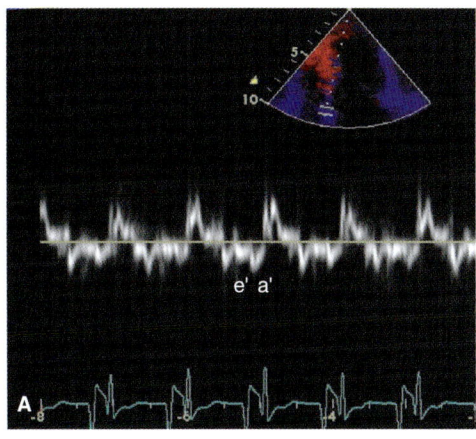

e' = 4 cm/s, a' = 4 cm/s
TDI medial annulus

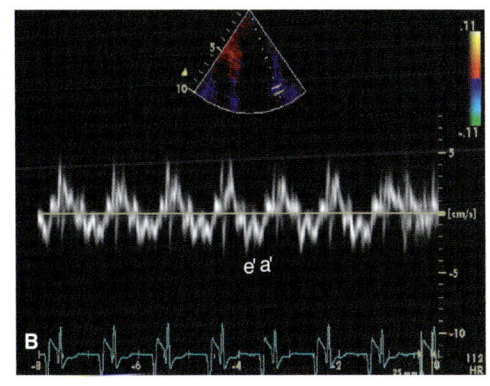

e' = 3.5 cm/s, a' = 3 cm/s
TDI lateral annulus

Figure 12.10. **A:** e' = 4 cm/s, a' = 4 cm/s. **B:** e' = 3.5 cm/s, a' = 3 cm/s. TDI, tissue Doppler imaging.

27. Based on the Doppler information in **Figure 12.11** and **Table 12.3**, which of the following statements is most consistent?
    A. The end-diastolic pressure–volume relationship in this patient is shifted downward and to the right.
    B. These findings can be explained by a process of progressive myocardial stiffening.

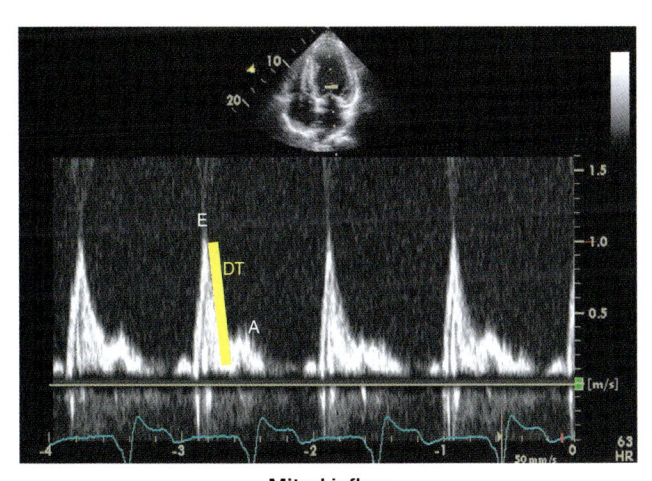

Mitral inflow
Figure 12.11

256 / Clinical Echocardiography Review

Table 12.3

E-wave velocity	80 cm/s
Deceleration time	106 ms
Tissue Doppler imaging medial annulus e′ velocity	4 cm/s

C. Cardiac catheterization will likely reveal a difference of 10 mm Hg between PCWP and RVEDP.
D. It is imperative to maintain sinus rhythm in this patient to improve his symptoms.

CASE 3

A 22-year-old woman presents with a 6-month history of intermittent palpitations without syncope. These are most notable when she is at her high stress job as a junior pilot. Physical examination is unremarkable. ECG reveals normal sinus rhythm with normal PR interval. Echocardiography shows a normal LVEF, normal wall thickness, E/e′ is 9, septal e′ is 11 cm/s and lateral e′ velocity is 14 cm/s, TR velocity is 180 cm/s, and LA volume index is 20 mL/m². Findings are shown in **Figure 12.12A-D**.

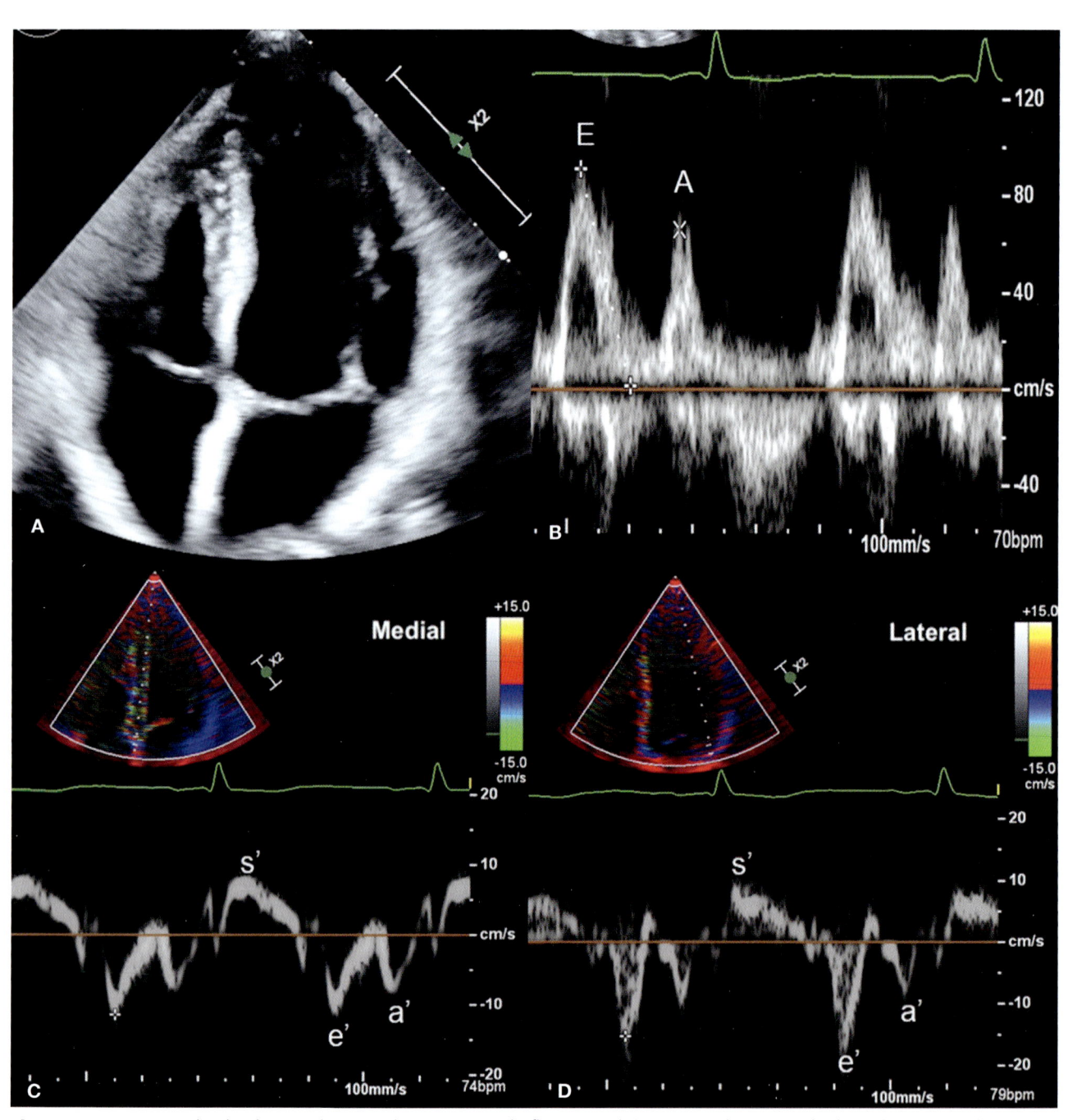

Figure 12.12. **A:** Apical 4-chamber two-dimensional image. **B:** Mitral inflow. **C:** Medial tissue Doppler imaging (TDI) annulus. **D:** Lateral TDI annulus.

28. Based on the Doppler information provided in **Case 3**, what is her diastolic function?
A. Normal diastolic function.
B. Indeterminate.
C. Cannot determine LAP and diastolic dysfunction grade.
D. Further information such as E/A is needed.
E. Grade I diastolic dysfunction.

29. From **Case 3**, what would be the next step in the patient's diastolic function assessment?
A. Left atrial strain.
B. Stress echocardiography.
C. Holter monitor.
D. Repeat study in 2 to 3 months.
E. No further testing needed as this is normal.

CASE 4

A 67-year-old man recently diagnosed with multiple myeloma has been complaining of worsening dyspnea with activity for approximately the last 6 weeks. In addition, he has been reporting intermittent episodes of chest discomfort that are not always associated with activity. His medical history is otherwise remarkable only for hyperlipidemia and prior tobacco abuse, which he quit more than 10 years ago.

Physical examination is notable for a 2/6 systolic ejection murmur at the left lower sternal border. No S3 or S4 is audible. Neck veins are mildly elevated at 10 cm. There is mild lower extremity pitting edema that extends to the mid-tibias.

The ECG is remarkable for relatively low voltage. In addition, there are Q waves present in the anteroseptal precordial leads.

An abdominal fat pad biopsy confirms the diagnosis of amyloidosis (type AL) with apple-green birefringence under a polarized light microscope after staining with Congo red.

30. Which of the findings listed is considered a classical finding on transthoracic echocardiography in patients with amyloidosis?
A. Normal LV wall thickness.
B. Uniformly reduced segmental global longitudinal myocardial strain.
C. Short deceleration time associated with worsening prognosis.
D. Increased systolic and early diastolic velocities of the mitral annulus on tissue Doppler imaging.
E. Interventricular septal "bounce."

31. In patients with more advanced stages of amyloidosis, a combined relaxation abnormality and a mild increase in left atrial filling pressure will result in which of the following?
A. Grade I diastolic dysfunction (impaired relaxation).
B. Grade II diastolic dysfunction (pseudonormalized).
C. Decreasing pulmonary venous AR wave velocity.
D. Decreasing LVEDP.

CASE 5

A 25-year-old male athlete presents with mild exertional lightheadedness. Physical exam reveals a harsh crescendo-decrescendo systolic murmur at the left lower sternal border. ECG reveals normal sinus rhythm with very high voltages suggestive of left ventricular hypertrophy. Echocardiography shows hyperdynamic LV function, E/A is 2.9, septal e' is 6 cm/s and lateral e' velocity is 7 cm/s, average E/e' 15.7, TR velocity is 290 cm/s, and LA volume index is 35 mL/m^2. Findings are shown in **Figure 12.13A-D** *and* ▶ **Video 12.2**.

32. Based on the Doppler information provided in **Case 5**, what is his left atrial pressure?
A. Grade I diastolic dysfunction.
B. Grade II diastolic dysfunction.
C. Grade III diastolic dysfunction.
D. Cannot assess diastolic dysfunction due to severe left ventricular hypertrophy.

258 / Clinical Echocardiography Review

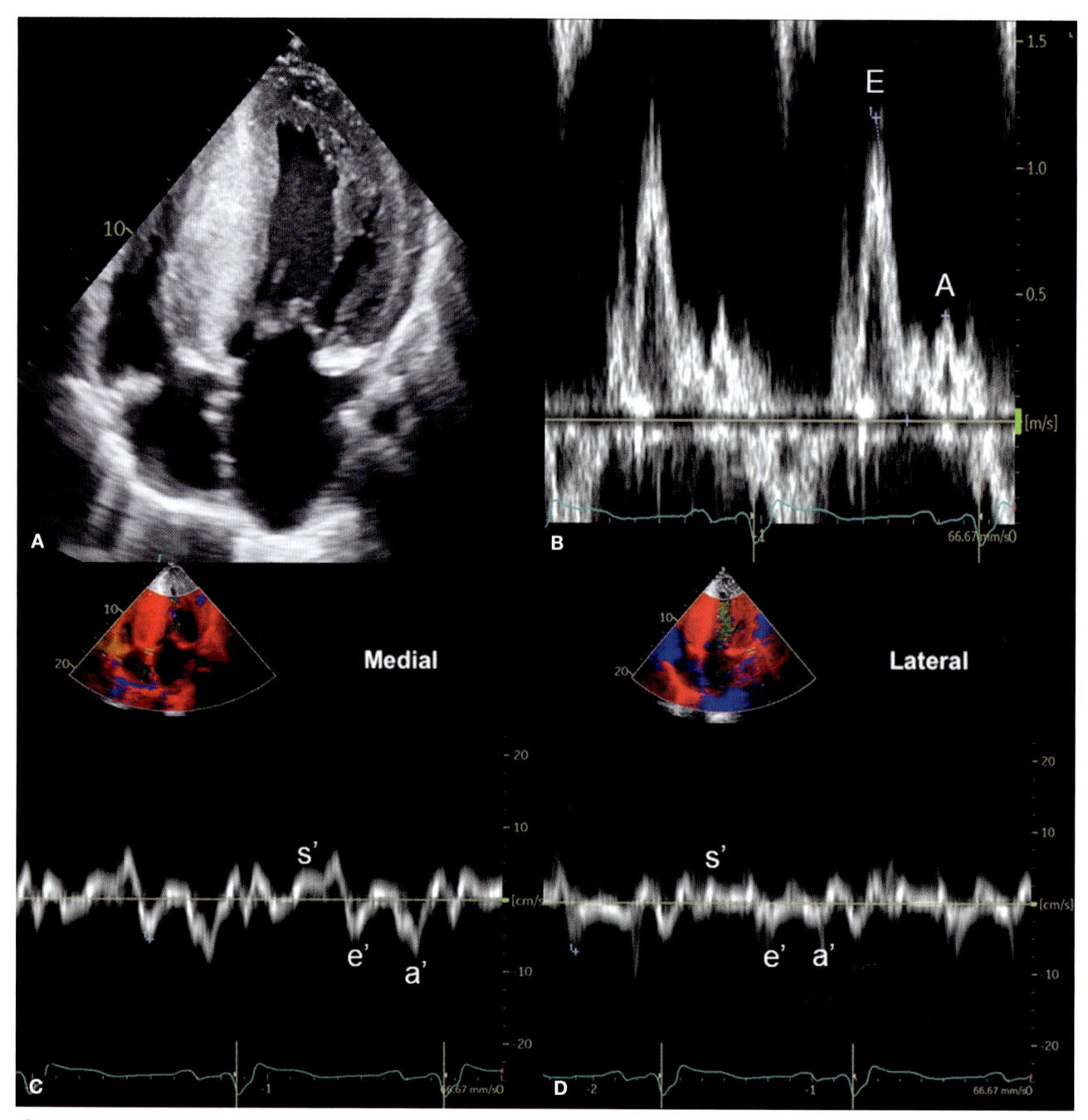

Figure 12.13. **A:** Apical 4-chamber two-dimensional image. **B:** Mitral inflow. **C:** Medial tissue Doppler imaging (TDI) annulus. **D:** Lateral TDI annulus.

CASE 6

A 58-year-old woman was admitted to the hospital with shortness of breath. Physical exam reveals bilateral pedal edema, abdominal distention, and jugular venous pressure is elevated to the level of the jaw. Echocardiography shows LV hypertrophy and LV function of 60%, E/A ratio of 1.3, E/e' ratio is not available, tricuspid regurgitation velocity is 200 cm/s, and left atrial volume is 44 mL/m². Findings are shown in **Figure 12.14A-D**.

33. Based on the findings in **Case 6**, what is the grade of diastolic function?
   A. Grade I diastolic dysfunction.
   B. Cannot determine LAP and diastolic dysfunction grade.
   C. Grade II diastolic dysfunction.
   D. Grade III diastolic dysfunction.

Chapter 12 Diastology / 259

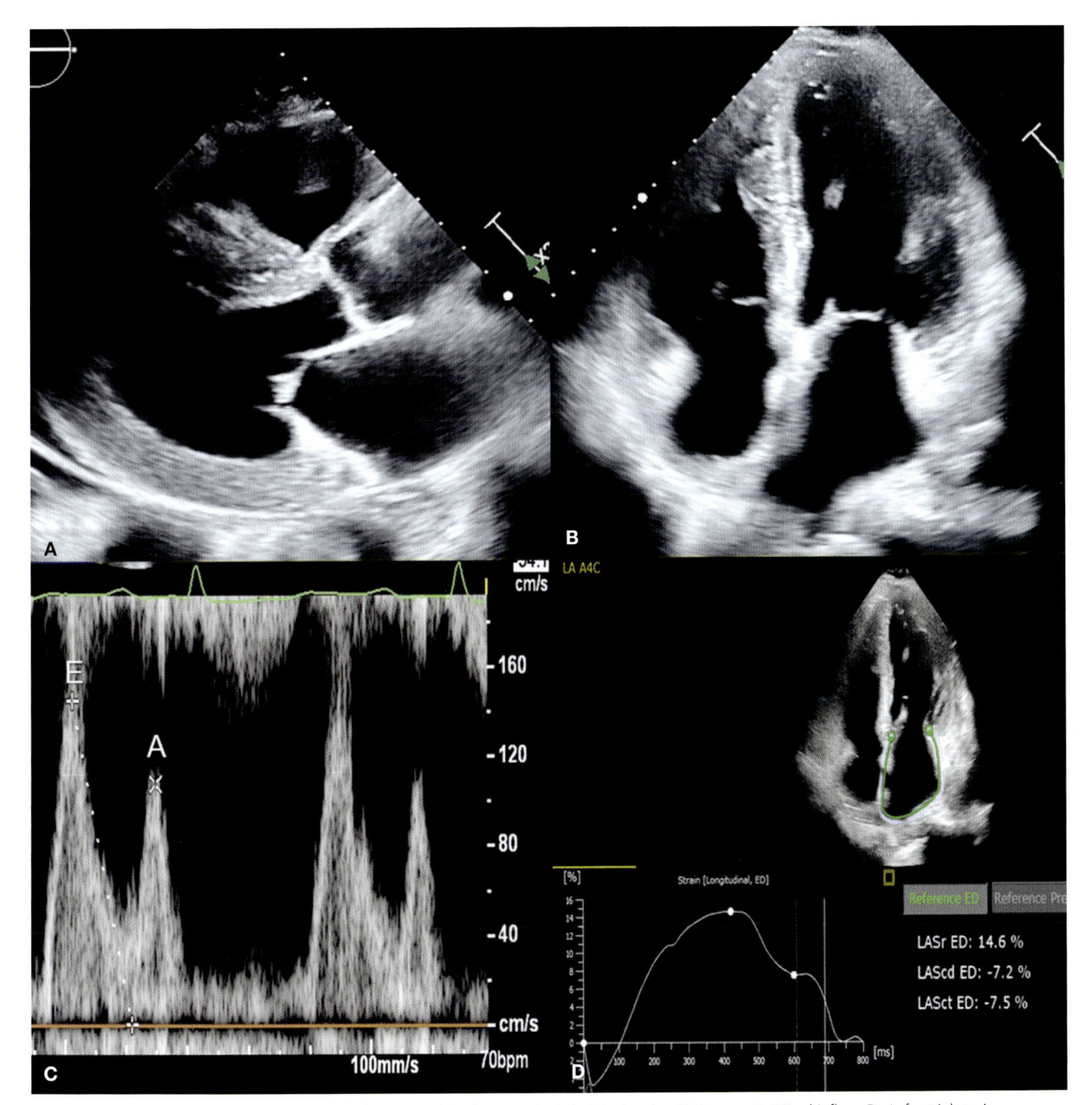

Figure 12.14. **A:** Parasternal long-axis two-dimensional (2D) image. **B:** Apical 4-chamber 2D image. **C:** Mitral inflow. **D:** Left atrial strain.

34. What does the left atrial strain suggest about left atrial pressure in this scenario?
   A. Left atrial strain is normal, suggesting normal left atrial pressures.
   B. Left atrial reservoir strain (LASr) is abnormal, suggesting elevated left atrial pressures.
   C. Grade II diastolic dysfunction.
   D. Grade III diastolic dysfunction.

CASE 7

A 66-year-old man presents with a 1-year history of progressive shortness of breath. Physical exam is notable for signs of pulmonary hypertension and loud S1. Echocardiographic images are shown in **Figure 12.15A-D**. *E/A ratio is 0.9, E/e' ratio of 25.6, LA volume index of 52 mL/m², and trivial TR. Echocardiographic findings are shown in* **Figure 12.15** *and* ▶ **Video 12.3**.

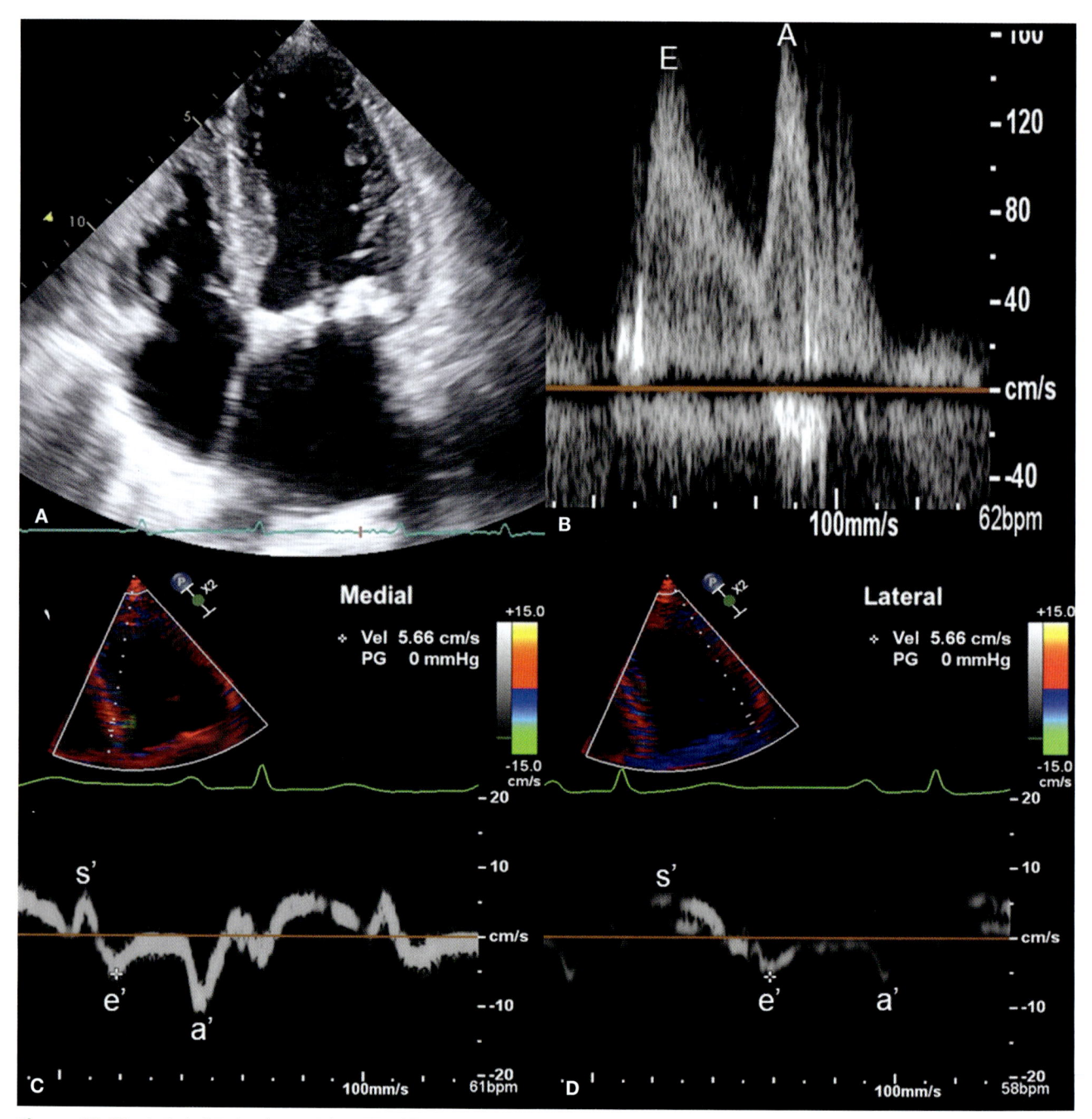

Figure 12.15. A: Apical 4-chamber two-dimensional image. **B:** Mitral inflow. **C:** Medial tissue Doppler imaging (TDI) annulus. **D:** Lateral TDI annulus.

35. What is the estimated diastolic function of the patient in **Case 7**?
   A. Diastolic function cannot be evaluated due to severe MAC.
   B. Diastolic function cannot be evaluated due to atrial fibrillation.
   C. Cannot determine LAP and diastolic dysfunction grade.
   D. Grade II diastolic dysfunction.
   E. Grade III diastolic dysfunction.

ANSWERS

1. **Answer: E.** Differentiating restrictive from constrictive pericarditis by echocardiography can be challenging. A mitral medial annular e' velocity >8 cm/s has been shown to be highly accurate in differentiating patients with constrictive pericarditis from those with restrictive cardiomyopathy, a point highlighted in the 2016 ASE/EACVI guideline document in an algorithmic form comparing constrictive pericarditis with restrictive cardiomyopathy (**Figure 12.16**).

   In particular, the presence of a normal annular e' velocity in a patient referred with a heart failure diagnosis should raise suspicion of pericardial constriction. The presence of grade I filling or absence of inferior cava dilation makes a diagnosis of constriction/restriction unlikely. Respirophasic ventricular septal shift is an echo correlate of ventricular interdependence, whereby one ventricle fills at the expense of the other and is generally present in constriction.

   Apart from 2D features that give clues to the differentiation of diseases, tissue Doppler imaging (TDI) can provide important specific information. In patients with restrictive cardiomyopathy, myocardial relaxation (e') will be severely impaired, whereas patients with constriction usually have preserved mitral annular vertical excursion. Of note, the lateral annular e' velocity could be decreased if the constrictive process involves the lateral mitral annulus.

   Figure 12.17A,B illustrates typical tissue Doppler tracings from a patient with constrictive pericarditis as compared to a patient with restrictive cardiomyopathy.

2. **Answer: B.** Diastolic function is particularly useful in left or right ventricular pressure overload where it may offer additional prognostic information. On the contrary, assessment of diastolic function may be limited by the presence of other comorbidities. For example, assessment of mitral inflow is limited in the presence of tachycardia due to E/A fusion (in patients with advanced cardiomyopathies, E/A fusion may even be seen with relatively normal heart rates [HRs]). Equally, the absence of coordinated atrial contraction in atrial fibrillation means an absent "A wave," while after the MAZE procedure or pulmonary vein isolation (PVI), atrial stunning or scar may result in an attenuated mechanical "A wave" despite the presence of an electrical "P wave." Exclusions special populations to assessment of diastolic function include scenarios where filling pressures are driven more by other confounding variables such as significant (>2+) mitral or aortic regurgitation or LVAD implantation. Atrial enlargement is a feature of all cardiac transplants while preset pacing parameters (such as the AV delay) can independently determine grade of diastolic function. Assessment of left ventricular filling pressures in special populations is summarized in **Table 12.4**.

Figure 12.16. Algorithm comparing constrictive pericarditis and restrictive cardiomyopathy. Note that restriction is associated with elevated E/A ratio, short deceleration time, and decreased mitral annular velocity (<6 cm/s). DT, deceleration time; E/A, ratio of peak mitral flow velocity of the early filling wave over peak mitral flow velocity of the late filling wave due to atrial contraction; mitral medial e' = tissue Doppler early diastolic mitral annular velocity; E/e', ratio of peak mitral flow velocity of the early filling wave over tissue Doppler early diastolic annular velocity; IVRT, isovolumic relaxation time; LAVI, left atrial volume index; PV, pulmonary vein; SVC, superior vena cava. (Based on data from Welch TD, Ling LH, Espinosa RE, et al. Echocardiographic diagnosis of constrictive pericarditis: Mayo Clinic criteria. *Circ Cardiovasc Imaging.* 2014;7:526-534 and reprinted from Nagueh SF, Smiseth OA, Appleton CP, et al. Recommendations for the evaluation of left ventricular diastolic function by echocardiography: an update from the American Society of Echocardiography and the European Association of Cardiovascular Imaging. *J Am Soc Echocardiogr.* 2016;29(4):277-314. Copyright © 2016 American Society of Echocardiography. With permission.)

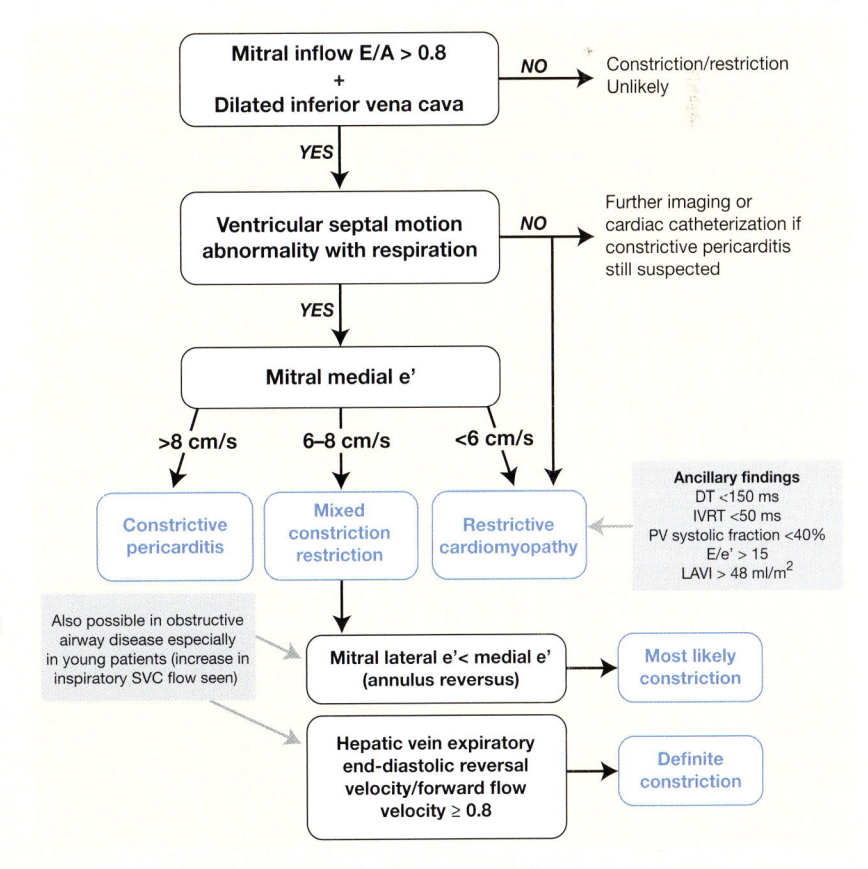

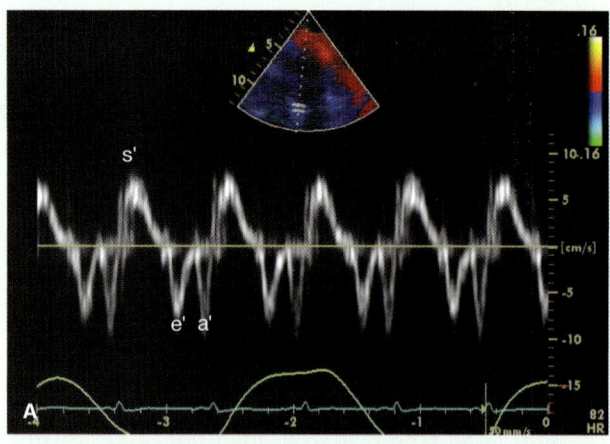

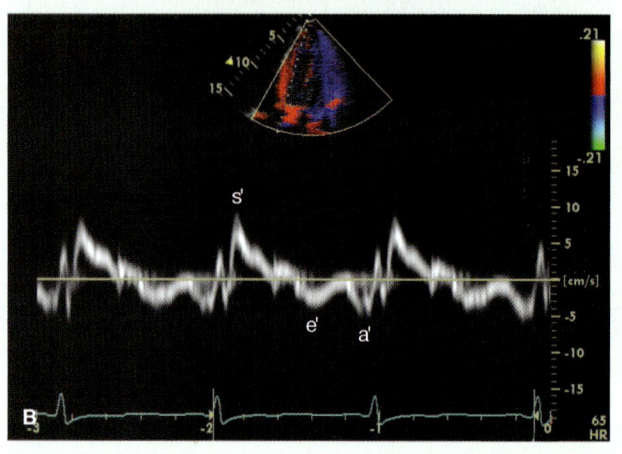

Figure 12.17. **A (Constrictive pericarditis)** and **B (Restrictive cardiomyopathy):** Tissue Doppler imaging medial annulus.

3. **Answer: D.** There are two systolic velocities (S1 and S2), mostly noticeable when there is a prolonged PR interval since S1 is related to atrial relaxation. S2 should be used to compute the ratio of peak systolic to peak diastolic velocity. S1 velocity is primarily influenced by changes in left atrial pressure and left atrial relaxation or contraction, whereas S2 is related to stroke volume and pulse wave propagation in the pulmonary arterial tree. The diastolic velocity D is influenced by changes in LV filling and compliance and changes in parallel with mitral E velocity. Pulmonary venous atrial flow reversal (AR) velocity and duration are influenced by LV late diastolic pressures, atrial preload, and left atrial contractility. Atrial fibrillation or atrial stunning will result in a blunted S wave, mainly due to a loss of S1 with a decreased systolic fraction and absence of AR velocity (**Figure 12.18**).

4. **Answer: A.** AR may increase with age, but AR >35 cm/s is usually consistent with elevated LV filling pressures particularly at end diastole. The diastolic velocity D is influenced by changes in LV filling and compliance and changes in parallel with mitral E velocity. Young and healthy individuals can therefore exhibit large D waves indicating forceful elastic recoil of the LV rather than high left atrial pressure. S1 velocity is primarily influenced by changes in left atrial pressure and left atrial relaxation or contraction, whereas S2 is related to LV contractility, stroke volume, mitral regurgitation, and pulse wave propagation in the pulmonary arterial tree. Mitral and pulmonary vein inflow patterns are

Table 12.4. Assessment of LV Filling Pressures in Special Populations

Disease	Echocardiographic Measurements and Cutoff Values
1. Atrial fibrillation	Peak acceleration rate of mitral E velocity (≥1900 cm/s^2), IVRT (≤65 ms), DT of pulmonary venous diastolic velocity (≤220 ms), E/Vp ratio (≥1.4), and septal E/e' ratio (≥11)
2. Sinus tachycardia	Mitral inflow pattern with predominant early LV filling in patients with EF <50%, IVRT ≤70 ms is specific (79%), systolic filling fraction ≤40% is specific (88%), and lateral E/e' >10 (a ratio >12 has highest specificity of 96%)
3. Hypertrophic cardiomyopathy	Lateral E/e' (≥10), Ar-A (≥30 ms), pulmonary artery pressures (>35 mm Hg), and LA volume (≥34 mL/m^2)
4. Restrictive cardiomyopathy	DT (<140 ms), mitral E/A (>2.5), IVRT (<50 ms has high specificity), and septal E/e' (>15)
5. Noncardiac pulmonary hypertension	Lateral E/e' can be applied to determine whether a cardiac etiology is the underlying reason for the increased pulmonary artery pressures (cardiac etiology: E/e' >10, noncardiac etiology: E/e' is <8)
6. Mitral stenosis	IVRT (<60 ms has high specificity), IVRT/TE-e' (<4.2), and mitral A velocity (>1.5 m/s)
7. Mitral regurgitation	Ar-A (≥30 ms), IVRT (<60 ms has high specificity), and IVRT/TE-e' (<5.6) may be applied for the prediction of LV filling pressures in patients with MR and normal EF, whereas average E/e' (>15) is applicable only in the presence of a depressed EF

Specificity comments refer to predicting filling pressures >15 mm Hg.
A, peak mitral flow velocity of the late filling wave due to atrial contraction; Ar-A, the time difference between duration of PV flow and mitral inflow during atrial contraction; DT, deceleration time; E, peak mitral flow velocity of the early filling wave; E/e', ratio of peak mitral flow velocity of the early filling wave over tissue Doppler early diastolic annular velocity; EF, ejection fraction; E/Vp, ratio of peak mitral flow velocity of the early filling wave over flow propagation velocity by color M-mode; IVRT, isovolumic relaxation time; LAVI, left atrial volume index; LV, left ventricle; TE-e', the time difference between the onset of e' velocity compared with onset of mitral E velocity. Adapted from Nagueh SF, Smiseth OA, Appleton CP, et al. Recommendations for the evaluation of Left ventricular diastolic function by echocardiography: an update from the American Society of Echocardiography and the European Association of Cardiovascular Imaging. *J Am Soc Echocardiogr.* 2016;29(4):277-314. Copyright © 2016 American Society of Echocardiography. With permission.

Chapter 12 Diastology / 263

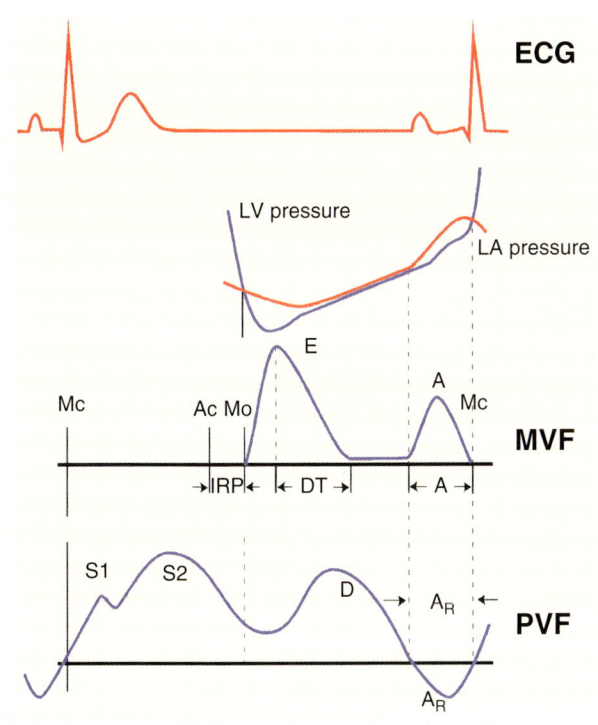

Figure 12.18. DT, deceleration time; IRP, isovolumic relaxation period; LA, left atrium; LV, left ventricle; MVF, mitral valve flow; PVF, pulmonary venous flow.

not very reliable for assessment of LV filling pressures in patients with an overall normal systolic function. AR dur–A dur >30 ms is, therefore, a more robust marker of elevated LVEDP in this group of patients. Pulmonary venous atrial reversal can be obtained in more than 70% of patients. A commercially available contrast ultrasonic enhancing agent injection can help enhance the Doppler tracing.

5. **Answer: A.** Although sometimes challenging, an estimate of LV filling pressures can be obtained in patients with atrial fibrillation using the E/e′ ratio. Different studies have shown good correlations in this population between filling pressures and the E/e′ ratio (a ratio ≥ 11 predicting LVEDP ≥ 15 mm Hg), the mitral deceleration time (<150 ms in the presence of LV systolic dysfunction), or the deceleration time (not the peak velocity) of the pulmonary venous diastolic velocity (≤220 ms associated with higher filling pressures).

6. **Answer: D. Figure 12.19** is an algorithm to help decide upon the absence or presence of diastolic dysfunction in the setting of normal LV systolic function and absence of myocardial disease. **Figure 12.20** is an algorithm that goes a step further to help decide upon the grade of diastolic dysfunction present and is the necessary algorithm to use if there is LV myocardial pathology such as decreased ejection fraction, cardiomyopathy, LVH, or coronary artery disease. This algorithm is used in most echo labs with patients who have a high likelihood of diastolic dysfunction and elevated LV filling pressures. This patient has LVH. **Table 12.5** shows typical diastology parameter values in a patient with grade I diastolic dysfunction. Thus, this patient has evidence of grade I diastolic function with normal to low LV filling pressures at rest with a BNP of 100 pg/mL; however, it can be useful to evaluate LV filling pressure not only at rest but with exercise using a supine bike or treadmill as well. The E/e′ ratio will remain unchanged in subjects with normal myocardial relaxation because both mitral E and e′ velocities increase proportionally. However, in patients

Diagnosis of diastolic dysfunction in patients with normal LVEF

1. Average E/e′ > 14
2. Septal e′ velocity < 7 cm/s or lateral e′ velocity < 10 cm/s
3. TR velocity > 2.8 m/s
4. LA volume index > 34 ml/m²

- 0 or 1 positive → Normal diastolic function
- 2 positive → Indeterminate
- 3 or 4 positive → Diastolic dysfunction

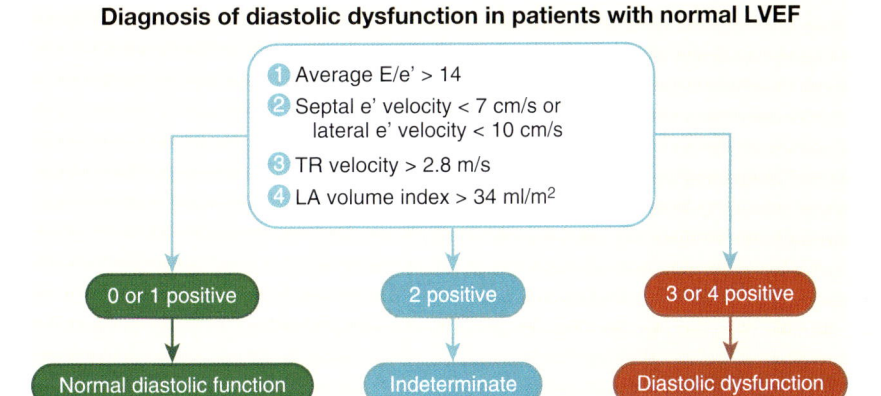

Figure 12.19. Algorithm for diagnosis of left ventricular diastolic dysfunction in subjects with normal LVEF. e′, tissue Doppler early diastolic annular velocity; E/e′, ratio of peak mitral flow velocity of the early filling wave over tissue Doppler early diastolic annular velocity; LA, left atrial; LVEF, left ventricular ejection fraction; TR, tricuspid regurgitation; . Note this diagram is used in patients with normal ejection fraction that do not have obvious pathology such as coronary artery disease with wall motion abnormalities, left ventricular hypertrophy, or cardiomyopathy. It also makes it more specific to call abnormal diastolic function since 3/4 criteria have to be satisfied. It applies to someone who may present with palpitations and no other cardiac pathology. An E/A <1 no longer means diastolic dysfunction. If only 50% of the criteria are positive, then it is called indeterminate. (Adapted from Nagueh SF, Smiseth OA, Appleton CP, et al. Recommendations for the evaluation of left ventricular diastolic function by echocardiography: an update from the American Society of Echocardiography and the European Association of Cardiovascular Imaging. *J Am Soc Echocardiogr.* 2016;29(4):277-314. Copyright © 2016 American Society of Echocardiography. With permission.)

Estimation of LV filling pressures in patients with depressed LVEF or normal EF and diastolic dysfunction

```
                ┌─────────────────────────┬─────────────────────────┐
                │                         │                         │
        E/A ≤ 0.8 + E ≤ 50 cm/s    E/A ≤ 0.8 + E > 50 cm/s      E/A ≥ 2
                                          or
                                    E/A > 0.8 – <2
                                          │
                                          ▼
                              3 criteria to be evaluated*
                              • Average E/e' > 14
                              • TR velocity > 2.8 m/s
                              • LA vol. index > 34 ml/m²
                                          │
                  ┌───────────────────────┼───────────────────────┐
            2 of 3 or                                       2 of 3 or
            3 of 3                                           3 of 3
            negative                                        positive

                              When only 2 criteria are available
                   ┌──────────────────────┼──────────────────────┐
              2 negative            1 positive and           2 positive
                                    1 negative

         Normal LAP,              Cannot determine        ↑ LAP, grade II    ↑ LAP, grade III
         grade I diastolic        LAP and diastolic       diastolic          diastolic
         dysfunction              dysfunction grade*      dysfunction        dysfunction

              │
        If symptomatic → Consider CAD, or proceed to diastolic stress test
```

*LAP indeterminate if only 1 of 3 parameters evaluation. Pulmonary vein S/D ratio <1 applicable to conclude elevated LAP in concert with depressed LVEF

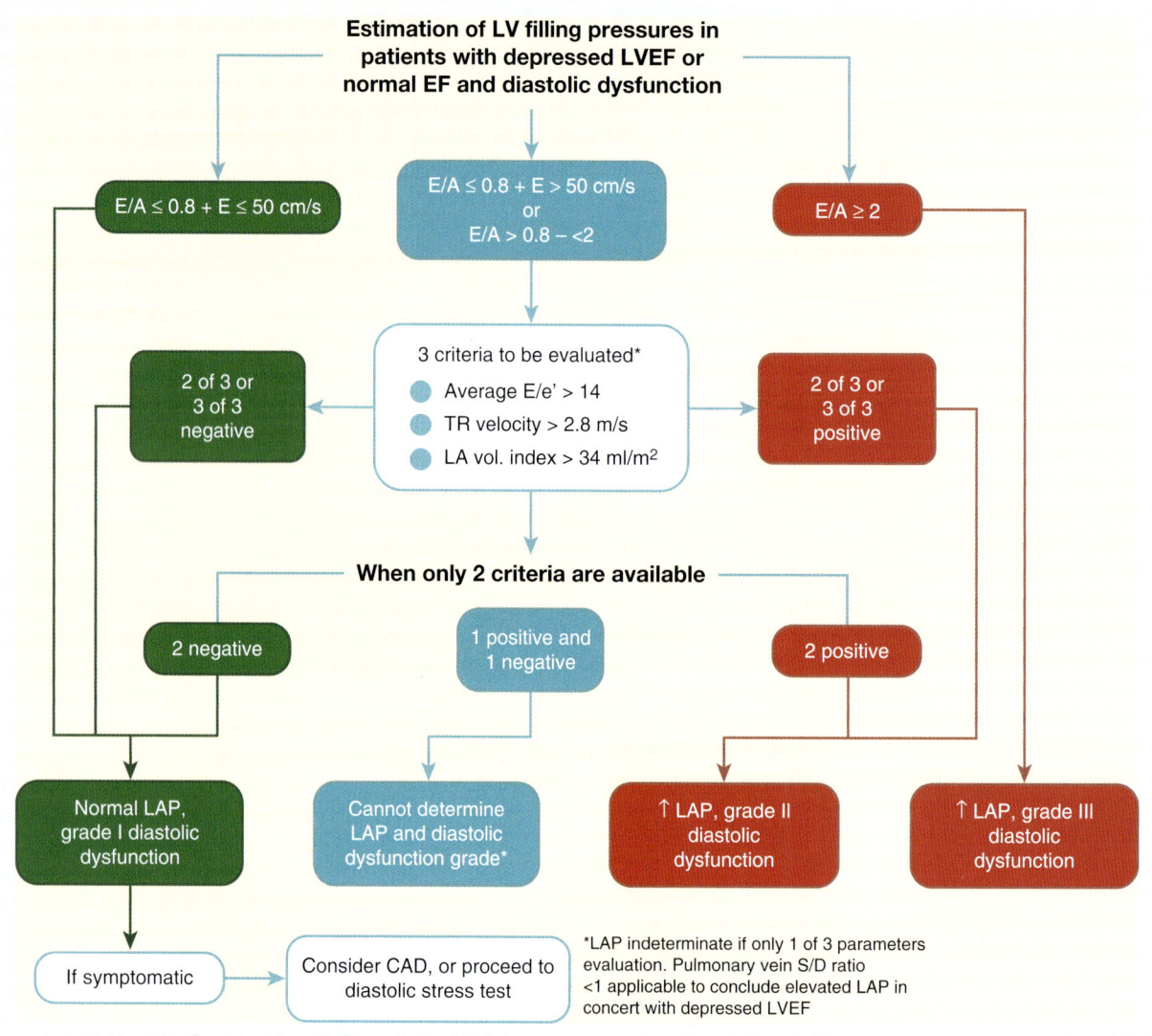

Figure 12.20. Algorithm for estimation of left ventricular (LV) filling pressures and grading LV diastolic function in patients with depressed LVEF and in patients with myocardial disease and normal LVEF. E/A, ratio of peak mitral flow velocity of the early filling wave over peak mitral flow velocity of the late filling wave due to atrial contraction; E/e', ratio of peak mitral flow velocity of the early filling wave over tissue Doppler early diastolic annular velocity; TR, tricuspid regurgitation; LA vol., left atrial volume; LAP, left atrial pressure; LVEF, left ventricular ejection fraction; CAD, coronary artery disease; pulmonary vein S/D, pulmonary vein systolic flow over pulmonary vein diastolic flow. Note this diagram applies to patients with depressed ejection fraction (EF) or normal EF and diastolic dysfunction as noted from the first diagram (**Figure 12.20**). This would usually apply to a patient with CAD and wall motion abnormalities, left ventricular hypertrophy, or cardiomyopathy. Also note for patients with a depressed EF, a pulmonary vein S/D ratio <1 may suggest elevated LAP. (Adapted from Nagueh SF, Smiseth OA, Appleton CP, et al. Recommendations for the evaluation of left ventricular diastolic function by echocardiography: an update from the American Society of Echocardiography and the European Association of Cardiovascular Imaging. *J Am Soc Echocardiogr.* 2016;29(4):277-314. Copyright © 2016 American Society of Echocardiography. With permission.)

with grade I diastolic dysfunction, the increase in e' with exercise is much less than that of mitral E velocity such that the E/e' ratio increases. Besides filling pressures, stress echocardiography also allows evaluation of systolic function in patients with coronary artery disease, of MR severity in patients with mitral valve disease, and of pulmonary artery pressures. Cardiac MRI is not warranted in mild LVH likely related to hypertension and without echo features of cardiomyopathy.

7. **Answer: E.** Estimation of LV filling pressure from the ratio of transmitral and annular velocities (E/e') after exercise echocardiography may identify diastolic dysfunction in patients who complain of exertional dyspnea. Elevated exercise E/e' (septal >14.5) is associated with cardiovascular hospitalization, independent of and incremental to inducible ischemia. Although the clinical implications of this finding have not yet been fully elucidated, one could consider starting therapy with a β-blocker, thereby preventing exercise-induced tachycardia

Table 12.5. LV Relaxation, Filling Pressures, and Two-Dimensional/Doppler Findings According to LV Diastolic Function

	Normal	Grade I	Grade II	Grade III
LV relaxation	Normal	Impaired	Impaired	Impaired
LAP	Normal	Low or normal	Elevated	Elevated
Mitral E/A ratio	≥0.8	≤0.8	>0.8-<2	>2
Average E/e' ratio	<10	<10	10-14	>14
Peak TR velocity (m/s)	<2.8	<2.8	>2.8	>2.8
LA volume index	Normal	Normal or increased	Increased	Increased

E/A, ratio of peak mitral flow velocity of the early filling wave over peak mitral flow velocity of the late filling wave due to atrial contraction; E/e', ratio of peak mitral flow velocity of the early filling wave over tissue Doppler early diastolic annular velocity; LA, left atrial; LAP, left atrial pressure; LV, left ventricle; TR, tricuspid regurgitation.
Adapted from Nagueh SF, Smiseth OA, Appleton CP, et al. Recommendations for the evaluation of left ventricular diastolic function by echocardiography: an update from the American Society of Echocardiography and the European Association of Cardiovascular Imaging. *J Am Soc Echocardiogr.* 2016;29(4):277-314. Copyright © 2016 American Society of Echocardiography. With permission.)

and maximizing the diastolic filling period in these patients.

8. **Answer: D.** The presence of V waves in the absence of significant MR in this type of patient suggests severely decreased left atrial compliance. Classically, the left atrium has been ascribed to three different functions throughout the cardiac cycle: (1) reservoir function during ventricular systole and isovolumic relaxation (reflected by the pulmonary venous S wave); (2) conduit phase from the moment the mitral valve opens until onset of atrial contraction (reflected by the pulmonary venous D wave); and (3) contractile phase during atrial systole (reflected by the pulmonary venous AR wave and the mitral A wave). LA enlargement may begin as an adaptive response with an initial increase in LA volume, and LA emptying fraction that serves to maintain LV stroke volume and cardiac output. LA enlargement may be considered pathologic when the optimal Frank-Starling relationship is exceeded, resulting in decreased LA compliance, reduced reservoir and contractile pump functions, and eventually increased incidence of atrial arrhythmias.

9. **Answer: A.** The sample volume should be positioned at or 1 cm within the septal and lateral insertion sites of the mitral leaflets and adjusted as necessary (usually 5-10 mm) to cover the longitudinal excursion of the mitral annulus in both systole and diastole. This contrasts with a sample volume size of 1 to 3 mm at mitral valve leaflet tips for optimal pulsed-wave Doppler assessment of mitral valve inflow, and a sample volume of 2 to 3 mm placed >0.5 cm into the pulmonary vein for optimal recording of pulmonary vein flow. Attention should be directed to Doppler spectral gain settings because annular velocities have high signal amplitude. Most current ultrasound systems have tissue Doppler presets for the proper velocity scale and Doppler wall filter settings to display the annular velocities. In general, the velocity scale should be set at ~20 cm/s above and below the zero-velocity baseline, although lower settings may be needed when there is severe LV dysfunction, and annular velocities are markedly reduced (scale set to 10-15 cm/s). Minimal angulation (<20°) should be present between the ultrasound beam and the plane of cardiac motion.

10. **Answer: B.** First-degree AV block may lead to fusion of the E and A wave and therefore has a similar effect on mitral inflow as sinus tachycardia. First-degree AV block results in delayed onset of ventricular contraction relative to atrial contraction but typically would not affect isovolumetric contraction (the time between mitral valve closure and aortic valve opening). A fused mitral inflow pattern can make an accurate interpretation of diastolic function impossible if no other information is available. In the presence of severely elevated LV filling pressures, first-degree AV block may lead to diastolic MR, as atrial contraction is not immediately followed by ventricular contraction, which is mandatory for complete mitral valve closure. Under these conditions, the atrioventricular pressure gradient may temporarily reverse during atrial relaxation, leading to diastolic MR. Fusion of E and A waves (leading to a decreased LV diastolic filling period) and diastolic MR may, in turn, have an adverse effect on cardiac output and filling pressures in patients with severe systolic dysfunction. Cardiac resynchronization therapy with restoration of optimal atrioventricular mechanical timing may improve LV filling in these patients. See **Figure 12.21A,B** for an illustration of the impact of PR prolongation on the mitral inflow pattern.

266 / Clinical Echocardiography Review

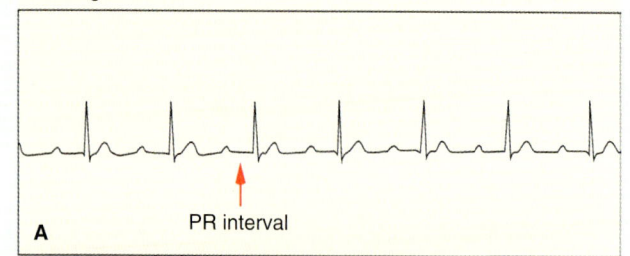

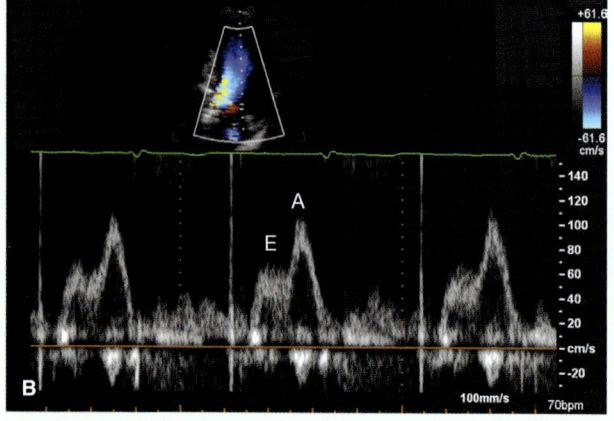

Figure 12.21. **A** and **B**: E/A fusion. Mitral inflow.

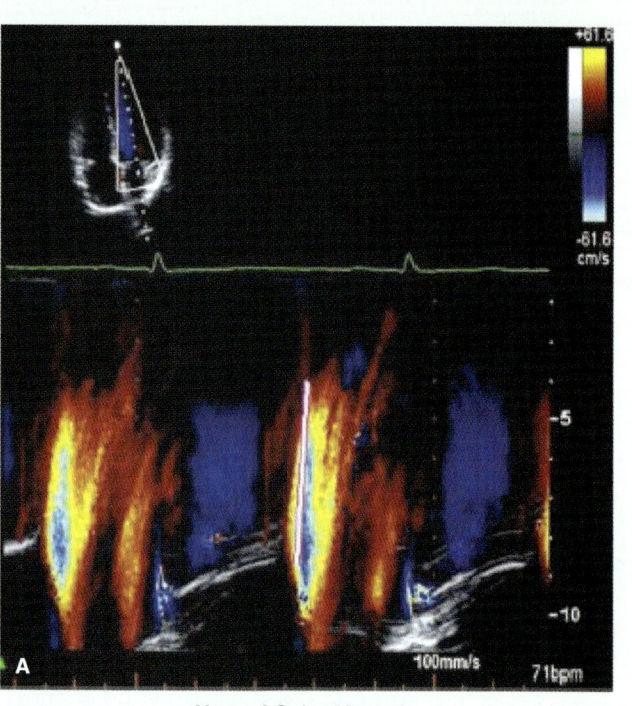

Normal Color M-mode
Figure 12.22A

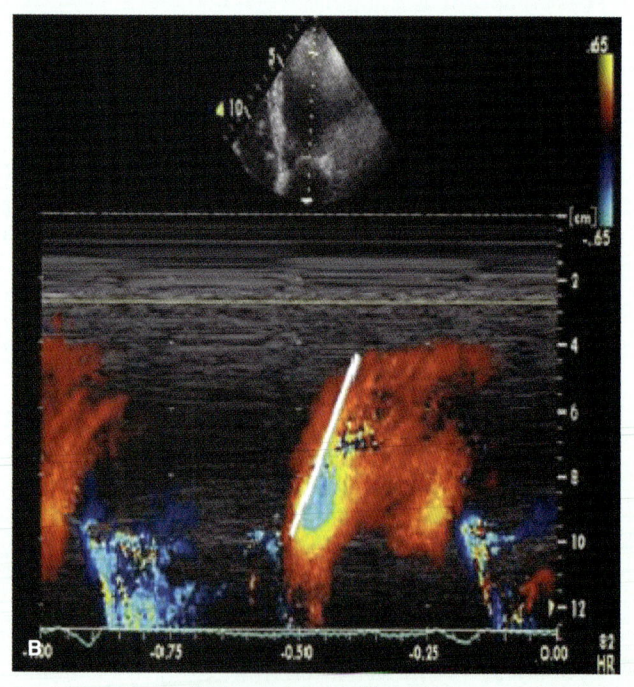

Prolonged Color M-mode
Figure 12.22B

11. **Answer: D.** Color Doppler M-mode (CMM) echocardiography provides a spatiotemporal map of blood distribution within the heart with a typical temporal resolution of 5 ms, a spatial resolution of 300 μm, and a velocity resolution of 3 cm/s. Assessment of diastolic flow propagation has offered novel information about LV filling dynamics. V_p is unique in that it appears to be relatively independent of loading conditions and therefore may overcome one of the main limitations of Doppler-based techniques. The earliest CMM velocities often occur during isovolumic relaxation. After the mitral valve opens, there is a rapid initial component (phase 1), often followed by a slower component (phase 2). Finally, the last component in late diastole is associated with atrial contraction. See **Figure 12.22A,B** for examples of CMM and determination of the V_p slope (normal V_p is ≥50 cm/s) (white line). In clinical practice, however, V_p has limited additive utility in that its predictive ability regarding filling pressures is predominantly in patients with systolic dysfunction (where E/V_p ≥ 2.5 predicts PCWP > 15 mm Hg with reasonable accuracy), a scenario where there are often multiple echocardiographic signs of impaired LV diastolic function already present. Often the CMM pattern provides a preview of the pulsed-wave Doppler mitral inflow pattern, that is, the higher E or A wave will have an increased aliasing velocity. In **Figure 12.22A**, this will be the E wave.

12. **Answer: B.** E-wave deceleration time is mostly influenced by the operating stiffness of the LV. Changes in LV compliance (ie, the relationship between LV pressure and volume) and also changes in ventricular relaxation or early (instead of late) diastolic ventricular pressures will affect the deceleration time. Left atrial mechanical function and ejection fraction are not or weakly and indirectly correlated with deceleration time (**Figure 12.23**).

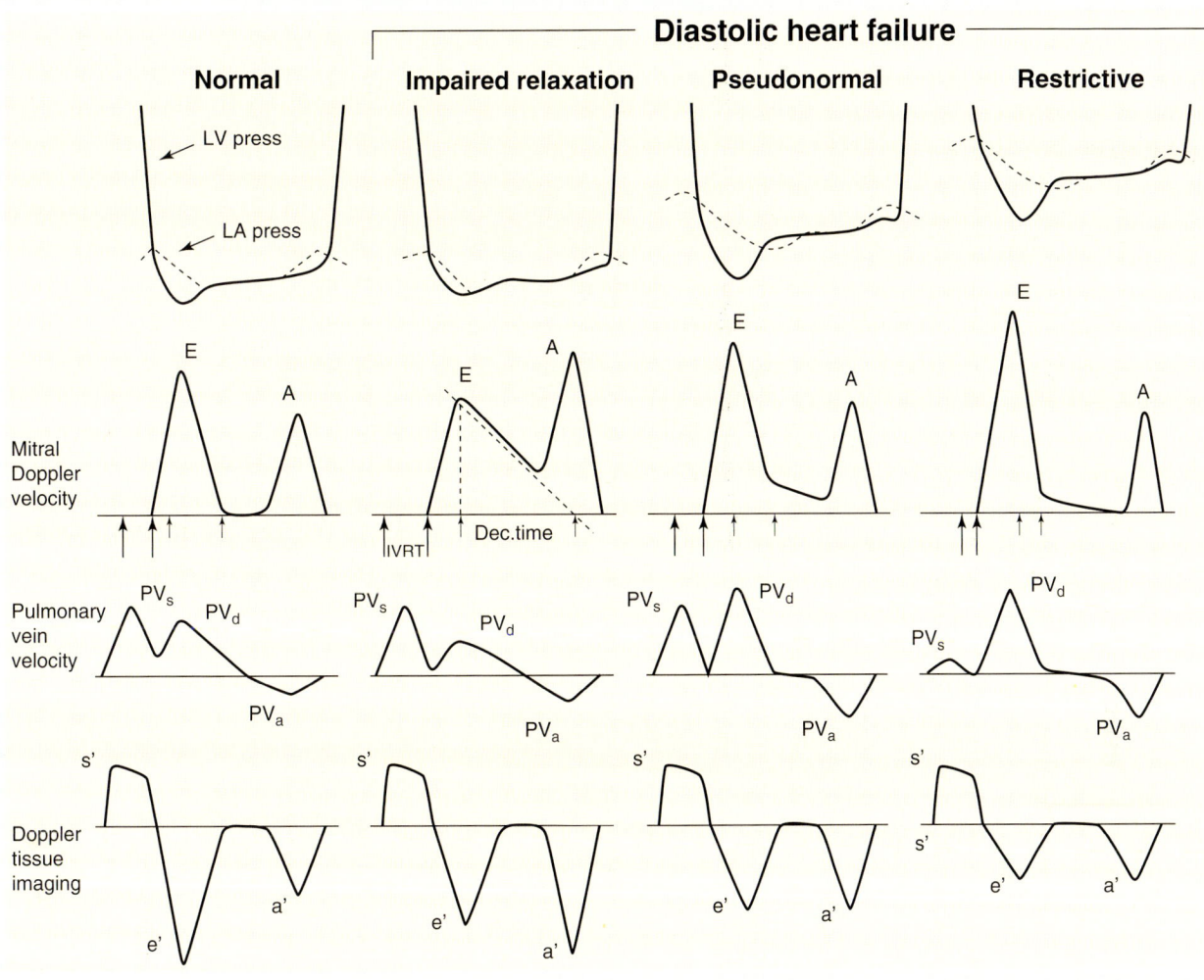

Figure 12.23. Impaired relaxation (Grade I diastolic dysfunction), pseudonormal (Grade II diastolic dysfunction) and restrictive (Grade III diastolic dysfunction). (Reprinted with permission from Zile MR, Brutsaert DL. New concepts in diastolic dysfunction and diastolic heart failure: part I—diagnosis, prognosis, and measurements of diastolic function. *Circulation*. 2002;105:1387-1393.)

13. **Answer: D.** In patients with dilated cardiomyopathies, pulsed-wave Doppler mitral flow velocity variables and filling patterns correlate better with cardiac filling pressures, functional class, and prognosis than does LV ejection fraction. Patients with impaired LV relaxation are the least symptomatic, while a short IVRT, short mitral deceleration time, and increased E- to A-wave velocity ratio characterize advanced diastolic dysfunction, increased left atrial pressure, and a worse functional class. A restrictive filling pattern is associated with a poor prognosis, especially if it persists after preload reduction. Likewise, a grade II or restrictive filling pattern associated with acute myocardial infarction indicates an increased risk of heart failure, unfavorable LV remodeling, and increased CV mortality, irrespective of ejection fraction (**Figure 12.24**). In addition to dilated cardiomyopathy, deceleration time has also been shown to be an important predictor of survival in restrictive cardiomyopathy (eg, cardiac amyloidosis).

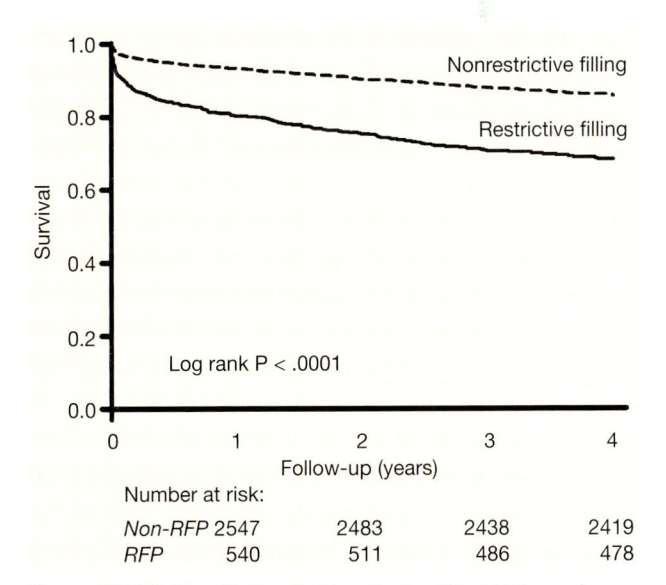

Figure 12.24. Event-free survival in patients with restrictive and nonrestrictive filling patterns (non-RFP). (Reprinted with permission from Meta-Analysis Research Group in Echocardiography [MeRGE] AMI Collaborators. Independent prognostic importance of a restrictive left ventricular filling pattern after myocardial infarction: an individual patient meta-analysis—Meta-analysis research group in echocardiography acute myocardial infarction. *Circulation*. 2008;117:2591-2598.)

14. **Answer: D.** In cardiac patients, a decrease of ≥50% in E/A ratio with application of the Valsalva maneuver is highly specific for increased LV filling pressure. However, a smaller magnitude of change does not always indicate normal diastolic function. One major limitation of the Valsalva maneuver is that not everyone is able to perform this maneuver adequately and it is not standardized. The Valsalva maneuver is performed by forceful expiration (about 40 mm Hg) against a closed nose and mouth. A decrease of 20 cm/s in mitral peak E velocity is usually considered an adequate effort in patients without restrictive filling. Lack of reversibility with Valsalva is imperfect as an indicator that the diastolic filling pattern is irreversible. In a busy clinical laboratory, the Valsalva maneuver can be reserved for patients in whom diastolic function assessment is not clear after mitral inflow and annulus velocity measurements. The Valsalva is obviously of little use in patients with grade I diastolic dysfunction but is useful to differentiate grade II diastolic function from normal (**Figure 12.25**). Currently, stages have been changed to grades of diastolic function. Also stages of 1B and 4 are not in current 2016 ASE diastology guidelines.

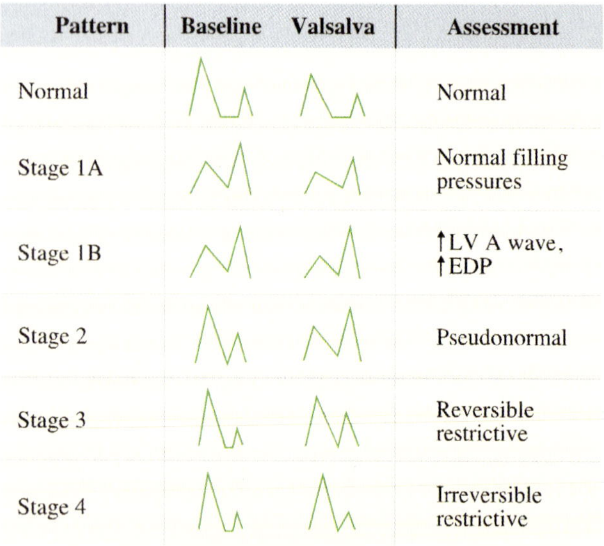

Pattern	Baseline	Valsalva	Assessment
Normal			Normal
Stage 1A			Normal filling pressures
Stage 1B			↑LV A wave, ↑EDP
Stage 2			Pseudonormal
Stage 3			Reversible restrictive
Stage 4			Irreversible restrictive

Figure 12.25

15. **Answer: A.** According to the grade of the disease progression, a spectrum of filling abnormalities can be seen in cardiac amyloidosis that varies from grade I diastolic function (delayed relaxation) (**Figure 12.1A**) to grade II diastolic function (pseudonormal) (**Figure 12.1B**) to grade III diastolic function (restrictive filling) (**Figure 12.1C**). Panels B and C in **Figure 12.1** represent these more advanced stages in the disease process where the operating stiffness of the LV becomes increasingly high due to a gradual loss in LV compliance. This is reflected in a short deceleration time (**Figure 12.1C**). In spite of the high left atrial pressure (suggested by a high E-wave velocity), atrial contraction itself hardly contributes to LV filling in the most advanced grades of diastolic dysfunction, as suggested by the diminutive A wave in restrictive filling. In contrast, although patients with delayed relaxation may be asymptomatic at rest or with mild exercise, their LV has become more dependent on atrial contraction (low E/A ratio). As such, these patients are most likely to feel a change in symptoms with sudden onset of atrial fibrillation due to loss of the atrial kick.

16. **Answer: D.** The Doppler tracing in **Figure 12.2** shows transmitral flow during diastasis, often referred to as a mitral "L wave." The result is a triphasic mitral inflow pattern that can be seen in patients without structural heart disease—particularly if the HR is relatively slow. It represents an advanced grade of diastolic dysfunction that is characterized by elevated filling pressures and loss of compliance (notice the high peak of early rapid filling and the short initial deceleration time) in combination with very delayed relaxation. The markedly prolonged relaxation, although not immediately obvious, results in a sudden decrease in LV diastolic pressure during mid-diastole, allowing further LV filling during mid-diastole. This explains the L wave. Preload reduction will decrease left atrial pressure as well as the operating stiffness of the LV and may unmask the underlying relaxation abnormality in the presence of pseudonormalization.

17. **Answer: C.** Athletes not uncommonly have resting bradycardia, mild concentric hypertrophy, and/or mild chamber dilation due to increased pressure and volume loads related to sustained increases in activity. An early diastolic velocity of the mitral annulus derived by tissue Doppler echocardiography (e′) <8 cm/s is, however, a markedly abnormal finding especially in a 35-year-old person.

Due to LVH, the algorithm shown in **Figure 12.20** will be used. This shows other findings that also suggest elevated left atrial filling pressures.

18. **Answer: D.** Although we have no information on the exact severity of LV dysfunction nor present hemodynamic state, Doppler findings show grade III diastolic dysfunction. Although these patients have a better long-term outcome if treated with beta-blocking agents, the echocardiographic findings also indicate that the current operating stiffness of the heart is probably very high. The cardiac output in these patients can therefore be very dependent on HR, as it is almost impossible to increase cardiac output by an augmentation of their stroke volume. Remember that cardiac output = HR multiplied by stroke volume. Careful titration of the β-blocker therapy dose in these patients is therefore warranted.

19. **Answer: A.** Figure 12.5 shows aortic regurgitation, with an end-diastolic velocity of 4.0 m/s. LVEDP can be estimated from diastolic blood pressure (78 mm Hg) minus the end-diastolic pressure gradient between the aorta and the left ventricle (which, using the simplified Bernoulli equation, equals here 4 Var^2 or 64 mm Hg). Similarly, in the absence of LV or aortic outflow tract obstruction, left atrial pressure can be estimated from systolic blood pressure minus 4 (Vmr)^2.

20. **Answer: C.** The Doppler findings demonstrate a large (>30 ms) difference between the duration of the mitral A-wave velocity and the duration of the late diastolic pulmonary venous flow reversal (AR), suggesting elevated end-diastolic LV filling pressures. This is usually seen in patients with grade II or grade III diastolic dysfunction, so that the most likely answer is the 60-year-old man with advanced hypertensive heart disease. A waves will be absent if atrial fibrillation is present. Reversal or at least blunting of the S wave would be expected if significant mitral regurgitation is present. Pulmonary venous inflow velocities are influenced by age: normal young subjects aged <40 years usually have prominent D velocities (reflecting their mitral E waves); the S/D ratio increases with increasing age. AR velocities also typically increase with age but usually do not exceed 35 cm/s without increased LVEDP.

21. **Answer: A.** The mitral inflow pattern can be used with relative accuracy to assess filling pressures in patients with depressed LV systolic function. In this population, changes in the inflow pattern will reflect changes in preload (eg, due to volume overload or changes in medical therapy). Confusion between normal and pseudonormal (grade II) filling should be absent as diastolic function is intrinsically disturbed in the presence of advanced systolic dysfunction.

    In contrast, additional information is needed in the presence of preserved ejection fraction as this Doppler pattern could equally represent normal or pseudonormal (grade II) filling. As mentioned earlier, the echocardiographer should assess tissue Doppler–derived e', Vp obtained by color M-mode Doppler, measure left atrial size, and finally evaluate the effect of Valsalva to detect an underlying relaxation abnormality in the case of pseudonormal (grade II) filling. Left atrial dilatation can merely represent atrial remodeling independent of filling pressures in the setting of atrial fibrillation. Moderate and severe MR usually leads to an elevation of peak E velocity, representing the increased flow rate during diastole with a normal deceleration time. However, particularly with chronic MR, the left atrium will dilate and the increased left atrial compliance may be sufficient to maintain filling pressures at a normal level. Finally, a high velocity tricuspid regurgitant jet may be suggestive of (but is not specific for) elevated left-sided filling pressures. Many other conditions may lead to pulmonary hypertension in the presence of normal diastolic function.

22. **Answer: C.** In patients with constrictive pericarditis, there are increased right ventricular and right atrial pressures, and characteristically, these patients demonstrate augmentation of diastolic flow reversals with expiration compared to diastolic forward flow. The hepatic vein expiratory diastolic reversal/forward diastolic flow ratio greater than and equal to 0.8 is highly suggestive of constriction. In normal patients, hepatic vein Doppler velocities reflect changes in pressure, volume, and compliance of the right atrium. Typically, hepatic vein Doppler velocities consist of four elements: (1) systolic forward flow (S), (2) diastolic forward flow (D), (3) systolic flow reversal (VR), and (4) atrial flow reversal (AR). In patients with normal hemodynamics, S is typically larger than D and there are no significant systolic or diastolic reversals. Typically, with myopathic conditions, flow reversals are accentuated with inspiration due to increased systemic venous return to the right heart. Diastolic flow reversal is seen most commonly in patients with pulmonary hypertension and constrictive pericarditis, and it is respiratory variation that helps to differentiate them from each other. Patients with pulmonary hypertension typically do not have augmentation of diastolic flow reversals with respiration. In addition, constrictive pericarditis can be differentiated from restrictive cardiomyopathy with hepatic venous Doppler recordings. In patients with restrictive cardiomyopathy, inspiratory diastolic flow reversal is larger than expiratory. Alternatively, patients with severe tricuspid regurgitation, which by definition is occurring during systole, will typically demonstrate prominent systolic flow reversals (**Figure 12.26**).

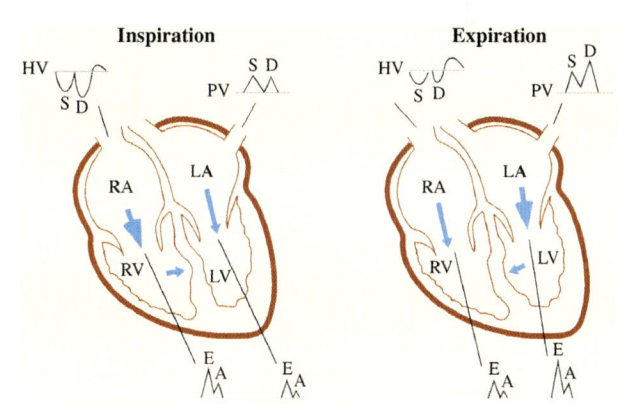

Figure 12.26

23. **Answer: D.** This patient has myocardial disease and normal LVEF. When myocardial disease such as ischemic heart disease is present, proceed to the algorithm shown in **Figure 12.20** rather than **Figure 12.19**. While additional parameters are provided here, it is important to note that before these are considered, the E/A ratio should be assessed. If E/A ratio is ≤0.8, this is grade I diastolic function. If E/A ratio is ≥2, this is grade III diastolic function. Thus, further information with the E/A is the next step for assessment.

24. **Answer: C.** The reduced septal and lateral e' velocities (3-4 cm/s) are consistent with a restrictive cardiomyopathy and the apical sparing bull's-eye ("cherry-on-top") pattern suggests it is likely cardiac amyloidosis. Red areas are normal longitudinal strain at the apex ("spared" or preserved apex), whereas pink/blue areas are abnormal longitudinal strain in the mid to basal segments. Other echocardiographic characteristics of cardiac amyloidosis include increased biventricular wall thickness, sparkling texture of the myocardium, biatrial enlargement, increased interatrial septal thickness, thickened mitral leaflets, and small pericardial effusion. In more advanced cardiac amyloidosis, the tissue Doppler imaging (TDI) shows the 5-5-5 sign (ie, s', e', and a' tissue velocities are all <5 cm/s). Isovolumic contraction and relaxation times are increased, whereas ejection time is decreased. (See Dorbala S, Ando Y, Bokhari S, et al. ASNC/AHA/ASE/EANM/HFSA/ISA/SCMR/SNMMI expert consensus recommendations for multimodality imaging in cardiac amyloidosis: Part 1 of 2-evidence base and standardized methods of imaging. *J Nucl Cardiol.* 2019;26(6):2065-2123).

25. **Answer: A.** The echocardiographic features and clinical findings including carpal tunnel syndrome, hypotension, and progressive blood pressure medication intolerance are suggestive of ATTR cardiac amyloidosis. It is important to note that not all features may be present clinically or on echocardiography, especially early in the disease process.

> **KEY POINTS**
> **Case 1**
> - Apical sparing bull's-eye ("cherry-on-top") pattern can be seen in cardiac amyloidosis. Red areas are normal longitudinal strain at the apex ("spared" or preserved apex), whereas pink/blue areas are abnormal longitudinal strain in the mid to basal segments.
> - Echocardiographic characteristics of cardiac amyloidosis include increased biventricular wall thickness, sparkling texture of the myocardium, biatrial enlargement, increased interatrial septal thickness, thickened mitral leaflets, small pericardial effusion.
> - In more advanced cardiac amyloidosis, the tissue Doppler imaging (TDI) shows the 5-5-5 sign (ie, s', e', and a' tissue velocities are all <5 cm/s).
> - Not all clinical or echocardiographic features may be present in cardiac amyloidosis, especially early in the disease process.

26. **Answer: D.** His symptoms can be explained by the constellation of preserved systolic function, normal ventricular size, and marked dilatation of both atria. These findings and a history of intermittent paroxysmal atrial fibrillation at an unusual young age suggest a form of restrictive cardiomyopathy.

27. **Answer: B.** Cardiac catheterization in this patient revealed normal coronary arteries but elevated filling pressures with a mean right atrial pressure of 20 mm Hg, pulmonary artery pressures of 57/25 mm Hg, right ventricular pressures of 56/22 mm Hg, PCWP of 26 mm Hg, and a cardiac output of 4 L/min. An endomyocardial biopsy showed focal nonspecific interstitial fibrosis with no evidence of amyloidosis, hemochromatosis, or sarcoidosis. The patient eventually died 3 months later from progressive heart failure and ventricular arrhythmias.

> **KEY POINTS**
> **Case 2**
> - An integrative Doppler assessment of diastolic function should be performed in every patient with unexplained shortness of breath. Advanced diastolic dysfunction and atrial dilatation in spite of normal LV size and function are the hallmarks of restrictive cardiomyopathy.
> - In idiopathic restrictive cardiomyopathy, the LV shows normal wall thickness with a preserved EF and biatrial enlargement.
> - Restrictive physiology is noted by the shortened mitral E wave deceleration time and the E/A ratio is markedly increased (typically ≥2.0).
> - Restrictive cardiomyopathy is notable for restrictive (grade III) diastolic filling with relatively normal systolic function.
> - As left atrial pressure increases with disease progression, the mitral valve opens at a higher pressure, which results in a decrease in the IVRT. In addition, there is increased transmitral pressure gradient, increased E velocity on pulsed-wave Doppler, and decreased systolic pulmonary venous flow velocity and pulmonary venous systolic/diastolic ratio <1.

28. **Answer: A.** This patient has normal diastolic function. The algorithm in **Figure 12.19** would be used given no myocardial pathology with normal LVEF and wall thickness. Her parameters fall within normal, that is, E/e' < 14, septal e' >7 cm/s and lateral e' velocity >10 cm/s, TR velocity is <2.8 m/s, and LA volume index is <34 mL/m^2.

29. **Answer: E.** No further testing is needed. The diastolic function is normal as per **Figure 12.19**.

> **KEY POINTS**
> **Case 3**
> - The initial step in determining diastolic function is assessment of LV function and assessing for the presence of myocardial pathology. If normal LV

function and no myocardial pathology, the algorithm should be used as shown in **Figure 12.19**.
- If there is normal LV function and no myocardial disease, four key parameters are assessed for abnormality: annular e' velocities (septal e' < 7 cm/s, lateral e' < 10 cm/s), average E/e' ratio >14, LA volume index >34 mL/m², and peak TR velocity >2.8 m/s. LV diastolic function is normal if more than half of the available variables are within the cutoff value. These parameters are normal in this case.

30. **Answer: C.** Deceleration time ≤150 ms in patients with biopsy-proven amyloidosis has been shown to correlate to a significantly worse prognosis and risk of cardiac death over an 18-month period with a relative risk for cardiac death nearly five times greater than those patients with a deceleration time >150 ms. Similarly, 1-year cardiac survival of patients with an increased E/A ratio (≥2.1) was less than that of patients with normal or decreased E/A ratio (<2.1) (**Figure 12.27**).

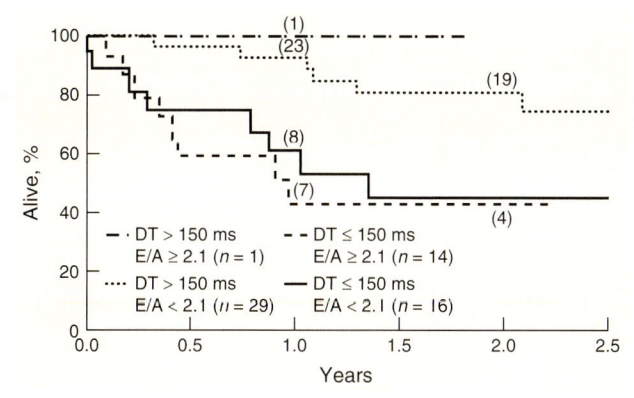

Figure 12.27. Reprinted with permission from Klein AL, Hatle LK, Taliercio CP, et al. Prognostic significance of Doppler measures of diastolic function in cardiac amyloidosis: a Doppler echocardiography study. *Circulation*. 1991;83:808-816.

31. **Answer: B.** In most, if not all, cardiac disease, as with cardiac amyloidosis, the initial diastolic dysfunction grade is impaired relaxation. With disease progression, continued impaired relaxation ultimately results in mild to moderate increases in left atrial pressure that can cause the mitral inflow velocity pattern to appear similar to a normal filling ("pseudonormal" or grade II) pattern. The E/A ratio is typically 1 to 1.5 and the E-wave deceleration time is usually between 160 and 220 ms. The best way to identify a grade II diastolic dysfunction or pseudonormal filling pattern is by demonstrating impaired myocardial relaxation by average E/e' >14, TR velocity >2.8 cm/s, and LAVI >34 mL/m² (see **Figure 12.20**) as per 2016 ASE diastology guidelines. In patients with known systolic dysfunction or abnormally increased wall thickness, a normal E/A ratio suggests that increased left atrial pressure is masking abnormal relaxation. By decreasing preload (ie, via the Valsalva maneuver), one may unmask the impaired LV relaxation by causing the E/A ratio to decrease by 0.5 or more and reversal of the E/A ratio. In addition, color M-mode of the mitral inflow can determine rate of flow propagation in the LV, and with worsening diastolic function, myocardial relaxation is always impaired and flow propagation is slow even when left atrial pressure and mitral E velocity are increased. Cardiac amyloidosis is characterized by regional variations in longitudinal strain with relative "apical sparing." This pattern is an easily recognizable, accurate, and reproducible method of differentiating cardiac amyloidosis from other causes of LV hypertrophy (see **Figure 12.28**).

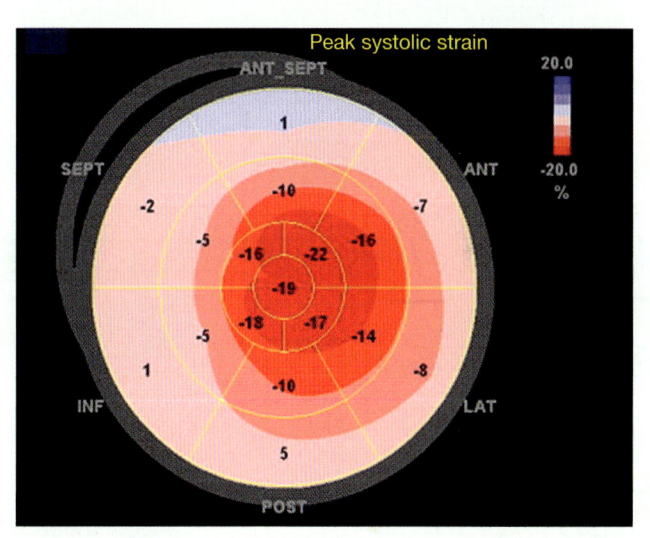

Figure 12.28. Bull's eye plot of segmental peak global longitudinal strain.

KEY POINTS
Case 4
- Deceleration time is an important prognostic factor in patients with cardiac amyloidosis.
- Grade II diastolic dysfunction ("pseudonormal" pattern) represents a moderate grade of diastolic dysfunction, combining mildly to moderately elevated left atrial pressures, and an LV relaxation abnormality.
- A relative "apical sparing" longitudinal strain pattern is an easily recognizable, accurate, and reproducible method of differentiating cardiac amyloidosis from other causes of LV hypertrophy.

32. **Answer: C.** This patient has grade III diastolic dysfunction with severe LVH due to hypertrophic cardiomyopathy. It is important to use the special population table for hypertrophic cardiomyopathy rather than **Figure 12.20**. There is elevated LV filling pressures with an elevated E/e' >14 and peak TR velocity >2.8 m/s and LAVI of > 34 mL/m²

KEY POINTS
Case 5

- In patients with hypertrophic cardiomyopathy, the usual algorithm approach should not be used. This is a special population
- Variables used to assess diastolic function in the algorithm shown in **Figure 12.20** include E/A ratio, average E/e' ratio (abnormal >14), LA volume index (abnormal >34 mL/m^2), pulmonary vein S/D ratio (abnormal <1), and peak velocity of TR jet by CW Doppler (abnormal >2.8 m/s). In this patient, there is elevated LV filling pressures with an elevated E/e' >14 and peak TR velocity >2.8 m/s and LAVI of > 34 mL/m^2
  For hypertrophic cardiomyopathy (special population) the following should be used:
  1. Average E/e' (>14)
  2. Ar-A (≥30 ms)
  3. Peak TR velocity (>2.8 m/s)
  4. LA maximum volume index (>34 mL/m^2)
- Diastolic function assessment in HCM is not recommended if there is more than moderate severity mitral regurgitation, usually due to systolic anterior motion (SAM) of the mitral valve.

33. **Answer: B.** Based on the ASE 2016 guidelines algorithm in **Figure 12.20**, although E/A is between 0.8 and 2, the absence of E/e' ratio means only two criteria are available. Here, the LA volume is abnormal and TR velocity is normal. Thus, the correct answer is cannot determine LAP and diastolic dysfunction grade. Often other paramaters such as pulmonary vein flow or left atrial reservoir strain can be used to further assess the grade of diastolic function.

34. **Answer: B.** The reduced LA reservoir strain can be a helpful marker of elevated left atrial pressures. The information in the figure reports three LA strain values: reservoir strain (LASr), which is peak longitudinal strain corresponding to atrial reservoir function; conduit strain (LAScd), which is during early diastole and reflects conduit function; and LA contraction strain (LASct), which is late diastole corresponding to atrial contraction. According to a 2022 consensus statement by Smiseth et al, if the LA reservoir strain (LASr) is <18%, this suggests elevated left atrial filling pressures and no longer indeterminate diastolic function (see **Figure 12.29**).

Estimation of left ventricular filling pressure

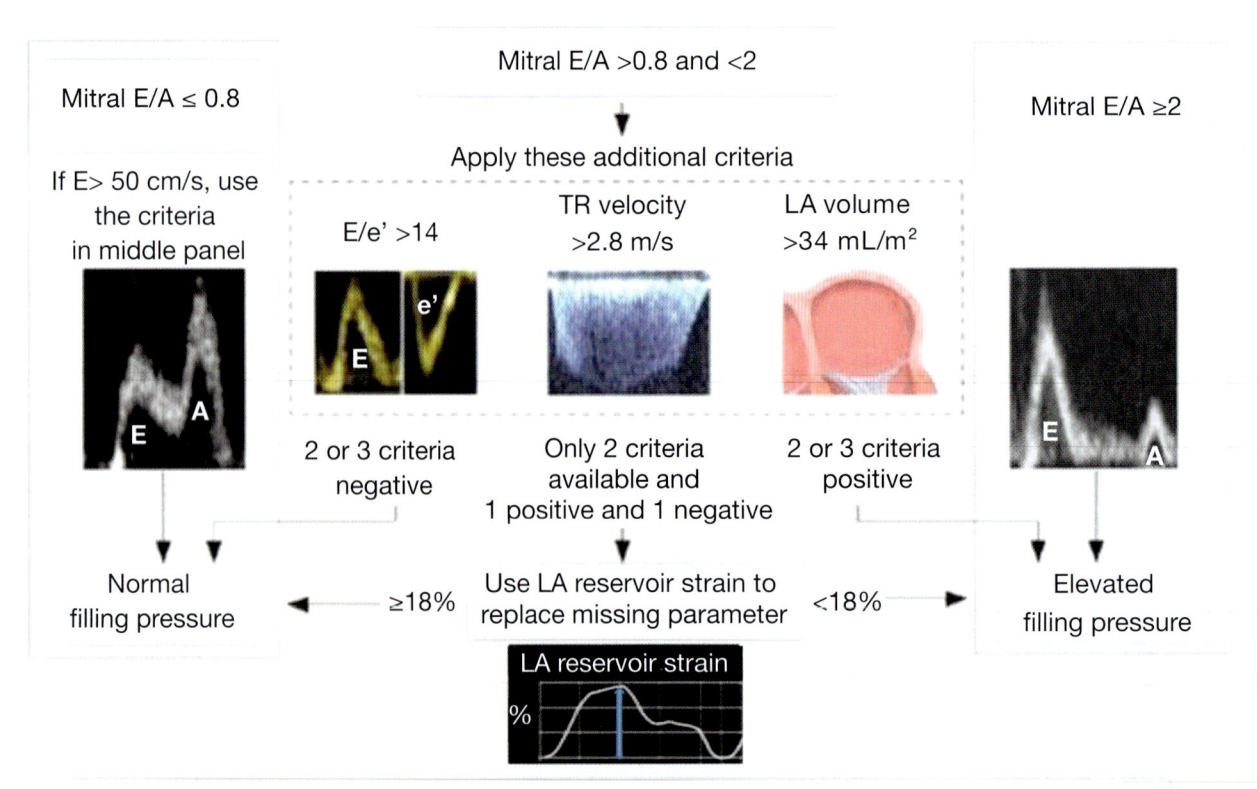

Caveat - Algorithm not to be applied in any of the following conditions:
no suspicion of heart disease; atrial fibrillation; LBBB/CRT/RV pacing; HCM; severe MR/MS/MAC; MV prosthesis or repair; high output HF; LV assist device

Figure 12.29. Reprinted with permission from Smiseth OA, Morris DA, Cardim N, et al. Multimodality imaging in patients with heart failure and preserved ejection fraction: an expert consensus document of the European Association of Cardiovascular Imaging. *Eur Heart J Cardiovasc Imaging.* 2022;23(2):e34-e61. Figure 15.

> **KEY POINTS**
> **Case 6**
> - Diastolic function assessment is generally indeterminate if there are one positive and one negative parameter, but missing the other one, that is, normal TR velocity and elevated LAVI, but no E/e' velocity available.
> - LA reservoir strain (LASr) <18% can be a useful adjunct to suggest elevated left atrial filling pressures. If it was >18%, this would suggest normal left atrial filling pressure.
> - LA reservoir strain (LASr) is peak longitudinal strain corresponding to atrial reservoir function; conduit strain (LAScd) is during early diastole and reflects conduit function; and LA contraction strain (LASct) is late diastole corresponding to atrial contraction.

35. **Answer: A.** Diastolic function cannot be evaluated due to severe MAC. In moderate to severe MAC, the mitral orifice is restricted, so lateral and posterior e' velocities can be decreased due to limited mitral leaflet movement. This can lead to an increased E/e' ratio due to the mitral annular calcification. Thus, the 2016 ASE diastolic function algorithms can only be applied in the absence of significant mitral valve disease.

> **KEY POINTS**
> **Case 7**
> - Diastolic function assessment relies on relatively healthy and functioning mitral valve leaflets. If there is significant mitral valve disease, parameters used for diastolic function assessment may not be reliable because the transmitral velocities and annular dynamics reflect valve disease rather than LV and LA pressures. In moderate to severe mitral annular calcification, the mitral leaflets are restricted due to the mechanical effect of the calcification process. For example, in MAC, the E/e' ratio increases unrelated to diastolic function, thus should not be used in significant MAC.
> - Abudiab et al showed that a high E/A ratio (>1.8) and short IVRT (<80 ms) were suggestive of elevated LAP in the setting of MAC (See Abudiab MM, Chebrolu LH, Schutt RC, et al. Doppler echocardiography for the estimation of LV filling pressure in patients with mitral annular calcification. *JACC Cardiovasc Imaging*. 2017;10(12):1411-1420).

Acknowledgments: We gratefully acknowledge the contributions of previous edition author(s), Andrew O. Zurick III and David Verhaert, as portions of their chapter have been retained in this revision.

SUGGESTED READINGS

Andersen OS, Smiseth OA, Dokainish H, et al. Estimating left ventricular filling pressure by echocardiography. *J Am Coll Cardiol*. 2017;69(15):1937-1948.

Chan N, Wang TKM, Anthony C, et al. Echocardiographic evaluation of diastolic function in special populations. *Am J Cardiol*. 2023;202:131-143.

Cohen GI, Pietrolungo JF, Thomas JD, Klein AL. A practical guide to assessment of ventricular diastolic function using Doppler echocardiography. *J Am Coll Cardiol*. 1996;27(7):1753-1760.

Inoue K, Khan FH, Remme EW, et al. Determinants of left atrial reservoir and pump strain and use of atrial strain for evaluation of left ventricular filling pressure. *Eur Heart J Cardiovasc Imaging*. 2021;23(1):61-70.

Klein AL, Abbara S, Agler DA, et al. American Society of Echocardiography clinical recommendations for multimodality cardiovascular imaging of patients with pericardial disease: endorsed by the Society for Cardiovascular Magnetic Resonance and Society of Cardiovascular Computed Tomography. *J Am Soc Echocardiogr*. 2013;26(9):965-1012.e15.

Klein AL, Garcia MJ, eds. *Diastology, Clinical Approach to Heart Failure and Preserved Ejection Fraction*. 2nd ed. Elsevier; 2021.

Klein AL, Ramchand J, Nagueh SF. Aortic stenosis and diastolic dysfunction: partners in crime. *J Am Coll Cardiol*. 2020;76(25):2952-2955.

Nagueh SF. Left ventricular diastolic function: understanding pathophysiology, diagnosis, and prognosis with echocardiography. *JACC Cardiovasc Imaging*. 2020;13(1 pt 2):228-244.

Nagueh SF. Heart failure with preserved ejection fraction: insights into diagnosis and pathophysiology. *Cardiovasc Res*. 2021;117(4):999-1014.

Nagueh SF, Khan SU. Left atrial strain for assessment of left ventricular diastolic function: focus on populations with normal LVEF. *JACC Cardiovasc Imaging*. 2023;16(5):691-707.

Nagueh SF, Smiseth OA, Appleton CP, et al. Recommendations for the evaluation of left ventricular diastolic function by echocardiography: an update from the American Society of Echocardiography and the European Association of Cardiovascular Imaging. *J Am Soc Echocardiogr*. 2016;29(4):277-314.

Obokata M, Reddy YNV, Borlaug BA. Diastolic dysfunction and heart failure with preserved ejection fraction: understanding mechanisms by using noninvasive methods. *JACC Cardiovasc Imaging*. 2020;13(1 pt 2):245-257.

Phelan D, Collier P, Thavendiranathan P, et al. Relative apical sparing of longitudinal strain using two-dimensional speckle-tracking echocardiography is both sensitive and specific for the diagnosis of cardiac amyloidosis. *Heart*. 2012;98(19):1442-1448.

Smiseth OA, Morris DA, Cardim N, et al. Multimodality imaging in patients with heart failure and preserved ejection fraction: an expert consensus document of the European Association of Cardiovascular Imaging. *Eur Heart J Cardiovasc Imaging*. 2022;23(2):e34-e61.

Welch TD, Ling LH, Espinosa RE, et al. Echocardiographic diagnosis of constrictive pericarditis: mayo clinic criteria. *Circ Cardiovasc Imaging*. 2014;7(3):526-534.

CHAPTER 13

Stress Echocardiography: Ischemic and Nonischemic

Edgar Argulian

QUESTIONS

1. A 77-year-old man with multiple cardiovascular risk factors complains of burning chest pain on exertion that is relieved by rest. During exercise echocardiography, which of the following is likely the latest event to be observed?
   A. Chest pain.
   B. Regional abnormality in myocardial relaxation.
   C. Regional wall motion abnormality.
   D. ST segment depression on electrocardiogram.
   E. None of the above.

2. Which of the following is normal global and regional response to dobutamine infusion during stress echocardiography?

3. A 54-year-old patient with chronic mild exertional shortness of breath and history of controlled hypertension is scheduled for dobutamine echocardiography. She has no history of coronary artery disease or prior ischemia testing. Her electrocardiogram shows normal sinus rhythm with left bundle branch block. Resting echocardiogram shows left ventricular ejection fraction of 54%. Which of the following is the most reliable indicator of normal, nonischemic regional response at peak dobutamine infusion rate compared to baseline?
   A. Exaggerated apical rocking.
   B. Improved wall thickening.
   C. Normalized endocardial excursion.
   D. Postsystolic segment shortening.
   E. None of the above.

	Endocardial Excursion		Left Ventricular End-Systolic Volume		Left Ventricular Ejection Fraction		Myocardial Thickening	
	Low Dose	Peak	Low Dose	Peak	Low Dose	Peak	Low Dose	Peak
A.	Inc	Inc	Dec	Dec	Inc	Inc	Inc	Inc
B.	Inc	Dec	Dec	Inc	Inc	Dec	Inc	Dec
C.	Inc	Inc	Inc	Inc	Inc	Inc	Inc	Inc
D.	Inc	Dec	Dec	Dec	Inc	Inc	Inc	Dec

Dec, decrease; Inc, increase.

4. Which of the following stress modalities is expected to demonstrate the highest degree of regional hyperkinesis in nonischemic segments?
A. Atrial pacing.
B. Dipyridamole.
C. Dobutamine.
D. Supine bicycle.
E. Treadmill exercise.

5. A 52-year-old patient with chronic exertional shortness of breath is referred for ischemia testing using dobutamine echocardiography. He is obese and has history of hyperlipidemia but no history of coronary artery disease. Resting echocardiogram shows normal left ventricular ejection fraction and no significant valvular abnormality. At dobutamine infusion rate of 20 µg/kg/min, the patient complains of dizziness and palpitations. His blood pressure is 75/50 mm Hg and heart rate is 100 bpm, from baseline of 135/75 mm Hg and 74 bpm, respectively. Dobutamine infusion is stopped. Immediate echocardiogram shows hyperdynamic left ventricle without regional wall motion abnormalities and normal right ventricular size. Which of the following additional echocardiographic interrogations is most likely to explain the hemodynamic response in this patient?
A. Continuous-wave Doppler through the left ventricular outflow.
B. Continuous-wave Doppler through the mitral valve.
C. Continuous-wave Doppler through the tricuspid valve.
D. Pulsed-wave Doppler at the mitral leaflet tips and mitral annular tissue Doppler.
E. Pulsed-wave Doppler at right ventricular outflow.

6. Which of the following is most likely to give a false-negative result during stress echocardiography?
A. Isolated left anterior descending artery disease.
B. Isolated left circumflex artery disease.
C. Marked increase in systolic blood pressure during stress.
D. Triple-vessel disease with "balanced" ischemia.
E. Use of atropine during dobutamine echocardiography.

7. Which of the following can decrease the specificity of stress echocardiography?
A. Apical foreshortening.
B. Delay on image acquisition.
C. Hypertensive response to exercise.
D. Inadequate exercise with suboptimal peak heart rate.
E. Use of a beta-blocker before stress testing.

8. Which of the following is the most appropriate reason to terminate the stress test during dobutamine echocardiography?
A. Chest discomfort.
B. New wall motion abnormalities.
C. T-wave inversions on electrocardiogram.
D. Upsloping ST segment depression on electrocardiogram.
E. Ventricular ectopic beats.

9. The sensitivity of stress echocardiography to detect ischemia is greatest in which of the following coronary artery distributions?
A. Left anterior descending artery.
B. Left circumflex artery.
C. Ramus intermedius.
D. Right coronary artery.
E. None of the above.

10. A 58-year-old woman complains of exertional shortness of breath and ankle swelling. She has no chest pain, cough, wheezing, palpitations, or syncope. She is treated for hypertension with hydrochlorothiazide and irbesartan. Pulmonary function testing is unremarkable. Resting transthoracic echocardiogram shows left atrial dilation, mild concentric left ventricular hypertrophy with left ventricular ejection fraction of 60%, and normal right ventricular size and function. The estimated pulmonary artery systolic pressure is 35 mm Hg. Which of the following postexercise parameters is most likely to explain this patient's symptoms?
A. Left ventricular ejection fraction.
B. Left ventricular outflow tract velocities.
C. Left ventricular wall motion analysis.
D. Right ventricular wall motion analysis.
E. Transmitral flow velocities and tissue Doppler velocities.

11. A 48-year-old woman complains of exertional dyspnea for the last several months. Her current exercise tolerance is about four blocks on a level ground, but she gets short of breath very easily when climbing stairs. Her past medical history is insignificant, but she has a strong family history of coronary artery disease. Electrocardiogram shows normal sinus rhythm with T-wave inversions in leads I, avL, and V6. Transthoracic echocardiogram shows left atrial enlargement, and dilated left ventricle with global hypokinesis and ejection fraction of 20%. The right ventricle is normal in size and function and the estimated pulmonary artery systolic pressure is 40 mm Hg. Which of the following is the best option in evaluating this patient?
  A. Dipyridamole echocardiography using 0.84 mg/kg.
  B. Dobutamine echocardiography using 2.5 to 40 µg/kg/min.
  C. Dobutamine echocardiography using 10 to 40 µg/kg/min.
  D. Treadmill exercise echocardiography using Bruce protocol.
  E. Treadmill exercise electrocardiogram using Bruce protocol.

12. A 44-year-old woman complains of exertional substernal chest discomfort that limits her exercise capacity. She has type 2 diabetes mellitus and hypertension. Her BMI is 29 kg/m². Coronary CT angiography shows no significant coronary atherosclerosis. Coronary flow reserve assessment is planned using flow velocity measurements in the left anterior descending artery interrogated with pulsed-wave Doppler during echocardiography examination. Which of the following is the stress modality of choice?
  A. Dipyridamole echocardiography using 0.84 mg/kg.
  B. Dobutamine echocardiography using 2.5 to 40 µg/kg/min.
  C. Dobutamine echocardiography using 10 to 40 µg/kg/min.
  D. Semisupine bicycle exercise electrocardiogram.
  E. Treadmill exercise echocardiography using Bruce protocol.

13. A 70-year-old man complains of progressive exertional dyspnea over the last 6 months. Cardiac catheterization shows no obstructive coronary disease. Echocardiogram shows left atrial dilation and left ventricular dilation with ejection fraction of 30%. Aortic valve appears calcified with restricted motion. Peak velocity across the aortic valve is 3 m/s, mean gradient is 28 mm Hg, and estimated aortic valve area is 0.8 cm². Which of the following findings during low-dose dobutamine infusion provide the strongest indication for the aortic valve replacement in this patient?
  A. Peak velocity across the aortic valve of 4.2 m/s and estimated aortic valve area of 0.8 cm².
  B. Mean gradient across the aortic valve of 35 mm Hg and estimated aortic valve area of 0.8 cm².
  C. Mean gradient across the aortic valve of 35 mm Hg and increase in stroke volume by 25%.
  D. Mean gradient across the aortic valve of 41 mm Hg and estimated aortic valve area of 1.2 cm².
  E. No increase in stroke volume and no increase in mean gradient across the aortic valve.

14. During myocardial perfusion echocardiography, a microbubble ultrasound-enhancing agent is infused at a constant rate. Echocardiographic images are acquired using low-power real-time imaging with intermittent high-energy bursts (flashes) aimed at destroying microbubbles. Which of the following curves best reflects normal replenishment of microbubble agent after a "flash" in segments not affected by flow-limiting coronary stenosis (**Figure 13.1**)?

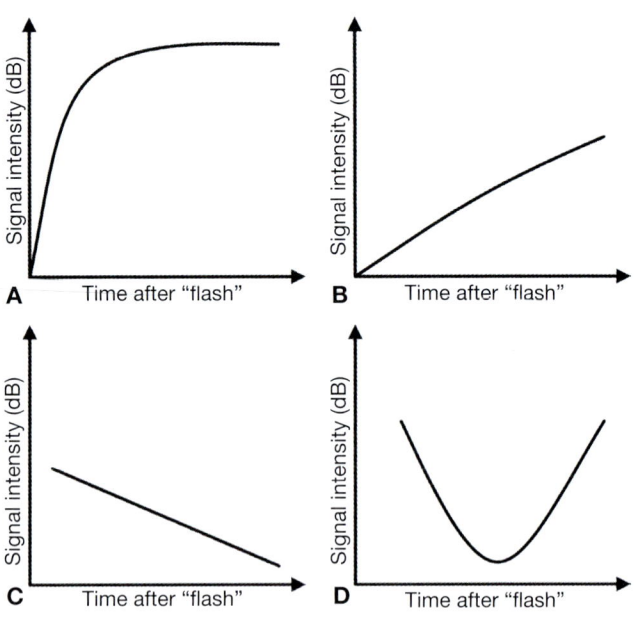

Figure 13.1

15. A patient with chronic exertional shortness of breath undergoes dobutamine echocardiography. She has known coronary artery disease and prior percutaneous coronary interventions. The beta-blocker therapy is appropriately held before the test. Her resting left ventricular ejection fraction is 36%. Her basal and mid-inferolateral and inferior walls are akinetic. During dobutamine infusion at low doses (2.5, 5, 10, and 20 µg/kg/min), the akinetic walls show no significant contractile reserve. At a high dose infusion (40 µg/kg/min), there is significant contractile reserve in the basal and mid-inferolateral segments. What **BEST** explains the latter finding in this patient?
A. Hibernating myocardium with critical coronary stenosis.
B. Nontransmural infarction of the inferolateral wall.
C. Stunned myocardium with open supplying coronary artery.
D. Tethering effect from the adjacent segments.
E. Transmural myocardial scarring.

16. A 64-year-old man presents with 5 months history of exertional dyspnea and intermittent chest pain. He has a strong family history of coronary artery disease. Transthoracic echocardiogram shows left atrial and left ventricular dilation with ejection fraction of 20%. The following peak longitudinal strain measurements are obtained with dobutamine infusion:

	Anterior Wall	Inferolateral Wall	Anterior Septum
Baseline	−10%	−12%	−9%
5 µg/kg/min	−14%	−10%	−13%
20 µg/kg/min (peak)	−9%	−9%	−15%

Which of the following is the **BEST** statement concerning the study results?
A. The anterior septum demonstrates ischemia.
B. The anterior septum is aneurysmal.
C. The anterior wall demonstrates ischemia.
D. The inferolateral wall demonstrates viability.
E. The findings are most consistent with nonischemic cardiomyopathy.

17. A 78-year-old patient with known coronary disease and prior percutaneous coronary interventions undergoes dobutamine echocardiography. He complains of exertional dyspnea and occasional chest tightness. His blood pressure is 115/75 mm Hg at rest and 155/85 mm Hg at peak. His only symptom during the test is "heart racing." Apical 3-chamber view during dobutamine infusion is shown (findings at 5 µg/kg/min, not shown, similar to 10 µg/kg/min) (**Figure 13.2** and ▶ **Video 13.1**).
Which of the following **BEST** describes the finding?
A. Marked viability in the apex.
B. Minimal viability in the inferolateral wall.
C. Ischemic regional response in the inferolateral wall.
D. Normal regional response in the anterior septum.
E. Normal regional response in the apex.

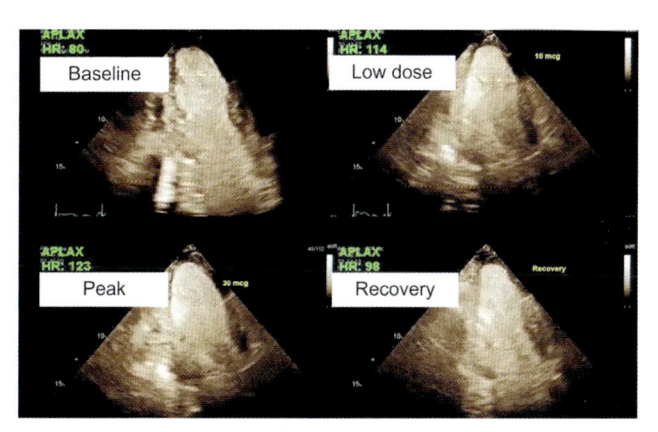

Figure 13.2

18. A 64-year-old patient with a history of hypertension and controlled HIV infection is referred for exercise echocardiography due to exertional chest discomfort. She exercises for 7 minutes and 20 seconds and has to stop due to chest tightness. She reaches 86% of her maximum predicted heart rate. The test findings (**Figure 13.3** and **Videos 13.2A-C**) are most consistent with which of the following coronary artery involvement?

A. Diagonal branch.
B. Left main coronary artery.
C. Proximal left anterior descending artery.
D. Posterior descending artery.
E. Right coronary artery.

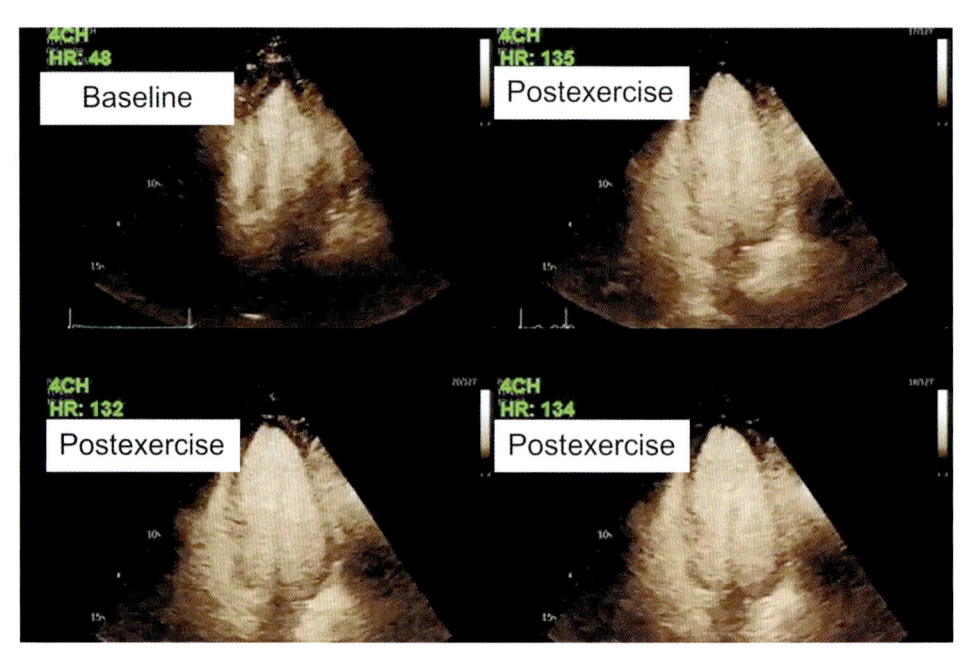

Figure 13.3

19. A 52-year-old female ex-smoker with a history of dyslipidemia and hypertension is referred for stress echocardiography due to exertional dyspnea and a recent episode of syncope. She exercises for 6 minutes on Bruce protocol and has to stop due to shortness of breath. She reaches 86% of her maximum predicted heart rate (**Figure 13.4** and **Video 13.3A-C**). What is the most likely cause of this patient's symptoms?

A. Dynamic pulmonary hypertension.
B. Hypertrophic obstructive cardiomyopathy.
C. Left anterior descending artery stenosis.
D. Multivessel coronary artery disease.
E. Right coronary artery stenosis.

Figure 13.4

20. A 50-year-old woman is referred for stress testing due to dyspnea on exertion. She jogs several times per week and rides a bicycle, but recently she has noticed heavy breathing and mild lightheadedness during her usual exercise. The resting echocardiogram shows left ventricular hypertrophy. She exercises for 10 minutes on Bruce protocol and has to stop due to fatigue and some dyspnea. Her heart rate and blood pressure are 74 beats per minute (bpm) and 135/80 mm Hg at rest and 131 bpm and 120/60 mm Hg, respectively, at peak exercise. A continuous-wave Doppler is done through the aortic valve post stress. Based on **Figure 13.5**, what would be the **BEST** next step in managing this patient?
   A. Aggressive blood pressure control with amlodipine.
   B. Aortic valve replacement.
   C. Coronary angiography with revascularization.
   D. Medical therapy with a beta-blocker.
   E. Right heart catheterization with adenosine infusion.

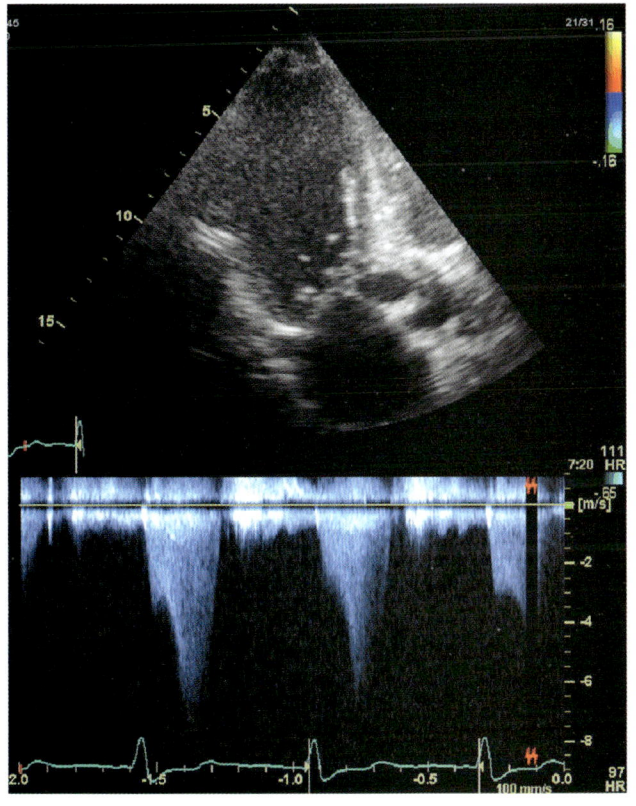

Figure 13.5

21. A 48-year-old human immunodeficiency virus (HIV)-positive man complains of progressive exertional shortness of breath for 6 months. He is a prior heavy alcohol drinker. He wants to establish medical care. Dobutamine echocardiography is performed and the target heart rate is achieved (**Figure 13.6** and ▶ **Video 13.4A-B**). He had no symptoms during the test.
Which of the following is the most accurate statement about this patient's condition?

   A. Cardiac magnetic resonance is likely to show extensive apical scarring.
   B. Early referral to cardiac transplantation center is advisable.
   C. The test is suggestive of isolated high-grade stenosis of the left circumflex coronary artery.
   D. The patient is likely to respond to beta-blocker therapy.
   E. The test is suggestive of triple-vessel severe coronary artery disease.

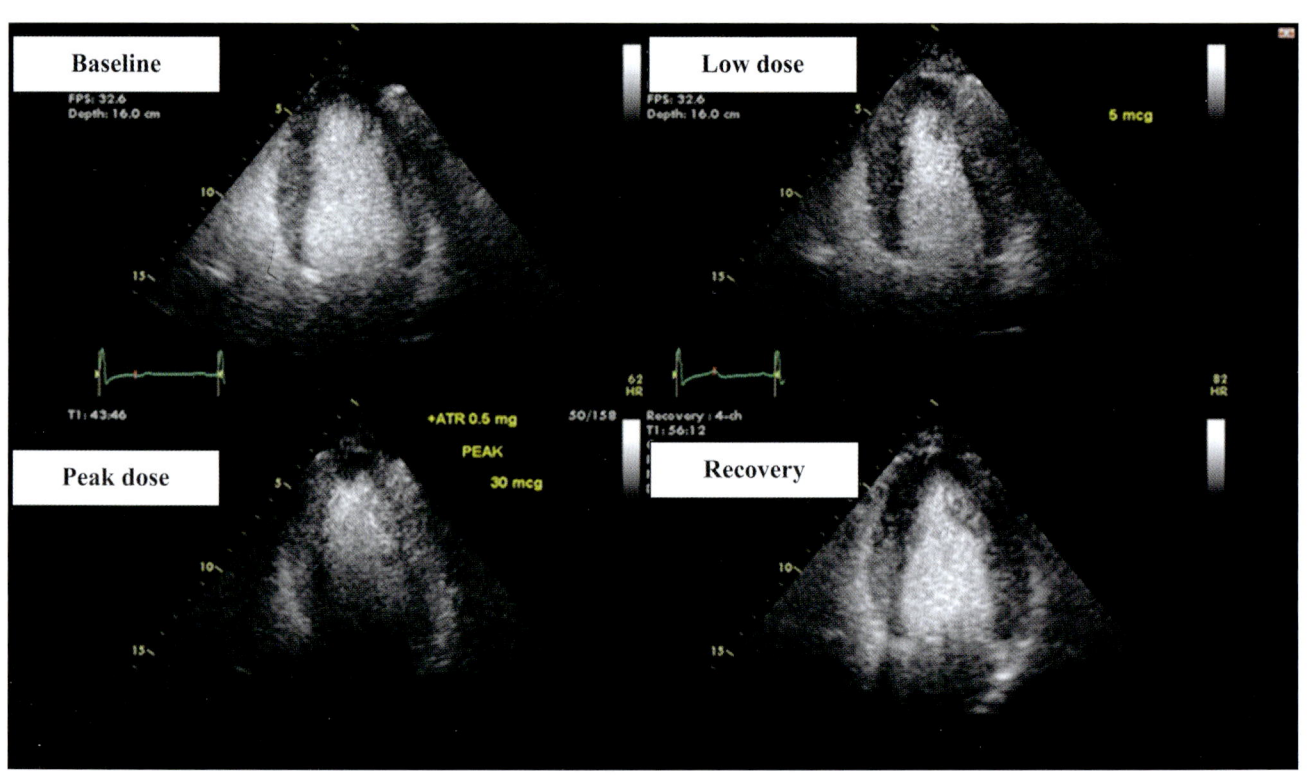

Figure 13.6

22. A 58-year-old man with a history of hypertension and smoking presents with recurrent chest pain for the last 3 weeks. He describes retrosternal pain, which has been recently occurring on mild exertion. The initial electrocardiogram and two sets of cardiac enzymes are normal. An exercise stress echocardiogram is performed. Which of the following are the most likely findings on coronary angiography (**Figure 13.7** and ▶ **Video 13.5A-C**).

   A. High-grade left anterior descending artery stenosis without distal collateral circulation.
   B. High-grade left anterior descending artery stenosis with distal collateral circulation.
   C. High-grade right coronary artery stenosis without distal collateral circulation.
   D. High-grade left circumflex artery stenosis without distal collateral circulation.
   E. High-grade left circumflex artery stenosis with distal collateral circulation.

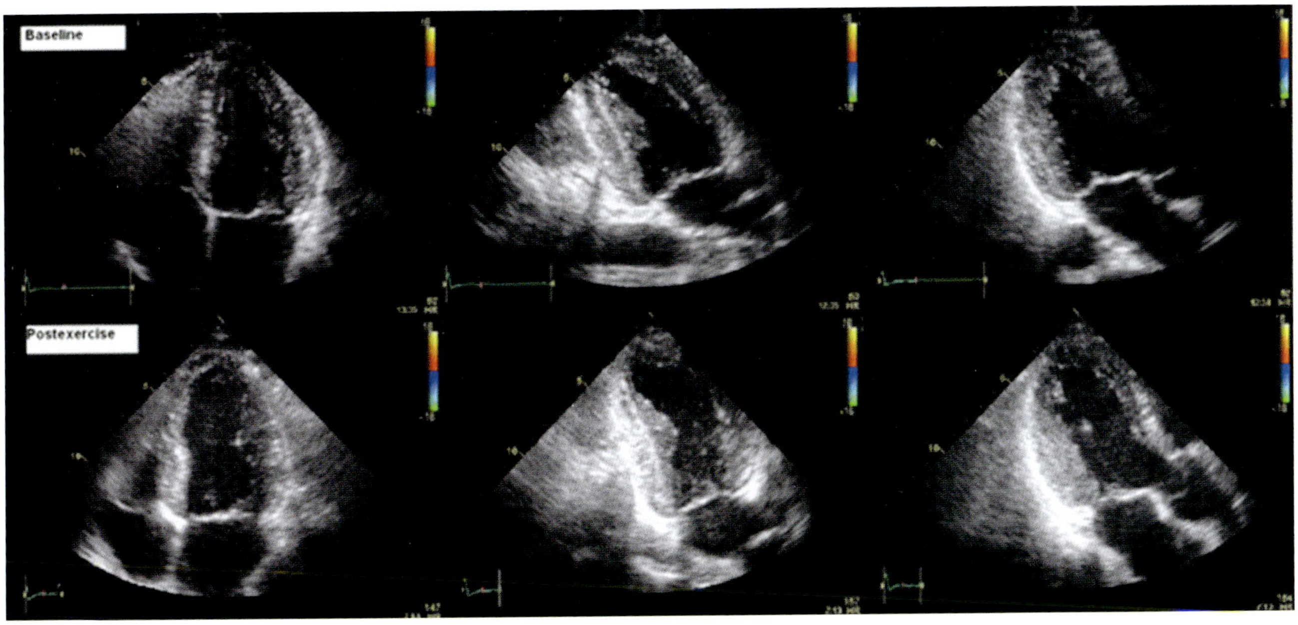

Chapter 13 Stress Echocardiography: Ischemic and Nonischemic / 281

Figure 13.7

23. A 71-year-old woman with a history of diet-controlled diabetes mellitus and hypertension presents with dyspnea on exertion. A dobutamine stress echocardiogram is performed (**Figure 13.8** and ▶ **Video 13.6A-F**). Which of the following are the most likely findings on coronary angiography?
   A. Flow-limiting left anterior descending artery stenosis.
   B. Flow-limiting left circumflex artery stenosis.
   C. Flow-limiting right coronary artery stenosis.
   D. Multivessel coronary artery stenosis.
   E. No high-grade stenosis in coronary arteries.

24. A 56-year-old asymptomatic male smoker with a history of dyslipidemia is referred for a stress echocardiogram prior to elective abdominal surgery. He has a strong family history of coronary artery disease. He has poor exercise tolerance and cannot exercise due to severe right knee osteoarthritis. The patient undergoes dobutamine stress echocardiography without chest pain or electrocardiographic changes (**Figure 13.9** and ▶ **Video 13.7A-D**). Based on the findings, which of the following is the most appropriate statement?
   A. Preoperative coronary angiogram should be considered.
   B. Further risk stratification using calcium scoring should be considered.
   C. The study is abnormal, but the preoperative risk is low.
   D. The study is abnormal due to nonischemic cardiomyopathy.
   E. The patient should be reassured since he has no evidence of coronary artery disease.

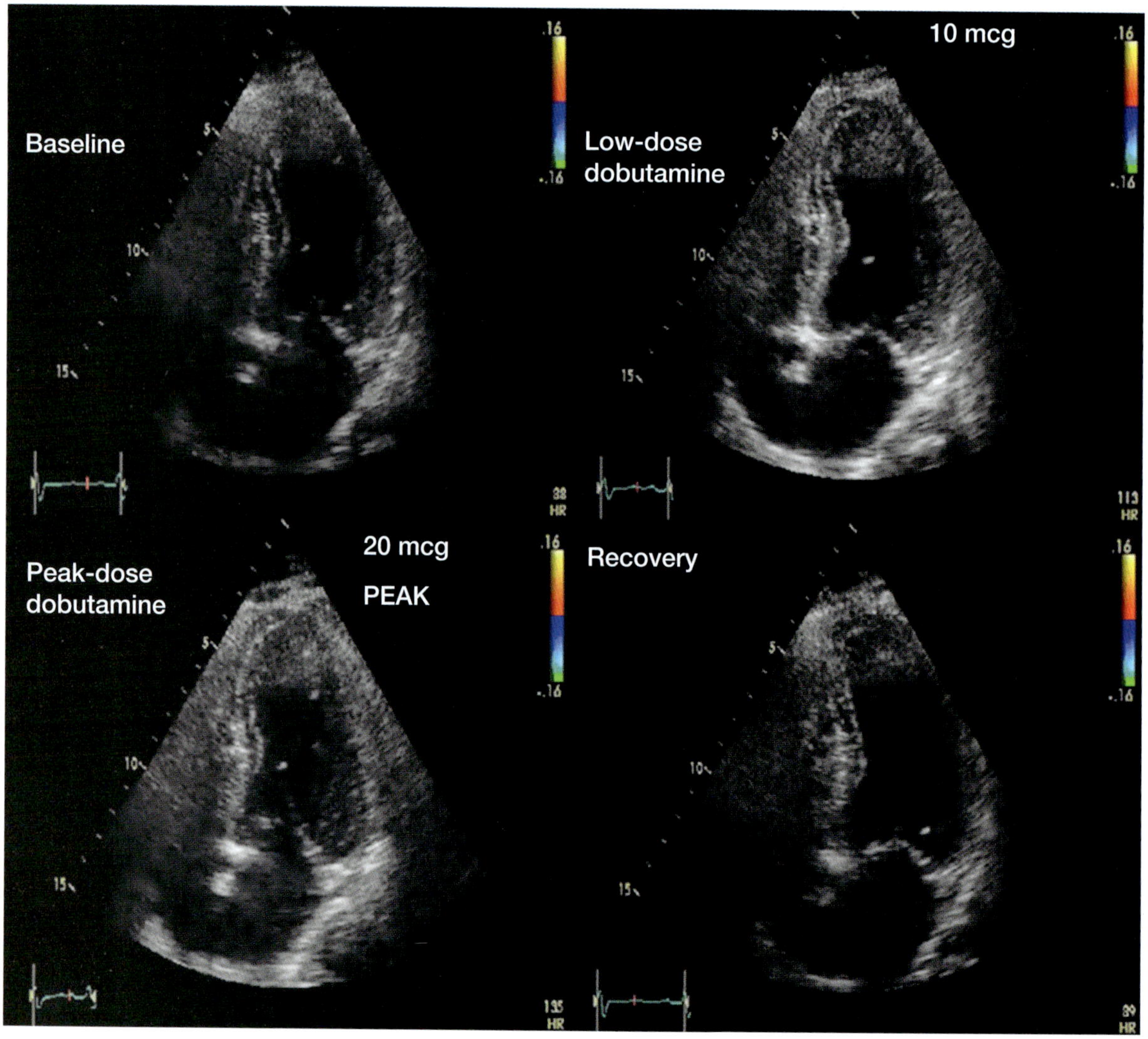

282 / Clinical Echocardiography Review

Figure 13.8

25. A 73-year-old woman with history of hypertension is evaluated for atypical chest pain. Her exercise capacity is limited by chronic knee pain. Her resting echocardiogram is normal. She undergoes dobutamine echocardiography, which shows moderate ischemia in the apical segments, anterior wall, and anteroseptum. Subsequent coronary angiography shows mild luminal irregularities, but no obstructive coronary artery disease. Her prognosis (overall survival) is most similar to which of the following patients?

A. Patient with markedly abnormal stress test and transient ischemic cavity dilation.
B. Patient with normal stress test and no significant (<50% stenosis) coronary disease.
C. Patient with similarly abnormal stress test and low baseline ejection fraction.
D. Patient with similarly abnormal stress test and obstructive (>50% stenosis) coronary disease.
E. Patient with similarly abnormal stress test undergoing exercise echocardiography.

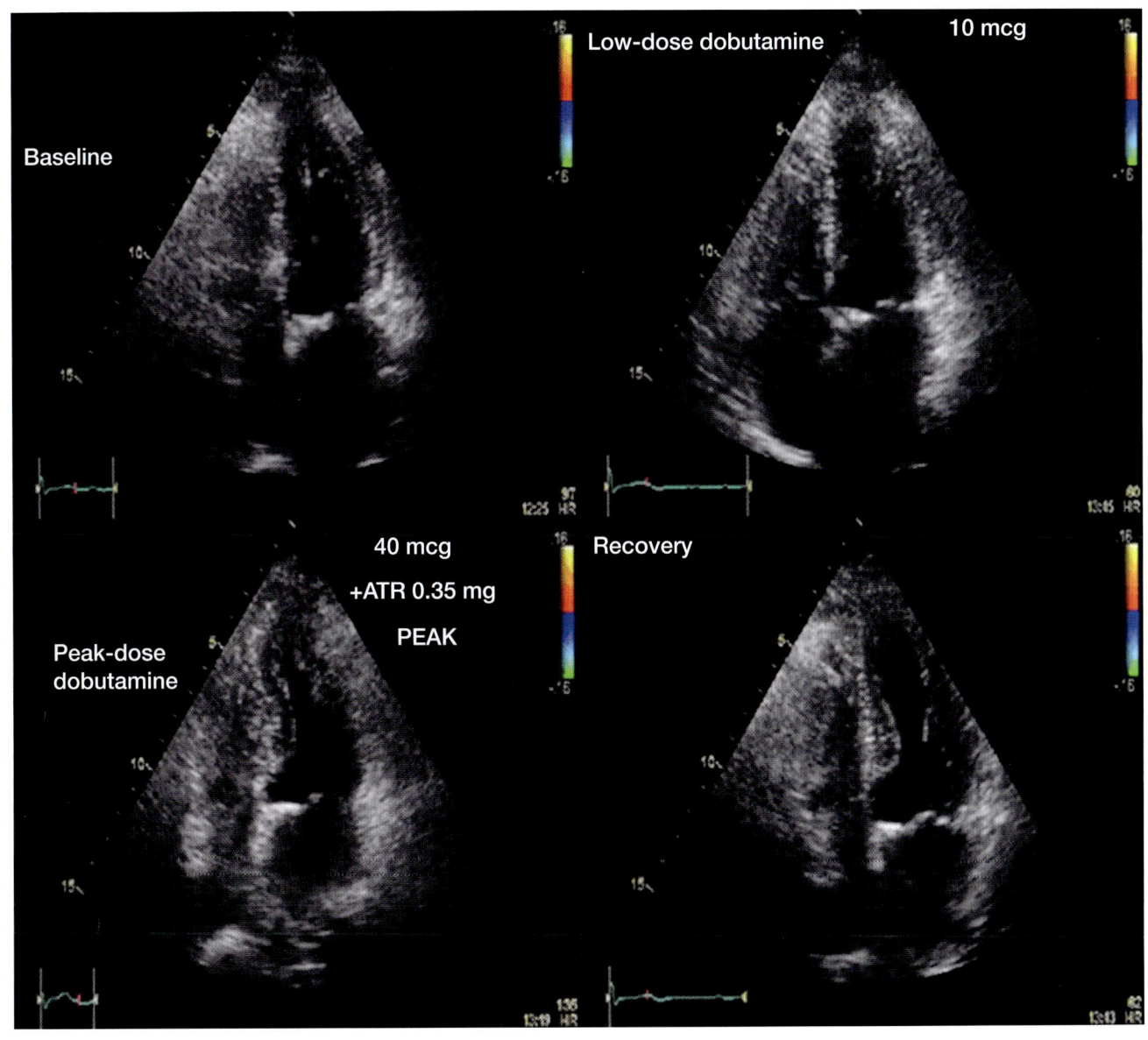

Figure 13.9

26. A 46-year-old woman complains of exertional dyspnea and occasional palpitations. Physical examination reveals a II/VI holosystolic murmur at the apex. Transthoracic echocardiogram shows mild left ventricular dilation, left ventricular ejection fraction of 65%, and mild to moderate mitral regurgitation. Exercise stress echocardiogram is performed and shows no evidence of myocardial ischemia (**Figure 13.10** and Video 13.8A-B). Which of the following is the **BEST** management for this patient?

A. Beta-blocker and vasodilator therapy.
B. Mitral valve repair.
C. Reassurance and clinical follow-up.
D. Treatment for primary pulmonary hypertension.
E. Tricuspid valve replacement.

284 / Clinical Echocardiography Review

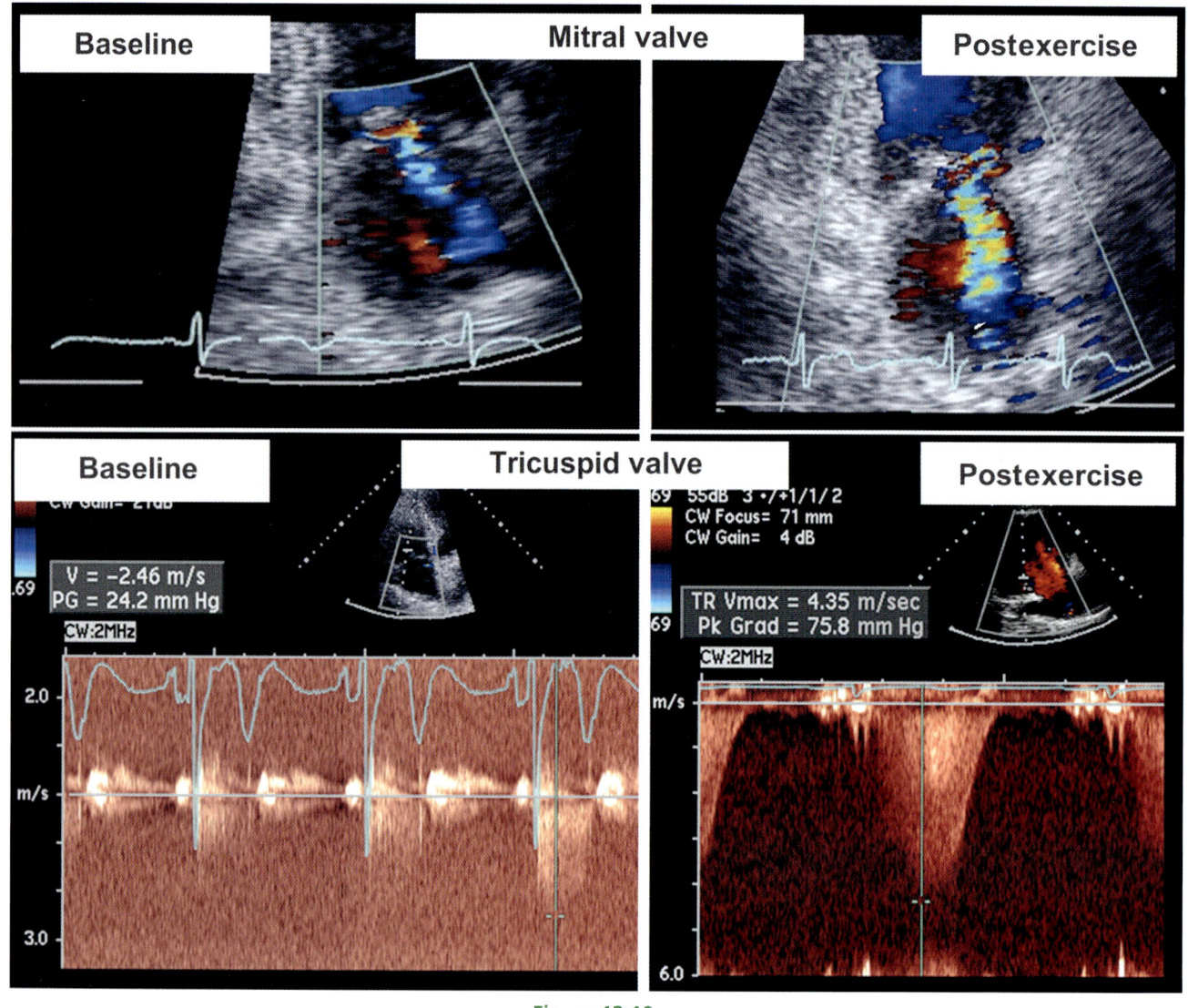

Figure 13.10

CASE 1

A 58-year-old woman with a history of hypertension presents to the emergency department with atypical left-sided chest discomfort. She is overweight but has no known history of diabetes mellitus or coronary artery disease. Her electrocardiogram is unremarkable and the initial set of cardiac biomarkers is negative. Her initial blood pressure is 152/90 mm Hg. A stress echocardiogram is performed with the use of an ultrasound-enhancing agent. She exercises on the treadmill reaching workload of 7 metabolic equivalents (METs) and her peak blood pressure is 170/90 mm Hg. Her target heart rate is achieved. The test is ended due to fatigue and mild dyspnea but no chest pain. Her electrocardiogram at peak heart rate reveals 2 mm downsloping ST segment depressions in leads II, III, AVf, V5, and V6 (**Figure 13.11** and ▶ **Video 13.9A-C**).

27. Which of the following statements about the stress echocardiogram on the patient in **Case 1** is **CORRECT**?
   A. Stress echocardiogram has a limited prognostic value in women.
   B. Stress electrocardiogram is more sensitive to subendocardial ischemia than stress echocardiography.
   C. The electrocardiographic changes represent a false-positive result.
   D. There is evidence of ischemia on electrocardiogram and imaging.
   E. There is global left ventricular hypokinesis postexercise due to hypertensive response.

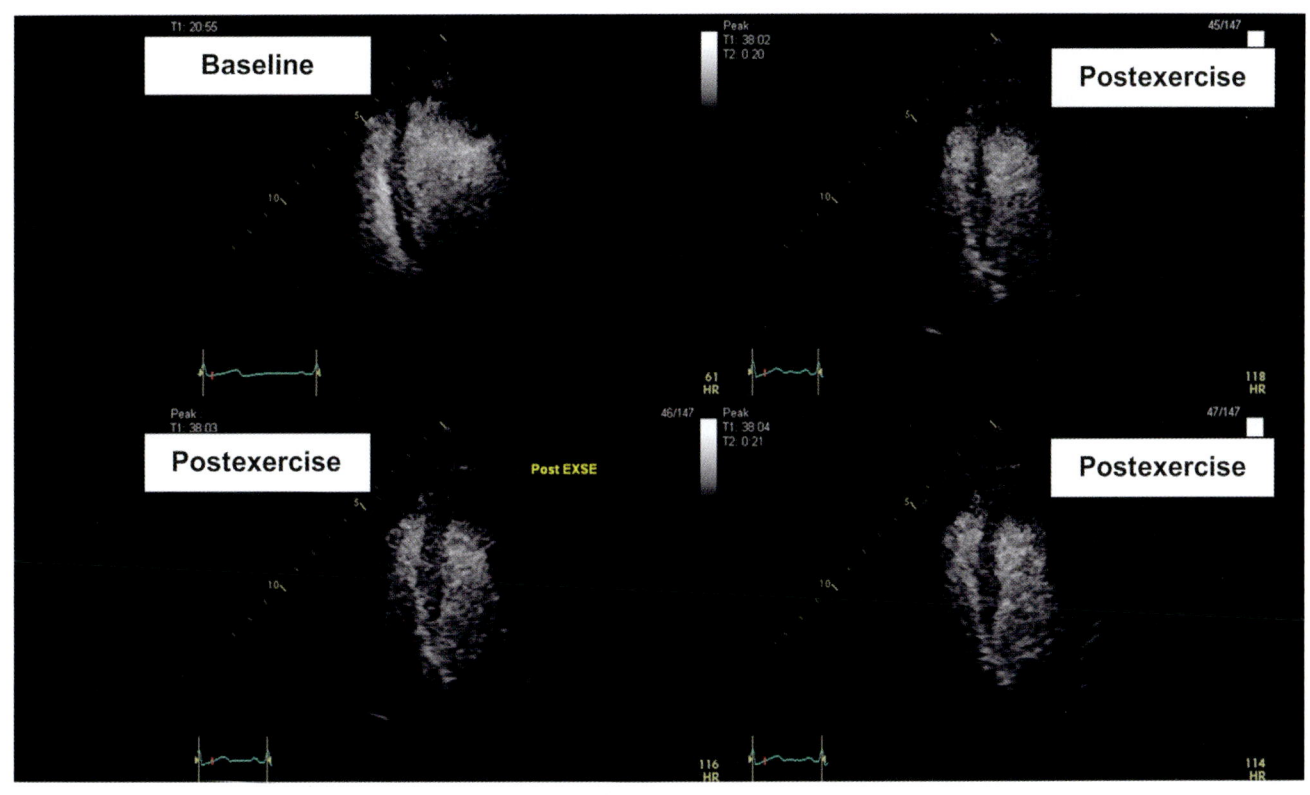

Figure 13.11

28. Based on the stress echocardiographic findings in **Case 1**, what would be the next step in managing this patient?
    A. Discharge home with outpatient follow-up.
    B. Refer for coronary angiography.
    C. Repeat stress echocardiogram after optimal blood pressure control.
    D. Order a coronary CT angiography.
    E. Order a vasodilator nuclear stress test.

CASE 2

*A 50-year-old man with known coronary artery disease who received a permanent pacemaker 3 years ago for syncope presents to the emergency department complaining of progressive shortness of breath. He is found to be in pulmonary edema and is admitted to the cardiac care unit. After diuresis, he experiences symptomatic improvement. A coronary angiogram reveals severe triple-vessel coronary artery disease. A dobutamine stress echocardiography is performed (**Figure 13.12** and ▶ **Video 13.10A-F**). The study also shows moderate mitral regurgitation.*

29. Which of the following statements **BEST** describes the stress echocardiography findings from the patient in **Case 2**?
    A. Biphasic response in the apical segments.
    B. Inferoseptal wall ischemia.
    C. Marked viability in the inferior wall.
    D. Mild viability in the inferolateral wall.
    E. Right ventricular ischemia.

30. Based on dobutamine echocardiography results in **Case 2**, which of the following statements is **CORRECT**?
    A. Cardiac magnetic resonance is likely to show mild apical scarring.
    B. Dobutamine echocardiography findings suggest a low risk for sudden cardiac death.
    C. The patient is likely to improve with high-dose beta-blocker therapy.
    D. The patient is likely to respond to cardiac resynchronization therapy if QRS complex duration is wide.
    E. The probability of left ventricular function improvement is low.

286 / Clinical Echocardiography Review

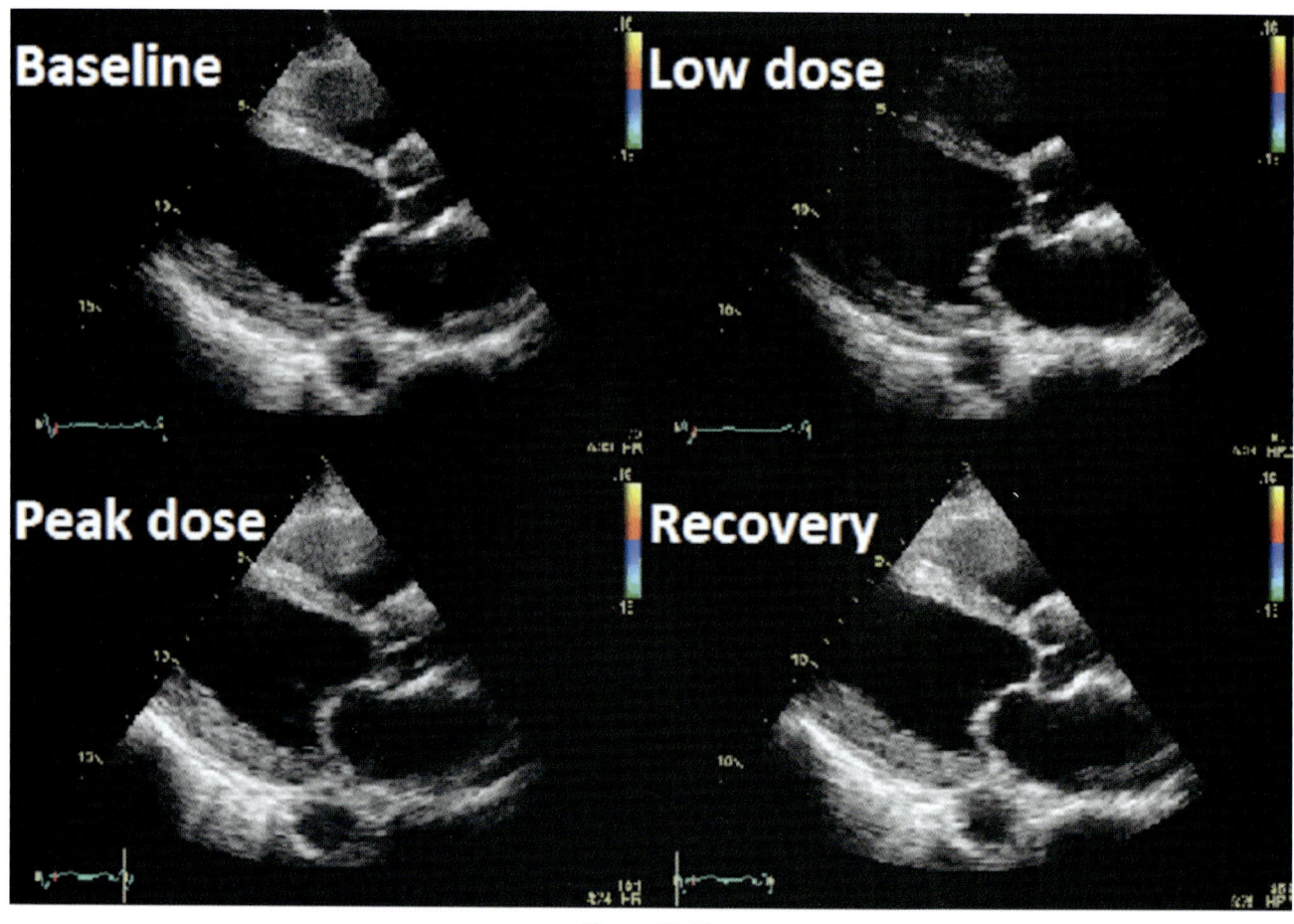

Figure 13.12

CASE 3

A 69-year-old woman with a history of type 2 diabetes mellitus, hypertension, and advanced renal disease presents to the emergency department with an episode of left-sided chest pain lasting 20 minutes. She is admitted and ruled out for acute myocardial infarction. A stress echocardiogram is requested. Her resting blood pressure is 220/100 mm Hg. A dipyridamole stress echocardiogram is performed due to elevated blood pressure. She experiences chest pressure during dipyridamole infusion, but the electrocardiogram does not show ischemic changes (Figure 13.13 and ▶ Video 13.11A-F).

31. Which of the following statements **BEST** describes the stress echocardiography findings from the patient in **Case 3**?
    A. Mild ischemia involving the anterolateral wall.
    B. Mild ischemia involving only apical septum.
    C. Moderate ischemia involving anteroseptal and anterior walls.
    D. Moderate ischemia involving inferior and inferolateral walls.
    E. No echocardiographic evidence of ischemia.

32. Which of the following statements is **CORRECT** about the stress echocardiogram from the patient in **Case 3**?
    A. Dipyridamole stress echocardiography has lower sensitivity compared to dobutamine echocardiography.
    B. Dipyridamole stress echocardiography has lower specificity compared to dobutamine echocardiography.
    C. In women, dipyridamole stress echocardiography is preferred to dobutamine echocardiography as it is less likely to produce a left ventricular outflow tract gradient.
    D. The chest pain in this patient is most likely a side effect of dipyridamole.
    E. The peak wall motion score index in this patient portends a low risk for cardiac events.

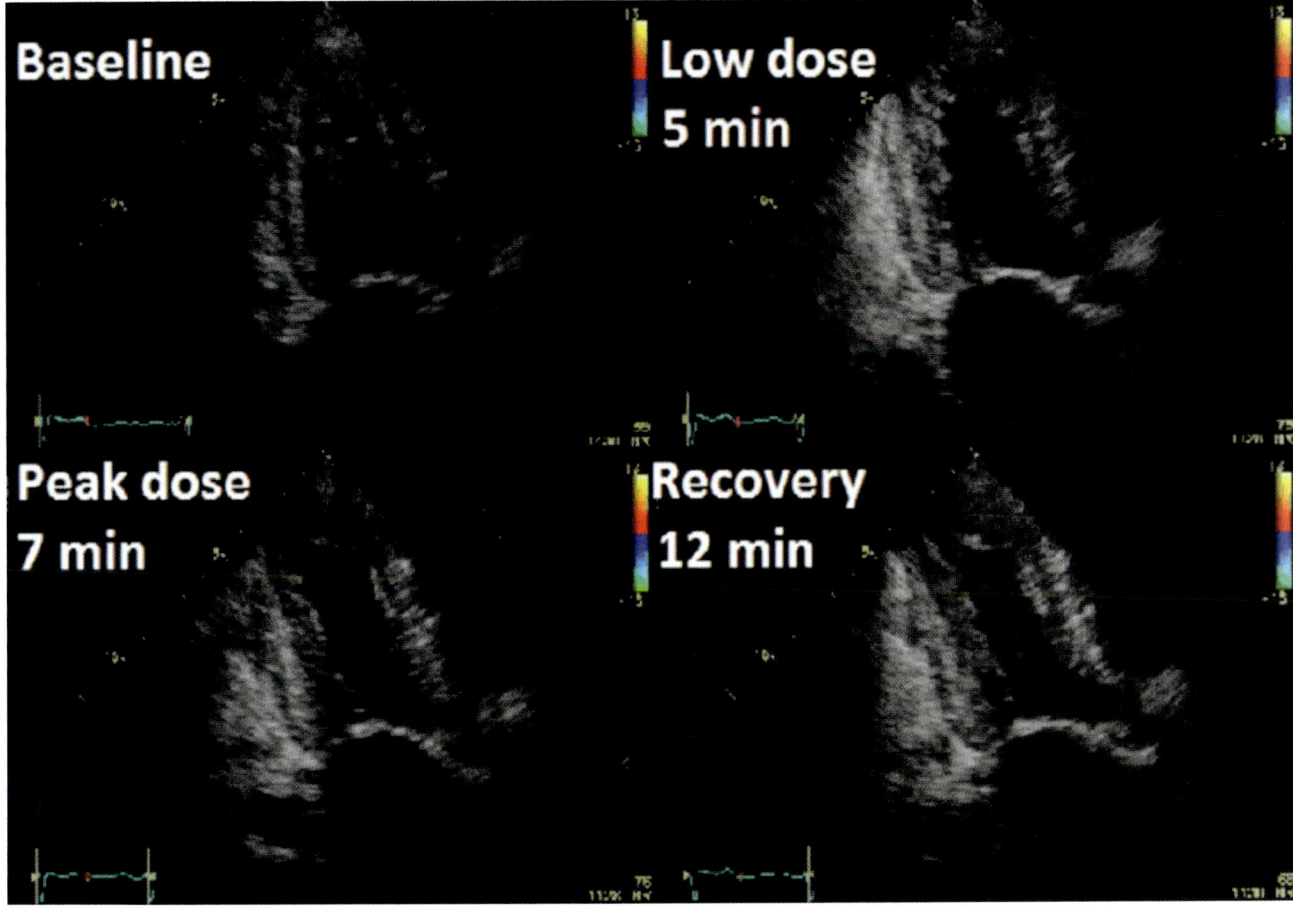

Figure 13.13

33. Based on the stress echocardiography results in **Case 3**, what would be the most likely finding on coronary angiogram in this patient?
    A. Diffuse disease involving distal left anterior descending artery.
    B. Flow-limiting mid left anterior descending artery stenosis.
    C. Flow-limiting obtuse marginal artery stenosis.
    D. Flow-limiting right coronary artery stenosis.
    E. No flow-limiting coronary artery disease.

CASE 4

A 72-year-old woman with hypertension and hyperlipidemia is evaluated for exertional dyspnea. She denies any chest pain, syncope, or palpitations. She is referred for exercise echocardiography. She exercises on treadmill using Bruce protocol for 7 METs and stops because of dyspnea. Her baseline blood pressure is 135/80 mm Hg and it increases to 165/90 mm Hg. Electrocardiogram shows borderline (0.5 mm) ST segment depression in inferolateral leads. The following echocardiographic images are obtained (Figure 13.14 and ▶ Video 13.12A-C). No significant pathology of the mitral and aortic valve is evident from Doppler studies.

34. Which of the following is the **BEST** interpretation of echocardiographic images of the patient in **Case 4**?
    A. Left anterior descending artery territory ischemia.
    B. Multivessel ischemia.
    C. Non–left anterior descending artery territory ischemia.
    D. No echocardiographic evidence of ischemia.

35. Which of the following is expected to remain relatively unchanged in response to exercise in healthy adults?
    A. E-wave velocity.
    B. Septal e' velocity.
    C. E/e' ratio.
    D. s' velocity.
    E. Left ventricular global longitudinal strain.

288 / Clinical Echocardiography Review

Mitral inflow | Tissue doppler imaging | Tricuspid regurgitation

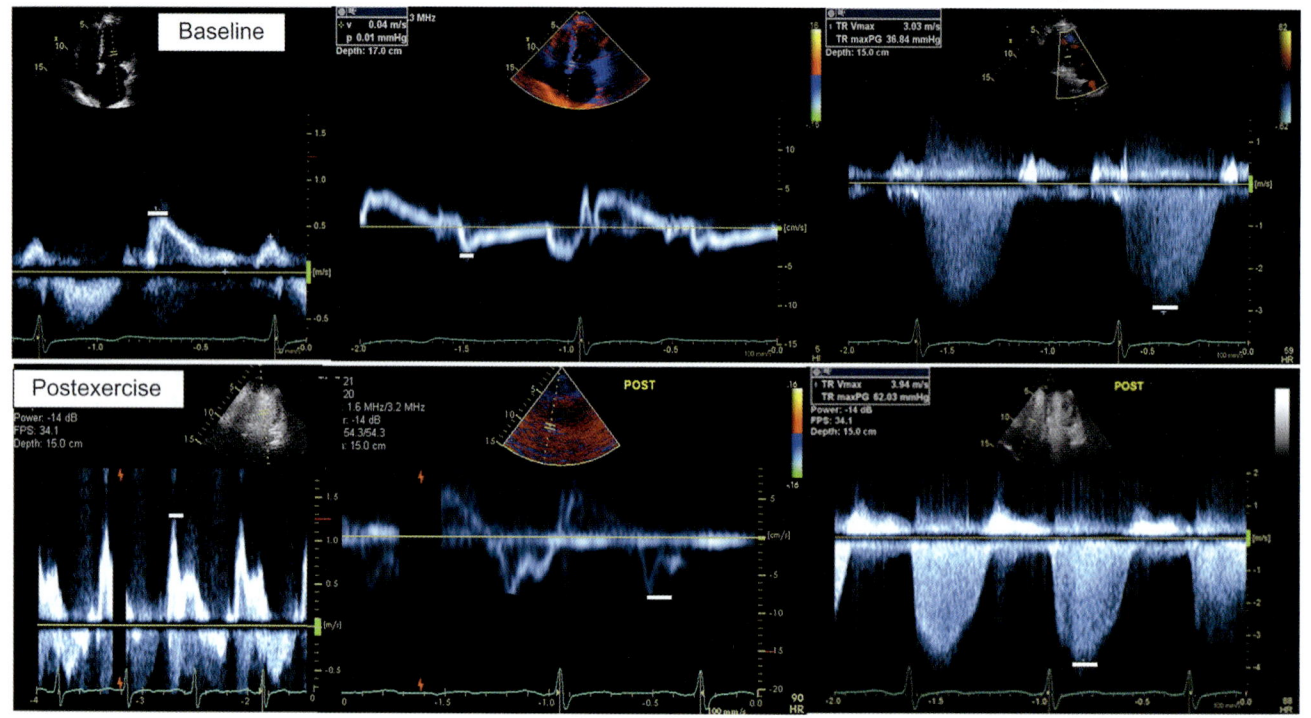

Figure 13.14

36. Based on echocardiographic data in **Case 4**, which of the following is most likely cause of this patient's symptoms?
    A. Deconditioning and muscle weakness without obvious cardiac cause.
    B. Increase in left ventricular filling pressures due to diastolic dysfunction.
    C. Increase in pulmonary artery pressures due to pulmonary disease.
    D. Increase in tricuspid regurgitation due to right ventricular failure.
    E. Systolic dysfunction due to exercise-induced ischemia.

CASE 5

*A 52-year-old man with a strong family history of coronary artery disease comes to the emergency room with intermittent chest pain. He has been having chest pain for the last several months, but the episodes are more frequent recently. The chest pain is not always related to exertion. He also noticed some shortness of breath that he attributes to anxiety. Electrocardiogram shows normal sinus rhythm and nonspecific T-wave changes. Cardiac enzymes are negative. A dobutamine stress echocardiogram is performed (**Figure 13.15** and ▶ Video 13.13A-C). During the test, the patient describes palpitations but no chest pain. Electrocardiogram shows borderline ST segment depression in inferior leads.*

37. Which of the following **BEST** describes echocardiographic findings of the patient in **Case 5**?
    A. Abnormal baseline wall motion, marked viability in affected segments, no ischemia.
    B. Abnormal baseline wall motion, no viability in affected segments, no ischemia.
    C. Abnormal peak wall motion with high-risk features.
    D. Normal baseline wall motion with normal peak wall motion.
    E. Normal baseline wall motion with abnormal peak wall motion.

38. Which of the following are most likely findings on coronary angiography of the patient from **Case 5**?
    A. Diffuse disease involving distal left anterior descending artery.
    B. Flow-limiting proximal left anterior descending artery stenosis.
    C. Flow-limiting right coronary artery stenosis.
    D. Multivessel obstructive coronary disease.
    E. No flow-limiting coronary artery disease.

Chapter 13 Stress Echocardiography: Ischemic and Nonischemic / 289

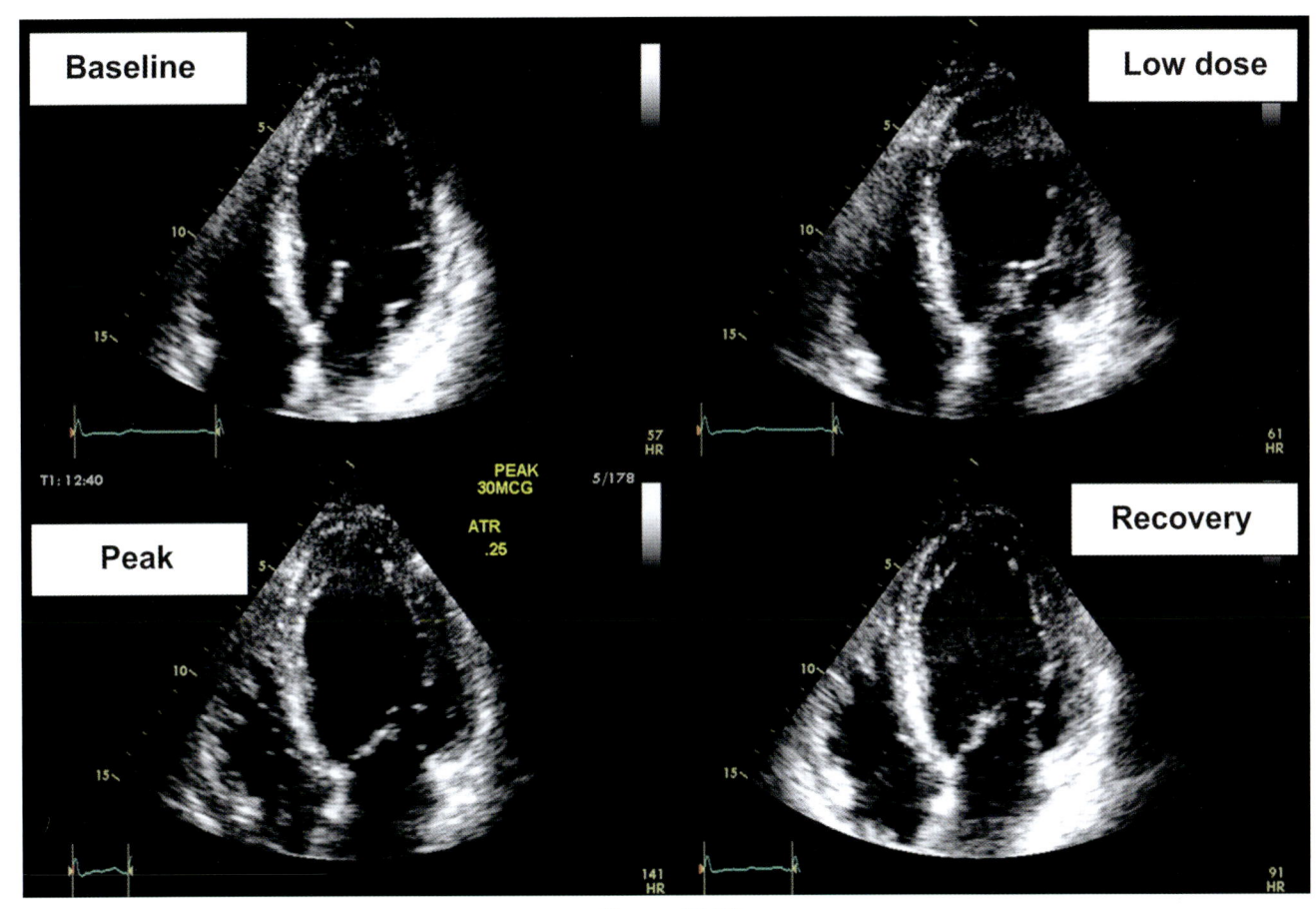

Figure 13.15

ANSWERS

1. **Answer: A.** The use of stress echocardiography to diagnose flow-limiting coronary artery disease is based on a sequence of events known as the ischemic cascade as shown in **Figure 13.16**. The decrease in blood flow initially produces a perfusion abnormality and diastolic and systolic dysfunction, in that order, and then hemodynamic abnormalities occur. Electrocardiographic changes and symptoms occur late in the ischemic cascade; hence, the sensitivity of these parameters to identify ischemia is lower.

2. **Answer: A.** A normal response to dobutamine infusion during stress echocardiography starting with a low dose is progressive increase in regional endocardial excursion, myocardial thickening, and left ventricular ejection fraction as well as decrease in end-systolic left ventricular volume. Decrease in regional endocardial excursion and myocardial thickening at peak dose compared to a low dose (as described in Option D) indicates myocardial ischemia. Cavity dilation and decrease in left ventricular ejection fraction at peak dose (as described in Option B) are uncommon and usually indicate a high ischemic burden.

3. **Answer: B.** Stress testing poses a challenge in patients with known left bundle branch block. Exercise electrocardiogram does not provide useful information regarding ischemia in these patients, and perfusion studies, specifically using exercise, have a high false-positivity rate. Stress echocardiography using

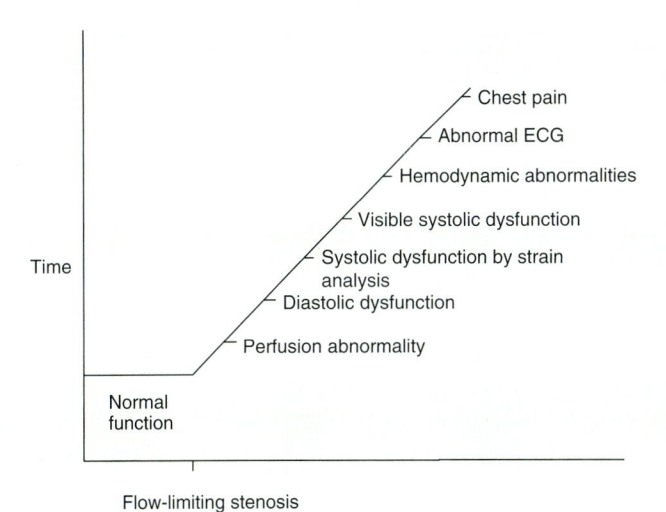

Figure 13.16. Ischemic cascade.

both exercise and dobutamine has demonstrated good accuracy in detecting angiographically significant coronary artery disease. In addition, stress echocardiography has an established prognostic value in patients with existing left bundle branch block. Interestingly, patients with left bundle branch block and nonischemic stress echocardiogram have mortality rates similar to nonischemic patients without left bundle branch block. The interpretation of stress echocardiogram in these patients is challenging due to abnormal septal motion and contraction dyssynchrony (Option A). At higher heart rates, these endocardial excursion abnormalities are exaggerated, not normalized (Option C). On the other hand, nonischemic patients demonstrate preserved wall thickening, which appears to be a more specific marker of nonischemic test compared to assessment of perfusion. Preserved myocardial thickening during stress testing may be easily appreciated if an ultrasound-enhancing agent is used during the test.

4. **Answer: C.** Regional and global response of the left ventricle to stress differs depending on the stress modality. It is critical to understand these modality-specific differences for correct interpretation of stress echocardiography. By definition, normal stress echocardiogram demonstrates appropriate regional and global left ventricular responses. In case of dobutamine echocardiography, marked hypercontractility of normal segments and a significant decrease in the left ventricular cavity size are observed. Treadmill exercise similarly produces regional hyperkinesis and overall decrease in end-systolic cavity size, but the response is less vigorous compared to dobutamine (Option E). Hyperkinesis is even less prominent with supine bicycle (Option D) and vasodilator stress (Option B), and it may be very mild with atrial pacing.

5. **Answer: A.** Hypotension during dobutamine infusion can be precipitated by a number of hemodynamic abnormalities. Sustained arrhythmias have been reported with dobutamine infusion, but they should be recognized on cardiac rhythm monitoring. Extensive, severe wall motion abnormalities due to ongoing ischemia can potentially decrease cardiac output and precipitate hypotension, but this is rare and can be detected during immediate echocardiographic imaging. Occasionally, vigorous left ventricular contraction and hyperkinetic state can precipitate paradoxical vagal response with hypotension and bradycardia, which is responsive to atropine administration. Finally, potent inotropic effect can precipitate dynamic mid-ventricular or left ventricular outflow obstruction in predisposed individuals. Dynamic left ventricular outflow obstruction has been reported in >10% of patients undergoing dobutamine echocardiography, and it can be conveniently documented and quantified using continuous-wave Doppler interrogation through the left ventricular outflow tract. Interestingly, dynamic left ventricular outflow obstruction provoked by dobutamine has been associated with future episodes of chest pain and syncope. Doppler interrogation is a valuable technique for hemodynamic assessment of stress-induced abnormalities. For instance, it can detect an increase in transmitral gradient in patients with mitral stenosis (Option B) or an increase in left ventricular filling pressures (Option D) and pulmonary artery systolic pressure (Option C) in patients with exercise-induced diastolic dysfunction. However, the expected abnormality in this patient is dynamic left ventricular outflow obstruction.

6. **Answer: B.** The sensitivity of stress echocardiography is proportionally related to the number of vessels involved, being the greatest for triple-vessel disease. This is especially true for left circumflex disease since it supplies smaller amount of myocardium. False-negative results due to "balanced" ischemia as seen during nuclear perfusion imaging are not characteristic for stress echocardiography (Option D). Hypertensive response to exercise can result in false-positive studies due to myocardial oxygen supply-demand mismatch (Option C). Atropine is frequently used during dobutamine stress echocardiography when the peak heart rate is suboptimal, to improve the sensitivity and thus decrease the rate of false-negative studies (Option E). Common causes of false-positive and false-negative results during stress echocardiography are listed in **Table 13.1**.

7. **Answer: C.** Specificity of stress echocardiography is affected by the presence of false-positive results (**Table 13.1**). The list of conditions that can cause wall motion abnormalities during stress in the absence of flow-limiting coronary stenosis includes hypertensive response to exercise, abnormal septal motion caused by left bundle branch block, and nonischemic cardiomyopathy. Other options listed can potentially cause false-negative results and therefore affect sensitivity of stress echocardiogram.

8. **Answer: B.** Dobutamine infusion can be associated with uncomfortable symptoms including chest discomfort and palpitations (Option A). Only if intolerable, these symptoms alone are an indication to terminate the test. Other end points for dobutamine echocardiography include attainment of the target heart rate (85% of the age-predicted maximum heart rate) or protocol completion, hypotension, new or worsening significant wall motion abnormalities, significant arrhythmias (not ventricular ectopic beats which are common during dobutamine infusion, Option E), and severe hypertension.

Table 13.1. Common Causes of False-Positive and False-Negative Results During Stress Echocardiography

False-Positive Results	False-Negative Results
Hypertensive response to stress	Inadequate level of stress including the use of beta-blockers before stress
Microvascular disease (syndrome X)	
Nonischemic cardiomyopathy	Single-vessel disease, especially left circumflex
Hypertrophic cardiomyopathy	Concentric left ventricular remodeling
Effect of tethering seen with mitral annular calcification or after mitral surgery	Apical foreshortening
Coronary vasospasm	Delays in image acquisition postexercise
Abnormal septal motion due to pacing, conduction abnormalities, prior surgery, or right ventricular volume overload	

9. **Answer: A.** The sensitivity of stress echocardiography to detect flow-limiting lesions depends not only on the degree of coronary stenosis but also on the number of vessels involved and the area of jeopardized myocardium. The sensitivity is higher for multivessel disease compared to single-vessel disease. Likewise, the sensitivity to detect stenosis in the left anterior descending artery and right coronary artery territory is superior to the sensitivity for the left circumflex. The highest sensitivity is for left anterior descending artery stenosis.

10. **Answer: E.** Exertional dyspnea is a ubiquitous complaint and a relatively common indication for stress echocardiography referral. A significant number of dyspneic patients have diastolic dysfunction. In recent years, it has been shown that stress-induced diastolic dysfunction can be diagnosed in these patients using postexercise transmitral flow velocities, tissue Doppler velocities, and tricuspid regurgitant velocity. Semisupine bicycle is commonly used, but treadmill exercise is an alternative. In patients with exercise-induced diastolic dysfunction, postexercise increase in E/e′ ratio (>15) and tricuspid regurgitant velocity are commonly observed. In this patient, resting mitral inflow pattern is A velocity dominant with decreased septal e′ velocity and s′ velocity. Resting septal E/e′ ratio is 12. Postexercise, the mitral inflow pattern is E dominant and septal E/e′ ratio increases to 18, suggestive of increase in left ventricular filling pressures. In addition, there is poor s′ reserve suggestive of impaired longitudinal systolic function (**Figure 13.17**). The diastology

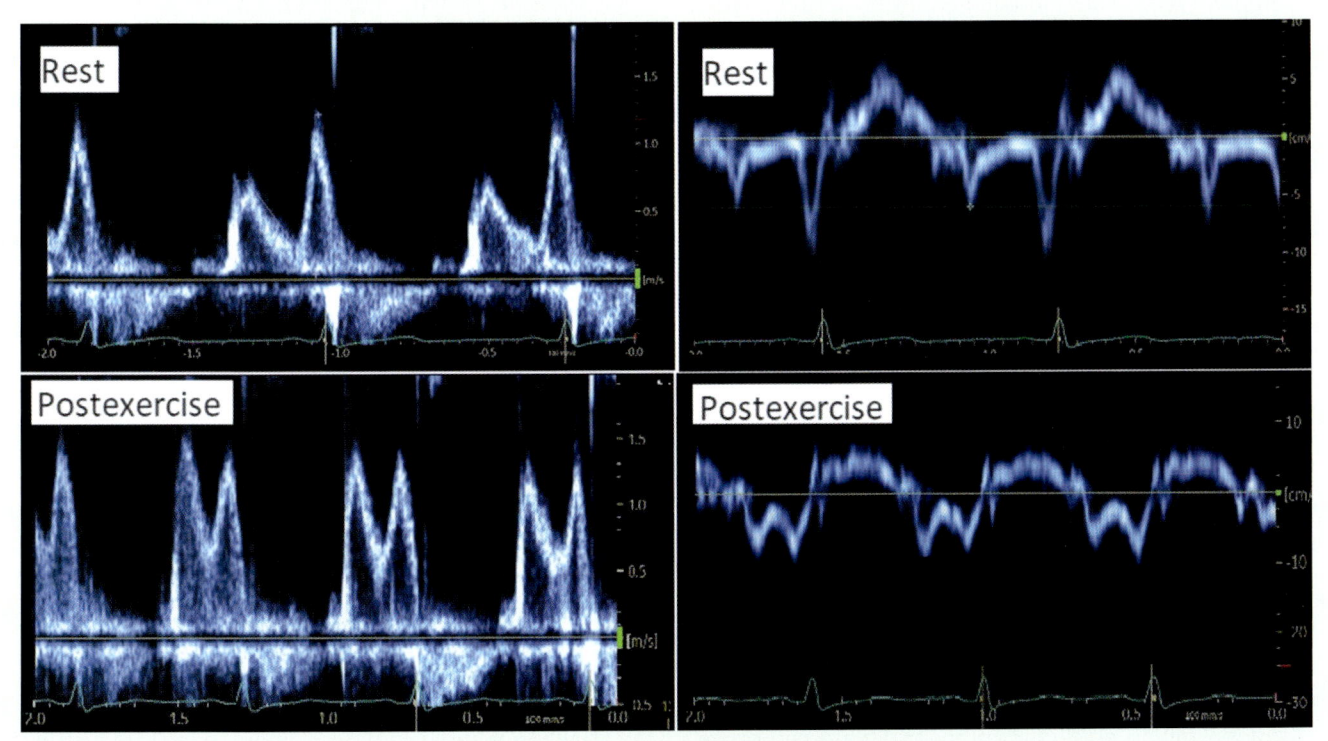

Figure 13.17. Exercise-induced diastolic dysfunction.

Table 13.2. Common Noncoronary Indications for Stress Echocardiography

Indication	Reason
Microvascular disease (diabetes mellitus, syndrome X, etc.)	Evaluation of coronary flow reserve
Dilated nonischemic cardiomyopathy	Assessment of inotropic contractile reserve
Hypertrophic cardiomyopathy	Gradient provocation and risk stratification
Valvular heart disease, native and prosthetic	Reconciliation of discrepancies between patient symptoms and echocardiographic severity of valve disease as assessed at rest Assessment of exercise tolerance, left ventricular performance, and hemodynamics including pressure gradients and tricuspid regurgitant velocity Differentiation of severe from "pseudosevere" aortic stenosis in patients with low left ventricular systolic function (dobutamine infusion)
Exertional dyspnea	Assessment of diastolic parameters and tricuspid regurgitant velocity
Postcardiac transplantation	Detection of transplant vasculopathy
Congenital heart disease	Assessment of exercise tolerance, ventricular performance, and hemodynamics including tricuspid regurgitant velocity

stress test according to ASE 2016 guidelines is considered definitely abnormal indicating diastolic dysfunction when all of the following 3 conditions are met: average E/e' > 14 or septal E/e' ratio >15 with exercise, peak TR velocity >2.8 m/sec with exercise and septal e' velocity is <7 cm/sec or if only lateral velocity is acquired, lateral e' < 10 cm/sec at baseline. Although coronary artery disease is a possibility in this patient, she reports no chest pain. Exertional dyspnea without chest pain is unlikely to be an angina equivalent in patients without known coronary artery disease or resting wall motion abnormalities (Option C). Common noncoronary indications for stress echocardiography are listed in **Table 13.2**.

11. **Answer: B.** Dobutamine echocardiography allows assessment of both viability and ischemia in patients with systolic left ventricular dysfunction and significant resting wall motion abnormalities. Dobutamine infusion is started at a lower dose (2.5 and 5 µg/kg/min) in these patients facilitating identification of viability in segment that are abnormal at rest. Viable segments will demonstrate inotropic contractile reserve. At higher doses, biphasic response can be elicited, which is indicative of ischemia. Thus, for many patients, the combination of low and high dose dobutamine is necessary to accurately define both viability and ischemia. Treadmill exercise electrocardiogram, treadmill echocardiography, and vasodilator stress echocardiography have poor sensitivity in identifying both viable and ischemic myocardium.

12. **Answer: A.** Microvascular dysfunction without flow-limiting epicardial coronary disease can cause angina-like exertional chest pain in different patient subgroups including patients with diabetes mellitus, hypertension, and syndrome X. During exercise testing, typical symptoms can be provoked along with ischemic ST segment changes. In contrast to coronary artery disease, wall motion abnormalities may not be an early event in these patients. Pulsed-wave Doppler examination of the mid-to-distal left anterior descending artery during vasodilator infusion (such as dipyridamole or adenosine) allows assessment of the coronary flow reserve. Absence of coronary flow augmentation during vasodilator stress is associated with worse long-term outcomes in patients with microvascular disease.

13. **Answer: A.** Dobutamine echocardiography is a useful diagnostic tool in patients with suspected severe aortic stenosis in the settings of severe left ventricular dysfunction. These patients typically have a depressed left ventricular ejection fraction, low mean aortic gradient (<40 mm Hg) and peak transvalvular velocity (<4 m/s), a calculated aortic valve area of <1.0 cm^2, and dimensionless index of <0.25. True severe aortic stenosis in this setting should be differentiated from "pseudosevere" aortic stenosis created by a low-flow state and moderate or mild aortic stenosis. If the aortic stenosis is severe, the peak transvalvular velocity and the mean gradient augment during low-dose dobutamine infusion, while the calculated aortic valve area does not change compared to baseline. Per current recommendations, aortic valve replacement should be considered in symptomatic patients with severe aortic stenosis with reduced left ventricular ejection fraction when a low-dose dobutamine stress study

shows an aortic velocity >4.0 m/s (or mean pressure gradient >40 mm Hg) with an estimated aortic valve area ≤1.0 cm² at any dobutamine dose. Also, dobutamine infusion can identify patients with lack of contractile reserve (increase of stroke volume <20%) who have poor prognosis (Option E).

14. **Answer: A.** A quick replenishment is observed in segments not affected by stenosis after a high-energy burst (flash) that destroys the microbubbles within the myocardium. This can be quantified by two parameters: the peak signal intensity and the rate of the signal intensity rise. Graph A is an example of normal rise of signal intensity to its peak level. Graph B, on the other hand, shows a slower rise and a lower peak intensity, which can be consistent with flow-limiting coronary stenosis.

15. **Answer: B.** Dobutamine is the preferred agent in the assessment of myocardial viability using stress echocardiography. The protocol should incorporate low-dose infusion rates to allow assessment of contractile reserve in dysfunctional segments. Different responses of dysfunctional segments to low and high doses of dobutamine in the right clinical context typically allow differentiation of stunning, hibernation, remodeling, and myocardial scarring (**Figure 13.18**). Similarly, response patterns to dobutamine infusion have been correlated with postrevascularization improvement

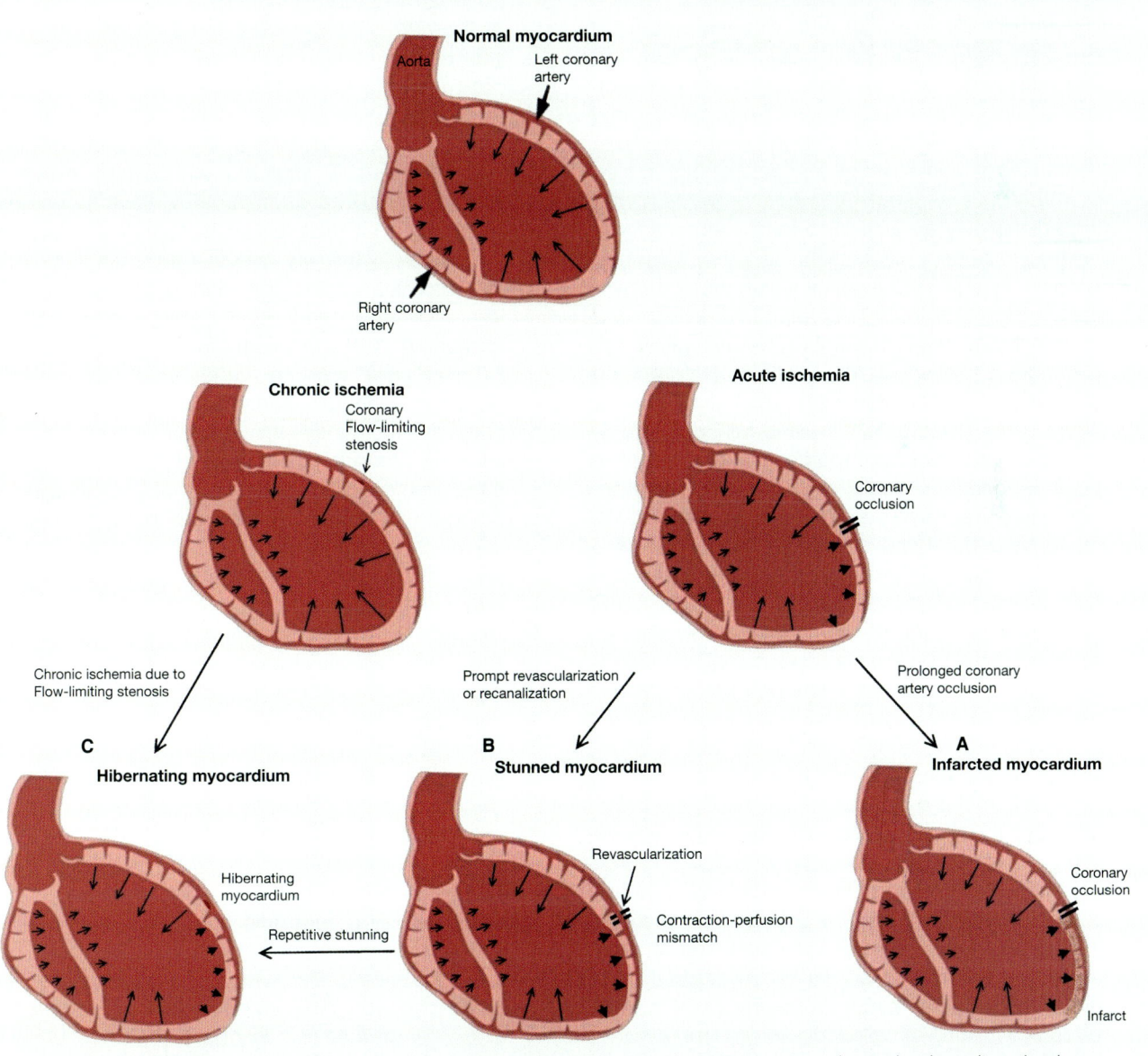

Figure 13.18. A normally perfused and functioning myocardium is depicted by normal coronary arteries and normal end-systolic and end-diastolic volumes. In the middle row on the right, a complete left coronary artery occlusion has occurred in the setting of plaque rupture with acute thrombosis. If the lack of perfusion is prolonged enough, a myocardial infarction ensues, with loss of function, depicted here by a regional increase in end-systolic volume **(A)**. If reperfusion occurs, due to either recanalization or revascularization, the contractility initially abnormal due to ischemia may remain impaired in the acute and subacute stages, with subsequent improvement. This phenomenon is called stunning **(B)**. Repetitive stunning leads to a state of chronic myocardial dysfunction called hibernation **(C)**. A chronic flow-limiting coronary artery occlusion leads to downregulation of the regional wall motion abnormality, leading to hibernating myocardium **(C)**.

in segmental and global myocardial dysfunction. Dysfunctional but viable myocardium in state of stunning or hibernation typically demonstrates contractile response to low-dose dobutamine infusion. Stunned myocardium with open vessel commonly demonstrates monophasic response (progressive improvement from low- to high-dose dobutamine, Option C), while hibernating myocardium with significant underlying coronary stenosis commonly demonstrates biphasic response (improvement in contractility with low dose and worsening with high dose, Option A). Caution should be taken differentiating tethering effect from contractile response: improved contractility in two adjacent segments is a more reliable indicator of contractile response compared to a single segment response (Option D). Transmural scarring and extensive damage demonstrate no contractile response at low and high doses (Option E). Nontransmural infarction can demonstrate improvement from rest at low dose; with more extensive nontransmural injury, contractile response can be seen only at high doses, as in this patient. Segments with improvement with high doses only are unlikely to show recovery with revascularization.

16. **Answer: C.** Peak longitudinal strain reflects myocardial shortening in longitudinal direction and therefore is a negative number. Normal values are commonly between −16% and −24%. Deformation analysis during dobutamine infusion can provide objective evidence of viability and ischemia. In this example, all described segments show reduced peak longitudinal strain at baseline. The anterior wall demonstrates increased deformation with low-dose dobutamine (longitudinal strain becomes more negative) followed by decreased deformation at the peak dose. This represents a biphasic response and is indicative of ischemia. The anterior septum demonstrates a continuous improvement in contractility across dobutamine doses (monophasic response), which is consistent with viable myocardium but not ischemia. Inferolateral wall demonstrates no viability.

17. **Answer: C.** In this patient with ischemic cardiomyopathy, dobutamine echocardiography allows assessment of viability and ischemia. At a low infusion dose (10 μg/kg/min shown, but similar response was demonstrated with 5 μg/kg/min), there is limited contractile reserve in the apex and anterior septum suggestive of significant myocardial scarring. On the other hand, inferolateral wall shows preserved resting contractility, which improves at low dose but decreases at peak dose. This response is typical for myocardial ischemia.

18. **Answer: A.** Exercise echocardiogram shows normal resting wall motion in this patient. On postexercise images, there is hypokinesis of the mid- and basal anterior wall seen on 2-chamber view. This is most consistent with a flow-limiting stenosis of the diagonal branch. Sparing of the apical segments and anterior septum is inconsistent with proximal left anterior descending artery stenosis (Option C). Similarly, significant stenosis of the left main coronary artery results in more extensive wall motion abnormalities typically involving apical, anterior, septal, and lateral segments (Option B).

19. **Answer: A.** This case illustrates the hemodynamic response to exercise in a patient with primary pulmonary hypertension who had only mild pulmonary hypertension at rest, with estimated pulmonary artery systolic pressure of 40 mm Hg that rose to 90 mm Hg during exercise (not shown). Post-stress images demonstrate marked right ventricular enlargement and hypokinesis due to a dynamic rise in the right-side pressures and D-shaped deformation of the interventricular septum with small and hyperdynamic left ventricle.

20. **Answer: D.** An exercise stress echocardiography is a useful tool to elicit a left ventricular outflow tract gradient in patients with latent hypertrophic obstructive cardiomyopathy. Patients without obstruction at rest or with resting provocation maneuvers (such as Valsalva or standing) may demonstrate obstruction during exercise as evidenced in this patient (peak instantaneous gradient exceeding 140 mm Hg). The continuous-wave Doppler signal through the left ventricular outflow tract has a dagger-shaped, late peaking envelope characteristic of dynamic obstruction as opposed to aortic stenosis where the envelope has a round shape and the gradient peaks in early to mid-systole. Symptomatic patients with hypertrophic obstructive cardiomyopathy commonly respond to beta-blocker and negative inotrope therapy, while vasodilators may worsen the obstruction (Option A).

21. **Answer: D.** The echocardiogram performed with the use of an ultrasound-enhancing agent shows severely decreased left ventricular ejection fraction with global hypokinesis at baseline. With dobutamine infusion, the wall motion starts to improve at low dose and continues to improve at peak in all segments (monophasic response). The end-systolic cavity size decreases at peak stress. This type of response is commonly seen in nonischemic cardiomyopathy and portends good prognosis due to presence of inotropic contractile reserve. The prognostic value of inotropic contractile reserve has been specifically demonstrated in patients with HIV cardiomyopathy. Studies have also shown that the presence of inotropic contractile reserve predicts good response to beta-blocker therapy.

22. **Answer: A.** The echocardiographic images show significant wall motion abnormalities postexercise affecting the mid to apical anterior wall, anteroseptum and inferoseptum, as well as the apex. This is typical of a left anterior descending artery

flow-limiting stenosis. There is also evidence of transient ischemic cavity dilatation: the end-systolic cavity size appears larger on postexercise images compared to resting images. Transient ischemic cavity dilatation predicts severe and extensive coronary artery disease and is most commonly seen in the absence of distal collateral circulation.

23. **Answer: D.** The echocardiographic images at peak dobutamine dose show wall motion abnormalities in multiple segments including apex, anterior, anterolateral, inferior, and inferolateral walls. This is consistent with extensive coronary artery disease affecting multiple coronary distribution territories.

24. **Answer: C.** The echocardiographic images reveal mild apical ischemia. Note on the apical long-axis view, the difference in cavity size between the stages of low dose and peak dose of dobutamine, at the level of the apex. During the low-dose stage, there is a normal hypercontractile response with complete cavity obliteration; while during the peak dose, there is apical hypokinesis without complete cavity obliteration that indicates ischemia in this region. The absence of symptoms and mild degree of ischemia (<3 segments) are factors that portend a low risk for perioperative cardiovascular events and further workup and delay in the surgical procedure are not warranted. Using pooled outcome data, a proposed threshold for moderate ischemia in stress echocardiography is based on identifying three or more ischemic segments.

25. **Answer: D.** "False-positive" results on stress echocardiography are not uncommon as judged by coronary angiography. One study estimated that 33% of patients with abnormal stress echocardiogram have no obstructive disease on coronary angiography. In that study, the mortality in patients with abnormal stress test was influenced by age, stress modality (dobutamine echocardiography carrying a higher mortality), and resting left ventricular ejection fraction (<50% carrying a higher mortality). Patients with markedly abnormal stress echocardiogram also carried a higher mortality. Presence or absence of obstructive coronary artery disease (>50% stenosis) had no influence on mortality.

26. **Answer: B.** This patient presents with symptoms not explained by the degree of mitral regurgitation seen on the resting echocardiogram. The exercise stress echocardiogram shows an increase in the severity of mitral regurgitation and a significant increase in the pulmonary artery systolic pressure, both consistent with hemodynamically significant mitral regurgitation. It is important to identify a subset of patients who have discrepancy between the degree of mitral regurgitation on resting echocardiogram, symptoms, and other findings (eg, left ventricular enlargement). Exercise echocardiography with emphasis of color and spectral Doppler findings (degree of mitral regurgitation and tricuspid regurgitant jet velocity) is an important tool in establishing the correct diagnosis.

27. **Answer: C.** The case illustrates a normal stress echocardiogram (as seen on the images) discordant with the stress electrocardiogram results. The specificity of the stress electrocardiogram can be affected by several factors including left ventricular hypertrophy, preexisting conduction abnormalities, drug therapy, etc. Also, the specificity of ST segment changes during exercise is lower in women than in men. The sensitivity and specificity of stress echocardiography are superior to that of stress electrocardiogram, and given the normal results of the stress echocardiographic images, it can be assumed that the results of electrocardiogram represent a false-positive one. Therefore, there is no need for additional inpatient workup and the patient can be safely discharged home.

KEY POINTS
- Specificity of ST segment changes during exercise is lower in women.
- The sensitivity of stress echocardiography is superior to that of stress electrocardiogram.
- A normal stress echocardiogram, even in the presence of electrocardiographic changes, portends a good prognosis.

28. **Answer: A.** See rationale for **Answer 27.**
29. **Answer: D.** This case illustrates a patient with ischemic cardiomyopathy and severe left ventricular dysfunction with minimal inotropic contractile reserve and without evidence of inducible ischemia. The absence of inotropic contractile reserve, consistent with a scarred myocardium, portends a poor prognosis. Patients with significant viability are likely to demonstrate improvement in left ventricular function after revascularization, beta-blocker therapy, and cardiac resynchronization therapy. This patient is unlikely to benefit from revascularization. Likewise, it is unlikely that this patient with minimal inotropic contractile reserve will respond to cardiac resynchronization therapy.

KEY POINTS
- Inotropic contractile reserve can predict left ventricular functional recovery after revascularization.
- Inotropic contractile reserve predicts response to beta-blocker therapy.
- Absence of inotropic contractile reserve portends a poor prognosis.

30. Answer: E. See rationale for **Answer 29**.

31. Answer: C. This case illustrates a patient with moderate ischemia in the mid and apical inferoseptal and anterior walls, as well as the mid-anteroseptum and apical inferior wall. Coronary angiography confirmed a severe mid left anterior descending artery stenosis. The sensitivity of dipyridamole stress echocardiography for single-vessel disease may be as low as 50%, but its specificity is excellent (88%-100%). Wall motion score index is a semiquantitative tool for the assessment of regional left ventricular systolic performance that can be computed at rest and with stress. A 16-segment model is commonly used for wall motion analysis (as opposed to 17-segment model used for perfusion imaging). Each segment is assigned a score from one to five and then the sum of all scores is divided by the number of visualized segments (**Table 13.3**). Wall motion score index of 1.0 is considered normal. The peak wall motion score index in this patient is about 1.7, which confers a high cardiovascular risk to this patient (>5%/year). Even though chest pain may represent a nonspecific symptom and a side effect of dipyridamole, the presence of new wall motion abnormalities indicates ischemia.

KEY POINTS

- Wall motion score index is a semiquantitative tool for the assessment of regional left ventricular systolic performance.
- Stress wall motion score index >1.7 confers a poor prognosis.
- Chest pain in conjunction with new wall motion abnormalities during stress echocardiography further supports ischemia.

Table 13.3. Wall Motion Scoring

Segment Score	Finding	Description
1	Normal or hyperkinetic	Normal systolic thickening, typically >50%
2[a]	Hypokinetic	Systolic thickening <40%
3	Akinetic	Systolic thickening <10%
4	Dyskinetic	Paradoxical outward systolic motion
5[b]	Aneurysmal	Diastolic deformation

[a]Some studies assigned a separate score to severe hypokinesis.
[b]Some experts advocate for not assigning a separate wall motion score for aneurysm.

32. Answer: A. See rationale for **Answer 31**.
33. Answer: B. See rationale for **Answer 31**.
34. Answer: D. This case describes a hypertensive woman with exertional shortness of breath, a commonly encountered clinical scenario. The differential diagnosis of dyspnea is broad and exercise echocardiography can provide important diagnostic information. Comprehensive echocardiography should focus on not only wall motion but also pre- and postexercise assessment of diastolic function by obtaining mitral inflow velocities, annular velocities by tissue Doppler, and tricuspid regurgitant jet velocity. Normal response to exercise includes increase in mitral inflow E velocity, e' and S' velocities, left ventricular ejection fraction, and global longitudinal strain, but E/e' ratio stays relatively constant. In this example, the postexercise wall motion analysis shows no evidence of myocardial ischemia. The resting E velocity is low (around 60 cm/s) and septal e' velocity is also decreased (around 4 cm/s) with E/e' ratio of 15. After exercise, there is a significant increase in E velocity reaching 135 cm/s, while the increase in septal e' velocity is small (around 7 cm/s). The postexercise E/e' ratio is 19, indicating high left ventricular filling pressures. Note that tricuspid regurgitation velocity also increases from around 3 to 4 m/s, indicating exercise-induced increase in pulmonary artery pressures due to left ventricular diastolic dysfunction.

KEY POINTS

- Diastolic stress echocardiography provides important diagnostic information in patients with exertional dyspnea.
- E/e' ratio remains relatively unchanged postexercise in normal adults.

35. Answer: C. See rationale for **Answer 34**.
36. Answer: B. See rationale for **Answer 34**.
37. Answer: C. This patient has resting wall motion abnormalities involving inferior, inferolateral, and anterolateral walls. At peak dobutamine infusion, he also develops wall motion abnormalities in the distribution of the left anterior descending artery as well as ischemic cavity dilation. The peak wall motion score index and the evidence of transient ischemic dilatation put this patient in a high-risk group for short-term cardiovascular events. Transient ischemic cavity dilatation denotes severe and extensive coronary artery disease. Coronary angiogram in this patient confirmed the presence of triple-vessel coronary artery disease.

> **KEY POINTS**
> - Transient ischemic cavity dilatation is a marker of severe and extensive coronary artery disease.
> - Transient ischemic cavity dilatation portends a poor prognosis.
> - Transient ischemic cavity dilatation appearance is affected by the presence of collateral circulation.

Acknowledgments: We gratefully acknowledge the contributions of previous edition author(s), Omar Wever-Pinzon, as portions of their chapter have been retained in this revision. The author would also like to acknowledge the contribution of the late Dr. Farooq Chaudhry to this chapter and in general to the field of stress echocardiography.

38. Answer: D. See rationale for **Answer 37.**

SUGGESTED READINGS

Argulian E, Chaudhry FA. Stress testing in patients with hypertrophic cardiomyopathy. *Prog Cardiovasc Dis*. 2012;54(6):477-482.

Argulian E, Halpern DG, Agarwal V, Agarwal SK, Chaudhry FA. Predictors of ischemia in patients referred for evaluation of exertional dyspnea: a stress echocardiography study. *J Am Soc Echocardiogr*. 2013;26(1):72-76.

From AM, Kane G, Bruce C, Pellikka PA, Scott C, McCully RB. Characteristics and outcomes of patients with abnormal stress echocardiograms and angiographically mild coronary artery disease (<50% stenoses) or normal coronary arteries. *J Am Soc Echocardiogr*. 2010;23(2):207-214.

Lancellotti P, Pellikka PA, Budts W, et al. The clinical use of stress echocardiography in non-ischaemic heart disease: recommendations from the European Association of cardiovascular imaging and the American Society of echocardiography. *J Am Soc Echocardiogr*. 2017;30(2):101-138.

Mahenthiran J, Bangalore S, Yao SS, Chaudhry FA. Comparison of prognostic value of stress echocardiography versus stress electrocardiography in patients with suspected coronary artery disease. *Am J Cardiol*. 2005;96(5):628-634.

Otto CM, Nishimura RA, Bonow RO, et al. 2020 ACC/AHA guideline for the management of patients with valvular heart disease: a report of the American College of Cardiology/American Heart Association Joint Committee on clinical practice guidelines. *Circulation*. 2021;143(5):e72-e227.

Pellikka PA, Arruda-Olson A, Chaudhry FA, et al. Guidelines for performance, interpretation, and application of stress echocardiography in ischemic heart disease: from the American Society of Echocardiography. *J Am Soc Echocardiogr*. 2020;33(1):1-41.e8.

Shaw LJ, Berman DS, Picard MH, et al. Comparative definitions for moderate-severe ischemia in stress nuclear, echocardiography, and magnetic resonance imaging. *JACC Cardiovasc Imaging*. 2014;7(6):593-604.

Wever-Pinzon O, Bangalore S, Romero J, Silva Enciso J, Chaudhry FA. Inotropic contractile reserve can risk-stratify patients with HIV cardiomyopathy: a dobutamine stress echocardiography study. *JACC Cardiovasc Imaging*. 2011;4(12):1231-1238.

Yao SS, Shah A, Bangalore S, Chaudhry FA. Transient ischemic left ventricular cavity dilation is a significant predictor of severe and extensive coronary artery disease and adverse outcome in patients undergoing stress echocardiography. *J Am Soc Echocardiogr*. 2007;20(4):352-358.

CHAPTER 14

Dyssynchrony Evaluation/ Atrioventricular Optimization

Pieter van der Bijl, Victoria Delgado, and Jeroen J. Bax

QUESTIONS

1. Which of the following statements about the echocardiographic assessment of cardiac dyssynchrony in patients with heart failure is **CORRECT**?
   A. Atrioventricular (AV) dyssynchrony can be identified by a long left ventricular (LV) filling time (LVFT) (>40%).
   B. Interventricular dyssynchrony is defined by a prolonged delay between the right ventricular (RV) and LV ejections as assessed with pulsed-wave Doppler echocardiography (≥40 ms).
   C. Early diastolic notching of the interventricular septum on M-mode in the LV parasternal long-axis can be observed in patients with left bundle branch block and indicates LV dyssynchrony.
   D. Intra-LV dyssynchrony is observed only in patients with left bundle branch block, whereas interventricular dyssynchrony is observed only in patients with right bundle branch block.

2. AV dyssynchrony is characterized by prolonged AV conduction. Which of the following echocardiographic signs can be observed?
   A. LV diastolic filling is reduced because atrial contraction occurs against a closed mitral valve.
   B. The diastolic LVFT lengthens as indicated by a relative early E wave on transmitral Doppler recordings.
   C. A truncated A wave is observed on transmitral Doppler recordings.
   D. The diastolic LVFT shortens with fusion of E and A waves.

3. Which echocardiographic method is used to measure interventricular dyssynchrony?
   A. M-mode echocardiography, measuring the time delay between peak systolic thickening of the interventricular septum and the RV free wall.
   B. Pulsed-wave Doppler echocardiography, measuring the time delay between the onset of LV ejection and RV ejection.
   C. Continuous-wave Doppler echocardiography, measuring the time difference between closure of the tricuspid valve and mitral valve.
   D. Tissue Doppler imaging (TDI), measuring the time delay between peak systolic velocity of the interventricular septum and the LV lateral wall.

4. LV dyssynchrony can be measured with M-mode echocardiography, obtaining the so-called septal-to-posterior wall motion delay (SPWMD) index. Which of the following statements about this method is **CORRECT**?
   A. This index is derived by measuring the time delay between the peak inward motion of the interventricular septum and the LV posterior wall.
   B. This index is measured by applying anatomic M-mode to the LV apical four-chamber view.
   C. A cutoff value of ≥65 ms predicts a favorable response to cardiac resynchronization therapy (CRT).
   D. This method is suitable for patients with ischemic heart failure with prior myocardial infarction of the posterolateral wall.

5. TDI techniques have been used extensively to quantify LV dyssynchrony. Which of the following statements about these methodologies is **CORRECT**?
   A. Pulsed-wave TDI allows simultaneous interrogation of two opposing LV walls in real time.
   B. TDI techniques permit angle-independent assessment of LV myocardial velocities.
   C. TDI data should be acquired with a frame rate of <90 frames per second.
   D. LV dyssynchrony can be measured by calculating the time delay between peak systolic velocities of two or four opposing walls.

6. Which of the following recommendations to measure LV dyssynchrony with color-coded TDI is **CORRECT**?
   A. Color-coded TDI data acquisition should be performed at a low frame rate (<90 frames per second).
   B. The timing of LV ejection should be determined from the beginning to the end of the pulsed-wave Doppler recording of the transmitral flow.
   C. LV dyssynchrony is calculated as the difference between time to isovolumic contraction in opposing walls.
   D. The components of the velocity signal include isovolumic contraction velocity, the systolic wave (S), the early diastolic wave (E), and the late-diastolic wave (A).

7. Which of the following statements about the measurement of LV dyssynchrony based on color-coded TDI is **CORRECT**?
   A. An opposing wall delay of ≥65 ms predicts a favorable response to CRT and long-term outcome.
   B. The standard deviation of time-to-peak systolic velocities of 12 segments of the LV apical two- and four-chamber views (basal, mid, and apical segments) yields the most accurate measurement of LV dyssynchrony.
   C. The standard deviation of the time-to-peak systolic velocities of 12 LV segments greater than 65 ms predicts clinical improvement after CRT.
   D. A septal-to-lateral wall delay of ≥31 ms predicts LV reverse remodeling after CRT.

8. TDI-derived strain rate imaging has been demonstrated to identify LV dyssynchrony. Which of the following statements is **CORRECT**?
   A. TDI-derived strain rate imaging evaluates myocardial displacement.
   B. TDI-derived strain rate imaging enables the measurement of time from QRS onset to peak strain in all LV segments (basal, mid, and apical) since this technique is not influenced by the insonation angle of the ultrasound beam.
   C. In patients with ischemic heart failure, TDI-derived strain rate imaging permits detection of myocardial segments with active contraction and segments that are passively tethered (myocardial scar).
   D. Applied to LV short-axis images, a time delay of ≥33 ms between peak systolic strain of the septal wall and the posterior wall predicts acute improvement in LV stroke volume after CRT.

9. Which of the following statements about LV dyssynchrony assessment with two-dimensional (2D) speckle tracking echocardiography is **TRUE**?
   A. The measurement of time-to-peak strain with 2D speckle tracking echocardiography is highly dependent on the angle of insonation of the ultrasound beam.
   B. 2D speckle tracking echocardiography permits the assessment of LV dyssynchrony in the radial, circumferential, and longitudinal directions.
   C. A peak radial strain–time delay between the (antero)septal and the (postero)lateral region of ≥31 ms predicts LV reverse remodeling.
   D. 2D speckle tracking echocardiography does not distinguish between myocardial segments with active contraction and myocardial segments that are passively tethered.

10. Three-dimensional (3D) echocardiography enables LV dyssynchrony assessment. Which of the following statements is **CORRECT**?
    A. Currently, the evaluation of LV dyssynchrony with 3D echocardiography techniques relies only on qualitative assessment of LV wall motion of 3D full volume data.
    B. With triplane tissue synchronization imaging (TSI), the standard deviation of time to minimum systolic volume of 16 segments (the so-called systolic dyssynchrony index [SDI]) is calculated to quantify LV dyssynchrony.
    C. With real-time 3D echocardiography, the time-to-peak systolic velocity of 16 segments is displayed in a polar map and time delays between two or four opposing walls as well as the standard deviation of 16 segments can be calculated.
    D. The presence of substantial LV dyssynchrony, defined by an SDI of ≥9.8% measured with real-time 3D echocardiography or ≥33 ms measured with triplane TSI, predicts response to CRT.

11. Which of the following statements about AV delay optimization is **CORRECT**?
    A. The optimal AV delay is the shortest AV interval without truncation of the A wave.
    B. Optimized AV synchrony is achieved by the shortest AV delay with fusion of the E and A waves.
    C. With an optimal AV delay, the end of left atrial contraction should coincide with the onset of the diastolic mitral regurgitation spectral signal.
    D. The optimal AV delay is the longest AV delay which permits a long LVFT, regardless of whether A wave truncation occurs.

12. Which of the following echocardiographic signs can be observed when a short AV delay is programmed?
    A. Diastolic mitral regurgitation.
    B. E and A wave fusion on transmitral pulsed-wave Doppler recordings.
    C. Reduced LVFT.
    D. A truncated A wave on transmitral, pulsed-wave Doppler recordings.

13. Which of the following echocardiographic methods can be used to optimize the AV delay?
    A. Pulsed-wave TDI, placing the sample volumes at the septal and lateral mitral annulus.
    B. M-mode recordings of the mitral annulus.
    C. Color-coded TDI, placing the sample volumes at the lateral wall of the left atrium and the LV lateral wall.
    D. Pulsed-wave Doppler recordings of the transmitral blood flow.

14. Which of the following statements about echocardiographic AV delay optimization is **TRUE**?
    A. The Ritter method can always be performed, regardless of the duration of the intrinsic PR interval.
    B. The iterative method involves programming a long AV delay and then shortening it by 20 ms decrements until the A wave is truncated.
    C. The peak rate of rise of LV pressure during isovolumic contraction, the so-called dP/dt_{max}, is the best method to optimize the AV delay.
    D. The shortest velocity-time integral of the flow across the LV outflow tract indicates the optimal AV delay.

15. Which of the following sentences about interventricular (VV) delay optimization is **TRUE**?
    A. The measurement of velocity-time integral of the LV outflow tract on pulsed-wave Doppler recordings can be used to optimize VV delay.
    B. Color-coded TDI is the most commonly used method to optimize VV delay, placing the sample volumes at the basal segments of the RV free wall and the LV lateral wall.
    C. VV delay optimization can be performed only by electrocardiographic methods.
    D. M-mode recording of the LV parasternal long-axis view, measuring the time delay between the peak inward motion of the septum and the posterior wall, is highly feasible in patients with ischemic heart failure.

16. Based on **Figure 14.1**, which of the following statements on AV dyssynchrony is **TRUE**?
   A. The AV delay is optimal and maximizes diastolic LVFT by starting the LV contraction at the end of the A wave.
   B. The AV delay is too short and the A wave is truncated.
   C. The AV delay is too long, and consequently, the E and A waves are fused, reducing the diastolic LVFT.
   D. The AV delay cannot be assessed because the patient is in atrial fibrillation.

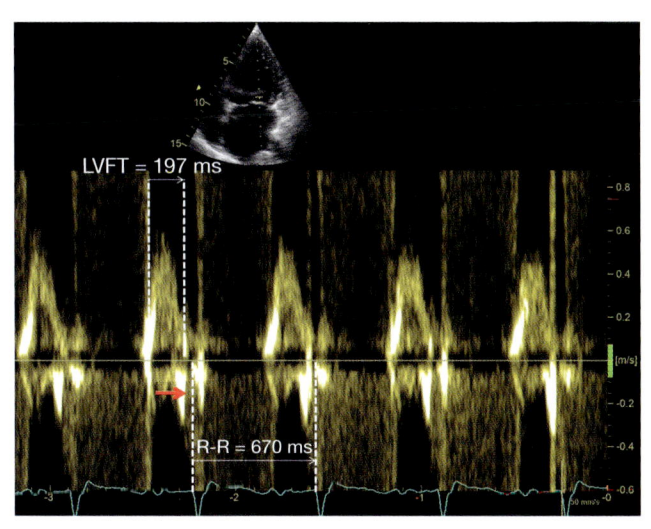

Figure 14.1

17. Figure 14.2 shows an example of LV dyssynchrony assessed with pulsed-wave TDI. Based on this example, which of the following statements is **CORRECT**?
   A. Time from the onset of the Q wave to the first positive deflection (isovolumic contraction) should be measured in the basal segments of the RV, septum, and LV lateral wall.
   B. There is substantial LV dyssynchrony, indicated by the difference in systolic velocities of the LV septal and lateral walls.
   C. Measurement of the electromechanical delay in the septal wall is incorrect because the ultrasound beam is not aligned well.
   D. There is substantial interventricular dyssynchrony (RV free wall to LV lateral wall delay of 90 ms) but not LV dyssynchrony, with a time delay of 25 ms between LV septal and lateral walls.

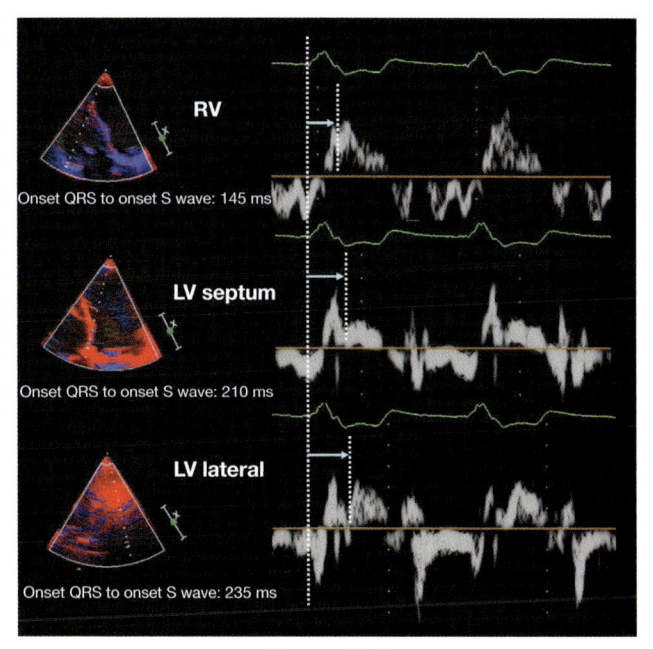

Figure 14.2

18. In **Figure 14.3A-C**, LV dyssynchrony is evaluated with color-coded TDI.
   What conclusion can be drawn from this example?
   A. The measured time difference between opposing walls is associated with no response to CRT.
   B. The timing of LV ejection does not include the first positive peak velocity, and therefore LV dyssynchrony cannot be evaluated.
   C. There is substantial LV dyssynchrony, with a maximum delay of 90 ms between two opposing walls, that has been associated with LV reverse remodeling at follow-up.
   D. The LV segments where the sample volumes are placed show very high systolic velocities, indicating active contraction.

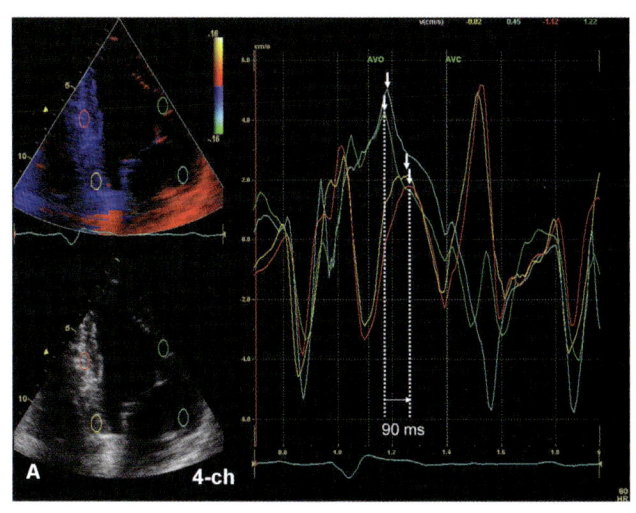

Figure 14.3A

Figure 14.3B

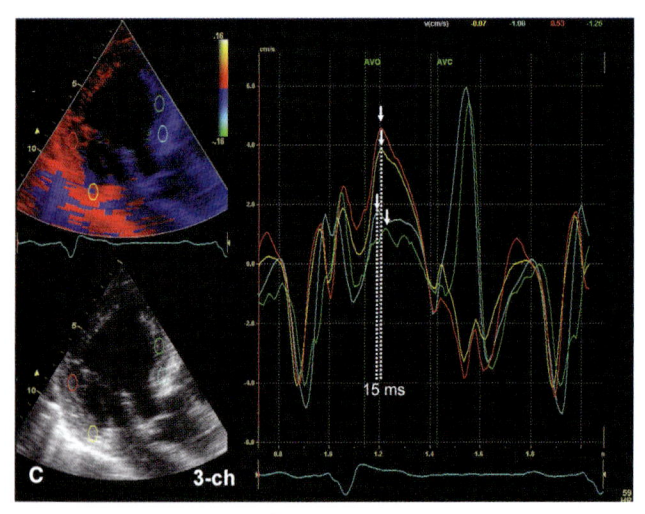

Figure 14.3C

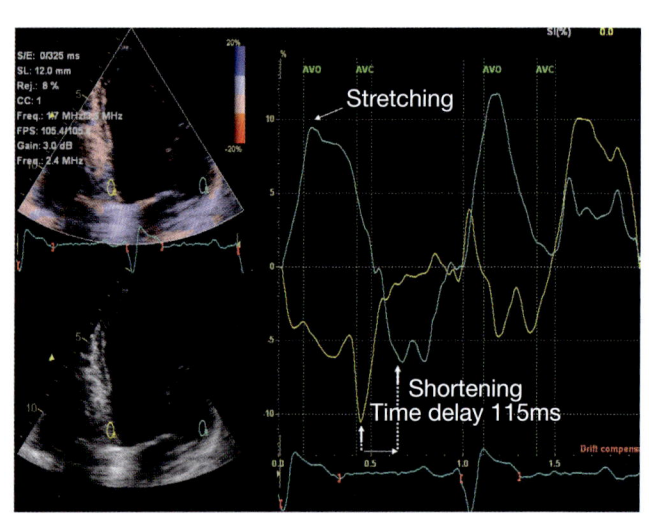

Figure 14.4

19. Doppler-derived strain imaging has been proposed to measure LV dyssynchrony. What is **INCORRECT** about **Figure 14.4**?
    A. There is substantial LV dyssynchrony with the lateral wall being stretched while the septal wall shortens.
    B. In this example, strain imaging is not the optimal method to assess LV dyssynchrony since the lateral wall appears tethered by the adjacent segments.
    C. There is substantial LV dyssynchrony with a peak systolic strain–time delay of 115 ms between the septal and lateral walls.
    D. Strain (rate) imaging enables the assessment of active myocardial contraction and therefore reflects viable myocardium.

20. LV dyssynchrony assessed with TDI-derived radial strain has been associated with improvement in LV stroke volume after CRT. Which sentence about **Figure 14.5** is **CORRECT**?
    A. The example shows circumferential strain–time curves and therefore LV dyssynchrony cannot be assessed.
    B. Peak septal radial strain occurs earlier than peak posterior radial strain indicating significant LV dyssynchrony.
    C. The sample volumes are incorrect and should be placed in the inferior and lateral walls.
    D. Radial strain–time curves in this example are too noisy and therefore LV dyssynchrony assessment is unreliable.

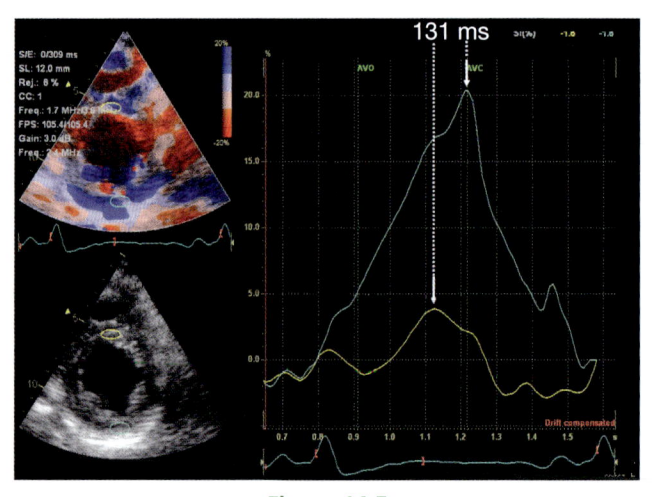

Figure 14.5

Chapter 14 Dyssynchrony Evaluation/Atrioventricular Optimization / 303

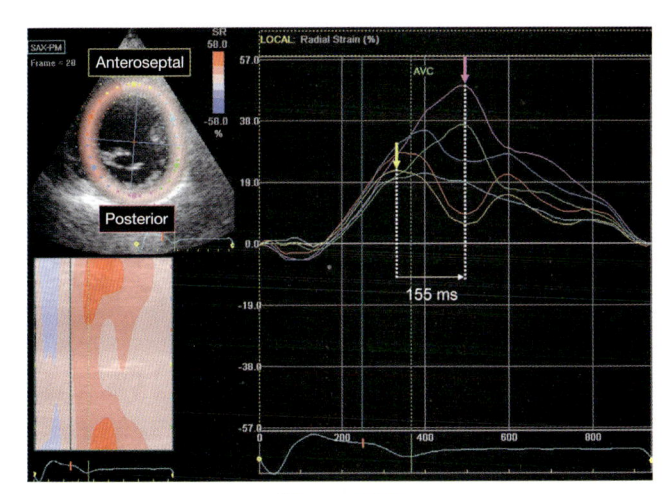

Figure 14.6

21. Based on **Figure 14.6**, which of the following sentences about 2D speckle tracking is **CORRECT**?
    A. LV dyssynchrony can be assessed only by measuring the time delay between peak radial strain of the anteroseptal segment and the posterior segment since those are the segments aligned along the direction of the ultrasound beam.
    B. With this method, the latest activated segment can be identified and may be useful to indicate where the LV pacing lead should be placed.
    C. There is no significant LV dyssynchrony, since the time delay between peak radial strain of the anteroseptal and posterior segments is <130 ms.
    D. The low values of radial strain of the septal, anteroseptal, and anterior segments indicate that these segments are tethered and do not contract actively.

22. Triplane TSI permits characterization of LV mechanical activation. Based on **Figure 14.7**, which of the following statements is **CORRECT**?
    A. In patients with ischemic heart failure, triplane TSI is the best tool to distinguish segments with active contraction from those that are passively tethered.
    B. Activation time intervals from 16 LV segments (six basal, six mid, and four apical segments) are obtained simultaneously during the same heartbeat.
    C. The site of maximal mechanical delay cannot be identified.
    D. The TSI algorithm calculates time-to-peak myocardial systolic velocities in 12 LV segments and converts these time intervals into color codes.

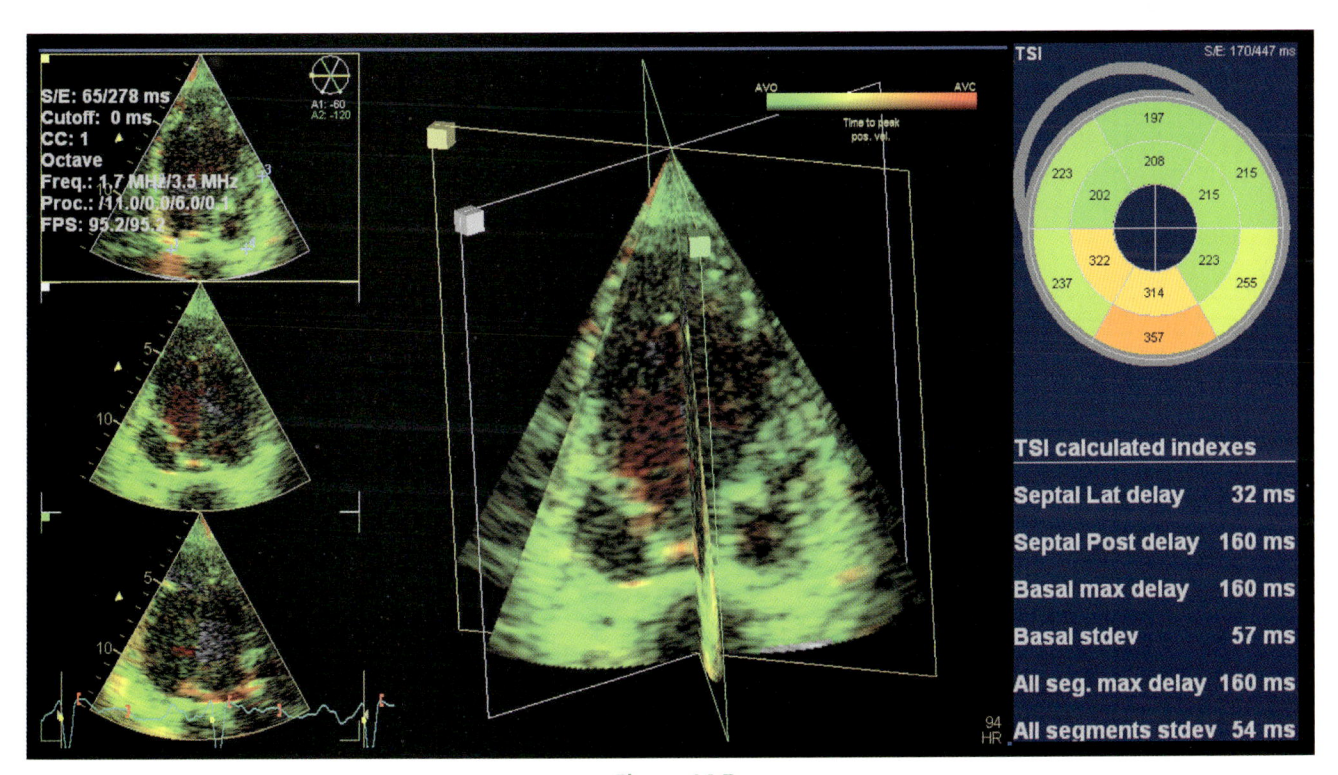

Figure 14.7

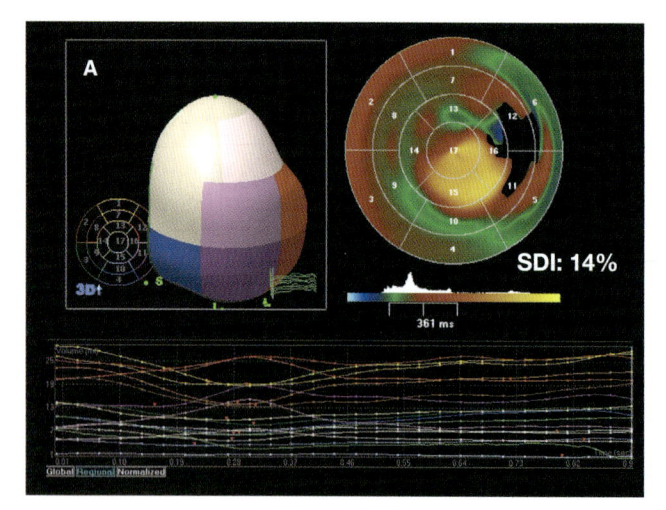

Figure 14.8A

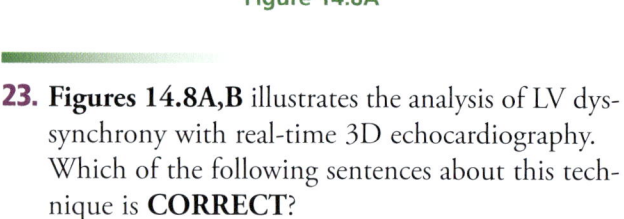

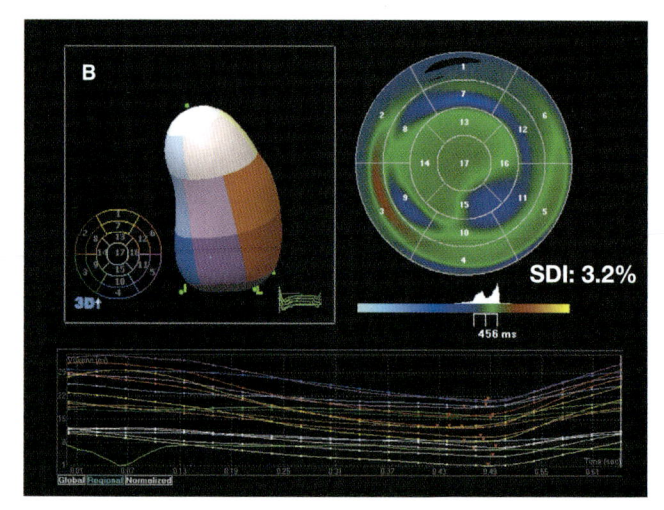

Figure 14.8B

23. **Figures 14.8A,B** illustrates the analysis of LV dyssynchrony with real-time 3D echocardiography. Which of the following sentences about this technique is **CORRECT**?
   A. LV dyssynchrony is quantified by calculating the standard deviation of time to minimum systolic volume of 16 LV subvolumes, the so-called SDI.
   B. The polar maps show the time to minimum systolic volume of the 15 to 17 LV subvolumes, but the latest activated region cannot be identified.
   C. The time-volume curves indicate which segments show active contraction and which segments are tethered by the adjacent segments.
   D. After 6-month follow-up (Panel B), substantial LV dyssynchrony remains.

24. The iterative method to optimize the AV delay has been used in several single-center and randomized multicenter CRT studies. Based on the sequence shown in **Figure 14.9**, which of the following statements is **CORRECT**?
   A. The sequence is incorrect since this method starts with the shortest AV delay, increasing by 10 ms increments until the E and A waves are fused.
   B. The optimal AV delay is 120 ms.
   C. The optimal AV delay is defined by the longest AV delay with truncation of the A wave.
   D. This method cannot be applied if there is no mitral regurgitation.

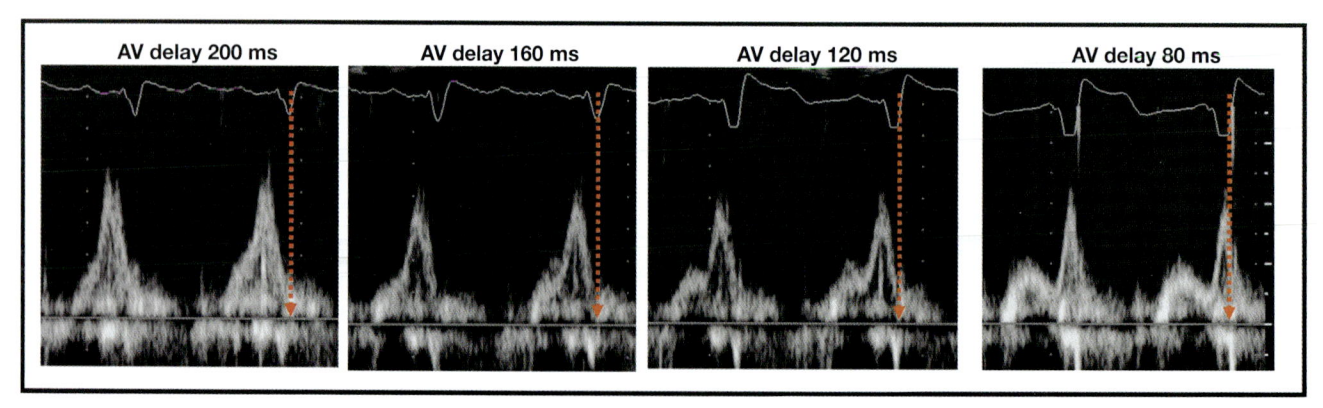

Figure 14.9

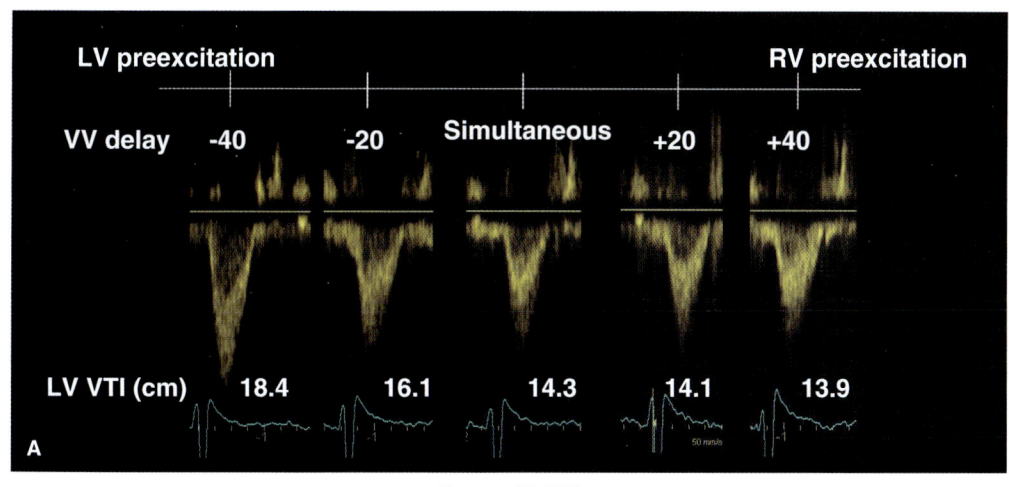

Figure 14.10A

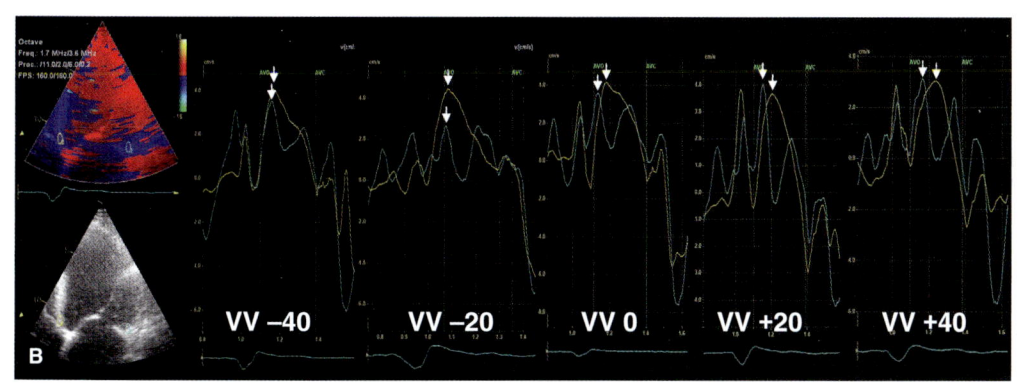

Figure 14.10B

25. Optimization of the VV delay can be performed with pulsed-wave Doppler recordings of the LV outflow tract by measuring the cardiac output, and with TDI by evaluating LV dyssynchrony. Based on **Figure 14.10A,B**, which of the following statements is **CORRECT**?
   A. The VV delay that provides the highest cardiac output does not necessarily have the least amount of LV dyssynchrony.
   B. Prestimulation of the RV usually provides the highest cardiac output.
   C. In this example, the optimal VV delay should be set at −40 ms (prestimulation of the LV) since it yields the highest cardiac output and the most synchronous LV contraction.
   D. Once the optimal VV delay is programmed, it remains stable and no further adjustments are needed.

CASE 1

A 56-year-old man with New York Heart Association heart failure functional class II was referred to the echocardiography laboratory to evaluate LV dimensions and function, mitral regurgitation, and dyssynchrony.

26. Based on **Figure 14.11** and **Case 1**, which conclusions can be drawn regarding cardiac dyssynchrony?
   A. The patient shows a normal LV diastolic filling pattern and optimal AV synchrony.
   B. There is a high degree of interventricular synchrony with the onset of RV ejection after the onset of LV ejection.
   C. The color-coded TDI image does not show LV dyssynchrony.
   D. The patient demonstrates a restrictive LV diastolic filling pattern with shortened diastolic LVFT (<40%) and significant interventricular and LV dyssynchrony.

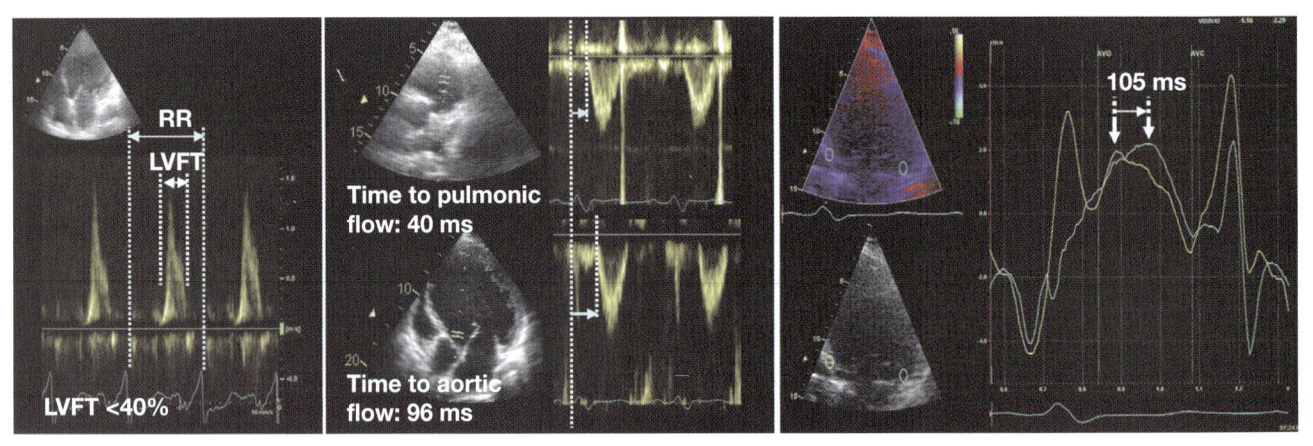

Figure 14.11

27. On color Doppler, severe functional mitral regurgitation was seen (**Figure 14.12A** and ▶ **Video 14.1A**). 2D speckle tracking echocardiography was used to evaluate mechanical dyssynchrony between the LV segments underlying the papillary muscles (**Figure 14.12B** and ▶ **Video 14.1B**). Which of the following statements regarding the assessment of mitral regurgitation in this patient is **CORRECT**?

   A. An ischemic etiology can be excluded because the most common cause of functional mitral regurgitation in patients with heart failure is atrial secondary mitral regurgitation.
   B. A significant reduction in mitral regurgitation can be observed by resynchronizing the LV segments underlying the papillary muscles.
   C. 2D speckle tracking echocardiography cannot distinguish between segments with active contraction and segments that are tethered and therefore an ischemic etiology cannot be excluded.
   D. The evaluation of LV dyssynchrony should be performed at the level of the mitral valve (basal short-axis view).

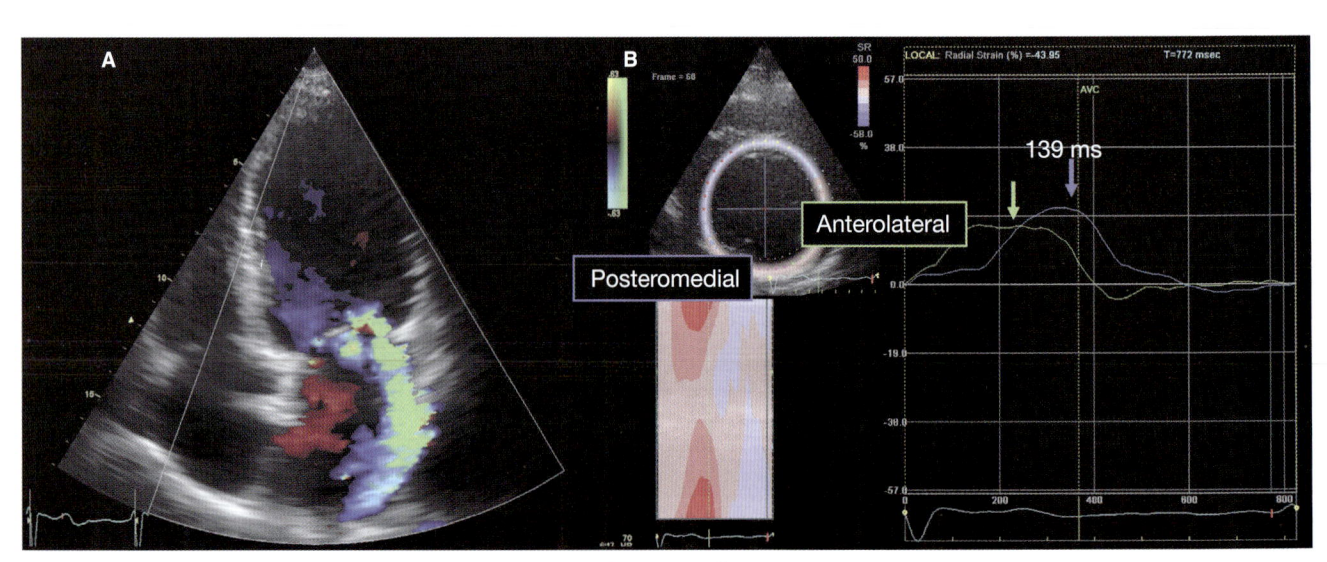

Figure 14.12

CASE 2

An 87-year-old man was admitted at the emergency department because of heart failure symptoms 1 week after dual-chamber pacemaker implantation. **Figure 14.13** *shows the pulsed-wave Doppler recording of the transmitral flow.*

28. Based on **Figure 14.13** in **Case 2**, which of the following statements about the transmitral flow pattern is **CORRECT**?
    A. The transmitral flow pattern demonstrates normal LV diastolic filling.
    B. The cardiac rhythm is atrial fibrillation and therefore only an E wave can be seen.
    C. The AV delay is programmed too short and therefore the A wave is truncated.
    D. The AV delay is programmed too long, and consequently, the E and A waves are fused, thereby reducing the LVFT.

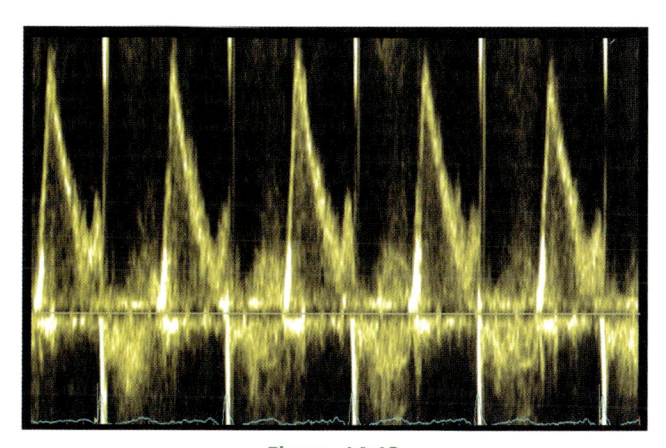

Figure 14.13

29. What would the **CORRECT** management of the patient in **Case 2** entail?
    A. Turn off the pacemaker because it can induce heart failure.
    B. A cardioversion is indicated because the patient is in atrial fibrillation.
    C. Program a longer AV delay to ensure completion of diastolic LV filling without truncation of the A wave.
    D. Program a shorter AV delay to lengthen the LVFT, thereby separating the E and A waves.

CASE 3

A 67-year-old man with a prior inferoposterior myocardial infarction was admitted to the cardiac care unit with acute pulmonary edema. After stabilization, a transthoracic echocardiogram was performed to evaluate LV volumes, ejection fraction, and LV dyssynchrony. When the sonographer applied M-mode to quantify SPWMD, **Figure 14.14** *was observed.*

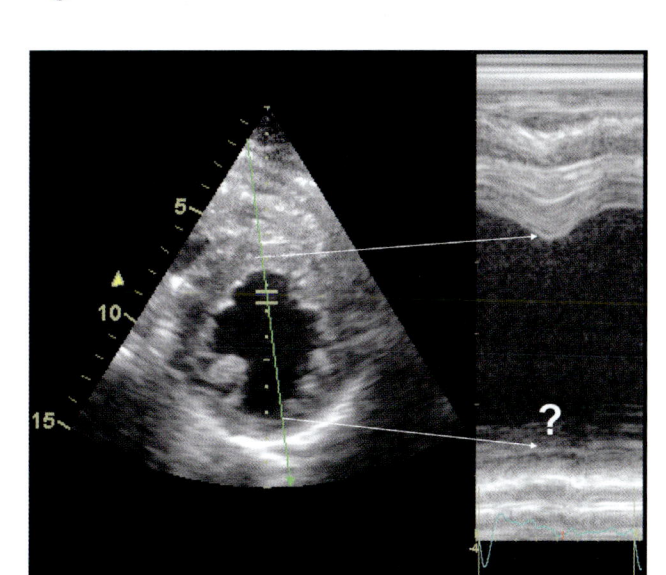

Figure 14.14

30. Based on **Figure 14.14** in **Case 3**, which of the following statements about LV dyssynchrony assessment with M-mode is **CORRECT**?
    A. In this patient, the degree of LV dyssynchrony is significant because the posterior wall does not demonstrate peak inward motion.
    B. LV dyssynchrony cannot be assessed with this method because the posterior wall may not contract actively and therefore peak inward motion cannot be appreciated.
    C. Myocardial velocities based on color-coded TDI have the ability to distinguish myocardial segments with active contraction from passively tethered segments and therefore may constitute a better tool to evaluate LV dyssynchrony.
    D. 2D speckle tracking echocardiography cannot evaluate LV dyssynchrony in this case due to the high angle dependency of the technique.

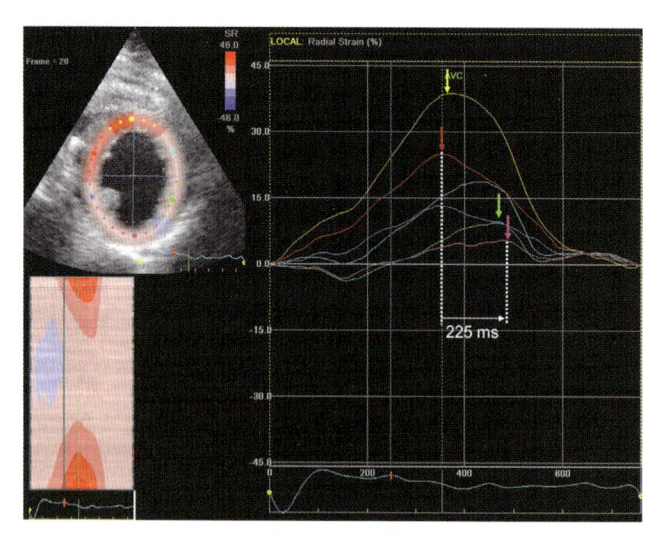

Figure 14.15

31. A second, more experienced sonographer performed 2D speckle tracking analysis on short-axis images to evaluate the LV mechanical activation pattern and obtained **Figure 14.15**.
    Which of the following sentences about this case is **CORRECT**?
    A. There is substantial LV dyssynchrony, as indicated by the radial strain–time curves with the earliest activated segments at the septal and anteroseptal walls and the latest activated segments at the lateral and posterior walls.
    B. The likelihood of a favorable response to CRT is high regardless of the location and extent of myocardial scar since there is substantial LV dyssynchrony.
    C. The analysis is incorrectly performed because the region of interest is not narrow enough to evaluate the endocardium.
    D. After CRT, a responder should demonstrate postsystolic thickening in the anteroseptal and septal segments.

CASE 4

A 54-year-old man with ischemic heart failure, a LV ejection fraction of 28%, and a left bundle branch block, received CRT. At 6-month follow-up, the patient did not experience any clinical or echocardiographic improvement.

32. According to **Figure 14.16**, which of the following statements is **CORRECT** regarding the patient in **Case 4**?
    A. The LV diastolic filling pattern is normal, as indicated by the transmitral pulsed-wave Doppler recordings, but there is substantial LV dyssynchrony as shown by the large septal-to-lateral wall delay on TDI data.
    B. LV diastolic filling is compromised by a long AV delay with fusion of the E and A waves.
    C. LV diastolic filling is compromised by a short AV delay with truncation of the A wave and there is still substantial LV dyssynchrony with a large septal-to-lateral wall delay on TDI recordings.
    D. LV dyssynchrony is incorrectly measured with misalignment of the ultrasound beam, very small sample volumes, and high noise-to-signal ratio in the time-velocity curves.

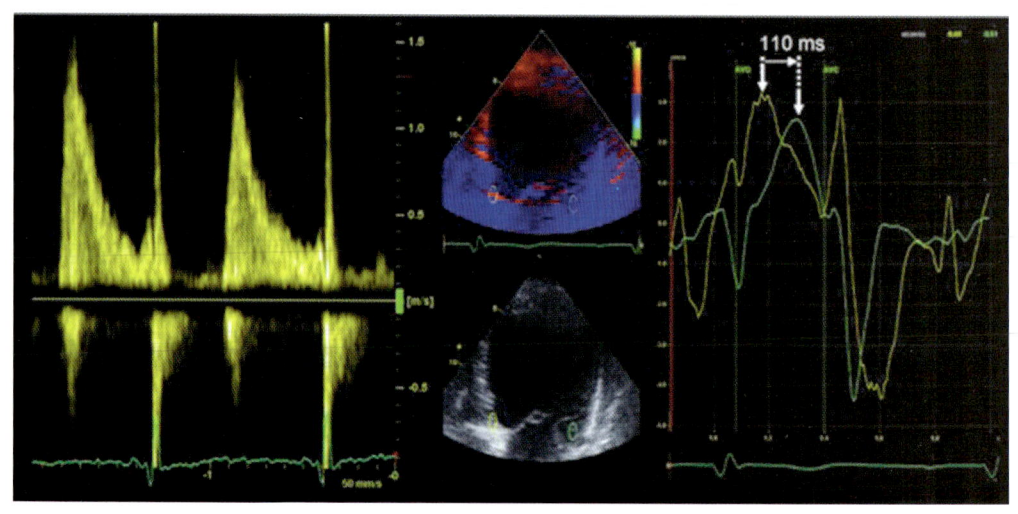

Figure 14.16

33. On color-coded TDI tracings, substantial diastolic LV dyssynchrony could also be observed (**Figure 14.17**).

The time delay between septal and lateral early diastolic peak velocities (E) was 98 ms. Which of the following statements about diastolic LV dyssynchrony is **CORRECT?**
   A. Diastolic LV dyssynchrony is uncommon in patients with heart failure.
   B. Diastolic LV dyssynchrony is strongly related to the QRS complex duration.
   C. After CRT, persistent diastolic LV dyssynchrony may explain the lack of clinical improvement despite systolic LV resynchronization.
   D. AV or VV delay optimizations do not affect diastolic LV dyssynchrony.

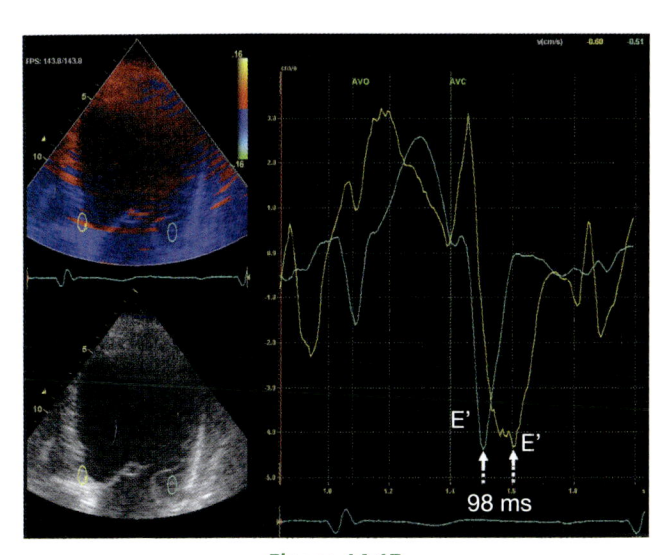

Figure 14.17

34. An AV delay optimization was performed (**Figure 14.18**).

Which of the following statements about AV delay optimization is **CORRECT?**
   A. AV delay optimization by the Ritter method requires continuous-wave Doppler recordings of the transmitral flow and the presence of mitral regurgitation to measure the dP/dt_{max}.
   B. The Ritter method is the most accurate method to optimize the AV delay and it is applicable in all patients, regardless of intrinsic AV conduction.
   C. The iterative method starts with a long AV delay and shortens by 20-ms decrements until the E and A waves are fused.
   D. The Ritter method calculates the optimal AV delay with the formula: AV short + ([AV long + QA long] − [AV short + QA short]). In this case, the optimal AV delay was 180 ms.

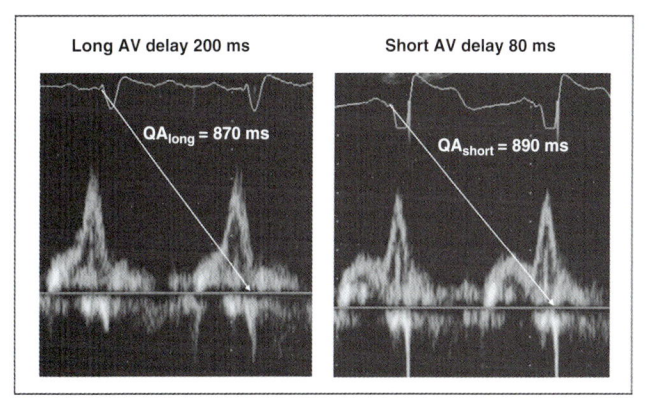

Figure 14.18

35. After AV delay optimization, the VV delay was optimized by measuring the velocity-time integral of the flow at the LV outflow tract (**Figure 14.19**). Which of the following statements about VV delay optimization is **CORRECT?**
   A. Optimization of the VV delay in this case is not necessary since changes in the AV delay may favorably affect interventricular and LV dyssynchrony.
   B. Preexcitation of the LV with a VV delay of −60 ms provides the highest cardiac output.
   C. Preexcitation of the RV, regardless of the VV delay programmed, usually yields the highest cardiac output.
   D. Changes in the angle of incidence between the outflow jet and the ultrasound beam do not affect the accuracy of the velocity-time integral measurement.

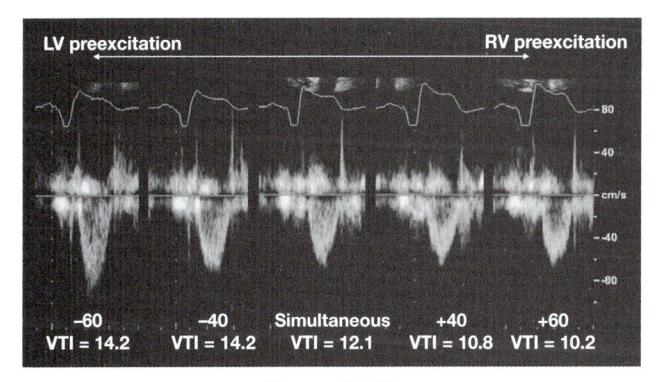

Figure 14.19

CASE 5

A CRT device was implanted in a 67-year-old woman with dilated cardiomyopathy, New York Heart Association heart failure functional class III, a LV ejection fraction of 30% (see ▶ **Video 14.2**), *and a QRS duration on the surface electrocardiogram of 120 ms.* **Figure 14.20** *shows the key information to evaluate cardiac dyssynchrony.*

Figure 14.20

36. Based on **Figure 14.20** in **Case 5**, which of the following statements about cardiac dyssynchrony is **CORRECT**?
    A. There is no AV, interventricular, or LV dyssynchrony.
    B. Only AV dyssynchrony is present, with a diastolic LVFT <40%.
    C. There is borderline LV dyssynchrony, as assessed with real-time 3D echocardiography, with the inferoposterior segments being most delayed.
    D. Pulsed-wave TDI does not indicate the presence of LV dyssynchrony because the ultrasound beam was not well aligned.

37. At 6-month follow-up, the patient in **Case 5** was in New York Heart Association functional class I and the LV ejection fraction improved to 38%. **Figure 14.21** illustrates the changes in cardiac dyssynchrony.
    In this particular case, which of the following statements about response to CRT is **CORRECT**?
    A. The patient showed improved LV synchronicity with a reduction in SDI, but the LV diastolic filling pattern was still impaired.
    B. LV dyssynchrony did not improve.
    C. The AV delay is too short and therefore the A wave is truncated.
    D. The improvement in LV ejection fraction may be secondary to improved AV and LV synchrony.

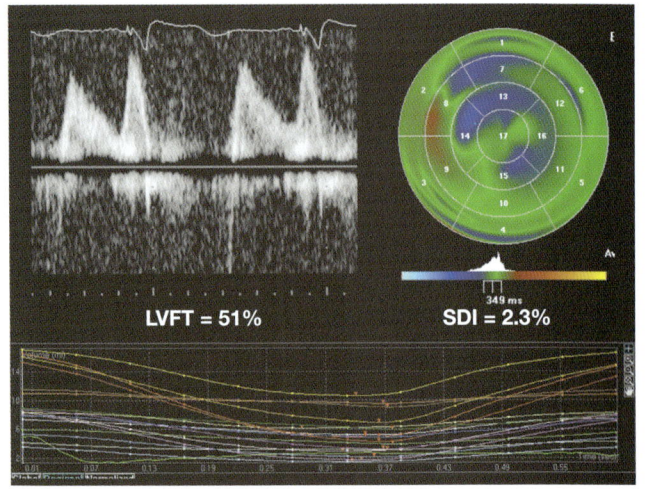

Figure 14.21

CASE 6

A 45-year-old patient with a dilated cardiomyopathy presents with New York Heart Association II dyspnea and an LV ejection fraction of 35%. Speckle tracking strain imaging was performed from the apical long-axis views.

38. A parametric map of LV global longitudinal strain is shown in **Figure 14.22** from the patient in **Case 6**. Which of the following statements is **CORRECT**?
    A. LV global longitudinal strain assessment demonstrates significant LV dyssynchrony.
    B. LV segmental strain analysis suggests that the underlying etiology is prior myocarditis.
    C. The global LV longitudinal strain is significantly impaired.
    D. LV global longitudinal strain <16% is a guideline-based indication for CRT.

Chapter 14 Dyssynchrony Evaluation/Atrioventricular Optimization / 311

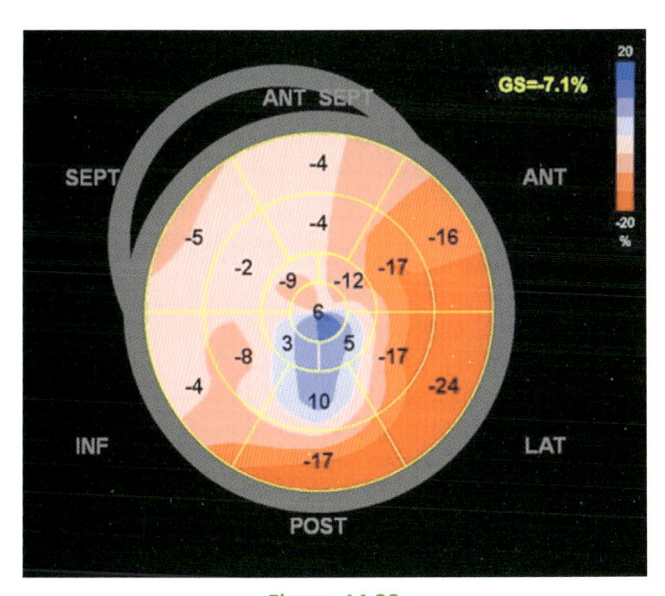

Figure 14.22

CASE 7

An 80-year-old patient presents to the outpatient clinic with New York Heart Association IV dyspnea and an LV ejection fraction of 20%. His 12-lead ECG demonstrates a broad left bundle branch block. Speckle tracking strain imaging was performed from the apical long-axis views, and noninvasive myocardial work derived from his brachial sphygmomanometric blood pressure and LV speckle tracking strain data.

39. A parametric map of noninvasive, LV myocardial work is shown in **Figure 14.23** of the patient in **Case 7**.
Which of the following statements is **CORRECT**?
A. Noninvasive speckle tracking strain, longitudinal strain-based LV myocardial work, reflects LV dyssynchrony in patients with a left bundle branch block.
B. LV noninvasive myocardial work values are more susceptible to afterload than LV global longitudinal strain.
C. Regional LV myocardial work distribution in this patient suggests that the underlying etiology of his LV systolic impairment is previous myocardial infarction.
D. Noninvasive myocardial work cannot predict CRT response.

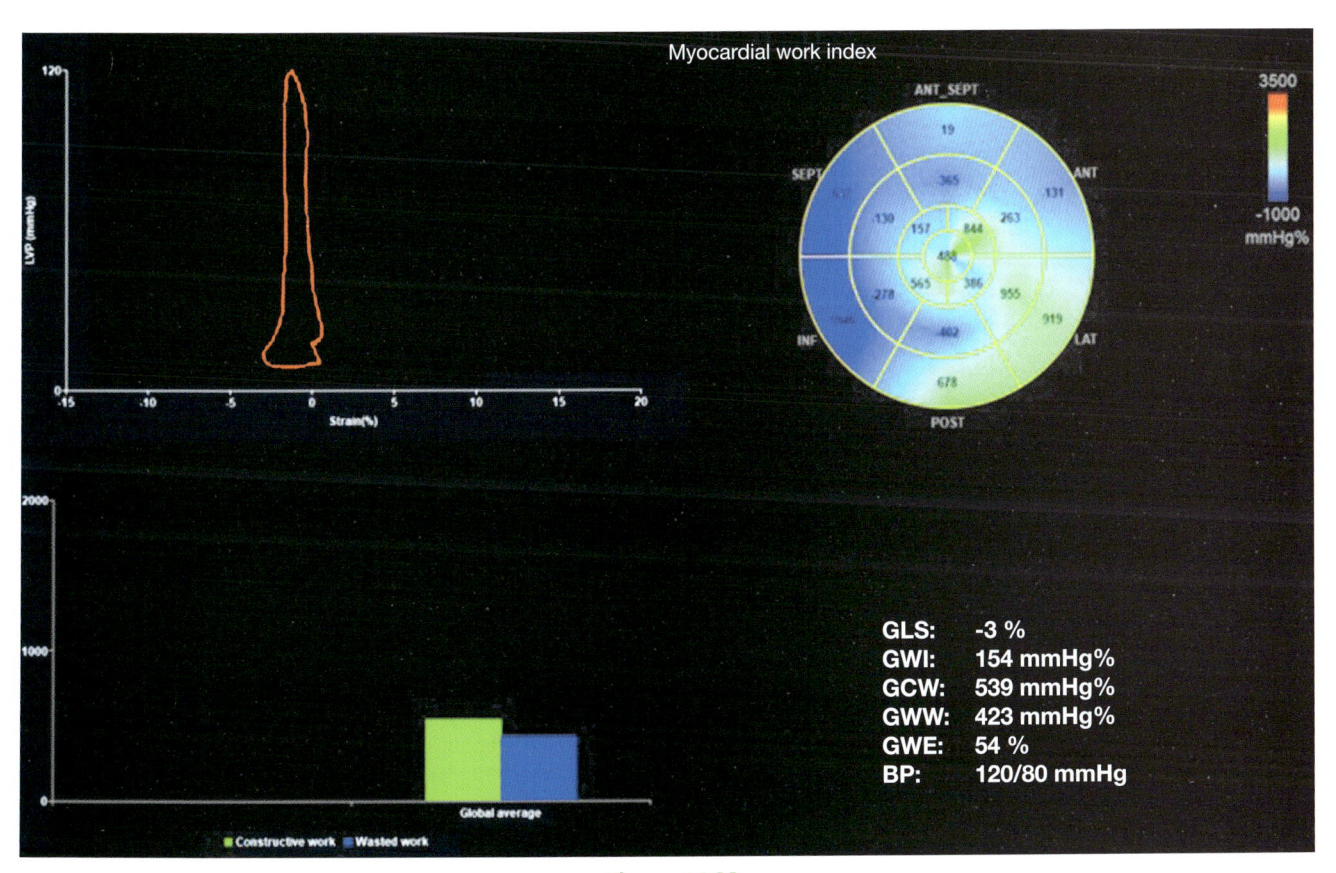

GLS: -3 %
GWI: 154 mmHg%
GCW: 539 mmHg%
GWW: 423 mmHg%
GWE: 54 %
BP: 120/80 mmHg

Figure 14.23

ANSWERS

1. **Answer: B.** Cardiac dyssynchrony can occur at three different levels: AV, interventricular, and LV dyssynchrony. Prolonged AV conduction (first-degree AV block) is commonly observed in patients with heart failure. On echocardiography, pulsed-wave Doppler recordings of the transmitral flow permit the evaluation of AV dyssynchrony and are defined by an LVFT (indexed to R-R interval) of ≤40% (**Figure 14.24A**). It is short due to the AV delay, allowing little filling time before the onset of LV contraction. Prolonged ventricular conduction, most commonly left bundle branch block, causes either interventricular dyssynchrony or LV dyssynchrony. Interventricular dyssynchrony is commonly assessed by measuring the time delay between the start of the QRS complex and the onset of RV and LV ejection, the so-called interventricular mechanical dyssynchrony (IVMD) index (**Figure 14.24B**). An interventricular mechanical index of ≥40 ms indicates substantial interventricular dyssynchrony and has been proposed as a predictive index of favorable response to CRT. Finally, LV dyssynchrony can be assessed with multiple and sophisticated echocardiographic techniques, and this parameter is most closely associated with response to CRT. On M-mode echocardiography, LV dyssynchrony is defined by a time delay between the systolic inward motion of the septum and the posterior wall ≥130 ms, the SPWMD index (**Figure 14.24C**).

2. **Answer: D.** Prolonged AV conduction is not uncommon in patients with heart failure, and in this situation, atrial contraction occurs relatively early in diastole, thereby shortening the effective LVFT. On pulsed-wave Doppler recordings of transmitral flow, fusion of the E and A waves is observed (**Figure 14.25**). In addition, following atrial contraction, the mitral valve remains open and late-diastolic mitral regurgitation may occur.

3. **Answer: B.** Interventricular dyssynchrony is usually quantified by using the IVMD index. This index is derived by calculating the time delay between the onset of the RV and LV ejection on pulsed-wave Doppler recordings of the pulmonic and aortic flows, respectively (**Figure 14.24B**). A cutoff value of ≥40 ms indicates substantial interventricular dyssynchrony and has been related to a favorable response to CRT. Interventricular dyssynchrony refers to the LV and is not reflected in the time delay between peak systolic thickening of the interventricular septum and the RV free wall. Closure of the tricuspid and mitral valves does not indicate the onset of RV and LV contraction. The time delay between peak systolic velocity of the interventricular septum and the LV lateral wall is a measure of intraventricular dyssynchrony, and not interventricular dyssynchrony.

4. **Answer: A.** M-mode echocardiography was one of the first techniques to assess LV dyssynchrony and to predict response to CRT. Applied to the midventricular short-axis view of the LV, M-mode recordings

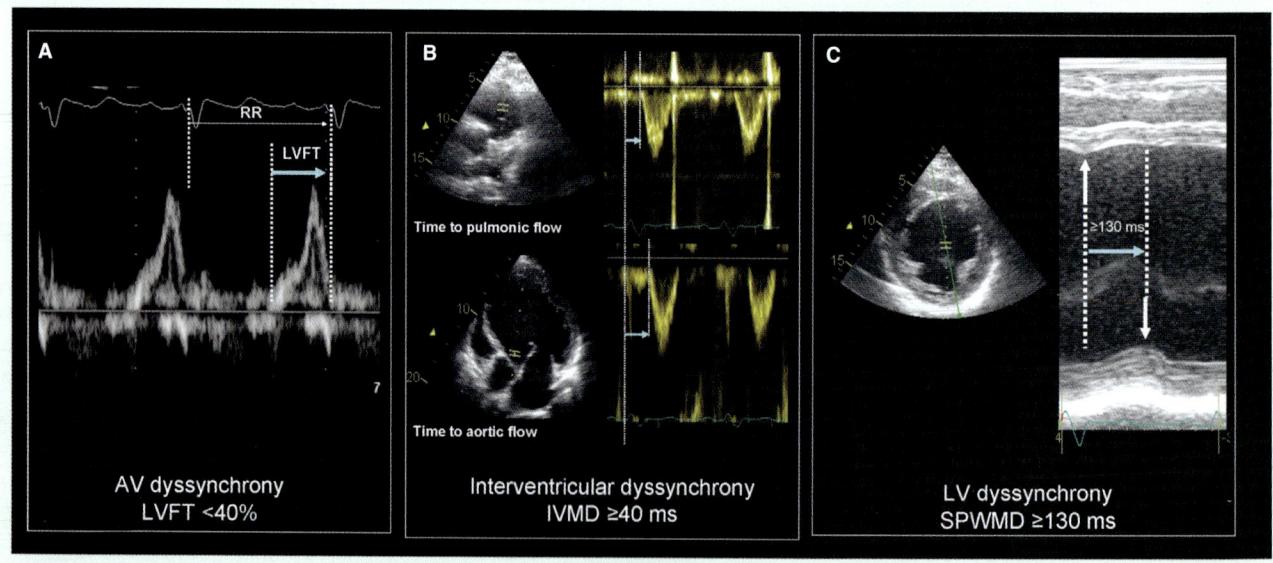

Figure 14.24. A: Example of atrioventricular (AV) dyssynchrony with a left ventricular (LV) filling time (LVFT) of <40% of the R-R interval. **B:** Assessment of interventricular dyssynchrony by measuring the time delay between the onset of the right and LV ejection on pulsed-wave Doppler recordings of the pulmonic and aortic flows. **C:** Assessment of LV dyssynchrony by one of the echocardiographic methods proposed, namely M-mode. The systolic septal inward motion occurs >130 ms earlier than posterior inward motion. IVMD, interventricular mechanical dyssynchrony; SPWMD, septal-to-posterior wall motion delay.

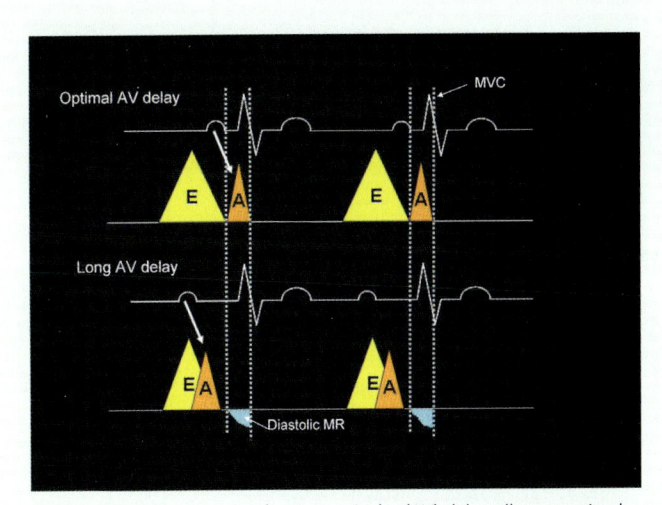

Figure 14.25. An optimal atrioventricular (AV) delay allows maximal atrial contribution to left ventricular (LV) filling and the mitral valve closes (mitral valve closure [MVC]) at the end of the A wave. However, a long AV delay results in relatively early atrial contraction, with subsequent fusion of the E and A waves and a shortening of LV diastolic filling. In addition, after atrial contraction, the mitral valve remains open and diastolic mitral regurgitation can occur. MR, mitral regurgitation.

display the motion of the septum and posterior wall through the cardiac cycle. The time delay between the inward motion of the septum and posterior wall yields the SPWMD index. A cutoff value of ≥130 ms indicates the presence of LV dyssynchrony and predicts response to CRT. The feasibility of M-mode to assess LV dyssynchrony, however, is limited in ischemic heart disease. A variety of echocardiographic techniques have been developed to quantify LV dyssynchrony and predict response to CRT. **Table 14.1** summarizes echocardiographic approaches to detect LV dyssynchrony and predict CRT response.

5. **Answer: D.** LV dyssynchrony has been extensively studied with TDI. Among several TDI modalities, assessment of LV longitudinal velocities is the principal method used in clinical practice. Pulsed-wave TDI and color-coded TDI are the main approaches to evaluate LV longitudinal velocities. Pulsed-wave TDI permits interrogation of only one region at a time and precludes simultaneous comparison of two opposite regions. This technical issue may reduce the accuracy of LV dyssynchrony assessment. In contrast, color-coded TDI permits the assessment of LV longitudinal velocities in multiple regions simultaneously. Myocardial velocities are obtained by postprocessing color-coded TDI data, and subsequently, LV dyssynchrony is evaluated by means of time delay to peak systolic velocity between two to four opposing regions or calculating the standard deviation of time-to-peak systolic velocity of six–12 LV segments. As with all Doppler-based techniques, TDI analysis is highly dependent on the angle of insonation of the ultrasound beam and therefore accurate LV dyssynchrony assessment requires proper alignment of the ultrasound beam with the direction of longitudinal motion.

6. **Answer: D.** To ensure proper analysis of LV dyssynchrony with TDI techniques, tissue Doppler data acquisition and postprocessing should follow these steps:
   - Acquire high frame rate color tissue Doppler (>90 frames per second).
   - Optimize gain and time gain control settings for myocardial definition.
   - Position the LV cavity in the center of the sector and align the Doppler ultrasound beam for optimal LV longitudinal motion assessment.
   - Have patients breath hold for 5 seconds while a three- to five-beat digital acquisition is performed.
   - Record standard apical two-, four-, and three-chamber views.
   - Measure the LV ejection interval from pulsed-wave Doppler recordings of the LV outflow tract, where the aortic valve opening and closure time can be identified.
   - Place the regions of interest (5 × 10 mm to 7 × 15 mm size) at the basal and midventricular segments of opposing LV walls to obtain time-velocity tracings.
   - Check the signal quality by identifying the components of the velocity curve: isovolumic contraction (<60 ms from the Q wave), the systolic wave (S), and the early (E) and late (A)-diastolic waves (**Figure 14.26**).
   - Adjust the regions of interest to obtain the most reproducible peak systolic velocity. Time from the onset of the QRS complex to the peak S wave should be measured for basal and midventricular segments of the three apical views (12 segments). Alternatively, the difference in time to the peak S wave from opposing walls can be used to quantify LV dyssynchrony.

7. **Answer: A.** Color-coded TDI is the technique most frequently used to evaluate LV dyssynchrony and to predict mid- and long-term prognosis after CRT. Several LV dyssynchrony parameters have been developed. The measurement of the time delay in peak systolic velocity between the basal septal and basal lateral segments of the apical four-chamber view is the simplest parameter to identify LV dyssynchrony. A cutoff value of ≥60 ms predicts a favorable echocardiographic response to CRT. In addition, LV dyssynchrony can be defined by the time delay between four opposing walls (basal segments of the anterior, inferior, septal, and lateral walls). A cutoff value of ≥65 ms predicts favorable clinical and echocardiographic response to CRT at midterm follow-up and improved long-term prognosis (**Table 14.1**). Finally, Yu et al. developed a LV dyssynchrony index that integrates information from the three apical views (two-chamber, four-chamber, and long-axis views). This index is derived by calculating the standard deviation of time-to-peak systolic velocity of 12 segments (basal and midventricular segments). A cutoff value of ≥31.4 ms predicts a favorable

Table 14.1. LV Dyssynchrony Assessment With Echocardiography

Measurement	Echocardiographic Technique	LV Dyssynchrony Threshold Value and Outcomes
Septal-to-posterior wall motion delay	M-mode	A value of ≥130 ms predicted response to CRT with a sensitivity and specificity of 100% and 63%, respectively.[a] Subsequent studies have demonstrated this measurement to be less feasible and accurate, particularly in patients with ischemic heart failure.
Sum of LV and VV dyssynchrony (pulsed-wave systolic velocities)	Pulsed-wave TDI	A value of >102 ms predicted response to CRT with a sensitivity and specificity of 96% and 77%, respectively.[b]
Delay in peak systolic velocities (four segments: basal septum, lateral, anterior, and inferior walls)	Color-coded TDI	A value of ≥65 ms predicted response to CRT with both a sensitivity and specificity of 92%.[c]
Standard deviation of time-to-peak systolic velocities (12 LV segments)	Color-coded TDI	A value of ≥31.4 ms predicted response to CRT with a sensitivity and specificity of 87% and 81%, respectively.[d]
Delay in peak radial strain (anteroseptal to posterior wall)	2D radial strain speckle tracking	A value of ≥130 ms predicted the response to CRT (≥15% reduction in LVESV) with a sensitivity and specificity of 83% and 80%, respectively.[e]
Strain delay index (sum of wasted energy calculated as the difference between end-systolic and peak longitudinal strain for 16 segments)	2D longitudinal speckle tracking	A cutoff value of ≥25% predicted response to CRT with a sensitivity and specificity of 82% and 92%, respectively.[f]
Systolic dyssynchrony index (standard deviation of time to minimum volume of 16 subvolumes)	Real-time 3D echocardiography	A value of >10.4% predicted response to CRT (≥15% reduction in LVESV) with a sensitivity and specificity of 90% and 67%, respectively.[g]
Systolic dyssynchrony index (standard deviation of time to minimum volume of 16 subvolumes)	Real-time 3D echocardiography	A value of >9.8% yielded a sensitivity of 93%, with a specificity of 75% to predict CRT response.[h]
Global myocardial constructive work	2D longitudinal speckle tracking	A value of <1057 mm Hg% demonstrated a positive predictive value of 88% and a negative predictive value of 51% for CRT nonresponse (≤15% reduction in LVESV).[i]

2D, two-dimensional; 3D, three-dimensional; CRT, cardiac resynchronization therapy; LV, left ventricular; LVESV, left ventricular end-systolic volume; TDI, tissue Doppler imaging; VV, interventricular.
[a]Pitzalis MV, et al. *J Am Coll Cardiol.* 2002;40:1615-1622.
[b]Penicka M, et al. *Circulation.* 2004;109:978-983.
[c]Bax JJ, et al. *J Am Coll Cardiol.* 2004;44:1834-1840.
[d]Yu CM, et al. *Am J Cardiol.* 2003;91:684-688.
[e]Delgado V, et al. *J Am Coll Cardiol.* 2008;51:1944-1952.
[f]Lim P, et al. *Circulation.* 2008;118:1130-1137.
[g]Kapetanakis S, et al. *JACC Cardiovasc Imaging.* 2011;4:16-26.
[h]Kleijn SA, et al. *Eur Heart J Cardiovasc Imaging.* 2012;13:763-775.
[i]Galli E, et al. *Eur Heart J Cardiovasc Imaging.* 2018;19:1010-1018.

response to CRT with a sensitivity and specificity of 87% and 81%, respectively (**Table 14.1**).

8. Answer: C. Strain and strain rate imaging evaluates myocardial deformation and permits distinction of myocardial segments with active contraction from segments that are passively tethered (scar segments). From TDI data, strain and strain rate–time curves can be obtained. As with all Doppler techniques, TDI-derived strain and strain rate measurements are highly dependent on the insonation angle of the ultrasound beam. On apical LV views, only longitudinal strain or strain rate can be measured, whereas from short-axis views, radial strain and strain rate can be measured at the (antero)

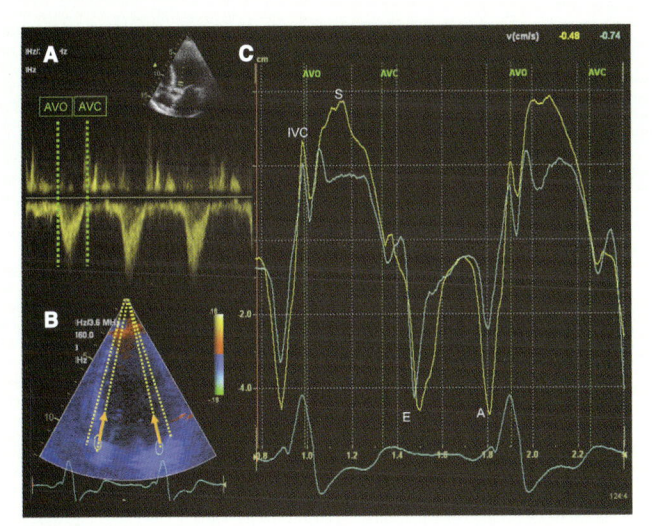

Figure 14.26. A-C: Left ventricular (LV) dyssynchrony assessment with color-coded tissue Doppler imaging (TDI). The LV ejection interval should be defined first (Panel A). TDI data acquisition requires proper alignment of the ultrasound beam along the direction of LV motion (Panel B). Postprocessing of TDI data provides velocity-time curves of two opposing LV walls. The components of the velocity-time curves should be identified (Panel C): isovolumic contraction (IVC), the systolic velocity (S), and early (E) and late (A)-diastolic velocities. Finally, the time delay between peak systolic velocities (S waves) can be measured to assess LV dyssynchrony.

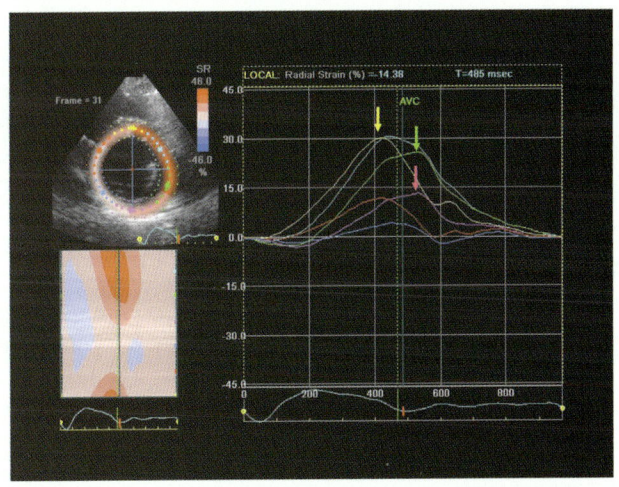

Figure 14.27. Left ventricular (LV) dyssynchrony assessed with two-dimensional (2D) speckle tracking analysis. From the midventricular LV parasternal short-axis view, time–radial strain tracings of six LV segments are obtained. A time delay of ≥130 ms between peak radial strain of the anteroseptal (*yellow arrow*) and the posterior (*pink arrow*) segments defines the presence of substantial LV dyssynchrony. In addition, the latest activated segments can be identified (*pink and green arrows*), indicating where the LV pacing lead should preferably be placed.

septal and posterior walls and circumferential strain and strain rate can be measured at the (infero)septal and lateral walls. Several studies have evaluated the role of strain and strain rate imaging to define LV dyssynchrony and in the prediction of CRT response. LV dyssynchrony can be evaluated with either longitudinal or radial strain and strain rate by measuring the time delay between the peak strain of two opposing walls. A time delay of ≥130 ms between the (antero)septal and the posterior walls measured on radial strain–time curves is predictive of acute improvement in stroke volume after CRT, while longitudinal strain does not predict LV reverse remodeling after CRT.

9. **Answer: B.** 2D speckle tracking echocardiography permits angle-independent myocardial strain and strain rate assessment in three orthogonal directions (radial, circumferential, and longitudinal) and in all LV segments. Strain analysis, based on this modality, also enables the differentiation of myocardial segments with active contraction from segments that are passively tethered by the adjacent segments. From radial strain–time curves, a time delay between peak strain of the anteroseptal and posterior walls of ≥130 ms predicts LV reverse remodeling after CRT (**Figure 14.27**). In addition, strain analysis based on 2D speckle tracking echocardiography permits the detection of the latest activated segment. This has important clinical implications since positioning the LV pacing lead at the latest activated site provides a high likelihood of favorable response to CRT and superior clinical outcome.

10. **Answer: D.** 3D echocardiography allows for the assessment of LV dyssynchrony in all LV segments in a single cardiac cycle. 3D echocardiographic analysis of LV dyssynchrony can be performed by direct volumetric analysis (real-time 3D echocardiography) or by triplane TSI analysis. With real-time 3D echocardiography, a LV full volume is obtained and divided into 17 subvolumes. LV dyssynchrony is calculated as the standard deviation of time-to-minimum regional systolic volume for 16 segments, the so-called SDI. A threshold of >9.8% predicts LV reverse remodeling after CRT. Triplane TSI automatically calculates time-to-peak systolic velocity in the basal and midventricular segments of the septal, lateral, inferior, anterior, posterior, and anteroseptal walls. This method selects a specific interval of the cardiac cycle to calculate time delays (only in the LV ejection interval) and excludes the early isovolumic contraction as well as late, postsystolic shortening. A color-coded overlay is added onto 2D images to visually identify regional mechanical delays. The earliest activated areas are coded in shades of green, whereas the latest activated areas are coded in shades of red. Time-to-peak systolic velocities are displayed in a 12-segment polar map and LV dyssynchrony is defined by the septum and lateral walls and the standard deviation of 12 segments. A standard deviation of time-to-peak systolic velocity of 12 segments ≥33 ms has been shown to predict a favorable clinical and echocardiographic response to CRT at midterm follow-up.

316 / Clinical Echocardiography Review

11. **Answer: A.** The optimal AV delay is defined by the shortest AV interval which does not compromise left atrial contribution to LV filling. On pulsed-wave Doppler recordings of transmitral flow, the end of the A wave should coincide with the onset of the rise in LV pressure. The optimal AV delay settings provide complete late-diastolic filling by atrial contraction and the maximum diastolic LVFT, which results in the largest LV stroke volume.

12. **Answer: D.** When the AV delay is programmed too short, LV contraction occurs relatively early and the mitral valve closes prematurely, compromising left atrial contribution to LV filling. On pulsed-wave Doppler recordings of transmitral flow, a truncated A wave is observed together with a relatively early E wave. As a consequence, LVFT lengthens, with widely separated E and A waves (**Figure 14.28**).

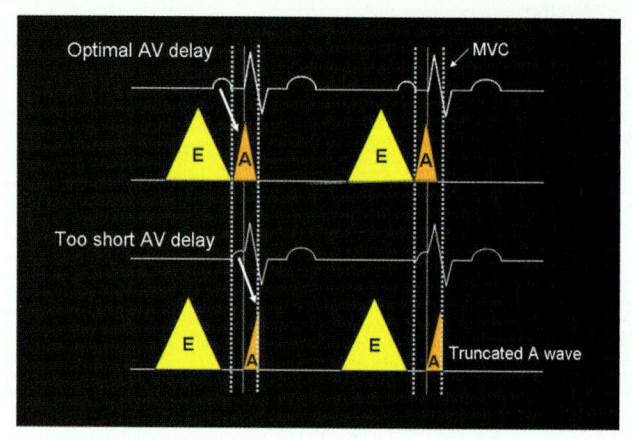

Figure 14.28. Too short atrioventricular (AV) delay compromises the left atrial contribution to left ventricular (LV) filling. Left atrial contraction is interrupted by early LV contraction. On transmitral, pulsed-wave Doppler recordings, the A wave is truncated and LV filling time increases, with widely separated E and A waves. MVC, mitral valve closure.

13. **Answer: D.** The echocardiographic methods used to optimize the AV delay aim to improve either diastolic LVFT or hemodynamic markers of LV systolic function. Diastolic LVFT is usually evaluated using pulsed-wave Doppler recordings of transmitral flow. LV hemodynamics are usually evaluated using the following: (1) continuous-wave or pulsed-wave Doppler recordings of the LV outflow tract, measuring the velocity-time integral of the flow and calculating the cardiac output, or (2) continuous-wave Doppler recordings of the mitral regurgitation spectral trace, measuring the rate of change of LV pressure during isovolumic contraction (dP/dt_{max}).

14. **Answer: B.** Echocardiographic AV optimization techniques aiming to improve LV diastolic filling include the iterative method, the Ritter method, the mitral inflow velocity–time integral method, and the simplified (Meluzin) mitral inflow method. Echocardiographic AV optimization methods aiming to improve LV hemodynamics include the assessment of aortic valve or LV outflow tract velocity–time integral, dP/dt_{max}, and myocardial performance index. **Figure 14.29** summarizes and illustrates these methods.

15. **Answer: A.** The most common echocardiographic methods to optimize the VV delay include the measurement of velocity-time integral on pulsed-wave Doppler recordings of the LV outflow tract and the evaluation of LV dyssynchrony on color-coded TDI data by measuring septal-to-lateral peak systolic velocity–time delay.

16. **Answer: C.** Prolonged AV conduction causes relatively late ventricular contraction. The early diastolic filling (E wave) occurs late in diastole, and on pulsed-wave Doppler recordings of the transmitral flow, the E and A waves appear fused (superimposition of atrial contraction on the early diastolic LV filling phase). Subsequently, diastolic LVFT is reduced. In addition, after left atrial contraction, the mitral valve remains open and diastolic mitral regurgitation can be observed (see **Figure 14.1**, red arrow).

17. **Answer: D.** Interventricular and LV dyssynchrony can be assessed with pulsed-wave TDI. Interventricular dyssynchrony is measured as the peak systolic velocity–time delay between the basal segment of the RV free wall and the most delayed basal LV segment. LV dyssynchrony is calculated as the peak systolic velocity–time delay between two, four, or six basal LV segments. The combination of both interventricular and LV dyssynchrony predicts a favorable response to CRT with high sensitivity and specificity (**Table 14.1**). In this case, the sum of both delays is 115 ms and therefore the likelihood of a favorable response to CRT is high.

18. **Answer: C.** Color-coded TDI is one of the most commonly used echocardiographic techniques to evaluate LV dyssynchrony. The time delay between two (septal-to-lateral) or four opposing walls (anterior, inferior, septal, and lateral) as well as the standard deviation of the time-to-peak systolic velocity of 12 segments defines LV dyssynchrony and predicts a favorable response to CRT (**Table 14.1**). In this case, a septal-to-lateral wall delay of 90 ms (≥65 ms) is present, which has been associated with LV reverse remodeling.

19. **Answer: B.** In this example, there is substantial LV dyssynchrony as assessed with TDI-derived longitudinal strain: the lateral wall stretches, whereas the septal wall shortens. Peak shortening of the lateral wall occurs after aortic valve closure. TDI-derived strain imaging is a valuable technique to evaluate patients with heart failure who are candidates for CRT since it provides information not only on LV dyssynchrony but also on active myocardial contraction. TDI-derived strain imaging permits

Echocardiographic optimization method		Technique
Optimization of LV diastolic filling		
	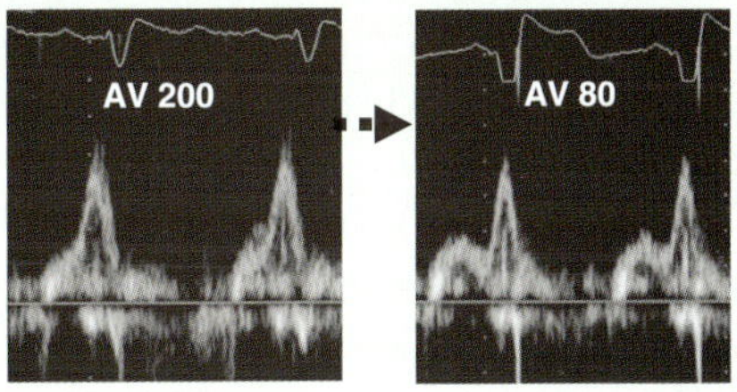 Iterative method	- Pulsed wave Doppler recordings of the transmitral flow. - A long AV delay is programmed and then it is shortened by 20 ms increments until truncation of the A wave. Then, the optimal AV delay is identified by lengthening the AV delay until the A wave is no longer truncated.

	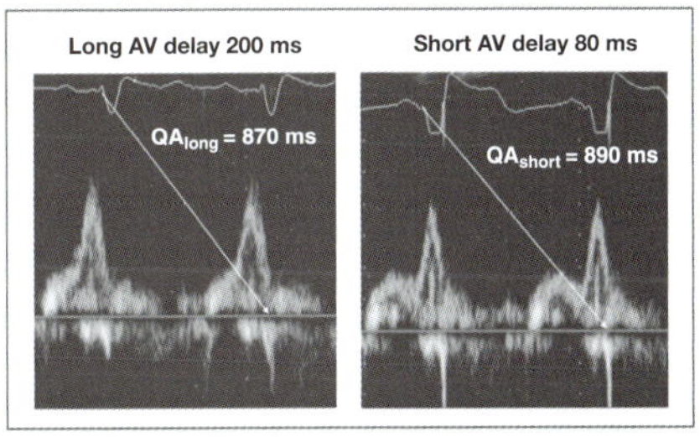 Ritter method	- Pulsed wave Doppler recordings of the transmitral flow.
		- Two extreme AV delays are programmed:
		  - Long AV delay without A wave attenuation (AV_{long})
		  - Short AV delay with truncation of A wave (AV_{short})
		- For each AV delay, the time between QRS onset and completion of the A wave is measured (QA_{long} and QA_{short}).
		- Optimal AV delay is calculated using the formula:
		$AV_{opt} = AV_{short} + [(AV_{long} + QA_{long}) - (AV_{short} + QA_{short})]$
		- Limitation: high heart rates, intrinsic AV conduction <150 ms.

	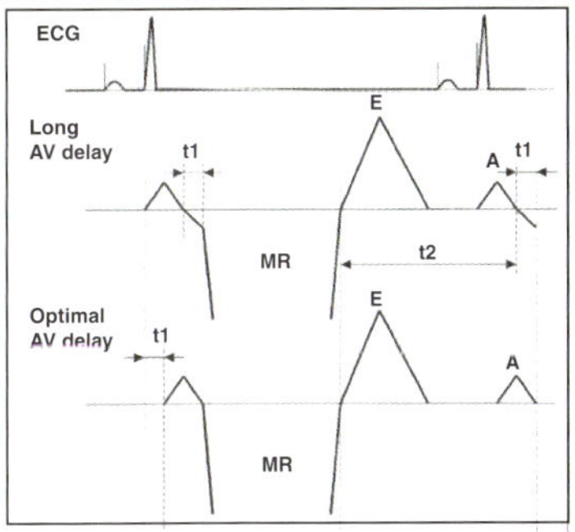 Simplified mitral inflow method	- Pulsed wave Doppler recordings of the transmitral flow for 5-10 s. - A long AV delay is defined as the maximum AV delay allowing full ventricular capture (lowered by 5-10 ms). - The time between the end of the A wave and the onset of mitral regurgitation spectral signal is measured (t1). - The optimal AV delay is calculated by subtracting t1 from the long AV delay and t1. - Limitation: detectable mitral regurgitation is needed.
Optimization of LV hemodynamics		
	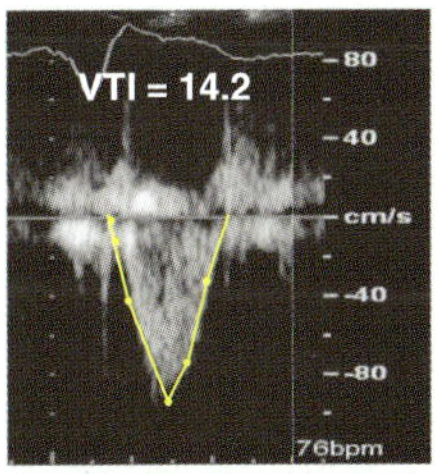 Aortic valve/LV outflow tract velocity—time integral	- Continuous-or pulsed-wave Doppler recordings of the aortic valve or LV outflow tract flow, respectively. - The product of LV outflow tract area and its velocity time integral yields stroke volume. - The optimal AV delay provides the optimal LV filling and the optimal stroke volume.
	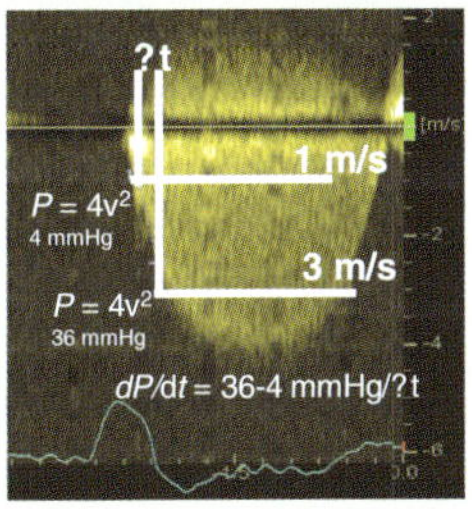 dP/dt_{max}	- The peak rate of rise of LV pressure during isovolumic contraction, or dP/dt_{max}, can be noninvasively assessed on mitral regurgitation continuous-wave Doppler recordings. - The time difference between two points on the continuous wave mitral regurgitation spectral signal (corresponding to 1 and 3 m/s) is measured. - The pressure gradient is calculated according to Bernoulli equation. - Limitation: detectable mitral regurgitation is needed.

Figure 14.29

differentiation of myocardial segments with active deformation or contraction (viable segments) from those segments with a substantial amount of scar tissue that are usually tethered by the adjacent segments. Previous studies have demonstrated the importance of assessing the extent and location of scar tissue before CRT implantation. Thus, when the LV pacing lead is placed in a region with transmural scar or when the LV content of scar tissue is excessive, the likelihood of a favorable response to CRT is reduced. In this example, the LV lateral wall shows active contraction, although delayed when compared to the septal wall.

20. **Answer: B.** From midventricular short-axis images of the LV, radial or circumferential strain can be assessed. Although TDI-derived strain is highly dependent on the ultrasound angle of incidence, radial strain can be assessed at the (antero)septal and posterior walls. With radial strain, myocardial thickening is expressed as positive values. Circumferential strain can be assessed only at the lateral and inferior (septal) walls and evaluates myocardial shortening along the curvature of the LV. Circumferential shortening is expressed as negative values. In this example, LV dyssynchrony is evaluated with TDI-derived radial strain and demonstrates the presence of substantial LV dyssynchrony with a peak radial strain–time delay between the septum and the posterior wall of ≥130 ms.

21. **Answer: B.** Strain imaging based on speckle tracking echocardiography has emerged as a powerful technique to evaluate patients with heart failure with reduced ejection fraction who are candidates for CRT. This imaging technique enables almost angle-independent, multidirectional LV strain and strain rate assessment. LV dyssynchrony can be assessed with radial strain speckle tracking analysis. In addition, the latest activated segment can be identified, which has important implications for CRT response. In patients with an LV pacing lead placed at the latest activated area, a higher CRT response rate and superior long-term outcome have been demonstrated. Viable LV segments, showing active contraction, may be identified and differentiated from scarred segments that are passively tethered.

22. **Answer: D.** The assessment of LV dyssynchrony can be performed with triplane TSI. First, the apical two-, four-, and three-chamber views of the LV are simultaneously acquired. Color-coded TSI is applied to the triplane view in order to assess myocardial longitudinal velocities. The time from onset of the QRS complex to peak systolic velocity in every segment of the LV is calculated automatically and LV dyssynchrony is expressed as time delays between the septum and the lateral wall, as well as the standard deviation of 12 segments. In addition, the TSI algorithm color codes the time delays ranging from the green (earliest activated) to yellow-orange to red (latest activated) within systole. The electromechanical activation times are presented as a polar map, allowing for the identification of the earliest and latest activated segments. **Figure 14.7** illustrates an example of a patient with substantial LV dyssynchrony, as indicated by a standard deviation of 54 ms, with the posterobasal segment being activated last.

Triplane TSI relies on myocardial velocity Doppler imaging and is highly dependent on ultrasound beam angle. It also has to be kept in mind that active contraction cannot be distinguished from passive tethering.

23. **Answer: A.** LV dyssynchrony analysis based on real-time 3D echocardiography is performed by calculating the SDI: standard deviation of time-to-minimum regional volume of 16 subvolumes in which the LV is divided. This time dispersion can be also displayed graphically in a color-coded polar map illustrating the most delayed areas. After CRT, the LV synchrony improves and the SDI decreases, as seen in **Figure 14.8B**. Consequently, the polar map shows homogeneous mechanical activation. Real-time 3D echocardiography evaluates the excursion or displacement of the 16 LV subvolumes but does not provide information on segmental active contraction, and therefore its accuracy may be limited in patients with ischemic heart failure.

24. **Answer: B.** The iterative method is one of the most commonly used echocardiographic methods to optimize the AV delay. With pulsed-wave Doppler recordings of the transmitral flow, the LVFT is evaluated at different AV delays. Starting with a long AV delay, the AV delay is shortened by 20 ms decrements until the A wave is truncated. Thereafter, the AV delay is lengthened by 10 ms increments until truncation of the A wave is no longer observed. Therefore, the shortest AV delay without truncation of the A wave is set as the optimal AV delay for LV filling. In **Figure 14.9**, an AV delay of 80 ms is associated with clear truncation of the A wave (red arrow indicates the onset of the LV ejection period). An AV delay of 120 ms shows the greatest LVFT without truncation of the A wave.

25. **Answer: C.** Echocardiographic optimization of the VV delay is usually performed by measuring the velocity-time integral on pulsed-wave Doppler recordings at the LV outflow tract or by TDI techniques evaluating the amount of LV dyssynchrony. Optimal VV delay aims to decrease LV dyssynchrony and improve LV hemodynamics. The role of VV delay optimization remains controversial. Two multicenter randomized trials (DECREASE-HF and RHYTHM II ICD) did not demonstrate any benefit, whereas the INSYNC III trial and other multiple single-center studies demonstrated slight but significant improvement in clinical status and stroke volume after VV optimization. The range of optimal VV delay is narrow but usually involves LV preexcitation by 20 to 40 ms. RV preexcitation may induce impairment in LV function and should be reserved for patients with

LV dyssynchrony in the septal and inferior walls. At follow-up, optimization of AV and VV delays may be necessary secondary to the effects of CRT on LV reverse remodeling and systolic function.

26. **Answer: D.** Cardiac dyssynchrony evaluation includes assessment of the following:
    - LVFT: On pulsed-wave Doppler recordings of the transmitral flow
    - Interventricular dyssynchrony: By calculating the time delay between the onset of RV and LV ejection on the pulsed-wave Doppler recordings of the LV outflow tract and the pulmonary flow
    - LV dyssynchrony: Preferably by TDI

    In the present case, there is substantial cardiac dyssynchrony at all three levels, indicated by a reduced LVFT (<40%), delayed LV ejection onset when compared to RV ejection onset (>40 ms), and significant time delay between the septal and the lateral wall (>60 ms).

27. **Answer: B.** Functional mitral regurgitation is commonly observed in patients with advanced heart failure. Dilated cardiomyopathy and ischemic heart disease manifest adverse remodeling, leading to dilatation of the LV cavity, displacement of the papillary muscles, dilatation of the mitral annulus, and malcoaptation of the mitral leaflets. In addition, ventricular conduction disturbances may have a detrimental effect on mitral regurgitation. Dyssynchronous mechanical activation of the LV segments underlying the papillary muscles can increase mitral regurgitation severity. The value of 2D speckle tracking echocardiography to evaluate the effect of LV dyssynchrony on mitral regurgitation has been demonstrated. The evaluation of mechanical activation with 2D speckle tracking echocardiography at the midventricular level provides invaluable information on mitral regurgitation pathophysiology. By resynchronizing the LV segments underlying the papillary muscles, mitral regurgitation can be significantly reduced.

    Figure 14.12A,B and ▶ **Video 14.1A,B** show an example of a patient with dilated cardiomyopathy and severe functional mitral regurgitation. 2D speckle tracking analysis was applied to midventricular short-axis images of the LV where the segments underlying the papillary muscles were visible. A substantial time delay between peak radial strain of the segment underlying the anterolateral (earliest) and the posteromedial (latest) papillary muscles was observed.

    ▶ **Video 14.1B** shows the mechanical activation pattern in the corresponding LV short-axis view. The region of interest includes the entire myocardial wall and tracks the movement of the speckles (natural acoustic markers) within the myocardium during the cardiac cycle. Myocardial thickening is coded in red, whereas myocardial thinning is coded in blue. The segment underlying the anterolateral papillary muscle reaches peak radial strain earlier than the segment underlying the posteromedial papillary muscle.

> **KEY POINTS**
> Echocardiographic evaluation of patients with heart failure who are candidates for CRT include the following:
> - LV dimensions and function
> - Cardiac dyssynchrony
> - AV dyssynchrony: LVFT < 40%
> - Interventricular dyssynchrony: Interventricular mechanical delay of >40 ms
> - LV dyssynchrony (latest activated segment): Different threshold values according to the echocardiographic method used
> - Mitral regurgitation severity (and presence of mechanical dyssynchrony in the LV segments underlying the papillary muscles)

28. **Answer: C. Figure 14.13** illustrates a restrictive LV filling pattern with an E/A ratio of >2 and E wave deceleration time of <160 ms. In addition, the A wave is truncated, indicating that the AV delay has been programmed too short.

29. **Answer: C.** In this case, the AV delay should be optimized. The iterative method or the Ritter method may be suitable echocardiographic methods to set the optimal AV delay. In particular, the Ritter method was derived from dual-chamber pacing studies.

> **KEY POINTS**
> Dual-chamber pacemakers may induce AV dyssynchrony, interventricular dyssynchrony, and LV dyssynchrony. In patients with pacemakers who experience their first episode of heart failure, cardiac dyssynchrony should be evaluated:
> - AV dyssynchrony: If present, the AV delay should be optimized. Echocardiographic methods to optimize AV delay include:
>   - Iterative method: A long AV delay is programmed and afterward the AV interval is shortened by 20 ms decrements until the A wave is truncated. Then, the AV delay is lengthened by 10 ms increments until truncation of the A wave is no longer observed.
>   - Ritter method: A long and a short AV delay are programmed. Time from QRS onset until the completion of the A wave (QA) is measured for each AV delay. By applying the formula: AV short + ([AV long + QA long] − [AV short + QA short]), the optimal AV delay is obtained.
> - Interventricular and LV dyssynchrony: Upgrade to biventricular pacing or conduction system pacing may be an option.

30. **Answer: B.** In patients with ischemic heart failure who are candidates for CRT, the accuracy of M-mode echocardiography to evaluate LV dyssynchrony is limited, as demonstrated in several studies. In these patients, echocardiographic techniques based on strain imaging to evaluate LV dyssynchrony may be of interest since they allow identification of those segments with active contraction. In particular, 2D speckle tracking echocardiography is a powerful technique to evaluate LV dyssynchrony in multiple segments and in the three orthogonal directions of LV deformation.

31. **Answer: A.** LV dyssynchrony assessment with radial strain 2D speckle tracking echocardiography is usually performed at the midventricular short-axis level. The region of interest is placed at an end-systolic frame and includes the entire myocardial wall. After checking for adequate tracking quality, radial strain–time curves are displayed for six LV segments (septal, anteroseptal, anterior, lateral, posterior, and inferior) and the earliest and latest activated segments can be identified. LV dyssynchrony is one of the most important determinants of CRT response. In addition, LV lead position (at the latest activated segment) and the extent and location of myocardial scar are also important determinants of CRT response. 2D speckle tracking echocardiography may be a suitable technique to guide LV lead position.

> **KEY POINTS**
> - In patients with ischemic heart failure who are candidates for CRT, LV dyssynchrony and latest activated segments as well as location and extent of myocardial scar are important determinants of CRT response.
> - 2D speckle tracking echocardiography may provide a comprehensive evaluation of all these parameters.

32. **Answer: C.** After CRT implantation, a lack of improvement in clinical status or echocardiographic parameters (LV systolic function and LV reverse remodeling) may indicate unoptimized device settings, such as AV and VV delay. Too short AV delay compromises the atrial contribution to LV filling. LV contraction occurs prematurely and the left atrium contracts against a closed mitral valve. On transmitral pulsed-wave Doppler recordings, this phenomenon is identified by truncation of the A wave. In addition, substantial LV dyssynchrony may remain, and VV delay optimization may provide a more synchronous LV activation, leading to an improved LV stroke volume.

33. **Answer: C.** Diastolic LV dyssynchrony is frequently observed in patients with heart failure. Studies have demonstrated that the incidence of diastolic LV dyssynchrony may be as high as systolic LV dyssynchrony (58%-69% vs 47%-73%, respectively). Similar to systolic LV dyssynchrony, diastolic LV dyssynchrony is weakly related to QRS complex duration on the surface electrocardiogram. Systolic dyssynchrony is one of the pathophysiologic mechanisms proposed to account for diastolic dyssynchrony: LV segments showing delayed contraction also show delayed relaxation. However, the severity of LV diastolic dysfunction has been shown to be strongly related to the presence of LV diastolic dyssynchrony. Finally, diastolic LV dyssynchrony can be improved by CRT, although to a lesser extent than systolic LV dyssynchrony. An optimal AV and VV delay may play a role in improving diastolic LV dyssynchrony by improving LV diastolic filling and systolic LV dyssynchrony. In this clinical example, after 6 months of CRT, the patient showed pronounced AV dyssynchrony on pulsed-wave Doppler recordings of the transmitral flow and systolic and diastolic LV dyssynchrony on color-coded TDI. All these parameters reflect a lack of resynchronization, which manifested as suboptimal clinical and echocardiographic improvement after CRT.

34. **Answer: D.** The Ritter method is one of the most commonly used methods to optimize the AV delay. Two extreme AV delays are programmed, and the time interval between the onset of the QRS and the completion of the A wave on transmitral pulsed-wave Doppler recordings is calculated for each AV delay. The clinical use of this method may be limited in patients with high heart rates or with an intrinsic AV interval <150 ms.

35. **Answer: B.** The combination of velocity-time integral, measured at the pulsed-wave Doppler recording at the LV outflow tract, and LV dyssynchrony assessment with color-coded TDI, may constitute a valuable approach to optimize the VV delay. Preexcitation of the LV (−20 to −60 ms) usually yields the highest stroke volume and reduces LV dyssynchrony.

> **KEY POINTS**
> - In patients with heart failure and reduced ejection fraction treated with CRT who do not show improvement in clinical status or echocardiographic parameters, persistent AV, systolic, and diastolic LV dyssynchrony must be evaluated. If the latter is present, CRT device settings should be checked, including the AV and VV delays.
> - Too short an AV delay can be identified on a transmitral pulsed-wave Doppler recording by truncation of the A wave.
> - Too long an AV delay can be identified by a short LVFT with fusion of the E and A waves.
> - The presence of LV dyssynchrony can be reduced by optimizing the VV delay.

36. **Answer: C.** Cardiac dyssynchrony can exist in the presence of heart failure with reduced ejection fraction and a narrow QRS complex. This example illustrates the presence of AV dyssynchrony and substantial LV dyssynchrony, as assessed with real-time 3D echocardiography. The left panel illustrates the pulsed-wave Doppler recording of the transmitral flow and indicates the presence of AV dyssynchrony with a reduced LVFT (<40% of the R-R interval). The middle panel shows the pulsed-wave TDI tracings of the basal segments of the RV free wall and the septal and lateral segments of the LV. Time from the onset of the QRS complex to peak systolic velocity is calculated in each region. Interventricular dyssynchrony is measured as the peak systolic velocity–time delay between the basal segment of the RV free wall and the most delayed basal LV segment. Dyssynchrony is calculated as the time difference between peak systolic velocity of the septum and the lateral wall. In this patient, borderline interventricular dyssynchrony was observed (40 ms), whereas no LV dyssynchrony with pulsed-wave TDI could be discerned (septal-to-lateral wall delay of 10 ms). However, one of the limitations of pulsed-wave TDI is that the interrogation of opposing LV walls cannot be performed simultaneously. In contrast, real-time 3D echocardiography allows for the assessment of LV dyssynchrony in the entire LV during a single cardiac cycle. Time to minimum systolic volume is automatically calculated for 16 LV segments and the SDI is subsequently derived. In addition, time to minimum systolic volume is displayed in polar map format, from which the latest activated segments can be identified. Borderline LV dyssynchrony is present with an SDI of 6.4%. The latest activated segments were the mid and apical inferoposterior segments (coded in red).

37. **Answer: D.** AV dyssynchrony can be corrected with CRT and LV diastolic filling improved. In addition, LV dyssynchrony can be reduced, as demonstrated in this patient, with induction of a more synchronous LV contraction pattern and improved LV hemodynamics.

KEY POINTS

- In patients with heart failure and a reduced ejection fraction and a narrow QRS (<120 ms), substantial cardiac dyssynchrony may exist.
- Echocardiography represents a suitable imaging technique to evaluate cardiac dyssynchrony in such patients, in whom current guidelines do not recommend CRT implantation.

38. **Answer: C.** Speckle tracking strain, presented as a parametric map of the LV, represents peak systolic longitudinal strain and does not reflect differences in timing between segments. It can therefore not easily be used to evaluate dyssynchrony (**Figure 14.30**).

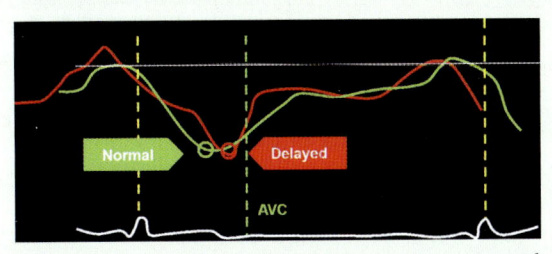

Figure 14.30. Segmental, longitudinal time-versus-strain curves from two theoretical, opposing left ventricular (LV) segments. Although peak systolic (before aortic valve closure [AVC]) strain occurs later in the red-coded curve than in the green-coded curve, the absolute value of peak strain achieved is identical in both segments and subsequently, will not reflect LV dyssynchrony on a parametric map of LV longitudinal strain.

The pattern of segmental strain in this patient does not suggest any specific underlying etiology but is significantly impaired. LV global longitudinal strain is not a parameter which can be used to determine if CRT is indicated, and is not a guideline-based indication for resynchronization therapy.

39. **Answer: A.** Noninvasive myocardial work is a novel echocardiographic parameter, where speckle tracking strain data are integrated with sphygmomanometric blood pressure values to obtain a pressure-strain loop, wherefrom LV myocardial work can be derived. Differences in septal and lateral myocardial work reflect LV dyssynchrony and have been shown to predict CRT response. Noninvasive myocardial work does generally not suggest the etiology of abnormal work distribution in the LV, and it is less susceptible to afterload than global longitudinal strain, since it integrates blood pressure into the metric.

KEY POINTS

- LV strain does not have practical utility in demonstrating LV dyssynchrony.
- Noninvasive myocardial work is a novel echocardiographic parameter, which is less load-dependent than longitudinal strain, and reflects LV dyssynchrony.

SUGGESTED READINGS

Auger D, Hoke U, Bax JJ, Boersma E, Delgado V. Effect of atrioventricular and ventriculoventricular delay optimization on clinical and echocardiographic outcomes of patients treated with cardiac resynchronization therapy: a meta-analysis. *Am Heart J.* 2013;166(1):20-29.

Donal E, Delgado V, Magne J, et al. Rational and design of EuroCRT: an international observational study on multi-modality imaging and cardiac resynchronization therapy. *Eur Heart J Cardiovasc Imaging.* 2017;18(10):1120-1127.

Galli E, Leclercq C, Hubert A, et al. Role of myocardial constructive work in the identification of responders to CRT of responders to CRT. *Eur Heart J Cardiovasc Imaging.* 2018;19(9):1010-1018.

Glikson M, Nielsen JC, Kronborg MB, et al. 2021 ESC Guidelines on cardiac pacing and cardiac resynchronization therapy: the Task Force on cardiac pacing and cardiac resynchronization therapy of the European Society of Cardiology (ESC). Developed in collaboration with the European Heart Rhythm Association (EHRA). *Eur Heart J.* 2021;42(35):3427-3520.

Khan FZ, Virdee MS, Palmer CR, et al. Targeted left ventricular lead placement to guide cardiac resynchronization therapy: the TARGET study—a randomized, controlled trial. *J Am Coll Cardiol.* 2012;59(17):1509-1518.

Kleijn SA, Aly MF, Knol DL, et al. A meta-analysis of left ventricular dyssynchrony assessment and prediction of response to cardiac resynchronization therapy by three-dimensional echocardiography. *Eur Heart J Cardiovasc Imaging.* 2012;13(9):763-775.

Mele D, Bertini M, Malagu M, Nardozza M, Ferrari R. Current role of echocardiography in cardiac resynchronization therapy. *Heart Fail Rev.* 2017;22(6):699-722.

Saba S, Marek J, Schwartzman D, et al. Echocardiography-guided left ventricular lead placement for cardiac resynchronization therapy: results of the Speckle Tracking Assisted Resynchronization Therapy for Electrode Region trial. *Circ Heart Fail.* 2013;6(3):427-434.

Van Bommel RJ, Marsan NA, Delgado V, et al. Cardiac resynchronization therapy as a therapeutic option in patients with moderate-severe functional mitral regurgitation and high operative risk. *Circulation.* 2011;124(8):912-919.

CHAPTER 15

Aortic Stenosis

Marie-Annick Clavel, Jordi S. Dahl, and Philippe Pibarot

QUESTIONS

1. A 72-year-old man is referred for a cardiology evaluation after his primary care physician noted the presence of a loud systolic ejection murmur. Transthoracic echocardiogram shows normal left ventricular size with a left ventricular ejection fraction (LVEF) of 65%. The left ventricular outflow tract (LVOT) diameter is 2 cm, and the LVOT time-velocity integral (TVI) is 15 cm with a peak velocity of 0.8 m/s. The peak aortic velocity is 4.8 m/sec and the aortic valve TVI is 100 cm. Your interpretation of the echocardiogram is?
   A. Severe aortic stenosis (AS), because the valve area is less than 1 cm^2.
   B. Severe AS, because the LVOT/aortic velocity ratio is less than 0.3.
   C. Severe AS, because the peak aortic velocity is greater than 3.5 m/s.
   D. The severity of the AS cannot be determined from the data presented.

2. In this asymptomatic patient in **Question 1**, the most appropriate recommendation is?
   A. Inform the patient that the chance of developing symptoms in the next 5 years is 20%.
   B. Recommend coronary angiography in anticipation of surgical intervention.
   C. Recommend transesophageal echocardiography.
   D. Recommend oxygen consumption treadmill test.
   E. Recommend repeat echocardiogram in 2 years.

3. Which of the following statements referring to the echocardiographic evaluation of AS is **CORRECT**?
   A. Echocardiographic maximum aortic gradient is usually higher than the pullback gradient obtained during left heart catheterization. This is due to overestimation of the true gradient by echocardiography.
   B. Echocardiographic assessment of mean aortic gradient correlates well with the mean gradient obtained in the cardiac catheterization laboratory.
   C. The usual echocardiographic measurement of the mean aortic gradient cannot overestimate the true gradient.
   D. The assessment of mean aortic gradient with a nonimaging probe is more accurate because these probes allow for better Doppler software processing.

4. A patient is evaluated for AS. Doppler measurements from all available windows show a highest peak aortic velocity of 5 m/s, and an LVOT velocity of 2 m/s. Which of the following calculations are **CORRECT**?
   A. Peak aortic valve gradient is 116 mm Hg.
   B. Peak aortic valve gradient is 100 mm Hg.
   C. Peak aortic valve gradient is 84 mm Hg.
   D. Peak aortic valve gradient is 36 mm Hg.

5. Two patients just had their follow-up echocardiographic assessments for known AS. They both are asymptomatic. In both patients, peak aortic jet velocity increased since the last evaluation. For the first patient, initials LL, LV ejection fraction was 75%, peak gradient 42 mm Hg, mean gradient 28 mm Hg, ejection time 300 ms, and acceleration time 70 ms. Aortic valve area was not calculable due to acceleration in the LV outflow tract. For the second patient, initials MM, LV ejection fraction was 75%, peak gradient 42 mm Hg, mean gradient 28 mm Hg, ejection time 300 ms, and acceleration time 110 ms. Aortic valve area was not calculable due to acceleration in the LV outflow tract.
Which of the following statement is **CORRECT**?
A. These patients have moderate AS and required echocardiographic follow-up in 1 to 3 years.
B. Aortic valve area is not calculable by continuity equation; however, planimetry of the valve area can be performed and should be used to assess severity of AS.
C. LL is at more at risk of adverse event because acceleration time is fast (ie, <100 ms).
D. MM is at more at risk of adverse event because the ratio of acceleration time divided by ejection time is high (ie, >0.32).

6. A 78-year-old patient has an echocardiographic evaluation for a mid-systolic murmur heard at the right upper sternal border. He is symptomatic with development of dyspnea at exercise this last month. He is known for hypertension (136/70 mm Hg) and mild coronary artery disease. At echocardiography, LV ejection fraction was 70%, peak aortic jet velocity 3.5 m/s, mean gradient 29 mm Hg, aortic valve area 0.8 cm^2 (indexed 0.45 cm^2/m^2), and stroke volume 64 mL (indexed 36 mL/m^2).
Which of the following statement is the most correct?
A. This patient has a low-flow, low-gradient aortic stenosis with preserved LV ejection fraction (ie, paradoxical low-flow AS).
B. This patient has a high risk for adverse outcomes due to its elevated valvulo-arterial impedance (ZVa).
C. The patient has a normal-flow, peak aortic jet velocity <4.0 m/s, and mean gradient <40 mm Hg; thus, stenosis is nonsevere and prognosis is good. Symptoms are related to concomitant disease.
D. The patient has a symptomatic severe AS and should be referred to aortic valve intervention.

7. A 30-year-old woman is referred for management of a newly diagnosed subaortic stenosis. She is asymptomatic, but during a routine physical examination, a loud systolic murmur was heard. An echocardiogram demonstrated a subaortic membrane with a gradient of 44 mm Hg and concomitant presence of moderate aortic valve regurgitation. The left ventricle is borderline enlarged, with an LVEF of 57%. On TEE, the aortic valve does not appear to be calcified. Which of the following statements are **CORRECT**?
A. This type of lesion responds well to balloon dilatation.
B. The patient should undergo resection of the subaortic membrane and aortic valve replacement.
C. Careful inspection of the pulmonary valve and pulmonary artery should be carried out during TEE.
D. Doppler interrogation of the abdominal aorta provides no information in this case.

8. Which is the most compatible with the aortic valve presented in **Figure 15.1**?
A. A 75-year-old man with tricuspid moderate AS.
B. A 35-year-old man with a bicuspid AS with fusion of the left and right coronary cusps.
C. A 35-year-old man with a bicuspid AS with fusion of the noncoronary and right coronary cusps.
D. A 35-year-old man with a bicuspid AS with fusion of the noncoronary and left coronary cusps.

9. Which of the following is the most accurate interpretation of the images of the aortic valve/left ventricular outflow tract/aortic root presented in **Figure 15.2**?
A. Severe AS.
B. Systolic motion of the anterior mitral valve leaflet.
C. Severe subaortic stenosis.
D. Severe supra-aortic stenosis.
E. The Doppler signal is that of mitral regurgitant flow and not that of transaortic flow.

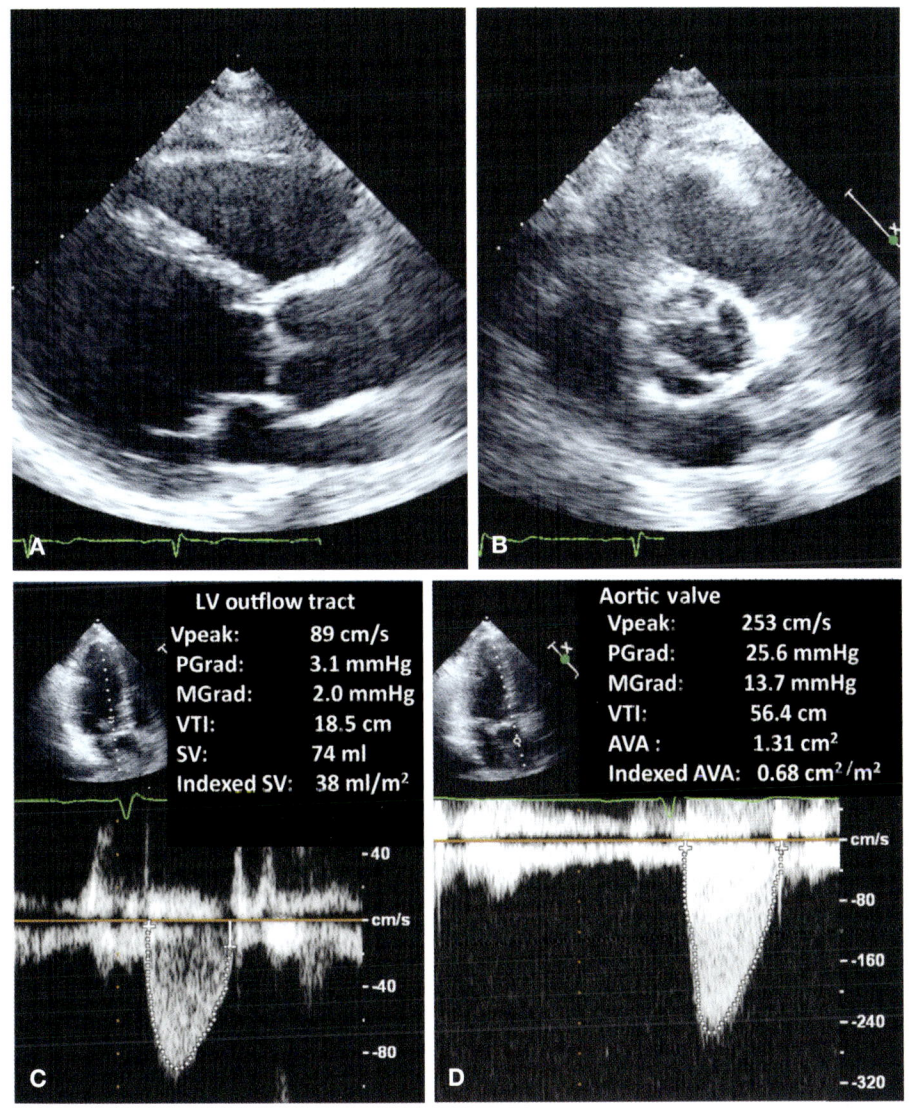

Figure 15.1. Doppler echocardiographic assessment of the aortic valve morphology and hemodyanmics. Parasternal long-axis view of left ventricle (LV) **(A)**; parasternal short-axis view of the aortic valve **(B)**; pulsed-wave Doppler in the LV outflow tract **(C)**; continuous-wave Doppler across aortic valve in the apical 3-chamber window **(D)**. AVA, aortic valve area; MGrad, mean gradient; PGrad, peak gradient; SV, stroke volume; VPeak, peak aortic jet velocity; VTI, velocity-time integral.

CASE 1

A 45-year-old patient known with hypertension presents for evaluation of a murmur. He has no previous medical conditions and has during the last 6 months been experiencing worsening in functional capacity. At TTE, the LV is borderline dilated with an LVEF of 40% and a stroke volume of 85 mL. **Figure 15.3** *shows the CW Doppler across the aortic valve (peak gradient 53 mm Hg, mean gradient 33 mm Hg). There were no signs of aortic regurgitation.*

10. What is the aortic valve area of the patient in **Case 1**?
    A. Cannot say, I need the LVOT diameter.
    B. Cannot say, I need the LVOT velocity.
    C. 1.13 cm².
    D. 0.88 cm².
    E. 1.01 cm².

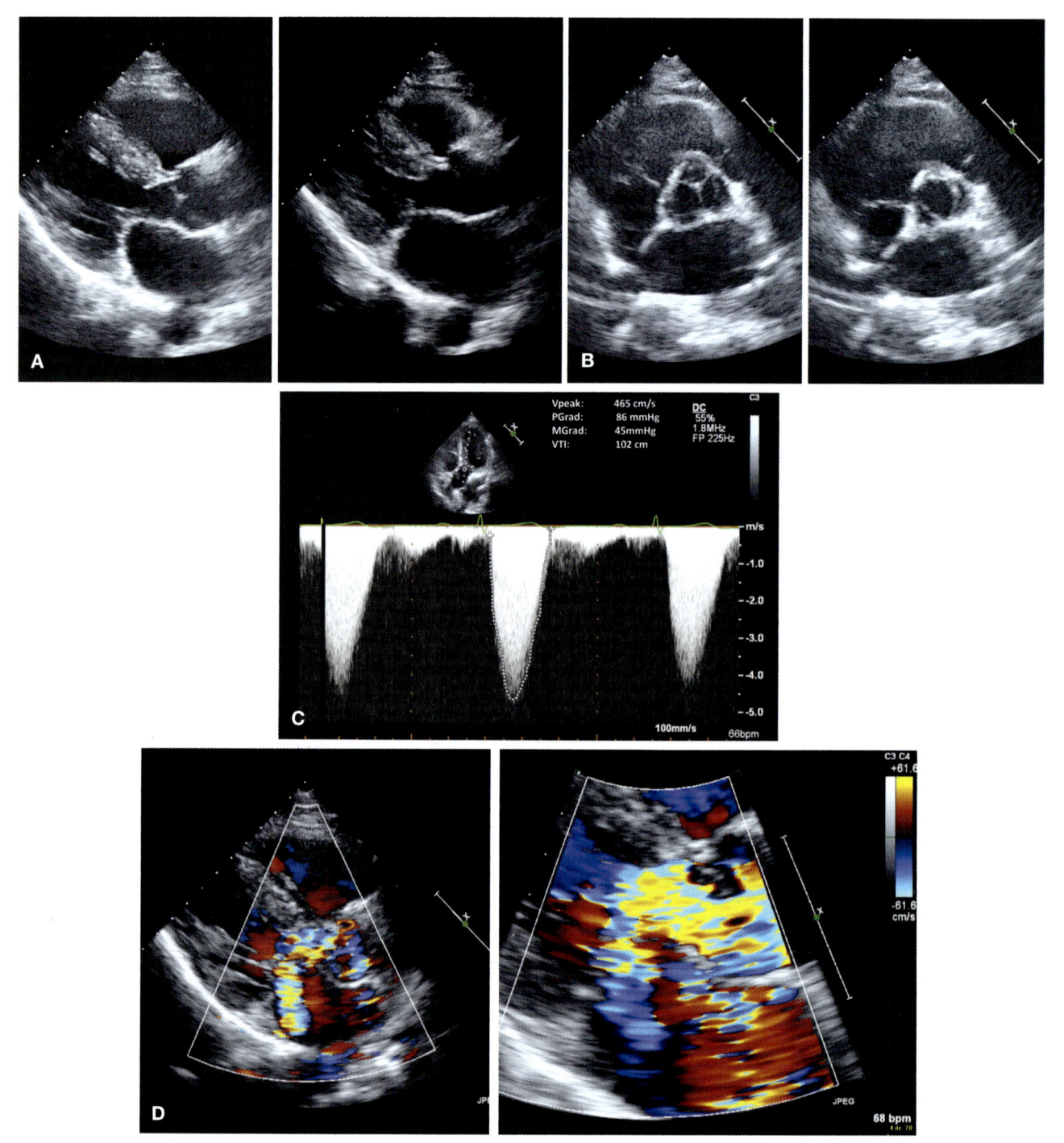

Figure 15.2. Doppler echocardiographic assessment of the aortic valve morphology and hemodyanmics. **A:** Parasternal long-axis view of the left ventricle (LV) in diastole and systole; **B:** parasternal short-axis view of the aortic valve in diastole and systole; **C:** continuous-wave Doppler across aortic valve in the apical 5-chamber window; **D:** parasternal long-axis with color Doppler, unzoomed and zoom image. MGrad, mean gradient; PGrad, peak gradient; VPeak, peak aortic jet velocity; VTI, velocity-time integral.

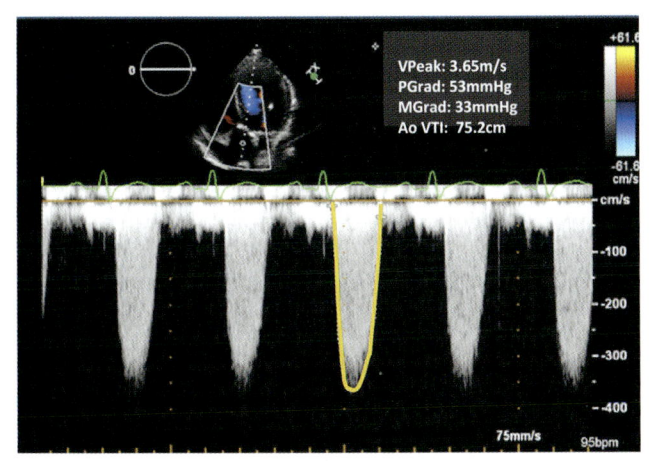

Figure 15.3. Continuous-wave Doppler across aortic valve in the apical 5-chamber window. Ao, aortic; MGrad, mean gradient; PGrad, peak gradient; VPeak, peak aortic jet velocity; VTI, velocity-time integral.

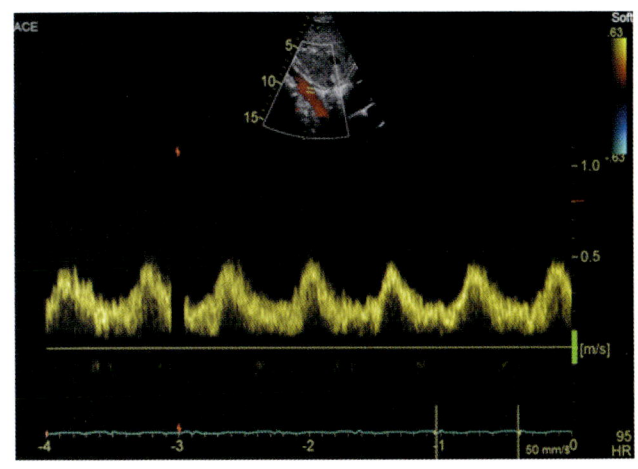

Figure 15.4. Doppler echocardiographic assessment of the flow of the abdominal aorta. Pulsed-wave Doppler in the abdominal aorta.

11. For the patient in **Case 1**, which of the following statements is the most **CORRECT**?
    A. The patient has low-gradient AS and should be referred for AVR because LVEF < 50%.
    B. Aortic stenosis severity cannot accurately be determined due to reduced LVEF. Dobutamine stress test should be performed to provide incremental information.
    C. Aortic stenosis severity is not possible to assess solely by echocardiography. CT should be performed to assess AV calcification and accurately estimate AS severity.
    D. This patient most likely has a moderate AS and something else. Further rest echocardiographic evaluation is required.
    E. Patient has symptoms due to combination of hypertension and moderate AS. Treat hypertension and follow-up evaluation in 6 months.

12. Figure 15.4 demonstrates the flow at the abdominal aorta.
    Which statements is the most **CORRECT**?
    A. Further evaluation of the aorta is required as it is highly probable that the patient has coarctation of the aorta.
    B. TEE should be performed as it is very probable that the patient has mixed aortic valve disease with concomitant moderate-severe aortic regurgitation.
    C. Abdominal flow indicates that there is no coarctation of the aorta; thus, AVR should be recommended.
    D. Abdominal flow does not provide additional information to this patient.

13. **Figure 15.5** demonstrates 3D reconstruction CT of the aorta. Blood pressure in the upper extremities is 160/80 mm Hg and in the lower extremities is 100/70 mm Hg.
    Which is the most likely statement?
    A. The patient has significant coarctation of the aorta. The patient should be referred for surgical repair or catheter-based stenting, treatment for hypertension, and subsequently being followed up for his moderate AS.
    B. Although there is a coarctation, blood pressure in lower extremities is preserved and patient should only be treated for hypertension, and subsequently followed up for AS.
    C. The patient should undergo surgical repair of the aorta with concomitant surgical AVR.
    D. As there are no reported limb symptoms, the patient should be treated conservatively with a echocardiographic follow-up in 6 months.

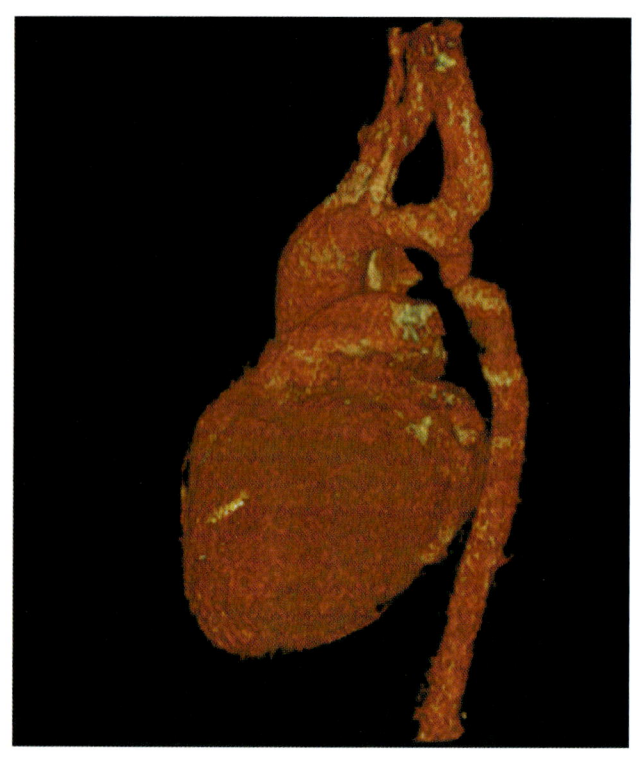

Figure 15.5. Three-dimensional reconstruction of a cardiac computed tomography.

CASE 2

An 81-year-old man presents for evaluation of AS. He has a history of hypertension, pacemaker implantation, and atrial fibrillation. He presents with dyspnea that worsened progressively during the last 3 months and a few episodes of angina during exercise.

Figure 15.6 shows the evaluation of the aortic valve hemodynamics. This patient has a normal LV outflow (stroke volume index: 50.7 mL/m^2; Figure 15.6A). In the apical 5-chamber view (Figure 15.6B), the peak aortic jet velocity is 3.7 m/s, the mean transvalvular gradient is 36 mm Hg, and the aortic valve area (AVA) is 1.01 cm^2. Figure 15.6C also shows the measurements of transvalvular gradient from the right parasternal window.

At Doppler echocardiography, the LV systolic function is preserved (▶ Videos 15.1 and 15.2) with a LV ejection fraction estimated by the biplane Simpson method of 60%. The LV end-diastolic diameter is 51 mm, LV outflow tract diameter 26 mm, and ascending aorta diameter 39 mm.

14. What would be the appropriate management of the patient in **Case 2**?
  A. The AS is moderate and a follow-up echocardiogram can be done in 1 to 2 years.
  B. The AS is severe but a "watchful waiting" strategy is appropriate and a follow-up echocardiogram can be done in 6 months to 1 year.
  C. The AS is severe, the patient is symptomatic, and surgical AVR is recommended.
  D. The AS is severe, the patient is symptomatic, but given the patient's age and comorbidities, transcatheter AVR is recommended.

15. The patient in **Case 2** underwent coronary angiography to assess presence and severity of coronary artery disease prior to AVR. At that time, should the interventional cardiologist systematically cross the aortic valve and reassess the valvular hemodynamics?
  A. Yes.
  B. No.
  C. Yes, with exceptions.
  D. No, with exceptions.

16. Coronary angiography of the patient in **Case 2** revealed a significant stenosis of the mid left circumflex artery. Although this was not necessary in this patient, the interventionalist measured the transvalvular gradient by the pullback method and obtained a gradient of 37 mm Hg. Which of the following statements most likely explains the discrepancy between catheterization versus echocardiography-derived transvalvular gradient?
  A. The phenomenon of pressure recovery downstream of the aortic valve is responsible for the lower gradient measured at catheterization versus at echocardiography.
  B. Hypertension during catheterization has resulted in an increase in LV afterload and a reduction in transvalvular flow and gradient.
  C. The pullback catheterization method underestimates the value of transvalvular gradients obtained by echocardiography.
  D. Doppler echocardiography from the right parasternal window overestimates the transvalvular gradient and only the gradient from the apical window should be used.

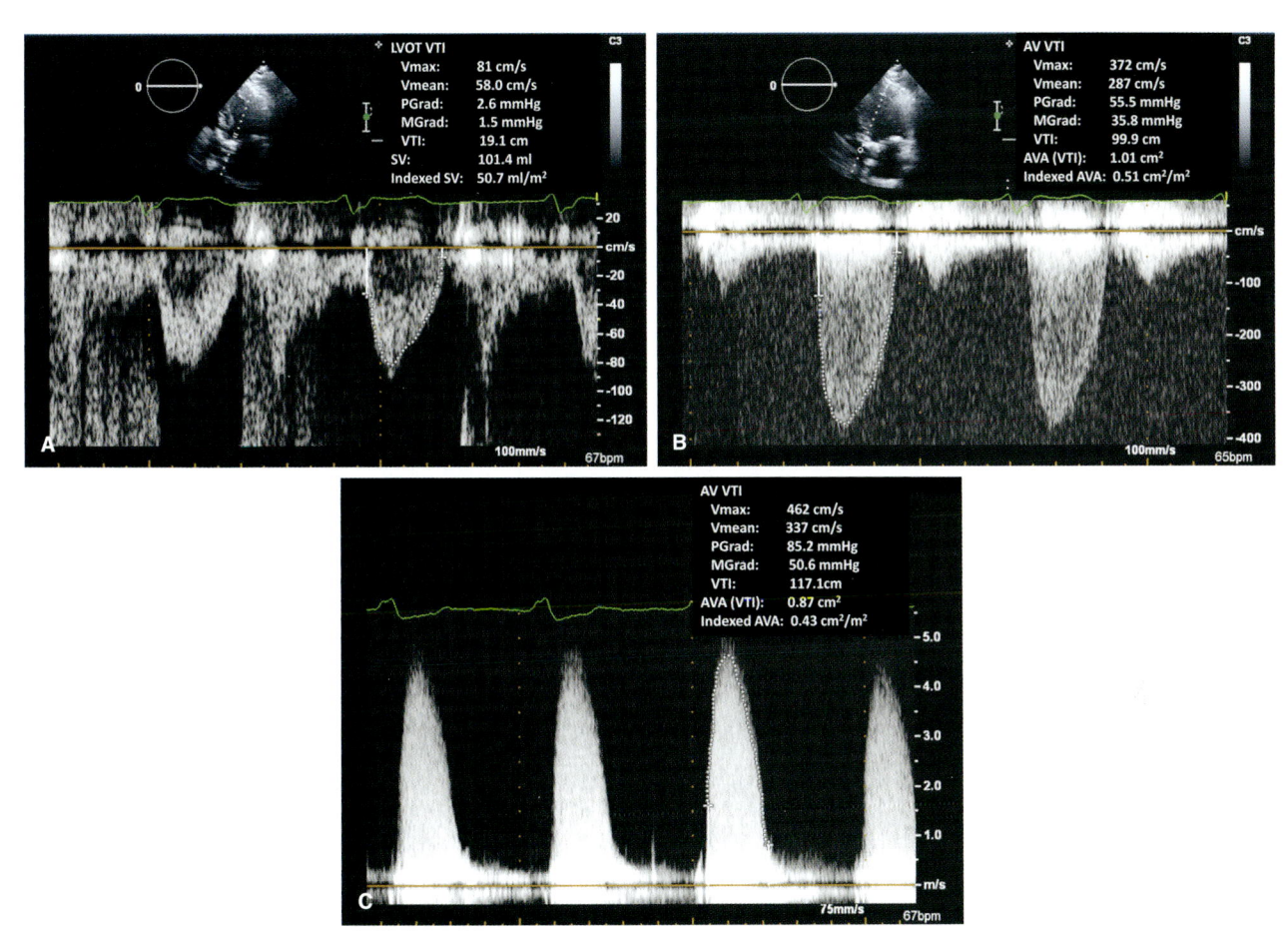

Figure 15.6. Doppler evaluation of aortic valve hemodynamics. **A:** Pulsed-wave Doppler in the left ventricle outflow tract; **B:** continuous-wave Doppler across aortic valve in the apical 5-chamber window; **C:** continuous-wave Doppler across aortic valve in the right parasternal window. AVA, aortic valve area; MGrad, mean gradient; PGrad, peak gradient; SV, stroke volume; VPeak, peak aortic jet velocity; VTI, velocity-time integral.

CASE 3

A 72-year-old man with a history of hypertension, previous myocardial infarction, coronary artery bypass graft surgery 12 years ago, and congestive heart failure is admitted at the hospital for worsening heart failure symptoms.

Doppler echocardiogram shows a reduced LVEF and dilated LV (▶ Video 15.3 and ▶ Video 15.4). The assessment of aortic valve hemodynamics reveals a peak aortic jet velocity of 3.6 m/s, a mean transvalvular gradient of 29 mm Hg, and an aortic valve area of 0.53 cm^2.

17. What is the diagnostic test that you would do next in patient in **Case 3**?
    A. Exercise stress echocardiography.
    B. Full-dose (up to 40 μg/kg/min) dobutamine stress echocardiography.
    C. Full-dose (up to 40 μg/kg/min) dobutamine stress echocardiography with contrast.
    D. Low-dose (up to 20 μg/kg/min) dobutamine stress echocardiography.
    E. Low-dose (up to 20 μg/kg/min) dobutamine stress echocardiography with contrast.

18. The patient in **Case 3** underwent a low-dose dobutamine echocardiography with contrast. The dobutamine infusion was stopped at 10 μg/kg/min. LV ejection fraction increased from 20% to 35% with dobutamine, stroke volume from 45 to 59 mL, mean gradient from 29 to 44 mm Hg, and aortic valve area from 0.53 to 0.60 cm^2 (**Figure 15.7**).
    How would you grade AS severity?
    A. Moderate AS because the resting mean gradient is <40 mm Hg.
    B. Severe AS because the resting aortic valve area is <1 cm^2.
    C. Severe AS because at the end of dobutamine infusion, mean gradient is >40 mm Hg.
    D. Severe AS because at the end of dobutamine infusion, mean gradient is >40 mm Hg and aortic valve area is <1 cm^2.

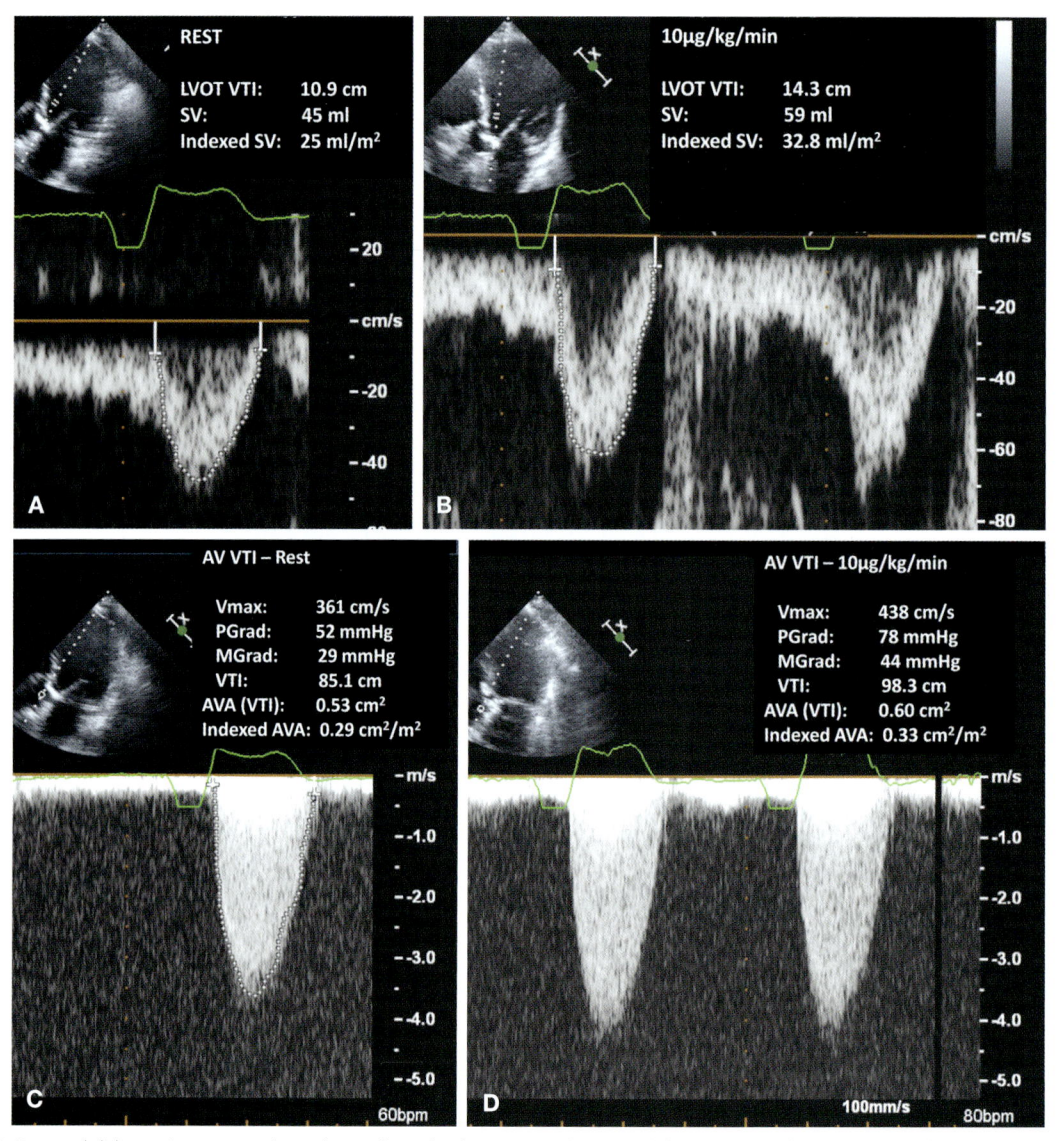

Figure 15.7. Rest and dobutamine stress echocardiography. Pulsed-wave Doppler in the left ventricle outflow tract **(A, B)** and continuous-wave Doppler across the aortic valve **(C, D)** at rest **(A, C)** and peak **(B, D)** dobutamine stress echocardiography. AVA, aortic valve area; LVOT, left ventricular outflow tract; MGrad, mean gradient; PGrad, peak gradient; SV, stroke volume; VPeak, peak aortic jet velocity; VTI, velocity-time integral.

19. The operative risk for surgical AVR in the patient from **Case 3** is?
   A. High risk (>8% risk of 30-day mortality) because rest LV ejection fraction is <50%.
   B. High risk (>8% risk of 30-day mortality) because of the absence of LV flow reserve during dobutamine stress.
   C. Intermediate risk (6%-8% risk of 30-day mortality) because rest LV ejection fraction is <50%, but there is significant LV flow reserve during dobutamine stress.
   D. Intermediate risk (6%-8% risk of 30-day mortality) because rest LV ejection fraction is <50%, but there is significant improvement in ejection fraction during dobutamine stress.

CASE 4

A 72-year-old woman with a history of hypertension and AS undergoes routine clinical and echocardiographic follow-up. Three years ago, Doppler echocardiogram showed a stroke volume of 71 mL (indexed stroke volume: 44 mL/m^2), an AVA of 1.20 cm^2 (indexed AVA of 0.75 cm^2/m^2), a mean gradient of 21 mm Hg, LV ejection fraction of 70%, and an LV end-diastolic diameter of 47 mm.

The echocardiogram performed today shows a stroke volume of 48 mL (indexed stroke volume: 30 mL/m^2), an AVA of 0.89 cm^2 (indexed AVA: 0.50 cm^2/m^2), a mean gradient of 24 mm Hg, an LV ejection fraction of 60%, and an LV end-diastolic diameter of 42 mm (▶ Video 15.5). The patient did not report any symptoms.

20. Your recommendation for the patient in **Case 4** is?
   A. Schedule a follow-up echocardiogram in 2 to 3 years.
   B. Perform an exercise test.
   C. Perform an exercise stress echocardiography.
   D. Perform a full-dose dobutamine echocardiography.
   E. Perform a low-dose dobutamine stress echocardiography.

21. The patient in **Case 4** underwent exercise stress echocardiography with a modified Bruce protocol. She stopped walking after only 4 minutes 39 seconds due to chest pain. She had moderate dyspnea at the time of test termination. Electrocardiogram and echocardiogram did not show any sign of ischemia. Percentage of the expected maximum heart rate was 72%. Stroke volume increased to 59 mL, mean gradient to 29 mm Hg, and an AVA to 0.92 cm^2. Projected aortic valve area at normal flow rate (250 mL/s) was calculated at 0.94 cm^2 with the use of the following formula (**Figure 15.8**).

$$\text{Projected AVA} = \text{AVA}_{rest} + \frac{\text{AVA}_{peak} - \text{AVA}_{rest}}{Q_{peak} - Q_{rest}} \times (250 - Q_{rest})$$

where AVA$_{rest}$ and Q$_{rest}$ are aortic valve area and flow rate (stroke volume divided by ejection time) at rest, and AVA$_{peak}$ and Q$_{peak}$ are AVA and Q during peak exercise.
Your recommendation is?

   A. Schedule follow-up echocardiogram in 2 to 3 years because AS is moderate.
   B. Schedule follow-up echocardiogram in 1 year or less because AS is severe but patient is asymptomatic.
   C. Confirm that AS is severe by multidetector computed tomography (MDCT) and refer the patient to AVR because AS is severe and the patient is symptomatic on exercise. Shared decision-making is recommended to choose between surgical and transcatheter AVR.
   D. Confirm that AS is severe by MDCT and refer the patient to transcatheter AVR and because AS is severe, the patient is symptomatic on exercise and is at high surgical risk.

CASE 5

A 62-year-old man underwent a clinical examination because of reduced exercise capacity and dyspnea. At cardiac auscultation, a loud (3/6) ejection murmur radiating to the neck vessels was noted. The patient underwent Doppler echocardiography, which shows mild LV hypertrophy, normal LV ejection fraction (60%), normal flow (stroke volume: 95 mL, stroke volume index: 47 mL/m^2), and a calcified aortic valve with a peak aortic jet velocity at 3.4 m/s, an AVA of 0.90 cm^2, and a mean gradient of 29 mm Hg.

22. How would you grade AS severity for the patient in **Case 5**?
   A. Moderate AS because peak aortic jet velocity is <4 m/s and mean gradient is <40 mm Hg and transvalvular flow is normal.
   B. Severe AS because AVA is <1 cm^2 and transvalvular flow is normal.
   C. Severe AS because aortic valve area is <1 cm^2 and indexed AVA is <0.60 cm^2/m^2.
   D. It is not possible to determine stenosis severity with rest echocardiography and we need to perform stress echocardiography.
   E. It is not possible to determine stenosis severity with rest echocardiography and we need to assess aortic valve calcification by MDCT.

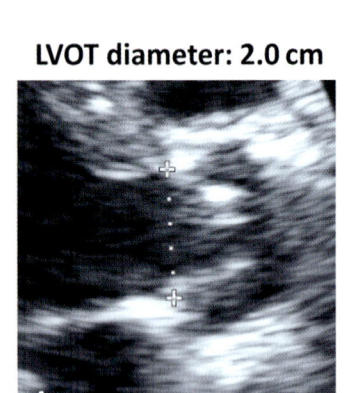

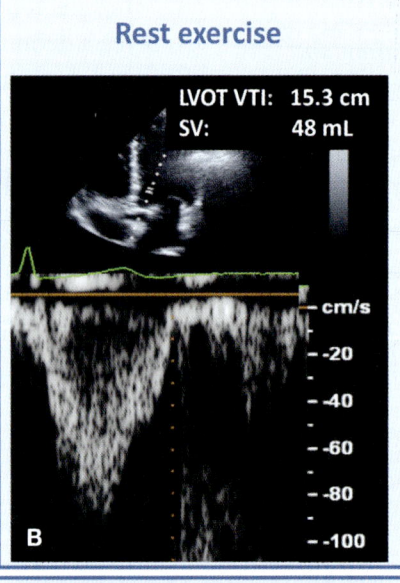

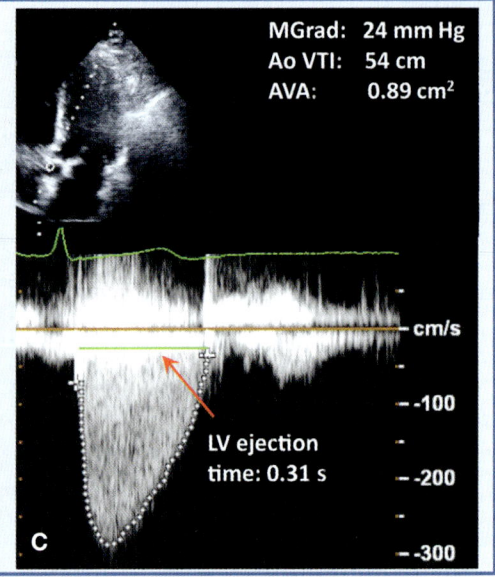

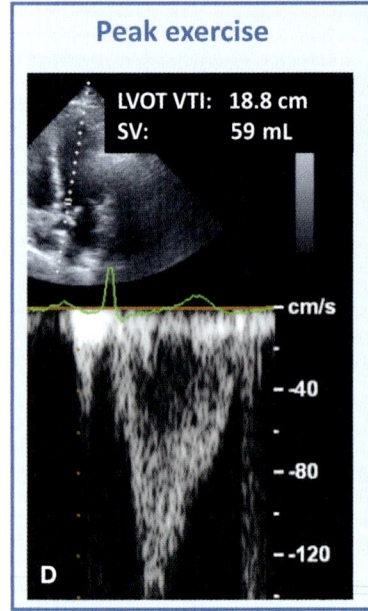

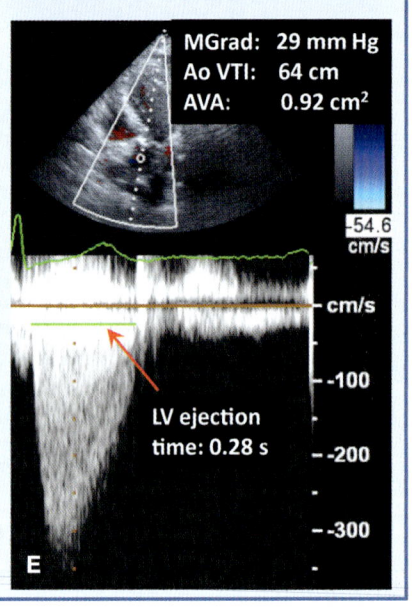

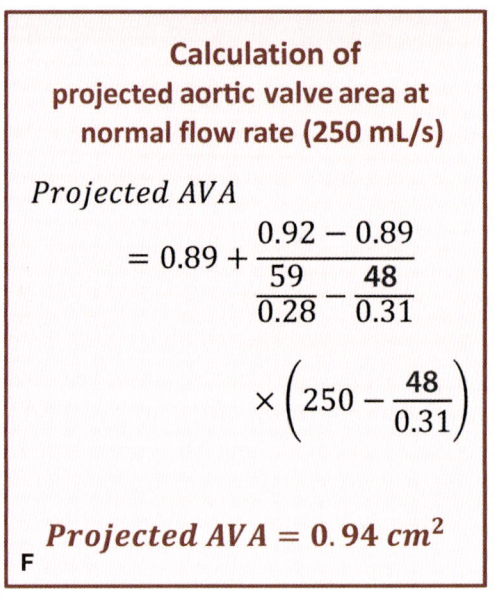

Figure 15.8. Rest and exercise stress echocardiography. Left ventricular (LV) outflow tract diameter measurement (**A**). Pulsed-wave Doppler in the LV outflow tract and continuous-wave Doppler across aortic valve at rest (**B**, **C**) and peak (**D**, **E**) dobutamine stress echocardiography. Calculation of the projected aortic valve area at normal flow rate (**F**). AVA, aortic valve area; LVOT, left ventricular outflow tract; MGrad, mean gradient; PGrad, peak gradient; Q, transvalvular flow rate; SV, stroke volume; VPeak, peak aortic jet velocity; VTI, velocity-time integral.

23. The patient in **Case 5** underwent an MDCT without contrast to assess aortic valve calcification (**Figure 15.9**). The aortic valve calcification score is 1810 AU.
Your recommendation is?
   A. Patient has severe AS and should be referred for AVR.
   B. Patients has severe AS but gradient is <40 mm Hg. A medical and echocardiographic follow-up should be planned in 6 months.
   C. Patient has moderate AS and should have clinical and echocardiographic follow-up in 1 year.
   D. Patient has moderate AS and other potential causes of symptoms should be investigated and treated.
   E. C and D.

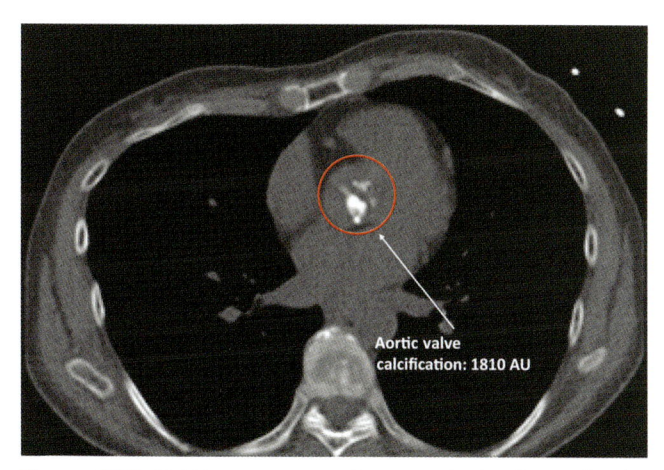

Figure 15.9. Multidetector computed tomography showing aortic valve calcification (red circle).

CASE 6

A 74-year-old man was referred for transcatheter aortic valve replacement with hypertension (treated) and history of carpal tunnel syndrome. The patient recently developed dyspnea at minimal exertion (walk). At echocardiography, LV is severely hypertrophied. Left ventricular ejection fraction was measured by Simpson method at 55%. Peak aortic jet velocity was 3.3 m/s, mean gradient 30 mm Hg, aortic valve area 0.8 cm², and stroke volume index 32 mL/m². Global longitudinal strain was −13% and there was a grade 2 diastolic dysfunction (Figure 15.10; ▶ *Videos 15.6 and 15.7).*

24. What should be the next evaluation step be for the patient in **Case 6**?
    A. Perform an exercise stress test to confirm symptoms.
    B. Perform a dobutamine stress echocardiography to confirm AS severity.
    C. Perform a CT scan to confirm AS severity.
    D. Refer the patient to transcatheter AVR.

25. The patient in **Case 6** underwent noncontrast and contrast CT scan as part of the pretranscatheter AVR evaluation (**Figure 15.11**). Aortic valve calcification was measured at 1864 AU.
    A. Calcification of the aortic valve is not severe, cancel transcatheter AVR. Follow-up should be scheduled in 12 months.
    B. Despite nonsevere aortic valve calcification, the aortic valve looks thickened at contrast CT. Moreover, echocardiography reveals global biventricular hypertrophy and impaired longitudinal systolic function with apical sparing. These findings raise suspicion for a concomitant infiltrative cardiomyopathy.
    C. Perform a dobutamine stress echocardiography to confirm AS severity.
    D. None of the above.

26. Patient underwent a scintigraphy with ⁹⁹mTc-labelled 3,3-diphosphono-1,2-propanodicarboxylic acid (DPD) (**Figure 15.12**) and was diagnosed with ATTR cardiac amyloidosis. What should be the course of treatment?
    A. Transcatheter AVR should be canceled and patient treated palliatively.
    B. Patient should undergo surgical AVR.
    C. Transcatheter AVR should be performed.
    D. Transcatheter AVR should be performed and tafamidis treatment should be considered.

CASE 7

A 45-year-old man with known bicuspid aortic stenosis is seen for a follow-up echocardiographic exam. The patient is asymptomatic. At echocardiography, LVOT diameter is 27 mm, peak aortic jet velocity 3.5 m/s, mean gradient 33 mm Hg, aortic valve area 0.8 cm², and stroke volume index 42 mL/m². Aortic root is normal size. The patient underwent a transesophageal echocardiography that confirms the bicuspid aortic valve (type 1 with left-right cusps fusion). The leaflets are moving well and raphe is calcified. Then patient underwent a noncontrast CT scan and aortic valve calcification was measured at 2100 AU.

27. What is the conclusion of the patient's evaluation and what should be the following step in his management?
    A. Moderate-to-severe AS. The patient should be medically followed up and seen in 6 to 12 months.
    B. Severe AS. The patient should be referred to transcatheter aortic valve replacement (AVR).
    C. Severe AS. The patient should be referred to surgical AVR.
    D. The echocardiographic and CT examinations are nonconclusive. The patient should undergo magnetic resonance imaging.

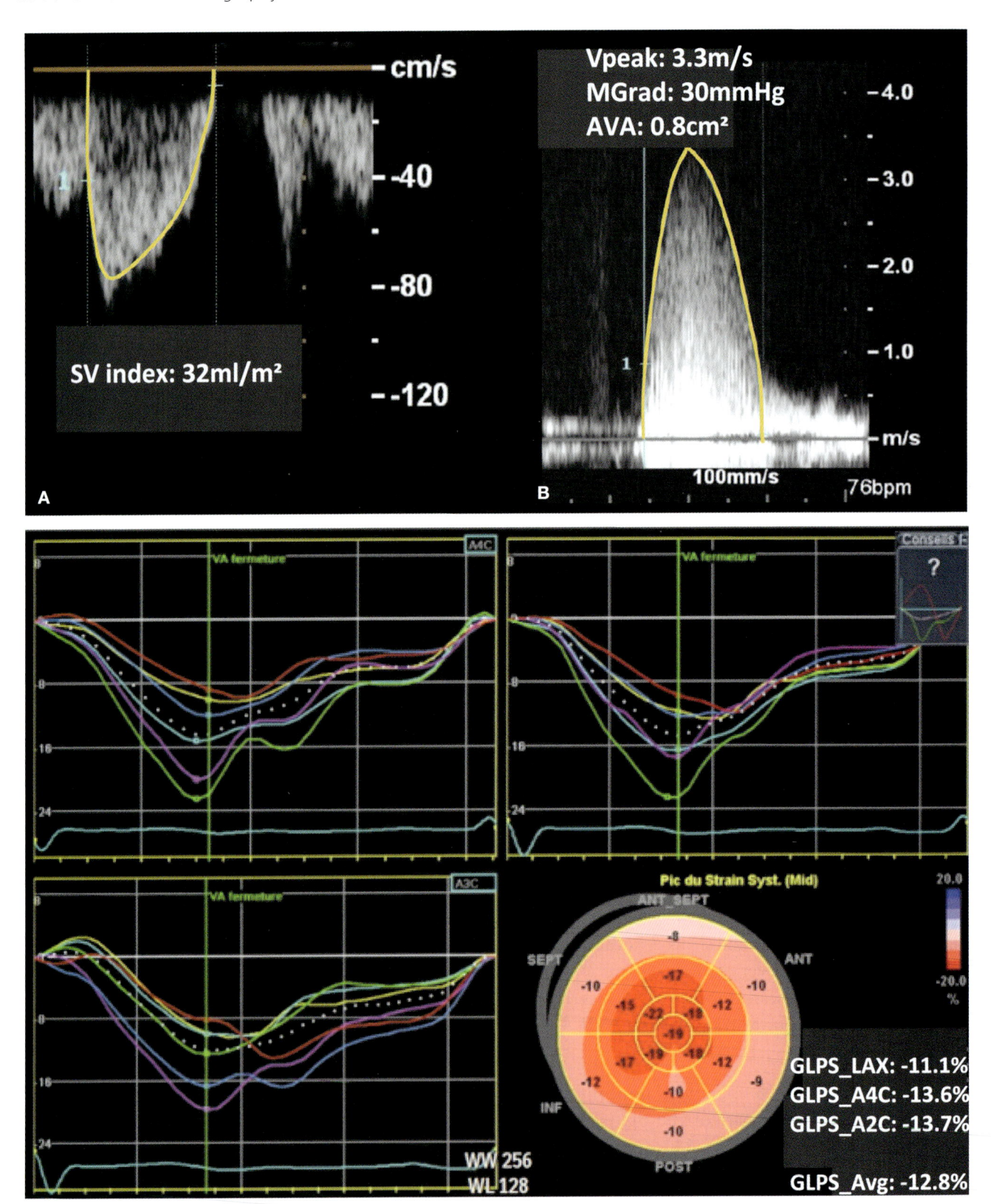

Figure 15.10. Doppler evaluation of aortic valve hemodynamics and global longitudinal strain. Pulsed-wave Doppler in the left ventricular outflow tract (upper left panel) and continuous-wave Doppler across the aortic valve (upper right panel). Global longitudinal strain assessment (bottom panel).

Figure 15.11. Noncontrast (**A**) and contrast (**B**) multidetector computed tomography of the aortic valve.

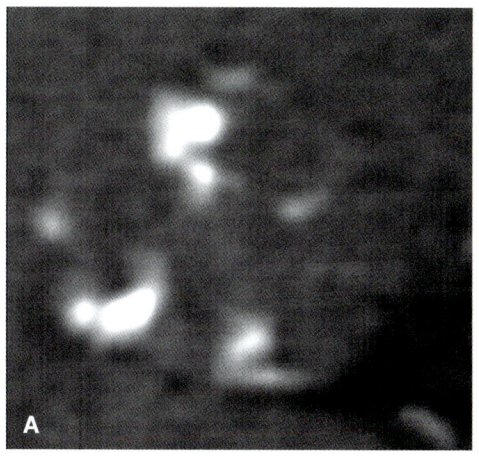

Noncontrast CT
Aortic valve calcification: 1864 AU

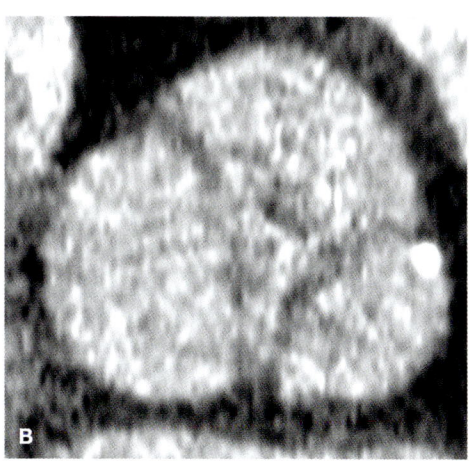

Contrast CT

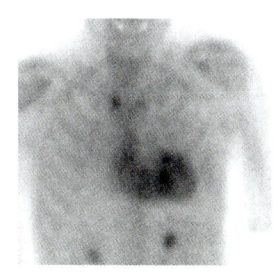

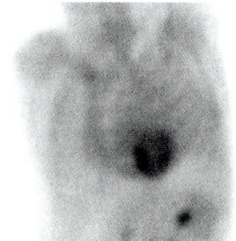

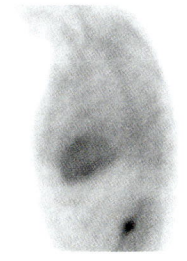

Figure 15.12. Technetium-99 m pyrophosphate imaging showing a pathological uptake.

ANSWERS

1. **Answer: A.** The Doppler findings are consistent with severe aortic stenosis (AS). Valve area can be calculated with the continuity equation. The basic formula is:

$$\text{LVOT flow} = \text{Aortic Valve flow}$$

$$\text{Area}_{LVOT} \times \text{TVI}_{LVOT} = \text{Aortic Valve area} \times \text{TVI}_{Aortic}$$

$$\pi \times \left(\frac{\text{LVOT}_{diameter}}{2}\right)^2 \times \text{TVI}_{LVOT} = \text{Aortic Valve area} \times \text{TVI}_{Aortic}$$

$$\frac{\pi}{4} \times \text{LVOT}^2_{diameter} \times \text{TVI}_{LVOT} = \text{Aortic Valve area} \times \text{TVI}_{Aortic}$$

$$\text{Aortic Valve area} = \frac{\pi}{4} \times \text{LVOT}^2_{diameter} \times \frac{\text{TVI}_{LVOT}}{\text{TVI}_{Aortic}}$$

In the example, the aortic valve area calculates at 0.47 cm². Choice B refers to the dimensionless index (LVOT/aortic TVI or velocity ratio), which is shown to accurately predict presence of severe aortic stenosis when the ratio is less than 0.25 (rather than 0.3). This measurement avoids the use of LVOT diameter, which is the largest source of errors in aortic valve area calculations. This is due to the inherent difficulty associated with the measurement in the presence of a heavily calcified valve; any error is further increased by using the squared value in the valve formula. Choice C is false; typical severe aortic stenosis has aortic velocities in excess of 4 m/s.

2. **Answer: D.** The evolution of completely asymptomatic AS is not benign. Several studies have shown that once the stenosis is severe, patients will inevitably develop symptoms. Rosenhek et al have shown that among 128 patients with asymptomatic severe AS, only 47% were free of death or aortic valve replacement after 2 years. Pellikka et al have shown that among asymptomatic AS patients with aortic velocities greater than 4 m/s at baseline, only 33% remain free of symptoms after 5 years. Therefore, Choice A is obviously false.

Available information in this question suggests presence of severe asymptomatic AS. While the patient is likely to require surgery, a decision cannot be made based solely on the information presented so far, and thus Choice B is false. Transesophageal echocardiography (TEE) can be used in the evaluation of aortic stenosis. Indeed, planimetry of the aortic valve area at TEE correlates well with aortic valve area by catheterization laboratory evaluation. However, this test is typically used as an incremental step only when the transthoracic study fails to establish disease severity (Choice C is false).

Exercise studies are useful in clinical decision-making for asymptomatic AS. Current AHA/ACC guidelines for management of valvular heart disease suggest their use in asymptomatic AS (class 2a). Development of symptoms or a decrease in blood pressure at peak exercise would suggest a more advanced disease state, and aortic valve replacement should be considered. Stress testing, either stress echocardiography or oxygen treadmill consumption test, can be used. In our experience, using oxygen treadmill consumption stress testing allows better quantification of patient's physical limitation; serial studies are also easier to compare to assess disease progression. Current ACC/AHA guidelines recommend every 6 to 12 months echocardiographic evaluations in patients with severe asymptomatic aortic stenosis who are not undergoing aortic valve replacement.

3. Answer: B. The peak-to-peak gradient typically evaluated at pullback in the cardiac catheterization laboratory does not reflect a true event, as the peak aortic pressure occurs after peak left ventricular pressure when AS is present. Echocardiographic estimation of the peak aortic gradient is more accurate as it reflects instantaneous pressure differences between aorta and left ventricle (Choice A is false). Choice B is correct in the vast majority of situations and has established echocardiography as the main diagnostic tool in valvular disease. A number of assumptions are made in echocardiographic assessment of valvular stenosis; if these are not accurate, Doppler-based estimations can be erroneously high (Choice C is false). The simplified Bernoulli equation estimates the pressure gradient according to the formula $\Delta p = 4V^2$; this in turn is a simplification of the convective acceleration term $\frac{1}{2}\rho(V_2^2 - V_1^2)$ in the original Bernoulli equation. The number 4 in the simplified formula is the approximation of the ½ ρ, converted for expressing pressure in mm Hg units; it assumes a blood mass density of 1060 kg/m³. However, blood mass density is lower when significant anemia is present, which would lead to overestimation of the pressure gradient if the same formula is applied. In addition, conditions with increased cardiac output (anemia, fever, subvalvular AS, significant valvular regurgitation) will increase the inflow velocity V_1, which is usually considered negligible. This also leads to overestimation of pressure gradients (Choice C is false).

The use of nonimaging probes is required in the assessment of AS not because of hardware or software properties, but because the smaller footprint allows ultrasound interrogation from a deeper position and better alignment of the Doppler signal with the direction of blood flow.

4. Answer: C. Since the aortic valve inflow velocity (LVOT velocity) is 2 m/s, the term V_1^2 cannot be ignored in the Bernoulli equation. The full formula $\Delta p = 4 \times (V_2^2 - V_1^2)$ has to be used. Therefore, the calculation using the Bernoulli equation would be 100 − 16 mm Hg or 84 mm Hg.

5. Answer: D. Although acceleration of flow in the LV outflow tract may make estimation of AVA difficult (uncertain LVOT VTI), AVA may still be below 1 cm² (Choice A is false). Aortic valve area measured by planimetry may be highly misleading, especially in patients with acceleration of flow in the LV outflow tract. Planimetered aortic valve area represents the geometric area of the valve, not the effective area of the valve, and these two measurements are different. Indeed, when the blood flow passes through a stenotic orifice, there is a contraction and acceleration of the flow, and the area where the flow jet is the smallest is called the vena contracta and is situated after the stenotic orifice. The ratio of the effective area and the geometric area is equal to the contraction coefficient. This coefficient is comprised between 0.61 and 1 (according to fluid dynamic) and depends on many factors including flow rate and shape of the valve. Thus, for a geometric aortic valve area of 1.3 cm², the effective area is comprised between 0.79 and 1.3 cm². Moreover, as flow is increased, the opening of the aortic valve (even the geometric one) could be higher than expected with normal flow. Thus, planimetered valve area cannot help in this case to assess the severity of the stenosis (Choice B is false). Severe AS has been associated with a delay (tardus) and reduction (parvus) in the upstroke of the aortic pressure, beginning at aortic valve opening, thus resulting in a delay to achieve the maximal instantaneous transvalvular gradient. Thus, acceleration time measured by continuous-wave Doppler is increased, not decreased, in severe AS and associated with adverse events (Choice C is false). Finally, as ejection time could be increased in AS too, the ratio of acceleration time over ejection time may be more accurate to identify severe AS and predict adverse events. A ratio ≥0.32 was found to be associated with increased occurrence of adverse events (Choice D is true).

6. **Answer: B.** The indexed stroke volume of the patient is 36 mL/m², thus not in the low-flow range (<35 mL/m²) (Choice A is false). As the patient is a man, flow could be considered low (sex-specific threshold in men <40 mL/m²); however, the sex-specific thresholds are not accepted by the current guidelines. The calculation of valvulo-arterial impedance (ZVa) is (systolic blood pressure + mean gradient)/stroke volume index. In this patient, ZVa = (136 + 29)/36 = 4.58 mm Hg/mL/m². ZVa is associated with worse outcome in patients with AS (ie, >4.5 mm Hg/mL/m²) (Choice B is true). The valvulo-arterial impedance gives an indication about outcomes; however, it does not evaluate the severity of the stenosis nor identifies the need for a valve intervention. Choice C is false because although it is suggested by European guidelines that patients with normal flow and a peak aortic jet velocity <4.0 m/s, and mean gradient <40 mm Hg probably, have nonsevere aortic stenosis, studies have suggested that 50% may have severe aortic stenosis and benefit from aortic valve replacement. However, not all patients with these echocardiographic findings have severe AS (indeed 50% have nonsevere AS) and the concomitant disease should be investigated/treated, such as hypertension and coronary artery disease (Choice D is false).

7. **Answer: C.** Subaortic stenosis does not respond well to balloon dilatation and surgical resection is recommended (class IIb) (Choice A is false). Presence of moderate aortic regurgitation is an indication for surgery, as further valve deterioration is expected due to a jet lesion from the subaortic acceleration. However, a noncalcified aortic valve is generally repaired rather than replaced in a young patient (Choice B is false). Associated lesions must be evaluated. The most common are patent ductus arteriosus, pulmonary valve stenosis (both can be diagnosed during TEE examination of the pulmonary artery and bifurcation; Choice C is correct), coarctation of the aorta (which can be diagnosed by pulsed-wave Doppler of the abdominal aorta; Choice D is false), and ventricular septal defect.

8. **Answer: B.** The parasternal long-axis view is not specific and Doppler measurements showed a moderate AS. The parasternal short-axis view reveals that the opening of the valve is asymmetric; thus, the valve is not tricuspid. Moreover, a raphe is visible between the right and left coronary cusps. Thus, Choice C is correct. This is the most frequent type of bicuspid valve as shown in **Figure 15.13**.

9. **Answer: C.** Parasternal long- and short-axis views show a normal aortic valve. Thus, Choice A is not correct. In the parasternal long-axis views, the distance between the anterior leaflet of the mitral valve and interventricular septum is sufficient and cannot explain the high gradient/velocity measured by continuous Doppler. Thus, Choice B is wrong. The continuous-wave Doppler jet shown in **Figure 15.2** has the contour shape and duration of transaortic flow and Choice E is thus not correct. Color Doppler shows aliasing of the velocity below the aortic valve, indicating that flow acceleration is at the subvalvular level. The correct answer is thus C. TEE confirms the presence of a membrane in the LV outflow tract causing the severe subvalvular stenosis (**Figure 15.14**).

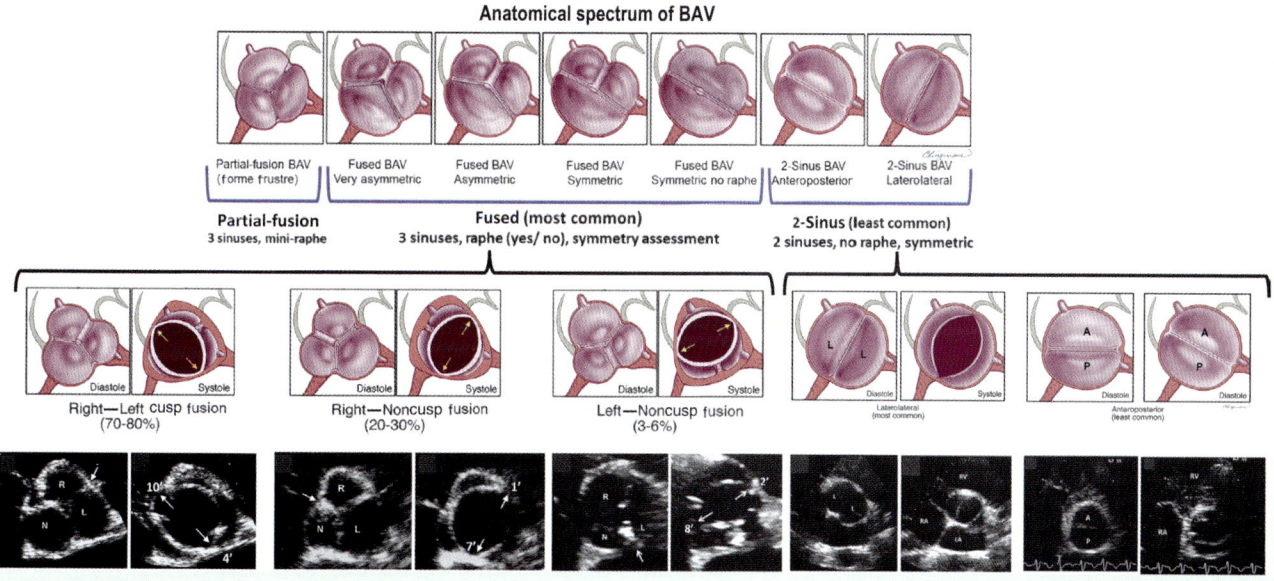

Figure 15.13. Schematic representation of the bicuspid aortic valve anatomical spectrum, fused bicuspid aortic valve phenotypes, and 2-sinus bicuspid aortic valve phenotypes as seen by parasternal short-axis transthoracic echocardiography as well as transthoracic echocardiography images.

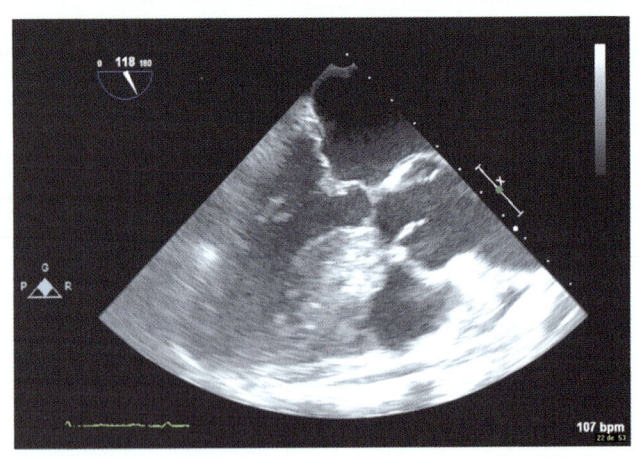

Figure 15.14. Transesophageal echocardiography. 3-chamber view centered on the left ventricular outflow tract showing a subvalvular membrane.

10. **Answer: C.** Choice A and B are wrong as the stroke volume could be used in the continuity equation:

$$Area_{LVOT} \times TVI_{LVOT} = Stroke\ Volume$$
$$= Aortic\ Valve\ area \times TVI_{Aortic}$$

$$Aortic\ Valve\ area = \frac{Stroke\ Volume}{TVI_{Aortic}}$$

$$= \frac{85}{75.2} = 1.13$$

Thus AVA = 1.13 cm² (Choice C).

11. **Answer: D.** The patient has an AVA > 1.0 cm² with a mean gradient of 33 mm Hg, thus the severity of AS is known: this is a moderate AS. Thus, Choices A, B, and C are false. Although a growing body of evidence indicates that patients with moderate AS and LVEF < 50% may benefit from AVR, we still have no randomized trials demonstrating this benefit. Although this patient indeed has moderate AS and hypertension, further evaluation of causes of symptoms and reduced LVEF should be explored; thus, Choice E is incorrect. The patient is young and thus most likely has a bicuspid valve. He thus could have concomitant aortic pathologies, which must be investigated.

12. **Answer: A.** The abdominal ultrasound demonstrates both systolic and diastolic flow in the abdominal aorta, indicating an aortic obstruction in the proximal part of the aorta. A normal flow pattern would require a brisk systolic upstroke and a rapid return to baseline at the end of systole. Thus, Choices C and D are incorrect. Further evaluation of the aorta is thus required.

Although this patient with a bicuspid aortic valve and a mildly dilated LV could have mixed aortic valve disease with a concomitant aortic regurgitation, the abdominal flow pattern is most indicative of obstruction rather than aortic regurgitation. Indeed, significant aortic regurgitation should demonstrate diastolic flow reversal. Thus, Choice B is incorrect. Moreover, the TEE examination should mainly be performed if aortic regurgitation was suspected by the TTE (which was not the case).

13. **Answer: A.** The difference in blood pressure between upper and lower limbs is significant. The best evidence to proceed with intervention for aortic coarctation includes systemic hypertension, upper extremity/lower extremity blood pressure gradient and echocardiography Doppler gradient, and anatomic evidence of coarctation (**Table 15.1**); thus, Choices B and D are incorrect as our patient presents all these features. Finally, the patient does not need an AVR as AS is moderate; thus, Choice C is incorrect.

14. **Answer: D.** This patient has severe stenosis as defined in ASE and ACC/AHA guidelines (**Table 15.2**). In this patient, the highest velocity and gradient were not recorded from the apical 5- or 3-chamber views, but from the right parasternal view. Indeed, in about 30% to 35% of patients, the highest velocity is obtained in views other than the apical ones. This raises the importance of performing multiple windows (apical 5-chamber, apical 3-chamber, right parasternal, suprasternal) for accurate measurement of transvalvular velocity and gradient in patients with AS.

Furthermore, the patient reports recent onset of symptoms (dyspnea and angina) likely related to AS. This patient thus has a class I indication for AVR according to the guidelines (**Table 15.3**). According to the most recent ESC and AHA/ACC guidelines,

Table 15.1. Therapeutic Recommendations for Coarctation of the Aorta

Recommendation	COR	LOE
Surgical repair/catheter-based stenting is recommended for adults with hypertension and significant native or recurrent coarctation of the aorta	I	B-NR
Balloon angioplasty for adults with native and recurrent coarctation of the aorta may be considered if stent placement is not feasible and surgical intervention is not an option	IIb	B-NR

COR, Class of recommendation; LOE, Level of evidence.

Table 15.2. Recommendations for the Grading of AS Severity

	Mild	Moderate	Severe
Echocardiography			
Peak aortic jet velocity (m/s)	2.6-2.9	3.0-3.9	≥4
Mean gradient (mm Hg)	<20	20-39	≥40
AVA (cm^2)	>1.5	1.1-1.5	≤1.0
Indexed AVA (cm^2/m^2)	>0.90	0.61-0.90	≤0.6
Velocity ratio[a]	>0.50	0.26-0.50	≤0.25
Computed Tomography			
Aortic valve calcium load (AU)			
Men	-	-	≥2000
Women	-	-	≥1200
Aortic valve calcium density (AU/cm^2)			
Men	-	-	≥500
Women	-	-	≥300

AS, aortic stenosis; AVA, aortic valve area.
The density is the calcium load divided by the cross-sectional area of the aortic annulus.
[a]Doppler velocity index = ratio of the LV outflow tract TVI to the aortic jet TVI, where TVI is the time-velocity integral.

this patient should be referred for TAVR, if transfemoral approach is feasible, as he is older than 75/80 years.

15. **Answer: B.** Doppler echocardiography may underestimate the transvalvular velocity and gradient (and so the severity of the stenosis) due to misalignment of the Doppler beam with transvalvular flow direction. However, Doppler rarely overestimates velocities and gradients. In this patient, the Doppler images are of good quality and those obtained from the right parasternal view clearly show a high gradient with severe stenosis. There is also no discordance between Doppler and two-dimensional echocardiography evaluation of stenosis severity and patient's symptomatic status. Therefore, there is no indication to perform an invasive assessment of aortic valve hemodynamics in this patient. Furthermore, crossing a stenotic aortic valve with a catheter is not without risk for the patient. Retrograde catheterization of the aortic valve has been shown to be associated with increased risk of cerebral emboli in patients with severe AS.

16. **Answer: B.** The most likely explanation for the discrepancies between Doppler echocardiography and catheterization for the measurement of transvalvular gradient is hypertension during catheterization. The pullback method generally overestimates the peak and mean gradients and thus the stenosis severity in patients with severe AS because of the space occupied by the catheter within the aortic valve orifice during the measurement of the LV systolic pressure. The simultaneous measurement of LV and aortic pressures is preferable for accurate measurement of peak and mean gradients by catheterization, particularly in patients with heart rhythm disorders, such as atrial fibrillation. It is also important to emphasize that the peak-to-peak gradient that can be measured by catheterization (but not by Doppler echocardiography) has no physiological relevance and is highly influenced by aortic compliance (ie, it is markedly reduced when compliance is low). This parameter should thus not be used for the assessment of AS severity.

The continuous Doppler interrogation of all windows, including the right parasternal window, allows more accurate estimation of transvalvular velocities and gradients and avoids underestimation of stenosis severity that may occur if only apical views are assessed. One should, however, pay attention not to mistake the mitral or tricuspid regurgitant flow velocity for the transaortic flow velocity in the right parasternal view. To overcome this pitfall, it is important to measure the duration of the flow in both the apical and right parasternal views. In this patient, the duration of the continuous-wave Doppler signals are very similar in both views (350 and 340 ms), thus confirming that the flow velocity recorded in the right parasternal view is indeed the transaortic velocity and this view shows the actual gradient.

Table 15.3. Recommendation for Intervention in AS

Recommendations	COR	LOE
AVR is recommended for patients with severe high-gradient AS who have symptoms by history or on exercise testing (stage D1)	I	B
AVR is recommended for asymptomatic patients with severe AS (stage C2) and LVEF < 50%	I	B-NR
AVR is indicated for patients with severe AS (stage C or D) when undergoing other cardiac surgery	I	B-NR
AVR is indicated for symptomatic patients with low-flow, low-gradient severe AS with reduced LVEF (stage D2)	I	B-NR
AVR is recommended for symptomatic patients with low-flow, low-gradient severe AS with normal LVEF (stage D3), if AS is the most likely cause of symptoms	I	B-NR
AVR is reasonable in apparently asymptomatic patients with severe AS (stage C1) and low surgical risk, when an exercise test demonstrates decreased exercise tolerance (normalized for age and sex) or a fall in systolic blood pressure of ≥10 mm Hg from baseline to peak exercise	IIa	B-NR
AVR is reasonable in asymptomatic patients with very severe AS (defined as an aortic velocity of ≥5 m/s) and low surgical risk	IIa	B-NR
AVR is reasonable in apparently asymptomatic patients with severe AS (stage C1) and low surgical risk; AVR is reasonable when the serum B-type natriuretic peptide level is >3 times normal	IIa	B-NR
AVR is reasonable in asymptomatic patients with high-gradient severe AS (stage C1) and low surgical risk; AVR is reasonable when serial testing shows an increase in aortic velocity >0.3 m/s per year	IIa	B-NR
AVR is reasonable in asymptomatic patients with severe high-gradient AS (Stage C1) and a progressive decrease in LVEF on at least three serial imaging studies to <60%	IIb	B-NR
AVR may be considered in patients with moderate AS (stage B) who are undergoing cardiac surgery for other indications	IIb	C-EO

AS, aortic stenosis; AVR, aortic valve area; COR, class of recommendation; LOE, level of evidence.
Adapted from Otto CM, Nishimura RA, et al. 2020 ACC/AHA guideline for the management of patients with valvular heart disease: executive summary: a report of the American College of Cardiology/American Heart Association Joint Committee on Clinical Practice Guidelines. *J Am Coll Cardiol.* 2021;77(4):450-500. Copyright © 2021 by the American College of Cardiology Foundation and the American Heart Association, Inc. With permission.

Doppler echocardiography and catheterization do not measure the transvalvular pressure gradient at the same location. Doppler echocardiography measures the velocity at the vena contracta where the pressure gradient is maximum, whereas catheterization measures the gradient at a few centimeters downstream of the vena contracta and so after pressure recovery has occurred. Downstream of the vena contracta, part of the pressure initially lost between the LV outflow tract and the vena contracta is recovered. Because of this pressure recovery phenomenon, the transvalvular pressure gradient is generally smaller at catheterization than at Doppler echocardiography. The magnitude of the pressure recovery is essentially determined by the ratio of the effective orifice area of the aortic valve and the cross-sectional area of the ascending aorta. The pressure recovery is clinically significant in patients with moderate or moderate to severe AS (AVA between 0.9 and 1.2 cm^2) and a small ascending aorta (diameter <30 mm). This patient has a severe stenosis and a medium size aorta. The pressure recovery in this patient is likely minimal and cannot explain the important discrepancy observed between the Doppler- and catheterization-derived gradients.

Left heart catheterization may be a stressful procedure for the patient and is thus often associated with hyperadrenergic response and acute increase in blood pressure. This patient already has a history of hypertension, which is only partially controlled by medication. The blood pressure was 148/70 mm Hg at the time of Doppler echocardiography versus 187/90 mm Hg at the time of catheterization. Previous studies have shown that acute hypertension may increase the LV afterload, which may in turn induce a decrease in LV outflow. Given that transvalvular gradients are highly flow dependent, even a modest reduction in flow may result in a major decrease in gradient.

> **KEY POINTS**
> - Doppler echocardiography is the first-line modality for the assessment of AS.
> - A multiwindow interrogation is key to obtain the maximum peak aortic jet velocity and gradients.
> - Surgical AVR is currently the recommended therapy in patients with severe AS and low or intermediate surgical risk and long life expectancy.

17. **Answer: E.** In patients with low LV ejection fraction, low-flow, low-gradient AS, a low-dose (up to 20 μg/kg/min) dobutamine stress echocardiography is useful (class IIa) to assess AS severity and evaluate LV contractile reserve. Exercise stress testing is contraindicated in symptomatic patients with severe AS (class III). Although rest echocardiography is inconclusive with regard to stenosis severity (ie, AVA is small suggesting severe stenosis but mean gradient is low suggesting moderate stenosis), right/left heart catheterization will not provide additional information beyond a resting echocardiogram because the patient will still be in low-flow state during catheterization. Hence, the AVA gradient discordance and uncertainty about stenosis severity will persist with rest catheterization and in fact a dobutamine stress catheterization would be required.

The use of contrast agents during dobutamine stress echocardiography is safe and may be helpful for myocardial visualization and assessment of LV ejection fraction. Contrast should be used in this patient given that two consecutive segments or less than 80% of myocardium were not visible. Contrast agents are also helpful for improving Doppler image quality (especially for the tricuspid regurgitant jet). The Doppler gain settings should be lowered when contrast is used, to reduce background noise. Hence, the optimal next step in this patient is to perform a low-dose dobutamine stress echocardiogram with injection of contrast (Choice E).

18. **Answer: D.** In low-flow state conditions, the valve may not be opened fully and so the AVA may be "pseudosevere" (ie, overestimates stenosis severity), whereas the gradient, which is highly flow-dependent, may be "pseudonormalized" (ie, underestimates stenosis severity). Hence, when there is a discordance between AVA (<1.0 cm^2) and mean gradient (<40 mm Hg) at rest Doppler exam, such as is the case in this patient, it is impossible to confirm the stenosis severity and a low-dose dobutamine stress echocardiogram should be performed to differentiate true- versus pseudosevere stenosis. Rest echocardiographic data cannot be used to confirm stenosis severity in such conditions and so Choices A and B are wrong.

Given that both gradient and AVA are flow-dependent but to various extents (gradient more flow dependent than AVA) and that the flow augmentation achieved by dobutamine stress may vary extensively from one patient to the other, it may be misleading to rely on only one parameter (gradient or AVA) to determine the stenosis severity during dobutamine stress echocardiography. The guidelines suggest a class IIa recommendation for AVR if dobutamine stress echocardiography shows a true-severe stenosis defined as a mean gradient ≥40 mm Hg and an AVA < 1.0 cm^2 at any dobutamine stage (not necessarily the maximum dose stage). In this patient, the gradient increased up to 44 mm Hg and the AVA remained below 1.0 cm^2 (ie, 0.60 cm^2) during dobutamine stress (**Figure 15.7**). Hence, the Choice C is wrong and the right Choice is D. If the AVA-gradient discordance persists with dobutamine stress (eg, stress AVA is 0.8 cm^2 and stress mean gradient is 35 mm Hg), one can calculate the projected aortic valve area at a normal flow rate.

19. **Answer: C.** In patients with low LV ejection fraction, operative risk would be at least intermediate. LV contractile reserve is however useful to further enhance operative risk stratification. LV contractile reserve has been defined as a percent increase in stroke volume ≥20% during dobutamine stress echocardiography. In the most recent guidelines, "LV contractile reserve" has been renamed "LV flow reserve" because the change in stroke volume during dobutamine stress echocardiography may be influenced by many other factors besides LV contractile reserve per se (ie, severity of AS, afterload mismatch, concomitant change in mitral regurgitation). This patient had a 31% increase in stroke volume with dobutamine stress and so would be considered at intermediate surgical risk. Previous studies reported 8% to 30% 30-day mortality following

surgical AVR versus 5% to 8% in those with flow reserve. A deterioration or absence of increase in LV ejection fraction during dobutamine stress echocardiography is often associated with worse prognosis. However, an improvement in ejection fraction, such as observed in this patient, has limited specificity because it may be due, in large part, to worsening of concomitant mitral regurgitation during dobutamine stress. Hence, Choices A, B, and D are wrong and Choice C is right. This patient has intermediate operative risk because he has reduced LVEF at rest and significant LV flow reserve during dobutamine stress echocardiography.

KEY POINTS
- In patients with low-LVEF, low-flow, low-gradient AS, low-dose dobutamine stress echocardiography is essential (i) to differentiate true vs pseudo severe stenosis and (ii) to assess the presence of LV flow reserve, which may be useful for surgical risk stratification. However, LV flow reserve is not associated with outcomes after transcatheter aortic valve replacement.
- Contrast should be used in patients with poor echogenicity (ie, two consecutive segments not visible).

20. **Answer: C.** Three years ago, this patient had a normal LV ejection fraction, a normal LV outflow, and moderate AS. Compared to this previous study, the patient had a significant decrease in LV ejection fraction, a reduction in LV end-diastolic diameter, and a marked decrease in stroke volume index. The stroke volume index measured on the current study is 30 mL/m², which is lower than the cut-point value of 35 mL/m² proposed in the guidelines to define low flow in patients with AS. The patient would thus be in a low-flow state although the LV ejection fraction (60%) is within normal range. The AVA has decreased markedly and is now in the severe range, whereas the gradient remains in the moderate range despite a mild increase compared to the previous study. The highest mean transvalvular gradient found after careful multiwindow interrogation by continuous-wave Doppler was 24 mm Hg.

The measurement of stroke volume in the LV outflow tract is subject to technical errors. In particular, the measurement of the LV outflow tract diameter may be challenging in patients with calcific AS. An underestimation of this diameter may result in an underestimation of stroke volume and AVA, and thus in a misclassification of the flow status (low vs normal) and stenosis severity (severe vs moderate). It is thus important to corroborate the measurement of LV outflow tract stroke volume by other methods. The biplane Simpson method is of limited utility for this purpose because it underestimates the LV volumes and thus the stroke volume, due to frequent foreshortening of the LV apex in the apical 4- and 2-chamber views. The assessment of LV volumes by three-dimensional echocardiography provides an accurate measure of LV stroke volume, but this imaging modality requires good-quality images. In this patient, three-dimensional echocardiography was not available. However, an estimation of LV stroke volume (SV) was obtained by multiplying the LV end-diastolic volume estimated by the Teichholz formula by the LV ejection fraction (LVEF):

$$SV = \frac{7 \times LVEDD^3}{2.4 + LVEDD} \times LVEF$$

$$SV = \frac{7 \times 4.2^3}{2.4 + 4.2} \times 0.60 = 47.1 \, mL$$

To avoid underestimation of the LV end-diastolic volume by Teichholz, it is important to measure the LV end-diastolic diameter (LVEDD) below the septal bulge (frequent in patients with AS), that is, where the LV cavity is the largest. In this patient, the LV stroke volume estimated by this method was very similar to the stroke volume measured in the LV outflow tract. Of note, this method cannot be used if ≥ moderate mitral regurgitation is present, which was not the case in this patient.

These data confirm that this patient has a low-flow state despite normal LV ejection fraction, an entity named "paradoxical low flow." This low-flow state is associated with a small AVA but a low gradient, and therefore, the stenosis severity remains undetermined with rest echocardiography. The patient reports no symptoms. However, about 30% of patients with severe AS claiming to be asymptomatic in fact have exercise-limiting symptoms at the time of exercise testing and these patients have a worse outcome. Hence, to guide the management of this patient, it is important to confirm both the symptomatic status and the stenosis severity. Exercise stress echocardiography fulfills these two objectives and the right answer is thus C. Exercise testing will determine the symptom status but not the stenosis severity, and dobutamine stress echocardiography will determine the stenosis severity but not the symptomatic status.

21. **Answer: C.** The patient had symptoms at a low level of exercise and the test was stopped prematurely. Hence, the patient is symptomatic. There was a minimal increase (+9%) in stroke volume with exercise stress echocardiogram and the discordance in AVA gradient that existed at rest (0.89 cm², 24 mm Hg) persisted at exercise (0.92 cm², 29 mm Hg). However, due to shortening in LV ejection time, the mean transvalvular flow rate increased by 20%,

which allowed the calculation of the projected AVA at a normal flow rate. This parameter provides an estimation of what the AVA would be at a standardized flow rate of 250 mL/s. In this patient, the projected AVA is 0.94 cm^2 (**Figure 15.8**), which would suggest a true-severe stenosis. Hence, Choices A and B are wrong.

This patient with paradoxical low-flow, low-gradient AS and preserved LVEF is symptomatic and has a severe stenosis according to the findings of exercise stress echocardiography. According to the ACC/AHA guidelines, AVR is recommended (class I) in patients who have low-flow/low-gradient severe AS (stage D3) with LVEF ≥ 50% if AS is the most likely cause of symptoms. For symptomatic patients who are 65 to 80 years of age and have no anatomic contraindication to transfemoral TAVI, either SAVR or transfemoral TAVI is recommended after shared decision-making. Thus, Choice C is right. This patient is however not at high surgical risk and thus Choice D is wrong.

Of note, in patients with discordant echocardiographic findings, it may be helpful to corroborate the stenosis severity using another imaging modality. Aortic valve scoring using multidetector computed tomography is the best modality for this purpose. The aortic valve calcification score measured in this patient was 3720 AU (**Figure 15.15**), thus corroborating the presence of severe stenosis. For a woman, the cut-point value of aortic valve calcium score to identify severe stenosis is >1200 AU.

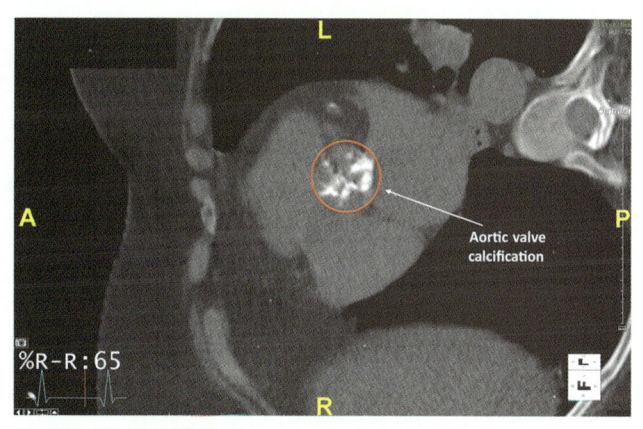

Figure 15.15. Multidetector computed tomography showing aortic valve calcification (red circle).

> **KEY POINTS**
> - Exercise stress testing is recommended to confirm symptomatic status in patients with severe (or possible severe) AS who claim to be asymptomatic.
> - Stress echocardiography and calculation of the projected AVA at normal flow rate may be useful to corroborate the stenosis severity in patients with paradoxical low-flow, low-gradient AS and preserved LVEF.
> - Assessment of aortic valve calcification load is a flow-independent marker of AS severity that may be useful in patients with paradoxical low-flow, low-gradient AS in whom stress echocardiography is not feasible or not conclusive.

22. **Answer: E.** This patient has a peak aortic jet velocity <4 m/s and a mean gradient <40 mm Hg with a normal LV ejection fraction and normal flow (stroke volume index >35 mL/m^2). According to the guidelines, he would thus be considered as most likely having moderate AS and no indication for AVR, even if he has a small AVA and he is symptomatic. However, it has been demonstrated that a substantial proportion of patients with discordant grading (ie, mean gradient < 40 mm Hg and AVA < 1 cm^2) and normal flow may have severely calcified aortic valves and may benefit from surgery. This subset of patients with normal-flow, low-gradient AS is highly heterogeneous and may include (i) patients with moderate AS and measurement error in the stroke volume and thus in the AVA; (ii) patients with moderate AS and small body surface area, in such case, AVA is small but indexed AVA is >0.6 cm^2/m^2, thus suggesting moderate stenosis; and (iii) patients with severe AS and discordant grading due to inconsistencies in the AVA gradient cut-point values used in the guidelines. Indeed, at a normal flow rate, the AVA cut-point value of 1.0 cm^2 generally used to define severe stenosis does not correspond to a gradient of 40 mm Hg, but rather to a value of 30 to 35 mm Hg.

In the patients with normal-flow, low-gradient but small AVA, it is difficult from the resting echocardiogram to be certain that stenosis is moderate or severe. Hence, Choices A, B, and C are wrong. The first step in these patients is to rule out errors in the measurement of stroke volume and AVA and ensure that the maximum velocity/gradient has been recorded by multiwindow interrogation. Once measurement errors have been ruled out, the next step, if the patient is symptomatic (such as is the case in this patient), is to confirm stenosis severity given that some of these patients (category iii described above) may have a severe stenosis despite the presence of low gradient and normal flow. Stress (exercise or dobutamine) echocardiography may not be the best approach in these patients because the transvalvular flow rate is already normal (Choice D is wrong). The assessment of aortic valve calcification load by MDCT may be helpful to corroborate the stenosis severity in the context of patients with normal-flow, low-gradient AS. The correct answer is thus E.

23. **Answer: E.** Recent studies emphasize that different cut-point values of aortic valve calcification load

should be used in women versus men to identify severe stenosis. Women reach hemodynamically severe stenosis with lower amount of aortic valve calcium, even after adjustment for smaller body size or annulus size (**Table 15.2**). In this male patient, aortic valve calcification load is 1810 AU and aortic valve calcification density is 426 AU/cm^2. The cut-point values that have been suggested to identify severe stenosis in men are >2000 AU for aortic valve calcium load and >500 AU/cm^2. Therefore, this patient likely has moderate AS and there is no indication for AVR. Hence, Choices A and B are wrong. This patient is symptomatic and should have a close clinical/echocardiographic follow-up. The symptoms in this patient may be related to other diseases including hypertension and coronary artery disease or the coexistence of severe disease (eg, moderate AS and moderate hypertension). Hypertension is often underdiagnosed and undertreated in patients with AS and it may contribute to the occurrence of symptoms and adverse events. Therefore, Choice E (C and D) is correct.

KEY POINTS

- In symptomatic patients with preserved LVEF, normal flow and discordant echocardiographic findings (eg, small AVA and low gradient), aortic valve calcium scoring with MDCT may be useful to corroborate the stenosis severity.
- Lower cutoff values of aortic valve calcification score should be used in women versus men to identify hemodynamically severe AS.

24. **Answer: C.** This patient is symptomatic; thus, exercise stress test is contraindicated; therefore, Choice A is false. As gradient and aortic valve area are discordant, the true severity of AS is unknown, thus another imaging test should be performed before undergoing AVR (Choice D is false). The LV ejection fraction of the patient is 55%; thus, dobutamine stress echocardiography is feasible, but not indicated by the guideline. The first-choice imaging test is computed tomography.

25. **Answer: B.** Aortic valve calcification is not severe, but the patient is symptomatic. Exercise stress testing is still contraindicated (Choice C is false). As a second test, dobutamine stress echocardiography could be considered. However, as the patient underwent noncontrast and contrast CT, the thickening of the valve could be assessed. According to the level of calcification and thickening of the valve, the stenosis could be considered severe. Actually, the aortic valve is infiltrated with amyloid substance as the patient had cardiac amyloidosis.

26. **Answer: D.** In patients with cardiac amyloidosis, transcatheter AVR has been shown to improve outcomes. Thus, Choice A is false. Given the impaired systolic and diastolic function, the patient is high risk for surgery; thus, transcatheter AVR should be preferred (Choice B is false). Finally, as ATTR cardiac amyloidosis has been diagnosed, tafamidis should be considered as it reduces all-cause mortality and cardiovascular-related hospitalizations, as well as reduces the decline in functional capacity and quality of life.

27. **Answer: A.** This patient has discordant echocardiographic findings with peak aortic jet velocity and mean gradient in the moderate range, while aortic valve area in the severe range. At TEE, the valve seems to open well and thus AS appears to be moderate. At CT evaluation, the valve calcification is borderline severe (ie, >2000 AU); however, the patient has a large valve (with an LVOT diameter at 27 mm). When indexed to the LVOT area, the aortic valve calcification density is only 367 AU/cm^2:

$$\text{AVC density} = \frac{\text{AVC}}{\pi \times \left(\frac{\text{LVOTd}}{2}\right)^2} = \frac{2100}{\pi \times 1.35^2} = 367$$

Despite not included in the current guidelines, AVC density has been shown to better predict outcomes. Threshold of AVC density to identify severe AS is 300 AU/cm^2 in women and 500 AU/cm^2 in men. These thresholds have been developed in tricuspid AS patients and then validated in bicuspid patients, in whom the use of AVC density has been shown to be superior to absolute AVC. In young bicuspid patients, especially women, fibrosis may be more preponderant than expected and false-negative patients by AVC density measurement are more frequent (ie, severe AS patients with low AVC density).

In our 45-year-old male patient, AVC density is in the moderate range and valve opens well at TEE. Thus, the stenosis is not severe (Choices B and C are false). Finally, regarding evaluation of AS severity, magnetic resonance imaging will not be helpful.

KEY POINTS

- In patients with small or large LVOT, aortic valve calcification should be indexed to the size of the aortic annulus to not over- (in large annulus) or under- (in small annulus) estimate the severity of AS.
- Aortic valve calcification was developed mostly in tricuspid patient. However, AVC density has been validated in bicuspid patients and is superior to absolute AVC. Thus, thresholds of AVC density could be used in bicuspid aortic stenosis, keeping in mind that young patients, especially women may have severe AS with low AVC density.

- AVC is probably not usable in rheumatic AS, as commissural fusion is the main process of stenosis, but could probably be used in radiation-induced AS, as calcification is the culprit of AS. In cardiac amyloidosis patients, aortic valve calcification could be less important than expected as amyloid substance may infiltrate the valve and thus participate to the obstruction. However, AVC was never tested in these types of AS.

SUGGESTED READINGS

Baumgartner H, Hung J, Bermejo J, et al. Echocardiographic assessment of valve stenosis: EAE/ASE recommendations for clinical practice. *J Am Soc Echocardiogr*. 2009;22:1-102.

Cartlidge TR, Bing R, Kwiecinski J, et al. Contrast-enhanced computed tomography assessment of aortic stenosis. *Heart*. 2021;107(23):1905-1911.

Clavel MA, Burwash IG, Mundigler G, et al. Validation of conventional and simplified methods to calculate projected valve area at normal flow rate in patients with low flow, low gradient aortic stenosis: the multicenter TOPAS (True or Pseudo Severe Aortic Stenosis) study. *J Am Soc Echocardiogr*. 2010;23(4):380-386.

Clavel MA, Ennezat PV, Maréchaux S, et al. Stress echocardiography to assess stenosis severity and predict outcome in patients with paradoxical low-flow, low-gradient aortic stenosis and preserved LVEF. *J Am Coll Cardiol Img*. 2013;6(2):175-183.

Clavel MA, Messika-Zeitoun D, Pibarot P, et al. The complex nature of discordant severe calcified aortic valve disease grading: new insights from combined Doppler-echocardiographic and computed tomographic study. *J Am Coll Cardiol*. 2013;62(24):2329-2338.

Clavel MA, Pibarot P, Messika-Zeitoun D, et al. Impact of aortic valve calcification, as measured by MDCT, on survival in patients with aortic stenosis: results of an international registry study. *J Am Coll Cardiol*. 2014;64(12):1202-1213.

Maurer MS, Schwartz JH, Gundapaneni B, et al. Tafamidis treatment for patients with transthyretin amyloid cardiomyopathy. *N Engl J Med*. 2018;379(11):1007-1016.

Michelena HI, Della Corte A, Evangelista A, et al. International consensus statement on nomenclature and classification of the congenital bicuspid aortic valve and its aortopathy, for clinical, surgical, interventional and research purposes. *Ann Thorac Surg*. 2021;112(3):e203-e235.

Pellikka PA, Sarano ME, Nishimura RA, et al. Outcome of 622 adults with asymptomatic, hemodynamically significant aortic stenosis during prolonged follow-up. *Circulation*. 2005;111(24):3290-3295.

Rosenhek R, Binder T, Porenta G, et al. Predictors of outcome in severe, asymptomatic aortic stenosis. *N Engl J Med*. 2000;343(9):611-617.

Shen M, Tastet L, Capoulade R, et al. Effect of age and aortic valve anatomy on calcification and haemodynamic severity of aortic stenosis. *Heart*. 2017;103(1):32-39.

Shen M, Oh JK, Guzzetti E, et al. Computed tomography aortic valve calcium scoring in patients with bicuspid aortic valve stenosis. *Struct Heart*. 2022;6(1):100027.

Stout KK, Daniels CJ, Aboulhosn JA, et al. 2018 AHA/ACC guideline for the management of adults with congenital heart disease: executive summary—a report of the American College of Cardiology/American Heart Association task force on clinical practice guidelines. *J Am Coll Cardiol*. 2019;73(12):1494-1563.

Writing Committee Members; Otto CM, Nishimura RA, Bonow RO, et al. 2020 ACC/AHA guideline for the management of patients with valvular heart disease: executive summary—a report of the American College of Cardiology/American Heart Association joint committee on clinical practice guidelines. *J Am Coll Cardiol*. 2021;77(4):450-500.

CHAPTER 16

Aortic Regurgitation

Joshua A. Cohen and Milind Desai

QUESTIONS

1. A 40-year-old man is referred for a cardiology evaluation after his primary care physician noted the presence of a blowing holodiastolic murmur. Transthoracic echocardiogram reveals a bicuspid aortic valve, a moderately dilated left ventricle (LVIDd 6.4 cm, LVIDs 4.5), and a left ventricular ejection fraction (LVEF) of 55%. There is a color Doppler jet from the aorta to the LV during diastole. The vena contracta is 0.7 cm, and the jet width/LVOT diameter is 65%. What quantitative echocardiographic findings would be consistent with the severity of aortic regurgitation suggested by data provided above?
   A. Regurgitant volume 50 mL/beat, regurgitant fraction 40%, EROA 0.25 cm^2.
   B. Regurgitant volume 70 mL/beat, regurgitant fraction 55%, EROA 0.4 cm^2.
   C. Regurgitant volume 40 mL/beat, regurgitant fraction 30%, EROA 0.2 cm^2.
   D. Regurgitant volume 55 mL/beat, regurgitant fraction 45%, EROA 0.25 cm^2.

2. In the asymptomatic patient in **Question 16.1**, the most appropriate recommendation is:
   A. Refer for aortic valve replacement.
   B. Follow up in 6 months with repeat echocardiogram.
   C. Recommend transesophageal echocardiography.
   D. Recommend exercise stress echocardiography.

3. Which of the following statements regarding aortic regurgitation (AR) is **CORRECT**?
   A. PISA radius of 0.8 cm with an aliasing velocity of 40 cm/s and a peak aortic regurgitant velocity of 4 m/s is consistent with severe AR.
   B. A pressure half-time greater than 200 ms is consistent with severe AR.
   C. Vena contracta is best evaluated from the apical long-axis view.
   D. The use of the suprasternal notch window is not useful in the assessment of AR.

4. What is the primary mechanism and severity of AR presented in **Figure 16.1**? Assume no concomitant cardiac pathology (isolated aortic valve disease) and an LVIDd of 6.6 cm.
   A. Moderate AR with aortic annulus dilatation and normal cusp motion.
   B. Severe AR with aortic annulus dilatation and normal cusp motion.
   C. Moderate AR with aortic cusp prolapse.
   D. Severe AR with aortic cusp prolapse.

5. An 85-year-old woman who underwent transcatheter aortic valve replacement (TAVR) 3 years ago presents for routine follow-up. Images from her echocardiogram are shown in **Figure 16.2**. The mechanism and severity of AR is **BEST** described by which of the following?
   A. Valvular AR, mild.
   B. Paravalvular AR, moderate.
   C. Paravalvular AR, mild.
   D. Valvular AR, severe.

Chapter 16 Aortic Regurgitation / 347

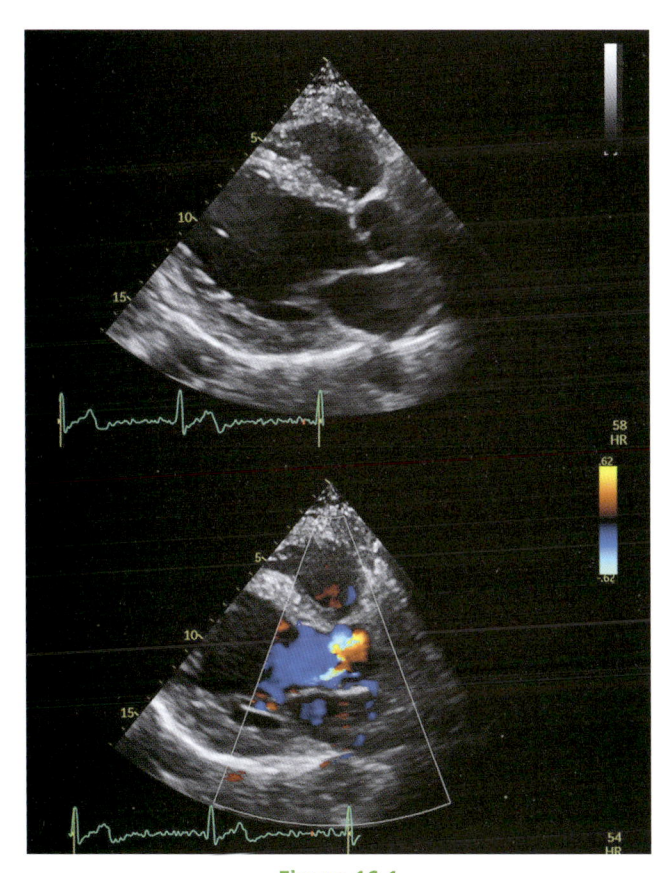

Figure 16.1

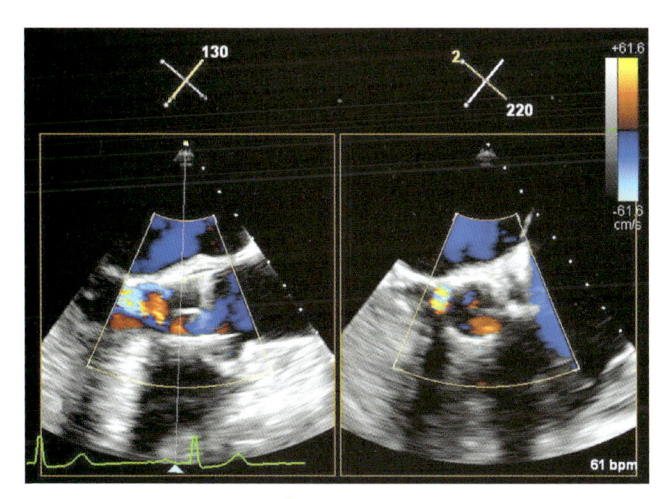

Figure 16.2

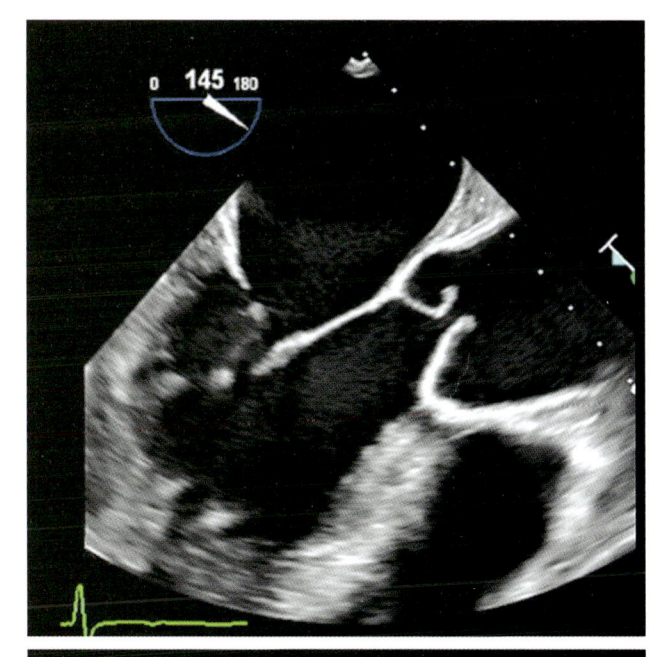

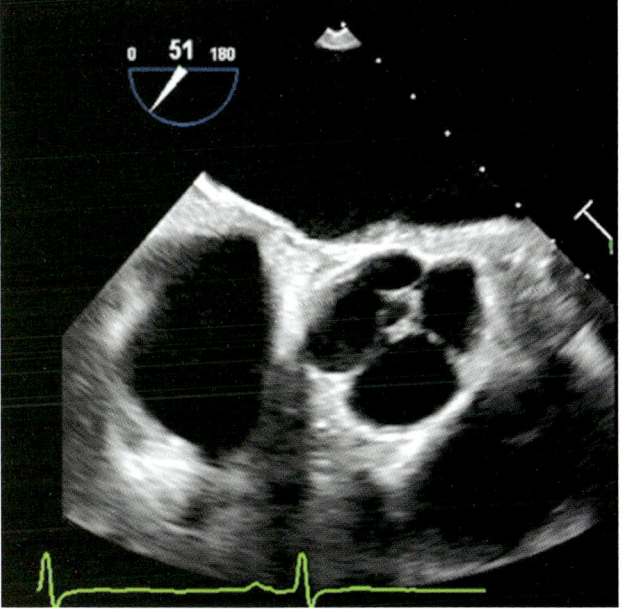

Figure 16.3

6. The anatomy of the valve shown in **Figure 16.3** is most commonly associated with what pathology?
   A. Aortic stenosis.
   B. Mitral regurgitation.
   C. Aortic regurgitation.
   D. Cleft mitral valve.

7. A 34-year-old asymptomatic man is referred for evaluation of AR. His Doppler echocardiogram shows a bicuspid aortic valve with AR (▶ Videos 16.1-16.4), a dilated LV (end-diastolic diameter 76 mm, end-systolic diameter 49 mm), an ascending aortic diameter of 4.6 cm, and an LV ejection fraction estimated at 45%. The effective regurgitant orifice area (EROA) measured by the PISA was 0.36 cm², and there was flow reversal in the descending aorta (**Figure 16.4A-C**). Which of the following statements regarding severity of AR is **CORRECT**?
   A. Aortic regurgitation is severe because the aortic regurgitant jet extends below the mid-ventricular level and the area of the jet is large.
   B. Aortic regurgitation is severe because EROA is >0.3 cm² and there is a holodiastolic flow reversal in the descending aorta.
   C. Aortic regurgitation is not severe because LV end-systolic diameter is <50 mm.
   D. Aortic regurgitation is severe because there is a holodiastolic flow reversal in the descending aorta and the LV ejection fraction is <50%.

8. The patient in **Question 16.7** is referred for surgery. At what size would it be indicated to also replace his ascending aorta?
   A. ≥4.5 cm.
   B. ≥4.2 cm.
   C. ≥5.0 cm.
   D. >5.5 cm.

CASE 1

A 65-year-old man presents with fever, acute hypoxemic respiratory failure, atrial fibrillation with rapid ventricular response (heart rate 120 bpm), and hypotension 2 weeks after a recent dental procedure. He is admitted to the intensive care unit.

Figure 16.5 shows key images from an emergent transesophageal echocardiogram (▶ Video 16.5).

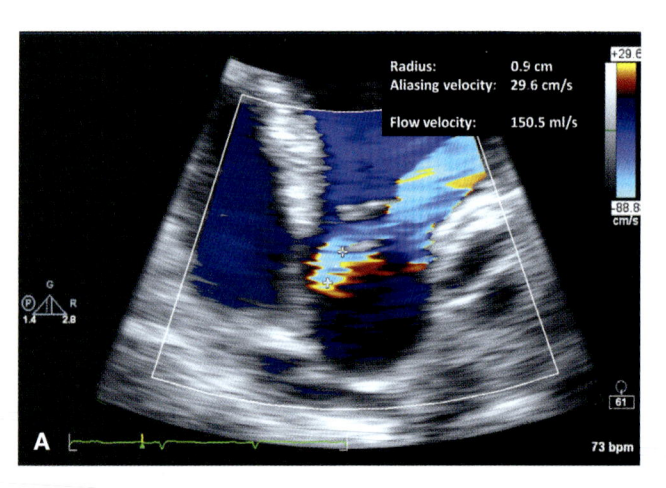

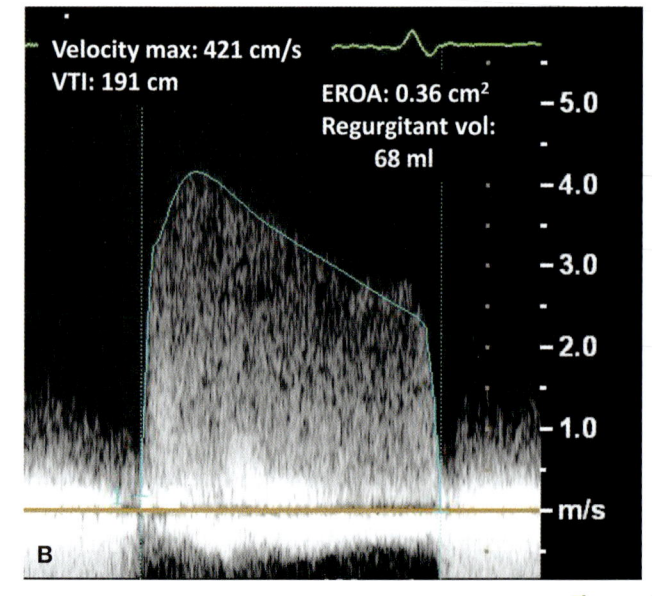

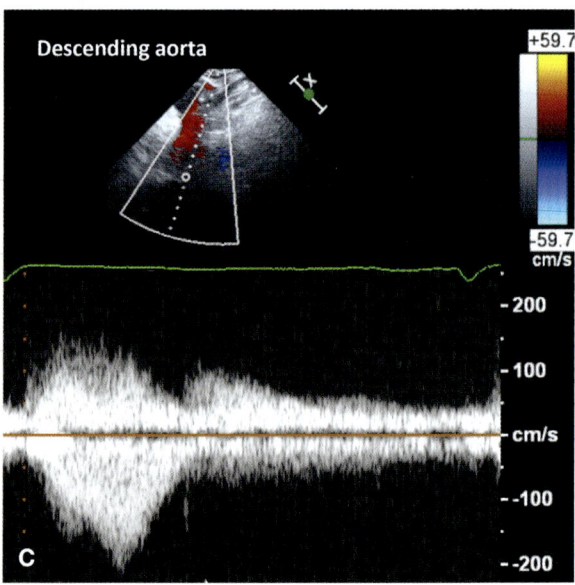

Figure 16.4

Chapter 16 Aortic Regurgitation / 349

9. What is the most appropriate management of the patient in **Case 1**?
   A. IV fluid administration for hypotension.
   B. Intra-aortic balloon pump insertion for hemodynamic support.
   C. Urgent cardiothoracic surgery consultation for aortic valve replacement.
   D. Beta-blockers for rate control in atrial fibrillation.

10. Additional images from **Case 1** are shown in **Figure 16.6**. The chronicity, severity, and mechanism of the aortic regurgitation are **BEST** described by which of the following answers?
    A. Chronic, severe aortic regurgitation due to prolapse and flail.
    B. Chronic, severe aortic regurgitation due to valve thrombosis.
    C. Acute, severe aortic regurgitation due to a large papillary fibroelastoma.
    D. Acute, severe aortic regurgitation due to infective endocarditis.

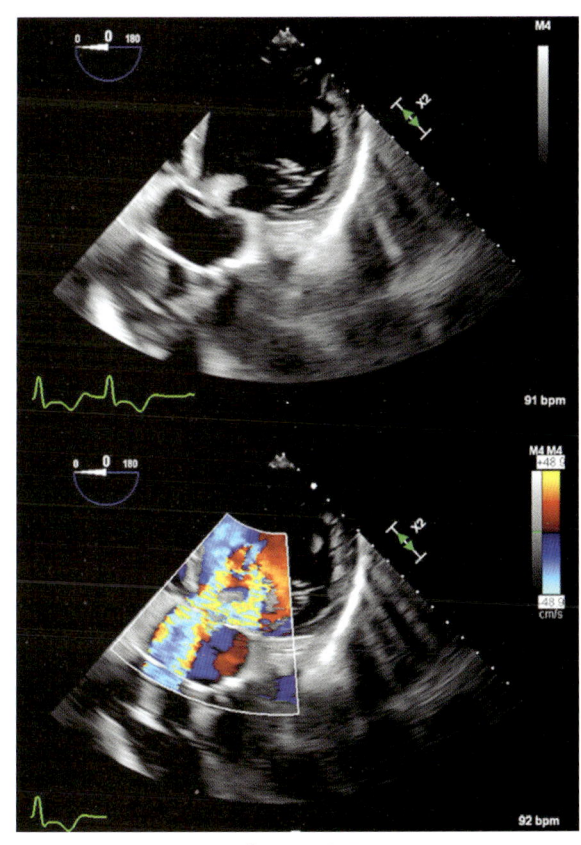

Figure 16.5

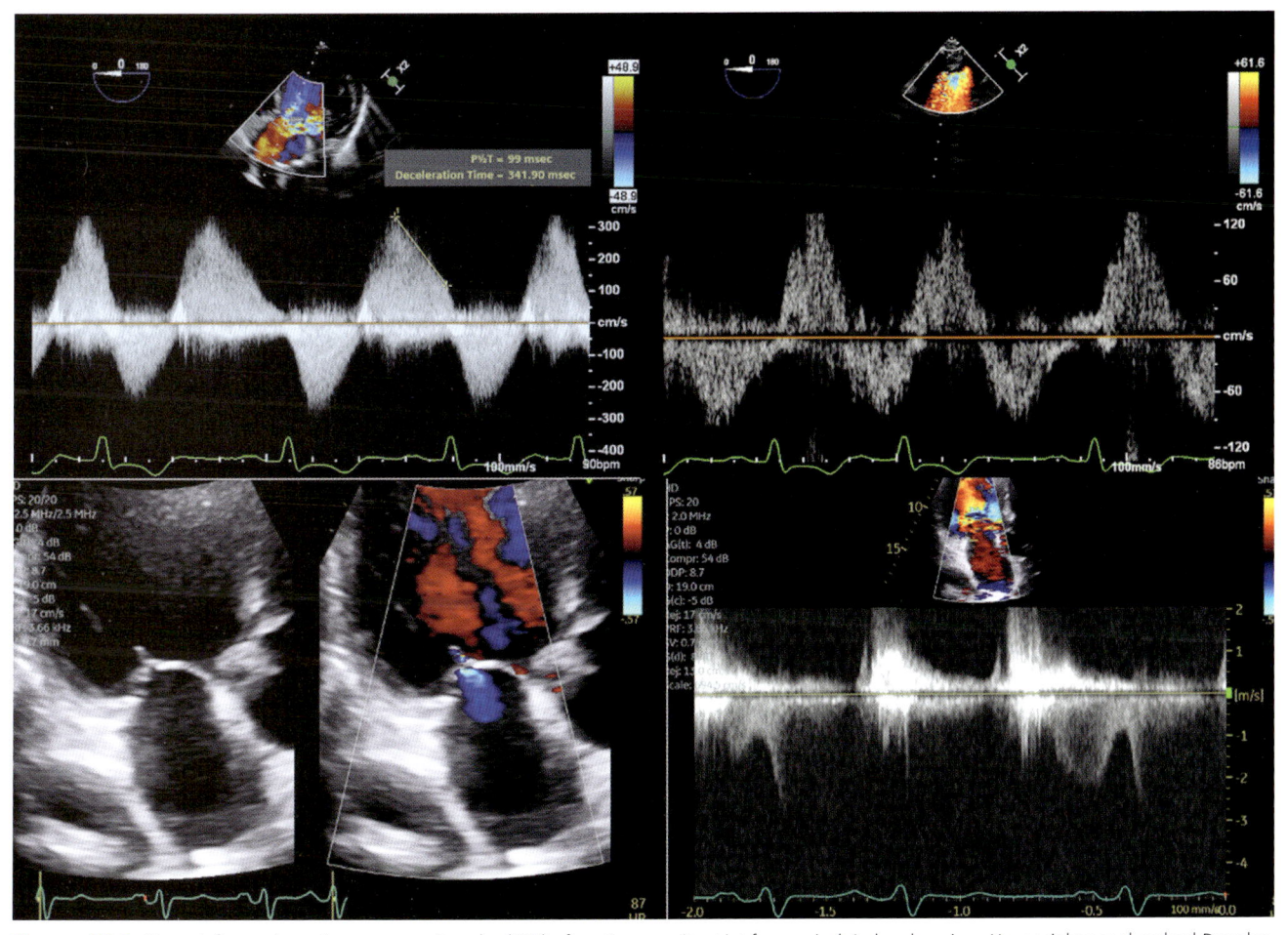

Figure 16.6. Upper left panel, continuous wave Doppler (CW) of aortic regurgitant jet from apical 4-chamber view; Upper right panel, pulsed Doppler ascending aorta; Lower left panel, apical 3-chamber view in systole; Lower right panel, CW Doppler apical 3-chamber view of mitral regurgitant jet.

CASE 2

A TEE is performed on a 65-year-old man after having a poor quality TTE reported as "suboptimal study due to limited windows, at least moderate aortic regurgitation." Key images are shown in **Figure 16.7**.

11. Based on the data provided in **Case 2**, what is the effective regurgitant orifice area (EROA)?
    A. 0.10 cm^2.
    B. 0.15 cm^2.
    C. 0.22 cm^2.
    D. 0.31 cm^2.

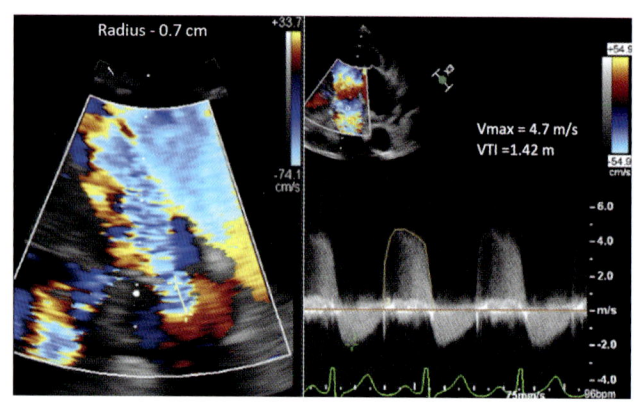

Figure 16.7

12. What are the regurgitant volume and regurgitant fraction for the patient in **Case 2**?
    A. RVol: 31 mL, RF: unable to be calculated with information provided.
    B. RVol: 38 mL, RF: 25%.
    C. RVol: 46 mL, RF: 36%.
    D. RVol: 61, RF: 55%.

13. From **Case 2**, the remainder of the patient's echocardiogram is within normal limits and the qualitative and semiquantitative data agree with the quantitative data above. As such, what is the severity of this patient's aortic regurgitation, and what is the most appropriate management moving forward?
    A. Mild aortic regurgitation, follow-up in 3 to 5 years.
    B. Moderate aortic regurgitation, follow-up in 1 to 2 years.
    C. Moderate aortic regurgitation, follow-up in 2 to 3 years.
    D. Severe aortic regurgitation, follow-up in 6 month to 1 year.

CASE 3

A 68-year-old man is referred to the cardiology clinic for a murmur appreciated on an annual physical exam. He reports an active lifestyle with no limitations. His LVEF is 65%, LVEDD 5.7 cm, LVEDV 191 mL, and LV EDVi 109 mL/m^2 (3D volumes). Images from his echocardiogram are shown in **Figure 16.8**

14. Based on the provided images provided in **Case 3** (**Figure 16.8**), What are the regurgitant volume and regurgitant fraction?
    A. RVol: 66 mL, RF: 52%.
    B. RVol: 46 mL, RF: 41%.
    C. RVol: 55 mL, RF: 48%.
    D. RVol: 70 mL, RF: 55%.

15. Under which condition would it be reasonable to recommend surgery for aortic valve replacement to the patient from **Case 3**?
    A. LVESD > 50 mm (LVESDi >25 mm/m^2).
    B. Undergoing other cardiac surgery.
    C. If serial echocardiography revealed EF decline to <55%, and LVEDD of >65 mm.
    D. All of the above.

16. Which of the following variables are not consistent with acute severe aortic regurgitation?
    A. Premature diastolic closure of the mitral valve.
    B. A flail cusp.
    C. Severely dilated left ventricle.
    D. EROA ≥ 0.3 cm^2.

17. Which of the following (from the Carpentier classification adapted for aortic regurgitation) best explains aortic regurgitation in patients with radiation-induced valvulitis?
    A. Type I: Normal cusp motion with aortic dilation or cusp perforation.
    B. Type II: Cusp prolapse.
    C. Type III: Cusp restriction.
    D. None of the above.

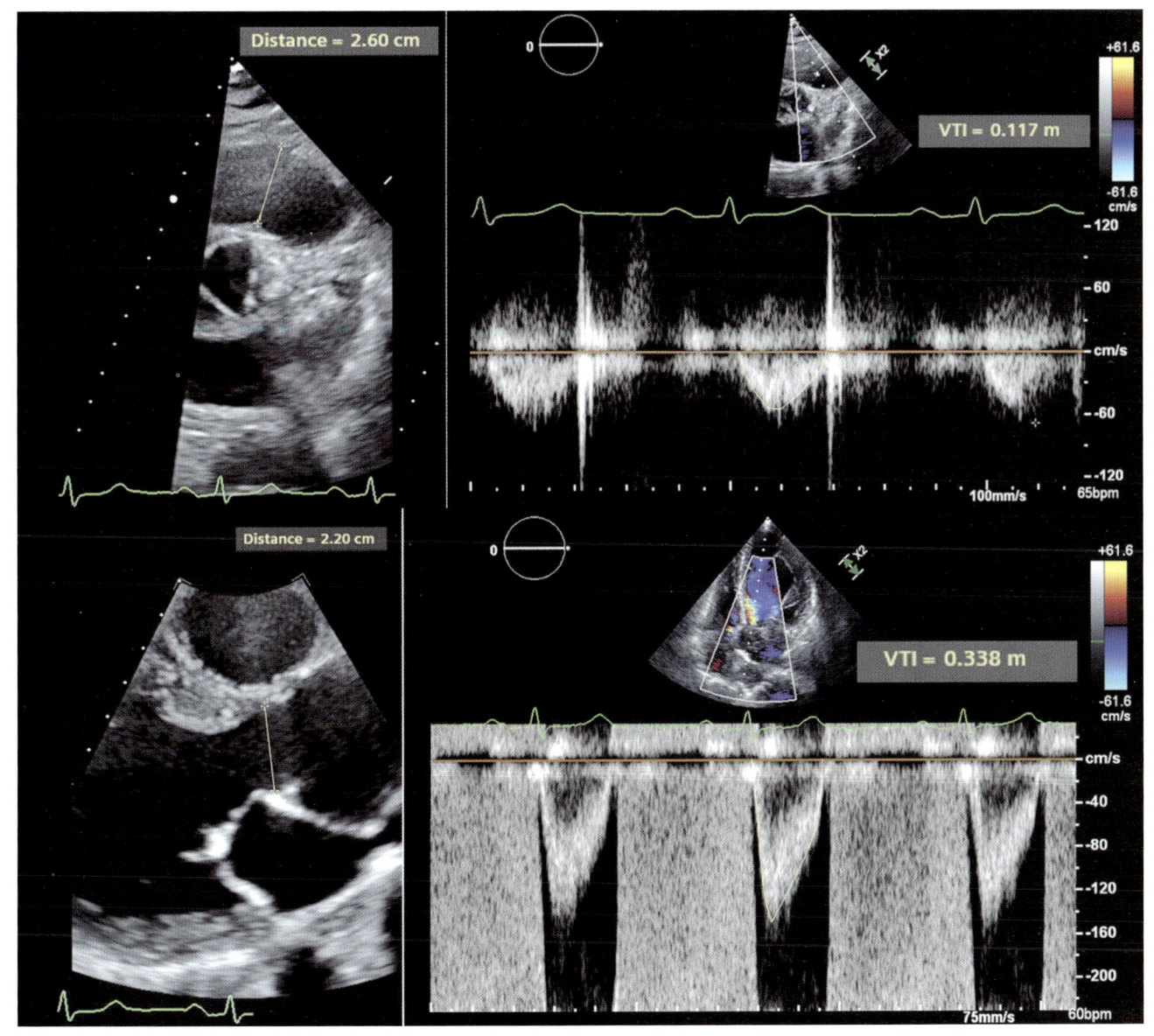

Figure 16.8. Upper left panel RVOT diameter; Upper right panel RVOT VTI; Lower left panel LVOT diameter; Lower right panel LVOT VTI.

18. Which of the following etiologies/mechanisms are not typically the cause of acute aortic regurgitation?
    A. Trauma.
    B. Endocarditis.
    C. Aortic dissection.
    D. Aortitis.

19. Which of the following is not a mechanism of aortic holodiastolic flow reversal in the upper descending aorta from echocardiographic images acquired from the suprasternal window?

    A. Moderate aortic regurgitation.
    B. Reduced aortic compliance in elderly patients.
    C. Rupture sinus of Valsalva aneurysm.
    D. Upper extremity AV fistula.

20. Which of the following asymptomatic patients with severe aortic regurgitation likely has the best prognosis if left unoperated?
    A. LVIDs 2.1 cm/m^2; GLS (−17%); LVEF 60%.
    B. LVIDs 2.6 cm/m^2; GLS (−19%); LVEF 56%.
    C. LVIDs 2.0 cm/m^2; GLS (−22%); LVEF 56%.
    D. LVIDs 2.3 cm/m^2; GLS (−22%); LVEF 50%.

352 / Clinical Echocardiography Review

21. Which of the following statements is most accurate when comparing patients with asymptomatic compensated severe mitral regurgitation to patients with severe aortic regurgitation undergoing valve surgery?
    A. Patients with mitral regurgitation typically have a drop in LVEF postoperatively.
    B. Patients with aortic regurgitation typically have a drop in EF postoperatively.
    C. Patients with aortic regurgitation typically have high afterload, and low preload before surgery.
    D. Patients with mitral regurgitation typically have high afterload, and low preload before surgery.

22. A patient with severe aortic regurgitation and congestive heart failure is given sodium nitroprusside awaiting surgical intervention. Which of the following statements is most accurate regarding the aortic regurgitant pressure half-time and regurgitant fraction?
    A. Regurgitant fraction will decrease; pressure half-time will shorten.
    B. Regurgitant fraction will decrease; pressure half-time will lengthen.
    C. Regurgitant volume will be unchanged; pressure half-time will lengthen.
    D. Cannot be determined.

ANSWERS

1. **Answer: B.** The patient in this question presents with the murmur of aortic regurgitation. The semiquantitative and qualitative findings on echo are consistent with severe AR. Quantitative echocardiographic measures utilizing the PISA method or volumetric assessment indicating severe aortic regurgitation would be regurgitant volume 60 mL/beat, regurgitant fraction 50%, and EROA 0.3 cm² (Answer B). It is important to note that these cutoffs mirror that of mitral regurgitation, except for the EROA (0.4 cm² in severe MR), as a smaller orifice area can produce similar regurgitant volume and fraction due to the longer length of diastole relative to systole. **Table 16.1** reveals the ASE criteria for grading severity of aortic regurgitation. Additionally, LV size can play a role in surgical decision making/timing. In asymptomatic patients with severe AR and normal LV function (LVEF > 55%), but LVESD >50 mm/LVESDi 25 mm/m² or progressive LV dilation with LVEDD >65 mm on serial echocardiography, it may be reasonable to consider aortic valve surgery.

2. **Answer: A.** The patient in Question 16.1 has severe aortic regurgitation with evidence of left ventricular remodeling as evidenced by moderate LV dilation, and relative LV systolic dysfunction (EF ≤ 55%). Despite having no symptoms, there is a class 1 indication for aortic valve replacement. The 2020 ACC/AHA guidelines for the management of patients with valvular heart disease increased the LVEF threshold from <50% to ≤55% in asymptomatic patients with chronic severe AR as evidence suggests the best outcomes when surgery is performed before LVEF drops below 55%. Answer B refers to a reasonable follow-up interval if following up a patient with chronic severe aortic regurgitation without a current surgical indication. Obtaining a TEE (Answer C) would be appropriate if the mechanism and/or severity were not clear from TTE. Exercise stress testing (Answer D) would be appropriate to illicit symptoms in an asymptomatic patient or to have an objective measure of exercise capacity to follow over time. **Table 16.2** reveals the indications for surgery in patients with aortic regurgitation.

3. **Answer: A.** This question refers to the quantification of aortic regurgitation utilizing the proximal isovelocity surface area (PISA) method to calculate the effective regurgitant orifice area (EROA). According to the continuity equation, the flow converging to the valve must be equal to the flow through the valve. As blood flow accelerates toward a narrowing orifice (in this case the regurgitant orifice), the spatial distribution of points in which the fluid has the same velocity (isovelocity surface) is approximated by a hemisphere.

   Based on this concept, one can transcribe the continuity equation as

   Isovelocity flow = regurgitant flow

   Isovelocity area × aliasing velocity
   $$= EROA \times \text{Regurgitant velocity}$$

   $2 \times \pi \times R^2 \times$ aliasing velocity
   $$= ERO \times \text{regurgitant velocity}$$

   $$EROA = \frac{2 \times \pi \times R^2 \times \text{aliasing velocity}}{\text{Regurgitant velocity}}$$

   Replacing the numbers, this becomes:

   $$EROA = \frac{2 \times \pi \times 0.8^2 \times 40}{400} = 0.40 \text{ cm}^2,$$

Table 16.1. Recommendations for the Grading of Aortic Regurgitation Severity

Parameters	Mild	Moderate	Severe
Qualitative			
Aortic valve morphology	Normal/abnormal	Normal/abnormal	Abnormal/flail/large coaptation defect
Color flow AR jet width[a]	Small in central jets	Intermediate	Large in central jet, variable in eccentric jets
CW signal of AR jet	Incomplete/faint	Dense	Dense
Diastolic flow reversal in the descending aorta	Brief, protodiastolic flow reversal	Intermediate	Holodiastolic flow reversal (end-diastolic velocity 0.20 cm/s)
Diastolic flow reversal in the abdominal aorta	Absent	Absent	Present
Semiquantitative			
Jet width (% of LVOT)	<25%	25%-64%	≥65%
VC width (mm)	<3	Intermediate	≥6
Pressure half-time (ms)[b]	>500	Intermediate	<200
Angiography grade	1+	2+	3+ and 4+
Quantitative			
Regurgitant fraction, %	<30%	30%-49%	≥50%
EROA (mm^2)	<10	10-29[c]	≥30
RVol (mL)	<30	30-44; 45-59[c]	≥60
LV size[d]	Normal	Normal/mild dilation	Dilated

AR, aortic regurgitation; CW, continuous wave; EROA, effective regurgitant orifice area; LV, left ventricle; LVOT, left ventricular outflow tract; RVol, regurgitant volume; VC, vena contracta.

Adapted from Zoghbi WA, Adams D, Bonow RO, et al. Recommendations for noninvasive evaluation of native valvular regurgitation: a report from the American Society of Echocardiography developed in Collaboration with the Society for Cardiovascular Magnetic Resonance. *J Am Soc Echocardiogr.* 2017;30(4):303-371. Copyright © 2017 by the American Society of Echocardiography. With permission; Otto CM, Nishimura RA, Bonow RO, et al. 2020 ACC/AHA Guideline for the management of patients with valvular heart disease: executive summary: a report of the American College of Cardiology/American Heart Association Joint Committee on Clinical Practice Guidelines. *Circulation.* 2021;143(5):e35-e71 and Nishimura RA, Otto CM, Bonow RO, et al. 2014 AHA/ACC guideline for the management of patients with valvular heart disease: a report of the American College of Cardiology/American Heart Association Task Force on Practice Guidelines. *J Am Coll Cardiol.* 2014;63(22):e57-e185.

[a]At a Nyquist limit of 50 to 60 cm/s.
[b]Pressure half-time is shortened with increasing LV diastolic pressure, with vasodilator therapy, and in patients with a dilated compliant aorta or lengthened in chronic AR.
[c]Grading of the severity of AR classifies regurgitation as mild, moderate, or severe and subclassifies the moderate regurgitation group into "mild to moderate" (EROA of 10-19 mm^2 or an RVol of 20-44 mL) and "moderate to severe" (EROA of 20-29 mm^2 or an RVol of 45-59 mL).
[d]LV size is generally normal in acute AR.

---

consistent with severe AR (Answer A is correct).

A pressure half-time of less than 200 ms is consistent with severe AR and will often be seen in acute severe AR. With ventricular remodeling secondary to the chronic volume loading in chronic severe AR, the pressure half-time will often lengthen. The vena contracta is best measured in the parasternal long axis (best axial resolution); in the apical long-axis view, the vena contracta will typically be parallel to the ultrasonic beam, reducing the spatial resolution (Answer C is incorrect). The suprasternal notch window allows Doppler evaluation for flow reversal in the descending thoracic aorta; holodiastolic flow reversal in the descending thoracic aorta or abdominal aorta is suggestive of severe AR (Answer D is incorrect).

4. **Answer: D.** The regurgitant jet (color Doppler) is eccentric and appears at least moderate. Additionally, the left ventricle in the parasternal long-axis view is at least moderately dilated (LVEDD ~6.6 cm). Hence, AR is likely severe. Answers A and C are wrong. As shown in the parasternal long-axis view, the aortic annulus is not dilated and the leaflets are not restricted; thus, Answers B is wrong. This mechanism of AR and regurgitant jet is better appreciated in the deep transgastric view on TEE

Table 16.2. Recommendation for Intervention in Chronic Aortic Regurgitation

Recommendations	COR	LOE
AVR is indicated for symptomatic patients with severe AR regardless of LV systolic function (stage D)	I	B-NR
AVR is indicated for asymptomatic patients with chronic severe AR and LV systolic dysfunction (LVEF ≤ 55%) (stage C2)	I	B-NR
AVR is indicated for patients with severe AR (stage C or D) while undergoing cardiac surgery for other indications	I	C-EO
AVR is reasonable for asymptomatic patients with severe AR with normal LV systolic function (LVEF > 55%) but with severe LV dilation (LVESD >50 mm/LVESDi 25 mm/m², stage C2)	IIa	B-NR
AVR is reasonable in patients with moderate AR (stage B) who are undergoing other cardiac surgery	IIa	C-EO
AVR may be considered for low-risk asymptomatic patients with severe AR and normal LV systolic function (LVEF >55%, stage C1) but with progressive decline in EF to the low-normal range (55%-60%) or progressive LV dilation to the severe range (LVEDD >65 mm) on at least three serial studies	IIb	B-NR

AR, aortic regurgitation; AVR, aortic valve replacement; EF, ejection fraction; EO, expert opinion; LV, left ventricular; LVEF, left ventricular ejection fraction; LVESD, LV end-systolic dimension; LVEDD, LV end-diastolic dimension; LVESDi, LV end-systolic dimension; NR, nonrandomized.
Adapted from Otto CM, Nishimura RA, Bonow RO, et al. 2020 ACC/AHA guideline for the management of patients with valvular heart disease: executive summary—a report of the American College of Cardiology/American Heart Association Joint Committee on Clinical Practice Guidelines. *Circulation.* 2021;143(5):e35.

(**Figure 16.9**). This patient had a bicuspid aortic valve (with RCC/LCC fusion) and prolapse of the fused leaflets in diastole. The 3D structure of this valve can be seen in **Figure 16.10**. Thus, the correct Answer is D.

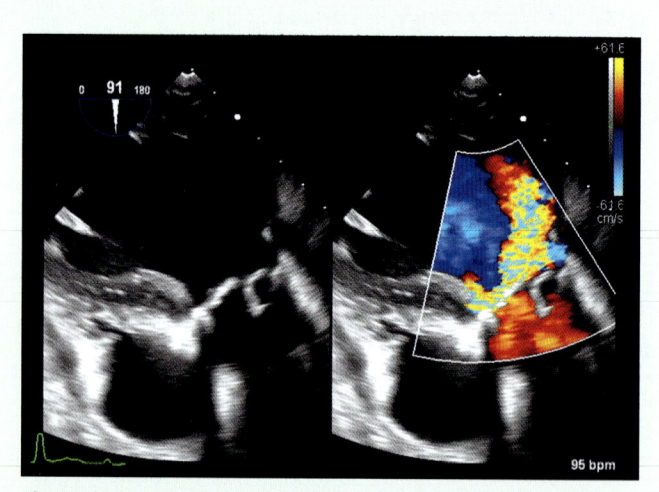

Figure 16.9. Transgastric transesophageal echocardiogram images demonstrating aortic valve cusp prolapse with a resultant severe posteriorly directed eccentric aortic regurgitant jet.

5. **Answer: B.** The figures in this question show long- and short-axis images of this patient's prosthetic aortic valve. The regurgitant jet passes around the stent frame of the transcatheter valve and is thus paravalvular. As with native valve regurgitation, multiple qualitative, semiquantitative, and quantitative parameters should be integrated to determine the severity of AR. Additional focus should be placed on prosthetic valve seating/positioning and leaflet structure/mobility. An additional semiquantitative parameter often used in the evaluation of paravalvular leak is the circumferential extent of the leak. Less than 10% of the circumference is considered mild, 10% to 29% moderate and ≥30% severe. This jet appears at least moderate with a circumferential extent of ~20% to 25%. Given this is the only information we are given, the best Answer choice is B. **Figure 16.11** helps in identifying the location and severity of paravalvular AR.

6. **Answer: C.** The valve shown in **Figure 16.3** is a quadricuspid aortic valve. Though a rare congenital anomaly, in the largest case series of patients with quadricuspid valves, the most common valvular pathology was aortic regurgitation with nearly one-third presenting with moderate or severe AR. **Figure 16.12** shows the same images as in **Figure 16.3** but with color Doppler (revealing severe aortic regurgitation). About one-third of these patients will have additional congenital anomalies and/or aortic dilation and as such should be screened appropriately. While the anatomy is well appreciated on the 2D images provided, the 3D structure of the quadricuspid valve referenced in the question can be seen in ▶ **Video 16.6**.

7. **Answer: B.** According to the 2020 ACC/AHA guidelines, and 2017 ASE guidelines for valvular regurgitation, the parameters and criteria that are proposed to define severe AR are a ratio of regurgitant jet width to LVOT diameter ≥65%, a vena contracta

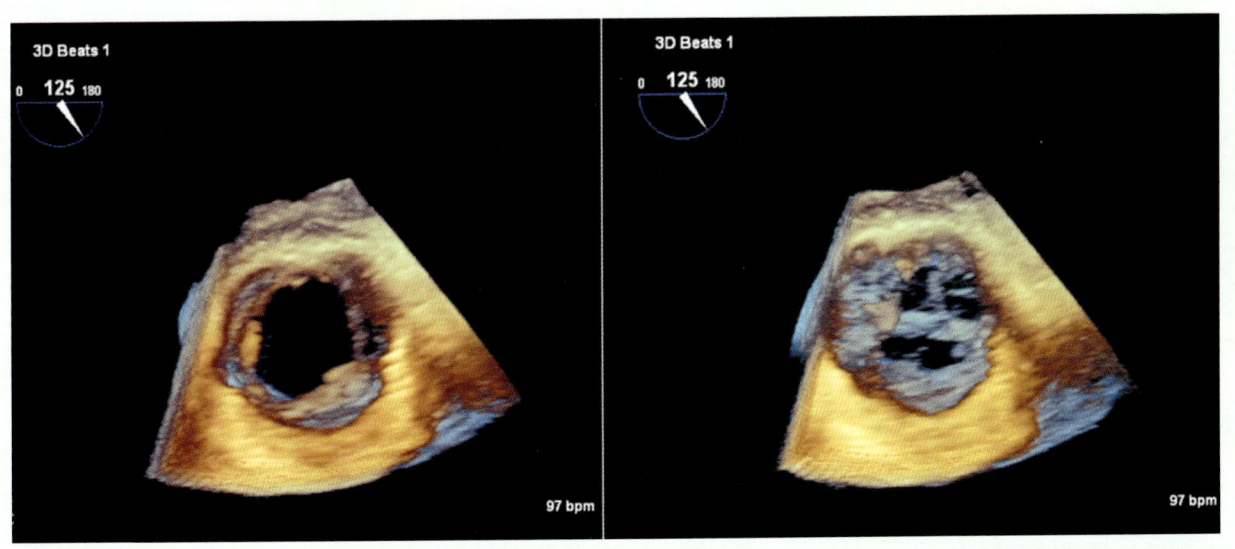

Figure 16.10. Three-dimensional images in systole (left) and diastole (right) showing bicuspid aortic valve with right/left coronary cusp fusion and prolapsing fused segment during diastole.

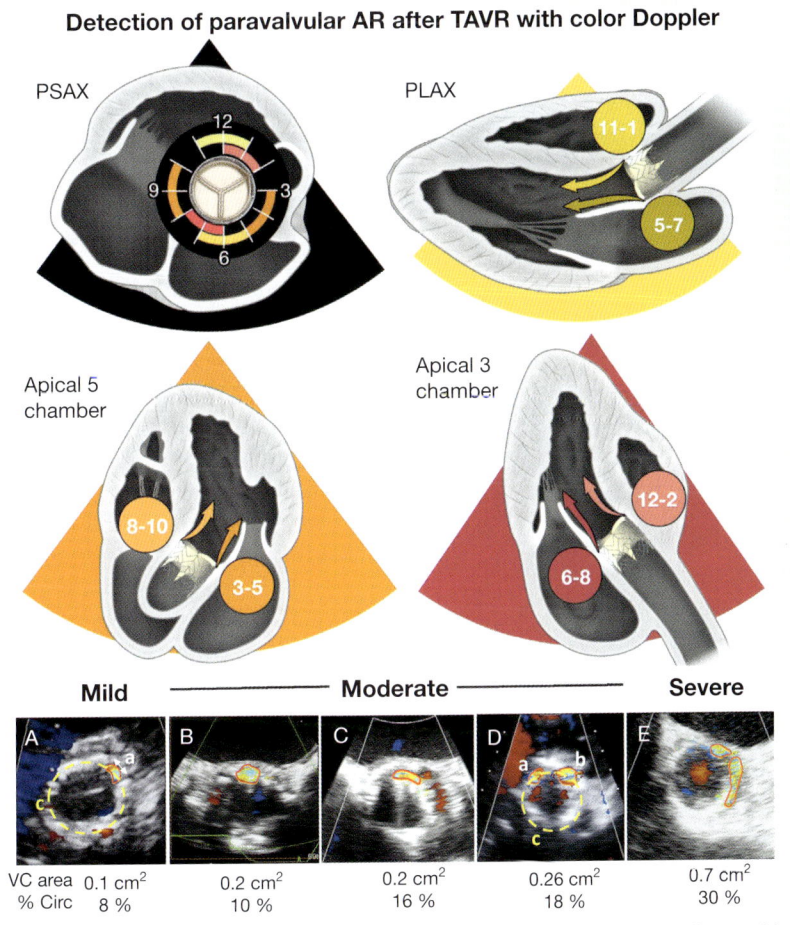

Figure 16.11. Detection of paravalvular leak location and quantification based on percentage of valve circumference (short axis). (Reprinted from Zoghbi WA, Asch FM, Bruce C, et al. Guidelines for the evaluation of valvular regurgitation after percutaneous valve repair or replacement: a report from the American Society of Echocardiography developed in collaboration with the Society for Cardiovascular Angiography and Interventions, Japanese Society of Echocardiography, and Society for Cardiovascular Magnetic Resonance. *J Am Soc Echocardiogr*. 2019;32(4):431-475. Copyright © 2019 by the American Society of Echocardiography. With permission.)

>0.6 cm, the presence of holodiastolic flow reversal in the descending aorta, an EROA ≥0.3 cm², a regurgitant volume ≥60 mL/beat, and a regurgitant fraction ≥50%. In addition, the diagnosis of chronic severe AR requires evidence of LV dilation.

The extent or area of the aortic regurgitant jet in the LV cavity is not reliable to assess the severity of AR and thus Answer A is wrong. The finding of LV end-systolic diameter >50 mm is a criterion used to identify LV systolic dysfunction and may prompt

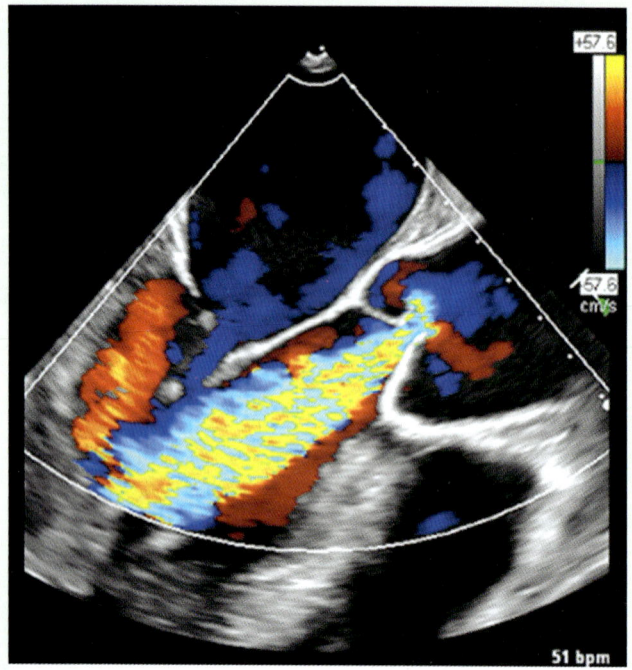

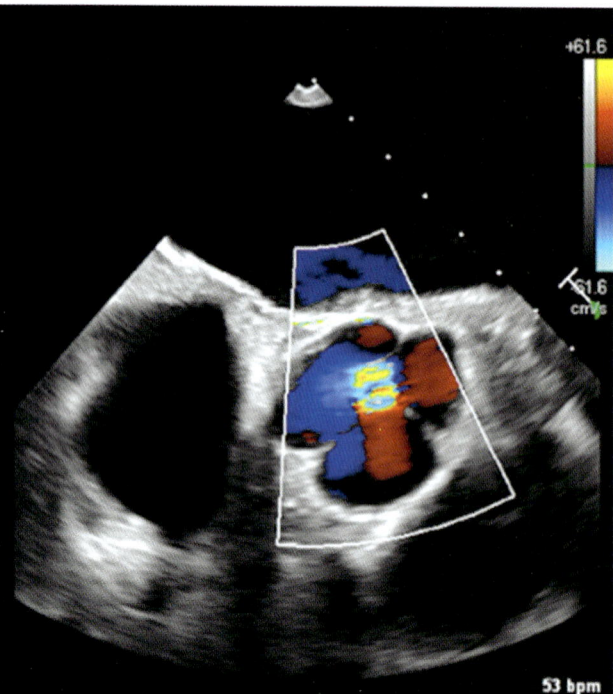

Figure 16.12. Color Doppler evaluation of both long- and short-axis view of quadricuspid aortic valve.

a recommendation for intervention in patients with severe AR despite an LVEF >55%; however, this finding is not a prerequisite to confirm the presence of severe AR. So Answer C is wrong. Holodiastolic flow reversal in the descending aorta is supportive of severe AR. However, this parameter cannot be used in isolation because there are often false positives, especially in patients with reduced aortic compliance such as is often the case in elderly patients. An LV ejection fraction <50% is a marker of LV dysfunction, but the decrease in LV ejection fraction may also be related to other concomitant diseases besides severe AR and vice versa, a large proportion of patients with severe AR have preserved LV ejection fraction. This parameter thus lacks sensitivity and specificity for the identification of severe AR. So Answer D is wrong.

In this patient, the EROA is ≥0.3 cm² and there is holodiastolic flow reversal in the descending aorta and significant LV dilation (LV end-diastolic diameter: 76 mm). The correct answer is B.

8. **Answer: A.** Based on the most recent ACC/AHA 2022 aortic disease guidelines, in patients with a bicuspid valve who are undergoing valve surgery and have an aortic root or ascending aorta ≥4.5 cm, it is reasonable to replace the aorta as well (class IIa) if at an experienced center. Thus, Answer A is correct. This situation is different from the primary indication for surgery being the aorta in a patient with a normally functioning bicuspid valve in which case thresholds are different at ≥5.5 cm (class I), ≥5.0 + additional risk factor for dissection (class IIa), and ≥5.0 and no additional risk factors for dissection (class IIb).

9. **Answer: C.** The patient described is critically ill and has endocarditis with a large aortic valve vegetation that can be seen prolapsing into the LVOT in diastole. There is associated torrential aortic valve regurgitation that has resulted in hemodynamic decompensation. Surgery is the appropriate definitive management (Answer C). Administering fluids when the patient is likely suffering from acute pulmonary edema is ill-advised and thus Answer A is incorrect. Insertion of an intra-aortic balloon pump is contraindicated in patients with aortic regurgitation and thus Answer B is incorrect. Despite the patient presenting in atrial fibrillation with rapid ventricular response, forward flow and cardiac output are heavily dependent on the elevated heart rate in this scenario and thus Answer D is incorrect.

10. **Answer: D.** The patient presents with acute severe aortic regurgitation in the context of infective endocarditis and a large aortic valve vegetation. The additional images provided reveal holodiastolic flow reversal in the ascending thoracic aorta (**Figure 16.6**, top right), a dense CW Doppler tracing with a very short pressure half-time (PHT < 200 ms) (**Figure 16.6**, top left), and diastolic mitral regurgitation (**Figure 16.6**, bottom two panels). The clinical history in conjunction with these findings support a diagnosis of acute severe AR. A very short PHT and diastolic MR are representative of a rapid and significant rise in LV diastolic pressure, which may happen more commonly in acute AR, though neither is necessarily specific to differentiate between acute and chronic AR. Prolapse and flail, valve thrombosis, and papillary fibroelastoma would not fit the clinical scenario described. Additionally, the echocardiographic appearance would be different from that of the images presented.

KEY POINTS
Case 1
- Doppler echocardiography is the first-line modality for the assessment of AR.
- Multiple parameters should be integrated to determine the acuity and severity of aortic regurgitation.
- The hemodynamic consequences of acute versus chronic severe AR are very different, and present differently. Acute severe AR often requires urgent if not emergent surgery/intervention.

11. Answer: C. The images provided supply all of the necessary information to perform quantification of aortic regurgitation utilizing the PISA method.

$$\text{Area(hemisphere)} \times \text{Velocity(Alias)} = \text{EROA} \times \text{AR peak velocity}$$

$$\left(2\pi \times (0.7\ \text{cm})^2 \times 33.7\ \text{cm/s}\right) / 470\ \text{cm/s} = \text{EROA}$$

$$\text{EROA} = 0.22\ \text{cm}^2$$

One must make sure to convert units of the aortic regurgitant peak velocity (from m/s to cm/s to obtain the correct value).

12. Answer: A. The regurgitant volume can be calculated by multiplying the EROA by the aortic regurgitant VTI, which is provided in the figure. Given that there is no LVOT VTI or volumetric assessment (for the purposes of calculating stroke volume) shown in the figure provided, one cannot calculate the regurgitant fraction. As such, Answer A is correct.

$$\text{EROA} = 0.22\ \text{cm}^2$$
$$\text{VTI AR} = 142\ \text{cm}$$
$$0.22\ \text{cm}^2 \times 142\ \text{cm} = 31\ \text{mL}$$

13. Answer: B. This patient has moderate aortic regurgitation based on a quantitative assessment with an EROA of 0.22 cm² and regurgitant volume of 31 mL. As shown in **Table 16.3**, the appropriate follow-up for AR of moderate severity would be in 1 to 2 years.

KEY POINTS
Case 2
- Quantitative assessment of AR can be performed utilizing the PISA method.
- The frequency of follow-up for patients with aortic regurgitation is based on the severity of aortic regurgitation and/or the interval development of symptoms.

14. Answer: A. This question provides all of the necessary information to calculate the regurgitant volume and fraction using volumetric data. This can be performed by subtracting mitral valve stroke volume from the LVOT stroke volume (RVol = SV LVOT − SV MV) or by subtracting the RVOT SV from the LVOT stroke volume. The latter method is also helpful if there is concomitant mitral regurgitation. Using these data:

$$\text{RVOT SV} : 0.785 \times (\text{RVOT diameter})^2 \times \text{RVOT VTI}$$

$$0.785 \times (2.6\ \text{cm})^2 \times 11.6\ \text{cm} = 62\ \text{mL}$$

$$\text{LVOT SV} = 0.785 \times (\text{LVOT diameter})^2 \times \text{LVOT VTI}$$

$$0.785 \times (2.2\ \text{cm})^2 \times 33.8\ \text{cm} = 128\ \text{mL}$$

$$\text{RVol} = \text{LVOT SV} - \text{RVOT SV}$$

$$\text{RVol} = 128 - 62 = 66\ \text{mL}$$

$$\text{RF} = \text{RVol}/\text{Total SV}$$

$$\text{RF} = 66/128 - 52\%$$

The regurgitant volume is 66 mL, and regurgitant fraction is 52% making A the correct answer.

15. Answer: D. This patient has asymptomatic severe aortic regurgitation. In the absence of symptoms, the 2020 ACC/AHA guidelines for management of patients with valvular heart disease list 2 class I indications and 2 class II indications for aortic valve replacement. These include LVEF ≤ 55% (class I), the need for other cardiac surgery (class I), LVESD > 50 mm, LVESDi > 25 mm/m² (class IIa), and progressive decline in EF to <55% to 60% and worsening LV dilation with LVEDD > 65 mm in at least three studies (class IIb). As such, all of the above are correct answers. See **Table 16.2**.

Table 16.3. Recommended Follow-Up for Aortic Regurgitation

Severity of Aortic Regurgitation	Follow-Up
Mild	q 3-5 y
Moderate	q 1-2 y
Severe	q 6 mo-1 y

Data from Otto CM, Nishimura RA, Bonow RO, et al. 2020 ACC/AHA guideline for the management of patients with valvular heart disease: executive summary—a report of the American College of Cardiology/American Heart Association Joint Committee on Clinical Practice Guidelines. *Circulation*. 2021;143(5):e35.

KEY POINTS
Case 3
- Quantitative assessment of AR can be performed utilizing the volumetric assessment through calculation of stroke volumes. Right-sided stroke volume should be used if there is concomitant left-sided valve disease (mitral regurgitation).
- LV size and function factor heavily into surgical indications in asymptomatic patients with severe aortic regurgitation.

16. **Answer: C.** A severely dilated left ventricle suggests chronicity with regard to aortic regurgitation and is not typically present in acute severe aortic regurgitation. The lack of LV remodeling typically leads to an acute presentation as the ventricle is not preconditioned to handle the massive volume load of severe aortic regurgitation. Premature closure of the mitral valve (Answer A) and even diastolic mitral regurgitation can occur due to rapid pressure rise with left ventricular diastolic pressure exceeding that of the left atrium. A flail cusp typically creates a physical defect that produces a large regurgitant orifice area leading to severe AR. Endocarditis is a typical reason for this to occur in the acute setting. EROA of ≥0.3 applies to both acute and chronic aortic regurgitation.

17. **Answer: C.** The modified Carpentier classification for aortic regurgitation classifies the mechanism of AR into three types. Type 1 can be further subdivided based on the location of aortic dilation responsible for AR. Types II and III are cusp prolapse and cusp restriction, respectively. Cusp prolapse can be seen in conditions with excess leaflet tissue or disruption of the commissures. Restriction is typically seen with any condition that causes calcification or thickening/fibrosis of the aortic valve leaflets. Radiation-induced aortic valve disease typically leads to both premature calcification and fibrosis of aortic valve leaflets. See **Figure 16.13**.

18. **Answer: D.** Aortic dissection, traumatic injury, and endocarditis typically lead to acute clinical presentations, all of which have the potential to involve the aortic valve and result in acute severe aortic regurgitation. Aortitis is typically a more chronic process (with intermittent flare-ups) that can lead to remodeling over time (subacute to chronic). **Table 16.4** reveals the most common mechanisms/etiologies of aortic regurgitation.

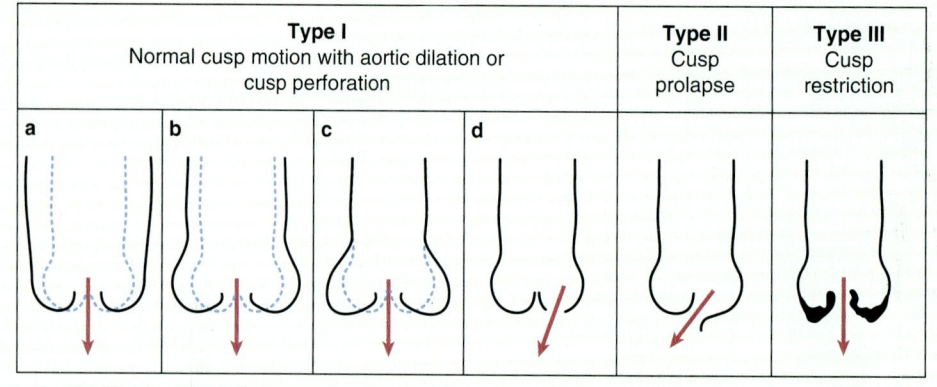

Figure 16.13. Carpentier classification of aortic regurgitation. (Reprinted from Zoghbi WA, Adams D, Bonow RO, et al. Recommendations for noninvasive evaluation of native valvular regurgitation: a report from the American Society of Echocardiography developed in collaboration with the Society for Cardiovascular Magnetic Resonance. *J Am Soc Echocardiogr*. 2017;30(4):303. Copyright © 2017 by the American Society of Echocardiography. With permission.)

Table 16.4. Classification of the Most Common Congenital and Acquired Etiologies of Aortic Regurgitation

Aortic Regurgitation Mechanism	Etiologies	
	Congenital	**Acquired**
Leaflet abnormalities	Bicuspid, unicuspid, quadricuspid aortic valve	Senile calcific Endocarditis[a] Rheumatic heart disease Radiation associated
Aortic root abnormalities	Connective tissue diseases (Loeys-Deitz, Ehlers-Danlos, Marfan syndrome), nonsyndromic heritable thoracic aortic disease	Systemic hypertension Aortitis/large vessel vasculitis Aortic dissection[a] Idiopathic aortic root dilatation Trauma[a]

Adapted from Zoghbi WA, Adams D, Bonow RO, et al. Recommendations for noninvasive evaluation of native valvular regurgitation: a report from the American Society of Echocardiography developed in collaboration with the Society for Cardiovascular Magnetic Resonance. *J Am Soc Echocardiogr*. 2017;30(4):303. Copyright © 2017 by the American Society of Echocardiography. With permission.
[a]Conditions that typically lead to acute aortic regurgitation.

19. **Answer: A.** Holodiastolic flow reversal in the descending thoracic aorta is a specific but insensitive sign of severe aortic regurgitation. Other conditions can indeed cause a similar phenomenon and should be ruled out. Reduced aortic compliance (typically in elderly patients), abnormal arteriovenous connections such as an upper extremity AV fistula, and a ruptured sinus of Valsalva aneurysm can all lead to holodiastolic flow reversal in the descending thoracic aorta. A patent ductus arteriosus (PDA) would be an additional cause (not listed in the answer choices). Moderate aortic regurgitation may produce some degree of aortic flow reversal though it should not extend throughout diastole.

20. **Answer: C.** The maladaptations of severe aortic regurgitation include progressive LV dilation and LV systolic dysfunction. These parameters are prognostic in asymptomatic patients and also predict surgical outcomes in both symptomatic and asymptomatic patients. There is some evidence (nonrandomized) to suggest that global longitudinal strain provides incremental value in the assessment of patients with asymptomatic severe AR with cutoff values less than ~ GLS −19%. Answer C is the only answer with normal LV dimensions, GLS, and EF; thus, this patient's prognosis without surgery is likely the best. Abnormal strain is present in Answer A (GLS = −16%), there is surgical threshold LV dilation in Answer B (LVIDs = 2.6 cm/m^2), and the LVEF is abnormal in Answer D (LVEF = 50%).

21. **Answer: A.** Severe aortic regurgitation is a high afterload, high preload condition, while severe mitral regurgitation is thought to be a low afterload, high preload condition. Following aortic valve surgery, EF will often improve as a result of correction of afterload mismatch and correction of unfavorable loading conditions. Following mitral valve surgery, however, there is generally a predictable decline in LVEF thought to be the result of correction of a low impedance LV-LA pathway resulting in an increase in afterload that may unmask and contribute to systolic dysfunction.

22. **Answer: A.** Pressure half-time and slope of the aortic regurgitant velocity profile as obtained by continuous-wave Doppler is an important measure of aortic regurgitation severity and correlates well with aortic regurgitant fraction. However, pressure half-time is also dependent on systemic vascular resistance and compliance of the aorta and left ventricle. Experimental studies have demonstrated that pressure half-time may not be a reliable indicator of aortic regurgitant severity in an individual patient when hemodynamic conditions are altered. When sodium nitroprusside is given, aortic regurgitant severity or aortic regurgitant fraction will decrease, associated with a reduction in systemic vascular resistance. In this case, despite a reduction in aortic regurgitant severity, the pressure half-time will usually shorten, not lengthen, as a result of faster equilibration between aortic diastolic and left ventricular diastolic pressures.

SUGGESTED READINGS

Addetia K, Miyoshi T, Amuthan V, et al; WASE Investigators. Normal values of left ventricular size and function on three-dimensional echocardiography: results of the world alliance societies of echocardiography study. *J Am Soc Echocardiogr*. 2022;35(5):449-459.

Lancellotti P, Pibarot P, Chambers J, et al; Scientific Document Committee of the European Association of Cardiovascular Imaging. Multi-modality imaging assessment of native valvular regurgitation: an EACVI and ESC council of valvular heart disease position paper. *Eur Heart J Cardiovasc Imaging*. 2022;23(5):e171-e232.

Otto CM, Nishimura RA, Bonow RO, et al. 2020 ACC/AHA guideline for the management of patients with valvular heart disease: executive summary—a report of the American College of Cardiology/American Heart Association Joint Committee on clinical Practice guidelines. *Circulation*. 2021;143(5):e35.

Vahanian A, Beyersdorf F, Praz F, et al; ESC/EACTS Scientific Document Group. 2021 ESC/EACTS guidelines for the management of valvular heart disease. *Eur Heart J*. 2022;43(7):561-632. Erratum in: *Eur Heart J*. 2022.

Zoghbi WA, Adams D, Bonow RO, et al. Recommendations for noninvasive evaluation of native valvular regurgitation: a report from the American Society of Echocardiography developed in collaboration with the Society for Cardiovascular Magnetic Resonance. *J Am Soc Echocardiogr*. 2017;30(4):303-371.

Zoghbi WA, Asch FM, Bruce C, et al. Guidelines for the evaluation of valvular regurgitation after percutaneous valve repair or replacement: a report from the American Society of Echocardiography developed in collaboration with the Society for Cardiovascular Angiography and Interventions, Japanese Society of Echocardiography, and Society for Cardiovascular Magnetic Resonance. *J Am Soc Echocardiogr*. 2019;32(4):431.

CHAPTER 17

Mitral Regurgitation

Maurice Enriquez-Sarano

QUESTIONS

1. A comprehensive echocardiogram is performed for assessment of isolated mitral regurgitation. The mitral annulus measures 4 cm and the VTI of the Doppler signal obtained from the plane of the mitral annulus is 10 cm. The LVOT diameter is 2 cm, with a VTI of 25 cm. The mitral regurgitant volume is:
   A. 125 mL.
   B. 47 mL.
   C. 78.5 mL.
   D. 30 mL.
   E. The regurgitant volume cannot be calculated based on presented data.

2. A cardiac surgeon calls you regarding an echocardiogram from an outside institution. He noticed presence of significant mitral regurgitation by color Doppler and asks you to help with formal quantification of the degree of regurgitation. The study shows clips for mitral regurgitant PISA (aliasing velocity 40 cm/s, PISA radius 1 cm), but there is no continuous-wave Doppler interrogation of the mitral regurgitant signal. You tell him that an exact measurement cannot be done without knowing the exact mitral regurgitant velocity and VTI; however, with some reasonable assumptions you can say that:
   A. Mitral regurgitation is severe because mitral effective regurgitant area is ~0.50 cm^2.
   B. Mitral regurgitation is nearly severe because effective regurgitant area is ~0.38 cm^2.
   C. Mitral regurgitation is severe because the regurgitant volume is ~76 mL.
   D. Mitral regurgitation cannot be quantified based on existing data.
   E. A and C.

3. Which of the following signs is consistent with severe mitral regurgitation?
   A. A vena contracta of the mitral regurgitant jet of 6 mm.
   B. Presence of a flail anterior scallop with a posteriorly directed wall hugging jet.
   C. A mitral inflow velocity of 1 m/sec on pulsed-wave Doppler.
   D. An area of the color Doppler regurgitant jet occupying 40% of the left atrium.
   E. A regurgitant fraction of 37%.

4. The Doppler echocardiogram of a patient with isolated mitral regurgitation provides the following data: PISA radius 0.8 cm, aliasing velocity 35 cm/s, regurgitant velocity 5.25 m/s, regurgitant VTI 131 cm, LVOT diameter 2 cm, LVOT VTI 20 cm, and peak aortic velocity 1.5 m/s. What is the regurgitant fraction?
   A. 55%.
   B. 45%.
   C. 35%.
   D. 25%.
   E. None of the above.

5. The left atrial area of a patient with MR is 20 cm² in the 4-chamber view and 16 cm² in the 2-chamber view with an LA length of 8 cm in systole. What is the LA systolic volume by the biplane area length method?
   A. 40 mL.
   B. 34 mL.
   C. 62 mL.
   D. 31 mL.
   E. None of the above.

6. What is the most frequent cause of moderate or severe mitral regurgitation?
   A. Secondary MR due to LV remodeling.
   B. Isolated annular enlargement due to atrial fibrillation.
   C. Mitral annular and/or valvular calcification.
   D. Mitral valve prolapse.
   E. None of the above.

7. A 55-year-old patient with hypertrophic obstructive cardiomyopathy presents with new shortness of breath on exertion and a peak velocity in the LVOT of 4 m/s and a jet of MR eccentric, thin and directed behind the anterior leaflet. What is the most appropriate conclusion?
   A. Maximize beta-blockade to control obstruction and MR.
   B. Treat with mavacamten to minimize the hypertrophy.
   C. Refer to interventional cardiology for alcohol septal ablation.
   D. Perform a TEE and refer to cardiac surgery for myectomy and mitral repair.
   E. None of the above.

8. A patient, former alcoholic with liver cirrhosis, presents with MR on an outside echocardiogram reporting the following data: BSA 2 m², LV end-diastolic volume index 120 mL/m², end-systolic volume index 55 mL/m², effective regurgitant orifice by PISA 0.50 cm², LVOT diameter 2.5 cm, and LVOT VTI 21 cm. Which of the following potential explanations is **INCORRECT**?
   A. The MR is definitely severe with enlarged LV, requiring mitral surgery or edge to edge repair.
   B. The LV volumes are underestimated. Verify by MRI.
   C. The MR is due to prolapse and late systolic. No intervention.
   D. The PISA radius was measured just after the QRS and the ERO is overestimated.
   E. None of the above.

9. To measure the flow convergence radius in the PISA formula, the **CORRECT** approach is:
   A. Measure the largest flow convergence.
   B. Measure in the first third of systole.
   C. Measure simultaneously to the T wave of the electrocardiogram.
   D. Measure simultaneously to the peak velocity of the MR.
   E. C and D.

10. In patients with mitral regurgitation due to mitral valve prolapse, which of the following statement is **CORRECT** about associated tricuspid regurgitation?
    A. Severe tricuspid regurgitation is often due to tricuspid valve prolapse.
    B. Patients in atrial fibrillation are as much at risk of developing severe TR as those in sinus rhythm.
    C. Women do not incur as much risk of severe TR as men.
    D. Even in the absence of TR, correction of tricuspid annular dilatation ≥4 cm by annuloplasty prevents progression of TR.
    E. None of the above.

11. Which of the following statements regarding the vena contracta width (VCW) is **NOT CORRECT**?
    A. VCW is valid when there are multiple jets.
    B. VCW is less influenced by loading conditions.
    C. VCW is reliable for both central and eccentric jets.
    D. In patients with mitral regurgitation in which the jet is elliptical (as opposed to circular), the VCW width of the regurgitant jet may appear abnormally broad or as a double jet.
    E. None of the above.

12. Which of the following statements regarding the benefits of cross-sectional 3D-derived vena contracta area (VCA) is **INCORRECT?**
    A. No assumptions are made regarding the shape of the regurgitant orifice.
    B. VCA can be used with multiple jets.
    C. Compared to flow convergence method, VCA yields lower values for effective regurgitant area (EROA).
    D. VCA provides a measure of EROA.
    E. None of the above.

13. An 80-year-old woman is admitted for her first episode of heart failure and responds well to diuresis. She has a history of paroxysmal atrial fibrillation but has remained in sinus rhythm recently. Her blood pressure is 130/80 mm Hg and she is in sinus bradycardia at 54/min. Her jugular veins are flat and cardiac auscultation reveals a 2/6 soft systolic murmur at the apex with an S4. There is no rumble or diastolic murmur. Doppler echocardiography demonstrates a left ventricular end-diastolic diameter of 52 mm with ejection fraction of 62% without detectable regional wall motion abnormality, enlarged left atrium, mitral E velocity is 80 cm/s with E/e' at 13, mild-moderate tricuspid regurgitation, and calculated right ventricular systolic pressure of 52 mm Hg. Mitral regurgitation is present and quantified as effective regurgitant orifice 0.30 cm^2 and regurgitant volume 45 mL/beat. The apical 4-chamber views (left: end-diastolic; middle: end-systolic; right: color zoom on left atrium) are shown in **Figure 17.1**. Your interpretation of the echocardiogram is:
    A. Takotsubo syndrome.
    B. Atrial functional mitral regurgitation.
    C. Restrictive cardiomyopathy.
    D. Amyloid cardiomyopathy with secondary mitral regurgitation.
    E. None of the above.

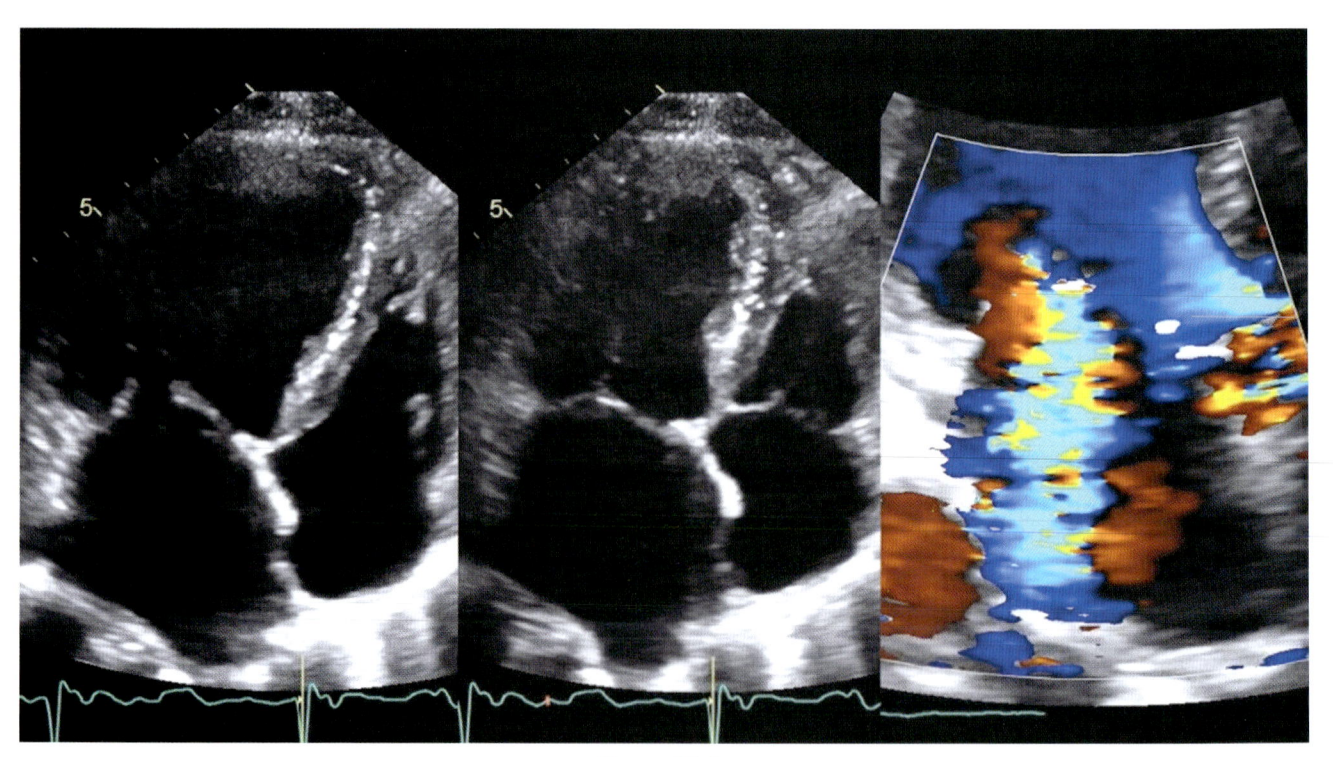

Figure 17.1

Chapter 17 Mitral Regurgitation / 363

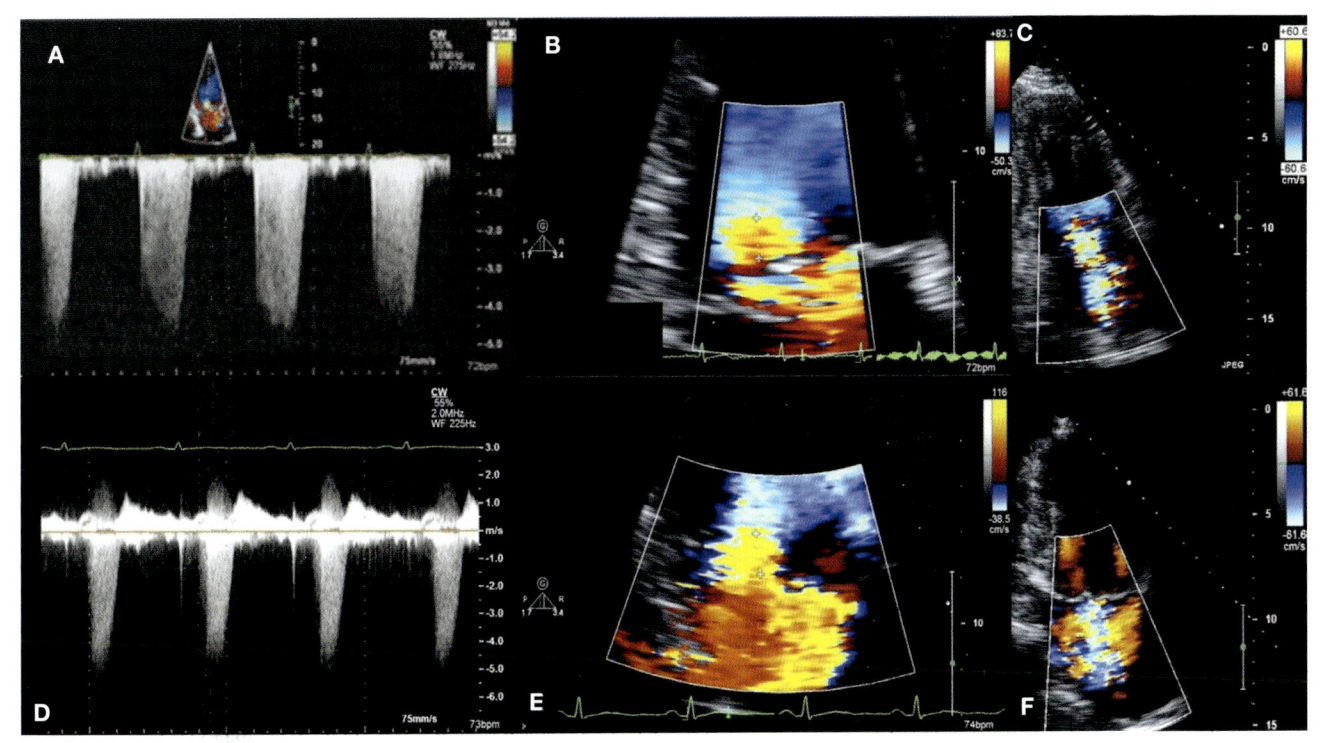

Figure 17.2

14. Two patients with degenerative mitral regurgitation are referred the same day to your clinic. Both have a 3/6 systolic murmur at the apex predominant in late systole and no overt sign of heart failure by symptoms or physical examination. Both echocardiograms reveal a bileaflet prolapse without flail segment with a large jet of regurgitation in the left atrium as shown above.
Patient 1 (**Figure 17.2**, top row, panels A, B, C) has a mild late systolic flow convergence radius of 0.8 cm and patient 2 (**Figure 17.2**, lower row, panels D, E, F) has a mid-late systolic flow convergence radius of 0.9 cm.
The following statements are **CORRECT** except:
A. In comparing these patients, the regurgitant volume may be more reflective of MR severity differences.
B. While the flow convergence is smaller in patient 1, because of the higher aliasing velocity, MR severity and outcome consequences are similar.
C. Watchful waiting management may be most appropriate in one of these patients.
D. Progression of MR has been reported in these patients between 7 and 10 mL/beat/y.
E. None of the above.

15. A 69-year-old woman presents with a known and asymptomatic bileaflet mitral valve prolapse. She is diminutive with body surface area of 1.5 cm^2 and body mass index of 22 kg/m^2 but is well nourished and quite active. She maintains a garden, and she can climb the three flights of stairs to her older sister's apartment without difficulty. The echocardiogram (**Figure 17.3**) shows a LV end-diastolic diameter of 49 mm, end-systolic diameter of 26 mm, and ejection fraction of 65%. The jet of the mitral regurgitation is shown below. The ERO area is 0.38 cm^2 with regurgitant volume of 68 mL/beat and left atrial volume of 98 mL. The forward left ventricular stroke volume index is maintained at 40 mL/m^2 and systolic pulmonary artery pressure is estimated at 32 mm Hg. Her estimated risk for mitral repair is 0.9%.
What is your interpretation?
A. The discordant estimation of "severe" MR with normal LV size shows that MR is overestimated.
B. She is asymptomatic and has no class I or II repair indication. Follow medically.
C. She has severe MR requiring transcatheter edge-to-edge repair.
D. The left atrial volume index (LAVI) of 98/1.5 = 65 mL/m^2 is a class II European guideline indication for repair. Consider surgical repair.
E. None of the above.

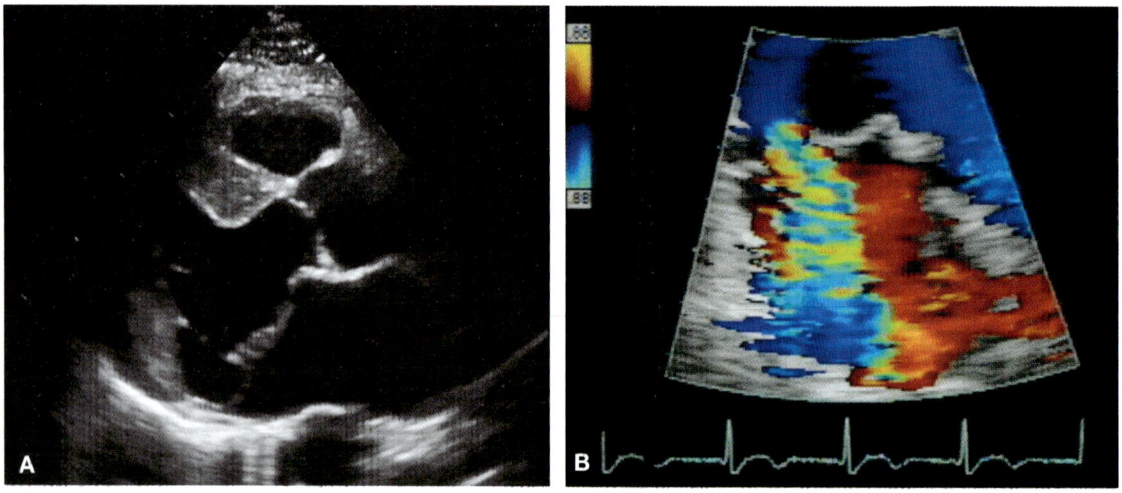

Figure 17.3. A: Parasternal long-axis view. **B:** Apical 3-chamber view with color Doppler.

16. A 61-year-old man was diagnosed 5 years ago with mitral valve prolapse associated with mild MR and was told that this condition is benign. Since he has been well, he can exercise as much as he likes with no shortness of breath and no palpitations and has remained asymptomatic. The electrocardiogram is in sinus rhythm and the Holter shows no episode of paroxysmal atrial fibrillation. He comes back for a systematic follow-up. The mitral regurgitation has progressed to moderate to severe, but the ejection fraction measured by LV volumes is 62% and hemodynamics remains acceptable with mild TR of peak velocity of 2.1 m/s. Selected images of the echocardiogram are presented in **Figure 17.4**. What is your recommendation?
   A. The mitral regurgitation is not yet severe. Follow-up assessment in 1 year.
   B. The patient is asymptomatic. Perform an exercise test and recommend accordingly.
   C. Recommend prompt valve repair.
   D. Perform a transesophageal echocardiography with 3D imaging and recommend accordingly.
   E. None of the above.

17. A 32-year-old man is referred for a systolic murmur. He is asymptomatic and can exercise without limitation. The examination shows an apical thrill with a 4/6 apical systolic murmur radiating to the axilla and the base, holosystolic with S3 and a short rumble. He has no sign of heart failure. The echocardiogram (**Figure 17.5**) shows a bileaflet mitral valve prolapse with a flail segment of P2 with severe MR with ERO 0.72 cm^2 and regurgitant volume 114 mL/beat. The LV is enlarged as shown below and LV volumes are 180 mL/m^2 at end diastole and 80 mL/m^2 at end systole with ejection fraction 55%. LA volume index (LAVI) is 90 mL/m^2. The patient models for clothing and bathing suits and does not want a chest scar unless he has a class I indication for valve repair. What is the rationale for valve repair?
   A. He has a flail leaflet with regurgitant volume ≥100 mL, a class I indication for valve repair.
   B. The end-systolic volume is ≥60 mL/m^2. It is a class I indication for repair.
   C. The LAVI is ≥60 mL/m^2. It is a class I indication for repair.
   D. The EF is <60%. It is a class I indication for repair.
   E. None of the above.

Chapter 17 Mitral Regurgitation / 365

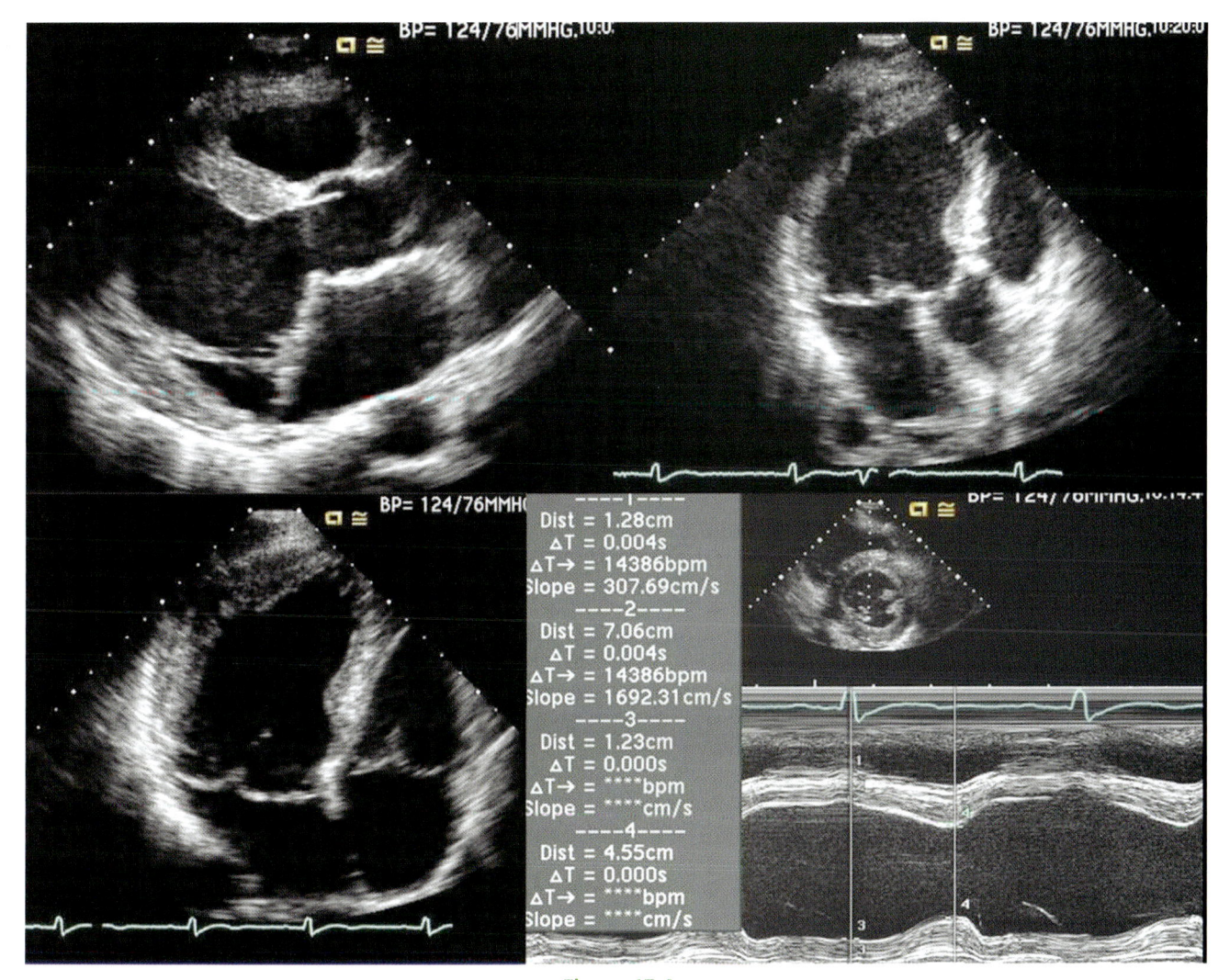

Figure 17.4

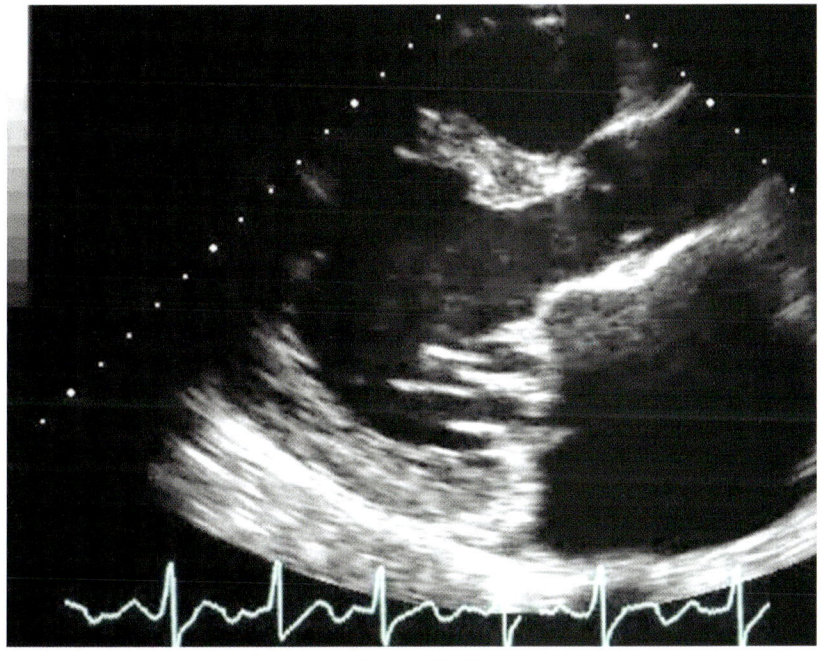

Figure 17.5

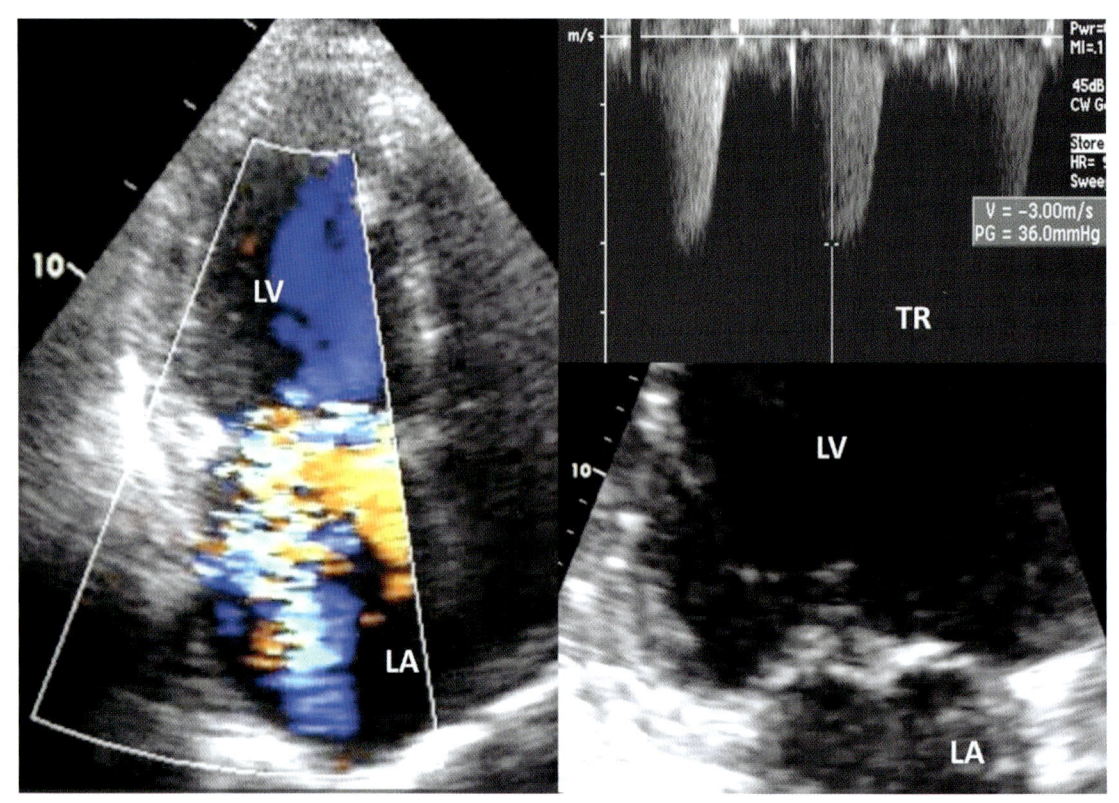

Figure 17.6

18. A 66-year-old woman is seen at the clinic for severe hip osteoarthritis preventing her from most physical activity. She is confined at home and has profound pain with moving from her room to her kitchen. However, she does not complain of any chest pain, dyspnea, snoring, or sudden nightly awakenings. She is noted to be obese with body mass index of 34 kg/m², and her blood pressure was 115/65 mm Hg with heart rate 64/min. A loud murmur is heard at the apex with S3 and short rumble. Lungs are clear.

By echocardiography, the LV is considered mildly enlarged at 59 mm with ejection fraction (EF) estimated as 65% (note 1 year earlier, the EF was 75%, and 6 months ago, the EF was 70%). There is a ruptured chord on the A2 portion of the anterior leaflet (**Figure 17.6**, bottom panel) with a large jet of MR (**Figure 17.6**, left panel). There is mild TR with continuous-wave Doppler signal in the top right panel. The RV and RA are somewhat enlarged with an enlarged IVC that collapses >50% with inspiration. No pericardial effusion is noted.

The patient should be considered for valve repair despite the lack of symptoms because:
A. A flail anterior leaflet usually yields severe regurgitation.
B. The LVEF is normal, but there is progressive decline in LVEF on three consecutive studies.
C. There is an elevated pulmonary artery systolic pressure.
D. The RV is dilated.
E. None of the above.

19. A 52-year-old man with a history of cardiac murmur presents after an episode of atrial fibrillation. He was transiently feeling weak while he was tachycardic but after rate control feels well. He has a loud murmur at the apex and the echocardiogram (**Figure 17.7**) shows a flail posterior leaflet with markedly enlarged left ventricle (end-diastolic diameter 79 mm).

MR quantitation should follow which of the following principles?
A. ERO = (6.28*130*1.48*1.48)/440 without correction = 4.1 cm².
B. ERO = (6.28*75*1.48*1.48)/440 without correction = 2.3 cm².
C. ERO = (6.28*130*1.48*1.48)/440 with correction for the angle of the flail, 200° (vs 360°), = 2.3 cm².
D. ERO = (6.28*75*1.48*1.48)/440 with correction for low MR velocity (4.4 m/s vs 5.0 m/s) = 2.0 cm².
E. None of the above.

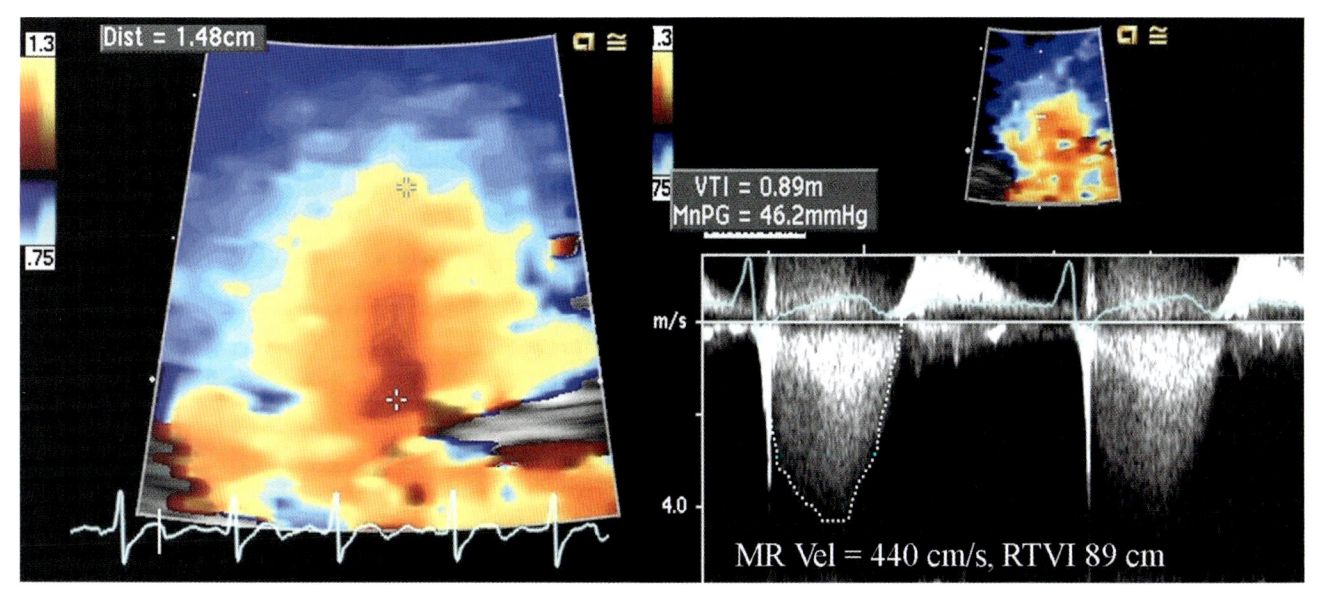

Figure 17.7

20. A 75-year-old man presents with new-onset symptomatic atrial fibrillation to the emergency room. The patients receives heparinization and prompt rate control and becomes asymptomatic (**Figure 17.8**).
A 4/6 holosystolic murmur is heard at the apex and an echocardiogram is done and demonstrates severe degenerative mitral regurgitation with marked enlargement of the left atrium as shown in **Figure 17.9**.
What is your **BEST** recommendation?
   A. At his age and with this degree of left atrial enlargement, return to sinus rhythm is unlikely and rate control is the most appropriate course.
   B. The atrial fibrillation is recent and catheter ablation is the most appropriate course before reassessing the mitral regurgitation.
   C. Refer to cardiac surgery for consideration of mitral repair and intraoperative ablation of the atrial fibrillation (MAZE-like).
   D. The safest course of action is TEE-guided cardioversion and reassessment after 6 months of antiarrhythmic treatment.
   E. None of the above.

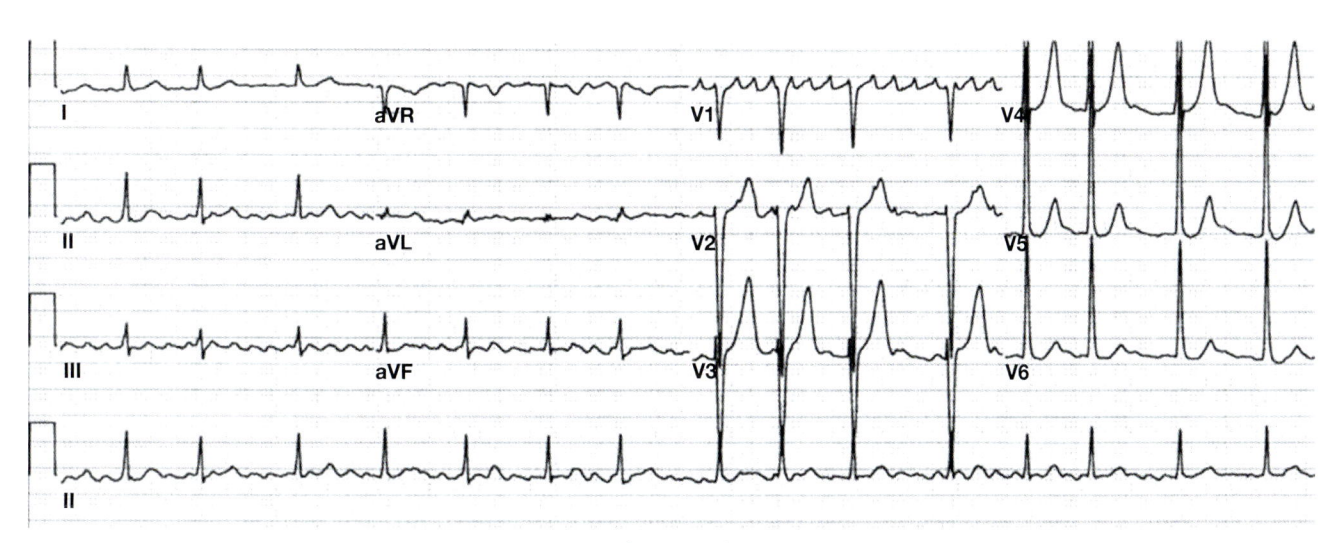

Figure 17.8

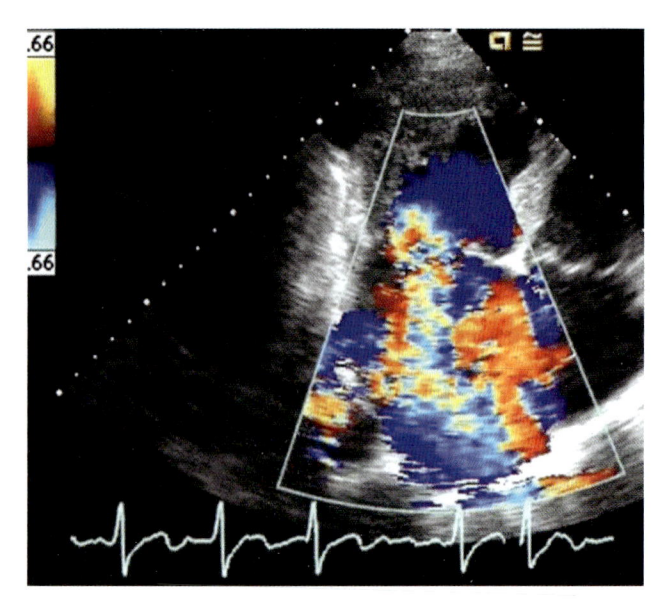

Figure 17.9

21. A 67-year-old patient with a history of mitral valve repair 6 years ago for severe degenerative mitral regurgitation using a restrictive annuloplasty is referred for evaluation. She had normal coronaries on the preoperative coronary angiogram. She presents now with worsening dyspnea on exertion over the past year. She also complains of cough with occasional blood-tinged sputum. An echocardiography is performed and shown in **Figure 17.10**. Which of the following statements is **CORRECT**?

A. Right ventricular dilatation reveals the development of precapillary pulmonary hypertension: Consider for pulmonary hypertension medical therapy.
B. Her symptomatic deterioration may reveal development of new coronary lesions: Consider coronary angiography and stenting.
C. Order a computed tomography to rule out pulmonary embolism.
D. Refer to an interventional cardiology colleague for consideration of transcatheter edge-to-edge repair.
E. Refer the patient to cardiac surgery for consideration of mitral valve replacement.

22. A 23-year-old woman is referred for a diagnosis of mitral valve prolapse based on **Figure 17.11**, obtained during screening echocardiography.
For a reliable diagnosis of mitral valve prolapse, which of the following imaging windows should be used?

A. Apical 4-chamber view.
B. Apical 2-chamber view.
C. Apical long-axis view.
D. Parasternal short-axis view.
E. Parasternal long-axis view.

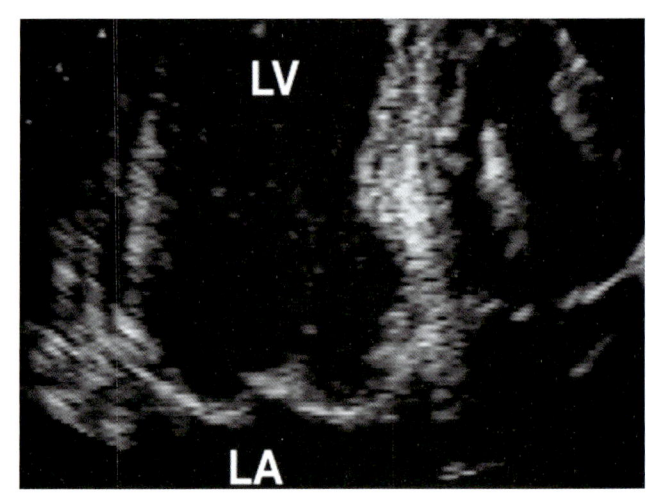

Figure 17.11

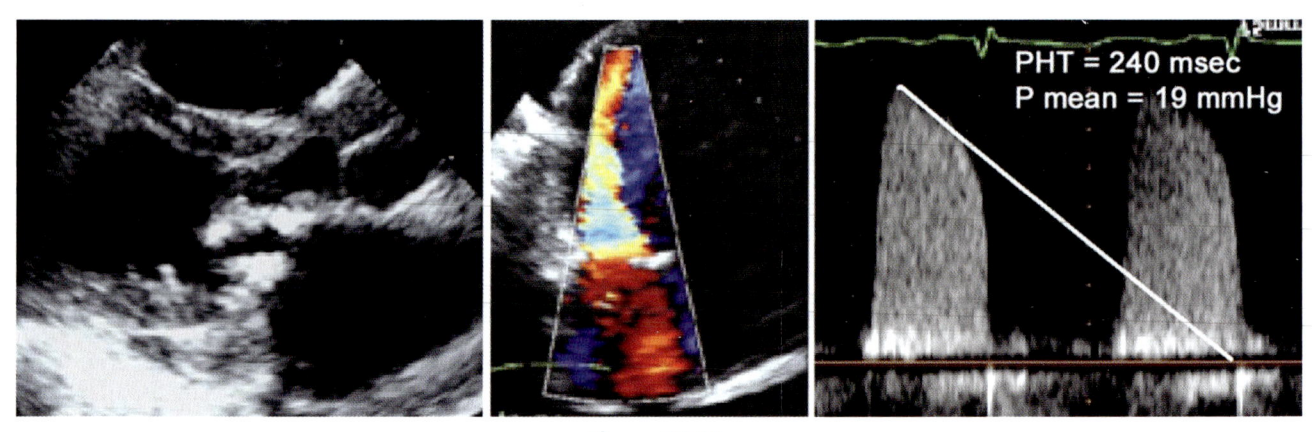

Figure 17.10

Chapter 17 Mitral Regurgitation / 369

23. A 54-year-old man is hospitalized with an acute myocardial infarction. He is taken emergently to the catheterization laboratory, where a completely occluded right coronary artery is found. He undergoes successful stenting. On the third day of hospitalization, he becomes short of breath and appears diaphoretic. There is no murmur on clinical examination. An emergency bedside echocardiogram shows hyperdynamic left ventricular function; there is no pericardial effusion. The mitral continuous-wave Doppler signal is shown in **Figure 17.12**. The most likely explanation for patient's symptoms is?
    A. Left ventricular pseudoaneurysm formation.
    B. Ventricular septal rupture with large ventricular septal defect.
    C. Acute severe mitral regurgitation due to papillary muscle rupture.
    D. Acute thrombosis of the coronary stent.
    E. None of the above.

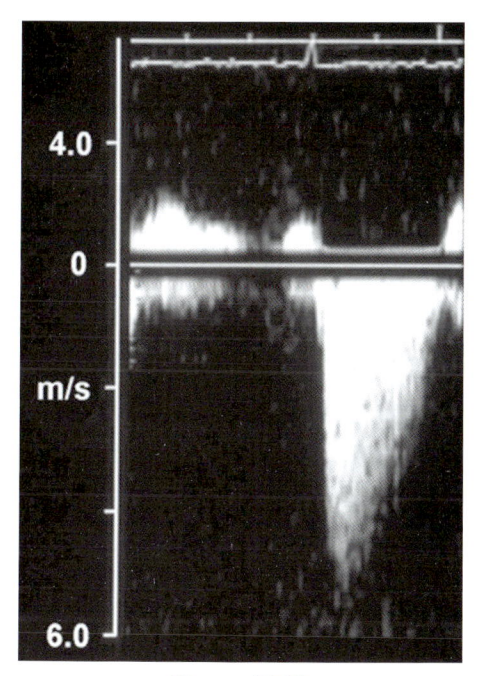

Figure 17.12

24. The echocardiographic images in **Figure 17.13** are suggestive of:
    A. Mitral regurgitation due to posterior leaflet prolapse.
    B. Mitral regurgitation due to ischemic tethering.
    C. Mitral regurgitation due to annular enlargement.
    D. Mitral regurgitation due to rheumatic valve disease.
    E. Mitral regurgitation due to ruptured posterior chord.

25. You are called to assist with an intraoperative transesophageal echocardiogram. Images are shown in **Figure 17.14**.
    You advise the surgeon that:
    A. The mitral regurgitation is severe, and he will need to perform a posterior leaflet repair.
    B. The mitral regurgitation is severe, and he will need to perform an anterior leaflet repair.
    C. The mitral regurgitation is severe, and he will need to be reassessed after coming off cardiopulmonary bypass.
    D. The mitral regurgitation is moderate-severe and does not require intervention.
    E. Medical therapy is unlikely to have an effect on the mitral regurgitation in this type of disease.

26. A 39-year-old woman is referred for evaluation of mitral regurgitation due to a very eccentric jet. The TEE findings in **Figure 17.15** are consistent with:
    A. The mitral regurgitation is severe.
    B. The mitral regurgitation is moderate.
    C. Eccentric jets are not reliably quantified by PISA.
    D. The regurgitant volume is less than 60 mL.
    E. The only definitive proof of severe regurgitation in the case of eccentric jets is demonstration of systolic flow reversals in the pulmonary veins.

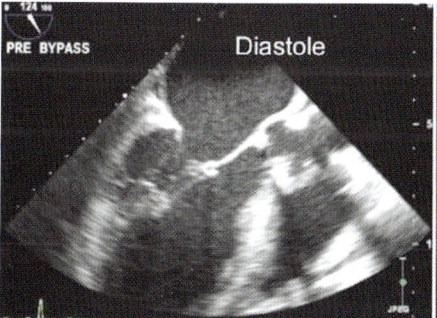

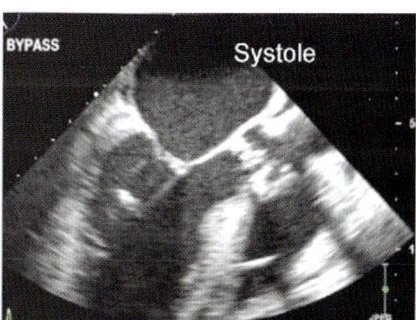

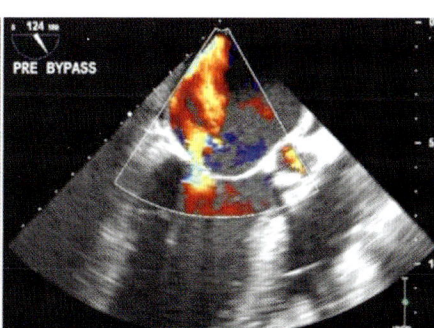

Figure 17.13

370 / Clinical Echocardiography Review

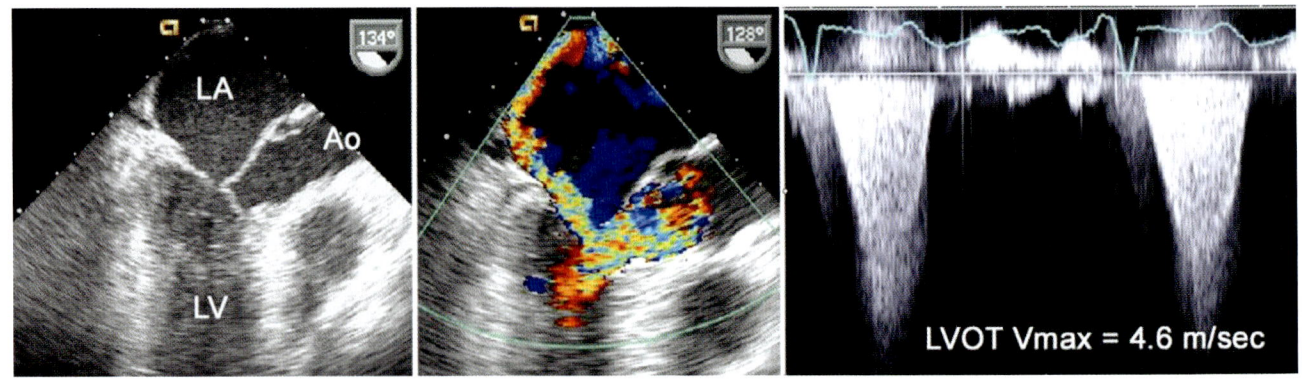

Figure 17.14

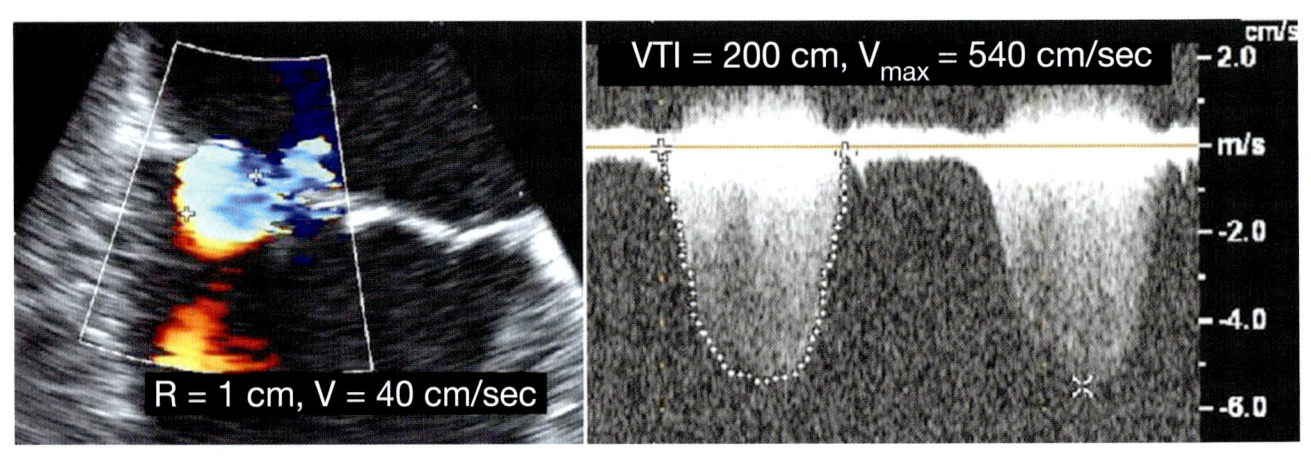

Figure 17.15

CASE 1

A 70-year-old man is admitted to the hospital for overt congestive heart failure. He has known LV dysfunction and was minimally symptomatic with shortness of breath and has had no angina after a myocardial infarction 4 years ago. The apical imaging of his initial echocardiogram is shown in **Figure 17.16**.

The ejection fraction is estimated at 25% with an enlarged cavity; the mitral regurgitation is graded as severe; and tricuspid regurgitation is mild with right ventricular systolic pressure estimated at 75 mm Hg. The QRS duration is 140 ms. The patients is treated with diuretics, sacubitril/valsartan, and empagliflozin and receives a cardioverter/defibrillator with biventricular pacing. Three months later, the patient returns and has had no new episode of congestive heart failure but remains symptomatic and cannot climb his one flight of stairs without stopping due to shortness of breath.

The repeated echocardiogram shows persistent LV dilatation with end-diastolic diameter at 75 mm with slightly improved ejection fraction at 28% and systolic right ventricular pressure at 62 mm Hg. The mitral leaflets remain markedly tenting, the MR is visually graded as moderate to severe, and quantification of the regurgitation is shown in **Figure 17.17**.

27. In regard to the mitral regurgitation quantification, which statement is accurate regarding the patient in **Case 1**?
    A. The measure is unreliable and not predictive of outcome because the peak velocity of MR occurs early in systole and is excluded from clinical trials.
    B. The measure of effective regurgitant orifice should be corrected for the angle of tenting, here 210°, ie, by a factor of 210/180 = 1.17 to calculate at 0.41 cm².
    C. The regurgitant volume is 47 mL/beat.
    D. Effective regurgitant orifice and volume need to be corrected for the LV end-systolic volume to account for disproportionate mitral regurgitation.
    E. None of the above.

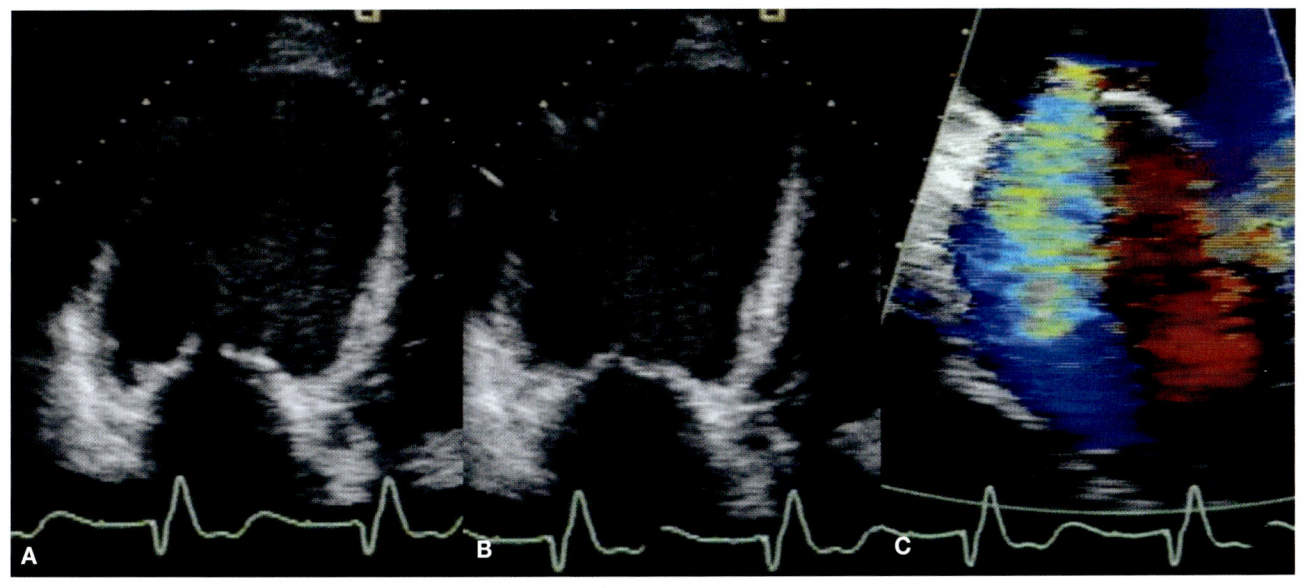

Figure 17.16

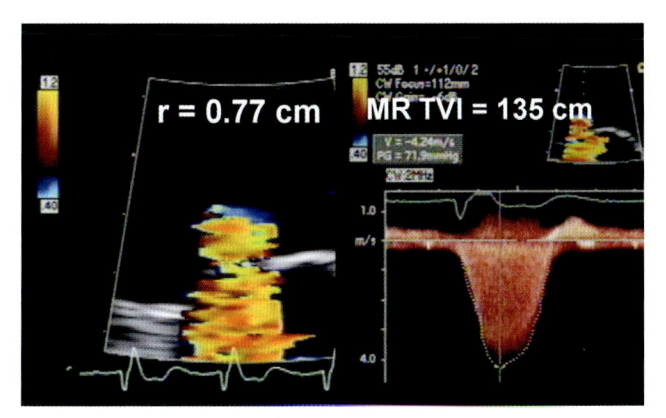

Figure 17.17

28. For the patient from **Case 1**, what statement is **CORRECT** in regard to surgical repair or transcatheter edge-to-edge repair (TEER)?
   A. The patient has a recommended indication for TEER because he remains symptomatic despite full guideline-based medical therapy.
   B. The patient is not within guideline-based indications for TEER due to RV systolic pressure that reached ≥70 mm Hg at presentation.
   C. The patient is not within guideline-based indications for TEER due to LV end-diastolic diameter remaining ≥70 mm despite treatment.
   D. Surgical repair provides improved outcomes over valve replacement for functional MR.
   E. None of the above.

CASE 2

A 23-year-old man is referred for mitral valve prolapse with mitral regurgitation. His symptoms are essentially fatigue with any physical or mental activity. His physical examination reveals an apical 2/6 holosystolic murmur, soft, blowing with no S3 or rumble. He has no peripheral signs of heart failure. The echocardiogram shows a left ventricular diastolic and systolic diameter of 55/32 mm, with calculated ejection fraction 60%, E/e' of 12, LA volume index of 36 mL/m^2, and mild tricuspid regurgitation with estimated systolic right ventricular pressure of 31 mm Hg. The mitral regurgitation involves two main jets covering a large proportion of the left atrium and quantification is shown in **Figure 17.18**.

The flow convergence radii of the two notable jets are measured at 0.65 and 0.45 cm in mid-late systole.

29. For the patient in **Case 2**, the effective regurgitant orifice and volume calculation is:
   A. 0.20 cm^2 and 40 mL.
   B. 0.25 cm^2 and 50 mL.
   C. 0.39 cm^2 and 78 mL.
   D. Inappropriate with multiple jets.
   E. None of the above.

Figure 17.18

30. For the patient in **Case 2**, in view of his symptomatic limitations, it is legitimate to consider:
    A. Watchful waiting with yearly assessment.
    B. Prompt reassessment in 3 months after initiation of low-dose ACE inhibitors.
    C. Transcatheter edge-to-edge repair.
    D. Surgical repair.
    E. None of the above.

CASE 3

A 40-year-old man who performs sustained and regular physical activity consults for palpitations. He denies shortness of breath. The 24-hour Holter shows frequent ventricular extrasystoles. The echocardiogram shows a left ventricle slightly enlarged with ejection fraction of 61%. The diastolic parameters are normal and the right ventricle is of normal size and function. The mitral valve has regurgitation detected and appears somewhat deformed and the long-axis parasternal view is shown in **Figure 17.19**.

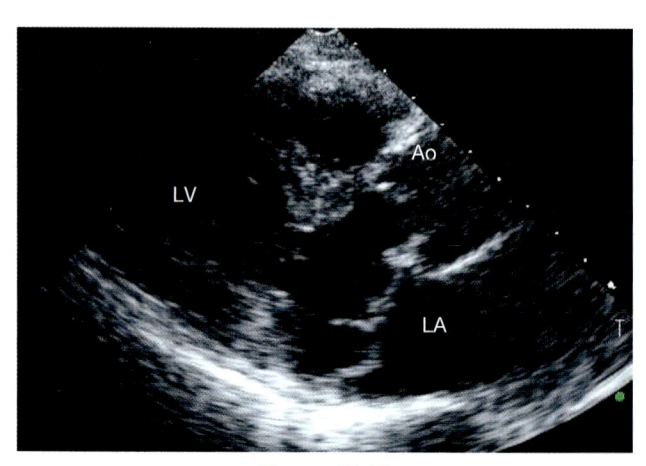

Figure 17.19

31. What is the anomaly detected in the patient from **Case 3**?
    A. Flail posterior leaflet.
    B. Hypertrophic cardiomyopathy.
    C. Subaortic stenosis with membrane.
    D. Mitral annular disjunction.
    E. None of the above.

32. The anomaly detected in the patient from **Case 3** is associated with the following outcomes **EXCEPT**:
    A. Occurrence of nonsustained VT.
    B. Syncope.
    C. Increased need for an implantation of internal cardioverter-defibrillator.
    D. Excess mortality.
    E. None of the above.

33. Among the three patients with mitral regurgitation (**Figure 17.20A-C**) using apical views in systole, the mechanisms of regurgitation according to Carpentier's classification are to be defined as:
    A. Type I, type II, type III.
    B. Type II, type III, type I.
    C. Type III, type I, type II.
    D. Type II, type II, type I.

34. In the patients from **Question 33**, what is the most likely distribution of ejection fraction?
    A. 55%, 75%, 35%.
    B. 75%, 35%, 55%.
    C. 75%, 55%, 35%.
    D. 75%, 55%, 65%.

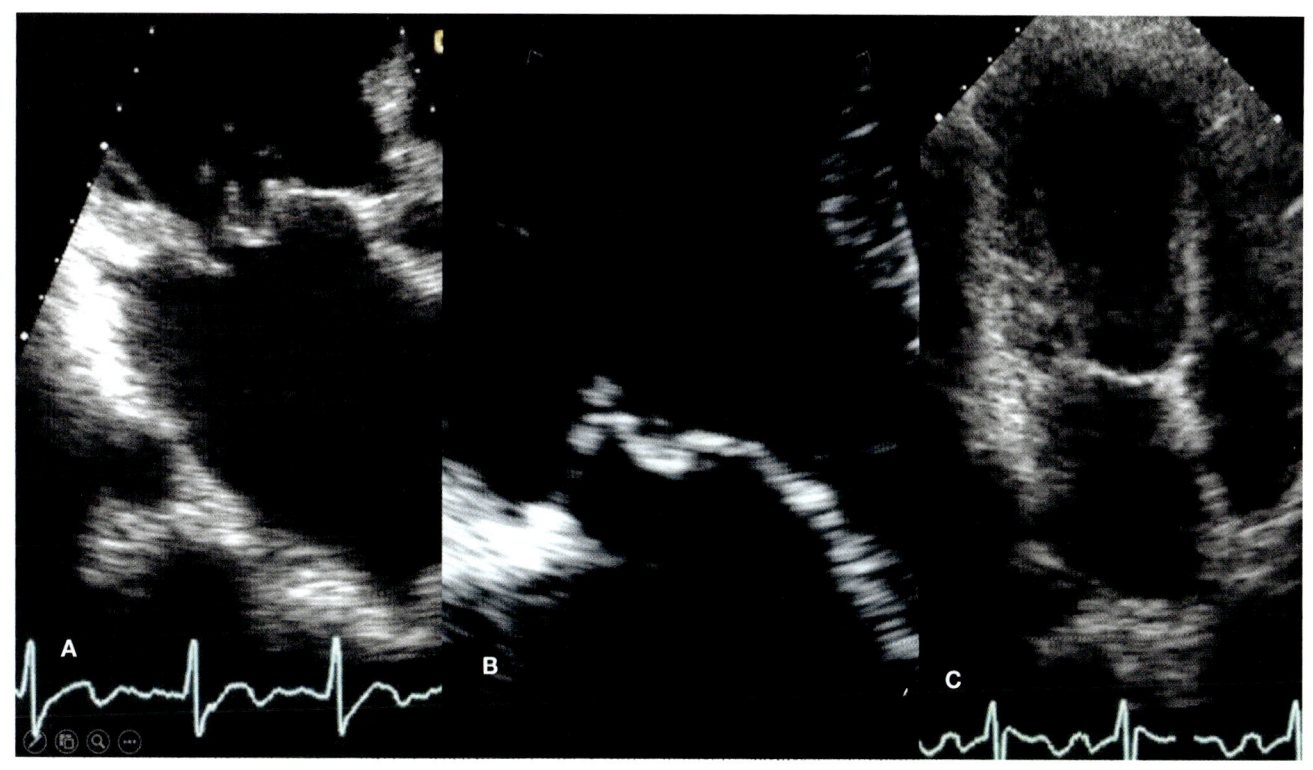

Figure 17.20

ANSWERS

1. **Answer: B.** The calculation of the regurgitant volume by quantitative Doppler involves the calculation of the mitral inflow stroke volume and the aortic outflow stroke volume. In normal subjects, these are equal, but in patients with MR, the mitral inflow stroke volume is higher due to the fact that in systole, the LA is overloaded by the regurgitant volume which returns to the LV in diastole. The calculation of these volumes is the following:

$$\text{Stroke volume} = \pi * R^2 * VTI = 3.14 * (D^2/4) * VTI$$
$$= 0.785 * D^2 * VTI$$

Mitral stroke volume = 0.785 * 4 * 4 * 10 = 126 mL
Aortic stroke volume = 0.785 * 2 * 2 * 25 = 79
Regurgitant volume = 126 − 79 = 47 mL

2. **Answer: E.** There are several simplified calculations that are commonly used in PISA evaluation of mitral regurgitation. They are all based on some presumptions, but their simplicity makes them attractive for rapid calculations in cases where the continuous-wave Doppler cannot be obtained.

Two simplifications are commonly used for ERO calculation. In the first one, the aliasing velocity is set at 40 cm/s. If the mitral regurgitant velocity is considered 500 cm/s (a reasonable assumption when systemic blood pressure is normal), calculation of the effective regurgitant orifice (ERO) is:

PISA surface × aliasing velocity = ERO × regurgitant velocity

$$ERO = (2 \times 3.14 \times R^2 \times 40 \text{ cm/s})/500 \text{ cm/s}$$
$$= 251 \times R^2/500 - R^2/2$$

Using this simplification, the ERO is 0.5 cm²

A second simplification for ERO is using an aliasing velocity of 30 cm/sec and assuming again that the mitral regurgitant velocity is 500 cm/s. With these numbers:

$$ERO = 2 \times 3.14 \times R^2 \times 30/500 = 0.38 \times R^2$$

It becomes that if PISA radius is over 1 cm, the ERO is over 0.38 cm², ie, the regurgitation is severe.

There is also a simplification for estimating the regurgitant volume (RV). This takes advantage of the observation that the ratio between mitral regurgitant VTI and velocity is relatively constant ~1/3.25.

RV = ERO × regurgitant VTI

$$RV = (2 \times 3.14 \times R^2 \times \text{aliasing velocity/mitral velocity}) \times \text{regurgitant VTI}$$

$$RV = 2 \times 3.14 \times R^2 \times \text{aliasing velocity}/3.25 = 1.9 \times R^2 \times \text{aliasing velocity}$$

Using the numbers provided in the question (aliasing velocity − 40 cm/s; PISA radius 1 cm) and the equation 1.9 × R² × aliasing velocity (1.9 × 1 × 40), the RV is 76 mL.

Chronic mitral regurgitation by Doppler echocardiography

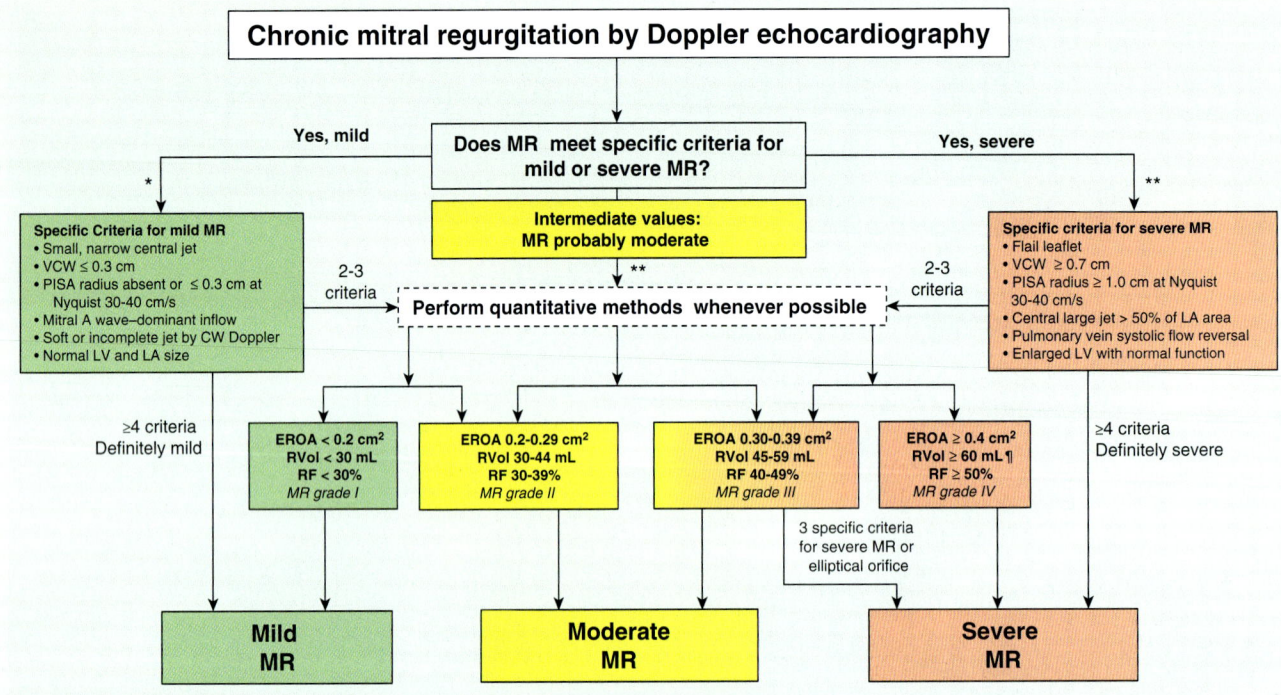

```
                    Does MR meet specific criteria for
    Yes, mild       mild or severe MR?                    Yes, severe
         *                   │                                **
         │           Intermediate values:                     │
Specific Criteria for mild MR  MR probably moderate      Specific criteria for severe MR
• Small, narrow central jet                              • Flail leaflet
• VCW ≤ 0.3 cm         2-3            **          2-3    • VCW ≥ 0.7 cm
• PISA radius absent or ≤ 0.3 cm at  criteria              • PISA radius ≥ 1.0 cm at Nyquist
  Nyquist 30-40 cm/s  Perform quantitative methods whenever possible  30-40 cm/s
• Mitral A wave–dominant inflow                          • Central large jet > 50% of LA area
• Soft or incomplete jet by CW Doppler                   • Pulmonary vein systolic flow reversal
• Normal LV and LA size                                  • Enlarged LV with normal function

 ≥4 criteria    EROA < 0.2 cm²   EROA 0.2-0.29 cm²  EROA 0.30-0.39 cm²  EROA ≥ 0.4 cm²   ≥4 criteria
 Definitely mild  RVol < 30 mL     RVol 30-44 mL      RVol 45-59 mL    RVol ≥ 60 mL ¶   Definitely severe
                  RF < 30%         RF 30-39%          RF 40-49%         RF ≥ 50%
                  MR grade I       MR grade II        MR grade III      MR grade IV

                                                   3 specific criteria
                                                   for severe MR or
                                                   elliptical orifice

       Mild              Moderate                                 Severe
        MR                  MR                                      MR
```

Figure 17.21. ASE recommendations for noninvasive evaluation of native valvular regurgitation. *Beware of underestimation of MR severity in eccentric, wall impinging jets; quantitation is advised. **All values for EROA by PISA assume holosystolic MR; single frame EROA by PISA and VCW overestimate non-holosystolic MR. (Reprinted from Zoghbi WA, Adams D, Bonow RO, et al. Recommendations for noninvasive evaluation of native valvular regurgitation: a report from the American Society of Echocardiography developed in collaboration with the Society for Cardiovascular Magnetic Resonance. *J Am Soc Echocardiogr.* 2017;30(4):303-371. Figure 18. Copyright © 2017 by the American Society of Echocardiography. With permission.)

3. Answer: B. There are multiple signs that can be interpreted for determining the grade (ie, mild, moderate or severe) of MR. Each quantitative sign has specific thresholds for being considered as specific of severe MR. These are summarized by the 2017 ASE guidelines for the grading of MR **(Figure 17.21)**.

As can be noted, vena contracta width ≥7 mm is considered as suggesting severe MR and Answer A is therefore incorrect. Mitral inflow velocity is not mentioned as a sign of severe MR and Answer C is incorrect. A jet to LA area ≥50% is considered suggestive of severe MR and thus Answer D is incorrect. Similarly, regurgitant fraction ≥50% is suggestive of severe MR and thus Answer E is incorrect. Conversely, a flail leaflet is a specific sign of severe MR irrespective of the size/nature of the jet (a flail anterior leaflet is generally associated with very large orifices) and therefore Answer B is correct.

4. Answer: C. The regurgitant fraction for isolated MR (no AR) is calculated as:

RF = (regurgitant volume)/(total LV stroke volume)

= (regurgitant volume)/(regurgitant volume + forward stroke volume)

In the presented case:

Regurgitant Volume = 0.8 * 0.8 * 6.28 * 35 * (131/525)

= 35 mL/beat

Forward stroke volume = 2 * 2 * 0.785 * 20

= 63 mL/beat

Regurgitant fraction = 35/(35 + 63) = 35%

5. Answer: B. The biplane area length formula to calculate a volume is:

Volume = Area1 * Area2 * 0.85/L

In this case:

LA volume = 20 * 16 * 0.85/8 = 34 mL

6. Answer: A. The current data in the community show that while the type I MR (normal leaflet movement) is the most frequent mechanism of moderate or severe MR, the isolated annular enlargement (so-called atrial functional MR) is encompassing only 27% of the total community burden and even less so with atrial fibrillation. Thus, Answer B is incorrect. Mitral valvular and annular calcification represents a small portion of organic (primary) MR. Thus, Answer C is incorrect. Degenerative MR due to mitral prolapse is the largest segment of organic MR but is smaller than the largest group, ie, MR due to LV remodeling. Thus, Answer C is incorrect and A is correct. Etiologies of MR are listed in **Table 17.1**.

7. Answer: D. While all answers have the potential to reduce LVOT obstruction, the present case is characterized by the association of LVOT obstruction to a jet of MR not typically associated with LVOT obstruction, directed not behind the posterior leaflet (typical for MR due to SAM) but behind the anterior leaflet highly suggestive of MR due to mitral prolapse/flail that is probably responsible for the symptom and requires specific treatment, ie, valve repair associated with the required myectomy.

Table 17.1. ASE Recommendations for Noninvasive Evaluation of Native Valvular Regurgitation

Etiology of Primary and Secondary MR

Primary MR (leaflet abnormality)

MVP myxomatous changes	Prolapse, flail, ruptured or elongated chordae
Degenerative changes	Calcification, thickening
Infectious	Endocarditis vegetations, perforations, aneurysm
Inflammatory	Rheumatic, collagen vascular disease, radiation, drugs
Congenital	Cleft leaflet, parachute MV

Secondary MR (ventricular remodeling)

Ischemic etiology secondary to coronary artery disease	
Nonischemic cardiomyopathy	
Annular dilation	Atrial fibrillation, restrictive cardiomyopathy

ASE, American Society of Echocardiography; MR, mitral regurgitation; MV, mitral valve; MVP, mitral valve prolapse
Reprinted from Zoghbi WA, Adams D, Bonow RO, et al. Recommendations for noninvasive evaluation of native valvular regurgitation: a report from the American Society of Echocardiography developed in collaboration with the Society for Cardiovascular Magnetic Resonance. *J Am Soc Echocardiogr.* 2017;30(4):303-371. Table 5. Copyright © 2017 by the American Society of Echocardiography. With permission.

8. **Answer: A.** The data provided in the question show that the patient has indeed a large stroke volume:

$$\text{Total LV stroke volume} = (\text{EDVI} - \text{ESVI}) * \text{BSA}$$
$$= (120 - 55) * 2 = 130 \text{ mL}$$

But the forward stroke volume is also large
$2.5 * 2.5 * 0.785 * 21 = 103$ mL

Thus, the regurgitant volume calculated is 130 − 103 = 27 mL and is discordant and incompatible with the ERO of 0.50 cm².

The potential explanations of this discordance are either underestimated LV volumes yielding underestimated total stroke volume and regurgitant volume or a late systolic MR whereby there is a large ERO but brief regurgitation which would yield a small regurgitant volume, or the PISA radius was measured incorrectly. Thus, the proposition in Answer A is incorrect (no certainty of severe MR whereby LV dilatation may be due to the liver disease) and therefore Answer A is the correct answer.

9. **Answer: E.** The largest flow convergence may not be concomitant with the peak velocity and may overestimate the MR, and a flow convergence measured in the first 1/3 of systole is incorrect to reflect the entire MR. Conversely, the flow convergence is usually measured simultaneously to the T wave of the electrocardiogram concomitant with the peak jet velocity, or if the peak is slightly earlier, it is correctly measured simultaneously to the peak velocity

10. **Answer: D.** The TR associated with MR is rarely due to valve prolapse and is generally functional, and more frequent in women and in atrial fibrillation. A randomized trial reported in NEJM in 2022 evaluated patients undergoing mitral valve surgery for degenerative MR and compared TV repair for those patients with moderate TR, or less than moderate TR with annular dilatation (defined as annular dilatation of 40 mm or more [or 21 m/m²]). The key finding was a decrease in progression of TR for those undergoing TV repair, though at the cost of an increased rate of pacemaker implant.

11. **Answer: A.** VCW is a semiquantitative measure of MR severity that assesses the regurgitant orifice in a linear dimension and is not accurate for multiple jets. VCW is a quick method of semiquantifying MR. The VCW is measured perpendicular to the flow direction at the narrowest diameter of the MR jet. One of the advantages of this measurement is that it is less influenced by loading conditions and is reliable for both central and eccentric jets. The main limitation of the VCW is the assumption that the regurgitant orifice is circular, which may not be correct. Therefore, the VCW may overestimate MR severity if there is a markedly elliptical (noncircular) orifice shape, as often seen in secondary MR. For example, a two-chamber view, which is oriented parallel to the line of leaflet coaptation, may show a wide vena contracta even in mild MR.

12. **Answer: C.** The VCA is a cross-sectional 3D direct measurement of the narrowest portion of the regurgitant flow that occurs at or immediately downstream from the regurgitant orifice (see **Figure 17.22**) and is slightly smaller than the anatomical regurgitant orifice. VCA is measured via 3D echocardiography using axial multiplanar reconstruction (MPR) analysis and provides a reliable measure of EROA; therefore, Answer D is correct. The

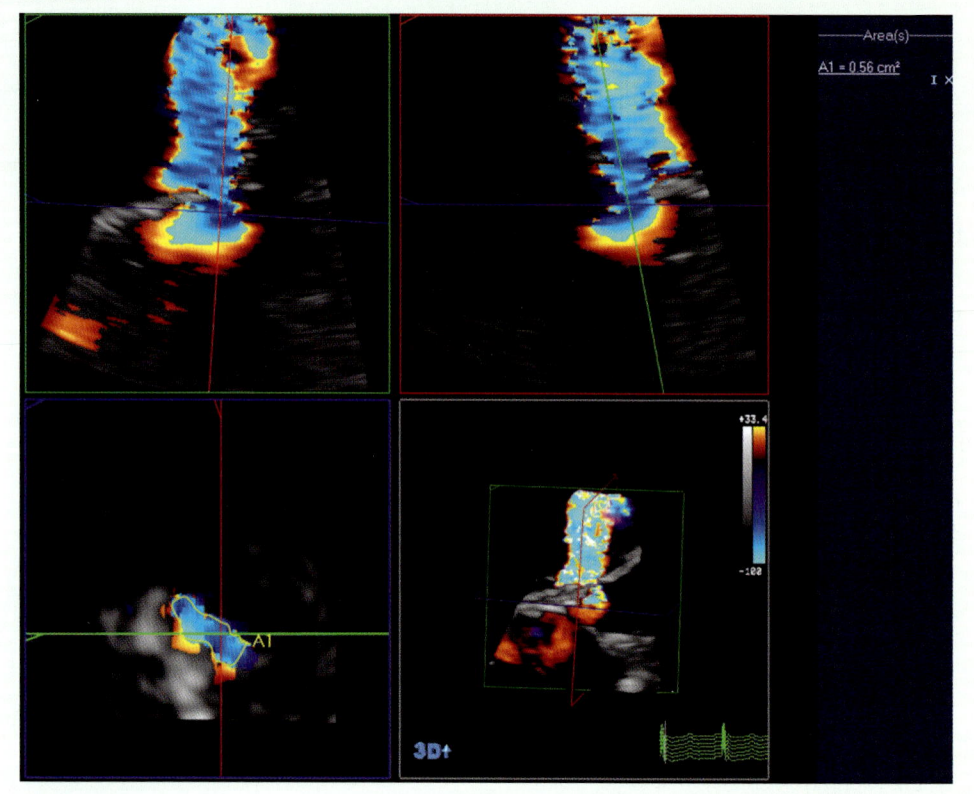

Figure 17.22. Measurement of vena contracta area by multiplanar reconstruction. Axial 3D images of the mitral valve with color Doppler imaging are shown. A late-systolic frame has been chosen for analysis. The top left panel shows a commissural 2D slice; the top right image shows a long-axis 2D slice; the bottom left panel shows a short-axis image at the level of the vena contracta; the bottom right panel shows a volume-rendered color 3D image in the surgical orientation from the left atrial aspect. In the commissural and long-axis quadrants, the red and green lines have been adjusted, so they are positioned through the center of the jet, and the blue lines have been adjusted so they pass through the narrowest part of the jet (ie, the vena contracta). The vena contracta area has then been measured with planimetry (bottom left panel). The value of 0.33 cm² indicates mild to moderate regurgitation. (From Sidebotham D, Merry AF, Legget ME, Wright IG, eds. *Practical Perioperative Transoesophageal Echocardiography.* 3rd ed. Oxford University Press; 2018:127. Reproduced with permission of the Oxford Publishing Limited through PLSclear.)

advantage of being able to manipulate a 3D dataset for proper image alignment and analysis eliminates assumptions regarding the shape (often noncircular) of the regurgitant orifice; therefore, Answer A is correct. The VCA can also be used when there are multiple jets and the VCA can be measured for each jet; therefore, Answer B is correct. Multiple VCAs can be used to identify severe functional MR, which is often underestimated by PISA. VCA yields higher values for EROA compared to the flow convergence method; therefore, Answer C is incorrect and the correct answer selection.

13. **Answer: B.** The patient has a normal LV size, EF, and wall thickness without obvious regional wall motion abnormalities and structural abnormalities of the mitral leaflets, and with only slightly elevated E/e'. Thus, the diagnosis of takotsubo syndrome of restrictive cardiomyopathy and of amyloid heart disease is highly unlikely. The images shown in **Figure 17.1** are highly suggestive of atrial functional MR.

14. **Answer: B.** Both patients have a large flow convergence and a large jet and thus have similar instantaneous regurgitant flow of MR. However, the bottom patient has only a mid-late systolic MR, while the top patient has holosystolic MR. The clinical consequences of MR are less in mid-late systolic MR, which has generally a better outcome than holosystolic MR. In patients with MVP and mid-late systolic MR, the regurgitant volume is more reflective of the true MR severity than ERO; watchful waiting is an appropriate course of action and MR may progress as in all patients with MVP and DMR. The statement B is incorrect.

15. **Answer: D.** In women with small body size, the LV appears within the normal range of size but maybe enlarged as compared to the small baseline of these small patients. Thus, judging that MR is overestimated based on this criterion is incorrect. The patient has a class II criterion for surgery based on LA size as proposed by European guidelines (LAVI ≥ 60 mL/m²) with statement D correct and statement B incorrect (see **Figure 17.23**). Of note, a highly repairable valve >95% likelihood, with low operative mortality <1%, is considered a 2a indication for repair in the ACC/AHA 2020 guidelines (see **Figure 17.24**). Transcatheter edge-to-edge repair in patients with organic MR is reserved to older patients at higher risk for surgical repair, which is low risk in this patient.

16. **Answer: C.** The patient is asymptomatic with EF > 60% and no atrial fibrillation and no evidence

Chapter 17 Mitral Regurgitation / 377

Management of patients with severe chronic primary mitral regurgitation

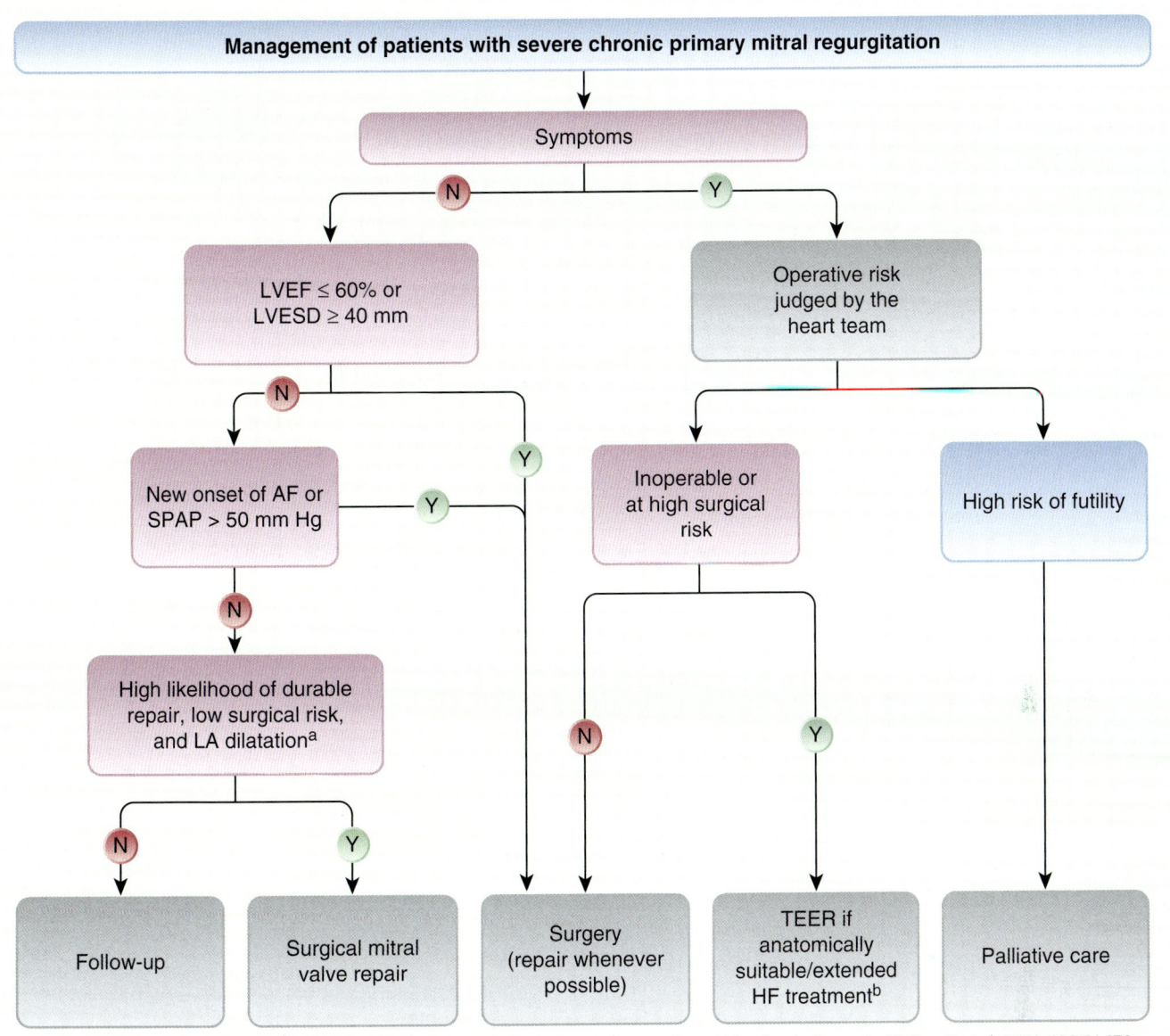

```
                              Symptoms
                           N ↙      ↘ Y
        LVEF ≤ 60% or              Operative risk
        LVESD ≥ 40 mm              judged by the
              │                     heart team
            N ↓                    ↙          ↘
    New onset of AF or      Inoperable or    High risk of futility
    SPAP > 50 mm Hg   —Y→   at high surgical
              │              risk
            N ↓              N ↙    ↘ Y
   High likelihood of durable
   repair, low surgical risk,
   and LA dilatation^a
         N ↙    ↘ Y
   Follow-up   Surgical mitral    Surgery        TEER if           Palliative care
               valve repair       (repair whenever  anatomically
                                  possible)      suitable/extended
                                                  HF treatment^b
```

Figure 17.23. ESC/EACTS guidelines for the management of valvular heart disease. (From Vahanian A, Beyersdorf F, Praz F, et al. 2021 ESC/EACTS guidelines for the management of valvular heart disease. *Eur Heart J.* 2022;43(7):561-632. Figure 5. Reproduced by permission of The European Society of Cardiology and the European Association for Cardio-Thoracic Surgery.)

of pulmonary hypertension. However, the measurements show that the LV end-systolic dimension is 45.5 mm, much larger than the guideline-based threshold of 40 mm and reflective of overt LV dysfunction. Thus, the patient has a class I criterion for referral to prompt mitral surgery

17. **Answer: D.** A large regurgitant volume is not a class I criterion for surgery. The LV end-systolic volume index is not part of the criteria for surgery as no large study has shown an association to outcome and the specific threshold currently. The LAVI indicated is a class II criterion for surgery. An LV EF < 60% is reflective of overt LV dysfunction and is a class I criterion for mitral surgery.

18. **Answer: B.** The patient has little mobility and cannot be judged based on the lack of shortness of breath. While a flail anterior leaflet is usually associated with severe MR, it would not be a class I indication for surgery. LV diastolic dimension reflects the MR severity but is not part of surgical criteria, rather LV systolic dimensions only are criterion. The RV status is concerning but also is not part of guideline-based criteria for surgery. The patient has a TR velocity of 3 m/s and the RAP is estimated as 8 mm Hg, giving an estimated pulmonary systolic pressure of 44 mm Hg. Pulmonary pressures are not considered criterion for surgery in current ACC/AHA guidelines but are considered in ESC guidelines. However, a progressive decline in LVEF over three consecutive studies is considered a 2b indication for surgery in ACC/AHA criteria.

19. **Answer: B.** The formula for the calculation of ERO in A is incorrect as it uses the wrong velocity at flow convergence border. The flow convergence is not constrained and does not require a correction for angle. The color flow map is adjusted to visualize the hemisphere where the first aliasing velocity is seen. This is generally done by shifting the color scale in the

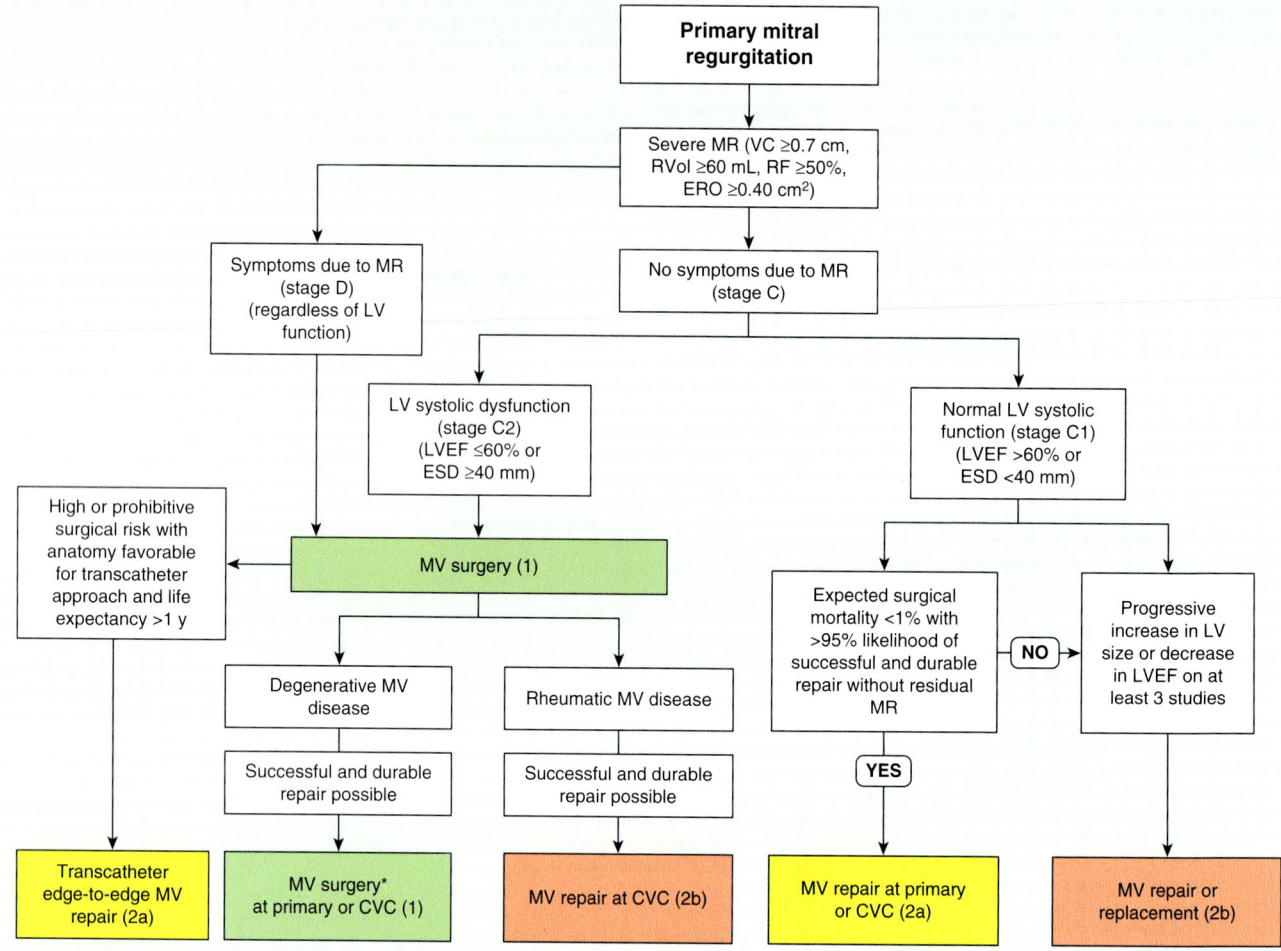

Figure 17.24. Reprinted with permission from Otto CM, Nishimura RA, Bonow RO, et al. 2020 ACC/AHA guideline for the management of patients with valvular heart disease: executive summary—a report of the American College of Cardiology/American Heart Association joint committee on clinical practice guidelines. *Circulation*. 2021;143(5):e72-e227. Copyright © 2020 by the American College of Cardiology Foundation and the American Heart Association, Inc.

direction of the regurgitant jet (downward on TTE where MR enters the LA, and upward on TEE). The radius of PISA is measured from the color Doppler aliasing of blue to yellow in this example. Correction for low peak jet velocity is not a correct answer.

20. **Answer: C.** The patient has severe degenerative MR complicated by atrial fibrillation. Rate control is not the preferred treatment of AF due to MR, similarly cardioversion or catheter ablation has a low probability to yield long-term sinus rhythm. In this case, a symptomatic presentation with AF is an indication for surgery and should be managed with mitral valve repair and MAZE procedure. The poor prognosis of patients with AF complicating DMR is improved after surgery and is the rationale for this indication.

21. **Answer: E.** The correct diagnosis is that the patient has calcific degeneration of the repaired mitral valve with severe stenosis. There is a restricted open of the mitral leaflets seen in diastole, color flow convergence on the atrial side of the mitral valve, a high peak and mean diastolic gradient, and a pressure halftime of >200 ms, all suggesting significant prosthetic mitral stenosis. Only the removal of the structural mitral defect will provide relief and outcome improvement. Transcatheter edge-to-edge repair is not indicated in patients with baseline mitral stenosis. The pulmonary hypertension is postcapillary and requires treatment of the left-sided valve disease.

22. **Answer: E.** The diagnosis of mitral valve prolapse (MVP) requires a movement of a mitral leaflet > 2 mm beyond the plane of the mitral annulus in the parasternal long-axis view. Images such as the one presented in the 4-chamber view do not allow to ascertain the diagnosis of MVP. This is because the mitral valve annulus has a saddle shape and MVP should only be diagnosed if there is prolapse beyond the superior plane of the saddle seen in the parasternal long-axis view.

23. **Answer: C.** Papillary muscle rupture occurs most often around the 5th day post MI and is generally associated with acute shortness of breath and orthopnea with a diminished or absent murmur due to the rapid equalization of pressure between LV and LA in systole. Pseudoaneurysm is a critical defect but generally does not cause hemodynamic distress without rupture into the pericardium. Ventricular septal defects are marked by signs of low cardiac output, prominent jugular venous pressure, and a loud sternal murmur. Stent thrombosis is often complicated by chest pain and LV function deterioration. The Doppler signal shows MR with a

triangular shape, early peaking, and dense profile, suggestive of a large V wave most consistent with papillary muscle rupture.

24. **Answer: B.** The echocardiogram shows an enlarged LV with little change in dimension between systole and diastole. The mitral leaflets show minimal thickening and no doming or prolapse and are pulled toward the apex of the LV and do not return to the level of the mitral annulus in systole. Thus, the diagnosis of MR due to leaflet tethering due to LV remodeling (possibly ischemic) is correct.

25. **Answer: C.** The echocardiogram shows LV hypertrophy with a basal septal bulge, systolic anterior motion of the mitral valve, (SAM) and by continuous-wave Doppler a double signal of MR and LVOT obstruction. The jet is posteriorly directed, suggestive that the MR is due to the SAM. Relief of the obstruction by myectomy will usually relieve the MR by eliminating the SAM.

26. **Answer: A.** Using the values obtained here, the ERO is 0.47 cm^2 and regurgitant volume is 93 mL, a calculation valid even with eccentric jets and irrespective of the presence of a systolic reversal in the pulmonary veins, which is related more to the presence of a V wave in the LA than by the severity of the MR.

27. **Answer: C.** The correction of PISA measurements proposed is incorrect and the MR quantified by the usual method is highly predictive of outcome. Thus, indeed the regurgitant volume is 47 mL/beat.

28. **Answer: A.** This patient fulfills the COAPT criteria of MR persistently severe with persistent symptoms despite full guideline-directed medical therapy. He has no contraindication based on COAPT criteria as the pulmonary pressure is currently below 70 mm Hg, and end-diastolic diameter >70 mm is not a COAPT criterion (end-systolic diameter >70 mm is a contraindication). Surgical repair does not provide improved outcomes versus valve replacement for severe functional MR. This was studied in randomized trial from the Cardiothoracic Surgical Network, and there was no difference in left ventricular reverse remodeling or survival but less recurrent moderate to severe regurgitation with replacement.

KEY POINTS
- EROA calculated by the PISA method provides assessment of severity of MR as well as prognostic information predictive of outcomes
- Based on the COAPT trial criteria, ACC/AHA 2020 Guidelines for Management of Valvular Heart Disease recommend that transcatheter edge-to-edge repair (TEER) is a 2a indication for severe secondary MR when there are persistent symptoms despite GDMT and anatomy is suitable with an LVEF of 20% to 50%, PASP ≤ 70 mm Hg, and LVESD≤70 mm.

29. **Answer: A.** In patients with two jets, both flow convergences need to be imaged if possible with the same aliasing velocity. The total regurgitant flow is the sum of the two regurgitant flows.

Flow 1 = 6.28 * 0.65 * 0.65 * 33
Flow 2 = 6.28 * 0.45 * 0.45 * 33
Total flow = 6.28 * 33 (0.65 * 0.65 + 0.45 * 0.45)
= 130 mL/s
ERO = 130/644 = 0.20 cm^2
RVol = 0.20 * 200 = 40 mL/beat

30. **Answer: A.** The patient has moderate MR without any criteria for surgery. Fatigue does not represent a symptom that can be causally linked to MR. He is not a candidate for any repair at this time but should be reevaluated for MR progression. ACE inhibitors are not a treatment of MR with normal blood pressure.

KEY POINTS
- When two separate flow convergence zones are visualized, they can be summed together to determine total EROA and total RV.
- Although prognostically important, there is no specific medical therapy or intervention recommended for moderate MR.

31. **Answer: D.** The patient has no sign of flail leaflet, hypertrophic cardiomyopathy, or subaortic stenosis. Conversely in late systole, the image shows a clear detachment of the posterior myocardium from the mitral annulus (see **arrow** in **Figure 17.25**) to which it is normally attached characteristic of mitral annular disjunction (MAD) associated with mitral valve prolapse.

32. **Answer: D.** MAD is associated with more frequent (than in MVP without MAD) occurrence of

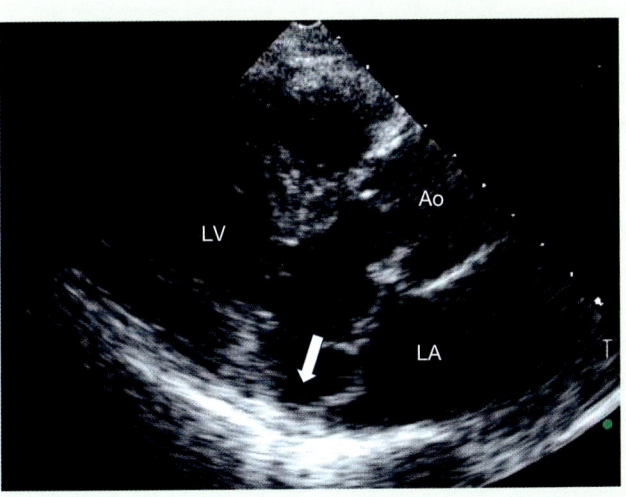

Figure 17.25

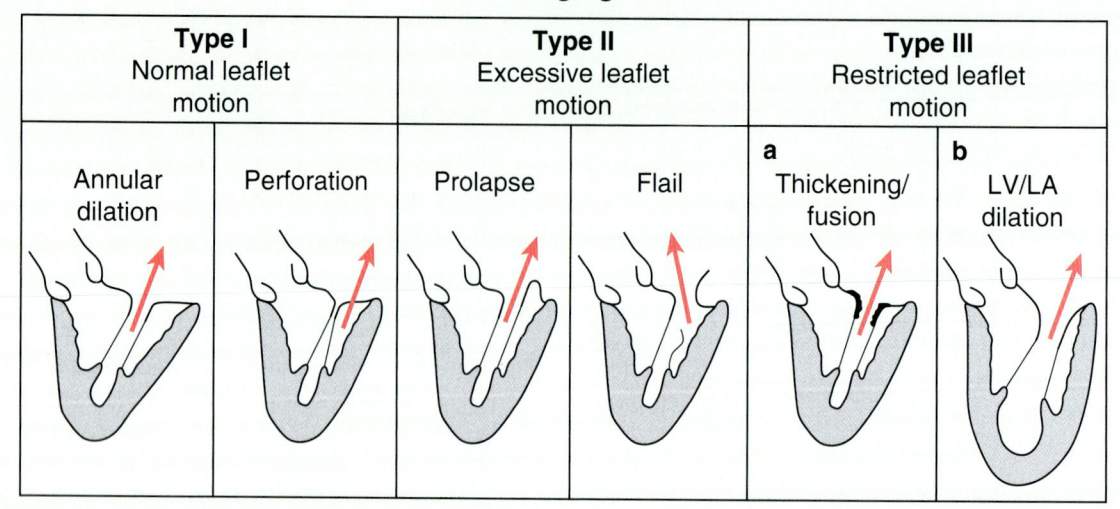

Figure 17.26. ASE Recommendations for Noninvasive Evaluation of Native Valvular Regurgitation. [a]Type IIIa, restriction in diastole. [b]Type IIIb, restriction in systole. (Reprinted from Zoghbi WA, Adams D, Bonow RO, et al. Recommendations for noninvasive evaluation of native valvular regurgitation: a report from the American Society of Echocardiography developed in collaboration with the Society for Cardiovascular Magnetic Resonance. *J Am Soc Echocardiogr.* 2017;30(4):303-371. Figure 10. Copyright © 2017 by the American Society of Echocardiography. With permission.)

ventricular tachycardia, syncope, and need for ICD, which are all observed at progressively increasing rates. However, within the first 10 years after diagnosis, MAD is not associated with excess mortality.

> **KEY POINTS**
> - MAD is a structural abnormality often associated with MVP, where there is detachment and separation of the posterior myocardium from the mitral annulus.
> - MAD may be associated with ventricular arrhythmias and sudden cardiac death.

33. **Answer: B.** The movement of leaflet is what determines the mechanistic type of MR. The first patient has excessive movement (type II), the second restrictive movement due to leaflet tethering in the ventricle (type IIIb), and the third normal movement (type I).

The fact that the second patient has an overshoot of the anterior leaflet behind the posterior does not qualify as excess movement or prolapse as the plane of the annulus is not broken. See **Figure 17.26**.

34. **Answer: B.** Type II is associated with a EF normal to high, type IIIb with reduced EF, and type I with normal to slightly low EF.

> **KEY POINTS**
> - The Carpentier classification is used to characterize leaflet dysfunction and the mechanism of mitral regurgitation.
> - Based on the Carpentier classification, success of interventional therapies (TEER, mitral repair or replacement) can better be selected.
> - The Carpentier classification is not specific to etiology of MR, though there is a general correlation between type and LVEF.

SUGGESTED READINGS

Doherty JU, Kort S, Mehran R, et al. ACC/AATS/AHA/ASE/ASNC/HRS/SCAI/SCCT/SCMR/STS 2017 appropriate use criteria for multimodality imaging in valvular heart disease. *J Am Soc Echocardiogr.* 2018;31(4):381-404.

Otto CM, Nishimura RA, Bonow RO, et al. 2020 ACC/AHA guideline for the management of patients with valvular heart disease: executive summary—a Report of the American College of Cardiology/American Heart Association Joint committee on clinical practice guidelines. *Circulation.* 2021;143(5):e35-e71.

Vahanian A, Beyersdorf F, Praz F, et al. 2021 ESC/EACTS guidelines for the management of valvular heart disease. *Eur Heart J.* 2022;43(7):561-632.

Zoghbi WA, Adams D, Bonow RO, et al. Recommendations for noninvasive evaluation of native valvular regurgitation: a report from the American Society of Echocardiography developed in collaboration with the Society for Cardiovascular Magnetic Resonance. *J Am Soc Echocardiogr.* 2017;30(4):303-371.

CHAPTER 18

Mitral Stenosis

Mary Philip and Igal A. Sebag

QUESTIONS

1. Which of the following statements regarding mitral valve planimetry for mitral stenosis is **TRUE?**
   A. 2D planimetry has been limited by technical demands, time, and observer variability.
   B. 3D-derived planimetry (when feasible) is the standard of care for the quantification of mitral stenosis.
   C. Planimetry of the mitral valve, whether by 2D or 3D, overcomes several limitations of hemodynamically derived parameters (pressure-half time, PHT and continuity equation) and should be attempted as part of an integrative approach to quantifying mitral stenosis.
   D. A and C.
   E. All statements are true.

2. What is the **CORRECT** measurement of the mean transmitral gradient of the mitral inflow signal shown in **Figure 18.1**?
   A. Trace 1.
   B. Trace 2.
   C. Trace 3.

3. Which of following parameter(s) is(are) the preferred parameter(s) for quantification of mitral valve area in calcific mitral stenosis?
   A. Continuity equation.
   B. PHT.
   C. Planimetry.
   D. A and C.
   E. None of the above.

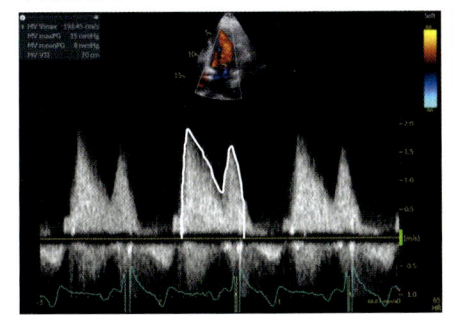

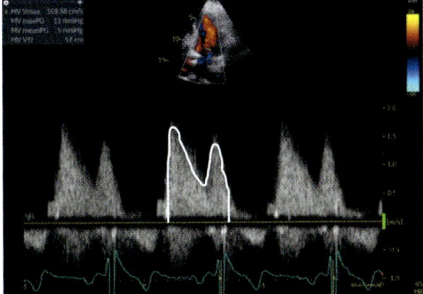

Trace 1   Trace 2   Trace 3

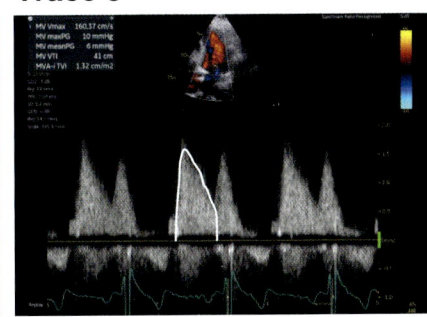

Figure 18.1

4. The incremental qualitative value of the *en face* view of the mitral valve by 3D TEE includes which of the following?
   A. It can further confirm the rheumatic nature of the mitral stenosis by clearly demonstrating commissural fusion (the hallmark of mitral stenosis).
   B. It can improve the selection of patients with rheumatic mitral stenosis for valvuloplasty.
   C. It can further guide intraprocedural mitral annuloplasty.
   D. All statements are true.
   E. None of the above.

5. Which of the following statements is **CORRECT** regarding MS severity grading?
   A. A mitral valve area (MVA) of 1.8 cm² generally corresponds to severe rheumatic MS.
   B. A mean gradient (MG) of 10 mm Hg at an HR of 110 bpm is indicative of severe rheumatic MS.
   C. A MVA ≥ 1.6 cm² is usually not associated with symptoms.
   D. B and C.
   E. None of the above.

6. Regarding differences between rheumatic and calcific MS, which one of the following statements is **CORRECT**?
   A. The rheumatic MV is characteristically funnel-shaped, mainly due to commissural fusion.
   B. The calcific MV is characteristically funnel-shaped, mainly due to the extension of calcium from the annulus into the base of the mitral leaflets.
   C. For a same MVA, the transmitral MG will be greater in calcific MS than in rheumatic MS.
   D. All the statements are incorrect.
   E. A and B are correct.

7. Which of the following are considered successful outcomes after balloon mitral valvuloplasty (BMV)?
   A. At least one commissure is open.
   B. MR grade is not increased by more than 1 grade (scale 1-4+).
   C. MVA is increased to ≥1.0 cm²/m².
   D. All statements are true.
   E. None of the above.

8. A 45-year-old patient is referred to your clinic for shortness of breath on exertion. Transthoracic echocardiography reveals rheumatic mitral valve involvement, with an MVA of 1.8 cm² and a transmitral mean gradient of 4 mm Hg. Otherwise, the echocardiogram showed a normal LVEF, no diastolic dysfunction, no other significant valvular disease, and no direct or indirect features of pulmonary HTN (PH). You request a stress echocardiogram. Which of the following statements are **CORRECT**?
   A. Stress echocardiography is indicated in this context.
   B. Exercise on a bicycle is preferable to exercise on a treadmill or a dobutamine infusion.
   C. You may consider an intervention on the mitral valve if the transmitral mean gradient (TMG) at peak exercise exceeds 15 mm Hg.
   D. All statements are true.
   E. None of the above.

9. Which one of the following statements is **TRUE** about pressure half time and the factors that potentially influence it?
   A. As ventricular compliance increases, PHT increases and MVA also increases.
   B. When ventricular compliance decreases, PHT decreases and MVA increases.
   C. When there is severe AR, PHT decreases and MVA also decreases.
   D. B and C are correct.
   E. None of the above.

10. Which of the following echocardiographic findings predicts favorable outcomes of mitral balloon valvuloplasty?
    A. Asymmetric commissural fusion.
    B. Highly mobile leaflets with only the tips restricted.
    C. Heavily calcified commissures.
    D. Moderate MR or less.
    E. None of the above.

11. During routine assessment of a patient with known valvular disease, the sonographer measures a mitral inflow deceleration time of 758 ms. Which of the following is a reasonable estimate of the mitral valve area?
A. 1.0 cm².
B. 0.3 cm².
C. 3.0 cm².
D. 1.5 cm².
E. 2.0 cm².

12. Which of the following mitral stenosis patients is likely to benefit from mitral balloon valvuloplasty?
A. An asymptomatic 29-year-old woman with a mitral valve area of 1.5 cm² and resting TR velocity of 4 m/s.
B. A 49-year-old man complaining of dyspnea and a mitral pressure half-time of 110 ms.
C. A 62-year-old woman complaining of dyspnea and evidence of heavily calcified mitral leaflets and subvalvular apparatus and a mitral valve mean gradient of 12 mm Hg.
D. An asymptomatic 35-year-old woman with a mitral valve mean gradient of 12 mm Hg and a loud apical holosystolic murmur.
E. None of the above.

13. A 34-year-old woman with a history of rheumatic heart disease presents for yearly evaluation. She is completely asymptomatic. An echocardiogram shows mitral valve doming in diastole, commissural fusion and chordal retraction, and the mitral valve area by both planimetry and pressure half-time is 1.3 cm² with a mean gradient of 9 mm Hg. The tricuspid regurgitant peak velocity is 3 m/s. In what disease stage is this patient?
A. Stage A.
B. Stage B.
C. Stage C.
D. Stage D.
E. Unable to determine by the data supplied.

14. A 78-year-old woman has been complaining of worsening dyspnea on exertion for the past 6 months. Her primary care physician noted a murmur and requested an echocardiogram. This shows presence of a mildly enlarged left ventricle, with calculated ejection fraction of 65%. The aortic valve is sclerotic, with a mean gradient of 10 mm Hg and moderate regurgitation. The mitral annulus and base of mitral valve leaflets are densely calcified, with a mean diastolic gradient of 9 mm Hg at a heart rate of 92 beats/min. The E velocity is 2.1 m/s, with a pressure half-time of 110 ms. The mitral valve area by planimetry in the short-axis parasternal view is 1.3 cm². Which of the following statements is **CORRECT**?
A. The mitral valve area is best estimated in this patient by the pressure half-time method.
B. Mitral balloon valvuloplasty is indicated in this symptomatic patient.
C. Mitral valve replacement is indicated in this symptomatic patient.
D. Mitral stenosis severity should be reassessed after blood pressure and heart rate are more optimally controlled.
E. None of the above.

15. What is the **CORRECT** measurement of the pressure half-time of the mitral inflow signal shown in **Figure 18.2**?
A. Trace 1.
B. Trace 2.
C. Trace 3.
D. All statements are true.
E. None of the above.

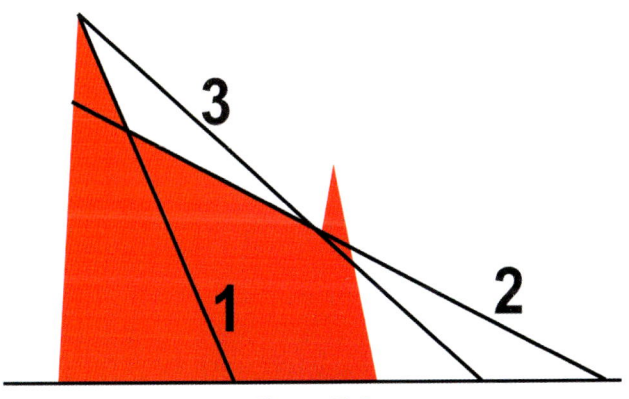

Figure 18.2

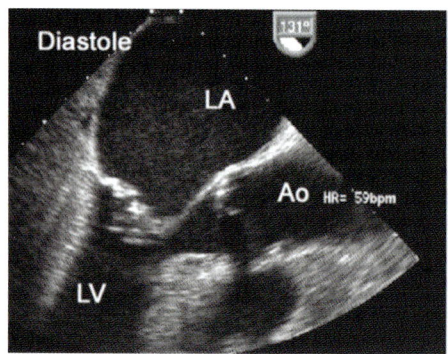

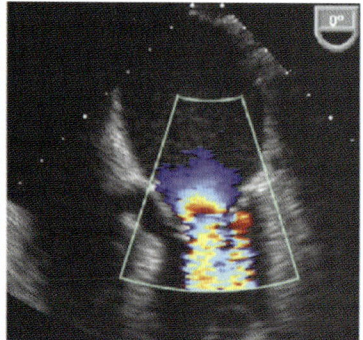

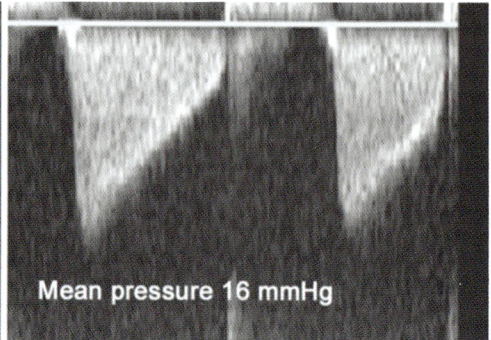

Figure 18.3

16. A 49-year-old woman presents with a history of progressively worsening dyspnea. She remembers having frequent throat infections as a child. The electrocardiogram shows atrial fibrillation with an average heart rate of 85 beats/min. A TEE is performed (see **Figure 18.3**).
Chest x-ray shows normal heart size. Clinical examination is most likely to show:
   A. Laterally displaced apical impulse.
   B. Opening snap occurring late after A_2.
   C. Opening snap occurring early after A_2.
   D. Apical diastolic rumble decreasing with leg exercise.
   E. None of the above.

17. A 67-year-old woman with a history of mitral valve repair 6 years ago for severe mitral regurgitation presents now with worsening dyspnea on exertion over the last 6 months. She also complains of cough with occasional blood-tinged sputum. An echocardiography is performed and shown in **Figure 18.4**.
Which of the following statements is **CORRECT**?

   A. Patient's symptoms are likely due to development of secondary pulmonary hypertension.
   B. The difference between diastolic LV pressure and pulmonary wedge pressure is the best estimate of a mitral gradient.
   C. Supine bicycle echocardiography is the best next step in evaluation.
   D. Mitral balloon valvuloplasty is likely to result in clinical improvement.
   E. All statements are correct.

CASE 1

A 28-year-old woman of Vietnamese origin is brought by her family with complaints of shortness of breath when walking at a fast pace. This has worsened over the last few months. She was not seen by a physician other than during her delivery 5 years ago. She is considering having another child but is concerned about her dyspnea.

On physical examination, she has a murmur, and an echocardiogram is performed (▶ Video 18.1). The gradient across the mitral valve is 14 mm Hg at a heart rate of 78 beats/min.

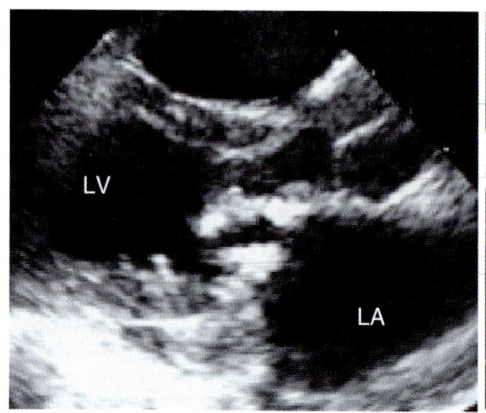

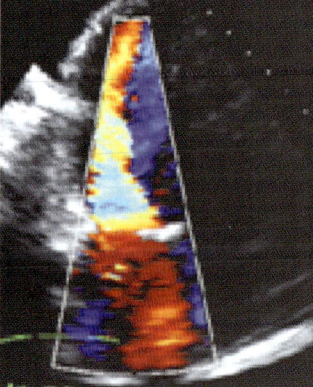

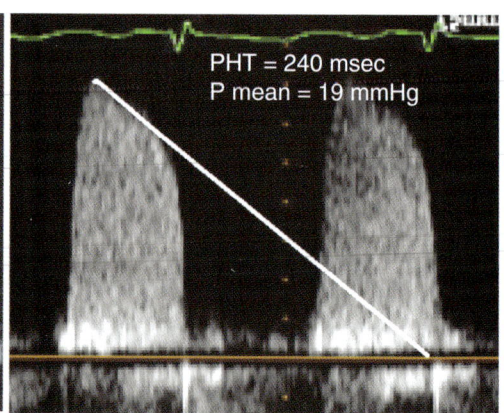

Figure 18.4

18. For the patient in **Case 1**, what would you advise her in regard to her planned pregnancy?
 A. Pregnancy is of great danger to her and should be avoided.
 B. She should consider percutaneous intervention before becoming pregnant.
 C. She should consider valve replacement with a biologic valve before becoming pregnant.
 D. She should consider valve replacement with a mechanical valve before becoming pregnant.
 E. None of the above.

19. As the patient from **Case 1** was considering a recommended therapeutic approach, she returns to your office 6 months later after being told that she is 18 weeks pregnant. She now experiences dyspnea upon minimal efforts (such as walking a few steps). The echocardiogram shows a mitral valve gradient of 16 mm Hg at a heart rate of 110 beats/min, and an estimated pulmonary artery systolic pressure of 64 mm Hg.
What is the **BEST** therapeutic strategy?
 A. Start beta-blocker therapy and titrate to a resting heart rate of less than 80 beats/min, then reassess the mitral valve.
 B. Perform mitral valve replacement.
 C. Perform surgical mitral commissurotomy.
 D. Perform percutaneous mitral balloon valvuloplasty.
 E. None of the above.

20. Which of the following conditions are causes of congenital mitral stenosis?
 A. Double outlet mitral valve.
 B. Parachute mitral valve.
 C. Supravalvular mitral ring.
 D. Mitral arcade.
 E. All of the above.

21. Which of the following statements regarding a supravalvular mitral ring is **CORRECT**?
 A. A supravalvular mitral ring divides the left atrium into a lateral and a medial chamber.
 B. A supravalvular mitral ring usually occurs in isolation.
 C. A supravalvular mitral ring is located inferiorly to the left atrial appendage.
 D. A supravalvular mitral ring is a variant of a cor triatriatum sinister.
 E. None of the above.

22. Which of the following statements is **CORRECT** regarding mitral stenosis related to radiation-induced heart disease?
 A. Commissural involvement is common.
 B. Associated aortic valve stenosis is uncommon.
 C. Leaflet tip calcification is common.
 D. Thickening and calcification of the mitral-aortic intervalvular fibrosa is common.
 E. None of the above.

23. Which of the following statements regarding the quantification of mitral valve area using the PISA method is **CORRECT**?
 A. The PISA method is not valid if mitral regurgitation is present.
 B. The method is validated for all forms of mitral stenosis.
 C. An angle correction is required.
 D. The formula is $\pi r^2 \times V_{aliasing}/V_{max\ MS\ velocity}$.
 E. None of the above.

24. Which of the following statements regarding echocardiographic risk scores to assess the likelihood of success of percutaneous balloon mitral valvuloplasty (PBMV) is **CORRECT**?
 A. The Padial score predicts post-PBMV mitral stenosis.
 B. A Wilkins score >8 is a contraindication to PBMV.
 C. The Wilkins score does not incorporate commissural calcification as a parameter.
 D. The Wilkins score can be used for all etiologies of mitral stenosis.
 E. None of the above.

25. Which of the following statements is most accurate regarding pressure half-time assessment of mitral valve area post-PBMV?
 A. The pressure half-time method is not accurate for the first 3 months post-PBMV.
 B. Pressure half-time is the preferred method for determining the mitral valve area post-PBMV.
 C. Pressure half-time is not accurate post-PBMV due to acute changes in atrial and ventricular compliance.
 D. Pressure half-time is not accurate post-PBMV due to the development of an iatrogenic septal defect, typically with left-to-right flow.
 E. None of the above.

26. Which of the following statements is **CORRECT** regarding the methods of pressure half-time (PHT) to assess mitral valve area?
    A. PHT equates to the time it takes for the velocity to decrease to 50% of peak velocity.
    B. PHT should be performed by pulsed Doppler, rather than continuous-wave Doppler mitral inflow pattern.
    C. PHT is accurate with atrial fibrillation.
    D. PHT determination of mitral valve area will be underestimated if Lutembacher syndrome is present.
    E. None of the above.

27. Which of the following findings are generally considered contraindications to percutaneous balloon mitral valvuloplasty?
    A. Mitral regurgitation ≥3+ at baseline.
    B. The presence of a left atrial appendage thrombus.
    C. Fixed pulmonary hypertension with right-to-left shunting.
    D. Calcific (degenerative) mitral stenosis.
    E. All of the above.

ANSWERS

1. **Answer: E.** Planimetry is considered the echocardiographic gold standard for measuring the mitral valve area largely because it is not subject to the various confounders that impact Doppler-based methods. Measurement of the mitral valve area is more accurate because navigation in 3-dimensional space allows identification of the limiting orifice. Three-dimensional methods include volumetric 3D acquisition (**Figure 18.5A**) or the simplified 3D-guided biplane method (**Figure 18.5B**), where the cursor is positioned across the tips of both leaflets in the parasternal long-axis view. In the latter case, the short-axis simultaneous orthogonal view is displayed, so that the narrowest opening of the MV is accurately identified and the MV area can be traced along its free margin.

2. **Answer: B.** The question refers to measuring the mean pressure gradient by tracing the mitral flow velocity. **Figure 18.1** shows a Doppler signal from a continuous-wave interrogation across the mitral inflow, with three different traces. A correct tracing should not include protrusions that do not represent red blood cells but rather hug the complete envelope. This has a real clinical impact since in this case the first tracing derives a MG of 8 mm Hg while the correct one derives a MG of 5 mm Hg. Therefore, trace 2 is correct. Trace 3 is incorrect since it does not include the mitral a wave.

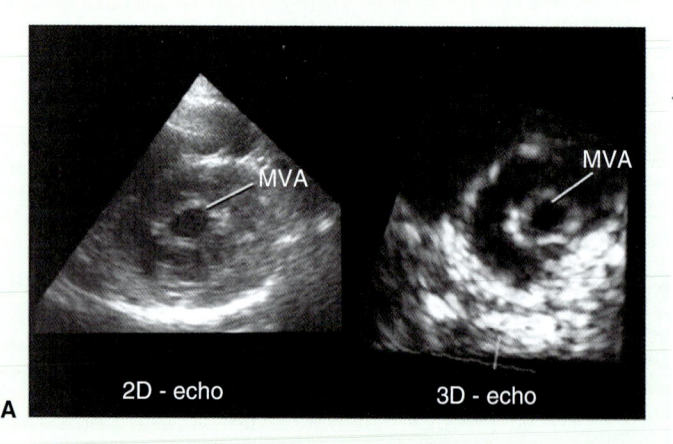

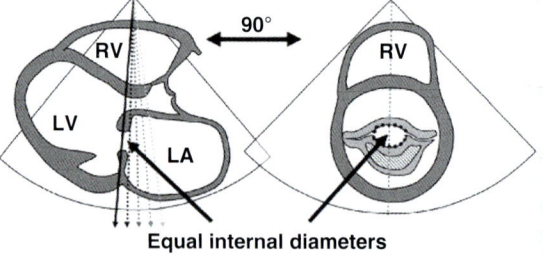

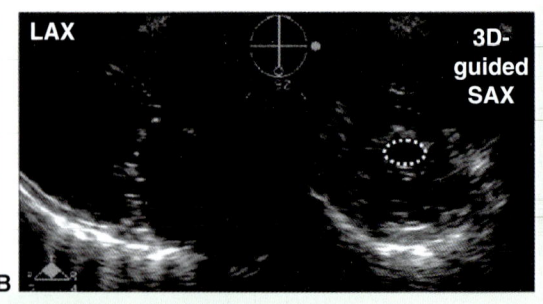

Figure 18.5. **A:** Reprinted from Binder TM, Rosenhek R, Porenta G, Maurer G, Baumgartner H. Improved assessment of mitral valve stenosis by volumetric real-time three-dimensional echocardiography. *J Am College Cardiol*. 2000;36:1355-1361. Copyright © 2000 American College of Cardiology. With permission. **B:** Reprinted from Sebag IA, Morgan JG, Handschumacher MD, et al. Usefulness of three-dimensionally guided assessment of mitral stenosis using matrix-array ultrasound. *Am J Cardiol*. 2005;96:1151-1156. Copyright © 2005 Elsevier. With permission.

3. **Answer: D.** The comorbidities associated with mitral annular calcifications decrease LV compliance and consequently shorten the PHT, which prevents using the Hatle formula to calculate MV area (only validated in rheumatic disease). In calcific MS, the relationship between the mean gradient and the MVA is less predictable than in rheumatic MS, due to numerous confounders (such as LV diastolic dysfunction or MR). The continuity equation (**Figure 18.6**) is one of the two preferred methods for measuring MV area in calcific MS. To be noted though, inaccuracies in this calculation may result from underestimating the diameter of the LVOT (particularly when the aorto-mitral curtain is heavily calcified) or from significant MR or AR. In addition, although limited by acoustic shadowing, 3D-derived planimetry of the mitral valve is also a preferred method because it overcomes several hemodynamic confounders and can locate the limiting mitral orifice (that is not at the tips of the leaflets).

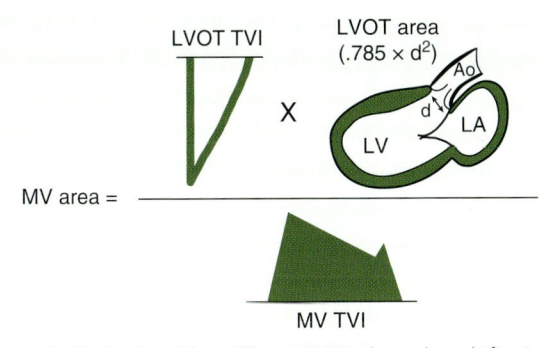

Figure 18.6. Reprinted from Silbiger JJ. Mitral annular calcification and calcific mitral stenosis: role of echocardiography in hemodynamic assessment and management. *J Am Soc Echocardiogr*. 2021;34:923-931. Copyright © 2021 by the American Society of Echocardiography. With permission.

4. **Answer: D.** The 3D-guided TEE *en face* view provides detailed visualization of the mitral valve commissures, and consequently a morphological evaluation and accurate assessment of commissural fusion (the pathognomonic feature of rheumatic MS). According to Anwar and its 3D adaptation of the historical Wilkins score, RT3DE can improve the selection of patients for BMV. 3D TEE provides valuable information beyond the Wilkins score features, such as commissural calcifications (one of the strongest predictors of outcomes after percutaneous BMV because it affects the degree of commissural splitting). The 3D TEE en face view also accurately detects the mechanism of new MR during valvuloplasty by mandating an interruption in the procedure in the event of MR secondary to a leaflet tear (**Figure 18.7**).

5. **Answer: C.** According to the most recent 2020 ACC/AHA guidelines on the management of valvular disease

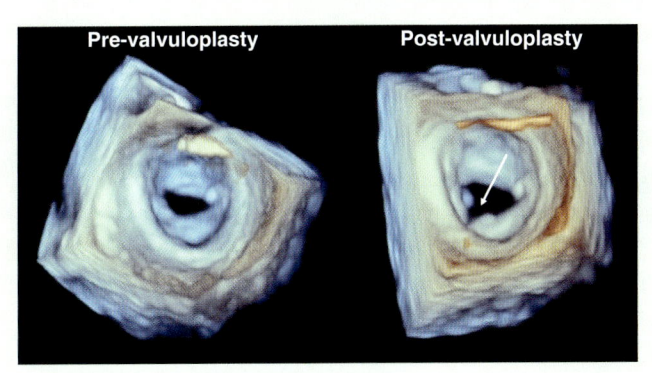

Figure 18.7. 3D TEE surgeon's view showing pre- and post-valvuloplasty images from a patient with rheumatic mitral stenosis. Post-valvuloplasty, arrow points to a leaflet tear associated with significant mitral regurgitation

(**Table 18.1**), the definition of "severe" rheumatic MS is based on the symptoms it produces, as well as the severity at which intervention will improve symptoms. An MV area between 1.6 and 2.0 cm^2 is not usually associated with symptoms and is referred to as "moderate" or "nonsevere" MS. Thus, an MVA ≤ 1.5 cm^2 is considered severe, which typically corresponds to a transmitral MG of ≥5 to 10 mm Hg at a normal HR (between 60 and 80 bpm). To be noted, the MG is indeed highly dependent on transvalvular flow rate, diastolic filling period, and heart rate (therefore the Answer B cannot be considered as correct, because of the tachycardia, in this case the MG must be reevaluated at a controlled HR, and be associated with other parameters of quantification such as planimetry).

6. **Answer: A.** Narrowing of the valve results from commissural fusion in rheumatic MS, leading to a characteristic funnel shape (**Figure 18.8A**) of the MV opening. On the other hand, the calcific MS is usually tunnel-shaped (**Figure 18.8B**), due to the extension of calcium from the annulus to the base of the MV leaflet(s) (the MV hinge point is displaced into the LV inlet, **Figure 18.8C**). These differences in MV geometry have important hemodynamic consequences. This is because rheumatic MV has lower coefficient of contraction and a greater pressure drop as blood passes from the annulus to the orifice. Thus, for a given MVA, the transmitral gradient will be greater in rheumatic than in calcific MS.

7. **Answer: D.** In multivariate analysis, the predictors of poor functional outcome include low valve area after BMV (<1.5 cm^2), high gradient after BMV, and mild to moderate or more (≥2+) mitral regurgitation after BMV. Typically, the MVA increases by 1 cm^2 and the MG is divided by 3. Complete commissural opening is associated with greater MVA, smaller gradients, and functional improvement. The degree of commissural opening provides important prognostic information and thus should therefore be systematically assessed during and after BMV. Postprocedural MR grades also independently predict long-term clinical outcomes after BMV.

Table 18.1. Stages of Rheumatic Mitral Stenosis

Stage	Definition	Valve Anatomy	Valve Hemodynamics	Hemodynamic Consequences	Symptoms
A	At risk of MS	Mild valve doming during diastole	Normal transmitral flow velocity	None	None
B	Progressive MS	Rheumatic valve changes with commissural fusion and diastolic doming of the mitral valve leaflets Planimetered mitral valve area >1.5 cm^2	Increased transmitral flow velocities Mitral valve area >1.5 cm^2 Diastolic pressure half-time <150 ms	Mild to moderate LA enlargement Normal pulmonary pressure at rest	None
C	Asymptomatic severe MS	Rheumatic valve changes with commissural fusion and diastolic doming of the mitral valve leaflets Planimetered mitral valve area ≤1.5 cm^2	Mitral valve area ≤1.5 cm^2 Diastolic pressure half-time ≥150 ms	Severe LA enlargement Elevated PASP >50 mm Hg	None
D	Symptomatic severe MS	Rheumatic valve changes with commissural fusion and diastolic doming of the mitral valve leaflets Planimetered mitral valve area ≤1.5 cm^2	Mitral valve area ≤1.5 cm^2 Diastolic pressure half-time ≥150 ms	Severe LA enlargement Elevated PASP >50 mm Hg	Decreased exercise tolerance Exertional dyspnea

LA, left atrium; MS, mitral stenosis; PASP, pulmonary artery systolic pressure
Reprinted with permission from Otto CM, Nishimura RA, Bonow RO, et al. 2020 ACC/AHA guideline for the management of patients with valvular heart disease: a report of the American College of Cardiology/American Heart Association Joint Committee on Clinical Practice Guidelines. *Circulation*. 2021;143(5):e72-e227. Copyright © 2020 by the American College of Cardiology Foundation and the American Heart Association, Inc.

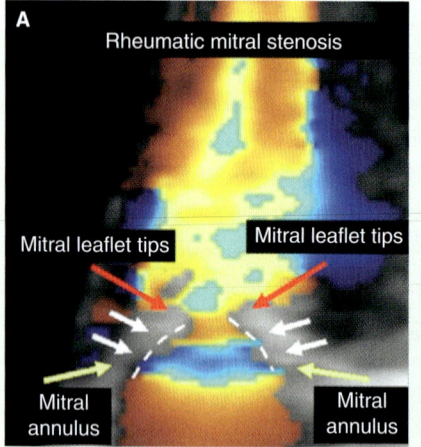

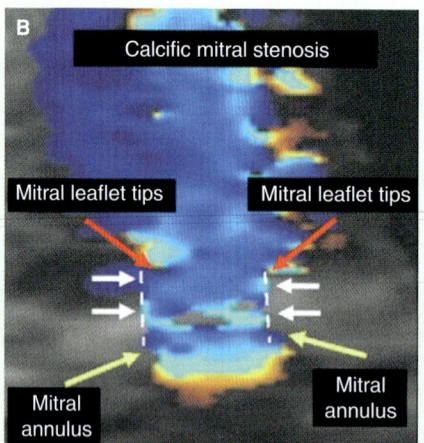

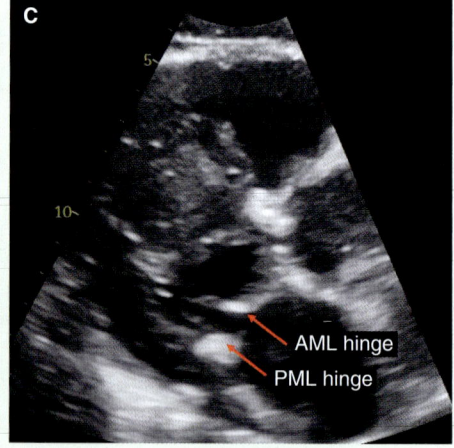

Figure 18.8. Reprinted from Chu JW, Levine RA, Chua S, et al. Assessing mitral valve area and orifice geometry in calcific mitral stenosis: a new solution by real-time three-dimensional echocardiography. *J Am Soc Echocardiogr*. 2008;21:1006-1009. Copyright © 2008 American Society of Echocardiography. With permission.

8. Answer: D. Stress testing is particularly useful in MS when there is a discordance between a patient's symptoms and the MVA. It can help guide the treatment of symptomatic patients with nonsevere MS on the resting echocardiogram. If these patients demonstrate an increasing transmitral MG during exercise to >15 mm Hg, mitral valve intervention may be considered per 2020 ACC/AHA guidelines (**Table 18.2**). An sPAP >60 mm Hg on exercise is another marker of hemodynamically significant marker of MS. Regarding the type of stress, exercise is preferred as the more physiological test (compared to dobutamine infusion). Most experience is with treadmill exercise, with images and Doppler obtained immediately after stress, but bicycle exercise allows data acquisition

Table 18.2. Recommendations for Medical Therapy and Intervention in Patients with Rheumatic MS

COR	LOE	Recommendations
1	C-LD	1. In patients with rheumatic MS and (1) AF, (2) a prior embolic event, or (3) a LA thrombus, anticoagulation with a VKA is indicated.
2a	C-LD	2. In patients with rheumatic MS and AF with a rapid ventricular response, heart rate control can be beneficial.
2a	A	3. In patients with rheumatic MS in normal sinus rhythm with symptomatic resting or exertional sinus tachycardia, heart rate control can be beneficial to manage symptoms.
2a	B-NR	3. In asymptomatic patients with severe rheumatic MS (mitral valve area ≤1.5 cm², stage C) and favorable valve morphology with less than 2+ MR in the absence of LA thrombus who have elevated pulmonary pressures (pulmonary artery systolic pressure >50 mm Hg), PMBC is reasonable if it can be performed at a Comprehensive Valve Center.
2b	C-LD	4. In asymptomatic patients with severe rheumatic MS (mitral valve area ≤1.5 cm², stage C) and favorable valve morphology with less than 2+/MR[a] in the absence of LA thrombus who have new onset of AF, PMBC may be considered if it can be performed at a Comprehensive Valve Center.
2b	C-LD	5. In symptomatic patients (NYHA class II, III, or IV) with rheumatic MS and a mitral valve area >1.5 cm², if there is evidence of hemodynamically significant rheumatic MS on the basis of a pulmonary artery wedge pressure >25 mm Hg or a mean mitral valve gradient >15 mm Hg during exercise, PMBC may be considered if it can be performed at a Comprehensive Valve Center.
2b	B-NR	6. In severely symptomatic patients (NYHA class III or IV) with severe rheumatic MS (mitral valve area ≤1.5 cm², stage D) who have a suboptimal valve anatomy and who are not candidates for surgery or are at high risk for surgery, PMBC may be considered if it can be performed at a Comprehensive Valve Center.

PMBC, percutaneous mitral balloon commissurotomy; VKA, vitamin K antagonist.
[a]2+ on a 0 to 4+ scale according to Sellar's criteria or less than moderate by Doppler echocardiography.
Source: American Heart Association, Inc.

at each step of increasing workload and measures parameters at the peak of exercise as opposed to postexercise. Of note, sPAP cannot be assessed by dobutamine infusion stress test, as the increase in sPAP usually seen during exercise is attenuated by dobutamine due to the beta2 effects on the pulmonary vasculature.

9. Answer: B. This question refers to PHT (pressure half-time) and the factors influencing its variations. PHT is determined by the rate at which falling LA pressure and rising LV diastolic pressures balance each other out. When this balance is achieved slowly, PHT is prolonged and MS is more severe (**Figure 18.9**). Therefore, PHT and MVA vary in opposite

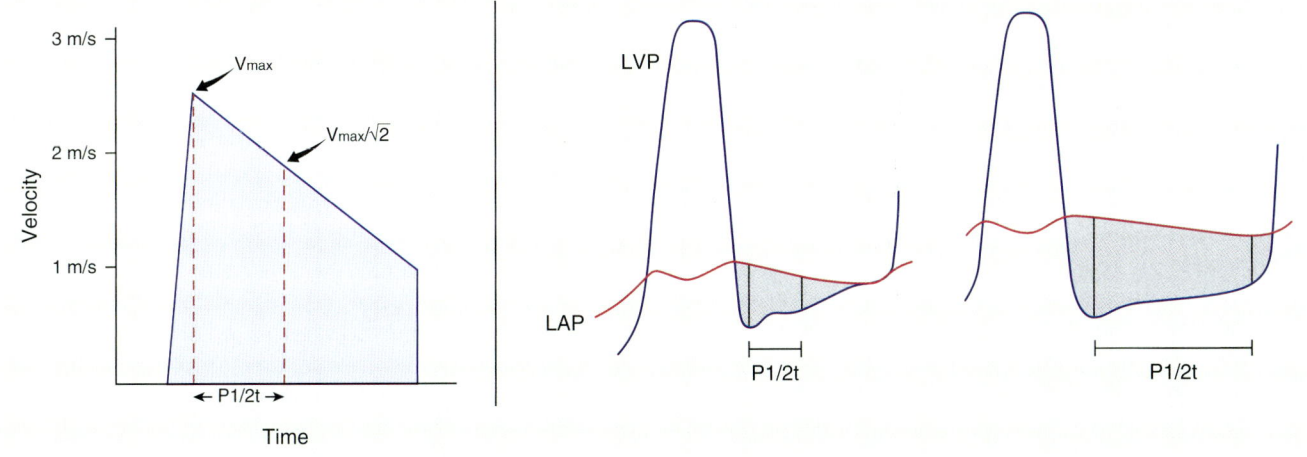

Figure 18.9. LAP, left atrial pressure; LVP, left ventricular pressure. (Reprinted from Silbiger JJ. Advances in rheumatic mitral stenosis: echocardiographic, pathophysiologic, and hemodynamic considerations. *J Am Soc Echocardiogr*. 2021;34:709-722.e1. Copyright © 2021 by the American Society of Echocardiography. With permission.)

directions (MVA is estimated according to the Hatle formula: MVA = 220/pressure half-time). Reduced ventricular compliance and significant aortic regurgitation increase LV diastolic pressures, resulting in shortened PHT.

10. **Answer: B.** The commissural ratio is a measure of the asymmetry of the commissural disease. A commissural ratio >1.25 independently predicts more than one grade increase in MR severity after BMV (**Figure 18.10**). Calcified fusion of the commissures resists splitting and balloon expansion can cause tissue rupture, potentially leading to significant MR. Finally, more than mild MR is associated with less favorable outcomes after BMV.

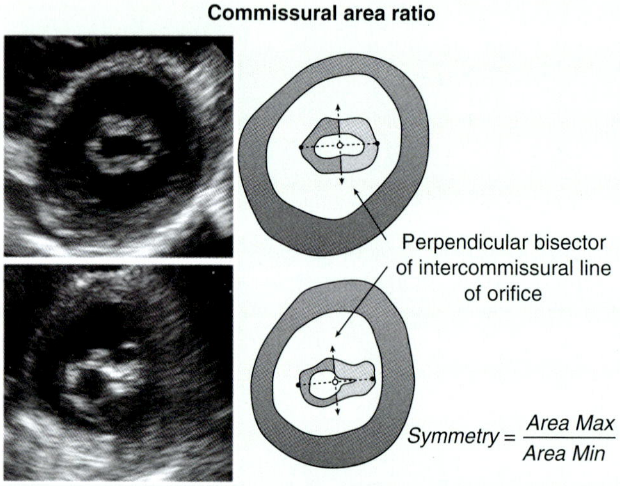

Commissural area ratio

$$Symmetry = \frac{Area\ Max}{Area\ Min}$$

Perpendicular bisector of intercommissural line of orifice

Figure 18.10. Reprinted with permission from Nunes MCP, Tan TC, Elmariah S, et al. The echo score revisited: impact of incorporating commissural morphology and leaflet displacement to the prediction of outcome for patients undergoing percutaneous mitral valvuloplasty. *Circulation*. 2014;129(8):886-895. Copyright © 2013 American Heart Association, Inc.

11. **Answer: A.** This question refers to mitral valve area calculation based on the pressure half-time. The relationship between pressure half-time and deceleration time is constant:

    Pressure half-time = 0.29 × deceleration time.

    Furthermore, the mitral valve area is estimated according to the formula:

    MVA = 220/pressure half-time.

    Using the numbers provided, MVA is 220/(0.29 × 758 ms) = 1.0 cm² (Answer A).

12. **Answer: A.** This question addresses the indications and contraindications for mitral balloon valvuloplasty. Case A is consistent with severe mitral stenosis (according to most recent 2020 ACC/AHA guidelines). While asymptomatic, a TR velocity of 4 m/s is suggestive of a markedly increased pulmonary artery systolic pressure (sPAP 64 mm Hg + RAP); therefore, this patient has a clear indication for balloon valvuloplasty (correct answer). See **Figure 18.11** on indications for intervention for mitral stenosis. In Case B, the mitral valve area is estimated at 2 cm² (220/pressure half-time), and therefore the etiology of dyspnea must be sought elsewhere. The mechanism of successful mitral valvuloplasty is commissural splitting; presence of heavy calcification of the commissures and subvalvular apparatus is associated with lower procedural success and higher incidence of significant mitral regurgitation (Answer C is incorrect). Presence of significant mitral regurgitation (suggested by clinical examination) is a contraindication for valvuloplasty (Answer D is incorrect).

13. **Answer: C.** Current ACC/AHA guidelines (**Table 18.1**) on valvular heart disease have focused on disease staging: at-risk patients (stage A), progressive mild–moderate disease (stage B), severe asymptomatic disease (stage C), and severe, symptomatic disease (stage D). Note that mitral stenosis is now considered severe when the valve area is ≤1.5 cm² (previously 1.0 cm²). Answer C is, therefore, the correct choice.

14. **Answer: D.** The grading of mitral stenosis severity in this patient is challenging. Pressure half-time is not reliable in the assessment of mitral valve area in elderly patients with degenerative calcific mitral stenosis, as it is influenced by coexisting diastolic dysfunction. In addition, the presence of moderate aortic regurgitation also impacts pressure half-time. The mean gradient is consistent with significant mitral stenosis, but the heart rate is fast. The patient's symptoms may also be related to uncontrolled hypertension. Although direct planimetry measurements are the preferred method for quantifying mitral stenosis, 2D planimetry is nevertheless challenging with a background of severe valvular calcification. Given all these findings, the next logical step is to optimize blood pressure control, reduce the heart rate, and then reassess mitral stenosis severity with 3D-guided planimetry and continuity.

15. **Answer: B.** The deceleration slope of the transmitral flow is sometimes bimodal, the decline of mitral inflow velocity being more rapid in early diastole than during the following part of the E wave. The first part of the signal is in fact reflective of both left atrial and ventricular pressure, not only mitral stenosis. Using trace 1 for measuring mitral valve pressure half-time is therefore a common mistake. Current ASE recommendations recommend that the deceleration slope in mid-diastole must be traced rather than the early deceleration slope.

Chapter 18 Mitral Stenosis / 391

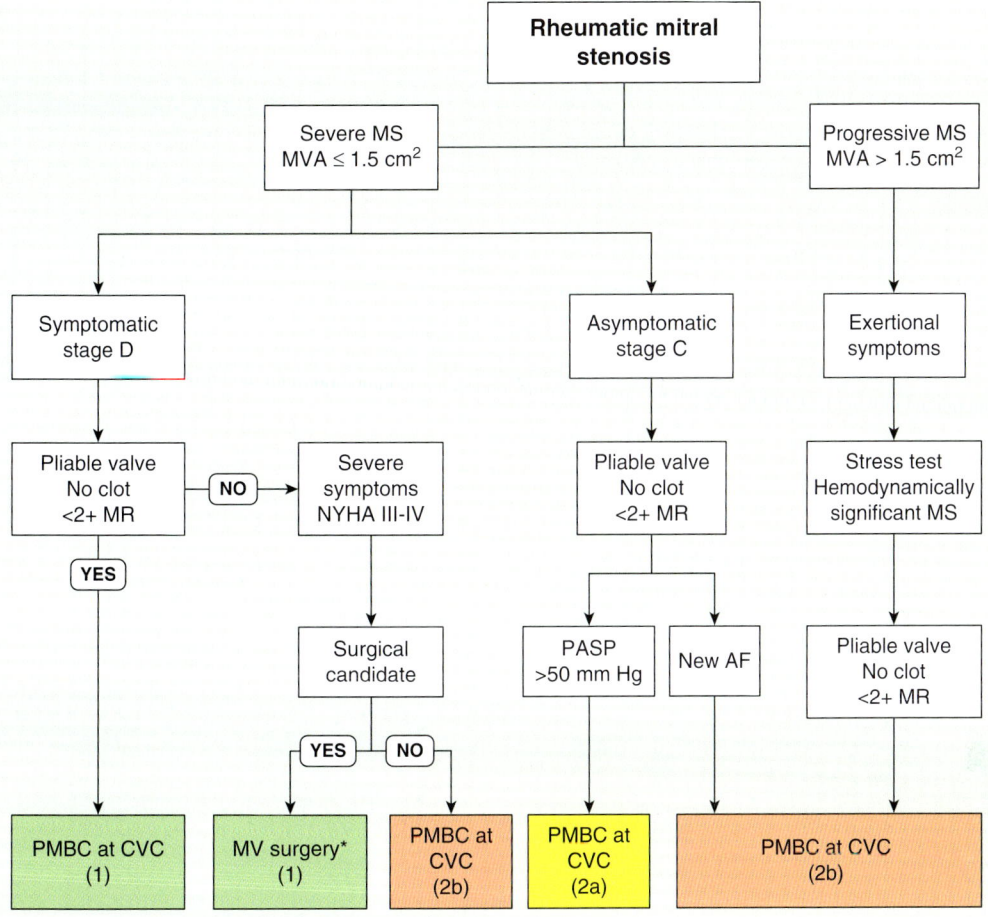

Figure 18.11. CVC, comprehensive valve center; PMBV, percutaneous mitral balloon commissurotomy. (Reprinted with permission from Otto CM, Nishimura RA, Bonow RO, et al. 2020 ACC/AHA guideline for the management of patients with valvular heart disease: a report of the American College of Cardiology/American Heart Association Joint Committee on Clinical Practice Guidelines. *Circulation*. 2021;143(5):e72-e227. Copyright © 2020 by the American College of Cardiology Foundation and the American Heart Association, Inc.)

16. **Answer: C.** The TEE images are diagnostic of rheumatic mitral stenosis. Note the hockey stick deformity of the anterior mitral leaflet and incomplete opening of the posterior leaflet. There is visible mitral inflow acceleration, and continuous-wave Doppler is consistent with severe mitral stenosis (a mean pressure gradient of 16 mm Hg). This condition in isolation is associated with a normal LV size (Answer A is incorrect). The interval between the second heart sound A_2 and the opening snap reflects the isovolumic relaxation time and is typically shorter with higher left atrial pressure (the shorter the A_2-opening snap interval, the more severe is the stenosis; Answer C is correct). The mitral gradient is significantly increased with increasing heart rates; presence of a diastolic rumble can be brought out with some physical activity at the time of examination (Answer D is incorrect).

17. **Answer: A.** The echocardiographic images show the hockey stick deformity with limited excursion of the anterior mitral leaflet. In this case, this is occurring after surgical repair with a posterior reduction annuloplasty. While uncommon, this is a known complication after mitral valve repair. The pathophysiologic mechanisms are similar to mitral stenosis of any other etiology, with left atrial hypertension leading to secondary pulmonary hypertension (Answer A is correct); hemoptysis is in this case a direct reflection of elevated postcapillary pulmonary pressure. Estimation of the left atrial pressure by catheterization with the use of the pulmonary capillary wedge pressure (to determine mitral gradients) may be inaccurate (overestimation of a gradient) and therefore the echocardiographic assessment of the mitral gradient is the preferred technique. An accurate transmitral gradient can be obtained at catheterization only by transseptal approach with direct measurement of the left atrial and left ventricular pressures (Answer B is incorrect). This patient has evidence of symptomatic severe mitral stenosis; an exercise echocardiogram will not provide additional information (Answer C is incorrect). Mitral balloon valvuloplasty cannot be used in patients who underwent mitral valve repair (Answer D is incorrect).

Table 18.3. Recommendations for Mitral Stenosis During Pregnancy

Recommendations	Class	Level
Pre-pregnancy evaluation, including echocardiography, and counseling is recommended for any woman with known or suspected valvular disease.	I	C
Mitral Stenosis		
In patients with symptoms or pulmonary hypertension, restricted activities and beta-1-selective blockers are recommended.	I	B
Diuretics are recommended when congestive symptoms persist despite beta-blockers.	I	B
Intervention is recommended before pregnancy in patients with MS and valve area <1.0 cm².	I	C
Therapeutic anticoagulation using heparins or VKA is recommended in case of atrial fibrillation, left atrial thrombosis, or prior embolism.	I	C
Intervention should be considered before pregnancy in patients with MS and valve area <1.5 cm².	IIa	C
Percutaneous mitral commissurotomy should be considered in pregnant patients with severe symptoms or systolic pulmonary artery pressure >50 mm Hg despite medical therapy.	IIa	C

MS, mitral stenosis; VKA, vitamin K antagonist
From Regitz-Zagrosek V, Roos-Hesselink JW, Bauersachs J, et al. 2018 ESC guidelines for the management of cardiovascular diseases during pregnancy. *Europ Heart J*. 2018;39(34):3165-3241. Reproduced by permission of The European Society of Cardiology and The European Society of Hypertension.

18. **Answer: B.** The echocardiogram demonstrates typical features of rheumatic mitral stenosis. Given that the MS is severe, that she is symptomatic, and that the valve appears amenable to percutaneous intervention, this is the preferred approach in this setting. Indeed, severe rheumatic MS presents a significant risk of maternal adverse outcome during pregnancy. Intervention before pregnancy is therefore recommended (**Table 18.3**) in symptomatic women on the basis of standard indications (class I). If the patient considers pregnancy but is asymptomatic, with MVA ≤ 1.5 cm², a BMV is also reasonable on the condition of suitable anatomy (class IIa).

19. **Answer: D.** Although percutaneous mitral balloon valvuloplasty represents a high-risk procedure during pregnancy for both the mother (risk for acute MR and need for valvular surgery) and the fetus (radiation exposure), it is indicated in this setting of a patient with prior symptomatic, severe MS and exacerbation of symptoms to NYHA IV during pregnancy. BMV improves hemodynamic tolerance and labor terms. The most appropriate time for the procedure is after the 4th month of the second trimester. By this time, organogenesis is complete, the fetal thyroid is still inactive, and the uterine volume is still small, so there is a greater distance between the fetus and the chest than in later months. Consequently, according to 2020 ACC/AHA Guidelines, BMV should be performed only if there is hemodynamic deterioration or if there are severe NYHA class III or IV HF symptoms. While open mitral valve replacement or commissurotomy may be considered, their risk is significantly higher than that of percutaneous intervention (30%-40% fetal mortality rate and up to 9% maternal mortality rate reported), and so should be reserved only for patients with severe, intractable symptoms unresponsive to bed rest and maximally tolerated medical therapy. Beta-blocker therapy is unlikely to help considering the normal increase in cardiac output and heart rate associated with pregnancy.

KEY POINTS
- Mitral stenosis (like other obstructive lesions) is not well tolerated during pregnancy.
- Percutaneous mitral balloon valvotomy can be performed safely and effectively during pregnancy, allowing for a subsequent uneventful pregnancy.

20. **Answer: E.** Congenital malformations of the mitral valve may be encountered in isolation or in association with other congenital heart defects. Each component of the mitral valve apparatus may be affected, according to the embryological development, which explains why these lesions are occasionally associated with each other. These lesions include anomalies of the leaflets (mitral valve prolapse, isolated cleft, double outlet mitral valve, supravalvular mitral ring as part of Shone syndrome, Ebstein malformation of the mitral valve) and anomalies of the subvalvular apparatus (mitral arcade, straddling mitral valve, parachute mitral valve). Severe hypoplasia or atresia of the mitral valve results in a hypoplastic LV cavity size that is not

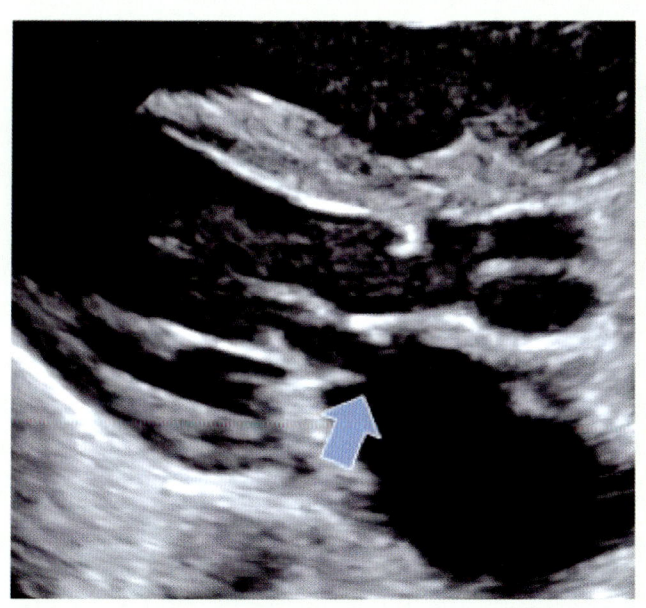

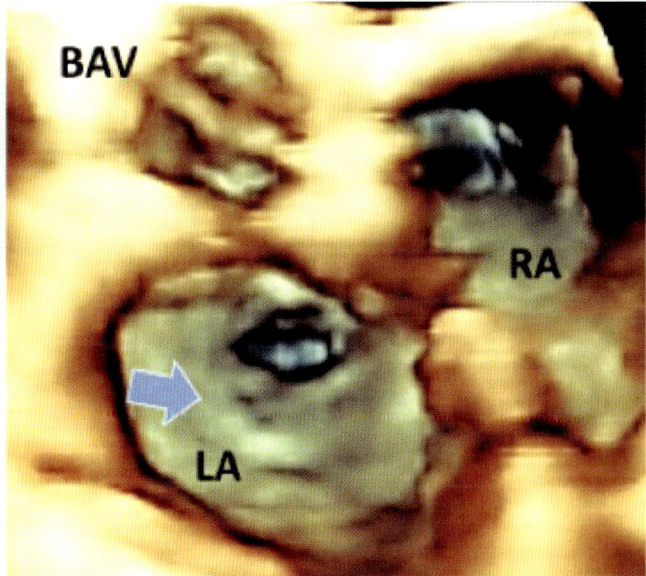

Figure 18.12. Blue arrow points to the supravalvar mitral ring. (Reprinted from Campbell M, Fuller S, Wang Y, et al. 3-Dimensional echocardiography provides incremental information in the diagnosis of supravalvar mitral ring. *J Am College Cardiol*. 2020;75(11):3022. Copyright © 2020 American College of Cardiology Foundation. With permission.)

capable of sustaining the systemic cardiac output. This situation is considered part of the spectrum of the hypoplastic left heart syndrome.

21. **Answer: C.** A supravalvular mitral ring, also called mitral ring or supramitral ring, is one of the components described in Shone syndrome. Occasionally isolated, this lesion is more often associated with other anomalies of the heart, mainly ventricular septal defect and left-sided obstructive lesions. The supramitral ring is a fibrous membrane originating just above the mitral annulus, beneath the orifice of the left atrial appendage, within the muscular atrial vestibule, not adhering to the leaflets and associated with a normal subvalvular apparatus (**Figure 18.12**). The supramitral ring must be distinguished from a cor triatriatum sinister, which is a fibromuscular membrane, distinct from the mitral valve (and proximal to the left atrial appendage) that divides the left atrium into two parts. This condition may be described as a valvar lesion rather than supravalvar because the annulus is an integral part of the mitral valve. Finally, the ring can be either complete, circumferential, or partial.

22. **Answer: D.** Radiation-induced valvular disease is uncommon (etiologies of MS in **Table 18.4**) and affects approximately 6% to 15% of patients exposed to mediastinal radiation therapy. The usual natural history starts with valvular regurgitation with later development of stenosis decades later often affecting the mitral and aortic valves. Typical echocardiographic features involve thickening and calcification of the mitral aortic intervalvular fibrosa (**Figure 18.13**) extending to the basal-to-mid anterior mitral leaflet and sparing the mitral commissures and posterior mitral leaflet. The calcification

Table 18.4. Etiologies of Mitral Stenosis

Common	Rheumatic
	Calcific
Uncommon	Radiation
	Systemic lupus erythematosus
	Endomyocardial fibrosis
	Carcinoid
Rare	Congenital
	Whipple disease
	Fabry disease
	Mucopolysaccharidoses type I and IV
Indirect cause	Infective endocarditis
	Left atrial myxoma

of the mitral-aortic intervalvular fibrosa commonly extends to the noncoronary cusp of the aortic valve causing aortic stenosis. Three-dimensional echocardiography provides an *en face* visualization of the mitral valve clearly demonstrating the absence of commissural fusion and obviating the need for balloon valvuloplasty. The pathophysiology of radiation-induced valvular disease is not fully understood. Over time, cellular injury combined with pressure-related trauma leads to valvular thickening, fibrosis, and calcification. Inflammation and fibrosis induce subvalvular deformities. Thus, radiation appears to initiate a degenerative process that ensues for many years.

394 / Clinical Echocardiography Review

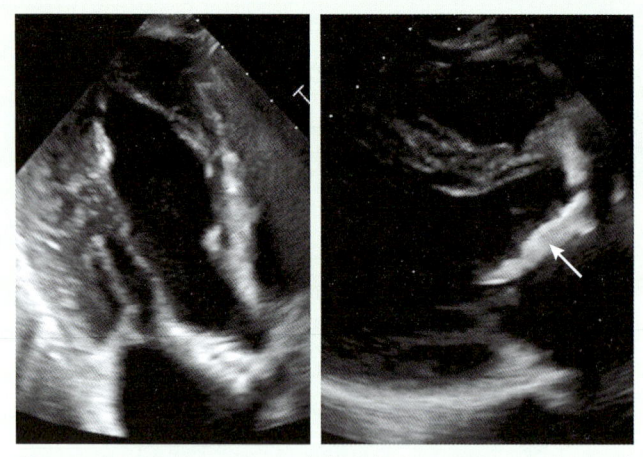

Figure 18.13. Arrow points to thickened aorto-mitral curtain seen with radiation heart disease.

23. **Answer: C.** The PISA method for calculation of the MVA assesses the mitral flow based on the hemispheric shape of the convergence zone of mitral flow in diastole on the left atrial side as depicted by color Doppler. Subsequently, the MVA is calculated by dividing the mitral volume flow by the maximum velocity of mitral flow in diastole, as assessed by continuous-wave Doppler: MVA = $2\pi r^2$ × (angle $\alpha/180$) × (V_{alias}/V_{max}), where r is the radius of the hemispheric convergence zone (in centimeters), V_{alias} is the aliasing velocity (in centimeters per second), peak V_{max} is the peak velocity of mitral inflow assessed by continuous-wave Doppler (in centimeters per second), and α is the opening angle of mitral leaflets relative to flow direction (example in **Figure 18.14**). The PISA method is technically challenging but can be used in the presence of severe mitral regurgitation. The integration of color M-mode, enabling simultaneous measurements of velocity and flow, improves the accuracy of this method. Moreover, correct visualization of the convergent zone is necessary to perform the PISA calculation, and thus, this method is not applicable for all etiologies of mitral stenosis, such as calcific MS where the calcifications often prevent accurate delineation of the hemispheric convergence zone.

24. **Answer: C.** The Wilkins score is the most widely used score, predicting the procedural success for balloon mitral valvuloplasty. This score integrates calcification, thickness, and mobility of the anterior mitral leaflet and the thickness of the chordal apparatus. Each of these four variables is assigned a score from 1 to 4, and these scores are summed. A total score

MVA = $2\pi r^2$ × (angle $\alpha/180$) × (V_{alias}/V_{max})

In this patient
With a radius of 0.55 cm and an angle of 155°
→ **MVA = 0.47 cm²**

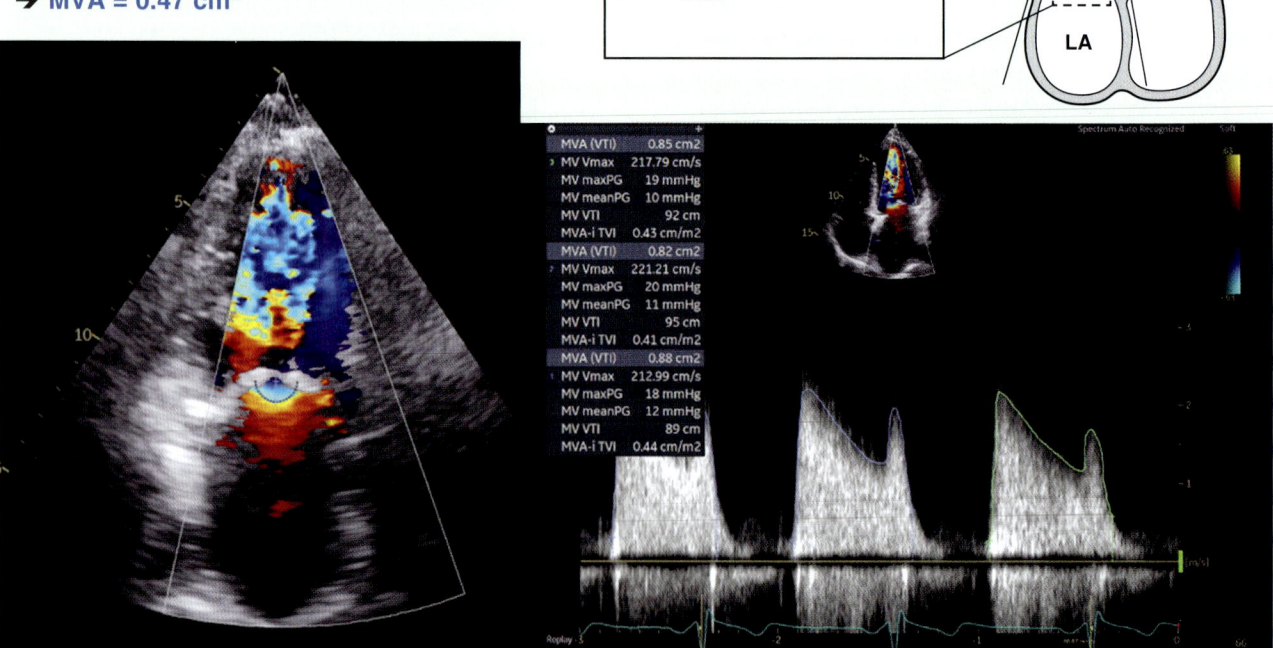

Figure 18.14

A Assessment of Mitral Valve Anatomy According to the Wilkins Score

Grade	Mobility	Subvalvular Thickening	Leaflet Thickening	Calcification
1	Highly mobile valve with only leaflet tips restricted	Minimal thickening just below the mitral leaflets	Leaflets near normal in thickness (4-5 mm)	A single area of increased echo brightness
2	Leaflet mid and basal portions have normal mobility	Thickening of chordal structures extending up to one-third of the chordal length	Mid-leaflets normal, considerable thickening of margins (5-8 mm)	Scattered areas of brightness confined to leaflet margins
3	Valve continues to move forward in diastole, mainly from the base	Thickening extending to the distal third of the chords	Thickening extending through the entire leaflet (5-8 mm)	Brightness extending into the midportion of the leaflets
4	No or minimal forward movement of the leaflets in diastole	Extensive thickening and shortening of all chordal structures extending down to the papillary muscles	Considerable thickening of all leaflet tissue (>8-10 mm)	Extensive brightness throughout much of the leaflet tissue

The total score is the sum of each of these echocardiographic features and ranges from 4-16.

B Assessment of Mitral Valve Anatomy According to the Padial Score

Grade	Leaflet Thickening (Score Each Valve separately.)	Commissure Calcification	Subvalvular Disease
1	Leaflet near normal (4-5 mm) or with only a thick segment	Fibrosis and/or calcium in only one commissure	Minimal thickening of chordal structures just below the valve
2	Leaflet fibrotic and/or calcified evenly; no thin areas	Both commissures mildly affected	Thickening of chordae extending up to one-third of chordal length
3	Leaflet fibrotic and/or calcified with uneven distribution; thinner segments are mildly thickened (5-8 mm)	Calcium in both commissures; one markedly affected	Thickening of the distal third of the chordae
4	Leaflet fibrotic and/or calcified with uneven distribution; thinner segments are near normal (4-5 mm)	Calcium in both commissures; both markedly affected	Extensive thickening and shortening of all chordae extending down to the papillary muscle

Figure 18.15. A: Wilkins Score. (Adapted from Wilkins GT, Weyman AE, Abascal VM, Block PC, Palacios IF. Percutaneous balloon dilatation of the mitral valve: an analysis of echocardiographic variables related to outcome and the mechanism of dilatation. *Br Heart J.* 1988;60(4):299-308, with permission from BMJ Publishing Group Ltd.) **B:** Padial Score. (Reprinted from Padial LR, Abascal VM, Moreno PR, Weyman AE, Levine RA, Palacios IF. Echocardiography can predict the development of severe mitral regurgitation after percutaneous mitral valvuloplasty by the Inoue technique. *Am J Cardiol.* 1999;83(8):1210-1213, with permission from Elsevier. Copyright © 1999 Elsevier. With permission.)

≤8 predicts favorable immediate and long-term outcomes, whereas a score >8 portends lesser likelihood of success. However, the score does not evaluate the anatomy of the commissures (particularly the presence of commissural calcifications) and therefore fails to predict the risk for developing mitral regurgitation. The MR echocardiographic score by Padial et al (**Figure 18.15**) is useful to predict significant regurgitation after BMV with high sensitivity and specificity using mitral valve morphology as the most important predictor for the development of significant MR after mitral balloon valvuloplasty.

25. Answer: C. The mitral PHT is inaccurate for determining valve area for approximately 24 to 48 hours after BMV, mostly due to the changes in pre- and afterload induced by the procedure on noncompliant cavities (LV and LA). LV diastolic dysfunction is a well-known consequence of long-standing mitral stenosis, which is related to atrophy of the chambers due to unloading, myocardial fibrosis from associated rheumatic myocarditis, internal restrictions due to the tethering of the thickened subvalvular apparatus, and/or the abnormal interactions between the abnormal right ventricular and LV interactions due to right ventricular pressure overload. After BMV, the sudden increase in LV preload therefore results in an increase in LV end-diastolic pressure without an increase in LV end-diastolic volume; this increases the mean LA pressure and therefore shortens the PHT. Despite the decrease in atrial volume after the BMV is performed, LA operational compliance remains reduced for 24 to 48 hours, further shortening the PHT. Because the accuracy of the PHT depends upon transmitral MG and LA compliance changing in opposite directions, PHT may remain inaccurate during this period. It is therefore recommended that MV area be measured using planimetry following BMV. It is useful to note that when planimetry cannot be accurately performed, a PHT < 130 ms reliably predicts a post-BMV MV area ≥1.5 cm² with high specificity but low sensitivity. Iatrogenic septal defects induced by the procedure are small and low in shunt ratio. They appear not to be associated with long-term adverse events.

26. **Answer: C.** The mitral PHT is the time it takes for the peak LA-LV pressure gradient to fall by 50%. This is determined by the rate at which falling LA and rising LV diastolic pressures come into equilibrium. When equilibrium is reached slowly, PHT is prolonged and mitral stenosis is severe, and vice versa. Empiric observations from invasive hemodynamic studies reveal that when PHT is 220 ms, MV area equals 1.0 cm². Hence, MV area can be calculated using the formula: 220/PHT (the Hatle formula). Doppler-derived PHT can be used to calculate MV area using the same formula, but it does not perform accurately unless the MV is stenotic and rheumatic. In general, the most optimal Doppler modality to use in mitral stenosis is continuous wave since it can record higher velocities than pulsed Doppler. Pressure half-time is influenced by several factors that render calculation of MV area inaccurate (especially in older patients) such as LV diastolic dysfunction (shortening the PHT by reducing ventricular compliance), significant AR (shortening the PHT also by increasing the rate of diastolic LV pressure rise), significant MR (lengthening the PHT by prolonging the time for transmitral velocity to decrease due to the marked rise in E-wave velocity), and presence of an ASD. In Lutembacher syndrome (the association of ASD and mitral stenosis), when MS is severe, and ASD is nonrestrictive, the left atrium finds another exit through the septum in addition to the mitral valve (LA decompression). Therefore, LA pressure does not rise in proportion to the severity of MS and PHT usually overestimates the mitral valve area. PHT is accurate with atrial fibrillation though it is recommended to average at least five cardiac cycles and avoid very short cycles where there is not time for the gradient to fall to one half of it original value. PHT equates to the time it takes for the velocity to decrease to 70% of peak velocity or $V_{t1/2} = V_{max}/\sqrt{2}$.

27. **Answer: E.** When the Wilkins score is >10, BMV is generally associated with a higher incidence of severe MR and not an optimal approach. The severity of preprocedural MR predicts the possibility of severe MR after the procedure that is associated with a poor long-term outcome post-BMV. Moderate to severe MR (≥3+) is considered a contraindication for BMV given that the procedure generally worsens MR severity. Interatrial septal and left atrial thrombi are absolute contraindications of transseptal puncture and BMV, whereas left appendage thrombi are considered a relative contraindication. Bicommissural and fluoroscopic valve calcification, such as in calcific MS, is associated with a poor outcome following BMV. When the commissural fusion is absent, BMV is ineffective and should be avoided.

SUGGESTED READINGS

Anwar AM, Attia WM, Nosir YFM, et al. Validation of a new score for the assessment of mitral stenosis using real-time three-dimensional echocardiography. *J Am Soc Echocardiogr*. 2010;23(1):13-22.

Ben-Farhat M, Betbout F, Gamra H, et al. Predictors of long-term event-free survival and of freedom from restenosis after percutaneous balloon mitral commissurotomy. *Am Heart J*. 2001;142(6):1072-1079.

Otto CM, Nishimura RA, Bonow RO, et al. 2020 ACC/AHA guideline for the management of patients with valvular heart disease: a report of the American College of Cardiology/American Heart Association Joint Committee on Clinical Practice Guidelines. *Circulation*. 2021;143(5):e72-e227.

Sebag IA, Morgan JG, Handschumacher MD, et al. Usefulness of three-dimensionally guided assessment of mitral stenosis using matrix-array ultrasound. *Am J Cardiol*. 2005;96(8):1151-1156.

Silbiger JJ. Advances in rheumatic mitral stenosis: echocardiographic, pathophysiologic, and hemodynamic considerations. *J Am Soc Echocardiogr*. 2021;34(7):709-722.e1.

Vahanian A, Beyersdorf F, Praz F, et al. 2021 ESC/EACTS guidelines for the management of valvular heart disease: developed by the task force for the management of valvular heart disease of the European Society of Cardiology (ESC) and the European Association for Cardio-Thoracic surgery (EACTS). *Rev Esp Cardiol*. 2022;75(6):524.

Wunderlich NC, Beigel R, Siegel RJ. Management of mitral stenosis using 2D and 3D echo-Doppler imaging. *JACC Cardiovasc Imaging*. 2013;6(11):1191-1205.

CHAPTER 19

Pulmonic and Tricuspid Valvular Disease

Diarmaid Hughes and Brian P. Griffin

QUESTIONS

1. In which of the following clinical scenarios is transesophageal echocardiography (TEE) usually indicated in addition to transthoracic echocardiography (TTE) in a diagnostic assessment?
   A. Pulmonary artery (PA) pressure in primary pulmonary hypertension.
   B. Inferior vena cava (IVC) thrombus.
   C. Suspected pacemaker endocarditis.
   D. Right ventricular (RV) function.
   E. Mild pulmonic stenosis.

2. The most common tricuspid valve anatomy consists of which of the following leaflets?
   A. Anterior, septal, lateral.
   B. Anterior, posterior, septal.
   C. Septal, lateral, posterior.
   D. Left, right, posterior.
   E. Left, right, anterior.

3. How often does the tricuspid valve have three leaflets?
   A. 95%.
   B. 85%.
   C. 75%.
   D. 65%.
   E. 55%.

4. A young man with mild pulmonary valve stenosis is seen. He has a peak gradient across the pulmonary valve of 20 mm Hg. His tricuspid regurgitant velocity is 3 m/s and his right atrial size is normal. His IVC is not enlarged and decreases further on sniffing. Which of the following is **TRUE**?
   A. His PA systolic pressure is normal.
   B. His PA systolic pressure is moderately elevated.
   C. His PA systolic pressure cannot be estimated when pulmonic stenosis is present.
   D. He has severe PA hypertension that will require treatment.
   E. None of the above.

5. An elderly woman is referred to your clinic for assessment. She has had progressive shortness of breath on exertion and lower limb edema over the last number of months. On examination, her JVP is elevated and her liver edge is palpable and pulsatile and there is a low frequency diastolic murmur present. Which of the following conditions is **NOT** associated with tricuspid stenosis?
   A. Carcinoid syndrome.
   B. Right-sided cardiac tumor.
   C. Rheumatic heart disease.
   D. Infective endocarditis.
   E. Tetralogy of Fallot.

6. A Gerbode defect is:
   A. Atrialization of the right ventricle in Ebstein anomaly.
   B. An unroofed coronary sinus with resultant bidirectional ASD at the level of the AV groove.
   C. A left-sided superior vena cava entering and enlarged coronary sinus.
   D. A communication between the right atrium and the left ventricle that may encompass the tricuspid valve leaflets.
   E. A sinus of Valsalva aneurysm that communicates with the right atrium.

7. A patient with prior rheumatic disease is seen. An echocardiogram is obtained. Which of the following is **TRUE** about the Doppler echocardiographic assessment of tricuspid stenosis in this condition?
   A. Doming and thickening of the valve in systole are seen.
   B. The mean pressure gradient is at least 10 mm Hg in severe stenosis.
   C. The valve area may be estimated by dividing 190 by the pressure halftime.
   D. Planimetry of the valve area is readily obtained.
   E. Tricuspid stenosis is clinically significant in 25% of patients with rheumatic mitral stenosis.

8. Pulmonary artery pressures cannot be estimated by measurement of a:
   A. Tricuspid regurgitation (TR) jet.
   B. Pulmonic insufficiency jet.
   C. Ventricular septal defect (VSD) jet.
   D. Atrial septal defect jet.
   E. Right ventricular outflow tract jet.

9. The most common cause of significant TR is:
   A. Myxomatous change or prolapse.
   B. Rheumatic disease.
   C. Endocarditis.
   D. Secondary to pulmonary hypertension and/or RV dilatation.
   E. Trauma.

10. Which of the following is consistent with the diagnosis of severe pulmonic stenosis?
    A. Peak velocity of >4 m/s across the pulmonic valve.
    B. Normal RV systolic pressure.
    C. RV wall thickness of 0.3 cm.
    D. Normal size of the PA.
    E. None of the above.

11. A 25-year-old asymptomatic man presents with a systolic murmur at the second left interspace. An echocardiogram is obtained and he is found to have pulmonic stenosis. A peak pressure gradient is measured and is 20 mm Hg. Which of the following statements about his condition is most likely to be **TRUE**?
    A. He is likely to require surgical or balloon valvuloplasty in the next decade.
    B. He should undergo yearly examination and echocardiography and a baseline transesophageal echocardiogram.
    C. Cardiac catheterization is indicated to more accurately determine his pulmonic pressure gradient.
    D. Systolic doming of the pulmonary valve is present.
    E. None of the above.

12. Which of the following statements about pulmonary insufficiency is **CORRECT**?
    A. Pulmonary insufficiency detected by Doppler of any degree is abnormal.
    B. Severe pulmonary insufficiency leads to a highly turbulent jet on color flow Doppler.
    C. Severe pulmonary insufficiency most commonly occurs in the setting of prior treatment of congenital heart disease.
    D. Pulmonary insufficiency may be used to measure the PA systolic pressure.
    E. None of the above.

13. Which of the following is the most likely cause of a mobile tricuspid valve mass?
    A. Sarcoma.
    B. Fibroelastoma.
    C. Myxoma.
    D. Chiari network.
    E. Carcinoid syndrome.

14. The normal pulmonic valve consists of which three cusps?
    A. Left, right, anterior.
    B. Anterior, posterior, left.
    C. Left, right, posterior.
    D. Anterior, posterior, septal.
    E. Anterior, posterior, right.

15. Which of the following statements about infundibular pulmonic stenosis is **CORRECT**?
    A. Infundibular pulmonic stenosis is always part of a congenital syndrome.
    B. Infundibular stenosis may cause a high-velocity jet that impinges on the pulmonary valve, causing pulmonary insufficiency.
    C. The site of stenosis is usually discrete.
    D. Doppler estimation of the pressure gradient across the infundibular stenosis is inaccurate except when valvular stenosis coexists.
    E. Infundibular stenosis is most easily assessed from a parasternal short-axis imaging plane.

16. A young man presents with fatigue and a history of occasional near syncope with onset of a fast heart rhythm. Based on the apical 4-chamber image in **Figure 19.1**, which is the least likely finding in this patient?
   A. Wolff-Parkinson-White pattern on electrocardiogram.
   B. Intracardiac shunt.
   C. Parchment-like RV wall.
   D. Severe TR.
   E. Atrialization of a portion of the RV.

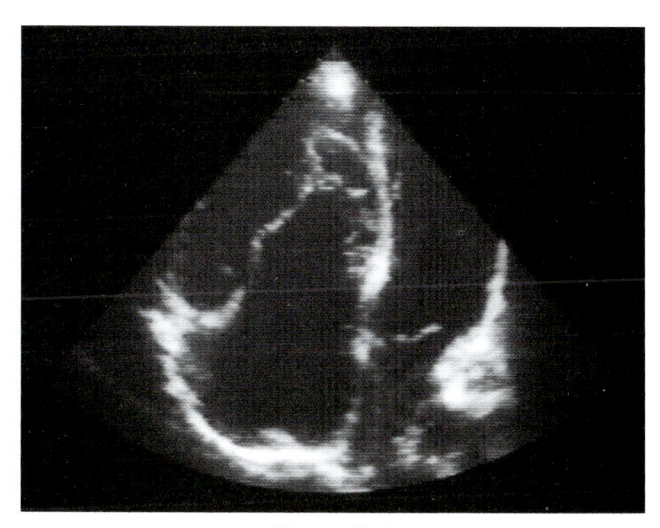

Figure 19.1

17. A young woman with a history of Noonan syndrome presents to your clinic to reestablish care after being lost to follow up. She is active, and enjoys hiking, though does get short of breath when hiking up steep inclines. There is no evidence of right heart failure on physical exam. The Doppler profile through her pulmonic valve from a parasternal short-axis view is shown in **Figure 19.2**. Which of the following statements regarding the Doppler profile is **TRUE**?
   A. There is at least moderate pulmonic stenosis.
   B. There is at least moderately elevated pulmonary artery pressure.
   C. There is significant pulmonary regurgitation.
   D. There is severe pulmonic stenosis.
   E. There is no significant pulmonic stenosis or regurgitation.

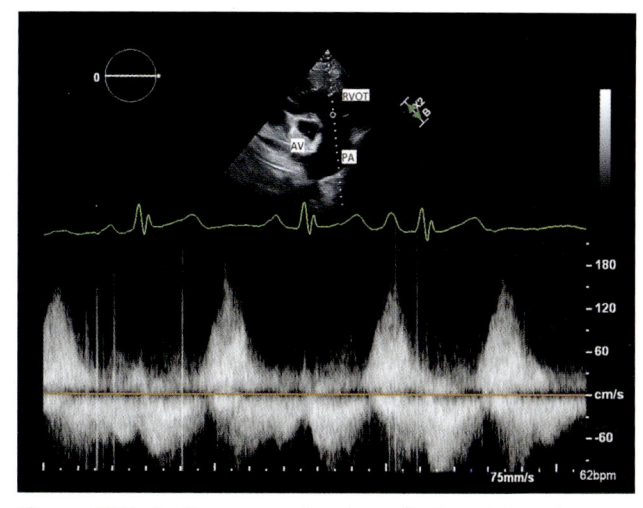

Figure 19.2. Continuous-wave Doppler profile through the pulmonary valve.

18. A 57-year-old man is undergoing mitral valve repair for severe mitral regurgitation from mitral valve prolapse. He has an intraoperative TEE before the surgical repair and you are asked to consult regarding the image of the TR and tricuspid valve in the mid-esophageal 4-chamber view (**Figure 19.3**). Which of the following is **CORRECT**?
   A. The degree of TR detected intraoperatively will likely overestimate that detected on routine ambulatory examination and should not be used in the decision-making regarding concomitant tricuspid valve surgery.
   B. Surgical intervention on the tricuspid valve is rarely required in this situation as it always improves after surgical correction of the mitral valve.
   C. Surgical correction of the tricuspid valve should be considered as the regurgitation appears severe with a significant flow convergence area, and TR is more likely underestimated in the operative setting.
   D. The most likely cause of severe TR in this situation is a flail tricuspid valve.
   E. TR occurs only in this situation in the presence of severe pulmonary hypertension.

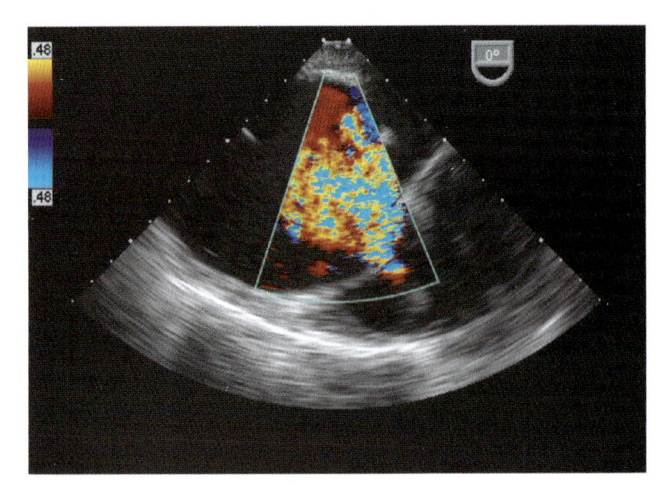

Figure 19.3

19. A 72-year-old woman with a history of hypertension, paroxysmal atrial fibrillation, and sick sinus syndrome, status post pacemaker insertion 4 years previously, is being worked up for progressive shortness of breath on exertion. A TTE shows new significant TR and so a TEE is performed. A mid-esophageal TEE image is shown in **Figure 19.4**. Which of the following is the most likely explanation for the new tricuspid regurgitation?
   A. Atrial functional tricuspid regurgitation.
   B. Pulmonary hypertension.
   C. RV dysfunction.
   D. Annular dilation.
   E. Pacing lead–induced tricuspid regurgitation.

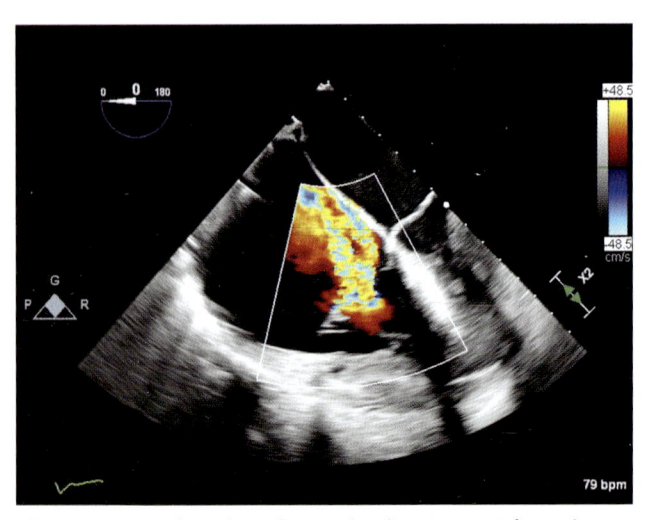

Figure 19.4. Mid-esophageal TEE 4-chamber view at 0° focused on the tricuspid valve.

20. The hepatic vein pulsed-wave Doppler profile shown in **Figure 19.5** is most likely associated with which of the following clinical profiles?
   A. Large "v" waves in the jugular venous profile.
   B. Pulsus paradoxus.
   C. Kussmaul sign.
   D. Pulsus alternans.
   E. Pulsus bisferiens.

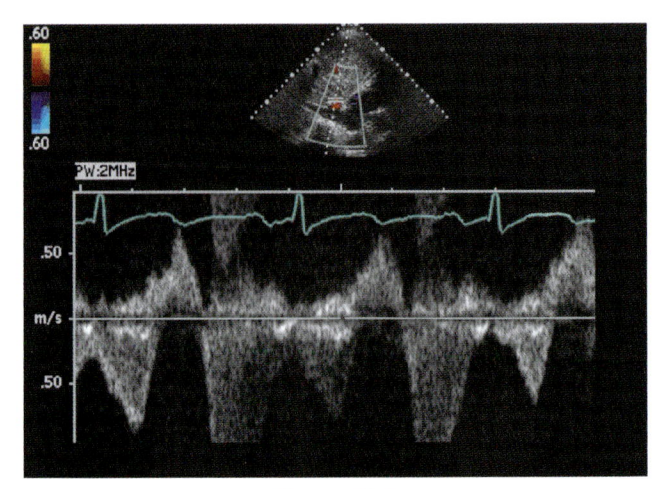

Figure 19.5

21. The RVOT pulsed-wave Doppler (note with arrow) in **Figure 19.6** is most likely associated with which of the following?
   A. Infundibular pulmonic stenosis.
   B. Elevated pulmonary artery pressures.
   C. Severe pulmonary regurgitation.
   D. Infective endocarditis.
   E. Pulmonic valve stenosis.

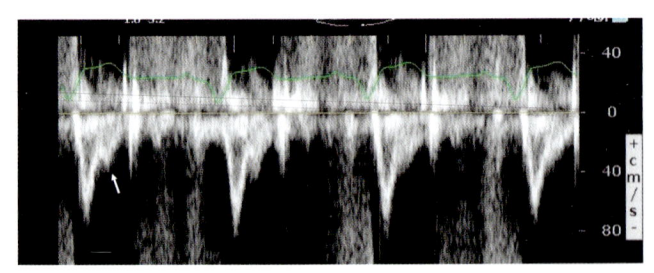

Figure 19.6. Pulsed-wave Doppler profile through the right ventricular outflow tract.

22. A 45-year-old woman status post kidney transplantation for lupus nephritis was referred for the evaluation of nonspecific chest pain. She has no fever or murmur. Which of the following diagnoses is most likely with regard to the image in **Figure 19.7**?
  A. Myxoma.
  B. Vegetation.
  C. Fibroma.
  D. Fibroelastoma.
  E. Thrombus.

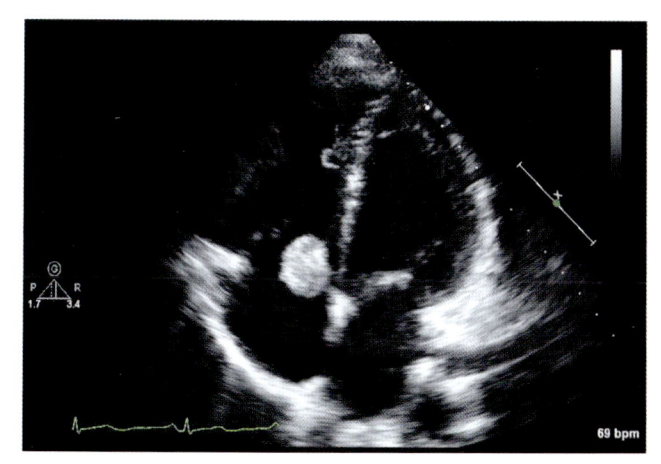

Figure 19.7

23. The Doppler velocity in **Figure 19.8** is through the pulmonary valve in the parasternal short-axis view of an 18-year-old man with chest pain. Which of the following statements is **CORRECT**?
  A. In the absence of chest pain, there is no indication for any intervention.
  B. He will likely benefit from a balloon valvuloplasty.
  C. Based on the Doppler profile, he has associated subvalvular stenosis.
  D. He most likely has a bicuspid pulmonic valve.
  E. His chest pain is unrelated to the valve lesion.

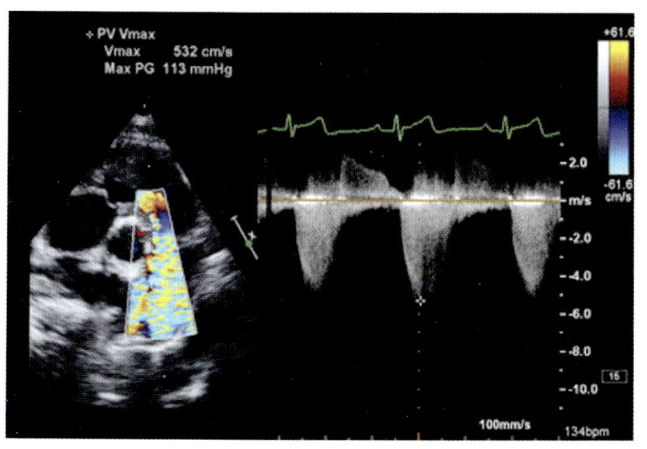

Figure 19.8

24. **Figure 19.9** illustrates a TEE transgastric view of the right atrium and right ventricle with the tricuspid valve open in diastole.
  The patient has been recently admitted with fevers 6 weeks after permanent pacemaker implantation. No obvious infection is evident at the site of the pacemaker insertion. Mild central TR is present. Which of the following statements is **TRUE** about this patient?
  A. The tricuspid valve will need to be replaced.
  B. Only antibiotic therapy is required.
  C. Surgical removal of the pacing wires followed by antibiotics is all that is required.
  D. Percutaneous removal of the pacing wires and antibiotic therapy is required.
  E. The patient will most likely require antibiotic treatment as well as surgical removal of the pacemaker wires and the pacemaker system including the generator.

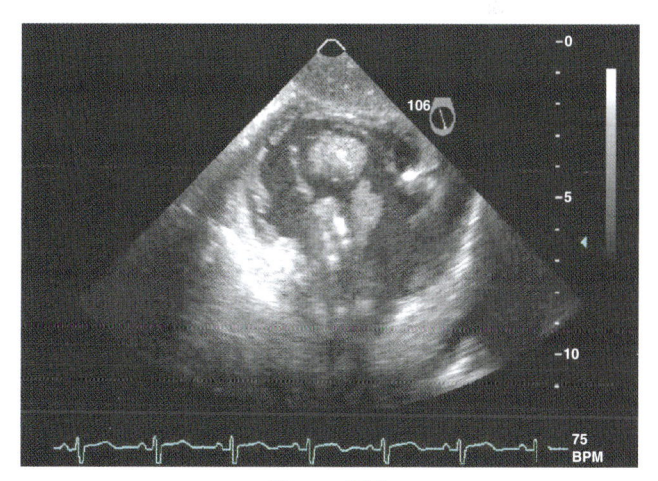

Figure 19.9

25. The pulmonary valve M-mode shown in **Figure 19.10** is most likely associated with which of the following?
  A. Endocarditis of the pulmonary valve.
  B. Infundibular pulmonic stenosis in a young man with prior repair of tetralogy of Fallot.
  C. A young woman with primary pulmonary hypertension being considered for therapeutic intervention.
  D. A retained PA catheter remnant in an elderly man with a prolonged hospital course.
  E. Severe pulmonic insufficiency.

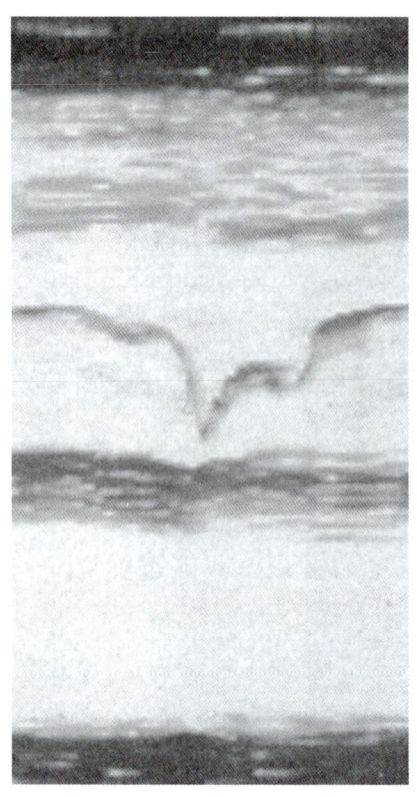

Figure 19.10. Pulmonary valve M-mode.

A. Tachycardia-mediated cardiomyopathy.
B. Severe TR.
C. Severe pulmonary hypertension.
D. Recent endocarditis.
E. Right-to-left shunt at the atrial level.

27. Which of the following statements about treatment of the patient in **Case 1** is **TRUE**?
    A. There is no indication for an electrophysiologic study as surgical correction of the condition will also eradicate the arrhythmia.
    B. Medical therapy is of little value in this condition and recourse to surgery is indicated.
    C. Tricuspid valve replacement is the surgical therapy of choice.
    D. The anterior leaflet is the most abnormal in this condition and should be removed if possible.
    E. The size of the functional right ventricle is important in defining the likelihood and type of surgery.

CASE 1

A 30-year-old woman presents with right-sided heart failure but without clubbing or cyanosis. She has had a murmur since childhood but has only recently complained of fatigue and ankle edema. On admission, she developed a wide complex tachycardia at a fast rate and required immediate cardioversion. An apical 4-chamber view of her heart is shown in ▶ Video 19.1 and Figure 19.11.

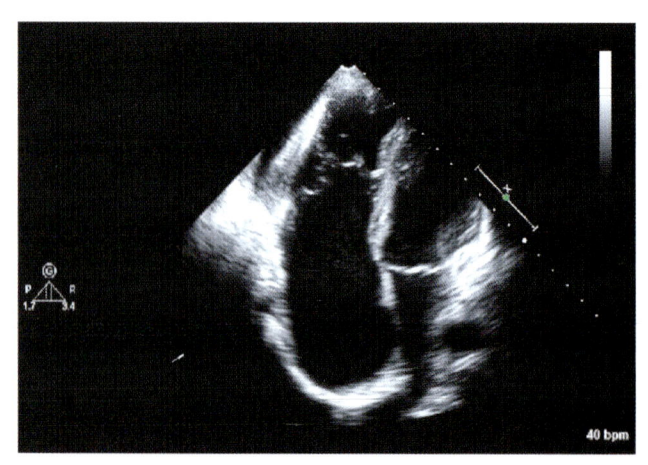

Figure 19.11

26. What is the most likely cause of the patient in **Case 1** (▶ Video 19.1, Figure 19.11) heart failure symptoms?

CASE 2

A 65-year-old man is readmitted 8 weeks following tricuspid and mitral valve repair for myxomatous disease of both valves. He has been feeling unwell and is anemic but has had no significant febrile illness. He has a white blood cell count of 12,000, with a leftward shift. A TEE is performed, an image of which is shown in ▶ Video 19.2 and Figure 19.12. He has no significant mitral regurgitation or TR.

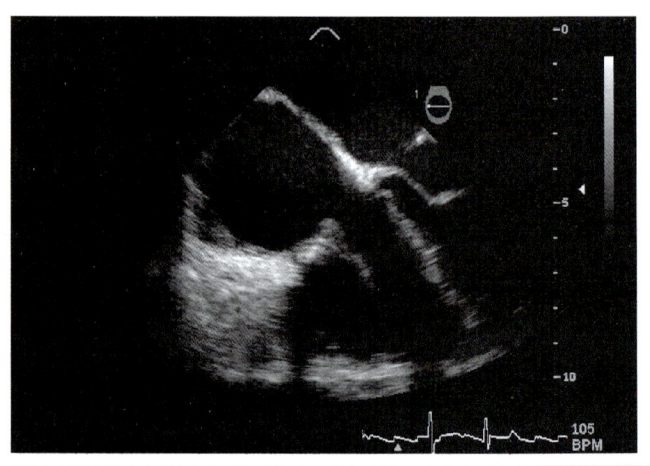

Figure 19.12

28. The most likely cause of the scenario in **Case 2** (▶ Video 19.2, Figure 19.12) is:
    A. Staphylococcal infection.
    B. Thrombus formation at the valve ring.
    C. Ring dehiscence.
    D. Embolus in transit.
    E. Fungal infection.

29. The **BEST** course of treatment for the patient in **Case 2** is:
    A. Immediate surgical exploration and removal of the mass.
    B. Intravenous thrombolysis.
    C. Blood cultures, broad-spectrum coverage pending cultures, and close monitoring of the valves by echocardiography.
    D. Replacement of both mitral and tricuspid valves.
    E. Heparin treatment followed by transition to warfarin (Coumadin).

CASE 3

A color Doppler video of the RV outflow tract in an asymptomatic young man found to have a murmur on routine physical examination is shown in ▶ Video 19.3. He has a right parasternal heave, an ejection click, and a loud ejection systolic murmur with a soft P2 heard on auscultation.

30. Based on the findings in **Case 3** (▶ Video 19.3), select the **CORRECT** statement from the following:
    A. He has a patent ductus arteriosus with Eisenmenger physiology.
    B. He has an ASD with Eisenmenger physiology.
    C. He has pulmonic stenosis, possibly severe, with mild pulmonic insufficiency.
    D. He has a high outflow state with a flow murmur.
    E. He has infundibular pulmonic stenosis.

31. The most appropriate next step in the management of the patient in **Case 3** is to:
    A. Perform balloon valvuloplasty of the pulmonic valve.
    B. Establish the pulmonic valve area by continuity.
    C. Measure the velocity and thus pressure across the RV outflow tract by continuous-wave Doppler.
    D. Assess the PA systolic pressure.
    E. Perform contrast echocardiography to define the presence and site of shunting.

CASE 4

A 42-year-old woman who is an immigrant from India presents to a cardiology clinic with new-onset right-sided heart failure. She has peripheral cyanosis, regular rhythm, a loud first heart sound, and an apical diastolic murmur. Her jugular venous pulse shows prominent pulsations that precede systole. She has an RV heave but normal P2 and a prominent abdomen and tender liver edge. A 4-chamber image is shown in ▶ Video 19.4.

32. Based on echocardiography and patient physical findings in **Case 4** (▶ Video 19.4), what is the most likely diagnosis giving rise to the patient's symptoms?
    A. Mitral stenosis and TR due to severe pulmonary hypertension.
    B. Tricuspid stenosis and regurgitation without significant mitral stenosis.
    C. Mitral stenosis and regurgitation.
    D. Tricuspid stenosis and mitral stenosis.
    E. Constrictive pericarditis.

33. What is the most appropriate treatment of the patient in **Case 4**?
    A. Medical therapy only.
    B. Balloon valvuloplasty of the mitral and tricuspid valve.
    C. Surgical replacement of both mitral and tricuspid valve.
    D. Surgical commissurotomy of both mitral and tricuspid valve.
    E. Balloon valvuloplasty of the mitral valve.

CASE 5

You are asked to perform a transesophageal echocardiogram (TEE) on a 55-year-old gentleman. He is 6 months post a heart transplant and has been admitted with symptoms of heart failure. A mid-esophageal TEE image is shown in ▶ Video 19.5.

34. What is the most likely cause of the appearance of the tricuspid valve abnormality in the patient from **Case 5** (▶ Video 19.5)?
    A. Acute allograft rejection.
    B. Postoperative complication.
    C. Transplant associated coronary artery disease.
    D. Post endomyocardial biopsy complication.
    E. Pulmonary hypertension.

35. Which of the following statements regarding the abnormality shown in ▶ Videos 19.6 and 19.7 is **CORRECT**?
    A. The mean pulmonary artery pressure can be estimated from the tricuspid regurgitation (TR) velocity in this case.
    B. There is a coaptation gap in systole consistent with severe TR.
    C. The tricuspid valve (TV) will likely be need to be replaced.
    D. There is concomitant tricuspid stenosis.
    E. There is evidence of infective endocarditis of the TV.

ANSWERS

1. **Answer: C.** Right-sided valve lesions are usually well identified by transthoracic imaging as these structures lie anterior in the chest and in the near field of the chest wall transducer. However, better resolution of pulmonary valve endocarditis or mass, embolus in transit in the right heart, and of vegetations involving a pacer wire have been reported with TEE than with TTE alone. TEE is not usually indicated in the assessment of PA pressures in primary pulmonary hypertension. When the tricuspid regurgitant velocity is difficult to measure by TTE, injection of agitated saline contrast has been shown to improve the spectral display of the regurgitant jet and is more likely to be helpful than a TEE in this situation.

2. **Answer: B.** The tricuspid valve consists most commonly of three leaflets: anterior, posterior, and septal. The leaflets are of unequal size with the anterior leaflet being the largest, the posterior leaflet is the smallest, and the septal leaflet is the shortest radially and least mobile. The leaflets are attached to the tricuspid valve annulus, which is an ellipsoid, saddle-shaped structure. The most common papillary muscle arrangement is to have an anterior, a posterior, and a septal papillary muscle, though the septal papillary muscle can be absent in up to 20% of people. It can be challenging to distinguish the individual leaflets on 2D echocardiography; however, standard views can help (see **Figures 19.13-19.15**). From the parasternal inflow view if the septum or coronary sinus is seen, then the leaflets imaged are the septal and anterior, while if no septum is seen, the leaflets imaged would be the anterior and posterior. From the parasternal short-axis view with the AV in view, a single anterior leaflet is seen; as the annulus dilates, the anterior and posterior leaflets may be seen, and with the transducer angled toward the LVOT, the septal leaflet may come into view. In the apical 4-chamber view, the septal leaflet can be identified attached to the septum, and the leaflet opposite is likely to be the anterior (if the AV is in view) or the posterior if coronary sinus is in view.

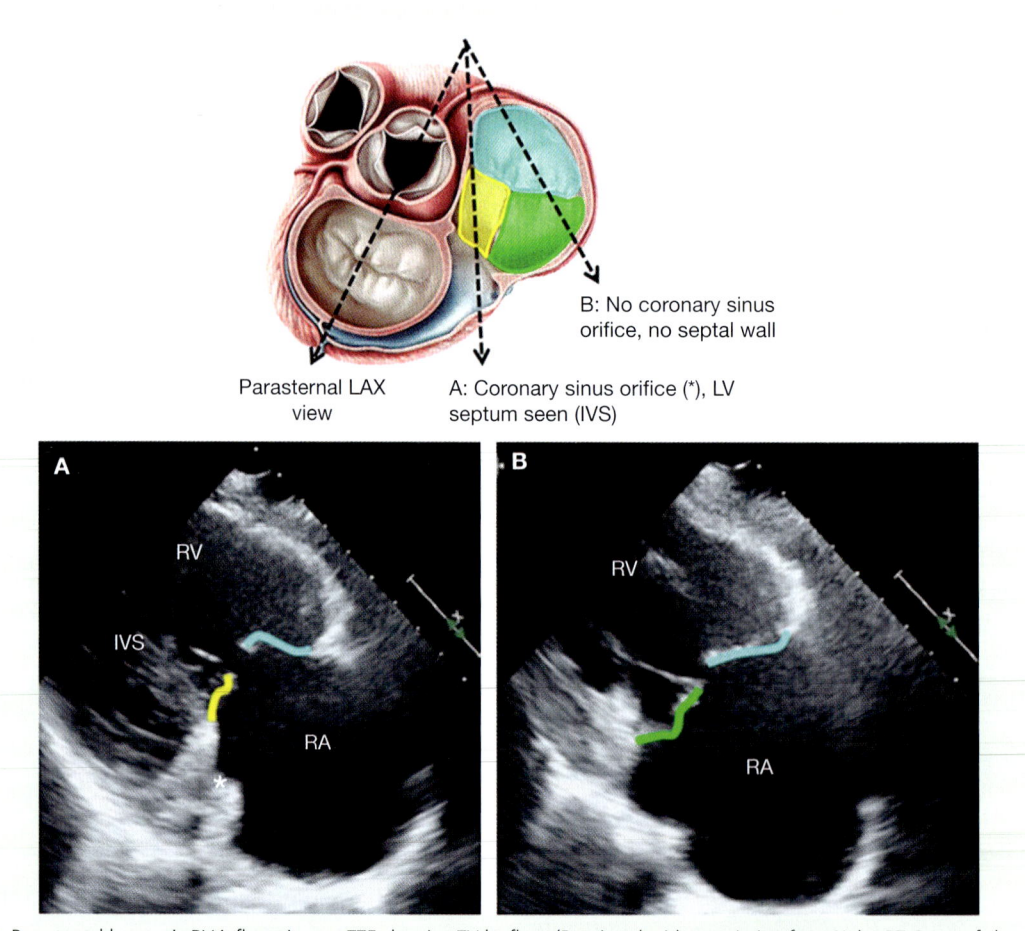

Figure 19.13. Parasternal long-axis RV inflow view on TTE showing TV leaflets. (Reprinted with permission from Hahn RT. State-of-the-art review of echocardiographic imaging in the evaluation and treatment of functional tricuspid regurgitation. *Circ Cardiovasc Imaging.* 2016;9(12):e005332. Figure 1. Copyright © 2016 American Heart Association, Inc.)

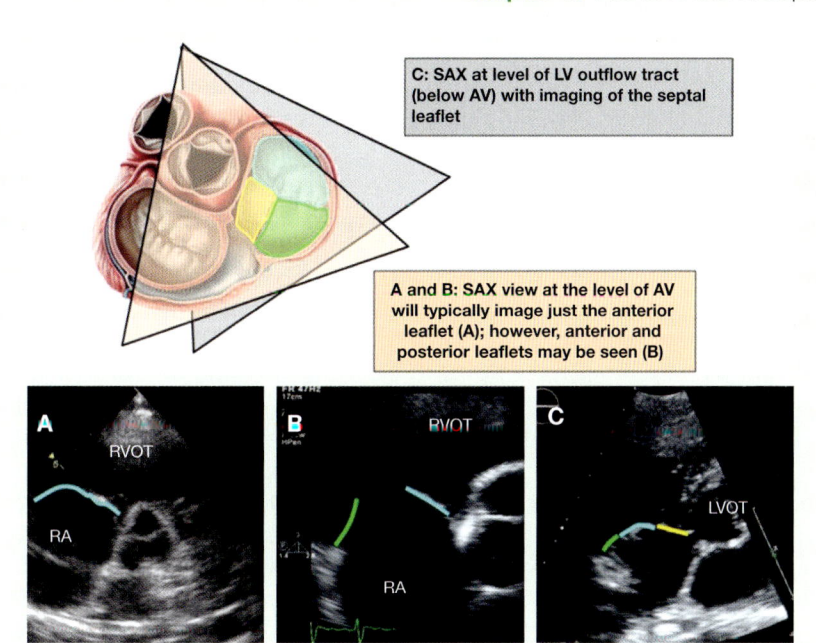

Figure 19.14. Parasternal short-axis (SAX) views on TTE showing TV leaflets. From the short-axis view at the level of the aortic valve (AV), a single anterior leaflet is typically imaged **(A)**. This in part is because of the lower (apical) position of the septal leaflet. As the lateral portion of the annulus dilates and loses its saddle shape, the anterior and posterior leaflets may be imaged **(B)**. As the transducer is angled toward the left ventricular outflow tract (LVOT), the septal leaflet may be seen **(C)**. RA, right atrial; RVOT, right ventricular outflow tract. (Reprinted with permission from Hahn RT. State-of-the-art review of echocardiographic imaging in the evaluation and treatment of functional tricuspid regurgitation. *Circ Cardiovasc Imaging*. 2016;9(12):e005332. Figure 2. Copyright © 2016 American Heart Association, Inc.)

3. **Answer: E.** There is a large amount of variability in tricuspid valve anatomy and there is actually only three leaflets in ~55% of individuals, with 40% having four leaflets, 5% having two leaflets, and 1% to 2% having five leaflets. Distinguishing a separate leaflet from a scallop can be challenging, though it can be identified when it has separate motion from the neighboring leaflet and color flow extending into the commissures around the leaflet. For multiple anterior leaflets, a proposed nomenclature is to call the leaflet at the anterior-septal commissure as A1 and the more lateral/inferior leaflet as A2. For multiple posterior leaflets, the numbering system starts at the anterior papillary muscle with P1, with P2 being more posterior. For multiple septal leaflets, the numbering starts with S1 at the anteroseptal commissure. For bicuspid valves, there is usually anterior/posterior fusion giving septal and lateral leaflets.

4. **Answer: A.** His PA systolic pressure is normal. The estimated RV systolic pressure from his tricuspid regurgitant velocity is 36 mm Hg + 5 mm Hg = 41 mm Hg, assuming a normal right atrial (RA) pressure (a reasonable assumption given normal RA size and IVC size). The peak systolic pressure across the pulmonary valve is 20 mm Hg. Therefore, the PA systolic pressure is approximately 41 − 20 mm Hg = 21 mm Hg or normal. PA systolic pressure can be estimated in pulmonary stenosis as long as the pressure gradient across the pulmonary valve is known.

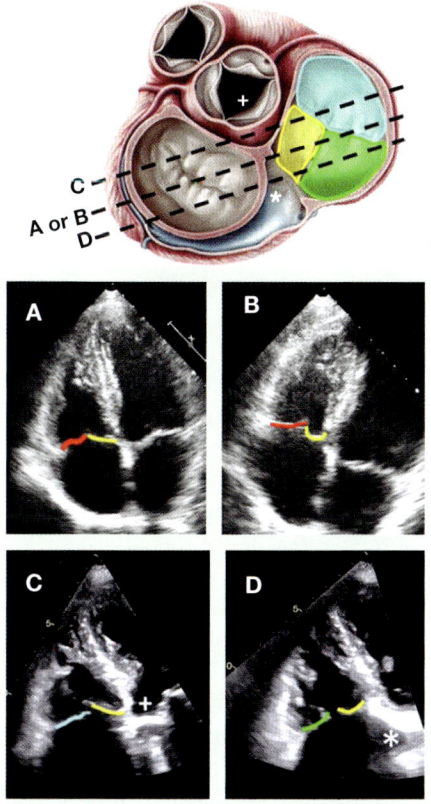

Figure 19.15. Apical 4-chamber views. From the 4-chamber views of the right ventricle (**A** and **B**), the septal leaflet can be clearly identified; however, the opposing leaflet can be the anterior or the posterior leaflet (red line). Angling the transducer anteriorly, so that a portion of the aorta (+) is imaged **(C)**, will image the septal and anterior leaflets. Angling the transducer posterior so that a portion of the coronary sinus (*) is imaged **(D)** will image the septal and posterior leaflets. (Reprinted with permission from Hahn RT. State-of-the-art review of echocardiographic imaging in the evaluation and treatment of functional tricuspid regurgitation. *Circ Cardiovasc Imaging*. 2016;9(12):e005332. Figure 3. Copyright © 2016 American Heart Association, Inc.)

5. **Answer: E.** Tricuspid stenosis (TS) is a rare valvular lesion and is commonly found in association with tricuspid regurgitation (TR). It causes elevated right atrial pressures, resulting in an elevated JVP and high venous pressure. Carcinoid syndrome commonly affects the right-sided valves and while TR is often the more significant lesion, TS can coexist. TS can be present in right-sided rheumatic disease, which will generally also affect the left-sided valves. Both malignant masses and large vegetations can cause physical obstruction and mechanical TS. The tetralogy of Fallot includes a ventricular septal defect, pulmonary stenosis, an overriding aorta, and right ventricular hypertrophy.

6. **Answer: D.** A Gerbode defect is a communication between the right atrium and left ventricle, often iatrogenic after surgery on the AV valves or following endocarditis of these valves. As the tricuspid valve is more apically situated under normal conditions in the heart than the mitral valve, the right atrium abuts the left ventricle over a small area. If a defect develops in this area, communication occurs between the right atrium and the left ventricle.

7. **Answer: C.** The constant used to estimate the valve area in tricuspid stenosis by pressure halftime is 190 not 220 (used in mitral stenosis). Doming of the valve is seen in tricuspid stenosis, but this is seen in diastole not systole. The mean gradient expected across the tricuspid valve in severe stenosis may be 5 mm Hg. Planimetry of the valve is difficult in tricuspid stenosis as it is difficult to get a true short-axis view of the valve; however, 3D TTE or 3D TEE may be useful for this. Although rheumatic involvement of the tricuspid valve occurs with some frequency, hemodynamically significant stenosis is relatively uncommon and is reported in about 5% of patients with rheumatic involvement of the mitral valve.

8. **Answer: D.** Pulmonary artery systolic pressure can be estimated using the TR jet using CW Doppler: $4(TR\ V_{max})^2$ plus estimated right atrial pressure (RAP). Mean and diastolic pulmonary artery pressures can be estimated using the pulmonic insufficiency jet using CW Doppler: $4(PI\ V_{max})^2$ + RAP and $4(PI\ \text{end-diastolic velocity})^2$ + RAP, respectively. Mean pulmonary artery pressure may also be estimated using the right ventricular outflow tract PW Doppler acceleration time (ms): $79 - (0.45 \times RVOT\ AT)$. A VSD may also be used to estimate right ventricular systolic pressure if a CW Doppler signal can be obtained coaxial with the direction of flow: systolic blood pressure $-4(VSD\ \text{velocity})^2$. An atrial septal defect cannot be utilized to estimate pulmonary artery pressures.

9. **Answer: D.** Secondary pulmonary hypertension and/or RV dilatation is the most common cause of significant TR. All of the other conditions may also lead to significant TR. Please see **Table 19.1** which lists the common primary and secondary causes of TR.

10. **Answer: A.** Normal RV systolic pressure should not occur with severe pulmonic stenosis as the RV systolic pressure must exceed the PA systolic pressure by the gradient across the pulmonary valve. RV hypertrophy (wall thickness of >0.5 cm) and post-stenotic dilatation are common in severe pulmonic stenosis. Severe pulmonic stenosis is defined by Doppler echocardiography as a peak velocity across the valve of ≥4 m/s, moderate 3 to 4 m/s, and mild <3 m/s. Of note: the PA systolic pressure is usually normal in the setting of severe pulmonic stenosis.

11. **Answer: D.** Mild stenosis is considered present when the Doppler velocity is <3 m/s or a pressure of <36 mm Hg. The prognosis is excellent and intervention is rarely necessary. It is appropriate to follow with yearly echocardiography, but cardiac catheterization or TEE is not indicated. Doming of the valve in systole is a common echocardiographic feature of pulmonic stenosis. Please see **Table 19.2** for a list of causes of congenital and acquired pulmonary stenosis.

12. **Answer: C.** Severe pulmonary insufficiency is usually seen in the setting of prior surgery on the RV outflow tract or pulmonary valve as part of the treatment of a congenital heart lesion. Pulmonary insufficiency is detected to be trivial or mild normally. Please see **Table 19.3** for a list of echocardiographic and Doppler parameters that are useful in grading the severity of PR (used with permission from Zoghbi et al). Severe pulmonary insufficiency is associated with a high end-diastolic pressure and a reduced pressure gradient across the pulmonic valve; thus, it is more often associated with laminar rather than turbulent velocity. The pulmonary insufficiency end-diastolic velocity (V) may be used to estimate the PA diastolic pressure as $4V^2$ + estimated RA pressure but is not used to estimate the PA systolic pressure. Pulmonary insufficiency may be graded using a number of parameters, at a Nyquist limit of 50 to 70 cm/s. Semiquantitative parameters and quantitative parameters such as vena contracta width, effective regurgitant orifice area, and regurgitant volume have not been well defined for PI. Qualitative parameters include an abnormal pulmonic valve morphology, a large jet with a wide origin, a dense jet by CW with steep deceleration/early termination of diastolic flow, and pulmonic flow > aortic flow by PW Doppler. Other suggestive findings include a dilated right ventricle.

13. **Answer: B.** A fibroelastoma is the most common cause of a mobile mass on the tricuspid valve among the choices provided. Myxoma and sarcoma of the valve are much less common. A Chiari network is a fenestrated membranous structure, which originates

Table 19.1. Etiology of Tricuspid Regurgitation

Morphologic Classification	Disease Subgroup	Specific Abnormality
Primary leaflet abnormality	Acquired disease	Degenerative, myxomatous Rheumatic Endocarditis Carcinoid Endomyocardial fibrosis Toxins Trauma Iatrogenic (pacing leads, RV biopsy) Other (eg, ischemic papillary muscle rupture)
	Congenital	Ebstein anomaly TV dysplasia TV tethering associated with perimembranous ventricular septal defect and ventricular septal aneurysm Repaired tetralogy of Fallot Congenitally corrected transposition of the great arteries Other (giant right atrium)
Secondary (functional) leaflet abnormality	Left heart disease	LV dysfunction or valve disease
	RV dysfunction	RV ischemia RV volume overload RV cardiomyopathy
	Pulmonary hypertension	Chronic lung disease Pulmonary thromboembolism Left-to-right shunt
	Right atrial abnormalities	Atrial fibrillation

Reprinted from Zoghbi WA, Adams D, Bonow RO, et al. Recommendations for noninvasive evaluation of native valvular regurgitation: a report from the American Society of Echocardiography Developed in Collaboration with the Society for Cardiovascular Magnetic Resonance. *J Am Soc Echocardiogr*. 2017;30(4):303-371. Copyright © 2017 by the American Society of Echocardiography. With permission.

Table 19.2. Causes of Congenital and Acquired Pulmonary Stenosis

Congenital	Acquired
Tetralogy of Fallot	Rheumatic heart disease
Noonan syndrome	Infective endocarditis
Maternal rubella	Carcinoid syndrome
Ehler-Danlos syndrome	Prior chest radiation
William syndrome	
Alagille syndrome	

at the orifice of the IVC and is an embryologic remnant. It may rarely float through the tricuspid valve but is usually confined to the right atrium and is not attached to the tricuspid valve. Carcinoid syndrome causes immobility of the valve leaflets such that they may remain in a partially open condition throughout the cardiac cycle.

14. **Answer: A.** The normal pulmonic valve (PV) consists of three leaflets: the anterior, the left, and the right leaflet. The PV is anatomically orthogonal to the aortic valve; thus, when one of these valves is seen in short axis, the other valve will be seen along its long axis. It can be imaged on TTE from the parasternal short-axis view, from a modified superiorly tilted parasternal long-axis view, or from the subcostal view. On TEE, the PV can be viewed from a mid-esophageal view (45°-60°), from an upper esophageal view (0°-20°), and from transgastric views (0°-20° or at 40°-60°).

15. **Answer: B.** Infundibular stenosis may give rise to a high-velocity jet that causes damage to the pulmonary valve leaflets and pulmonary insufficiency in a manner similar to subaortic stenosis. Infundibular stenosis may be either congenital or acquired. It occurs not only in congenital heart disease syndromes such as tetralogy of Fallot but also in hypertrophic cardiomyopathy, in tumors of the RV outflow tract, or in infiltrative disorders. It may be discrete or consist of a more extensive region of fibromuscular thickening. It is often best imaged

Table 19.3. Echocardiographic and Doppler Parameters That are Useful in Grading the Severity of PR

Parameter	Mild	Moderate	Severe
Pulmonic valve	Normal	Normal or abnormal	Abnormal and may not be visible
RV size	Normal*	Normal or dilated	Dilated[†]
Jet size, color Doppler[‡]	Thin (usually <10 mm in length) with a narrow origin	Intermediate	Broad origin; variable depth of penetration
Ratio of PR jet width/pulmonary annulus			>0.7[§]
Jet density and contour (CW)	Soft	Dense	Dense; early termination of diastolic flow
Deceleration time of the PR spectral Doppler signal			Short, <260 ms
Pressure halftime of PR jet			<100 ms[‖]
PR index[¶]		<0.77	<0.77
Diastolic flow reversal in the main or branch PAs (PW)			Prominent
Pulmonic systolic flow (VTI) compared to systemic flow (LVOT VTI) by PW[#]	Slightly increased	Intermediate	Greatly increased
RF**	<20%	20%-40%	>40%

CW, continuous-wave; LVOT, left ventricular outflow tract; PR, pulmonary regurgitation; *PW,* pulsed-wave Doppler; RV, right ventricular; VTI, velocity-time integral.
Reprinted from Zoghbi WA, Adams D, Bonow RO, et al. Recommendations for noninvasive evaluation of native valvular regurgitation: a report from the American Society of Echocardiography Developed in Collaboration with the Society for Cardiovascular Magnetic Resonance. *J Am Soc Echocardiogr.* 2017;30(4):303-371. Copyright © 2017 by the American Society of Echocardiography. With permission.
*Unless there are other reasons for RV enlargement.
[†]Exception: Acute PR.
[‡]At a Nyquist limit of 50 to 70 cm/s.
[§]Identifies a CMR-derived PR fraction ≥40%.
[¶]Defined as the duration of the PR signal divided by the total duration of diastole, with this cutoff identifying a CMR-derived PR fraction >25%.
[‖]Not reliable in the presence of high RV end-diastolic pressure.
[#]Cutoff values for RVol and fraction are not well validated.
**RF data primarily derived from CMR with limited application with echocardiography.

and evaluated from a parasternal short-axis view or from the subcostal window. Pressure gradients measured by Doppler across the infundibular stenosis are reasonably accurate. When concomitant pulmonic valvular stenosis is present, it is usually impossible to isolate the precise contribution of the pulmonic valve and infundibulum to the total gradient measured by continuous-wave Doppler across the RV outflow tract.

16. **Answer: C.** The image (**Figure 19.1**) is characteristic of Ebstein anomaly of the tricuspid valve with displacement of the septal leaflet into the right ventricle so that a portion of the right ventricle is "atrialized." The diagnostic criteria for diagnosing Ebstein anomaly from an echocardiogram is the apical displacement of the insertion of the septal leaflet from the insertion of the anterior leaflet of the mitral valve by ≥8 mm/m². Ebstein anomaly is associated with accelerated conduction via accessory pathways (Wolff-Parkinson-White), and severe TR but not with a parchment-like RV wall. This is seen in dysplastic RV or Uhl syndrome, which may be associated with ventricular arrhythmias.

17. **Answer: C.** The Doppler profile is consistent with significant pulmonary regurgitation (PR). From the parasternal short-axis view on TTE, color flow can be used to identify PR, which will be seen as a diastolic jet toward the probe in the right ventricular outflow tract. In severe PR, there is rapid equalization of diastolic pressures between the pulmonary artery

and the right ventricle, which results in a narrow, short-lived regurgitant jet. This can be misleading and cause the degree of PR to be underestimated. Red flow seen in the pulmonary artery is a sign of flow reversal and is consistent with severe PR. The most common cause of pulmonary regurgitation is prior surgical intervention for congenital heart disease, in this case, surgery to repair the congenital pulmonic stenosis from Noonan syndrome. Though the forward flow is not well seen on the image, there is no indication of increased gradients to suggest pulmonic stenosis. Pulmonary pressures can be estimated from the PR Doppler profile but are not elevated in this case.

18. **Answer: C.** There is severe TR present with a flow convergence area and dilation of the right atrium. Intraoperative TEE is more likely to underestimate the degree of regurgitation compared with the ambulatory setting due to decreased intravascular volume and change in loading consequent to anesthesia and mechanical ventilation. Severe TR occurs in mitral valve prolapse as a result of prolapse of the tricuspid valve or secondary to pulmonary hypertension from severe mitral regurgitation but rarely due to a concomitant flail of the tricuspid valve leaflet. Severe pulmonary hypertension is not necessary to cause this degree of TR; prolapse or secondary changes in the tricuspid annulus or valve may alone cause it. TR may improve after surgical repair of the mitral valve, especially if the pulmonary pressures fall, but this is less likely when the TR is severe preoperatively as in this case. Guideline recommendations are that severe or progressive TR be addressed at the time of left-sided valve surgery. It should be also noted that concomitant tricuspid annuloplasty at the time of mitral valve surgery can improve the progression of subsequent TR even in patients without significant TR preoperatively; however, this comes at the expense of an increased rate of pacemaker insertion (Gammie et al., 2022).

19. **Answer: E.** The image (**Figure 19.4**) shows a mid-esophageal 4-chamber view at 0° focused on the tricuspid valve. There is an eccentric jet of significant tricuspid regurgitation that is medially directed. This would be most in keeping with pacing lead induced tricuspid regurgitation. Cardiac implantable electronic device (CIED)-related TR is an increasingly recognized complication that can affect up to 45% of devices. There are three recognized mechanisms of CIED-related TR: implantation related, pacing related, and device related. With device/lead-related TR, there is often impingement/restriction of one of the leaflets (most commonly the septal leaflet, as in this case), resulting in an eccentric jet of TR that is medially directed. In all the other options, the TR would be more likely to be central/functional.

20. **Answer: A.** High-velocity systolic reversal in the hepatic veins can be seen in severe TR, which also gives rise to large "v" waves in the jugular venous profile (**Figure 19.16**). In this case, we see mid-systolic hepatic vein flow reversal, with increasing TR, the flow profile may progress to holosystolic flow reversal. Overall, the sensitivity of hepatic flow reversal for severe TR is approximately 80%. Pulsus paradoxus, an abnormally large reduction in systolic blood pressure by ≥10 mm Hg during inspiration, is most characteristic of cardiac tamponade (with a pericardial effusion, the sensitivity is >80%), although it is typically absent in occult (low pressure) or regional tamponade. Kussmaul sign with an increase in the venous pressure on inspiration is most characteristic of constrictive pericarditis. Pulsus alternans, alternating strong and weak peripheral pulses, is seen in end-stage LV systolic dysfunction. Pulsus bisferiens is a characteristic double-peaked high-amplitude pulse felt in the setting of both significant aortic stenosis and regurgitation.

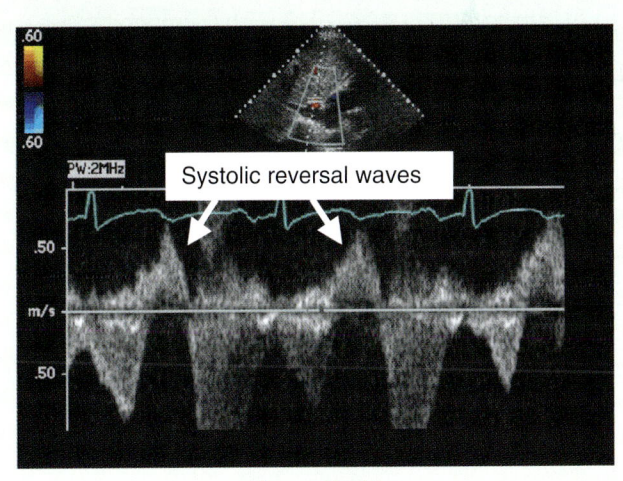

Figure 19.16

21. **Answer: B.** Elevated pulmonary artery pressure can be associated with "notching" of the Doppler profile of the right ventricular outflow tract signal (white arrow points to notch). This notching is thought to be related in part to transient flow deceleration from premature systolic arterial wave reflection, due to the elevated pulmonary artery pressure. In severe pulmonary hypertension, mid-systolic closure of the pulmonary valve can also occur. This appearance is not associated with the other lesions described. The image (**Figure 19.6**) shows an example of mid-systolic notching, which has been shown to be associated with more significant pulmonary hypertension. Early systolic notching is a relatively new description, which has been associated with large pulmonary emboli.

22. **Answer: D.** This well-circumscribed oval mass appears attached to the septal leaflet of the tricuspid valve by a narrow stalk. It is heterogeneous, with areas of echolucency, and most suggestive of a papillary fibroelastoma, the third most common primary tumor of the heart. These must be differentiated from other cardiac mass–like lesions such as myxomas, fibromas, infective vegetations, Libman-Sacks vegetations, Lambl excrescences, or thrombi. Libman-Sacks vegetations are possible given a history of lupus nephritis; however, the findings are more classic of fibroelastoma. Myxomas are usually located in the left atrium and originate from the mid interatrial septum. Infective vegetations are usually associated with clinical signs of endocarditis and valvular destruction often with a new regurgitant murmur. Fibromas are almost always single, located in the ventricular myocardium, frequently in the ventricular septum, often with central calcification (by contrast, rhabdomyomas rarely calcify). Thrombus is unlikely because of the location and rounded features of the mass.

23. **Answer: B.** The 2018 ACC/AHA Guidelines for the Management of Adults with Congenital Heart Disease recommend that balloon valvuloplasty is indicated for symptomatic patients with moderate or severe PS. Moderate stenosis = peak instantaneous Doppler gradient >36 mm Hg and severe stenosis = peak gradient >64 mm Hg across the pulmonary valve. Intervention is also reasonable in asymptomatic patients with severe PS. Subvalvular stenosis may be present, but is not evident on the Doppler profile. Two systolic velocity spectral displays are evident. A low-velocity (~1 m/s) jet with a dense spectral pattern is consistent with flow in the RV outflow tract. This suggests a relatively low velocity in the RV outflow tract but does not entirely exclude some degree of subvalvular stenosis. The high-velocity (532 cm/s) jet reflects the stenosis at the valve itself. Most pulmonary stenosis is congenital associated with dysplastic, unicuspid, bicuspid or tricuspid valves. Chest pain is common in severe pulmonic stenosis and likely reflects reduced cardiac outflow and flow to the coronaries and/or subendocardial ischemia in the hypertrophied right ventricle.

24. **Answer: E.** The patient has large mass lesions consistent with vegetations involving the pacing wires, which spare the tricuspid valve. Given the size of the apparent vegetations, the risk of pulmonary embolism is high and an open surgical approach will likely be needed. Antibiotic coverage will be required, and removal of the whole system including the generator is indicated to remove all potential sources of infection. Unless the tricuspid valve has been destroyed in the infective process, tricuspid valve replacement is not indicated.

25. **Answer: C.** Pulmonary hypertension is associated with abrupt mid-systolic closure of the pulmonary valve in about 50% of cases especially when severe. The appearance is thought to occur from transient reversal of the PA-RV outflow tract gradient due to impaired PA compliance. It is not associated with the other lesions previously described.

26. **Answer: B.** This is Ebstein anomaly. The usual cause of right-sided heart failure, at least with a later presentation, is TR. ASD occurs in many patients with Ebstein anomaly but would have been expected to present somewhat earlier if associated with significant shunting. Severe pulmonary hypertension is relatively rare. There is no evidence of endocarditis, and although tachycardia may occur in this condition (due to associated accessory pathways), there is no evidence of cardiomyopathy on the images.

27. **Answer: E.** An electrophysiologic study is indicated in the setting of suspected accessory pathway tachycardia, which occurs in about 10% to 25% of these patients and especially if surgery is being contemplated. Medical therapy is often sufficient in many patients with mild to moderate lesions for the effective control of symptoms. Tricuspid repair is the initial surgical treatment of choice. Its feasibility depends on the degree of tethering of the leaflets and the size of the functional right ventricle. The smaller the functional right ventricle, the less likely tricuspid repair is to be successful. The septal leaflet is usually the one most tethered, and the anterior leaflet is the least likely to be affected. It may have a sail-like configuration and float into the RV outflow tract, causing obstruction in some individuals.

> **KEY POINTS**
> - Ebstein anomaly of the tricuspid valve is associated with TR, right-sided heart failure, accessory pathways, and ASDs.
> - When tricuspid repair is required, it is dependent on the degree of septal leaflet tethering and the size and functionality of the right ventricle.

28. **Answer: A.** The patient has typical findings of endocarditis except fever, and fever occasionally does not supervene in this setting. The most likely cause of infection here is staphylococcal, perhaps from the time of implantation. Both thrombus formation and ring dehiscence are also possibilities, although somewhat less likely. Dehiscence is also less likely in the absence of associated regurgitation. The lesion is obviously attached to the tricuspid valve and thus is unlikely to be an embolus in transit.

29. **Answer: C.** Tricuspid valve endocarditis is usually amenable to antibiotic treatment and should be attempted before surgical consideration.

> **KEY POINTS**
> - *Staphylococcus* is a common cause of early-onset prosthetic valve endocarditis.
> - Tricuspid valve endocarditis is usually amenable to antibiotic treatment.

30. **Answer: C.** The physical examination suggests valvular pulmonic stenosis with an ejection click and ejection murmur and associated RV hypertrophy. With more severe stenosis, the P2 becomes softer. The Doppler shows turbulent flow just beyond the pulmonary valve, with also mild pulmonary insufficiency. Patent ductus arteriosus usually leads to continuous flow in the PA, but this may be attenuated in Eisenmenger physiology. Pulmonary hypertension as part of Eisenmenger syndrome will lead to a loud P2. Infundibular pulmonic stenosis will not have the ejection click of a mobile but dysplastic valve, and the turbulent velocity will be proximal to the valve.

31. **Answer: C.** The next step is to assess how severe the stenosis is by continuous-wave Doppler. Doppler measurements correlate well with those made by cardiac catheterization. Balloon valvuloplasty is indicated for symptomatic patients with moderate PS (peak gradient of >36 mm Hg) and is considered reasonable in asymptomatic patients with severe stenosis (peak gradient of >64 mm Hg). Although the pulmonic valve area may be assessed by the continuity equation, in practice, this is not usually performed. The various guidelines, on which decisions concerning intervention are based, use the pressure gradient rather than the area. Although pulmonary artery systolic pressure should be measured, it is usually low in this setting. Contrast injection is reasonable if a shunt is suspected. Most often valvular pulmonic stenosis is an isolated abnormality.

> **KEY POINTS**
> - Valvular pulmonary stenosis is generally graded on the basis of the gradient through the valve.
> - Valvular pulmonary stenosis when presenting as an isolated lesion is usually amenable to balloon valvuloplasty.

32. **Answer: D.** Both mitral stenosis and tricuspid stenosis are present in ▶ **Video 19.4**. The physical findings of an apical diastolic murmur and loud S1 suggest mitral stenosis, whereas the accentuated venous pulse in presystole is consistent with a large "a" wave seen with tricuspid stenosis. The absence of a loud P2 suggests that pulmonary hypertension has not occurred. Significant tricuspid stenosis (when it complicates mitral stenosis) may give rise to right-sided heart failure and ascites that may simulate constrictive pericarditis.

33. **Answer: B.** Assuming significant stenosis of both valves, suggested by the images and physical examination, balloon valvuloplasty of both valves is the ideal approach if the lesions are suitable. Otherwise, surgical commissurotomy is appropriate given the symptomatic state.

> **KEY POINTS**
> - Mitral and tricuspid stenosis may coexist especially in patients with rheumatic heart disease and simulate constrictive pericarditis.
> - Both mitral and tricuspid stenosis may be amenable to balloon valvuloplasty in many patients.

34. **Answer: D.** ▶ **Video 19.5** shows a flail segment of the tricuspid valve (TV). This is a well-known complication of an endomyocardial biopsy procedure, in which a transvenous catheter retrieves a tiny portion of the right ventricle for histological investigation. This can result in leaflet/chordal damage, particularly postcardiac transplant when multiple biopsy procedures are common. This complication can result in severe tricuspid regurgitation, particularly if it results in a flail segment of a leaflet. It would unlikely be related to the surgery, as the patient is now 6 months postoperative. Transplant coronary artery disease is usually a late complication, while acute allograft rejection would result in the echocardiographic findings of depressed myocardial function. While pulmonary hypertension is a possibility, the fact that there is a visible flail segment would point more to Answer D.

35. **Answer: B.** The severity of TR is assessed both with qualitative and quantitative methods. Please see **Figure 19.17** which shows an algorithm from the 2017 ASE guidelines on valvular regurgitation to assist in classifying the severity of TR.

The quantitative measures of jet area, vena contracta width, and proximal flow convergence are used routinely. A small jet area (<5 cm^2) suggests mild TR, while a large area (>10 cm^2) suggests severe TR. A TR vena contracta (VC) ≥ 0.7 cm is diagnostic of severe TR. A regurgitant volume of ≥45 mL or an effective regurgitant orifice area of ≥0.40 cm^2 also suggests severe TR. Other imaging features that suggest severe TR would be dilated right-sided chambers, a dilated IVC, and systolic flow reversal in the hepatic veins. In addition, a flail segment with

```
                  Chronic tricuspid regurgitation by Doppler echocardiography
```

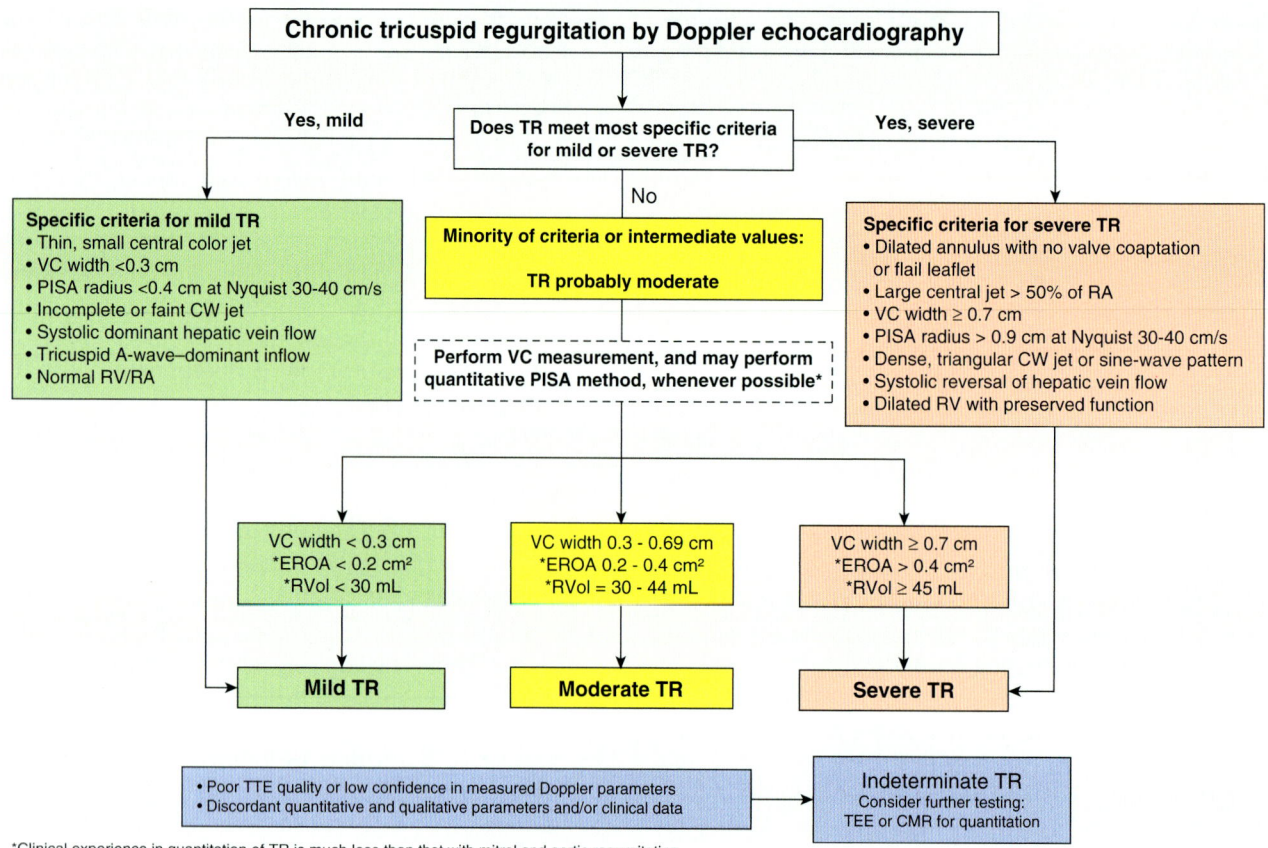

```
                            Does TR meet most specific criteria
        Yes, mild                  for mild or severe TR?                Yes, severe
                                           No
```

Specific criteria for mild TR
- Thin, small central color jet
- VC width <0.3 cm
- PISA radius <0.4 cm at Nyquist 30-40 cm/s
- Incomplete or faint CW jet
- Systolic dominant hepatic vein flow
- Tricuspid A-wave–dominant inflow
- Normal RV/RA

Minority of criteria or intermediate values:
TR probably moderate

Perform VC measurement, and may perform quantitative PISA method, whenever possible*

Specific criteria for severe TR
- Dilated annulus with no valve coaptation or flail leaflet
- Large central jet > 50% of RA
- VC width ≥ 0.7 cm
- PISA radius > 0.9 cm at Nyquist 30-40 cm/s
- Dense, triangular CW jet or sine-wave pattern
- Systolic reversal of hepatic vein flow
- Dilated RV with preserved function

VC width < 0.3 cm
*EROA < 0.2 cm²
*RVol < 30 mL

VC width 0.3 - 0.69 cm
*EROA 0.2 - 0.4 cm²
*RVol = 30 - 44 mL

VC width ≥ 0.7 cm
*EROA > 0.4 cm²
*RVol ≥ 45 mL

Mild TR | **Moderate TR** | **Severe TR**

- Poor TTE quality or low confidence in measured Doppler parameters
- Discordant quantitative and qualitative parameters and/or clinical data

Indeterminate TR
Consider further testing:
TEE or CMR for quantitation

*Clinical experience in quantitation of TR is much less than that with mitral and aortic regurgitation

Figure 19.17. Algorithm to assist in classifying the severity of TR.

a large coaptation gap is diagnostic of severe TR. Due to the wide range of severe TR, there are also now new classifications proposed of massive and torrential TR. Massive TR corresponds to a VC of 14 to 20 mm, an EROA of 60 to 79 mm², and a 3D VC of 95 to 114 mm³. Torrential TR corresponds to a VC of ≥21 mm, an EROA of ≥80 mm², and a 3D VC of ≥115 mm³. In most cases of TR, the right ventricular systolic pressure can be estimated from the TV velocity with the Bernoulli equation (4 × velocity²). However, in acute severe TR with laminar flow through the valve, the right atrium and right ventricle operate as a common chamber and the Bernoulli equation, which estimates flow through narrowed or restricted orifices, is not valid. In this example, there is no tricuspid stenosis seen, and no vegetation to suggest infective endocarditis. Given the focal defect, there is a good change of valvular repair.

> **KEY POINTS**
> - Severe TR from tricuspid valve apparatus trauma is a known complication of endomyocardial biopsy, a common procedure post heart transplant.
> - The severity of TR is assessed with a combination of qualitative and quantitative methods, with new classifications of massive and torrential being proposed.

SUGGESTED READINGS

Addetia K, Harb SC, Hahn RT, Kapadia S, Lang RM. Cardiac implantable electronic device lead-induced tricuspid regurgitation. *JACC Cardiovasc Imaging*. 2019;12(4):622-636.

Baumgartner H, De Backer J, Babu-Narayan SV, et al; ESC Scientific Document Group. 2020 ESC guidelines for the management of adult congenital heart disease: the task force for the management of adult congenital heart disease of the European Society of Cardiology (ESC). Endorsed by—association for European Paediatric and congenital cardiology (AEPC), International Society for Adult Congenital Heart Disease (ISACHD). *Eur Heart J*. 2021;42(6):563-645.

Casazza F, Bongarzoni A, Capozi A, Agostoni O. Regional right ventricular dysfunction in acute pulmonary embolism and right ventricular infarction. *Eur J Echocardiogr*. 2005;6(1):11-14.

Gammie JS, Chu MW, Falk V, et al; CTSN Investigators. Concomitant tricuspid repair in patients with degenerative mitral regurgitation. *N Engl J Med*. 2022;386(4):327-339.

Pellikka PA, Tajik AJ, Khandheria BK, et al. Carcinoid heart disease. Clinical and echocardiographic spectrum in 74 patients. *Circulation*. 1993;87(4):1188-1196.

Vahanian A, Beyersdorf F, Praz F, et al; ESC/EACTS Scientific Document Group. 2021 ESC/EACTS guidelines for the management of valvular heart disease: developed by the task force for the management of valvular heart disease of the European Society of Cardiology (ESC) and the European Association for Cardio-Thoracic Surgery (EACTS). *Eur Heart J*. 2022;43(7):561-632.

Hahn RT, Saric M, Faletra FF, et al. Recommended standards for the performance of transesophageal echocardiographic screening for structural heart intervention: from the American Society of Echocardiography. *J Am Soc Echocardiogr*. 2022;35(1):1-76.

Hahn RT, Weckbach LT, Noack T, et al. Proposal for a standard echocardiographic tricuspid valve nomenclature. *JACC Cardiovasc Imaging*. 2021;14(7):1299-1305.

Hahn RT. State-of-the-art review of echocardiographic imaging in the evaluation and treatment of functional tricuspid regurgitation. *Circ Cardiovasc Imaging*. 2016;9(12):e005332.

Stout K, Daniels CJ, Aboulhosn J, et al. 2018 AHA/ACC guideline for the management of adults with congenital heart disease: a report of the American College of Cardiology/American Heart Association task force on clinical practice guidelines. *Circulation*. 2019;139(14):e698-e800.

Zaidi A, Oxborough D, Augustine DX, et al. Echocardiographic assessment of the tricuspid and pulmonary valves: a practical guideline from the British Society of Echocardiography. *Echo Res Pract*. 2020;7(4):G95-G122.

Zoghbi WA, Adams D, Bonow RO, et al. Recommendations for noninvasive evaluation of native valvular regurgitation: a report from the American Society of Echocardiography developed in collaboration with the Society for Cardiovascular Magnetic Resonance. *J Am Soc Echocardiogr*. 2017;30(4):303-371.

CHAPTER 20

Prosthetic Valves

Linda D. Gillam, Leo Marcoff, and Konstantinos P. Koulogiannis

QUESTIONS

1. A diagnosis of patient-prosthesis mismatch is made in a 32-year-old woman with prior aortic valve replacement for severe aortic regurgitation on the basis of a congenitally bicuspid aortic valve. She is an active rock climber. The basis for this diagnosis is?
   A. A mechanical valve has been selected for a female patient in whom pregnancy is planned.
   B. A mechanical valve has been selected for a patient at increased risk for bleeding complications.
   C. The valve implanted is too small for this patient.
   D. The valve implanted is too large for this patient.
   E. A bioprosthesis has been selected for a young patient.

2. A 55-year-old man with prior aortic valve replacement presents with dyspnea on exertion which has been present since his surgery. Patient-prosthesis mismatch is suspected. Which of the following criteria is used to define this syndrome?
      Effective orifice area corrected for body surface area:
   A. ≤0.55 cm^2/m^2.
   B. ≤0.65 cm^2/m^2.
   C. ≤0.75 cm^2/m^2.
   D. ≤0.85 cm^2/m^2.
   E. ≤0.95 cm^2/m^2.

3. An 11-year-old boy had a 19 mm bileaflet mechanical aortic valve implanted for severe aortic stenosis on the basis of a congenitally bicuspid valve. On echocardiographic evaluation, the peak transvalvular velocity was 3.5 m/s. However, at catheterization, the left ventricle (reached by transseptal puncture) to aortic gradient was only 25 mm Hg. What is the most likely explanation for this discrepancy?
   A. At catheterization, the aortic valve gradient could not be measured by pullback.
   B. The cardiac output was higher at the time of catheterization than at the time of the echocardiogram.
   C. The pressure recovery phenomenon has resulted in overestimation of the aortic valve gradients by Doppler.
   D. The aortic valve gradients have been overestimated because a mitral regurgitant spectrum was confused with the aortic valve spectrum.
   E. The valve is too small for this patient.

4. A 72-year-old man who had a ball and cage (Starr-Edwards) mitral valve implanted 20 years ago is followed echocardiographically. In echocardiograms of patients with this type of prosthesis, the size of the ball is?
   A. Overestimated due to faster propagation of sound in the ball relative to that in tissue.
   B. Overestimated due to slower propagation of sound in the ball relative to that in tissue.
   C. Underestimated due to faster propagation of sound in the ball relative to that in tissue.
   D. Underestimated due to slower propagation of sound in the ball relative to that in tissue.
   E. Accurately represented.

5. A 55-year-old man with a recent aortic valve replacement undergoes postoperative echocardiography to establish baseline values for the valve. A peak velocity of 2.5 m/s is recorded. This value is?
   A. Abnormally high suggesting patient-prosthesis mismatch.
   B. Abnormally high suggesting prosthetic valve stenosis.
   C. May be normal depending on the size and type of the valve.
   D. Low suggesting that the valve is a homograft valve.
   E. Abnormally low suggesting that the patient has a reduced cardiac output.

6. A 63-year-old patient with prior bioprosthetic mitral valve replacement undergoes echocardiographic evaluation. The mean transvalvular gradient is 10 mm Hg. To interpret this result, which of the following patient information is most important?
   A. Height.
   B. Weight.
   C. Heart rate.
   D. Blood pressure.
   E. Gender.

7. A 71-year-old patient with a bileaflet mitral valve prosthesis undergoes transthoracic echocardiographic evaluation with harmonic imaging. In the apical views, microcavitations (spontaneous microbubbles) are seen in the left ventricle. This finding is most consistent with?
   A. Hemolysis.
   B. Paravalvular regurgitation.
   C. Imaging artifact.
   D. A patent foramen ovalis.
   E. Normal prosthetic function.

8. An 82-year-old man with a bioprosthetic aortic valve undergoes an echocardiographic evaluation. Which of the following is the formula for calculating effective orifice area?
   A. Stroke volume/prosthetic VTI.
   B. (Stroke volume × heart rate)/peak transvalvular velocity.
   C. Subvalvular VTI/prosthetic VTI.
   D. Subvalvular peak velocity/peak transvalvular velocity.
   E. (Subvalvular VTI × stroke volume)/prosthetic VTI.

9. A 12-year-old boy with a history of aortic valve replacement undergoes echocardiographic evaluation. The peak velocity across the prosthesis is 3.5 m/s. In which of the following valves is pressure recovery most likely to be a consideration?
   A. Bileaflet.
   B. Tilting disc.
   C. Homograft.
   D. Bovine stented bioprosthesis.
   E. Stentless bioprosthesis.

10. A 15-year-old boy who had bioprosthetic aortic valve replacement for a congenitally bicuspid aortic valve undergoes echocardiographic evaluation. The peak velocity across the prosthesis is 3.5 m/s. Which of the following is most supportive of the diagnosis of prosthetic valve stenosis?
    A. The bioprosthetic cusps are thickened with reduced mobility.
    B. The size of the valve is 19 mm.
    C. The aortic root is dilated.
    D. The patient's hematocrit is 45%.
    E. The patient's left ventricular ejection fraction is 32%.

11. A 72-year-old woman with a mitral bioprosthesis undergoes echocardiographic evaluation. Which of the following statements is **TRUE**?
    A. EOA calculated as 220/pressure half-time provides the best single measurement of functional valve area.
    B. EOA calculated as 270/pressure half-time provides the best single measurement of functional valve area.
    C. EOA calculated as 1.5 × (220/pressure half-time) provides the best single measurement of functional valve area.
    D. EOA calculated as 150/pressure half-time provides the best single measurement of functional valve area.
    E. EOA calculated by the pressure half-time method is inaccurate in patients with mitral prostheses.

12. A 63-year-old patient with prior mitral valve replacement undergoes echocardiographic evaluation. In which of the following valves is a large central jet most consistent with normal valve function?
A. Starr-Edwards ball and cage valve.
B. St. Jude bileaflet valve.
C. Medtronic-Hall single disc valve.
D. Bovine pericardial bioprosthesis.
E. Porcine bioprosthesis.

13. A 63-year-old patient with prior aortic valve replacement undergoes echocardiographic evaluation for new symptoms of dyspnea. In addition to recording peak and mean gradients, the Doppler velocity index (DVI) is calculated as:
A. Stroke volume/prosthetic VTI.
B. (Stroke volume × heart rate)/peak transvalvular velocity.
C. Subvalvular VTI/prosthetic VTI.
D. (Subvalvular VTI × stroke volume)/prosthetic VTI.
E. Calculated effective orifice area/factory-specified normal effective orifice area.

14. An 81-year-old woman with prior bioprosthetic mitral valve replacement is noted to have a new systolic murmur and evidence of congestive heart failure. Transthoracic echocardiography evaluation reveals only trace central mitral regurgitation. Which of the following statements is **CORRECT**?
A. TEE is essential to evaluate the patient for paravalvular regurgitation.
B. A peak transmitral velocity of 2 m/s argues against undetected paravalvular regurgitation.
C. A mean transmitral gradient of 10 mm Hg argues against undetected paravalvular regurgitation.
D. Normal (S dominant) pulmonary venous flow excludes the possibility of paravalvular regurgitation.
E. Paravalvular regurgitation is best detected in the apical three-chamber view.

15. A 22-year-old man presents for echocardiographic follow-up 10 years after a Ross procedure. A grade 3 murmur is heard. What complication is the echocardiogram most likely to demonstrate?

A. Aortic homograft stenosis.
B. Aortic homograft regurgitation.
C. Aortic (pulmonary autograft) stenosis.
D. Aortic (pulmonary autograft) regurgitation.
E. Pulmonary homograft regurgitation.

16. A 72-year-old woman with prior mitral valve replacement is noted to have a new systolic murmur. An echocardiogram is performed. Based on **Figure 20.1**, what is the diagnosis?
A. Bioprosthesis with paravalvular mitral regurgitation.
B. Bileaflet prosthesis with paravalvular mitral regurgitation.
C. Bioprosthesis with valvular mitral regurgitation.
D. Bileaflet prosthesis with normal closure jets.
E. Bileaflet prosthesis with valvular regurgitation.

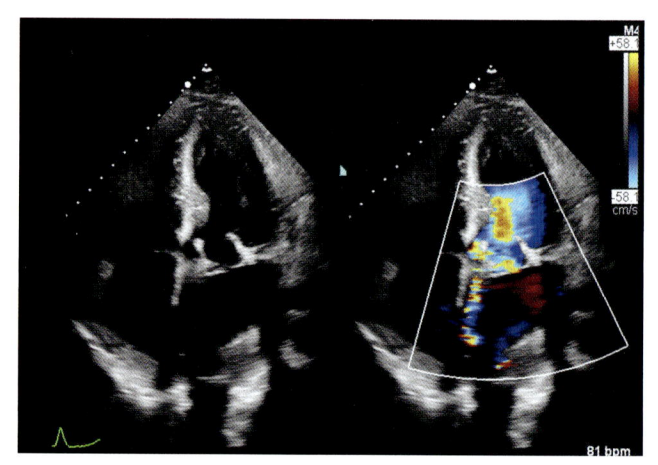

Figure 20.1. Apical 4 chamber transthoracic echocardiogram.

17. A patient with recent bioprosthetic mitral valve replacement for endocarditis undergoes echocardiographic evaluation because of persistent fatigue and a loud murmur. Based on this systolic frame (**Figure 20.2**), what is the most likely diagnosis?
A. Severe paravalvular mitral regurgitation.
B. Severe valvular mitral regurgitation.
C. Left ventricular outflow tract obstruction due to mitral systolic anterior motion.
D. Left ventricular outflow tract obstruction due to the mitral prosthesis.
E. Prosthetic mitral stenosis.

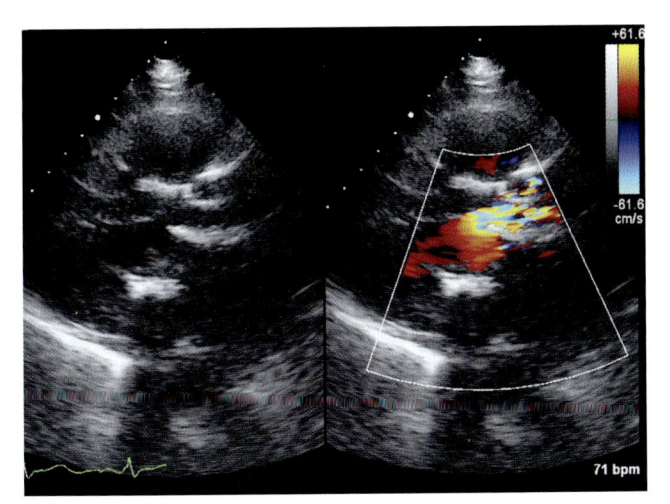

Figure 20.2. Transthoracic echocardiogram, parasternal long-axis view with and without color Doppler (systole).

18. A 65-year-old woman underwent tricuspid valve replacement for a traumatic flail tricuspid valve caused by acceleration-deceleration injury in a car accident. Two years later, she presented with peripheral edema. Transthoracic echocardiography was performed. The images in **Figure 20.3** were recorded at a heart rate of 55 bpm and a blood pressure of 120/75 mm Hg.
   Which of the following diagnoses is most consistent with these findings?
   A. Normal tricuspid prosthetic function with high output state.
   B. Normal tricuspid prosthetic function with pressure recovery.
   C. Mild tricuspid prosthetic stenosis.
   D. Moderate tricuspid prosthetic stenosis.
   E. Severe tricuspid prosthetic stenosis.

19. A 52-year-old man with prior mitral valve surgery undergoes three-dimensional (3D) transesophageal echocardiography following a suspected neuro-embolic event (**Figure 20.4**).
   What type of procedure has the patient undergone?
   A. Mitral ring annuloplasty.
   B. Alfieri stitch valvuloplasty.
   C. Bioprosthetic mitral valve replacement.
   D. Bileaflet mechanical mitral valve replacement.
   E. Mitral homograft replacement.

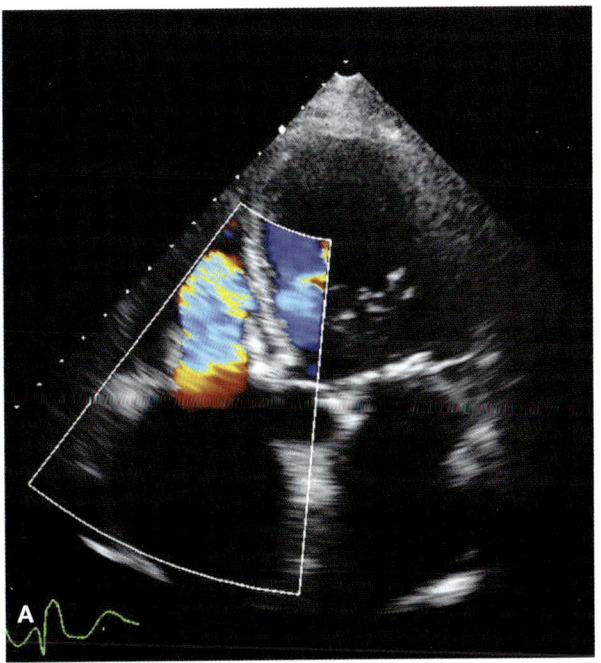

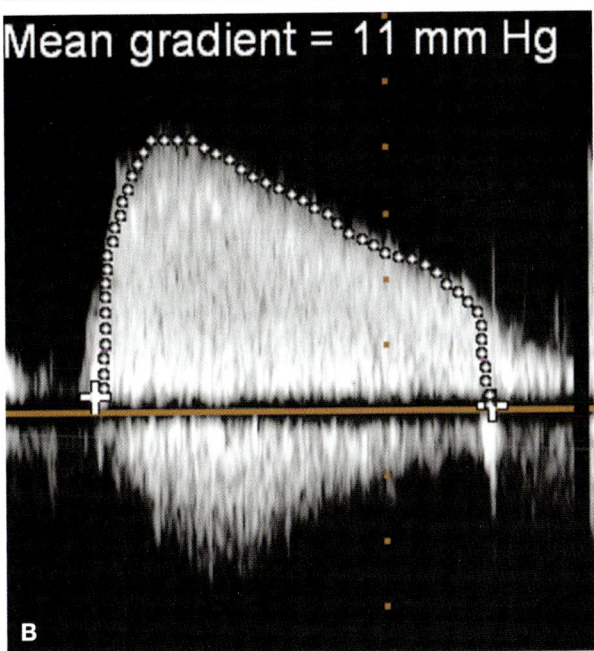

Figure 20.3. **A:** Transthoracic echocardiogram (TTE), apical 5-chamber view with color Doppler. **B:** TTE, tricuspid valve continuous-wave Doppler.

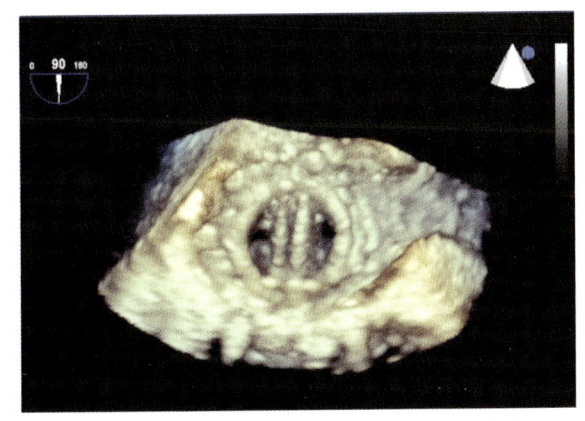

Figure 20.4. Transesophageal echocardiogram, mitral valve 3D view (left atrial perspective).

418 / Clinical Echocardiography Review

20. A 67-year-old man has undergone prior valve surgery. Based on the echocardiogram in **Figure 20.5**, what is the most likely diagnosis?
   A. Normal mitral and tricuspid ring repair.
   B. Normal mitral bioprosthesis, tricuspid ring dehiscence.
   C. Normal mitral bioprosthesis and tricuspid ring.
   D. Normal mitral bioprosthesis, pacer lead in the right ventricle.
   E. Normal mitral bioprosthesis, tricuspid vegetation.

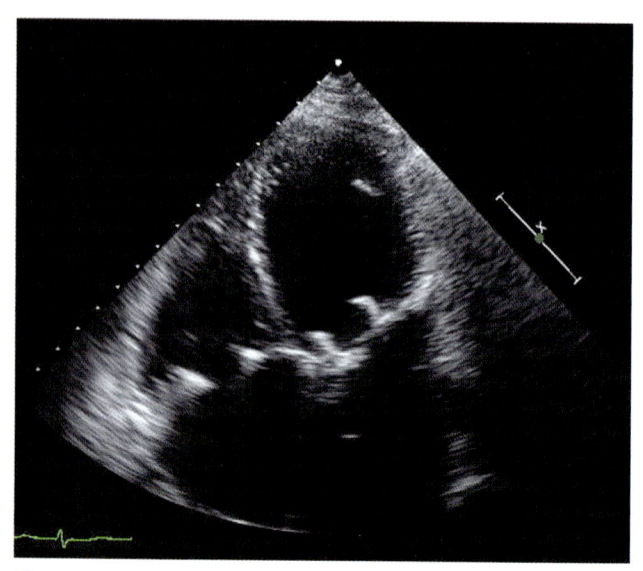

Figure 20.5. Apical 4 chamber transthoracic echocardiogram.

21. A 21-year-old man with recent aortic homograft valve replacement experiences a headache preceded by visual field deficits and undergoes a transesophageal echocardiogram to rule out a cardiac source of embolus. He has been afebrile and has negative blood cultures. Doppler evaluation reveals only trace aortic regurgitation. Based on the echocardiographic image in **Figure 20.6**, what would be an appropriate next step in management?

   A. Initiate broad spectrum antibiotics.
   B. Urgent reoperation.
   C. Refer for cardiothoracic surgery evaluation.
   D. Refer for coronary angiography.
   E. Provide reassurance that the appearance of the valve is normal.

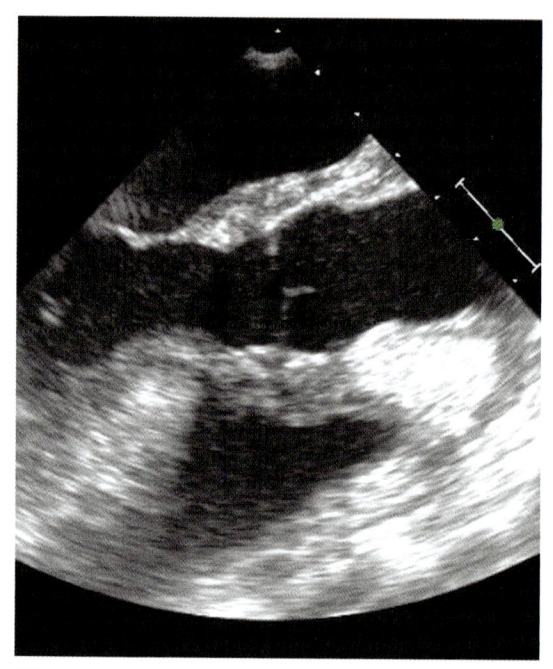

Figure 20.6. Transesophageal echocardiogram, midesophageal long-axis view.

22. A 62-year-old woman undergoes mitral valve surgery. What type of prosthesis is shown in the perioperative transesophageal echocardiogram in **Figure 20.7** and ▶ **Video 20.1**?
   A. Single tilting disc.
   B. Bileaflet disc.
   C. Trileaflet disc.
   D. Ball and cage.
   E. Disc and cage.

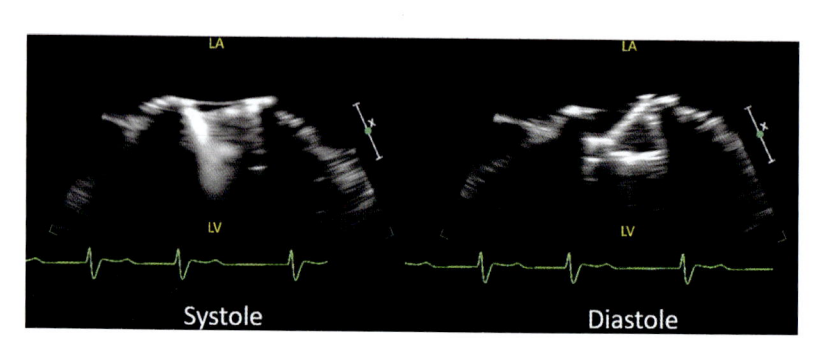

Figure 20.7. Transesophageal echocardiogram, midesophageal view.

23. A 75-year-old man with prior aortic valve replacement undergoes echocardiographic evaluation because of dyspnea on exertion (**Figure 20.8**). Pulsed-wave (PW) Doppler spectrum recorded in the left ventricular outflow tract yields a VTI of 10 cm. Continuous-wave (CW) Doppler recorded across the left ventricular outflow tract (and valve) yields a VTI of 67 cm. The LVOT diameter is 2.0 cm. What is the calculated Doppler velocity index?
   A. 3.0
   B. 1.05
   C. 0.75
   D. 0.5
   E. 0.15

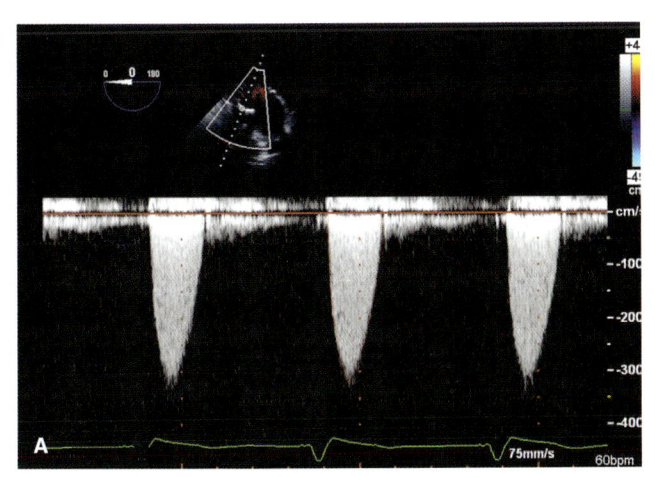

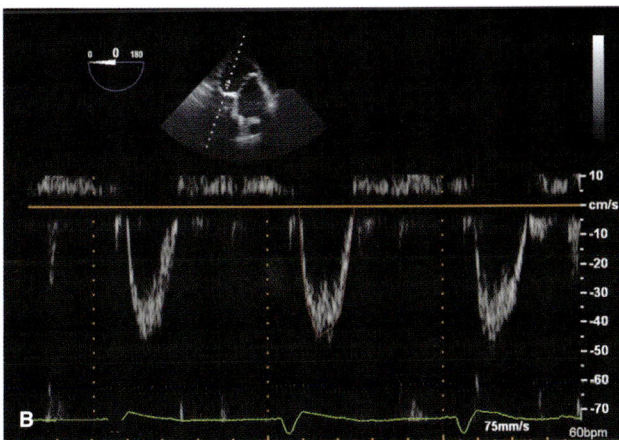

Figure 20.8. A: Continuous wave Doppler of transvalvular aortic flow (apical window). **B:** Pulsed-wave Doppler, left ventricular outflow tract.

24. A 32-year-old man with a prior history of aortic valve surgery undergoes echocardiographic evaluation because of suspected aortic dissection. Based on the echocardiographic image in **Figure 20.9**, what type of procedure was performed?

   A. Stentless bioprosthesis replacement.
   B. Aortic homograft replacement.
   C. Pulmonic autograft replacement.
   D. Stented bioprosthesis replacement.
   E. Aortic valve repair.

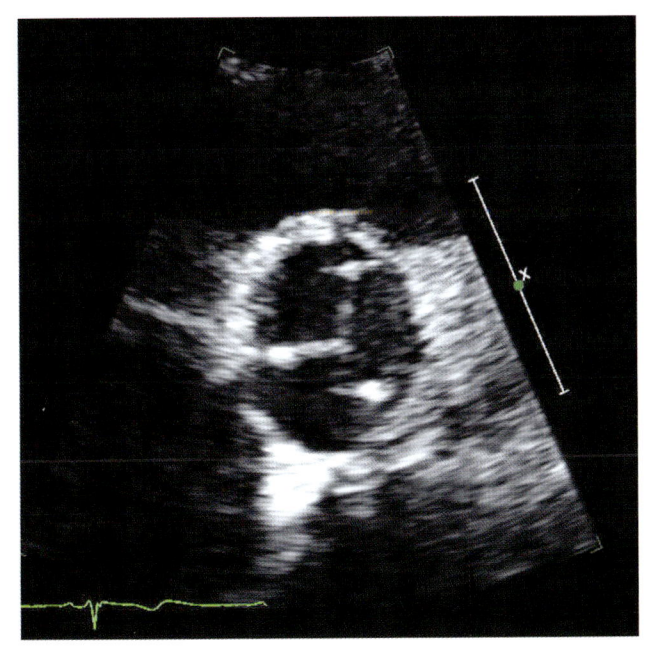

Figure 20.9. Transthoracic echocardiogram, parasternal short-axis view.

25. A 66-year-old woman undergoes resting transthoracic echocardiographic evaluation following an episode of chest pain. What is the most likely explanation for the echodensity identified by the arrow in **Figure 20.10**?
   A. Aortic prosthesis reverberation artifact.
   B. Aneurysm of the interatrial septum.
   C. Biventricular pacing lead.
   D. Alfieri stitch.
   E. Dehisced mitral ring.

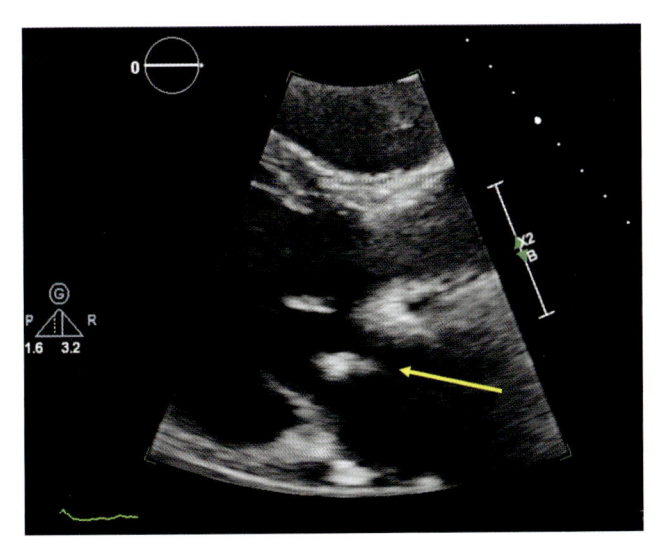

Figure 20.10. Parasternal long axis view.

CASE 1

A 62-year-old obese woman with prior mechanical mitral valve replacement is admitted with acute onset dyspnea. She is afebrile and blood cultures are negative. A transesophageal echocardiogram is performed (Figure 20.11, ▶ Video 20.2).

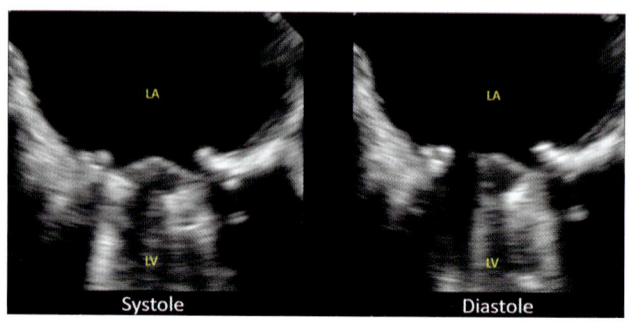

Figure 20.11. Systole (left) and diastole (right). LA, left atrium; LV, left ventricle.

26. Based on **Figure 20.11** in **Case 1** (and ▶ Video 20.2), what is the most likely diagnosis?
    A. Mitral prosthetic endocarditis.
    B. Mitral prosthetic thrombosis.
    C. Mitral pannus ingrowth.
    D. Normal tilting disc mitral prosthesis.
    E. Normal St. Jude mitral prosthesis.

27. Mitral prosthetic function in **Case 1** is most likely characterized as:
    A. Paravalvular regurgitation.
    B. Valvular regurgitation.
    C. Valvular stenosis.
    D. Valvular stenosis and valvular regurgitation.
    E. Normal valve function.

CASE 2

An 88-year-old woman with progressive dyspnea is referred for evaluation by the valve team and undergoes a percutaneous procedure. 3D TEE images recorded before (left panel) and after (right panel) the procedure are shown in Figure 20.12 and ▶ Video 20.3.

28. In **Case 2** (**Figure 20.12**, ▶ Video 20.3), what is the initial diagnosis and what mitral procedure has been performed?
    A. Tilting disc mechanical valve thrombosis—thrombolysis.
    B. Bioprosthetic valve stenosis—valve-in-valve replacement.

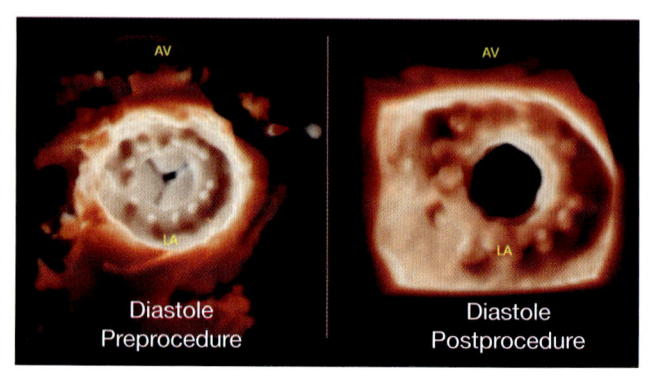

Figure 20.12. Three-dimensional transthoracic echocardiogram volume-rendered image, en face view of the mitral valve (atrial perspective) before (left) and after (right) intervention. AV, aortic valve; LV, left ventricle.

   C. Bileaflet mechanical valve pannus—valve-in-valve replacement.
   D. Native rheumatic valve disease—balloon valvuloplasty.
   E. Undersized mitral valve ring—balloon valvuloplasty.

CASE 3

A 36-year-old man with prior aortic valve replacement presents with a painful left toe. A transesophageal echocardiogram is performed to rule out a cardiac source of embolus (Figure 20.13 and ▶ Video 20.4).

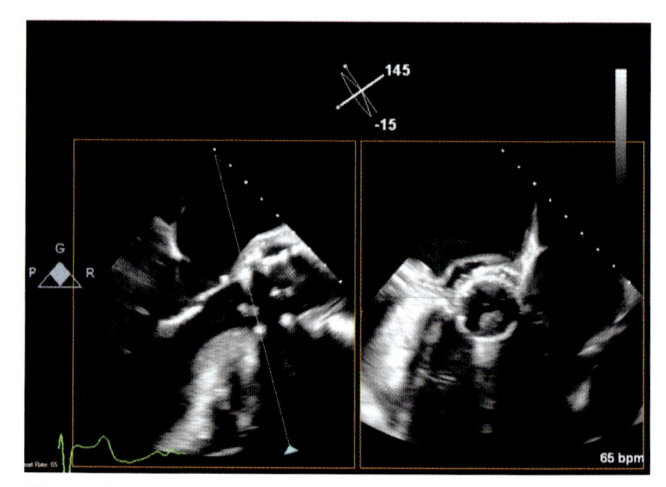

Figure 20.13. Transesophageal echocardiogram, mid-esophageal long- (left) and short-axis (right) views.

29. Based on the images in **Figure 20.13** and ▶ Video 20.4 in **Case 3**, what is the most appropriate next step in management?
    A. Initiate anticoagulation.
    B. Initiate antibiotics.
    C. Perform coronary angiography.
    D. Perform femoral arteriography.
    E. Schedule urgent cardiac surgery.

30. In addition to peripheral embolus, what other complication might commonly be encountered in the setting from **Case 3**?
   A. Acute myocardial infarction.
   B. Ventricular tachycardia.
   C. Aortic regurgitation.
   D. Aortic dissection.
   E. Pericardial effusion.

CASE 4

*A 77-year-old woman undergoes TEE evaluation (***Figure 20.14**, ▶ **Videos 20.5A,B***) following a transient ischemic attack.*

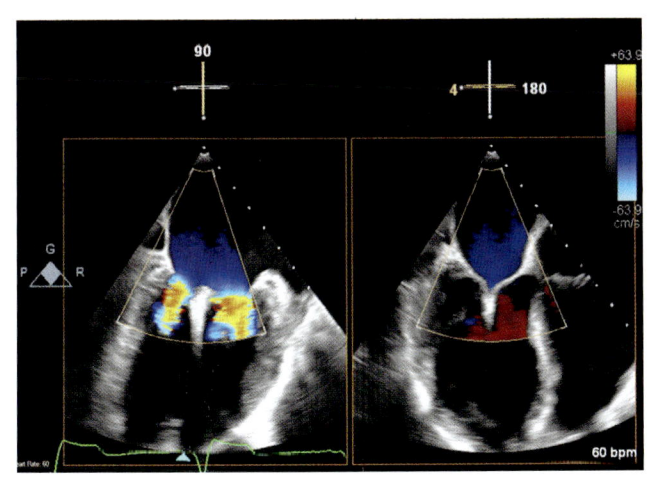

Figure 20.14. Transesophageal echocardiogram, diastolic mid-esophageal 2-chamber (left) and reverse 4-chamber (right) views with color Doppler.

31. Based on the images in **Figure 20.14** and ▶ **Videos 20.5A,B** from **Case 4**, what is the most likely diagnosis?
   A. Mitral balloon valvuloplasty.
   B. Transcatheter mitral valve replacement.
   C. Transcatheter mitral edge-to-edge repair.
   D. Surgical mitral Alfieri stitch repair with ring.
   E. Congenital double orifice mitral valve.

CASE 5

A 42-year-old man with a prior history of mitral valve replacement presents with fever and dyspnea. Blood cultures are positive for methicillin-sensitive Staphylococcus aureus. *A transesophageal echocardiogram is performed (***Figure 20.15** *and* ▶ **Video 20.6***).*

32. Based on the findings shown in the images in **Figure 20.15A,B** and ▶ **Video 20.6** from **Case 5**, what is the most likely basis for the patient's dyspnea?
   A. Left ventricular systolic dysfunction.
   B. Left ventricular diastolic dysfunction.
   C. Multiple septic pulmonary emboli.
   D. Right ventricular systolic dysfunction.
   E. Severe prosthetic mitral stenosis.

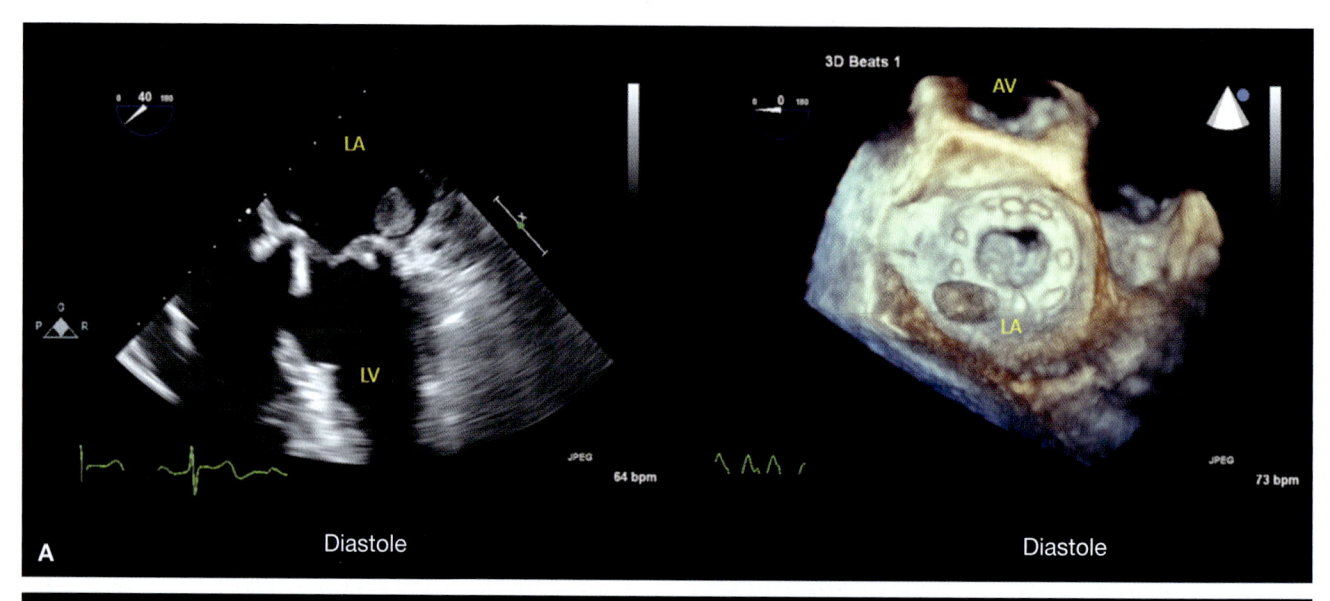

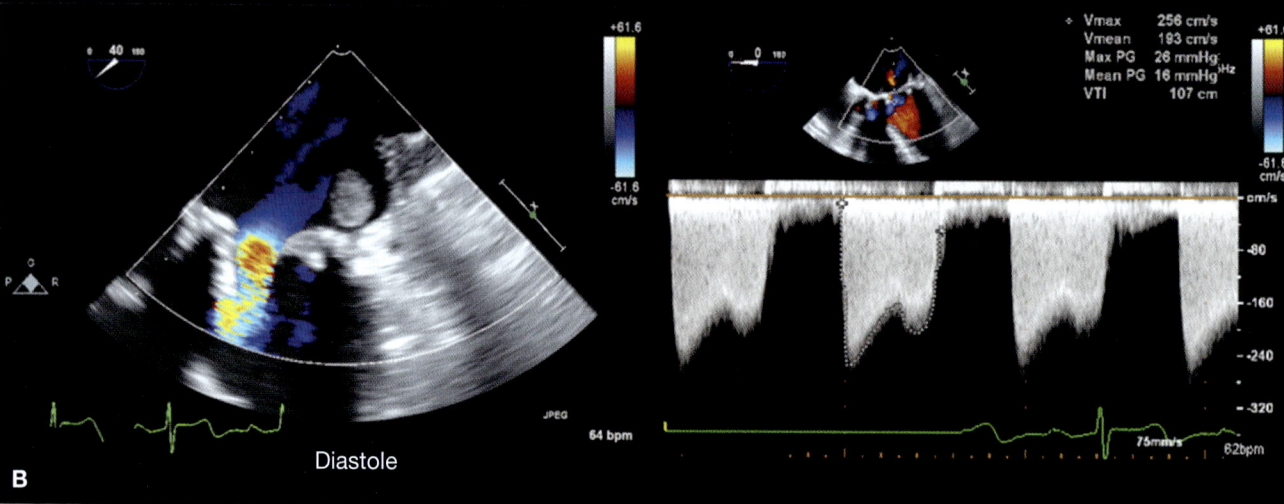

Figure 20.15. A: Transesophageal echocardiogram (TEE), mid-esophageal 4-chamber view (left) and three-dimensional en face view of the mitral valve from an atrial perspective (right). **B:** TEE, mid-esophageal 4-chamber view with color (left) and CW Doppler (right).

CASE 6

*An 82-year-old man with a past history of heart disease undergoes TEE (**Figure 20.16**) for perioperative monitoring for noncardiac surgery.*

---

33. Based on **Figure 20.16** in **Case 6**, what cardiac procedure has he undergone?
    A. Self-expanding transcatheter aortic valve replacement.
    B. Balloon expandable transcatheter aortic valve replacement.
    C. Surgical aortic valve replacement.
    D. Endovascular aortic root reconstruction.
    E. None of the above.

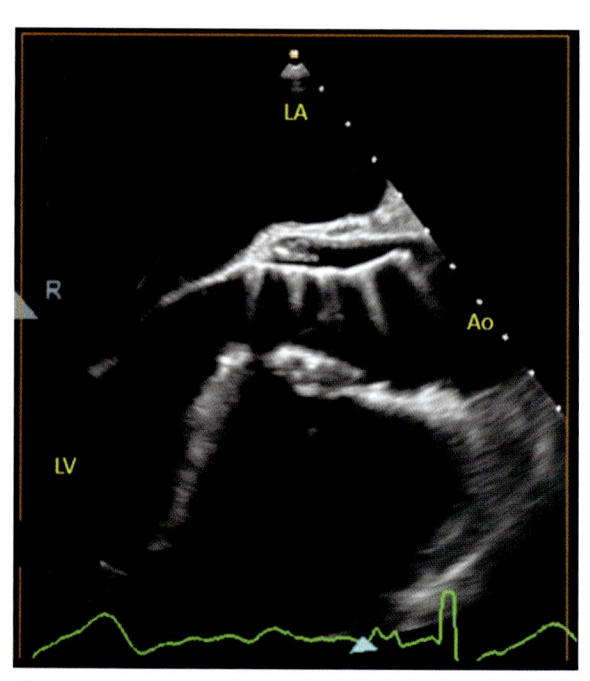

Figure 20.16. Transesophageal echocardiogram, mid-esophageal long-axis view. Ao, aorta; LA, left atrium; LV, left ventricle.

ANSWERS

1. **Answer: C.** The term patient-prosthesis mismatch (PPM) refers to the situation in which the effective orifice area (EOA) of a prosthesis is too small relative to the patient's body size, resulting in abnormally high postoperative gradients. Although bioprostheses rather than mechanical valves may be selected for women anticipating pregnancy as well as for patients at increased risk of bleeding complications due to anticoagulation, these situations are not considered PPM. Children with prosthetic valves may outgrow their valves and develop PPM, but this may be unavoidable regardless of whether a mechanical or a bioprosthetic valve is implanted.

2. **Answer: D.** Patient-prosthesis mismatch (PPM) refers to the situation in which the effective orifice area (EOA) of a prosthesis is too small relative to the patient's body size, resulting in abnormally high postoperative gradients. For prostheses in the aortic position, the cutoff for PPM has been established to be a BSA-indexed EOA of ≤0.85 cm²/m² based on the observation that at smaller areas there is a rapid increase in transvalvular gradients. BSA-corrected aortic prosthetic EOA ≤ 0.65 cm²/m² is considered severe PPM. The major adverse outcomes associated with PPM are reduced short-term and long-term survival, particularly if associated with LV dysfunction. The high gradients associated with PPM may be distinguished echocardiographically from prosthetic valve dysfunction by comparing the echo-calculated EOA with published normal values for individual valves and by excluding imaging evidence of valve dysfunction. Additionally, with PPM, the acceleration time is typically <100 ms and the Doppler velocity index (DVI) is usually ≥0.30.

3. **Answer: C.** Pressure recovery refers to the situation in which there is a localized pressure drop at the central orifice of a bileaflet mechanical valve that is partially recovered distally as flow from the lateral two orifices merges with the central flow jet (**Figure 20.16**). Since Doppler records the maximal pressure drop, it will yield a gradient higher than that measured at catheterization with catheters placed proximal and distal to the valve. Clinically significant pressure recovery is most often encountered in the setting of small bileaflet mechanical valves in the aortic position particularly when the cardiac output is increased. Answer A is incorrect because the direct measure of LV to aorta gradients used in this patient is superior to the pullback approach. It would be dangerous to attempt to cross this valve retrograde. Answer B is incorrect because a relatively higher cardiac output at catheterization would result in a relatively higher (not lower) transvalvular gradient. Answer D is incorrect. Although it is possible to mistake a mitral regurgitant for a transaortic Doppler spectrum, the peak MR velocities are typically much higher than 3.5 m/s (peak gradient = 49 mm Hg), reflecting large gradients from the left ventricle to left atrium. Answer E is incorrect. In the case of patient-prosthesis mismatch, elevated gradients are noted both by echocardiography and catheterization. Clinically significant pressure recovery is not commonly observed unless the ascending aorta diameter is less than 3 cm (**Figure 20.17**).

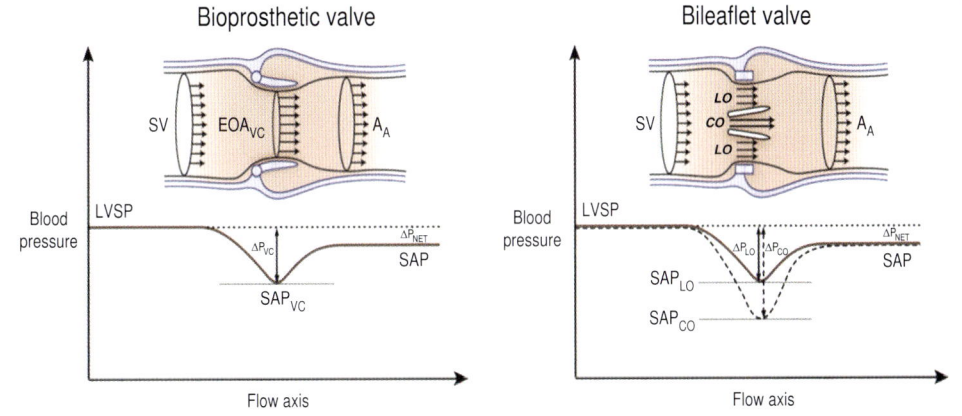

Figure 20.17. Pressure recovery. Schematic representation of velocity and pressure changes from the left ventricular outflow (LVO) tract to the ascending aorta (A_A) in the presence of a stented bioprosthesis and a bileaflet mechanical valve illustrating the phenomenon of pressure recovery. Because of pressure recovery, velocities are lower and systolic arterial pressure (SAP) is higher at the distal aorta than at the level of the vena contracta (VC). This is further exaggerated in the case of a bileaflet valve, in which the velocity is higher in the central orifice (CO) and thus pressure drop is higher at that level. Doppler gradients are estimated from maximal velocity at the level of the vena contracta and represent the maximal pressure drop, whereas invasive estimation of gradients usually reflect net pressure difference (ΔP) between left ventricular systolic pressure (LVSP) and ascending aorta. EOA, effective orifice area; LO, lateral orifice; SV, stroke volume in LVO. (Reprinted from Zoghbi WA, Chambers JB, Dumesnil JG, et al. Recommendations for evaluation of prosthetic valves with echocardiography and doppler ultrasound: a report From the American Society of Echocardiography's Guidelines and Standards Committee and the Task Force on Prosthetic Valves, developed in conjunction with the American College of Cardiology Cardiovascular Imaging Committee, Cardiac Imaging Committee of the American Heart Association, the European Association of Echocardiography, a registered branch of the European Society of Cardiology, the Japanese Society of Echocardiography and the Canadian Society of Echocardiography, endorsed by the American College of Cardiology Foundation, American Heart Association, European Association of Echocardiography, a registered branch of the European Society of Cardiology, the Japanese Society of Echocardiography, and Canadian Society of Echocardiography. *J Am Soc Echocardiogr*. 2009;22(9):975-1014; quiz 1082-1084. Copyright © 2009 by the American Society of Echocardiography. With permission.)

4. **Answer: B.** Echocardiographic displays are calibrated based on the velocity of sound through tissue and the assumption that only tissue will be encountered by the ultrasound beam. The speed of sound in a Starr-Edwards valve ball is slower than that in tissue. Consequently, the ball is misrepresented echocardiographically as being larger than it actually is.

5. **Answer: C.** Depending on size and valve type, there is significant variability in the normal values reported for aortic prosthetic valves. A peak velocity of 2.5 m/s is well within the normal range for many valves, and as such, would not be helpful in determining the type of prosthesis that has been implanted. In general, velocities >3.0 m/s prompt concern about pathologic elevation due to a variety of causes including patient-prosthesis mismatch and intrinsic valve pathology. However, velocities of >3.0 m/s may be normal for some valves (**Figure 20.18**). Stroke volume as an index of cardiac output is measured by multiplying the velocity-time integral of the pulsed-wave Doppler spectrum of the left ventricular outflow tract by the left ventricular outflow tract cross-sectional area (**Figure 20.18**).

6. **Answer: C.** Gradients across mitral and tricuspid prostheses are very heart rate dependent. Although a mean gradient of 10 mm Hg at a heart rate of 60 bpm would be abnormal, the same gradient at a heart rate of 120 bpm may be normal for most mitral prostheses. While height and weight (Choices A and B) and calculated BSA are important in evaluating patients for patient-prosthesis mismatch (BSA-indexed EOA < 1.2 cm²/m² for mitral prostheses), this assessment requires the calculation of effective orifice area, which is not possible with mean gradient only. It is important to record blood pressure (Choice D) at the time of echocardiography for patients with mitral disease; however, its major impact is on regurgitation rather than stenosis. Gender has no direct impact on valve gradients.

7. **Answer: E.** With harmonic imaging, microcavitations are frequently seen with normally functioning mechanical valves. While their origin is uncertain, they are not imaging artifacts. In the era of fundamental imaging, microcavitations were reported as markers of hemolysis, which may be a feature of paravalvular regurgitation. In the absence of intravenously injected microbubbles, a patent foramen ovalis and associated right-to-left shunt will not result in left-sided microbubbles.

8. **Answer: A.** Effective orifice area (EOA) is calculated using the continuity equation and is equivalent to the calculation of valve area in native valves. Thus:

$$EOA = \frac{CSA_{LVOT} \times VTI_{LVOT}}{Prosthetic\ VTI} = \frac{Stroke\ volume}{Prosthetic\ VTI}$$

Choices C and D are variations on the same approach used to calculate the Doppler velocity index (DVI) or dimensionless index (DI). By comparing calculated EOA with published norms, the diagnosis of prosthetic stenosis can be established (**Table 20.1**). Note that prosthetic valve size should not be used as a surrogate for measured left ventricular outflow tract diameter (**Table 20.1**).

9. **Answer: A.** See also discussion of **Question 20.3**. Pressure recovery is typically encountered in small bileaflet or ball and cage valves implanted in individuals with small aortas.

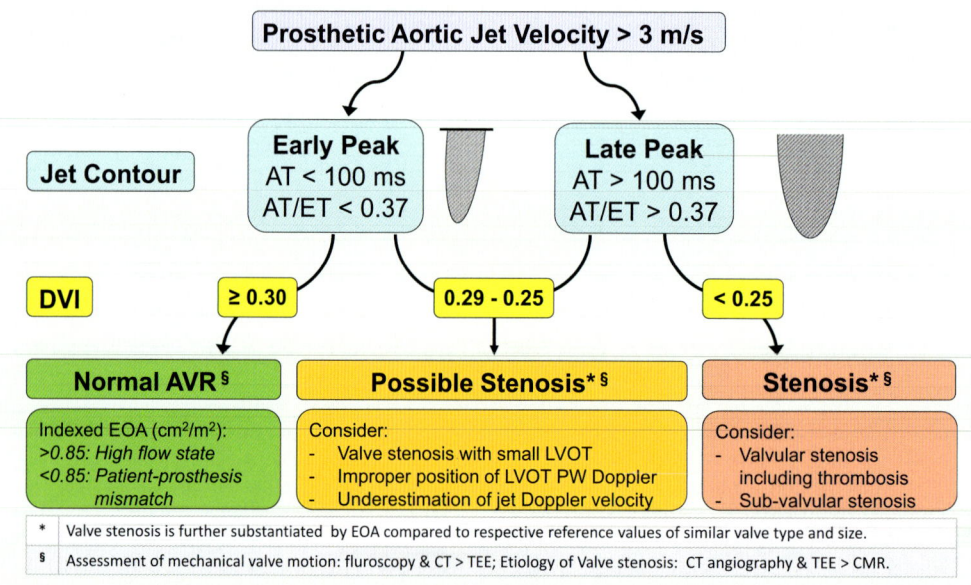

Figure 20.18. Algorithm for initial evaluation of elevated peak prosthetic aortic jet velocity incorporating DVI, jet contour, and measures of acceleration time (AT) and the ratio of AT to ejection time (ET). Improper PW Doppler sample volume influences both DVI and EOA calculations: too close to the valve will increase DVI and EOA, while too far (apical) will decrease them. AVR, aortic valve replacement. (Reprinted from Zoghbi WA, Jone PN, Chamsi-Pasha MA, et al. Guidelines for the evaluation of prosthetic valve function with cardiovascular imaging: a report from the American Society of Echocardiography Developed in Collaboration with the Society for Cardiovascular Magnetic Resonance and the Society of Cardiovascular Computed Tomography. *J Am Soc Echocardiogr.* 2024;37(1):2-63. Figure 13. Copyright © 2023 by the American Society of Echocardiography. With permission.)

Table 20.1. Doppler Parameters of Prosthetic Valves in the Aortic Valve Position

	Normal	**Possible Stenosis**	**Suggests Significant Stenosis**
Appropriate for All Prosthetic Aortic Valves			
Jet velocity contour[a]	Triangular, early peaking	Triangular to intermediate	Rounded, symmetric
Acceleration time, msec[a]	<80	80-100	>100
Acceleration time/LV ejection time ratio	<0.32	0.32-0.37	>0.37
Peak velocity, m/sec[b,c]	<3	3-4	≥4
Specific AVR Considerations			
SAVR			
Mean gradient, mm Hg[b]	<20	20-34	≥35
DVI[d]	>0.35	0.25-0.35	<0.25
EOA[d]	Reference EOA ± 1 SD	1 SD smaller than reference EOA	2 SDs smaller than reference EOA
TAVI (change from baseline)			
Mean gradient[t]	Change <10 mm Hg from baseline[b]	Increase of 10-19 mm Hg from baseline	Increase ≥20 mm Hg from baseline
DVI[d,e]	Change <0.1 or 20% from baseline[f]	Decrease 0.1-0.19 or 20%-39% from baseline[f]	Decrease ≥0.2 or ≥40% from baseline[f]
EOA[d]	Change <0.3 cm² or 25% from baseline[f]	Decrease of 0.3-0.59 cm² or 25%-49% from baseline[f]	Decrease ≥0.6 cm² or ≥50% from baseline[f]

AVR, Aortic valve replacement.
Significant stenosis should meet at least one flow-dependent (ie, velocity and mean gradient) and one flow-independent (ie, EOA or DVI) parameter.
Adapted from Zoghbi WA, Jone P-N, Chamsi-Pasha MA, et al. Guidelines for the evaluation of prosthetic valve function with cardiovascular imaging: a report from the American Society of Echocardiography developed in collaboration with the Society for Cardiovascular Magnetic Resonance and the Society of Cardiovascular Computed Tomography. J Am Soc Echocardiogr. 2024;37:2-63. Copyright © 2023 by the American Society of Echocardiography. With permission.
[a]This can be affected by LV function and heart rate.
[b]Flow dependent.
[c]Valid with normal stroke volume (50-90 mL) and flow rates (200-300 mL).
[d]Flow independent.
[e]DVI calculated using VTI.
[f]Baseline defined as TTE performed under stable hemodynamic conditions.

10. Answer: A. Imaging features of restricted thickened cusps support the diagnosis of prosthetic stenosis as the basis for the elevated gradients. A small valve (19 mm) as in Choice B may be associated with elevated gradients even in a structurally normal valve if there is patient-prosthesis mismatch (the valve is too small for the patient). The aortic root may be dilated (Choice C) in patients with native aortic valve disease and does not regress following aortic valve replacement in the absence of aortic reconstructive surgery. Choice D: The normal hematocrit excludes anemia-associated high output, which may be associated with elevated gradients in structurally normal valves. Choice E: Reduced LVEF is typically associated with low gradients and provides no explanation for the elevated gradients noted here.

11. Answer: E. The pressure half-time should not be used to calculate effective orifice area in patients with prosthetic valves. The pressure half-time measurement may be used on serial studies to monitor for development of prosthetic valve stenosis. Significant increases in pressure half-time may be associated with prosthetic valve obstruction.

12. Answer: C. All mechanical prosthetic valves have physiologic "regurgitation" that consists of a closing volume (a displacement of blood caused by the motion of the occluder) and leakage at the perimeter of or at hinge points of the occluders. Studies have shown bileaflet mechanical valves (eg, St. Jude) to have the largest degree of physiologic regurgitation with central as well as peripheral jets.

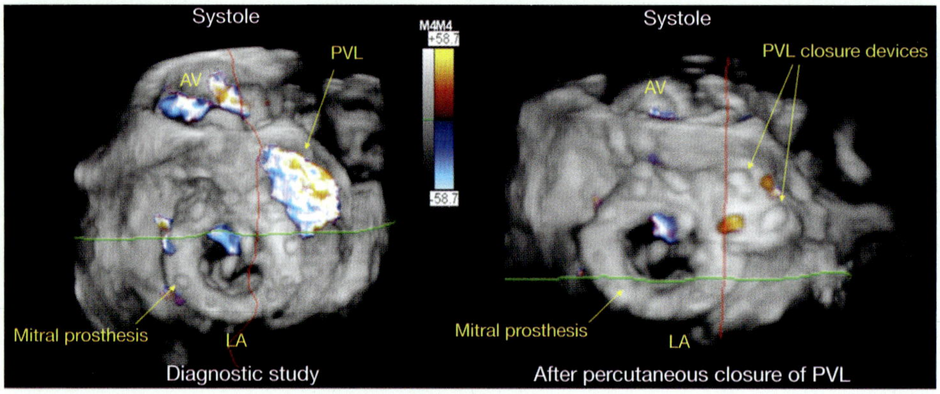

Figure 20.19. Three-dimensional transesophageal echocardiogram en face view of the mitral valve (atrial perspective) before (left) and after (right) paravalvular leak repair. AV, aortic valve; LA, left atrium; PVL, paravalvular leak.

While Medtronic-Hall single tilting disc valves have the most prominent central jets, the total amount of regurgitation is less when compared to mechanical bileaflet valves.

13. **Answer: C.** The Doppler velocity index is defined as the ratio of aortic subvalvular VTI or peak velocity to prosthetic VTI or peak velocity (ie, subvalvular VTI/prosthetic VTI or subvalvular peak velocity/prosthetic peak velocity), respectively. It is particularly useful when image quality precludes accurate measurement of the left ventricular outflow tract as is needed to calculate effective orifice area. A Doppler velocity index of <0.25 is suggestive of prosthetic aortic stenosis (**Table 20.1**).

14. **Answer: A.** Due to acoustic shadowing and the eccentricity of paravalvular jets, transthoracic echocardiography is relatively insensitive for paravalvular regurgitation. Thus, TEE is indicated whenever paravalvular regurgitation is suspected. Elevated mitral gradients (Choices B and C) favor mitral regurgitation. When jets are eccentric, normal (S dominant) flow may be preserved in pulmonary veins remote from the jet. All apical views should be used to assess for paravalvular regurgitation, but no single view is ideal.

15. **Answer: D.** The Ross procedure consists of moving the patient's pulmonary valve to the aortic position (pulmonary autograft) and placing an allograft (also termed homograft) cadaveric valve in the pulmonic position (pulmonary homograft). Of the possible correct answers, aortic (pulmonary autograft) regurgitation is the most common.

16. **Answer: A.** The prosthesis is identifiable as a stented bioprosthesis by the presence of clearly demarcated stents. There is a mitral regurgitant jet which clearly originates outside the sewing ring and extends toward the back of the left atrium: this is paravalvular regurgitation. Although the image has not been optimized for PISA-based quantitation, note the clearly demarcated PISA shell. Note also that the spatial extent of the regurgitant jet is difficult to assess due to acoustic shadowing (▶ **Video 20.7A**). While spontaneous valve dehiscence may occur, hemodynamically significant new paravalvular jets raise the possibility of endocarditis as the cause. **Figure 20.19** shows the 3D TEE appearance of the mitral valve from an atrial perspective before (left panel) and after (right panel) transcatheter paravalvular leak repair. ▶ **Video 20.7B** provides the corresponding moving images.

17. **Answer: D.** The mitral bioprosthetic struts are seen angled toward the interventricular septum and the systolic frame shows turbulent flow in the left ventricular outflow tract at the level of the mitral struts. While rare, high-profile mitral prostheses may cause significant left ventricular outflow tract obstruction. Patients at greatest risk are those with small hypertrophied ventricles. Mitral systolic anterior motion and LVOT obstruction may be a complication of mitral repair but not mitral valve replacement. Notably, in patients with MV replacement for active endocarditis, the mitral chords and leaflets are typically not preserved. Mitral stenosis would be associated with high velocity flow in diastole not systole. There is no evidence of mitral regurgitation (high-velocity flow is in the left ventricular outflow tract not left atrium.)

18. **Answer: E.** Although there are no large series of published normal values for tricuspid prosthetic gradients, the existing literature supports the diagnosis of prosthetic tricuspid stenosis whenever the mean gradients are ≥6 mm Hg. The mean gradient of 11 mm Hg at a slow heart rate is consistent with severe prosthetic stenosis. It is unlikely that this patient has a high output state with a heart rate of 55 bpm, and even a significantly elevated stroke volume would typically not be associated with gradient elevation of this degree at a heart rate of 55 bpm. Pressure recovery does not occur with large bioprosthetic valves in the tricuspid position. Note that the pressure half-time method has not been validated as a means of calculating effective orifice area for prosthetic tricuspid valves, but a pressure half-time ≥200 ms is supportive of bioprosthetic tricuspid stenosis.

19. **Answer: D.** This is the typical three-dimensional view of a bileaflet mechanical mitral prosthesis as seen from the atrial perspective. Two orifices are identified in this diastolic frame with the occluders in the open position.
20. **Answer: B.** Mitral struts are clearly seen, identifying this valve as a mitral bioprosthesis. In the right heart, the septal leaflet of the tricuspid valve is seen in the open position with the dehisced portion of a tricuspid ring (arrows, **Figure 20.20**) seen floating in the tricuspid inlet. The ring is appropriately attached laterally. This helps prevent mistaking the dehisced portion for either a vegetation or pacemaker lead. The echodensity of the dehisced ring also distinguishes it from a vegetation. This patient had severe tricuspid regurgitation.

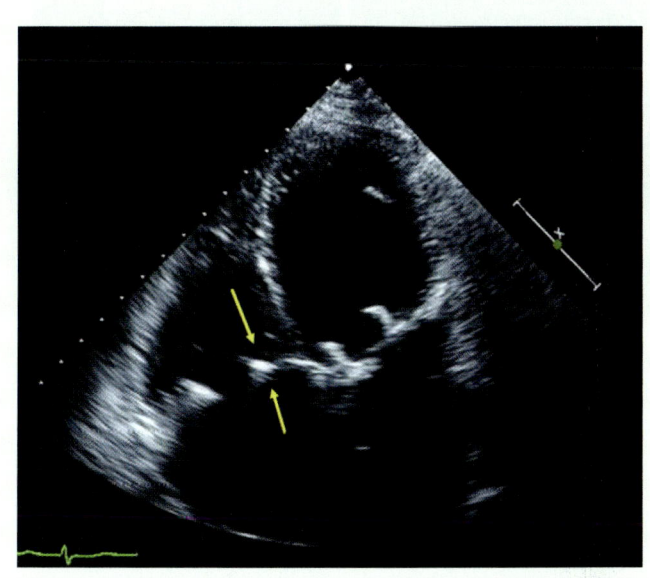

Figure 20.20. Transthoracic echocardiogram, apical 4-chamber view; arrows point to the dehisced tricuspid ring, no longer attached to the tricuspid annulus.

21. **Answer: E.** Aortic homografts are treated cadaveric aortic roots and valves, and portions of the tubular segment of the ascending aorta into which the native coronary arteries are reimplanted. The native aorta may be used to wrap the homograft aorta (the inclusion technique) or resected. Particularly when the inclusion technique is used, the normal postoperative appearance is one of a variably thickened root that may in part be due to hematoma. Over time, this resorbs and the appearance of the valve resembles that of the native aortic valve. In a clinical scenario suggestive of endocarditis, it may be impossible to differentiate a normal homograft from abscess. Comparison with the postimplantation perioperative TEE can be very helpful in resolving this dilemma. In the absence of clinical features of infection, the appearance shown here can be interpreted as normal.
22. **Answer: A.** This is a typical appearance for a single tilting disc mechanical mitral prosthesis. The disc pivots from an eccentric pivot point and closure is associated with a prominent central jet. This valve should not be confused with bileaflet or ball and cage valves (**Figure 20.21**). There are no trileaflet mechanical valves.
23. **Answer: E.** The Doppler velocity index is the ratio of aortic subvalvular VTI to prosthetic VTI (=10 cm/67 cm = 0.15). Peak velocity measurements may be used in place of VTI. The Doppler velocity index is easily calculated and may be used as an alternative to effective orifice area as a means of evaluating prosthetic valve function when the LVOT diameter is difficult to measure.
24. **Answer: D.** This short-axis image (**Figure 20.9**) shows three stents and cusps in the closed position. This appearance is typical of a stented bioprosthesis. Stents are not elements of homografts or autografts, which are human valves, or stentless heterograft bioprostheses. Aortic repairs are also not associated with stents. Stented valves are the most common type of bioprosthesis.
25. **Answer: E.** The arrow indicates a dehisced mitral ring (**Figure 20.10**). The anterior rim of the ring is seen in a normal position adjacent to the aortic root. This patient had severe posteriorly directed mitral regurgitation (not shown). Alfieri stitch is used in edge-to-edge mitral valve repair tying together the A2 and P2 scallops. The left ventricular lead in biventricular pacing is placed in the coronary sinus. The aortic valve in this patient is a native valve. Although atrial septal aneurysms may project into the left atrium and be visible from this window, they do not appear as discrete echodensities as is seen here. **Figure 20.22** shows the corresponding 3D TEE multiplanar reconstruction from this patient with the arrow pointing to the dehisced ring and the asterisk identifying the large gap between the ring and mitral annulus.
26. **Answer: B.** This patient has a bileaflet mechanical prosthesis in which one of the discs does not move and is stuck in the closed position. This is associated with severe prosthetic stenosis. While this may occur on the basis of either pannus ingrowth or thrombus, the acuity of the symptoms in this case favors the diagnosis of mitral prosthetic thrombosis. A history of inadequate anticoagulation would also support the diagnosis. Vegetations may also interfere with disc function; however, the clinical information (absence of fever and negative blood cultures) argues against active endocarditis. When the disc sticks in the open position, there is severe regurgitation. Both stenosis and regurgitation can occur when the occluder is stuck in an intermediate position.

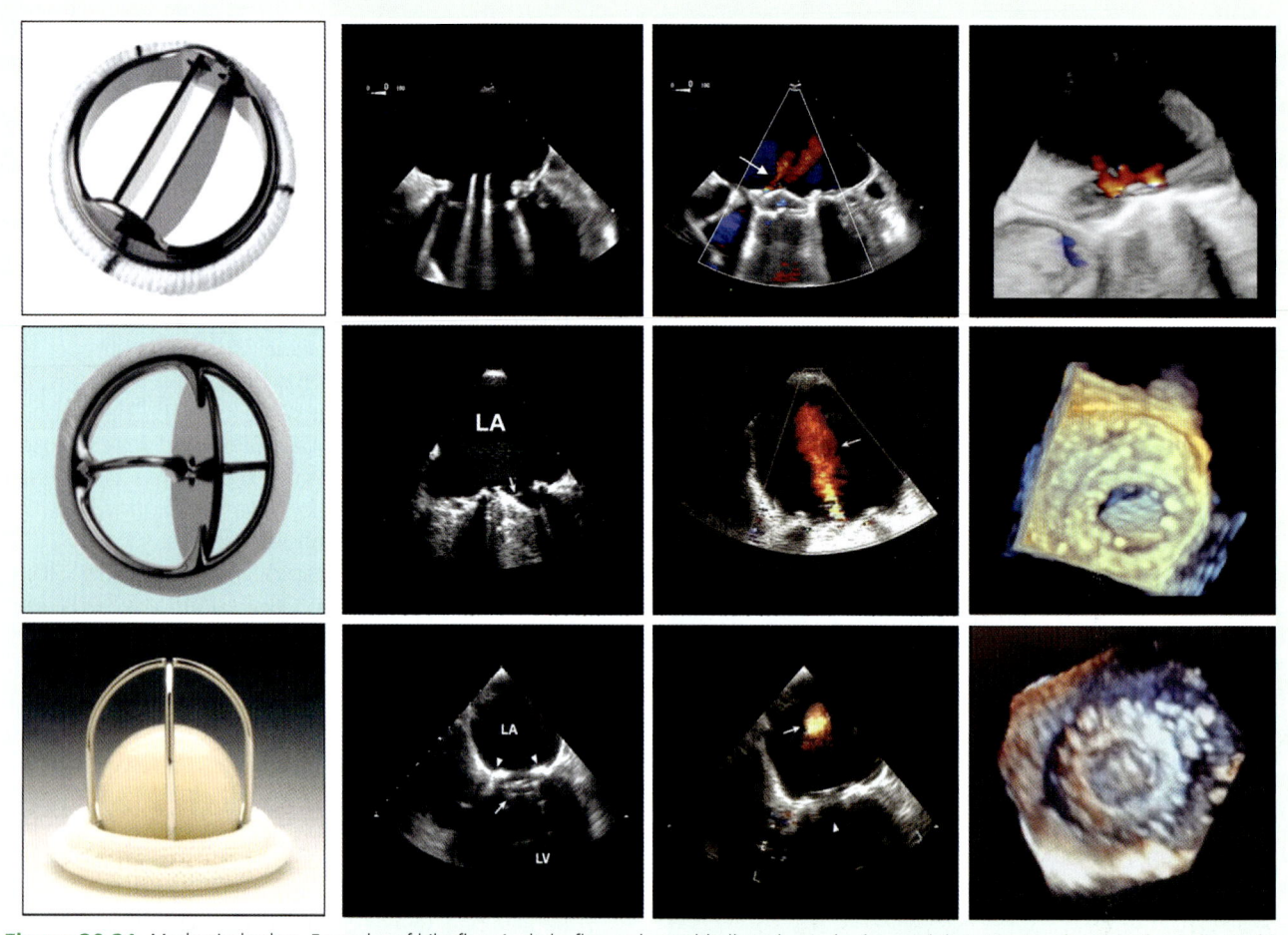

Figure 20.21. Mechanical valves. Examples of bileaflet, single-leaflet, and caged-ball mechanical valves and their transesophageal echocardiographic characteristics taken in the mitral position in diastole (middle) and in systole (right). The arrows in diastole point to the occluder mechanism of the valve and in systole to the characteristic physiologic regurgitation observed with each valve. LA, left atrium; LV, left ventricle. (Reprinted from Zoghbi WA, Jone P-N, Chamsi-Pasha MA, et al. Guidelines for the evaluation of prosthetic valve function with cardiovascular imaging: A report from the American Society of Echocardiography developed in collaboration with the Society for Cardiovascular Magnetic Resonance and the Society of Cardiovascular Computed Tomography. *J Am Soc Echocardiogr.* 2024;37:2-63. Copyright © 2023 by the American Society of Echocardiography. With permission.)

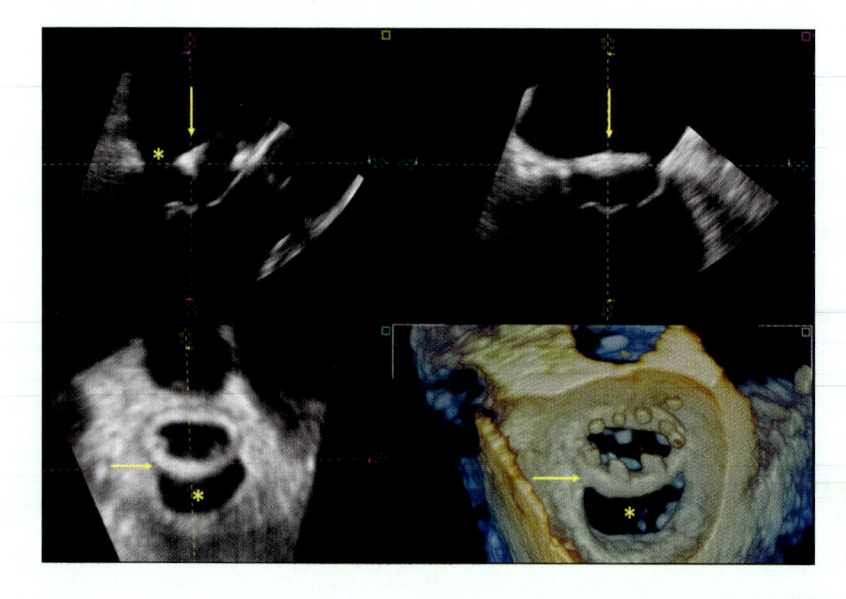

Figure 20.22. Three-dimensional (3D) transesophageal echocardiogram mid-esophageal volumes with 3D multiplanar reconstruction.

27. **Answer: C.** See **Answer 20.26**.

> **KEY POINTS**
> **Case 1**
> - Bileaflet mechanical prosthetic valve dysfunction can include valvular and paravalvular regurgitation (with variable degrees of dehiscence) and valve stenosis.
> - Valve stenosis is typically due to restricted motion of one or both occluders on the basis of either thrombus or pannus ingrowth. Less commonly, in the setting of infective endocarditis, critically placed vegetations may also limit occluder motion.
> - A history of inadequate anticoagulation and sudden onset of symptoms favors the diagnosis of thrombus.
> - The position of the restricted occluder will determine whether the outcome will be valve stenosis, regurgitation of a combination of the two.

28. **Answer: B.** This appearance on the left is typical for prosthetic mitral valve stenosis most likely due to leaflet degeneration. The sewing ring and three clearly seen leaflets identify this as a bioprosthesis. The valve area is markedly reduced due to severely reduced leaflet mobility. The absence of mechanical elements eliminates the possibility that this is a mechanical valve and the general appearance as well as three leaflets are inconsistent with prior ring repair. The image on the right was recorded after successful valve-in-valve replacement with a balloon-expandable valve.

> **KEY POINTS**
> **Case 2**
> - Bioprosthetic and mechanical valves have pathognomonic imaging features as do most mitral repairs that are anchored with a ring.
> - Bioprosthetic valve stenosis most commonly is the result of degenerative changes, often with calcific elements, that limit cusp motion. Less common causes include valve rejection and superimposed vegetation or thrombus.
> - Transcatheter redo valve replacement using a valve-in-valve technique provides an alternative to redo surgery in high-risk patients

29. **Answer: E.** These images show valvular vegetations as well as a large aortic root abscess and likely pseudoaneurysm with communication between the aortic blood pool and the abscess. While the communication would be best seen with color Doppler (not shown), the pulsatile expansion of the echolucent space suggests that blood is flowing in and out. Aortic root pseudoaneurysm and root abscess are indications for urgent surgery. There is no indication for anticoagulation as the painful toe can be attributed to a septic embolus. Coronary arteriography is contraindicated in the presence of large aortic valve vegetations and a friable root. Since the source of embolus has been identified, there is no need for femoral arteriography.

30. **Answer: C.** These images from **Case 3** (▶ **Video 20.4, Figure 20.13**) are consistent with bioprosthetic aortic valve vegetations (thin arrow) with associated abscess and likely pseudoaneurysm (*blunt arrows*, **Figure 20.23**). Aortic regurgitation (valvular and/or paravalvular) and stenosis may commonly be encountered in this clinical scenario. Coronary embolization leading to acute myocardial infarction can occur but is uncommon. Ventricular tachycardia is not commonly seen with aortic root abscess; conduction disturbances (ie, varying degrees of heart block) are more commonly observed. Aortic dissection and pericardial effusion are not commonly encountered complications of bioprosthetic aortic valve endocarditis and abscess or pseudoaneurysm.

> **KEY POINTS**
> **Case 3**
> - Complications of prosthetic valve endocarditis include root abscess, pseudoaneurysm (characterized by communication between the abscess and adjacent blood pool), and fistula in which infection results in a tract that connects two blood pools that would not normally connect (eg, the aorta and left atrium).
> - These complications are indications for urgent surgical intervention.

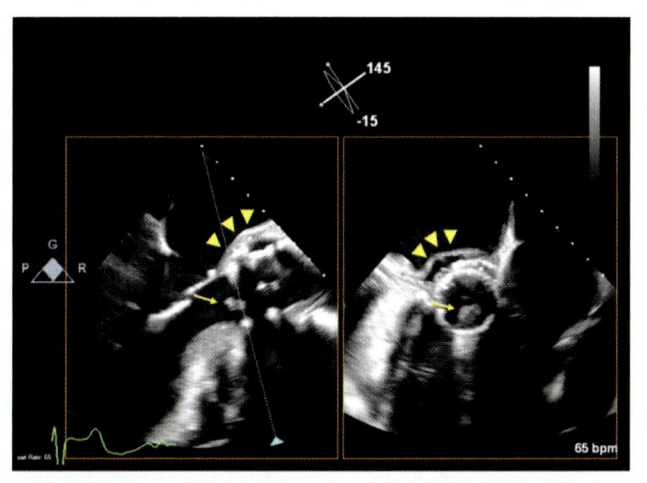

Figure 20.23. Transthoracic echocardiogram mid-esophageal long- (left) and short (right)-axis views.

31. Answer: C. These images in **Case 4** (▶ **Videos 20.5A,B, Figure 20.14**) demonstrate stable central positioning of a transcatheter edge-to-edge repair system (clip) that has created a bridge between A2 and P2 scallops and created a double orifice. This is patterned on the Alfieri stitch mitral repair that is performed surgically but does not employ a clip device. The features are highlighted by the labeled images (**Figure 20.24A,B**). Similarly, the presence of a clip device easily distinguishes this from a congenital double orifice valve.

> **KEY POINTS**
> **Case 4**
> - Transcatheter edge-to-edge repair (TEER) is based on the Alfieri stitch approach to surgical mitral valve repair.
> - TEER uses devices that connect opposing segments of the anterior and posterior leaflets to create a double orifice.
> - While the optimum site for mitral TEER is central (A2 and P2), TEER can be successfully used in other locations.
> - Multiple devices may be required for successful reduction in the severity of mitral regurgitation with recognition of the need to avoid mitral stenosis.

32. Answer: E. At a heart rate of 62 bpm, a mean gradient of 16 mm Hg is severely elevated and consistent with severe prosthetic mitral valve stenosis attributable to obstruction of the prosthesis by vegetations (see **Table 20.2**). While prosthetic mitral endocarditis is associated with peripheral emboli, septic pulmonary emboli are not a complication in the absence of concomitant right-sided endocarditis. While images of the left and right ventricles are limited, function does not appear to be severely impaired and it is not possible to attribute the patient's dyspnea to left or right ventricular systolic dysfunction. In the presence of an abnormal mitral prosthesis, it is impossible to assess left ventricular diastolic function on the basis of an isolated mitral inflow spectrum. **Table 20.2** and **Figure 20.25** provide an approach to the patient with elevated mitral prosthetic gradients.

> **KEY POINTS**
> **Case 5**
> - In the setting of prosthetic valve endocarditis, bulky and/or critically positioned vegetations can interfere with bioprosthetic cusp or mechanical valve occluder function, causing significant stenosis.
> - Transesophageal echocardiography is critical in the evaluation of patients with prosthetic valve endocarditis and may require nonstandard views.

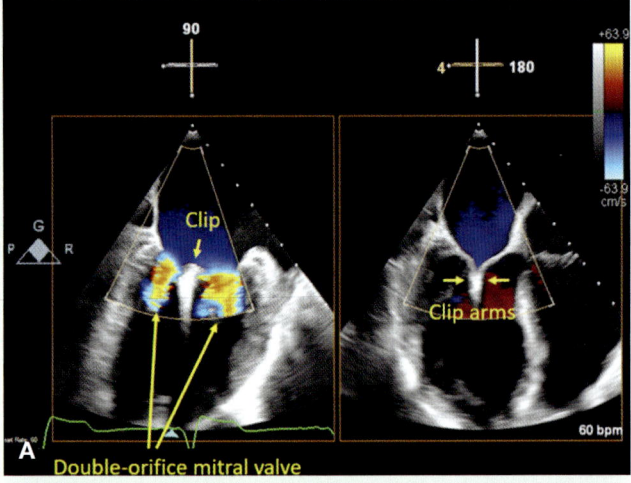

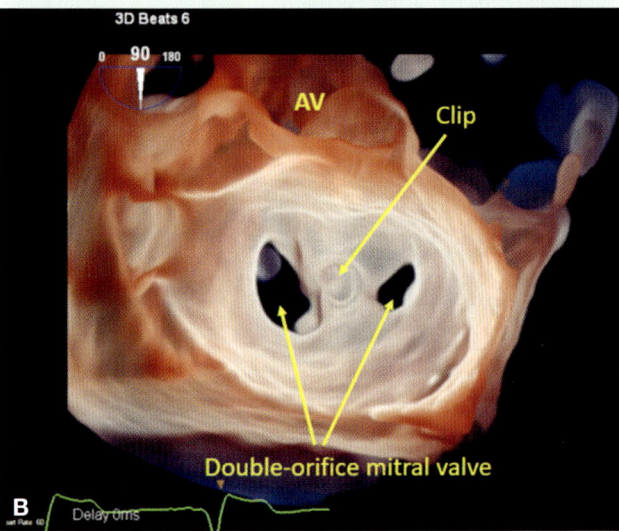

Figure 20.24. A transesophageal echocardiogram (TEE), diastolic mid-esophageal 2-chamber (left) and reverse 4-chamber view with color Doppler. B Three-dimensional TEE volume-rendered image, en face view of the mitral valve (atrial perspective). AV, aortic valve.

33. Answer: A. This is the typical appearance of a self-expanding transcatheter aortic valve replacement, identifiable by its "hourglass" shape and supra-annular position. The displaced native aortic cusps can be seen. Endovascular aortic procedures are not used for the root.

> **KEY POINTS**
> **Case 6**
> - Transcatheter aortic valves implantation (TAVI) has surpassed surgical aortic valve replacement for the treatment of symptomatic severe aortic stenosis, making it important for the echocardiographer to recognize characteristic TAVI valve appearance.
> - TAVI valves fall into two categories: self-expanding with a long hourglass contour and the more uniformly cylindrical and shorter balloon-expandable valves.
> - Echocardiography can typically identify the TAVI frame and may be able to delineate the cusps.

Table 20.2. Doppler Parameters of Prosthetic Mitral Valve Function

	Normal[a]	Possible Stenosis[b]	Suggests Significant Stenosis[a,b]
Peak velocity (m/s)[c,d]	<1.9	1.9-2.5	≥2.5
Mean gradient (mm Hg)[c,d]	≤5	6-10	>10
VTIPrMv/VTILVOT[c,d]	<2.2	2.2-2.5	>2.5
EOA (cm²)	≥2.0	1-2	<1
PHT (ms)	<130	130-200	>200

EOA, effective orifice area; LVOT, left ventricular outflow tract; PHT, pressure half-time; PrMV, prosthetic mitral valve; VTI, velocity-time integral.
[a]Best specificity for normality or abnormality is seen if the majority of the parameters listed are normal or abnormal, respectively.
[b]Values of the parameters should prompt a closer evaluation of valve function and/or other considerations such as increased flow, increased heart rate, or patient-prosthesis mismatch.
[c]Slightly higher cutoff values than shown may be seen in some bioprosthetic valves.
[d]These parameters are also abnormal in the presence of significant prosthetic mitral regurgitation.
Reprinted from Zoghbi WA, Chambers JB, Dumesnil JG, et al. Recommendations for evaluation of prosthetic valves with echocardiography and doppler ultrasound: a report From the American Society of Echocardiography's Guidelines and Standards Committee and the Task Force on Prosthetic Valves, developed in conjunction with the American College of Cardiology Cardiovascular Imaging Committee, Cardiac Imaging Committee of the American Heart Association, the European Association of Echocardiography, a registered branch of the European Society of Cardiology, the Japanese Society of Echocardiography and the Canadian Society of Echocardiography, endorsed by the American College of Cardiology Foundation, American Heart Association, European Association of Echocardiography, a registered branch of the European Society of Cardiology, the Japanese Society of Echocardiography, and Canadian Society of Echocardiography. *J Am Soc Echocardiogr*. 2009;22(9):975-1014; quiz 1082-1084. Copyright © 2009 by the American Society of Echocardiography. With permission.

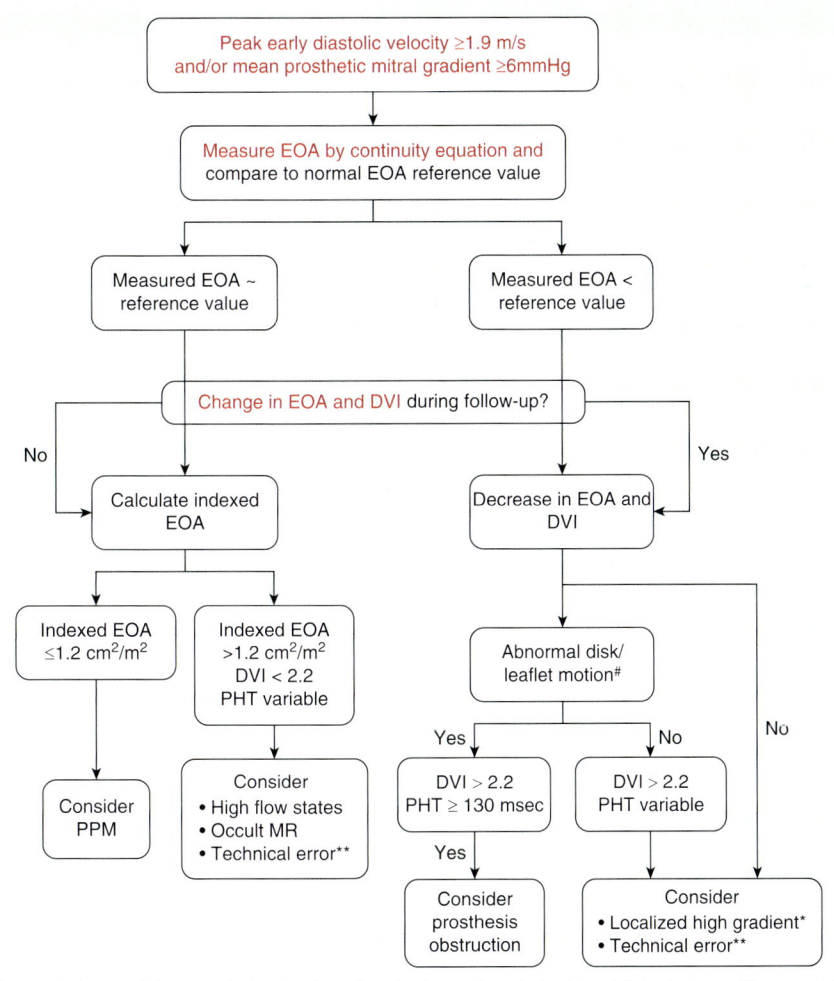

Figure 20.25. Algorithm for evaluation of high transvalvular mitral gradient. DVI, Doppler velocity index; EOA, effective orifice area; PHT, pressure half-time; PPM, patient-prosthesis mismatch. *Bileaflet valves only. **Consider underestimation of left ventricular outflow tract (LVOT) diameter and/or LVOT velocity-time integral (VTI). # If leaflet/disc motion unclear by transthoracic or transesophageal echocardiogram, consider cinefluoroscopy or cardiac CT. ## Consider overestimation of LVOT diameter and/or LVOT VTI. (Reprinted with permission from Lancellotti P, Pibarot P, Chambers J, et al. Recommendations for the imaging assessment of prosthetic heart valves: a report from the European Association of Cardiovascular Imaging endorsed by the Chinese Society of Echocardiography, the Inter-American Society of Echocardiography, and the Brazilian Department of Cardiovascular Imaging. *Eur Heart J Cardiovasc Imaging*. 2016; 17(6):589-590. Figure 24.)

SUGGESTED READINGS

Baumgartner H, Stefenelli T, Niederberger J, Schima H, Maurer G. "Overestimation" of catheter gradients by Doppler ultrasound in patients with aortic stenosis: a predictable manifestation of pressure recovery. *J Am Coll Cardiol*. 1999;33(6):1655-1661.

Eleid MF, Cabalka AK, Malouf JF, Sanon S, Hagler DJ, Rihal CS. Techniques and outcomes for the treatment of paravalvular leak. *Circ Cardiovasc Interv*. 2015;8:e001945.

Habib G, Badano L, Tribouilloy C, et al. Recommendations for the practice of echocardiography in infective endocarditis. *Eur J Echocardiogr*. 2010;11(2):202-219.

Hamid NB, Khalique OK, Monaghan MJ, et al. Transcatheter valve implantation in failed surgically inserted bioprosthesis: review and practical guide to echocardiographic imaging in valve-in-valve procedures. *JACC Cardiovasc Imaging*. 2015;8:960-979.

Horgan SJ, Mediratta A, Gillam LD. Cardiovascular imaging in infective endocarditis: a multimodality approach. *Circ Cardiovasc Imaging*. 2020;13(7):e008956.

Lancellotti P, Pibarot P, Chambers J, et al. Recommendations for the imaging assessment of prosthetic heart valves: a report from the European association of cardiovascular imaging endorsed by the Chinese Society of Echocardiography and Brazilian Department of Cardiovascular Imaging. *Eur Heart J Cardiovasc Imaging*. 2016;17(6):589-590.

Nicoara A, Skubas N, Ad N, et al. Guidelines for the use of transesophageal echocardiography to assist with surgical decision-making in the operating room: a surgery-based approach—from the American Society of Echocardiography in collaboration with the Society of Cardiovascular Anesthesiologists and the Society of Thoracic Surgeons. *J Am Soc Echocardiogr*. 2020;33(6):692-734.

Pibarot P, Magne J, Leipsic J, et al. Imaging for predicting and assessing prosthesis-patient mismatch after aortic valve replacement. *JACC Cardiovasc Imaging*. 2019;12(1):149-162.

Zamorano JL, Badano LP, Bruce C, et al. EAE/ASE recommendations for the use of echocardiography in new transcatheter interventions for valvular heart disease. *J Am Soc Echocardiogr*. 2011;24(9):937-965.

Zoghbi WA, Jone P-N, Chamsi-Pasha MA, et al. Guidelines for the evaluation of prosthetic valve function with cardiovascular imaging: A report from the American Society of Echocardiography developed in collaboration with the Society for Cardiovascular Magnetic Resonance and the Society of Cardiovascular Computed Tomography. *J Am Soc Echocardiogr*. 2024;37:2-63.

CHAPTER 21

Endocarditis

Lawrence Lau and Kwan Leung Chan

QUESTIONS

1. What is the negative predictive value of multiplane transesophageal echocardiography (TEE) for ruling out infective endocarditis (IE)?
   A. 50%.
   B. 60%.
   C. 70%.
   D. 80%.
   E. >85%.

2. A patient has *Staphylococcus aureus* bacteremia but a negative transthoracic echocardiogram (TTE) and no clinical signs of IE according to the modified Duke criteria. What is the likelihood that the diagnosis of IE would be missed if TEE is not performed?
   A. 1%.
   B. 5%.
   C. 15%.
   D. 50%.
   E. None of the above.

3. What is the most frequent location of an abscess in patients presenting with IE?
   A. Mitral valve annulus.
   B. Tricuspid valve annulus.
   C. Aortic root.
   D. Myocardium.
   E. Pericardial space.

4. Which of the following represents an early sign of an aortic root abscess in the setting of native aortic valve IE?
   A. An abnormal flow between the aorta and right atrium.
   B. An echolucent space at the aortic root without drainage into the aortic lumen.
   C. An abnormal thickness of the aortic root (>10 mm).
   D. An abnormal aortic root dilation (>42 mm).
   E. None of the above.

5. A 49-year-old man presents with IE. The TEE shows a 10 × 15 mm vegetation on the left atrial aspect of the posterior mitral valve leaflet without mitral regurgitation. The patient has been given intravenous antibiotics. He remains stable during his 4 weeks' course of therapy. A repeat TEE reveals a persistent vegetation on the mitral valve with similar dimension but without significant mitral regurgitation. Which of the following statements is **TRUE** regarding this patient?
   A. After 4 weeks of therapy, the size of the vegetation and the degree of mitral regurgitation is unlikely to change.
   B. After 4 weeks of therapy, if the brightness of the vegetation increases, there is an increased risk of complications related to endocarditis.
   C. After 4 weeks of therapy, persistence of the vegetation in the absence of significant valvular regurgitation is associated with no increased risk of complications related to endocarditis.
   D. After 4 weeks of therapy, rapid reduction of the vegetation size has been shown to correlate with an increased risk of embolic events.
   E. None of the above.

6. After complete resolution of a vegetation, what proportion of affected valves retain normal structure and function?
   A. 10%.
   B. 15%.
   C. 20%.
   D. 25%.
   E. 30%.

7. A mitral valve aneurysm has the following characteristics?
   A. A localized bulging of mitral leaflet toward the left atrium (LA) with expansion throughout the cardiac cycle.
   B. A localized bulging of mitral leaflet toward the LA with systolic expansion and diastolic collapse.
   C. A localized bulging of mitral leaflet toward the left ventricle (LV) with expansion throughout the cardiac cycle.
   D. A localized bulging of mitral leaflet toward the LV with systolic expansion and diastolic collapse.
   E. None of the above.

8. After a TTE showing no vegetations, it is inappropriate to proceed with a TEE in which of the following patients?
   A. 75-year-old woman with a bioprosthetic mitral valve, urinary tract infection, and *Escherichia coli* bacteremia.
   B. 35-year-old man with a bicuspid aortic valve and *Staphylococcus aureus* bacteremia.
   C. 40-year-old woman injection drug user with *S. aureus* bacteremia.
   D. 50-year-old man with a mechanical aortic valve and *Streptococcus mitis* bacteremia.
   E. None of the above.

9. A valvular mass can be detected in patients with the antiphospholipid antibody (APLA) syndrome. Which echocardiographic feature of a valvular mass suggests IE and not APLA syndrome?
   A. A larger size of the mass.
   B. The presence of multiple masses.
   C. Heterogeneous echogenicity of the mass.
   D. The presence of associated thickening of the leaflets.
   E. The presence of valvular tissue destruction.

10. A 66-year-old man is diagnosed with streptococcal IE of his native mitral valve. TEE shows that the maximal vegetation length is 13 mm and there is severe mitral regurgitation. However, no paravalvular complications are detected, the patient has no congestive heart failure, and there is no conduction block on the electrocardiogram. What would be the preferred management strategy?
    A. Medical treatment alone.
    B. Medical treatment with a rapid surgical referral if he develops heart failure, conduction block, destructive lesions, or paravalvular complications.
    C. Surgery within the next 48 hours.
    D. Emergent surgery if a systemic embolic event occurs.
    E. None of the above.

11. Which of the following conditions has not been associated with the finding seen in **Figure 21.1** in a patient with IE? TEE view obtained at the gastroesophageal junction.
    A. A coronary sinus lead in patients with cardiac resynchronization therapy.
    B. A coronary artery fistula to the coronary sinus.
    C. A tunneled permanent hemodialysis catheter.
    D. A persistent left superior vena cava.

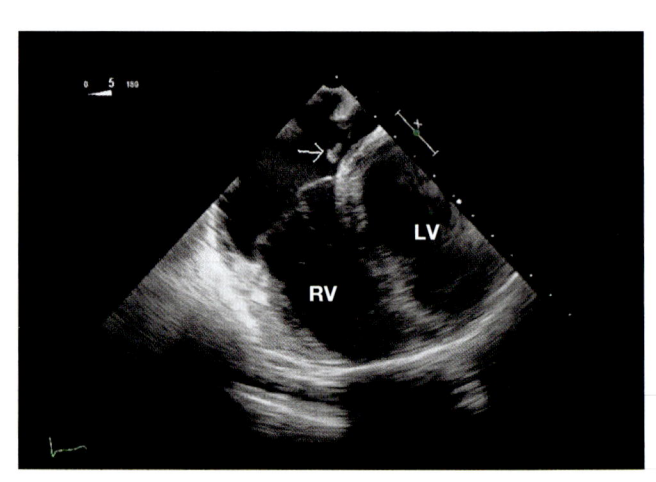

Figure 21.1

12. A patient with Behçet disease presents with new symptoms and signs suggesting right-sided heart failure. A TEE is performed (**Figure 21.2**). What is the most likely explanation for the TEE finding in the context of Behçet disease?
  A. A right atrial thrombus protruding into the right ventricle during diastole.
  B. A vegetation involving the atrial aspect of the tricuspid valve.
  C. Extension of renal cell carcinoma.
  D. A right-sided myxoma.
  E. None of the above.

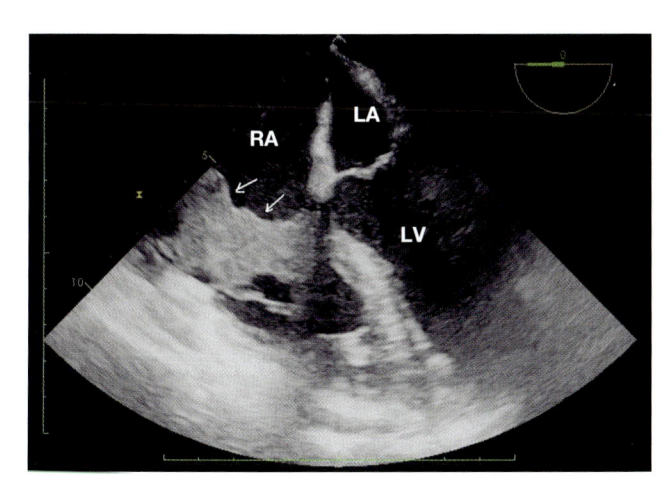

Figure 21.2

13. A patient with a right ventricular pacemaker lead infection undergoes lead removal. Following the procedure, a TEE is performed (**Figure 21.3**). What is the structure in the right atrium given the clinical context?

  A. A residual vegetation.
  B. A "ghost."
  C. A thrombus.
  D. A benign cardiac tumor.
  E. None of the above.

14. One year ago, this 70-year-old woman had successful medical treatment for IE. She has remained well and free of heart failure. A follow-up TTE is performed. A large echolucent mass is detected in the left atrium (**Figure 21.4** and ▶ **Video 21.1A,B**). Which of the following statements is **CORRECT**?
  A. She had mitral valve IE 1 year ago.
  B. She had an aortic annular abscess 1 year ago.
  C. She has recurrent mitral valve IE.
  D. Annular abscess is more common with mitral valve IE than with aortic valve IE.
  E. Urgent surgical intervention is needed.

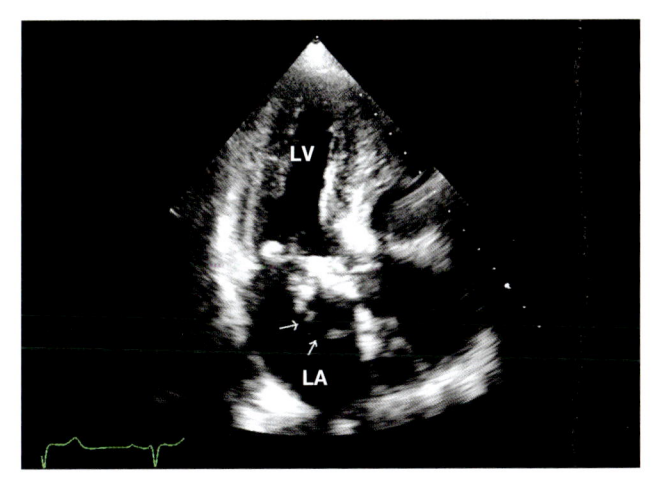

Figure 21.4

15. In patients with a second episode of infective endocarditis following successful treatment of the first episode, which clinical feature does not predict higher in-hospital mortality?
  A. Heart failure.
  B. Renal disease.
  C. Septic shock.
  D. Recurrence of infective endocarditis following successful treatment of the first episode.
  E. Cardiac surgery indicated but not performed.

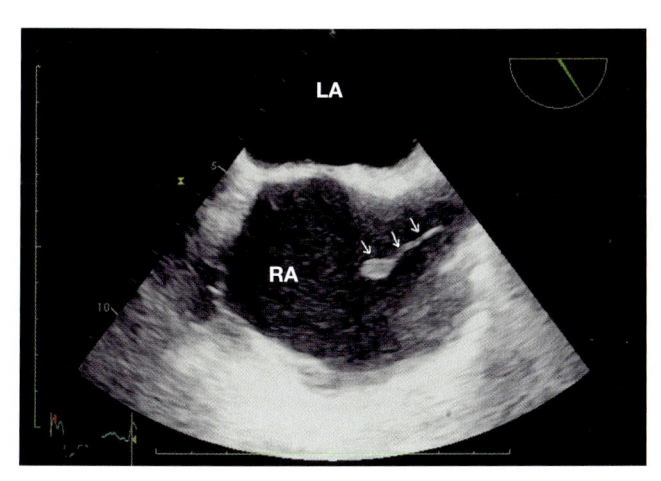

Figure 21.3

16. Which abnormality is the result of a satellite lesion in this patient with endocarditis (**Figure 21.5** and ▶ **Video 21.2**)?
  A. Aortic root abscess.
  B. Anterior mitral valve aneurysm.
  C. Aortic cusp perforation.
  D. Aorta to right ventricular outflow tract (RVOT) fistula.
  E. None of the above.

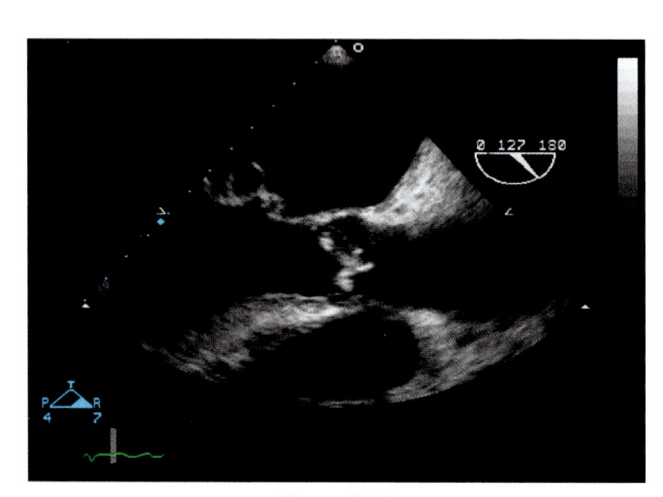

Figure 21.5

17. Based on the TEE image (**Figure 21.5** and ▶ **Video 21.2**), the vegetation on the aortic valve appears to affect more than one cusp. What is the best view to assess the extent of the lesion on the aortic valve?
  A. Short-axis view of the aortic valve (40°-60°).
  B. Short-axis view of the LVOT (40°-60°).
  C. Long-axis view of the LVOT and aortic valve (110°-140°).
  D. Five-chamber view of the LVOT and aortic valve (0°).
  E. Deep transgastric five-chamber view (0°).

18. Based on the TEE findings (**Figure 21.5** and ▶ **Video 21.2**), what is the prognosis of the patient?
  A. Low risk of embolic event, low risk of mortality, high likelihood to require valve replacement.
  B. High risk of embolic event, low risk of mortality, high likelihood to require valve replacement.
  C. High risk of embolic event, high risk of mortality, high likelihood to require valve replacement.
  D. High risk of embolic event, high risk of mortality, low likelihood to require valve replacement.

19. An 85-year-old man presented to the hospital with *Enterococcus faecalis* bacteremia, for which a TEE was performed (**Figure 21.6**, ▶ **Video 21.3**). What is the most frequent echocardiographic finding of infective endocarditis in a patient with this type of valve?
  A. Vegetation on prosthetic valve leaflets.
  B. Vegetation on stent frame.
  C. Vegetation on native mitral valve.
  D. New significant aortic regurgitation.
  E. Periannular complication.

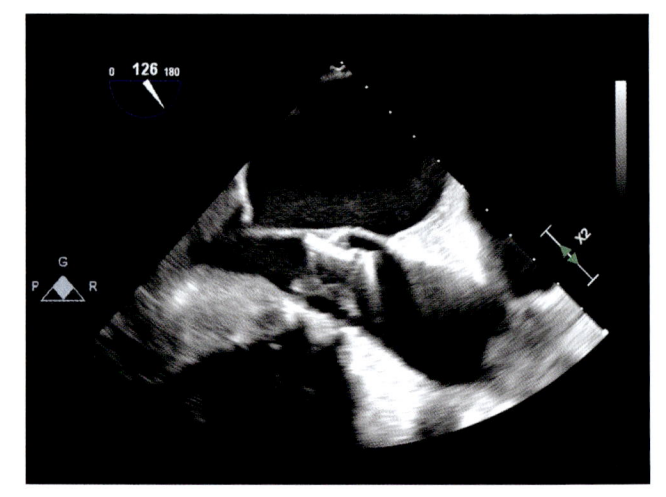

Figure 21.6

20. Which of the following is a risk factor for endocarditis following TAVR?
  A. Balloon-expandable TAVR.
  B. Balloon aortic valvuloplasty before TAVR.
  C. Older age.
  D. Moderate to severe residual aortic regurgitation post TAVR.
  E. None of the above.

21. A 65-year-old man presents with fever and transient loss of right eye vision. He has had a previous valve replacement. Four weeks ago, he had a dental extraction and received prophylactic antibiotic therapy. An echocardiogram is performed and shows vegetations on the aortic valve (**Figure 21.7** and ▶ **Video 21.4**). What type of prosthesis does the patient have?
   A. Aortic homograft.
   B. Aortic bioprosthesis.
   C. Aortic stentless prosthesis.
   D. Aortic mechanical prosthesis.
   E. None of the above.

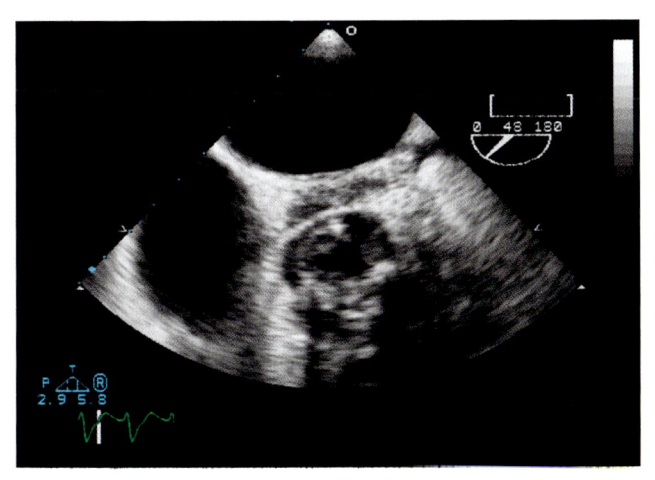

Figure 21.7

22. What is the other complication related to endocarditis, present in this patient (**Figure 21.7** and ▶ **Video 21.4**)?
   A. Aortic cusp rupture.
   B. Aortic root abscess.
   C. Aortic root pseudoaneurysm.
   D. Aortic root-LVOT fistula.
   E. None of the above.

23. Where is the aortic root pathology located (**Figure 21.7**)?
   A. Anterior and medial.
   B. Medial.
   C. Lateral.
   D. Posterior and lateral.
   E. None of the above.

24. In the same patient described in the previous question, color Doppler of the aortic prosthesis is performed (**Figure 21.8** and ▶ **Video 21.5**). What additional complication is present?
   A. Severe aortic regurgitation.
   B. Left main compression by the abscess.
   C. Aortic root to RVOT fistula.
   D. Sinus of Valsalva rupture.
   E. None of the above.

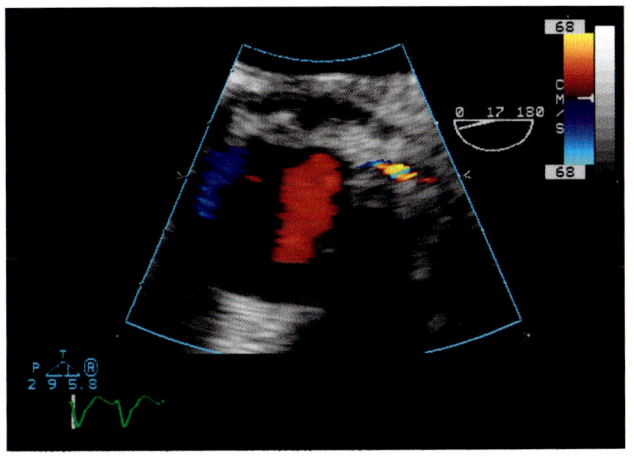

Figure 21.8

25. A patient presents with mitral valve endocarditis. He had been treated with antibiotics for 4 weeks. **Figure 21.9** shows a parasternal short-axis view of the mitral valve (▶ **Video 21.6**). What is the site of the attachment of the vegetation on the mitral valve?
   A. A1.
   B. A2.
   C. A3.
   D. P3.
   E. None of the above.

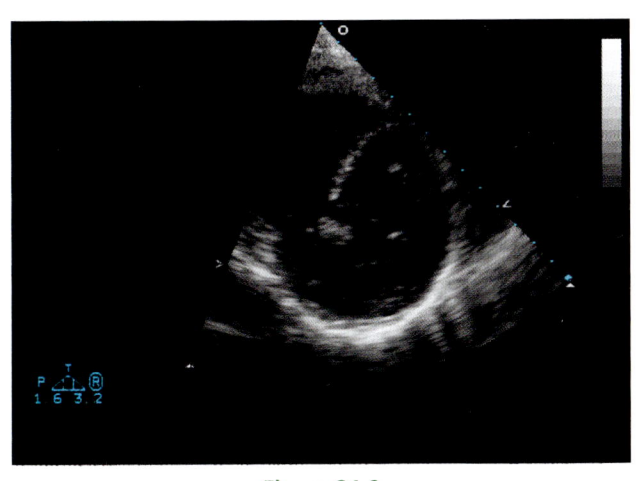

Figure 21.9

26. A patient with a previous mitral valve replacement is admitted for jaundice and shortness of breath. A zoomed apical four-chamber view is shown in **Figure 21.10** and ▶ **Video 21.7**. What is abnormal in the image shown?
   A. There is a large left atrial mass.
   B. There is dehiscence of the prosthesis.
   C. There is a fistula between the LA and aorta.
   D. There is no abnormality.
   E. None of the above.

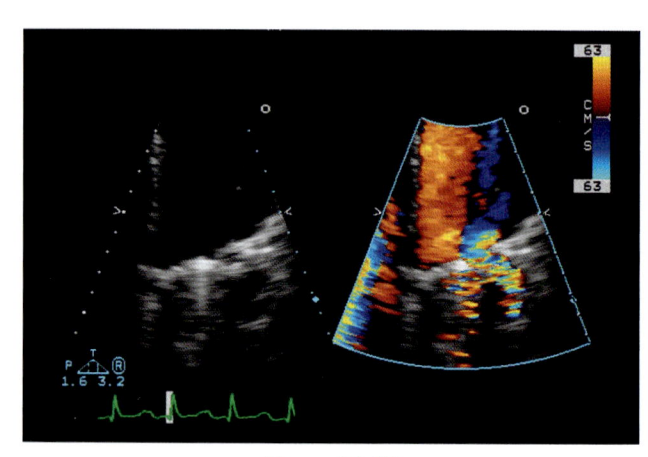

Figure 21.10

27. What findings would be expected for the peak and mean gradients in this patient?
   A. They would both be normal for the type and size of valve prosthesis.
   B. They would both be increased to a similar degree.
   C. They would both be decreased to a similar degree.
   D. The peak gradient would be increased more than the mean gradient.
   E. None of the above.

28. A patient with a previous aortic valve replacement is admitted for increased dyspnea. A TEE is performed, and the long-axis view of the LVOT is shown in ▶ **Video 21.8**. The primary abnormality seen in this image is:
   A. Dehiscence of the aortic prosthesis.
   B. Severe mitral regurgitation.
   C. Flail prosthetic leaflet.
   D. Severe aortic stenosis.
   E. None of the above.

29. What other lesion is also present in ▶ **Video 21.8**?
   A. Abscess of the aortic root.
   B. Pseudoaneurysm of the aortic root.
   C. Localized aortic dissection.
   D. No other lesion is noted.
   E. None of the above.

30. Demonstration of this finding on the parasternal long-axis view of the corresponding echocardiogram shown in ▶ **Video 21.9**, implies involvement of what percentage of the annular circumference?
   A. 5% to 10%
   B. 10% to 20%
   C. 20% to 40%
   D. 40% to 95%
   E. None of the above.

31. A 28-year-old woman with tetralogy of Fallot repaired as a neonate underwent transcatheter pulmonary valve implantation with a Melody valve 18 months ago. She presents with fever for 10 days. An echocardiogram shows a peak RVOT gradient of 60 mm Hg, but no vegetation is detected. **Figure 21.11A** demonstrates a parasternal short-axis view of the Melody valve, and **Figure 21.11B** is the continuous wave Doppler signal through the Melody valve. Which of the following is **CORRECT**?
   A. The risk of endocarditis diminishes after the first year of implantation.
   B. Endocarditis is unlikely given the negative echocardiogram.
   C. The outcome is worse when there is RVOT obstruction.
   D. Reintervention is seldom necessary.
   E. None of the above.

Chapter 21 Endocarditis / 439

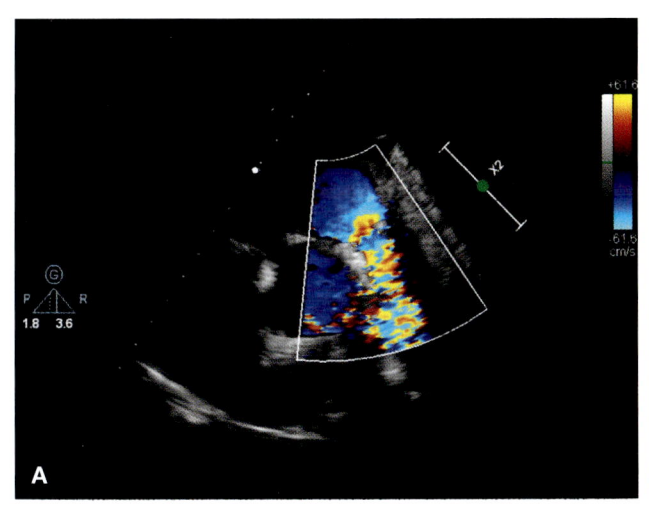

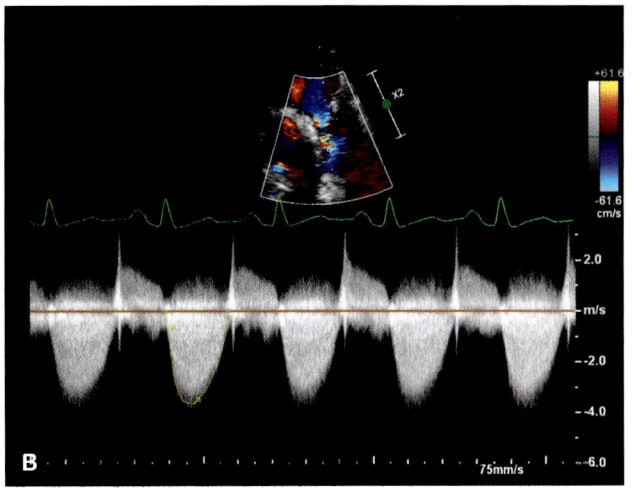

Figure 21.11

32. A 65-year-old man has been treated with 4 weeks of antibiotics for endocarditis in the aortic position. A repeat TEE was performed prior to discontinuation of antibiotics. Based on the images shown in **Figure 21.12A,B** and ▶ **Video 21.10A,B**, which of the following is true about the mitral valve?
   A. There are two long vegetations on the posterior mitral valve leaflet.
   B. There is a mitral valve aneurysm on the posterior mitral valve leaflet.
   C. There is a fistula between the LV and LA.
   D. There is a rupture of the mitral papillary muscle.
   E. None of the above.

CASE 1

A 75-year-old man presents with progressive shortness of breath and fever. On physical examination, a systolic and a diastolic murmur are present. ▶ *Video 21.11A,B (with and without color-flow imaging) show a midesophageal three-chamber view (120°) of the aortic valve. Color-flow imaging of the aortic valve in short axis is shown in* ▶ *Video 21.11C.*

33. Which of the following statements about the aortic valve is **CORRECT** regarding the patient in **Case 1** (▶ **Video 21.11**)?
   A. There are vegetations on the right coronary cusp (RCC) and noncoronary cusp (NCC) of the aortic valve. There is severe prolapse of the RCC.
   B. There is a perforation of the RCC of the aortic valve.
   C. There are vegetations on the RCC and NCC of the aortic valve. There is severe prolapse of the RCC and a perforation of the NCC.
   D. There is prolapse of the NCC of the aortic valve.
   E. None of the above.

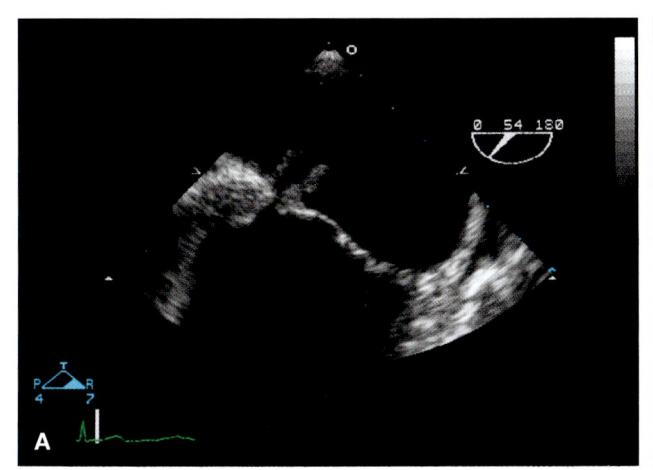

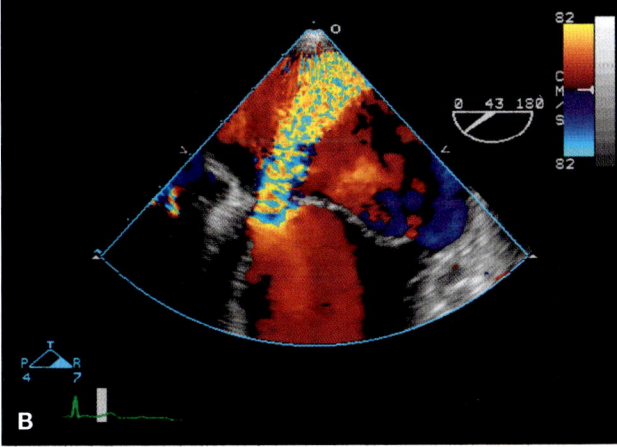

Figure 21.12

34. In addition to aortic regurgitation, what is the other finding on the color-flow imaging of the short-axis view of the aortic valve for the patient in **Case 1**?
   A. A fistula between the left sinus of Valsalva and LA.
   B. A fistula between the right sinus of Valsalva and RA.
   C. A fistula between the left sinus of Valsalva and RA.
   D. A fistula between the right sinus of Valsalva and LA.
   E. A fistula between the left sinus of Valsalva and RV.

35. Which of the following statements regarding the aortic regurgitation is **CORRECT**?
   A. There is severe aortic regurgitation.
   B. There is moderate aortic regurgitation.
   C. There is mild aortic regurgitation.

CASE 2

A 27-year-old man with a history of active intravenous drug use presented to hospital with fevers and malaise and was found to have S. aureus *bacteremia. A transthoracic echocardiogram was performed.* **Figure 21.13A** *and* **Video 21.12A** *show a large bulky vegetation attached to the anterior tricuspid valve leaflet in the right ventricular inflow view.* **Figure 21.13B** *and* **Video 21.12B** *show the same vegetation in a modified apical view.*

36. According to established guidelines, which of the following is an indication for surgery for the patient in **Case 2**?
   A. Vegetation 15 mm in length with high mobility.
   B. Tricuspid valve vegetation greater than 20 mm in length with recurrent septic pulmonary emboli despite appropriate antibiotic therapy.
   C. Severe valvular regurgitation in absence of heart failure symptoms.
   D. Methicillin-sensitive *Staphylococcus aureus* as the infecting organism.
   E. None of the above.

37. The patient from **Case 2** is discussed on Heart Team rounds, and it is felt that he may be a good candidate for transcatheter vacuum-assisted aspiration (AngioVac) as a bridge to valve replacement surgery. Which statement is **TRUE** of this procedure?
   A. The degree of tricuspid regurgitation is likely to decrease postprocedurally.
   B. The primary indication is to debulk the vegetation.
   C. There is a low probability of procedural success.
   D. It will obviate his need for surgical valve replacement.
   E. None of the above.

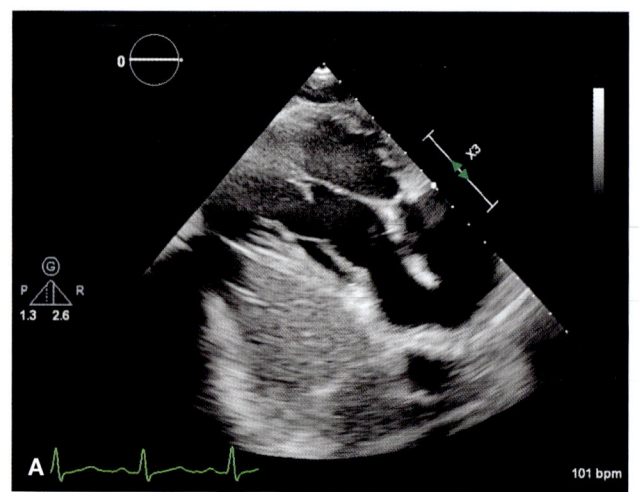

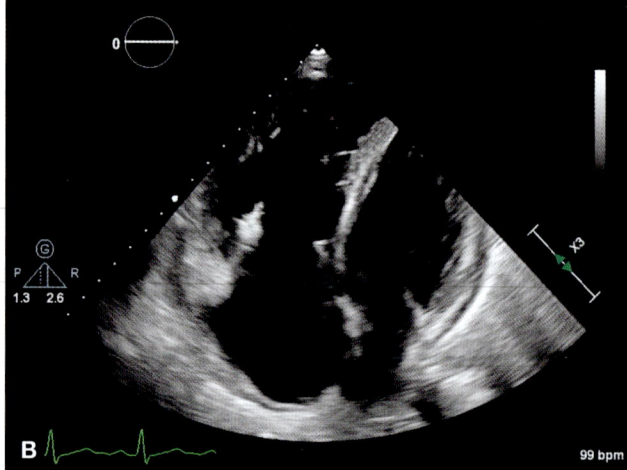

Figure 21.13

38. Which of the following features is **TRUE** of right-sided endocarditis?
A. Lower in-hospital mortality compared to patients with left-sided endocarditis.
B. Pulmonic and tricuspid valves are equally affected.
C. Higher rate of perivalvular abscess.
D. Viridans streptococci are the dominant infecting organism.
E. None of the above.

CASE 3

A 42-year-old man has been treated as an outpatient for pneumonia. After 3 days of antibiotics, he remains febrile and becomes progressively weaker. At presentation to the hospital, the patient appears toxic. A systolic murmur is present on physical examination. Two sets of blood cultures are positive for gram-positive cocci. A TTE and TEE are performed. ▶ *Video 21.13A,B show a midesophageal 65° view of the mitral valve and the same view with color-flow imaging, respectively.* ▶ *Video 21.13C shows a midesophageal four-chamber view.*

39. What lesion is being illustrated in ▶ Video 21.13A,B for the patient in **Case 3**?
A. There is a vegetation on the anterior mitral leaflet.
B. There is an aneurysm on the anterior mitral leaflet, which is perforated.
C. There is a vegetation on the posterior mitral valve leaflet.
D. There is an aneurysm on the posterior mitral valve leaflet, which is perforated.
E. None of the above.

40. What other lesion is shown in ▶ Video 21.13C for the patient in **Case 3**?
A. There is a mural thrombus attached to the lateral wall.
B. There is a mural vegetation attached to the lateral wall.
C. There is an abscess attached to the lateral wall.
D. There is a mural vegetation attached to the posterior wall.
E. None of the above.

CASE 4

A 65-year-old woman presents with progressive shortness of breath. Four weeks ago, she was diagnosed with endocarditis and is being treated with antibiotics. ▶ *Video 21.14A,B represent TTE parasternal long-axis views of the mitral valve and the same view with color-flow imaging, respectively.* ▶ *Video 21.14C illustrates TTE parasternal short-axis view of the mitral valve with color-flow imaging.*

41. Which of the following statements is **TRUE** about the mitral valve of the patient in **Case 4** (▶ Video 21.14)?
A. A vegetation is present on the mitral valve.
B. There is an anterior mitral leaflet perforation associated with significant mitral regurgitation.
C. There is mitral valve prolapse.
D. There is a cleft of the anterior mitral leaflet with significant mitral regurgitation.
E. None of the above.

42. You review the images from **Case 4** with a cardiac surgeon who asks you where the origin of the mitral regurgitant jet is located.
A. The regurgitant jet is located at P1.
B. The regurgitant jet is located at A1.
C. The regurgitant jet is located at A2.
D. The regurgitant jet is located at the junction of P2 and P1.
E. None of the above.

CASE 5

A 68-year-old man with a history of atrial fibrillation, nonischemic cardiomyopathy, and subsequent CRT-P implantation presents with 2 weeks of constitutional symptoms. Blood cultures showed methicillin-sensitive Staphylococcus aureus *(MSSA) in multiple bottles. A transthoracic echocardiogram was performed showing no vegetations.*

43. What is the next best step for the patient in **Case 5**?
A. A search for an alternate source of infection, as endocarditis has been ruled out.
B. TEE.
C. Repeat TTE.
D. 18F-fluorodeoxyglucose positron emission tomography (18F-FDG PET).
E. Cardiac CT.

44. A TEE was performed for the patient in **Case 5**. **Figure 21.14** and ▶ **Video 21.15** demonstrate biplane midesophageal views. What is the mass, and where is its attachment?
    A. Thrombus on right atrial lead.
    B. Fibrin strand on coronary sinus lead.
    C. Invagination of pericardial fat into the right atrium.
    D. Vegetation on the right ventricular lead adjacent to the anteroseptal commissure.
    E. Vegetation on coronary sinus lead adjacent to the posteroseptal commissure.

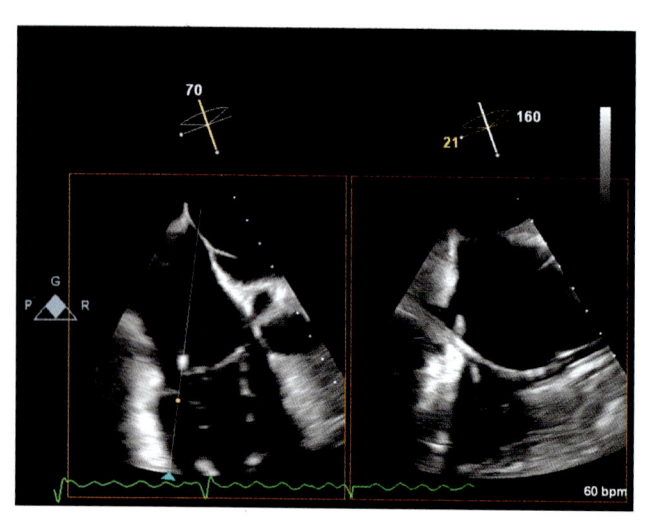

Figure 21.14

45. What is the most appropriate treatment for the mass of the patient in **Case 5** to ensure adequate eradication of the infection?
    A. Antibiotic treatment for 6 weeks.
    B. Antibiotic treatment and removal of pacemaker pulse generator and leads only if 18F-FDG PET/CT is positive.
    C. Antibiotic treatment and removal of pacemaker pulse generator and leads only if TEE shows vegetation present on the endocardial leads.
    D. Antibiotic treatment and removal of pacemaker pulse generator and leads.
    E. None of the above.

CASE 6

A 67-year-old man with a history of endocarditis was successfully treated with antibiotic therapy 6 months ago. He has no known complications related to endocarditis. His family physician orders a routine echocardiogram for follow-up. TTE shows severe mitral regurgitation. A TEE is then performed. See ▶ **Video 21.16A,B** *and* **Figure 21.15**.

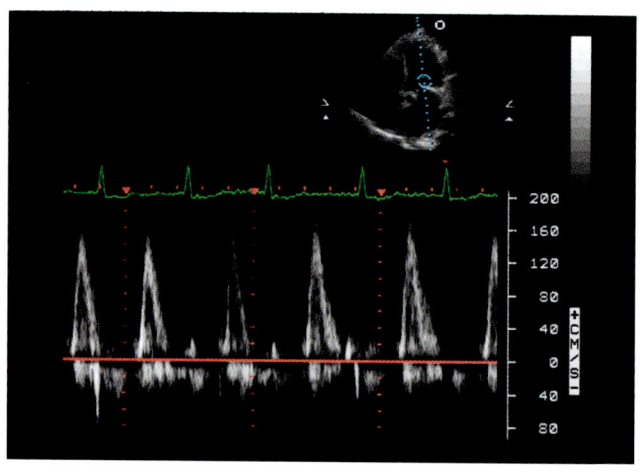

Figure 21.15

46. What is the abnormality of the mitral valve of the patient in **Case 6**?
    A. A calcified vegetation on the posterior mitral valve leaflet with valve disruption, leading to a coaptation defect.
    B. A fistula of the posterior mitral valve annulus between the LV and LA.
    C. An abscess of the posterior mitral valve annulus with a posterior mitral valve perforation.
    D. A ruptured chordae with flail of the posterior mitral leaflet.
    E. None of the above.

47. Pulsed wave Doppler tracing of the pulmonary veins do not show systolic flow reversal for the patient in **Case 6**. The E velocity of mitral valve inflow is illustrated in **Figure 21.15**. Based on these images, how would you grade the mitral regurgitation?
    A. Mild mitral regurgitation.
    B. Mild to moderate mitral regurgitation.
    C. Moderate mitral regurgitation.
    D. Severe mitral regurgitation.
    E. None of the above.

48. The absence of the systolic flow reversal in the pulmonary veins despite the presence of severe mitral regurgitation is least likely explained by which of the following?
   A. High left atrial compliance.
   B. Inadequate sampling of the pulmonary veins.
   C. Severe enlargement of the left atrium.
   D. Low left atrial compliance.
   E. None of the above.

CASE 7

A 24-year-old woman with a history of intravenous drug abuse presents with fever, fatigue, and shortness of breath. Two sets of blood cultures are positive for gram-positive cocci within 24 hours. A chest radiograph shows multiple small infiltrates in both lungs, highly suggestive of septic emboli. An initial TTE revealed two echogenic masses; one is on the tricuspid valve and the other is ill-defined and is in the LA. A TEE is then performed. See ▶ Video 21.17A–D.

49. For the patient in **Case 7**, what is the involvement on the tricuspid valve?
   A. There are vegetations on the anterior and posterior leaflets of the tricuspid valve.
   B. There are vegetations on the anterior and septal leaflets of the tricuspid valve.
   C. There are vegetations on all three tricuspid leaflets.
   D. There is an annular abscess.
   E. None of the above.

50. How severe is the tricuspid regurgitation for the patient in **Case 7**?
   A. Mild tricuspid regurgitation.
   B. Moderate tricuspid regurgitation.
   C. Severe tricuspid regurgitation.
   D. None of the above.

51. There is a large mobile left atrial mass attached to the posterior left atrial wall. This mass is likely?
   A. A vegetation.
   B. A thrombus.
   C. An angiosarcoma.
   D. A myxoma.
   E. None of the above.

CASE 8

A 22-year-old man with a history of injection drug use presents with fever, severe dyspnea, and hypotension. An urgent TEE is performed (Figure 21.16A,B and ▶ Video 21.18A,B). The cardiac surgeon schedules him for an emergency aortic valve and ascending aorta replacement (Bentall procedure).

52. Based on the TEE findings of the patient in **Case 8** (Figure 21.16, ▶ Video 21.18), in addition to the planned Bentall procedure, what is your advice to the surgeon about the surgery?
   A. Perform mitral valve repair.
   B. Perform mitral valve replacement.
   C. Perform coronary angiogram to exclude left coronary artery involvement.
   D. A and C.
   E. None of the above.

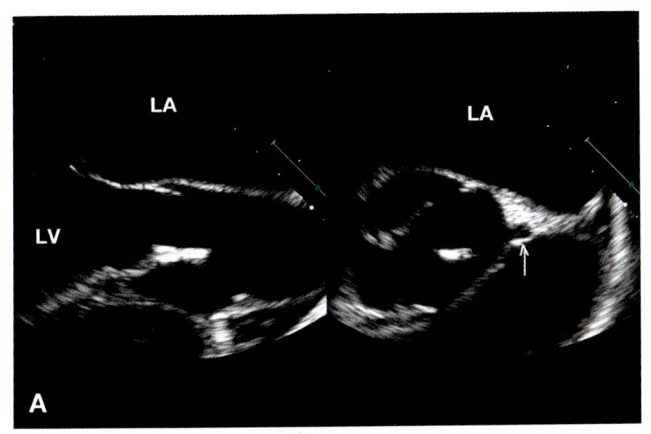

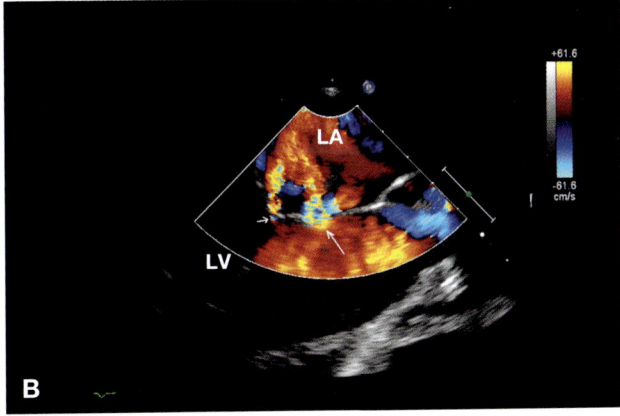

Figure 21.16

53. Which of the following statements is **TRUE** regarding the valvular complication seen in the patient in **Case 8**?
  A. It is usually associated with a specific bacteriologic profile.
  B. It is more common in injection drug users.
  C. It is associated with a higher in-hospital mortality.
  D. It is associated with less severe valvular regurgitation.
  E. None of the above.

CASE 9

A 65-year-old woman with cirrhosis, type 1 diabetes mellitus, and hypertension presented to the emergency department with left leg cellulitis. She was found to have methicillin-sensitive Staphylococcus aureus *bacteremia and underwent transesophageal echocardiogram (TEE), which demonstrated a highly mobile echodense mass on the closing margin of the P1 scallop of the mitral valve* (**Figure 21.17A** *and* ▶ *Video 21.19A), as well as a fixed, echodense mass at the base of the A3 scallop* (**Figure 21.17B** *and* ▶ *Video 21.19B). Both masses are demonstrated on a 3D rendering of the mitral valve viewed from the left atrium* (**Figure 21.17C** *and* ▶ *Video 21.19C).*

54. Based on **Case 9**, what is the definition of a typical vegetation during the acute phase of endocarditis?
  A. A discrete echolucent mass adherent to native valves or intracardiac prosthetic devices with high-frequency motion independent of the underlying cardiac structure. The mass cannot be imaged in multiple views throughout the cardiac cycle.
  B. A discrete echogenic dense mass adherent to native valves or intracardiac prosthetic devices with high-frequency motion independent of the underlying cardiac structure. The mass cannot be imaged in multiple views throughout the cardiac cycle.
  C. A discrete echogenic mass adherent to the native valves or intracardiac prosthetic devices with high-frequency motion related to the underlying cardiac structure. The mass can be imaged in multiple views throughout the cardiac cycle.
  D. A discrete echogenic mass adherent to the native valves or intracardiac prosthetic devices with high-frequency motion independent of the underlying cardiac structure. The mass can be imaged in multiple views throughout the cardiac cycle.
  E. None of the above.

55. The patient from **Case 9** was admitted to hospital with continuous cardiac rhythm monitoring. She was treated with intravenous cloxacillin. She defervesced after 4 days, and subsequent blood cultures were negative for growth. She did not have heart failure. On the seventh day of admission, she was noted to have a new first-degree AV block. What is the appropriate next step?
  A. TTE.
  B. TEE.
  C. 18F-FDG PET.
  D. Ongoing observation alone.
  E. None of the above.

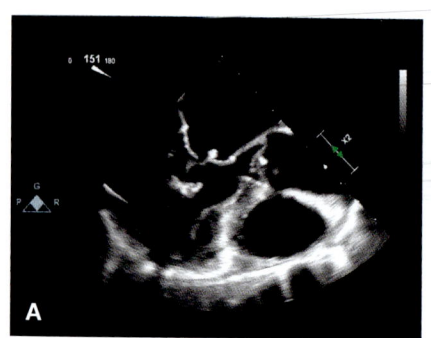

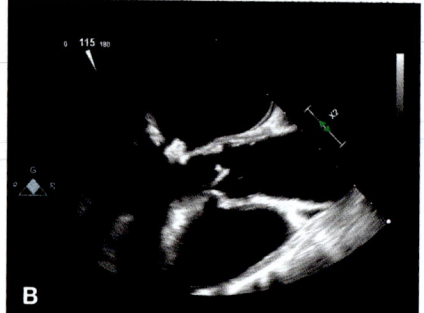

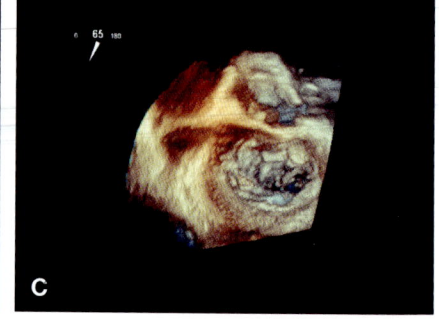

Figure 21.17

Chapter 21 Endocarditis / 445

56. A repeat TEE was performed for the patient in **Case 9**. The previously visualized fixed echodense mass on the base of the A3 scallop now demonstrated superimposed mobile fronds (**Figure 21.18**, ▶ Video 21.20). Particular attention was paid to rule out perivalvular extension from this mass on A3. Of the following, which view on TEE best visualizes the area where such an abscess may extend into the anatomic region containing the AV node?
   A. Midesophageal long-axis view at 120° to 140°.
   B. Midesophageal mitral commissural view at 50° to 70°.
   C. Transgastric two-chamber view mitral valve at 90° to 110°.
   D. Transgastric long-axis view of aortic root at 100° to 120°.
   E. None of the above.

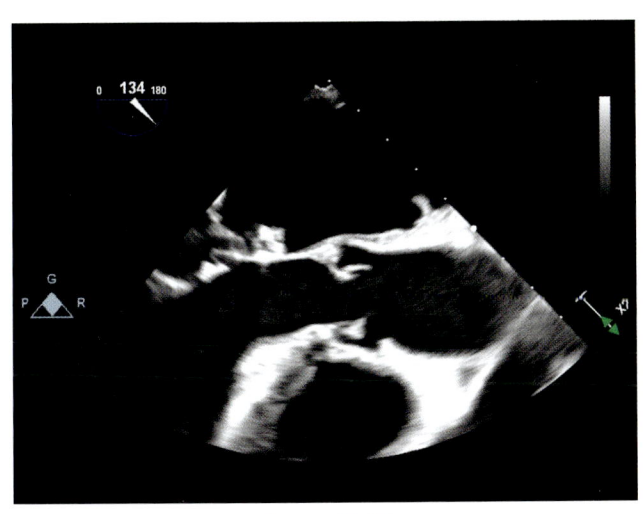

Figure 21.18

CASE 10

*A 32-year-old injection drug user without previously known cardiovascular disease is diagnosed with definite IE (**Figure 21.19**, ▶ Video 21.21A,B).*

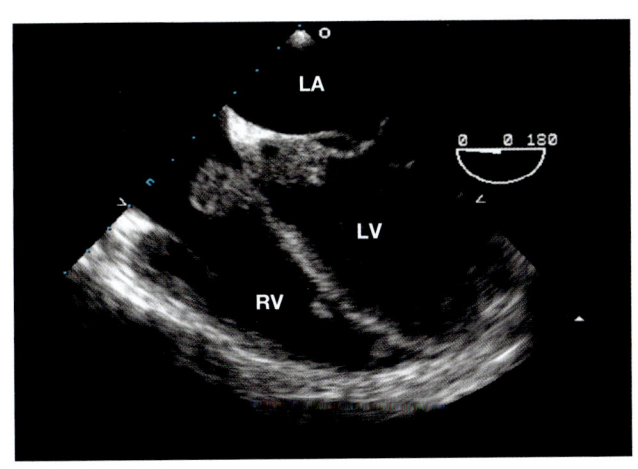

Figure 21.19

57. What is the most likely explanation for the TEE findings of the patient in **Case 10**?
   A. An atrial septal defect with left-to-right shunt and a vegetation on the atrial aspect of the tricuspid valve.
   B. A Gerbode-type shunt with a vegetation on the ventricular side of the septal tricuspid leaflet.
   C. A Gerbode-type shunt with vegetations on both the tricuspid and mitral valves.
   D. An RV-to-LA shunt with vegetations on both the tricuspid and mitral valves.

58. The patient in the previous question undergoes a cardiac catheterization with blood sampling from multiple sites. A mixed venous oxygen saturation sample from the inferior vena cava is 69%. What is the most plausible venous oxygen saturation value in the right atrium?
   A. 69%.
   B. 80%.
   C. 55%.
   D. 100%.
   E. None of the above.

ANSWERS

1. **Answer: E.** Multiplane TEE has been reported as a highly diagnostic tool with a negative predictive value varying from 87% to 98% in IE, depending on the clinical setting and the criteria used to define IE (native valve vs prosthetic valve, modified Duke criteria vs pathologic confirmation). The negative predictive value of TEE can be further increased if a repeat TEE 7 to 10 days later remains negative.

2. **Answer: C.** TEE detects vegetation(s) in about a third of all patients with *Staphylococcus aureus* bacteremia. In patients with insufficient criteria for IE based on the Duke criteria, which include the TTE findings, 15% of the patients will be reclassified to have possible or definite IE following TEE.

3. **Answer: C.** On echocardiography, an abscess is identified as a localized abnormal thickening of the perivalvular tissue or echolucent space within the

perivalvular tissue that does not communicate with surrounding cardiac chambers. It is predominantly located at the aortic root and aortomitral intervalvular fibrosa. Myocardial abscesses are associated with very high mortality. The development of heart block in this setting is an indication of abscess formation involving the ventricular septum. A pericardial abscess usually represents a fistula formation between an annular abscess and the pericardial space.

4. **Answer: C.** Abnormal thickness of the aortic wall of >10 mm is suspicious for an aortic root abscess in native aortic valve endocarditis. If present, serial echocardiograms can follow the evolution of this thickening and identify formation of an echolucent space over time. This criterion cannot be used in patients with recent aortic valve or aortic root replacement, as postoperative inflammation can contribute to thickening of the aortic wall. Prosthetic valvular thrombosis and pannus formation can be differentiated from an abscess by their predilection to involve the sewing ring encroaching onto the prosthetic orifice instead of the surrounding annulus. A pseudoaneurysm can be recognized by the presence of an echolucent cavity that communicates with a single neighboring cardiac chamber.

5. **Answer: C.** Vegetations evolve during successful antibiotic treatment. Reduction in vegetation size and increase in density are common. Persistence of vegetations alone does not predict a worse outcome. The lack of regression of vegetation size after 4 to 6 weeks of antibiotic therapy is associated with an increased risk of mortality and complications related to endocarditis. However, this occurs only in patients with progressive valve disruption and dysfunction. In contrast, in patients with endocarditis but without significant valve dysfunction, the mortality and morbidity rate is not increased despite the lack of reduction in the vegetation size.

6. **Answer: A.** After healing from endocarditis, <10% of affected valves regain their normal structure. The majority of affected valves show nodular changes, thickening, or disruption of the leaflets after healing. No reliable predictors for complete healing have been identified.

7. **Answer: B.** A mitral valve aneurysm is characterized by a localized bulging of the mitral leaflet toward the left atrium, with systolic expansion and diastolic collapse (**Figure 21.5** and ▶ **Video 21.2**). Mitral valve aneurysms are usually due to endocarditis. Surgical repair is frequently indicated because of the concomitant presence of perforation involving the aneurysm resulting in significant mitral regurgitation (▶ **Video 21.22**.)

8. **Answer: A.** According to the Appropriate Use Guidelines, TEE is indicated when there is a moderate to high pretest probability of IE such as is the case with a prosthetic heart valve, fungemia, or *Staphylococcus aureus* bacteremia. Despite a negative TTE for IE, about 15% of patients with *S. aureus* bacteremia are diagnosed to have possible or definite IE based on TEE findings. In patients with mechanical heart valves, a false-negative TTE is common and it is reasonable to perform TEE to exclude IE. TEE is inappropriate when the pretest probability is low such as transient fever, a known alternative source of infection, and negative blood culture or positive blood culture with an atypical pathogen for IE such as *Escherichia coli*. **Figure 21.20** shows an algorithm proposed by the ACC/AHA 2020 Valve Guidelines outlining when to consider TEE and other cardiac imaging modalities.

9. **Answer: E.** There is a wide spectrum of cardiac manifestations of APLA syndrome, ranging from valvular abnormalities to pulmonary hypertension. Large valvular masses can be detected in 10% to 40% of patients and may be difficult to differentiate from infective vegetations in patients with IE. The valvular masses in APLA syndrome can be mobile, pedunculated, or immobile and broad based in the setting of leaflet thickening. They may have heterogeneous echogenicity and often can present as multiple lesions (kissing vegetations) at any location on the leaflets (base to tip). However, tissue destruction is usually absent with APLA syndrome and when present should raise the suspicion for IE.

10. **Answer: C.** According to the current guidelines, patients with IE should undergo early surgery if there is valve dysfunction associated with heart failure; if there is a left-sided IE caused by a resistant organism, including *Staphylococcus aureus* and fungal organisms; or if periannular complications such as abscesses are present. An early surgery should also be performed if persistent signs of bacteremia are present following 5 to 7 days of targeted antimicrobial therapy, and in patients with recurrent embolic events and persistent vegetations. This patient does not meet any of these indications for surgery. However, the Early Surgery versus Conventional Treatment for Infective Endocarditis (EASE) trial, published in 2012, suggested that patients with a vegetation >10 mm and severe valvular disease benefited from early surgery, which was associated with a reduced risk of embolic events, although mortality was not reduced. This indication receives a 2b recommendation in the 2020 ACC/AHA Guidelines. Early surgery within 48 hours of diagnosis may be considered in this patient.

11. **Answer: D.** The TEE view shows a vegetation (arrow) at the orifice of the coronary sinus. Isolated coronary sinus IE is a rare occurrence that has not been reported in structurally normal hearts without prosthetic devices. The presence of a coronary sinus lead is associated with the development of a coronary

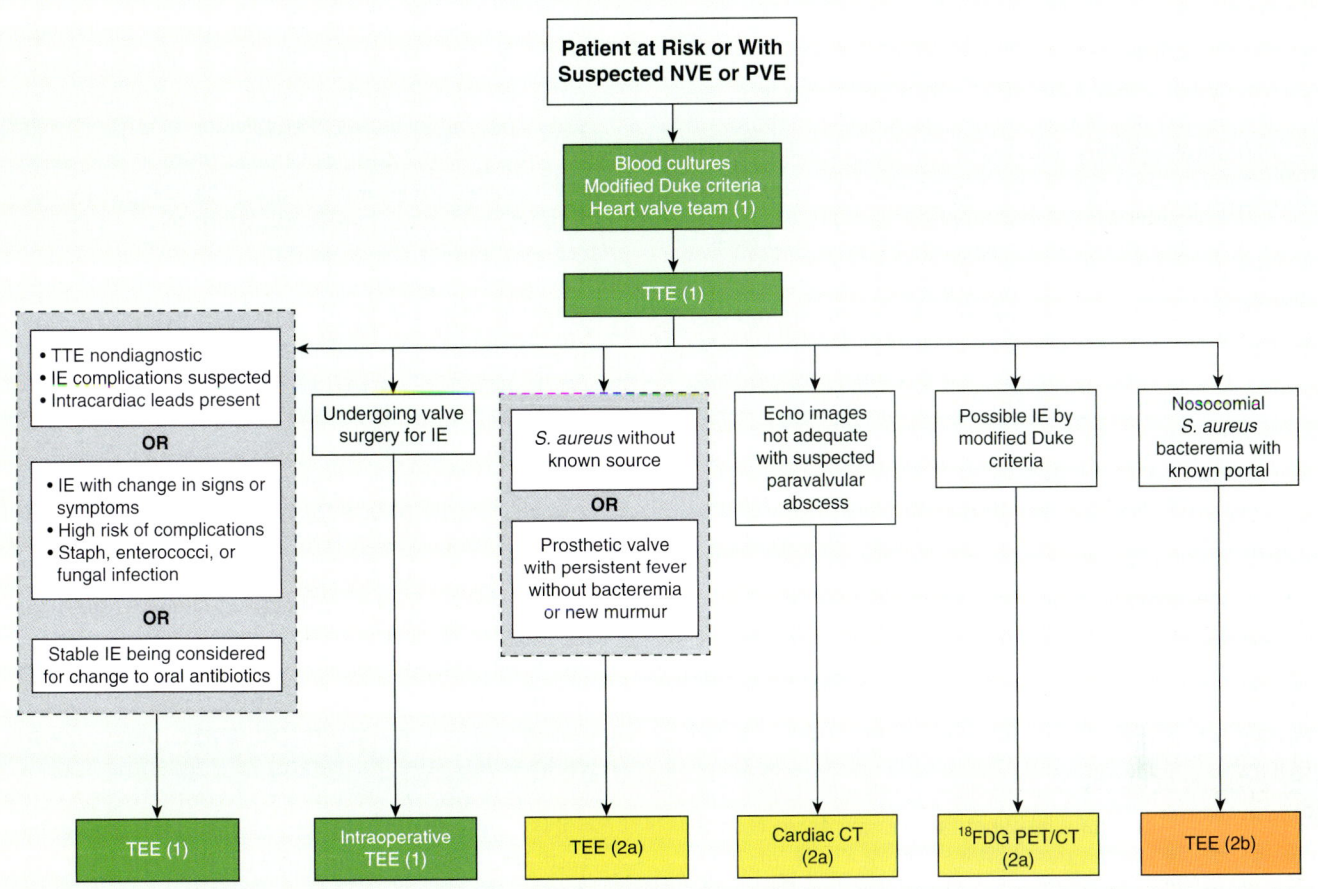

```
                    ┌─────────────────────────┐
                    │  Patient at Risk or With│
                    │  Suspected NVE or PVE   │
                    └───────────┬─────────────┘
                                │
                    ┌───────────▼─────────────┐
                    │  Blood cultures         │
                    │  Modified Duke criteria │
                    │  Heart valve team (1)   │
                    └───────────┬─────────────┘
                                │
                            ┌───▼───┐
                            │TTE (1)│
                            └───┬───┘
```

Figure 21.20. NVE, native valve endocarditis; PVE, prosthetic valve endocarditis. (Reprinted with permission from Otto CM, Nishimura RA, Bonow RO, et al. 2020 ACC/AHA guideline for the management of patients with valvular heart disease: executive summary—a report of the American College of Cardiology/American Heart Association Joint Committee on Clinical Practice Guidelines. *Circulation.* 2021;143(5):e72-e227. Copyright © 2020 by the American College of Cardiology Foundation and the American Heart Association, Inc.)

sinus vegetation. Coronary sinus vegetations have also been reported in patients with tunneled hemodialysis catheters or congenital coronary artery fistulas to the coronary sinus, but not in patients with persistent left superior vena cava.

12. **Answer: A.** Behçet disease is a vasculitis affecting multiple organ systems. Cardiac involvement is rare, and pericarditis is the most common finding. Other manifestations include valvular insufficiency (mostly aortic), myocardial infarction, and endomyocardial fibrosis. Intracardiac thrombi account for 19% of cardiac involvement in Behçet disease, always in the right-sided cavities. Right atrial thrombus extends into the vena cava in 40% of cases. Renal cell carcinoma involves the right cardiac chambers by extension via the inferior vena cava. In this patient, the large mobile mass (arrows) is attached to the lateral wall of the right atrium. Cardiac tumors are not features of cardiac involvement in Behçet disease. IE is rare in Behçet disease and would be less likely than a thrombus in this context.

13. **Answer: B.** A "ghost" is a tubular, mobile mass in the path of an intracardiac lead following lead extraction. It seldom occurs following lead extraction for a noninfective reason. It is believed to consist of fibrous sheaths mixed with vegetations in most cases. Ghosts have been reported in 8% to 19% of all patients following lead removal. The incidence rises to 16% in the setting of cardiac device–related IE, but only 5% if there is only local device pocket infection. Cardiac device–related IE and positive lead cultures, but not positive blood cultures, have been reported to be associated with the presence of a ghost after lead removal. Prospective data suggest an independent association between the presence of ghosts and mortality following lead removal.

A vegetation is an oscillating intracardiac mass usually attached to a cardiac valve. It may be pedunculated or sessile. Benign cardiac tumors do not arise from an implanted lead. Thrombus can develop on an intracardiac lead, but it is usually dislodged and embolized upon removal of the lead and unlikely to stay in situ.

14. **Answer: B.** This patient has a pseudoaneurysm of the intervalvular fibrosa, which communicates with the left ventricular outflow tract and protrudes into the left atrium. This is a known long-term complication of an aortic annular abscess, which this patient had 1 year ago. Annular abscess is much more common

in aortic valve IE than in mitral valve IE. Rupture of the pseudoaneurysm is rare, and thus urgent surgery is not indicated. The patient needs to be followed for worsening aortic valvular function and progressive enlargement of the pseudoaneurysm.

15. **Answer: D.** In a large international registry of IE, the incidence of recurrence was about 8.6%. Among patients with recurrent IE, about one in five (21%) were relapsed (defined as recurrence within 6 months of a previous episode) and the remainder (79%) were reinfection (recurrence >6 months after a previous episode). Recurrent IE was not found to be a risk factor for in-hospital death and showed similar in-hospital and long-term mortality in comparison with first-episode IE. On the other hand, occurrence of complications (eg, heart failure, renal failure, septic shock) at admission and while on therapy and failure to undertake surgery when indicated were independent predictors of in-hospital mortality in this population.

16. **Answer: B.** Aortic valve endocarditis usually leads to valve disruption and aortic regurgitation. The regurgitant jet can either be directed anteriorly against the septum or posteriorly against the anterior mitral valve leaflet. If aortic regurgitation is directed posteriorly, a satellite vegetation may form on the anterior mitral valve leaflet. This localized infection destroys the endothelium and fibrosa of the valve. If the infection is not controlled, aneurysm (diverticulum) formation and perforation of the anterior mitral leaflet may ensue, as demonstrated in **Figure 21.5** and ▶ **Video 21.23**.

17. **Answer: A.** On TEE, the short-axis view of the aortic valve allows the best visualization of the location of a vegetation on its three cusps. This view provides a 360-degree spatial orientation of the aortic root and aortic valve leaflet from the aspect of the aorta. To better assess the LVOT aspect of the aortic valve, real-time three-dimensional imaging may be very helpful.

18. **Answer: C.** The patient has double valve lesions, multiple mobile aortic vegetations, and severe aortic valve disruption with severe aortic regurgitation. These findings suggest a high risk of embolic events, a strong indication for surgical intervention, and a poor outcome.

19. **Answer: A.** The valve demonstrated in this case is a transcatheter aortic valve replacement (TAVR). The incidence of early endocarditis following TAVR is 0.3 to 2.0 per 100 patient-years and is similar to that of surgical aortic valve replacement (SAVR) and increases according to baseline surgical risk. The combined sensitivity of TTE and TEE for diagnosing endocarditis is 68%, in contrast to 73% in patients with prosthetic endocarditis of surgically implanted valves and 90% in native valve endocarditis. Vegetations located on the TAVR valve leaflets are the most common finding in both balloon-expandable and self-expandable valves. Vegetations anchored to the stent frame are generally less common but occur more frequently in self-expandable valves. Perivalvular extension with or without significant valve regurgitation and satellite involvement of the mitral valve are less common findings but nevertheless important to consider in a comprehensive TEE evaluation.

20. **Answer: D.** Procedural risk factors for IE following TAVR include moderate or severe residual aortic regurgitation, low TAVR placement, lack of balloon aortic valvuloplasty before TAVR, an elevated residual gradient, valve-in-valve TAVR, and vascular or bleeding complications. Patient-related risk factors include younger age, male sex, presence of chronic kidney disease, prior endocarditis before TAVR, and elevated BMI.

21. **Answer: B.** The detection of biologic leaflets excludes a mechanical prosthesis. Because of the presence of struts (stents), it is a bioprosthesis. A homograft or stentless prosthesis does not have struts on its sewing ring.

22. **Answer: B.** In the setting of aortic bioprosthesis endocarditis, the thickening of the aortic root is highly suggestive of an aortic root abscess. The thickening seems to have several ill-defined echolucent areas that further support this diagnosis.

23. **Answer: D.** The abscess is located posteriorly as it is close to the LA and laterally as it is away from the interatrial septum. The anterior aspect of the sewing ring is shadowed and not well seen.

24. **Answer: B.** As shown by the color Doppler, there is high-velocity flow in the left main coronary artery during diastole with evidence of extrinsic compression by the abscess.

25. **Answer: C.** The scallops of the mitral leaflet can be classified as lateral (A1), middle (A2), and medial (A3) of the anterior mitral leaflet, and lateral (P1), middle (P2), and medial (P3) of the posterior mitral leaflet.

    The vegetation is attached to the medial aspect of the anterior mitral leaflet, which is the A3 scallop.

26. **Answer: B.** Dehiscence of the prosthetic valve is present, as there is a large perivalvular regurgitation jet at the lateral sewing ring indicated by the large flow convergence. Most valvular dehiscences are due to infection. A mechanical mitral valve can produce a reverberation artifact in the LA simulating a mass, although no mass is present in these images.

27. **Answer: D.** In the setting of severe prosthetic mitral regurgitation and normal LV function, the peak early diastolic velocity (pressure gradient) is more significantly increased than the mean gradient. It should be noted that a small amount of regurgitation is normal for many types of mechanical prosthesis, particularly the bileaflet type. The normal mitral prosthetic regurgitant flow has a regurgitant jet area of <2 cm^2 and jet length of <2.5 cm. However,

with TTE it is usually difficult to detect mitral regurgitation by color-flow imaging because of shielding of the LA by the mitral prosthesis.

28. **Answer: A.** The posterior sewing ring (arrow, **Figure 21.21**) of the aortic prosthesis is dehisced from the aortic annulus and demonstrates rocking motion, which is not appreciated in the still images. Severe aortic regurgitation is expected when there is dehiscence of the prosthesis. A large pedunculated vegetation is present. No definite flail prosthetic leaflet is detected.

29. **Answer: B.** A pseudoaneurysm is demonstrated by the localized bulging at the posterior aortic root that is better seen in systole (▶ **Video 21.8**) and is a sequela of an aortic root abscess.

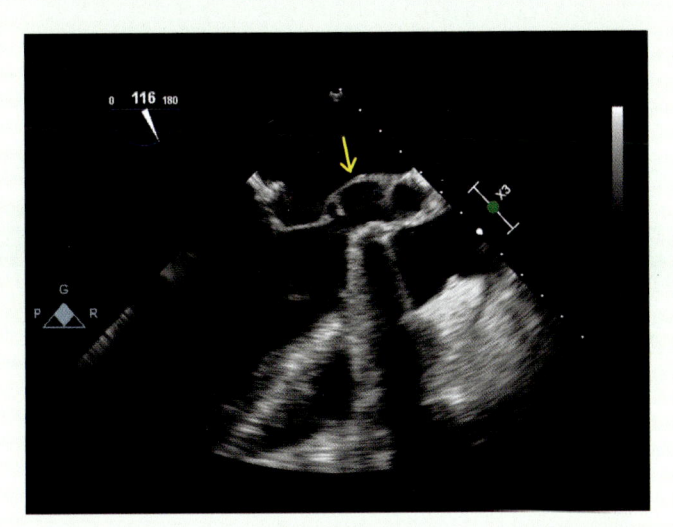

Figure 21.21

30. **Answer: D.** In a study correlating anatomic and echocardiographic findings in prosthetic valve endocarditis, cases with aortic valve dehiscence estimated at 40% to 95% of the annular circumference by direct observation correlated with demonstrable detachment on the parasternal long-axis view. Frame-by-frame analysis shows early systolic movement of the prosthesis upward into the aorta, which was not observed when the degree of dehiscence was less extensive or absent.

31. **Answer: C.** The annualized incidence of IE following implantation of a transcatheter pulmonic valve (Melody valve) is 1.8%, with a median time interval of 5 years between intervention and IE episode. *Staphylococcus aureus* and *Streptococcus* species are the predominant infecting organisms. A high residual transpulmonary gradient is a significant risk factor for IE; achieving a low RVOT gradient following implantation is critical. Owing to the anterior position of prosthetic material, leaflets of the Melody valve are difficult to visualize and neither TTE nor TEE is sensitive in detecting vegetations. Rather, endocarditis may present as RVOT obstruction and is more common than new valve regurgitation. Multimodality imaging such as 18F-FDG PET/CT may offer incremental diagnostic benefit when the diagnosis is in question. Surgery is required in patients with heart failure with hemodynamically significant obstruction, uncontrolled infections, or perivalvular complications. The cumulative incidence of reintervention is 4.8% at 5 years and 10.3% at 8 years.

32. **Answer: B.** After 4 weeks of antibiotic therapy and a favorable clinical response, it is unlikely to still have large vegetations. The two linear "vegetations" move in unison, and the mitral regurgitant jet is confined within these linear masses, which are in fact the walls of the mitral valve aneurysm. This aneurysm is defined as a localized bulging of mitral leaflet toward the LA with expansion during systole. In addition to mitral valve endocarditis, this condition can be encountered in the setting of aortic valve endocarditis with an aortic regurgitant jet impinging on the anterior mitral valve leaflet leading to a satellite infection. Acquired mitral valve aneurysm is invariably due to endocarditis, whereas a congenital mitral valve aneurysm is rare.

33. **Answer: C.** There are vegetations on the right coronary cusp (RCC) and noncoronary cusp (NCC) of the aortic valve. There is severe prolapse of the RCC. The midesophageal long-axis view of the aortic valve usually shows the RCC (anterior) and NCC (posterior) in patients with a tricuspid aortic valve. The two cusps are embedded by vegetations. Color-flow imaging shows that the posterior aortic regurgitant jet arises from the base of the NCC, which is consistent with a perforation.

34. **Answer: B.** Vegetations on the aortic valve are frequently associated with aortic root abscesses. The abscess erodes the aortic root wall and eventually ruptures. This results in a communication with other chambers. If the abscess has communication with the aortic lumen, it is called a pseudoaneurysm. If the abscess has communication with two chambers, it is then called a fistula. As illustrated by the color-flow imaging, there is a diastolic flow from the right coronary sinus of Valsalva (at the 7-o'clock position) to the right atrium (the flow is above the tricuspid valve). This flow results from a fistula between these two chambers.

35. **Answer: A.** Based on the two-dimensional images, the severe prolapse of the RCC of the aortic valve leads to a severe coaptation defect, resulting in severe valvular aortic insufficiency. This can be expected even if there is no other color-flow imaging or Doppler interrogation.

Table 21.1. Surgical Indications in Right-Sided Infective Endocarditis

Fastidious organism (eg, fungi, multidrug-resistant organisms)

Large (>20 mm), persistent tricuspid valve vegetations

Right-sided heart failure secondary to tricuspid regurgitation with poor response to medical therapy

Sustained infection despite appropriate antimicrobial therapy

Recurrent pulmonary emboli with or without concomitant right-sided heart failure

Abscess (more common in the setting of prosthetic valve)

Adapted from Shmueli H, Thomas F, Flint N, Setia G, Janjic A, Siegel RJ. Right-sided infective endocarditis 2020: challenges and updates in diagnosis and treatment. *J Am Heart Assoc.* 2020;9:e017293 and Baddour LM, Wilson WR, Bayer AS, et al. Infective endocarditis in adults: diagnosis, antimicrobial therapy, and management of complications—a scientific statement for healthcare professionals from the American Heart Association. *Circulation.* 2015;132(15):1435-1486.

KEY POINTS
- Endocarditis can cause valvular regurgitation by different mechanisms including leaflet erosion, retraction, perforation, and flail leaflet.
- Leaflet perforation should be suspected when the origin of the regurgitant jet is located away from the site of leaflet coaptation.
- Perivalvular complications including abscess and fistula formation are more common in aortic valve endocarditis.

---

36. **Answer: B.** The echocardiogram demonstrates a large vegetation attached to the anterior leaflet of the tricuspid valve, in addition to a very large coaptation gap and a dilated right ventricle. According to the American Heart Association Guidelines on Infective Endocarditis, intervention is reasonable for patients with right-sided heart failure secondary to severe tricuspid regurgitation with poor response to medical therapy, sustained infection caused by difficult-to-treat organisms (ie, fungi, multidrug-resistant bacteria) or lack of response to appropriate antimicrobial therapy, and tricuspid valve vegetations that are ≥20 mm in diameter with recurrent pulmonary embolism despite antimicrobial therapy (**Table 21.1**). *S. aureus* is a common infecting organism and so long as there is adequate response to antibiotic therapy is not in itself an indication for intervention. Additionally, treatment of the underlying substance use disorder is paramount.

37. **Answer: B.** Transcatheter vacuum-assisted aspiration is a relatively new strategy used to debulk vegetations. The system consists of an inflow (suction) cannula and a venovenous extracorporeal bypass circuit that provides suction-assisted removal of endovascular masses, including thrombi, tumors, and vegetation (**Figure 21.22**). The distal tip of the inflow cannula is funnel shaped and can be maneuvered under real-time fluoroscopic and echocardiographic guidance. A filter attached to the circuit traps suctioned debris and returns blood to the patient. Excellent procedural and clinical success has been demonstrated in tricuspid valve endocarditis in vegetations larger than 1.5 cm. Importantly, this intervention only debulks vegetation to reduce embolic risk and help achieve source control. It does not address tricuspid regurgitation, which may increase postprocedurally; it does not obviate the need for surgical debridement and valve repair or replacement when necessary.

38. **Answer: A.** The tricuspid valve is involved in 90% of cases of right-sided endocarditis; the pulmonic valve

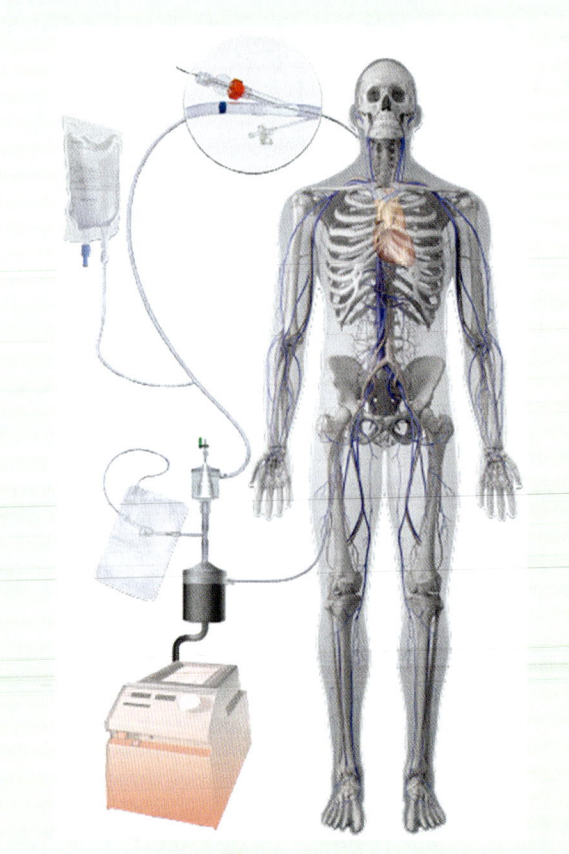

Figure 21.22

is involved in <2%. *Staphylococcus aureus* is the most common infecting organism. Right-sided endocarditis is associated with better outcomes compared with left-sided endocarditis. One study found an in-hospital mortality of 2.6% in right-sided endocarditis, compared with 17% in left-sided involvement. Factors that may contribute to this finding in right-sided endocarditis include younger age, a lower rate of perivalvular abscess, and fewer hemodynamic consequences from tricuspid valve involvement.

KEY POINTS

- The indications for surgery in right-sided endocarditis include right-sided heart failure secondary to severe tricuspid regurgitation, sustained infection caused by difficult-to-treat organisms, and large tricuspid valve vegetations with recurrent pulmonary emboli.
- Transcatheter vacuum-assisted aspiration may be considered to debulk right-sided vegetations larger than 1.5 cm with good clinical and procedural success.
- Right-sided endocarditis is associated with better outcomes compared with left-sided endocarditis.

39. Answer: D. Vegetations are not detected on either the anterior or posterior mitral valve leaflets. An aneurysm is seen on the posterior mitral valve leaflet. Color-flow imaging shows systolic flow traversing the aneurysm into the LA, consistent with perforation at the base of the aneurysm. An aneurysm of the mitral valve leaflet is usually a rare condition. Its incidence has been reported as low as 0.29%. It is almost always associated with IE, but rare cases can occur in patients with connective tissue disease without endocarditis. It is mostly located on the anterior mitral valve leaflet, which is frequently impinged on by an aortic regurgitant jet. The size of the aneurysm varies, with the largest reported being 30 mm. Perforation of the aneurysm can occur and is the main mechanism of mitral regurgitation.

40. Answer: B. In the setting of a mitral valve aneurysm, a satellite lesion should be sought. The mass attached to the lateral wall of the LV is most likely a vegetation, which is probably "seeded" from the mitral valve vegetation.

KEY POINTS

- Endocarditis is the most common cause of valvular diverticula or aneurysms.
- Leaflet perforation frequently coexists with valvular diverticula or aneurysms.
- Satellite vegetations should be sought along the path of the "infected" flow jet.

41. Answer: B. The mitral leaflets appear normal without prolapse, but color-flow imaging shows a perforation at the lateral scallop (A1) of the anterior leaflet. The regurgitant jet does not originate from the coaptation site but rather from the leaflet suggesting a perforation. The perforation is not well seen on the two-dimensional imaging. Based on the jet size with color-flow imaging, the mitral regurgitation is significant. No mitral valve cleft is present.

42. Answer: B. The regurgitant jet is located at the A1 segment of the mitral leaflet. The parasternal short-axis view with color-flow imaging clearly demonstrated that the jet is located laterally at the A1 scallop and is directed posteriorly.

KEY POINTS

- The short-axis view of the mitral valve allows precise localization of the abnormality involving the individual scallops of the mitral leaflets responsible for mitral regurgitation.
- Valvular dysfunction is common even after successful medical treatment of endocarditis.
- Valvular perforations may result from active or treated endocarditis.

43. Answer: B. Various prediction models have been developed to risk stratify patients with *S. aureus* bacteremia in the setting of a negative initial TTE. Factors that increase the pretest probability of endocarditis, and predict the need for TEE in diagnosis, include community-acquired *S. aureus*, presence of intracardiac prosthetic material, wires, or indwelling catheters, duration of symptoms >4 days, indeterminate TTE, and intravenous drug use.

44. Answer: E. The TEE demonstrates a mass attached to the coronary sinus lead adjacent to the tricuspid annulus at the posteroseptal commissure, which is at the entrance of the coronary sinus (as demonstrated in the biplane view). The differential for this finding includes thrombus and much less likely fibrin strands. The prevalence of fibrin strands increases with the age of the lead. Thrombi are also common, occurring in up to 25% of patients when TEE was routinely performed on average of 4 months following ICD insertion, and are most frequently located on leads within the junction between the right atrium and superior vena cava, right atrial body, or at the tricuspid valve annulus (**Figure 21.23**). Thrombi are common but cannot be distinguished from vegetations based on echocardiographic imaging alone. In the setting of MSSA bacteremia, the diagnosis of exclusion is a vegetation and it must be treated as such.

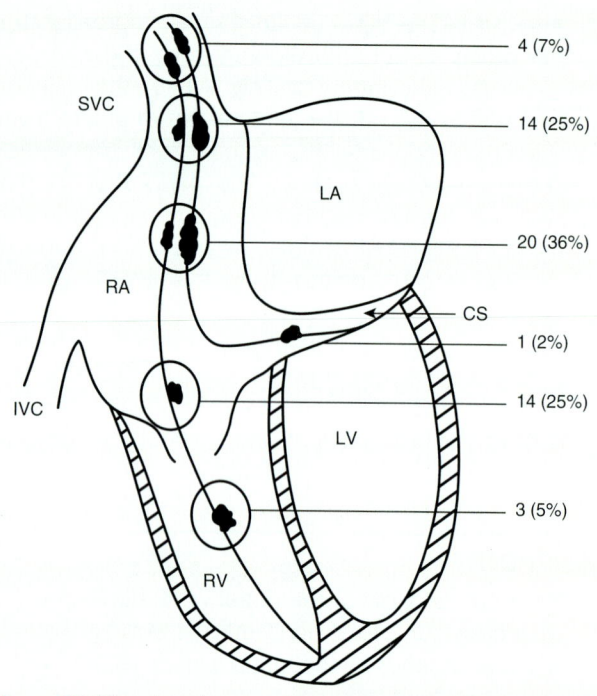

Figure 21.23. Relative locations of lead thrombi attached to device leads. (Reprinted from Chow BJ, Hassan AH, Chan KL, Tang AS. Prevalence and significance of lead-related thrombi in patients with implantable cardioverter defibrillators. *Am J Cardiol.* 2003;91(1):88-90. Copyright © 2003 Elsevier. With permission.)

KEY POINTS

- A TEE should be strongly considered in the presence of *S. aureus* bacteremia when there is a high index of suspicion for endocarditis.
- Fibrin strands and thrombi are relatively common on cardiac implantable electronic device leads; the diagnosis of vegetation is based on clinical suspicion.
- Successful treatment of definite pacemaker infections include complete removal of the pulse generator and leads.

45. **Answer: D.** The Novel 2019 International Cardiac Implantable Electronic Device (CIED) Infection Criteria propose criteria to make a diagnosis of definite infection, based on the modified Duke and ESC 2015 Guidelines criteria for infective endocarditis (**Tables 21.2** and **21.3**). In this case, the diagnosis of a lead vegetation implies infection of the pacemaker; while further imaging may be important to rule out perivalvular extension (eg, abscess), it will not change the diagnosis of CIED infection. Once a diagnosis of definite pacemaker infection has been made, successful treatment requires complete removal of pulse generator and leads. Extraction should not be delayed; extraction within 3 days of admission is associated with lower in-hospital mortality.

46. **Answer: B.** There is a fistula at the posterior mitral valve annulus between the LV and LA. The vegetation induces a cascade of structural complications including abscess, pseudoaneurysm, and fistula formation. The extension of necrosis forms an abscess. Drainage of the abscess into one chamber is called a pseudoaneurysm. A fistula is formed as a result of communication of abscess with two chambers. In this case, the mitral annular abscess led to formation of a fistula between the LV and LA and caused paravalvular mitral regurgitation. Infrequently, in patients with an annular abscess, the infection may respond to antibiotic therapy alone.

47. **Answer: D.** The dimension of the fistula on two-dimensional images, the size of the color jet, and the high mitral valve inflow E velocity all suggest severe mitral regurgitation.

48. **Answer: D.** Systolic flow reversal in the pulmonary veins may not be present in the setting of severe mitral regurgitation when the LA is severely dilated or highly compliant and when the regurgitant jet is highly eccentric and directed away from the pulmonary veins. The systolic flow reversal in the pulmonary veins is highly indicative of severe mitral

Table 21.2

Summary of Modified Duke Criteria for the Diagnosis of IE

Major Criteria

Blood Culture
- Two positive blood cultures with a typical organism in the absence of a known source, or persistently positive blood cultures, or single positive blood culture or positive serology for *Coxiella burnetii*

Endocardial Involvement
- Positive echocardiographic findings of vegetation, abscess or new dehiscence of prosthetic valve, or new valvular regurgitation

Minor Criteria

- Predisposing heart condition or intravenous drug use
- Fever (>38 °C)
- Vascular phenomena
- Immunologic phenomena
- Positive blood culture not meeting the major criterion, or positive serology of organism consistent with IE

regurgitation but its absence does not exclude severe mitral regurgitation.

> **KEY POINTS**
> - Perivalvular abscess is a dynamic process and can lead to long-term sequelae such as fistula and pseudoaneurysm formation.
> - Color-flow imaging can demonstrate the path of the fistula.
> - Flow reversal in the pulmonary veins is not present in all patients with severe mitral regurgitation.

49. **Answer: C.** There are vegetations on all three leaflets of the tricuspid valve. The anterior and the septal leaflets are retracted, causing a coaptation defect.

50. **Answer: C.** The lack of leaflet coaptation results in severe tricuspid regurgitation. The color-flow imaging is confirmatory.

51. **Answer: A.** In this clinical setting, the left atrial mass is likely a vegetation. In many injection drug users, vegetations can be present on the left-sided valves as well as the right-sided valves and can be seen in unusual locations. Tumor (myxoma or angiosarcoma) is less likely in this case.

> **KEY POINTS**
> - Intravenous drug users are at risk to develop right-sided and left-sided endocarditis, although the presence of right-sided endocarditis strongly suggests intravenous drug use.
> - Isolated right-sided endocarditis has a better prognosis compared with left-sided endocarditis.
> - Vegetations in right-sided endocarditis are frequently large regardless of the etiologic agent.
> - TTE is usually adequate to detect vegetations in right-sided endocarditis.

52. **Answer: A.** There is at least moderate mitral regurgitation largely due to a perforation at the anterior mitral leaflet, likely a result of a satellite vegetation. Mitral valve repair of the perforation using a pericardial patch is generally feasible. Mitral valve repair is preferred to replacement because of better long-term outcome with repair. The aortic valve is bicuspid with severe tissue destruction leading to flail of the anterior cusp and severe aortic regurgitation. Aortic valve repair is unlikely to be possible. Despite aortic root involvement, the left coronary artery is well seen (arrow, **Figure 21.16A,B**) and not affected by IE. Coronary angiogram is not indicated given his young age and the TEE findings.

53. **Answer: C.** Valvular perforation is associated with more severe regurgitation and a higher in-hospital mortality. This complication appears to be less common in injection drug users, and the bacteriologic profile is similar to that of patients with IE without this complication.

> **KEY POINTS**
> - Different mechanisms of valvular regurgitation may be present in patients with IE.
> - Valve repair is an option if the regurgitation is a result of leaflet perforation.

54. **Answer: D.** Initially, M-mode was used to detect vegetations. With two-dimensional TTE, better spatial definition of vegetations can now be obtained. An active vegetation is an echogenic mass with an irregular shape. It is usually located at or near the lines of valve closure at the low-pressure end of the jet lesion with high-frequency motion independent of the underlying cardiac structure. The mass can be associated with valve dysfunction. Chronic healed vegetations become echodense masses due to fibrin, collagen, and calcium deposition. The echocardiographic identification of vegetation or abscess is considered a major criterion for IE in the widely used Duke criteria (**Table 21.2**). A definite diagnosis of IE requires the presence of two major criteria, or one major and three minor criteria, or five minor criteria. According to the modified Duke criteria, a vegetation is "an oscillating intracardiac mass on valves or supporting structures, or in the path of regurgitant jets, or on implanted material, in the absence of an alternative anatomical explanation." Compared with infective vegetations, noninfective vegetations from marantic or Libman-Sacks endocarditis have similar morphologic features and can only be differentiated from infective vegetations on the basis of the clinical findings.

55. **Answer: B.** Evolutionary changes are common in infective endocarditis; repeat imaging should always be considered if there is a clinical change that may indicate a destructive process. *S. aureus* is notoriously destructive and is independently associated with increased mortality, owing to a host of virulence factors and propensity to embolize and rapidly form abscess cavities. Although abscesses are generally associated with aortic valve involvement, they may occasionally be seen when the mitral valve is involved. As TTE has poor sensitivity in detecting perivalvular complications, TEE is the modality of choice. A cardiac CT may be a complementary imaging modality to evaluate for these complications. 18F-FDG PET is useful to confirm the diagnosis of endocarditis, particularly when the diagnosis

Table 21.3. The Novel 2019 International Cardiac Implantable Electronic Device (CIED) Infection Criteria

Major Criteria

Microbiology

A. Blood cultures positive for typical microorganisms found in CIED infection and/or infective endocarditis (IE) (coagulase-negative staphylococci, *Staphylococcus aureus*)
B. Microorganisms consistent with IE from two separate blood cultures
    a. Viridans streptococci, *Streptococcus bovis*, HACEK group, *S. aureus*, or
    b. Community-acquired enterococci, in absence of a primary focus
C. Microorganisms consistent with IE from persistently positive blood cultures
    a. ≥2 positive blood cultures of blood samples drawn >12 h apart; or
    b. All of three or a majority of ≥4 separate blood cultures (first and last samples drawn ≥1 h apart); or
    c. Single positive blood cultures for *Coxiella burnetii* or phase I IgG antibody titer >1:800

Imaging

A. Echocardiogram positive for:
    a. CIED infection, including clinical pocket/generator infection or lead vegetation
    b. Valvular infection, including vegetation, abscess, pseudoaneurysm, intracardiac fistula; valvular perforations or aneurysm; or new partial dehiscence of a prosthetic valve
B. 18F-FDG PET/CT or radiolabeled WBC SPECT/CT
    a. Detection of abnormal activity at pocket/generator site, along leads, or at valve site
C. Cardiac CT
    a. Definite paravalvular involvement

Minor criteria

A. Predisposition (eg, predisposing heart condition, injection drug use)
B. Fever (temperature >38 °C)
C. Vascular phenomena, including those detected only by imaging: major arterial emboli, septic pulmonary emboli, infectious (mycotic) aneurysm, intracranial hemorrhage, conjunctival hemorrhage, Janeway lesions
D. Microbiological evidence: positive blood culture that does not meet a major criterion as noted above or serological evidence of active infection with organism consistent with IE or pocket/lead culture (extracted through a noninfected pocket)

Adapted from Blomström-Lundqvist C, Traykov V, Erba PA, et al. European Heart Rhythm Association (EHRA) international consensus document on how to prevent, diagnose, and treat cardiac implantable electronic device infections-endorsed by the Heart Rhythm Society (HRS), the Asia Pacific Heart Rhythm Society (APHRS), the Latin American Heart Rhythm Society (LAHRS), International Society for Cardiovascular Infectious Diseases (ISCVID) and the European Society of Clinical Microbiology and Infectious Diseases (ESCMID) in collaboration with the European Association for Cardio-Thoracic Surgery (EACTS). *Eur J Cardiothorac Surg*. 2020;57(1):e1-e31. Reproduced by permission of European Heart Rhythm Association.

---

is "possible" by modified Duke criteria in the setting of a prosthetic valve. In this case, the diagnosis of definite endocarditis has already been made.

56. Answer: D. When the index of suspicion for an abscess is high, oblique and nonstandard views are often necessary to adequately rule out perivalvular extension. A vegetation on the medial aspect of the mitral valve may extend posteromedially into the mitral annulus to invade into the anatomic space posterior to the central fibrous trigone, which contains the AV node. With further extension, the septal leaflet of the tricuspid valve may also be involved. Of the choices provided, the transgastric long-axis view of the aortic root at 100° to 120° visualizes all these important structures simultaneously (**Figure 21.24** and **Video 21.22**). It is important to sweep the probe in multiple directions to ensure that any hidden abscesses are identified. Three-dimensional data sets may also help to identify abscesses in unusual locations using postprocessing multiplanar reconstruction.

KEY POINTS

- Evolutionary changes are common in infective endocarditis; repeat imaging should always be considered if there is a clinical change that may indicate a destructive process.
- When the index of suspicion for an abscess is high, oblique and nonstandard views are often necessary to adequately rule out perivalvular extension.
- Alternate imaging such as cardiac CT and/or 18F-FDG PET may be useful to confirm a diagnosis of endocarditis, particularly when the diagnosis is "possible" by modified Duke criteria in the setting of a prosthetic valve.

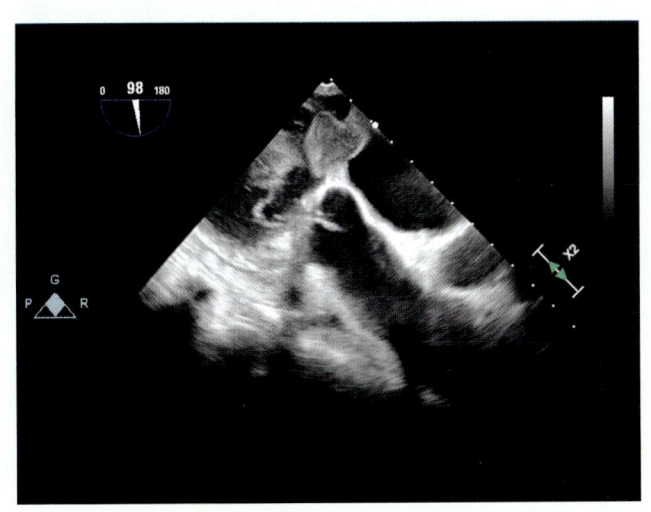

Figure 21.24

57. **Answer: C.** An acquired Gerbode defect (LV-to-RA shunt through the membranous interventricular septum) is a rare complication of IE. They can be diagnosed using color Doppler, which shows high-velocity flow between the two chambers. In the provided clips, the location of the vegetation on the ventricular aspect of the mitral valve is unusual. There is a satellite vegetation on the atrial aspect of the septal tricuspid leaflet. In injection drug users, left-sided valvular involvement has become increasingly common, in addition to involvement of the right-sided valves.

58. **Answer: B.** In this patient, there is an LV-to-RA shunt, which creates a step-up of oxygen saturation in the right atrium due to the highly oxygenated blood from the left ventricle. Venous oxygen saturation in this cardiac chamber should thus be higher than the mixed venous oxygen from the vena cava but lower than the oxygen saturation of the normal arterial blood. Atrial septal defect with shunting between the left and right atria also causes a step-up of oxygen saturation in the right atrium.

KEY POINTS

- Vegetations located at the atrioventricular junction may extend to involve the central fibrous body.
- Erosion at the central fibrous body can lead to shunting between the left and right ventricles, or between the left ventricle and the right atrium.
- An intracardiac shunt should be sought when a vegetation involves the central fibrous body.

SUGGESTED READINGS

Baddour LM, Wilson WR, Bayer AS, et al; American Heart Association Committee on Rheumatic Fever, Endocarditis, and Kawasaki Disease of the Council on Cardiovascular Disease in the Young, Council on Clinical Cardiology, Council on Cardiovascular Surgery and Anesthesia, and Stroke Council. Infective endocarditis in adults: diagnosis, antimicrobial therapy, and management of complications—a scientific statement for Healthcare Professionals from the American Heart Association. *Circulation.* 2015;132(15):1435-1486.

Blomström-Lundqvist C, Traykov V, Erba PA, et al. European Heart Rhythm Association (EHRA) international consensus document on how to prevent, diagnose, and treat cardiac implantable electronic device infections. *Eur J Cardio Thorac Surg.* 2020;57(1):e1-e31.

Bos D, De Wolf D, Cools B, et al. Infective endocarditis in patients after percutaneous pulmonary valve implantation with the stent-mounted bovine jugular vein valve: clinical experience and evaluation of the modified Duke criteria. *Int J Cardiol.* 2021;323:40-46.

Citro R, Chan KL, Miglioranza MH, et al; EURO ENDO Investigators Group. Clinical profile and outcome of recurrent infective endocarditis. *Heart.* 2022;108(21):1729-1736.

Del Val D, Panagides V, Mestres CA, Miro JM, Rodés-Cabau J. Infective endocarditis after transcatheter aortic valve replacement: JACC state-of-the-art review. *J Am Coll Cardiol.* 2023;81(4):394-412.

Incani A, Hair C, Purnell P, et al. *Staphylococcus aureus* bacteraemia: evaluation of the role of transoesophageal echocardiography in identifying clinically unsuspected endocarditis. *Eur J Clin Microbiol Infect Dis.* 2013;32(8):1003-1008.

Kang DH, Kim YJ, Kim SH, et al. Early surgery versus conventional treatment for infective endocarditis. *NEJM.* 2012;366(26):2466-2473.

Mhanna M, Beran A, Al-Abdouh A, et al. AngioVac for vegetation debulking in right-sided infective endocarditis: a systematic review and meta-analysis. *Curr Probl Cardiol.* 2022;47(11):101353.

San Roman JA, Vilacosta I, Lopez J, et al. Role of transthoracic and transesophageal echocardiography in right-sided endocarditis: one echocardiographic modality does not fit all. *J Am Soc Echocardiogr.* 2012;25(8):807-814.

Shmueli H, Thomas F, Flint N, Setia G, Janjic A, Siegel RJ. Right-sided infective endocarditis 2020: Challenges and Updates in diagnosis and treatment. *J Am Heart Assoc.* 2020;9(15):e017293.

Thuny F, Di Salvo G, Belliard O, et al. Risk of embolism and death in infective endocarditis: prognostic value of echocardiography—a prospective multicenter study. *Circulation.* 2005;112(1):69-75.

Interventional Echocardiography: Mitral, Aortic, and Prosthetic Valve Interventions

CHAPTER 22

Stephen H. Little, Priscilla Wessly, and Nadeen N. Faza

QUESTIONS

1. Which of the following are predictors of significant paravalvular regurgitation after transcatheter aortic valve implantation (TAVI)?
   A. Implantation depth.
   B. Valve under sizing.
   C. Calcium location and burden.
   D. All of the above.

2. Which of the following statements is/are **TRUE** regarding assessment of paravalvular leak post transcatheter aortic valve implantation (TAVI)?
   A. The regurgitant jet must enter the left ventricle.
   B. Color flow is seen around the transcatheter heart valve (THV) and above the annular valve skirt.
   C. Measure the ratio of jet width to left ventricular outflow tract (LVOT) width to assess severity.
   D. All the above.

3. Percutaneous closure of paravalvular regurgitation may avoid the risk of reoperation. Which of the following are American College of Cardiology (ACC)/American Heart Association (AHA) indications for percutaneous paravalvular leak (PVL) closure?
   A. Symptomatic heart failure.
   B. Prosthetic valve endocarditis with PVL.
   C. PVL involving more than one-third of the valve ring.
   D. All of the above.

4. Recommended timeline of transthoracic echocardiography (TTE) examinations for transcatheter aortic valve replacement include which of the following?
   A. Baseline between 1 and 3 months.
   B. 1 year.
   C. Annually beyond 1 year.
   D. All of the above.

5. Which of the following are risk factors for obstruction of coronary arteries after transcatheter aortic valve implantation (TAVI)?
   A. Height of the left main above the annulus >14 mm.
   B. The outer frame of the transcatheter heart valve (THV).
   C. Aortic root diameter on echo >30 mm.
   D. Female sex.

6. The key anatomic exclusion criteria for the transcatheter mitral valve edge-to-edge repair with MitraClip in the original EVEREST trial include which of the following?
   A. Regurgitant jet origin associated with A2-P2 segments of the mitral valve.
   B. Coaptation depth of ≤11 mm.
   C. A flail gap of >10 mm.
   D. A flail width of <15 mm.

7. Which of the following catheter-based mitral valve interventions is approved by the United States Food and Drug Administration (USFDA)?
   A. Transcatheter edge-to-edge repair (TEER) of the mitral valve.
   B. Placement of artificial chords.
   C. Mitral annuloplasty.
   D. All of the above.

8. What parameters are assessed intraprocedurally by TEE post mitral valve transcatheter edge-to-edge repair (TEER) deployment?
   A. Adequate leaflet insertion and a stable tissue bridge.
   B. Transmitral diastolic gradients.
   C. Residual mitral regurgitation (MR).
   D. All of the above.

9. Post transcatheter aortic valve implantation (TAVI) deployment, which of the following should be assessed using echocardiography?
   A. Aortic regurgitation.
   B. Mitral regurgitation.
   C. New wall motion abnormalities.
   D. All of the above.

10. Prior to mitral balloon valvuloplasty, preprocedural assessment should include evaluation for:
    A. Left atrial (LA) size.
    B. Presence or absence of left atrial appendage (LAA) thrombus.
    C. Tricuspid regurgitation (TR) severity.
    D. All of the above.

11. Which of the following echocardiographic parameters are used to assess mitral regurgitation (MR) severity after transcatheter edge-to-edge mitral valve repair?
    A. Improvement or normalization of pulmonary vein flow.
    B. Improvement in left ventricle outflow tract (LVOT) stroke volume.
    C. New-onset spontaneous contrast within left atrial (LA) or left atrial appendage (LAA).
    D. All of the above.

12. Which coronary artery is at an increased risk of obstruction during transcatheter aortic valve implantation (TAVI)?
    A. Left coronary ostium.
    B. Right coronary ostium.
    C. All of the above.
    D. None of the above.

13. Which of the following steps in the transcatheter mitral valve edge-to-edge repair (TEER) procedure are typically guided by echocardiography?
    A. Transseptal puncture.
    B. Guide catheter positioning.
    C. Device orientation.
    D. All of the above.

14. In a patient with severe symptomatic functional mitral regurgitation while on optimal guideline-directed medical therapy (GDMT), mitral valve transcatheter edge-to-edge repair (TEER) is reasonable in patients with which of the following parameters?
    A. LVEF 20% to 50%.
    B. Left ventricular end-systolic diameter (LVESD) > 70 mm.
    C. Pulmonary artery systolic pressure (PASP) > 70 mm Hg.
    D. All of the above.

15. To calculate the left ventricular outflow tract (LVOT) stroke volume in a patient with transcatheter aortic valve implantation (TAVI), which of the steps below is the preferred approach?
    A. Measure the LVOT diameter from outer-to-outer border of the stented valve at its ventricular tip.
    B. PW Doppler placed proximal to the site of flow acceleration.
    C. Stroke volume is calculated assuming a circular geometry of the LVOT.
    D. All of the above.

16. Which of the following statements describes the relation of structures to the mitral valve in this 3D TEE surgical view (**Figure 22.1**)?
    A. The aortic valve is medial, the interatrial septum is posterior, and left atrial appendage (LAA) is anterior.
    B. The aortic valve is lateral, the interatrial septum is anterior, and the LAA is posterior.
    C. The aortic valve is posterior, the interatrial septum is lateral, and the LAA is medial.
    D. The aortic valve is anterior, the interatrial septum is medial, and the LAA is lateral.

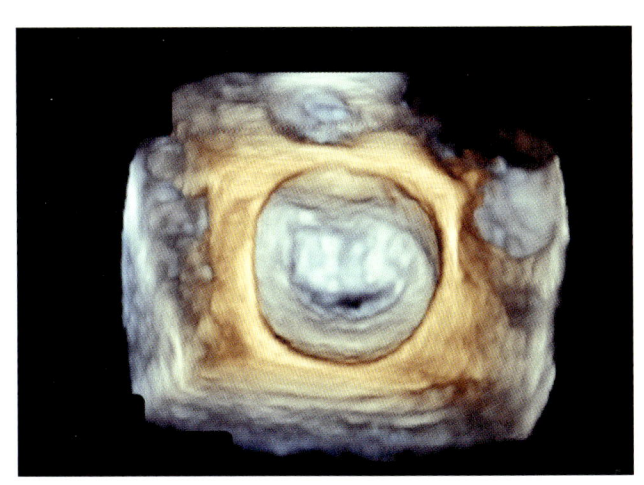

Figure 22.1. Three-dimensional transesophageal echocardiogram view of the mitral valve in the surgical view in systole.

458 / Clinical Echocardiography Review

17. The mitral valve (MV) transcatheter edge-to-edge repair (TEER) device angle in relation to the coaptation line should be:
  A. Perpendicular.
  B. Parallel.
  C. At any angle.
  D. None of the above.

18. The panels in **Figure 22.2** represent four patients with severe symptomatic mitral regurgitation. Which of the following would not be an appropriate candidate for transcatheter mitral valve repair (TEER)?
  A. P2 flail.
  B. Severe mitral annular calcification.
  C. Functional mitral regurgitation.
  D. All of the above.

19. A 75-year-old woman with severe symptomatic functional mitral regurgitation is referred for transcatheter mitral valve repair. The interventionalist asks you to perform a transesophageal echocardiogram (TEE) and guide the transseptal puncture. Which of the following is the preferred transseptal access site for crossing into the left atrium for this procedure?

  A. Through the foramen ovale.
  B. Superior and posterior of the fossa ovalis.
  C. Inferior limbus of the fossa ovalis.
  D. Anterior limbus of the fossa ovalis.

20. Aortic prosthetic paravalvular regurgitation is approached retrograde from the aorta. In the images in **Figure 22.3**, which of the following statements is **TRUE**?
  A. The posterior para-aortic jets are easiest to see on transthoracic imaging.
  B. Echocardiography must ensure that catheter crosses the paravalvular defect and not across the valve leaflets.
  C. Para-aortic regurgitation more commonly presents with hemolysis compared to paramitral regurgitation.
  D. Paravalvular jets associated with aortic prosthesis are typically large and multiple.

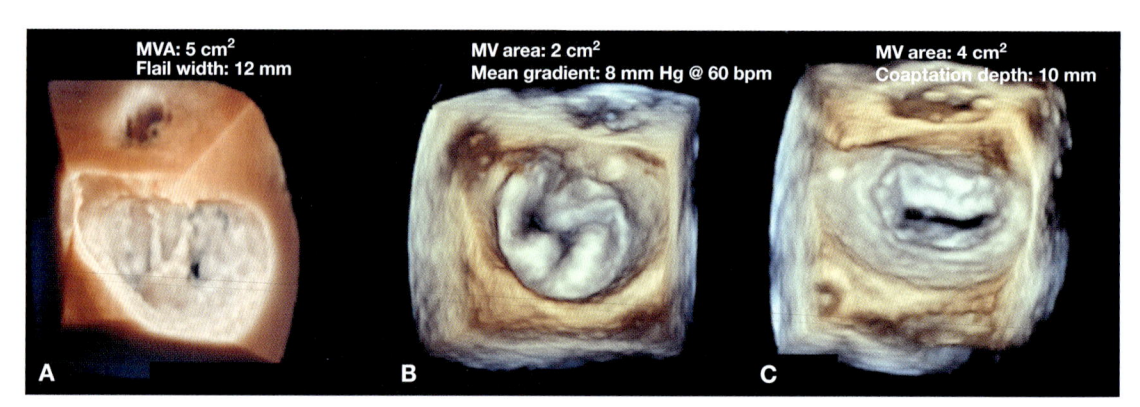

Figure 22.2. Three-dimensional still transesophageal echocardiogram images of the mitral valve in anatomic/surgical view during systole in three different patients presenting for mitral valve (MV) transcatheter edge-to-edge repair.

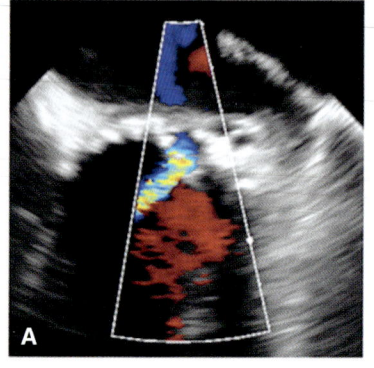

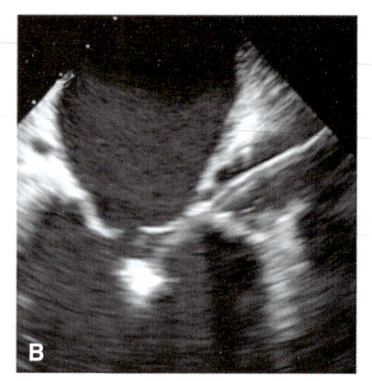

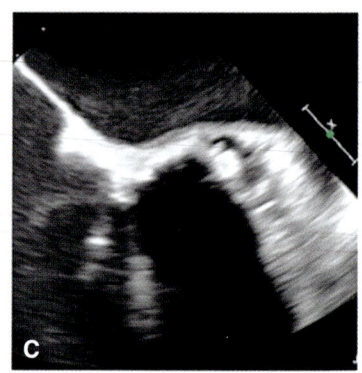

Figure 22.3. Intraprocedural imaging. **A:** Color Doppler of an aortic prosthesis on short axis. **B:** Procedural imaging of the aortic prosthesis on long axis. **C:** Postprocedural imaging of the aortic prosthesis on short axis.

21. The following images in **Figure 22.4** are simultaneous hemodynamic tracings and continuous-wave Doppler tracings from a symptomatic patient undergoing percutaneous balloon mitral valvuloplasty for mitral stenosis. Panel A is the baseline hemodynamics. Panel B is following percutaneous balloon mitral valvuloplasty. Which of the following statements is **TRUE**?
   A. The baseline mitral valve area and mean gradient do not fulfill class I indications for intervention.
   B. The final area is 1.5 cm² by pressure half-time calculation.
   C. The magnitude of mean gradient reduction defines procedural success.
   D. Planimetered valve areas are more accurate than pressure halftime following balloon valvuloplasty.

22. A 79-year-old hypertensive diabetic woman with advanced chronic renal failure presented for transcatheter aortic valve replacement (TAVR) with a balloon expandable valve. She underwent a successful procedure, but immediately following implantation, her blood pressure increased to 190/110 mm Hg. The intraprocedural TEE image in **Figure 22.5** was obtained. What would be the appropriate management be?
   A. Immediate open repair of the annular rupture.
   B. Balloon redilatation of an underdeployed transcatheter valve.
   C. Aggressive treatment of her hypertension.
   D. Valve-in-valve therapy for malpositioned transcatheter valve.

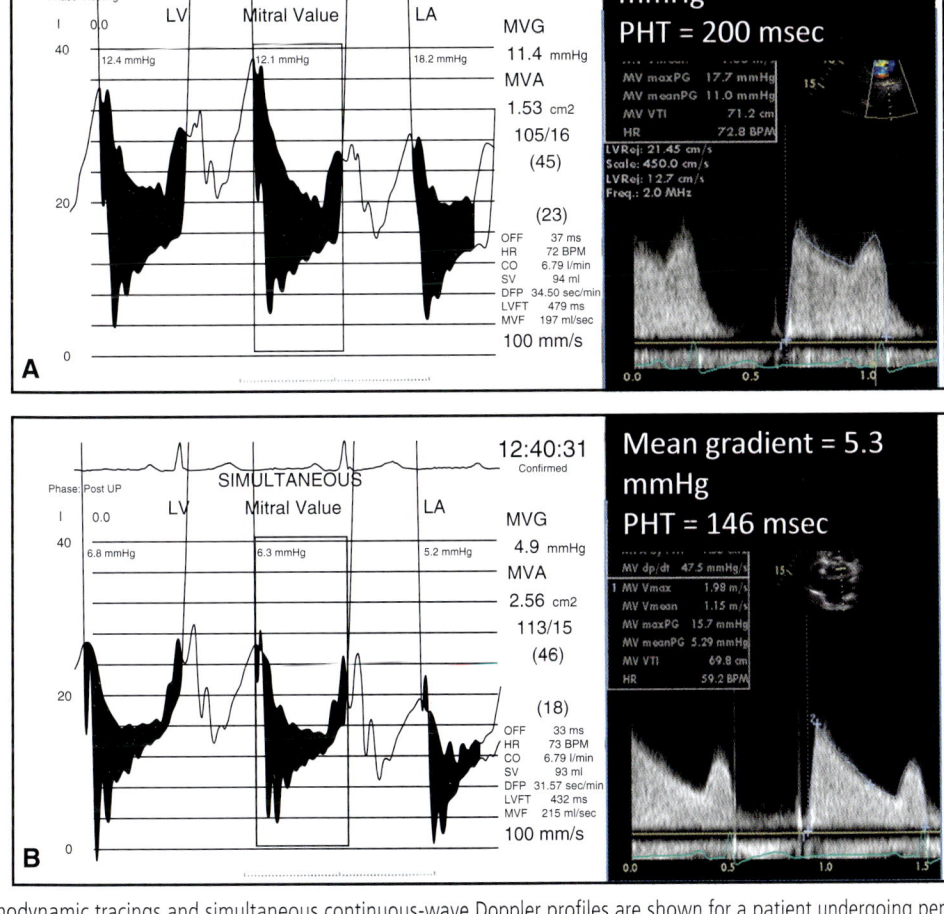

Figure 22.4. Hemodynamic tracings and simultaneous continuous-wave Doppler profiles are shown for a patient undergoing percutaneous mitral balloon valvuloplasty. **A:** Baseline hemodynamics. **B:** Following percutaneous mitral balloon valvuloplasty.

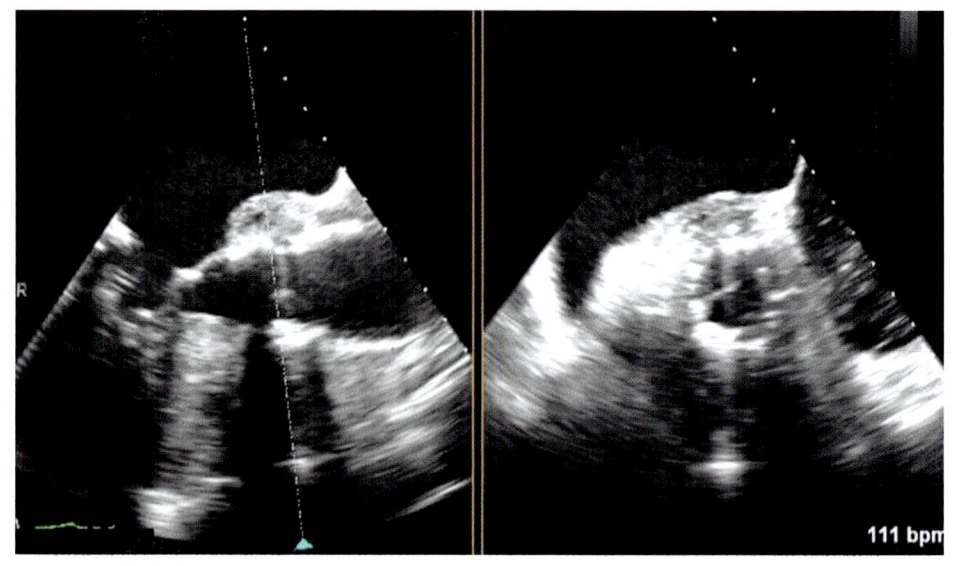

Figure 22.5. Simultaneous multiplane imaging soon after transcatheter aortic valve replacement.

23. A 79-year-old patient, status post bioprosthetic mitral valve replacement 8 years ago, presents with progressive shortness of breath over the last year. **Figure 22.6** shows the three-dimensional diastolic images in the surgical view from the left atrial side of the prosthesis at presentation (Panel A) and following a procedure (Panel B). What is the cause of the patient's shortness of breath and how was it treated?
   A. Flail bioprosthetic mitral valve; open replacement with a smaller bioprosthesis.
   B. Stenosis of the bioprosthetic mitral valve; transcatheter valve-in-valve procedure.
   C. Thrombus formation on the bioprosthetic mitral valve; aggressive anticoagulation.
   D. Vegetations on the bioprosthetic mitral valve; aggressive antibiotics administered.

CASE 1

A 94-year-old woman presents for transcatheter aortic valve implantation (TAVI) with a balloon expandable valve. She has a society for thoracic surgery risk score of 15 for surgical AVR, and a history of renal failure, diabetes, and hypertension. An intraprocedural transesophageal echocardiogram (TEE) is performed and the three-dimensional volume of the aortic root is reconstructed as shown in **Figure 22.7**, ▶ **Video 22.1** *and* **Video 22.2**. *From the multiplanar reconstruction, the coronal plane in Panel B is obtained. Imaging was then performed during the balloon aortic valvuloplasty.*

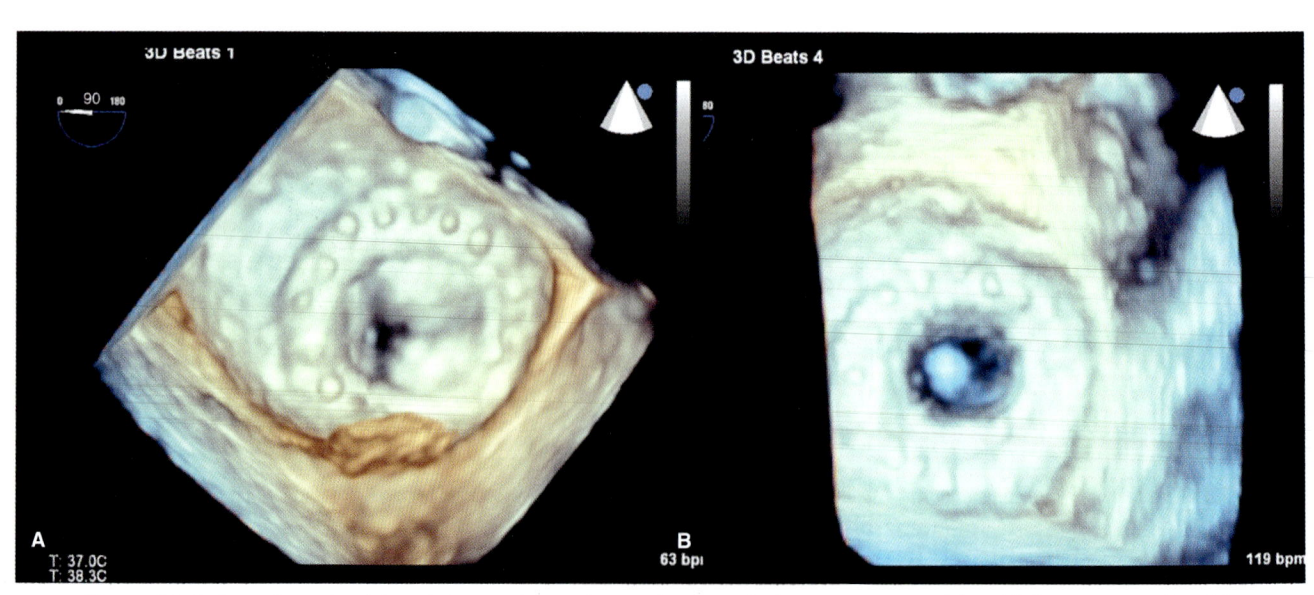

Figure 22.6. Three-dimensional diastolic image of a # 30 bioprosthetic mitral valve at presentation (**A**) and following a procedure (**B**).

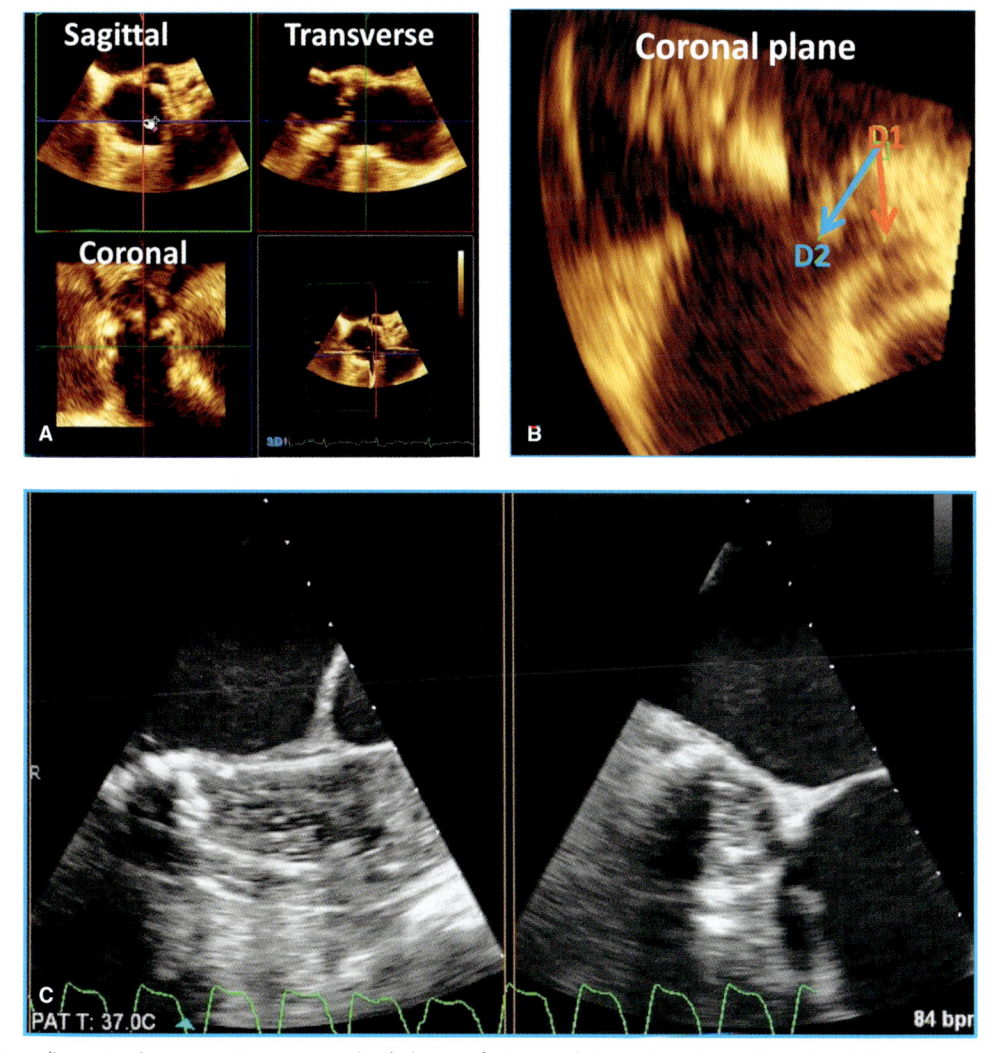

Figure 22.7. Three-dimensional reconstruction preprocedural planning for transcatheter aortic valve implantation. **A:** Three-dimensional echocardiographic reconstruction of aortic root in sagittal, transverse and coronal plane. **B:** Three-dimensional echocardiographic reconstruction of aortic root in coronal plane. **C:** Two-dimensional simultaneous biplane imaging during balloon aortic valvuloplasty.

24. Regarding the patient in **Case 1**, which of the following statements is **TRUE**?
    A. The linear measurement D1 is the distance from the annulus to the right coronary ostium.
    B. The linear measurement D1 is the distance from the annulus to the left coronary ostium.
    C. The linear measurement D1 is the distance from the annulus to the right coronary cusp tip.
    D. The linear measurement D1 is the distance from the annulus to the left coronary cusp.

25. For the patient in **Case 1**, after the balloon aortic valvuloplasty what is the most appropriate procedural approach?
    A. Proceed directly to the transcatheter AVR with a balloon expandable valve.
    B. Stent the left coronary artery prior to transcatheter AVR.
    C. Abort the transcatheter AVR and initiate a surgical consult for surgical AVR.
    D. Protect the left main with a wire and proceed with transcatheter aortic valve implantation (TAVI).

CASE 2

A 65-year-old woman, status post 25 mm St. Jude mechanical valve replacement for mitral stenosis, presented with recurrent hospitalizations for congestive heart failure. She has a history of diabetes mellitus (DM), hypertension (HTN), atrial fibrillation (Afib), and chronic renal insufficiency. A transesophageal echocardiogram (TEE) is shown in **Figure 22.8** *(▶ Videos 22.3 and 22.4).*

26. Which of the following statements describes the location of the defect in **Figure 22.8A** (▶ **Video 22.3**) for the patient in **Case 2**?
    A. Lateral sewing ring.
    B. Medial sewing ring.
    C. Anterior sewing ring.
    D. Posterior sewing ring.

27. What complication of paravalvular closure is imaged in **Figure 22.8B** (▶ **Video 22.4**) for the patient in **Case 2**?
    A. Distal embolization.
    B. Coronary obstruction.
    C. Obstruction of the prosthesis.
    D. All of the above.

CASE 3

A 74-year-old woman with history of severe symptomatic calcific mitral stenosis status post transcatheter valve replacement (TMVR) in mitral annular calcification presented with fatigue and lethargy. Laboratory investigation revealed hemolytic anemia. A transesophageal echocardiogram (TEE) is shown in **Figure 22.9** *(▶ Video 22.5).*

28. Which of the following statements is **TRUE** regarding the patient in **Case 3**?
    A. Mitral paravalvular leak (PVL) most commonly occurs in the anterolateral and posteromedial location.
    B. The patient has an indication for PVL closure.
    C. A lower transseptal puncture site is appropriate for lateral PVL site and while higher transseptal sites are needed for medial PVL site.
    D. All of the above.

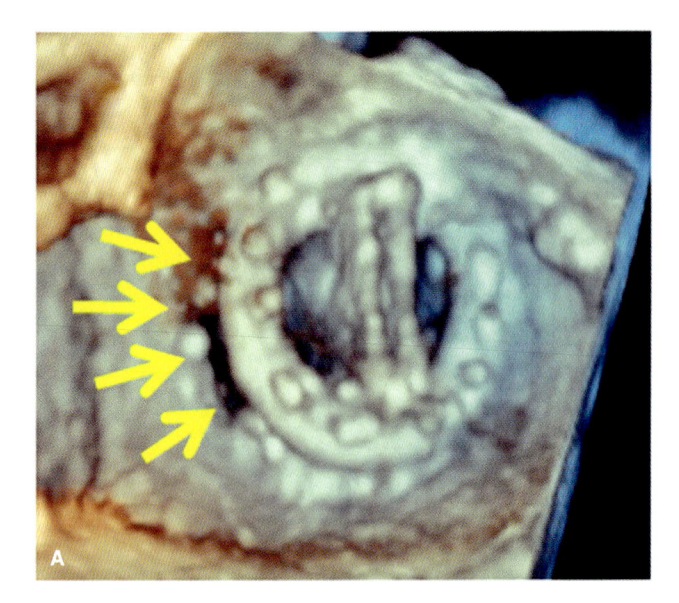

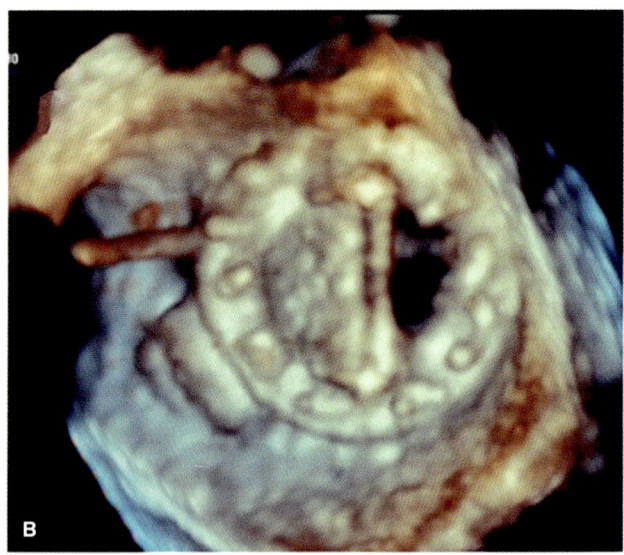

Figure 22.8. Three-dimensional images of a mechanical prosthetic mitral valve shown in the surgical anatomic view. **A:** Pre intervention image (yellow arrows showing defect). **B:** Intra-procedural image.

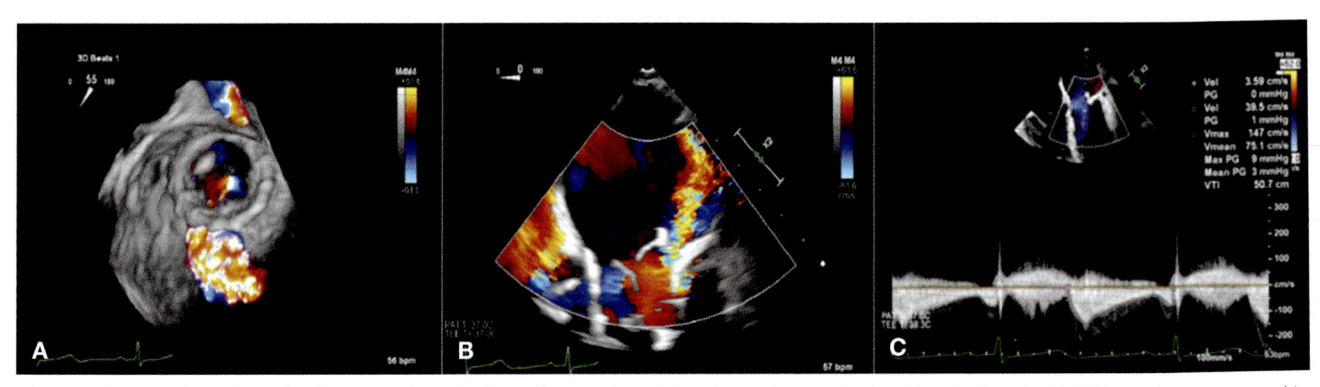

Figure 22.9. A: Three-dimensional transesophageal echocardiogram view of the mitral valve prosthesis with color Doppler. **B:** Mid-esophageal zoomed in view of the mitral prosthesis in systole with color Doppler. **C:** Transmitral continuous-wave Doppler with mean gradient across the mitral valve.

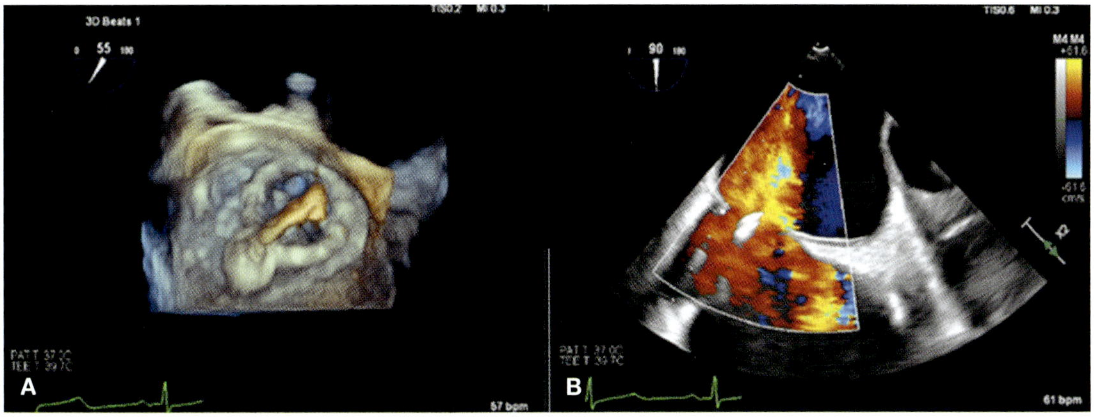

Figure 22.10. A: Catheter with paravalvular leak plug posterolateral to the transcatheter mitral valve prosthesis. **B:** Interatrial septum on transesophageal echocardiogram with color Doppler during the procedure.

29. During the procedure for PVL closure, the patient from **Case 3** became hypoxic. TEE images are shown in **Figure 22.10** and ▶ **Video 22.6**. Which of the following statements is **CORRECT**?
  A. There is significant right-to-left shunt through the iatrogenic atrial septal defect (iASD) causing hypoxia.
  B. Routine iASD closure is not warranted in all patients.
  C. iASD closure is warranted in patients with right-to-left or bidirectional shunting and hypoxia or left-to-right shunts with high-risk features.
  D. All of the above.

CASE 4

A 58-year-old woman was referred for management of severe symptomatic rheumatic mitral stenosis. The following transesophageal echocardiogram (Figure 22.11; ▶ Videos 22.7 and 22.8) was obtained on admission to the hospital. The planimetered valve area is 1.25 cm² and pulmonary artery systolic pressure was 91 mm Hg.

30. For the patient from **Case 4**, which of the following statements is **TRUE**?
  A. Planimetry is a direct measurement of mitral valve area (MVA) and is ideal for estimating valve area.
  B. Excessive gain setting may cause overestimation of valve area.
  C. Percutaneous mitral balloon valvuloplasty can be done in calcific MS.
  D. The optimal timing of the cardiac cycle to measure planimetry is end diastole.

CASE 5

The 58-year-old woman (from CASE 4) has worsening symptoms of dyspnea on exertion (NYHA 3). The decision is made to proceed with percutaneous balloon valvuloplasty (PBMV). Pre and post PBMV images (Figure 22.12 and ▶ Videos 22.9 and 22.10) are shown.

31. For the patient in **Case 5**, which of the following statements is **TRUE**?
  A. The magnitude of mean gradient defines procedural success.
  B. Pressure halftime (PHT) will accurately estimate valve area post mitral balloon valvuloplasty.
  C. The patient should have an emergent surgical consult with placement of intra-aortic balloon pump (IABP).
  D. The patient should be treated medically with guideline-directed medical therapy (GDMT).

464 / Clinical Echocardiography Review

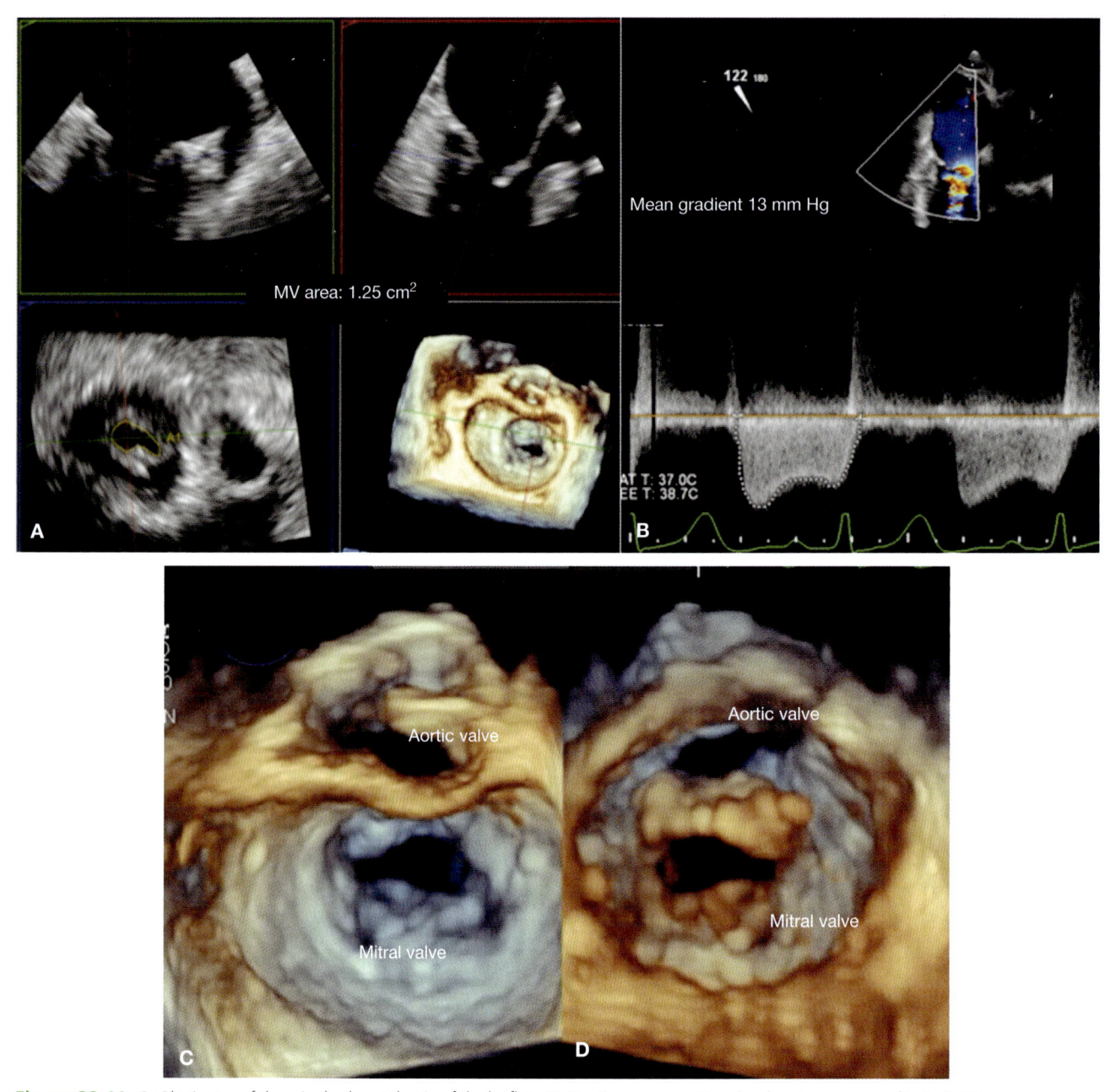

Figure 22.11. A: Planimetry of the mitral valve at the tip of the leaflets. **B:** Continuous-wave Doppler showing mean gradient. **C:** 3D transesophageal echocardiogram (TEE) surgical view of the mitral valve in diastole. **D:** 3D TEE view of the mitral valve in diastole when looking from the left ventricle looking into the mitral valve.

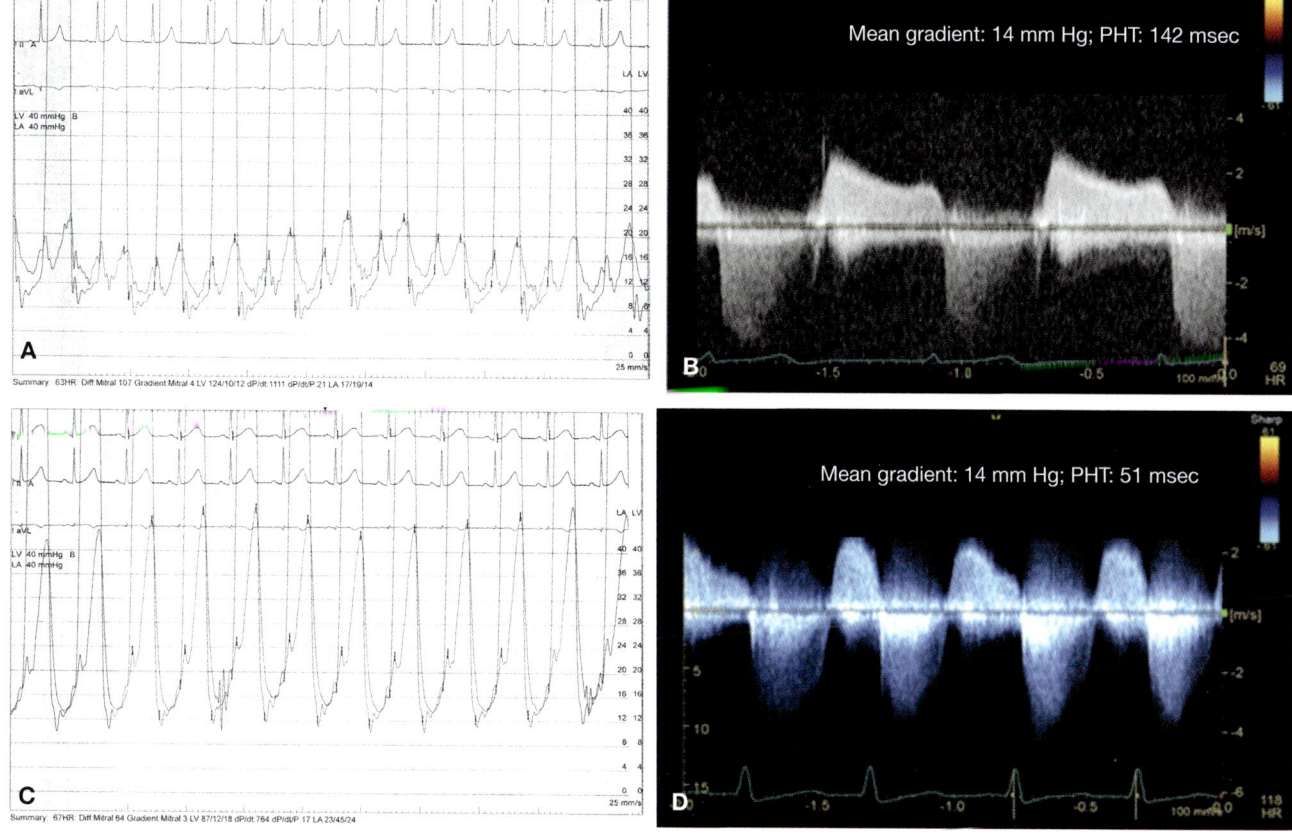

Figure 22.12. Hemodynamic tracings and simultaneous Continuous-wave (CW) Doppler profiles are shown for a patient undergoing percutaneous mitral balloon valvuloplasty (PBMV). **A** and **B:** Baseline hemodynamics. **C** and **D:** Following percutaneous balloon mitral valvuloplasty.

CASE 6

An 84-year-old woman was referred with severe aortic stenosis, LVEF = 50%, and significant heart failure. She had multiple comorbidities and unfavorable frailty parameters, hence was deemed to be inoperable. She was brought to the catheterization lab for TAVI with a balloon expandable valve. Transesophageal imaging from the procedure is shown in **Figure 22.13** *and* ▶ **Videos 22.11, 22.12,** *and* **22.13.**

32. Which statement most likely represents the sequence of events during the procedure for the patient in **Case 6**?

A. Pre-TAVI imaging would predict the possible annular rupture, seen in **Figure 22.13B**, which was successfully treated with a second valve deployment with final result seen in **Figure 22.13C**.
B. Pre-TAVI imaging would predict the paravalvular regurgitant jets in **Figure 22.13B**, which was successfully treated with postdilatation with final result seen in **Figure 22.13C**.
C. Pre-TAVI imaging would predict the paravalvular regurgitant jets in **Figure 22.13B**, which was successfully treated with watchful waiting with final result seen in **Figure 22.13C**.
D. One cannot determine the sequence of events.

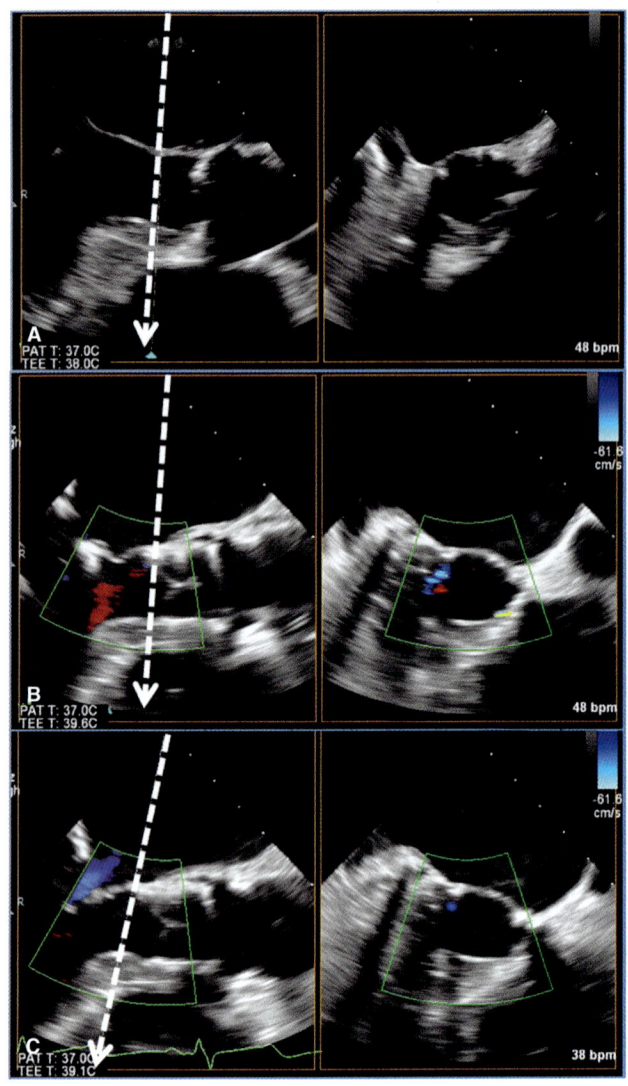

Figure 22.13. Simultaneous biplane imaging during intraprocedural imaging for transcatheter aortic valve replacement prior to implantation (**A**, ▶ Video 22.11), immediately following implantation (**B**: ▶ Video 22.12), and at the end of the procedure (**C**: ▶ Video 22.13).

33. Which of the imaging planes would be most helpful in predicting the occurrence of paravalvular regurgitation following TAVI for the patient in **Case 6**?
    A. Simultaneous biplane imaging at the level of the left ventricular outflow tract.
    B. Simultaneous biplane imaging at the level of the left main coronary artery.
    C. Simultaneous biplane imaging at the level of the aortic valve.
    D. None of the above.

ANSWERS

1. **Answer: D.** Meta-analyses have shown that all the risk factors listed predict significant paravalvular regurgitation. Low or high implantation, low cover index, and greater degrees of calcium were in most studies associated with severity of paravalvular regurgitation (PVR). The amount and location of calcium within the landing zone of the valve also play a key role in the incidence and severity of PVR following TAVI. Another risk factor is the valve type. In the only randomized comparison of balloon expandable and self-expanding valve implantation, the self-expanding valve had a higher incidence of significant PVR.

2. **Answer: A.** Central prosthetic aortic regurgitation (AR) jets will occur at the level of leaflet coaptation, whereas paravalvular regurgitation (PVL) will be seen at the proximal (ventricular) edge of the valve. Importantly, the jet must enter the left ventricle (LV) to be considered true regurgitation, thus imaging just below the edge of the stent will confirm the presence of true PVL; however, the vena contracta of the jet should be measured at its narrowest region. Color flow around the THV within the sinuses of Valsalva but above the annular valve skirt should not be mistaken for PVL. Flow in the sinuses has low velocity and does not connect with the LVOT in diastole. Scanning through the long axis of the valve is useful in distinguishing color flow

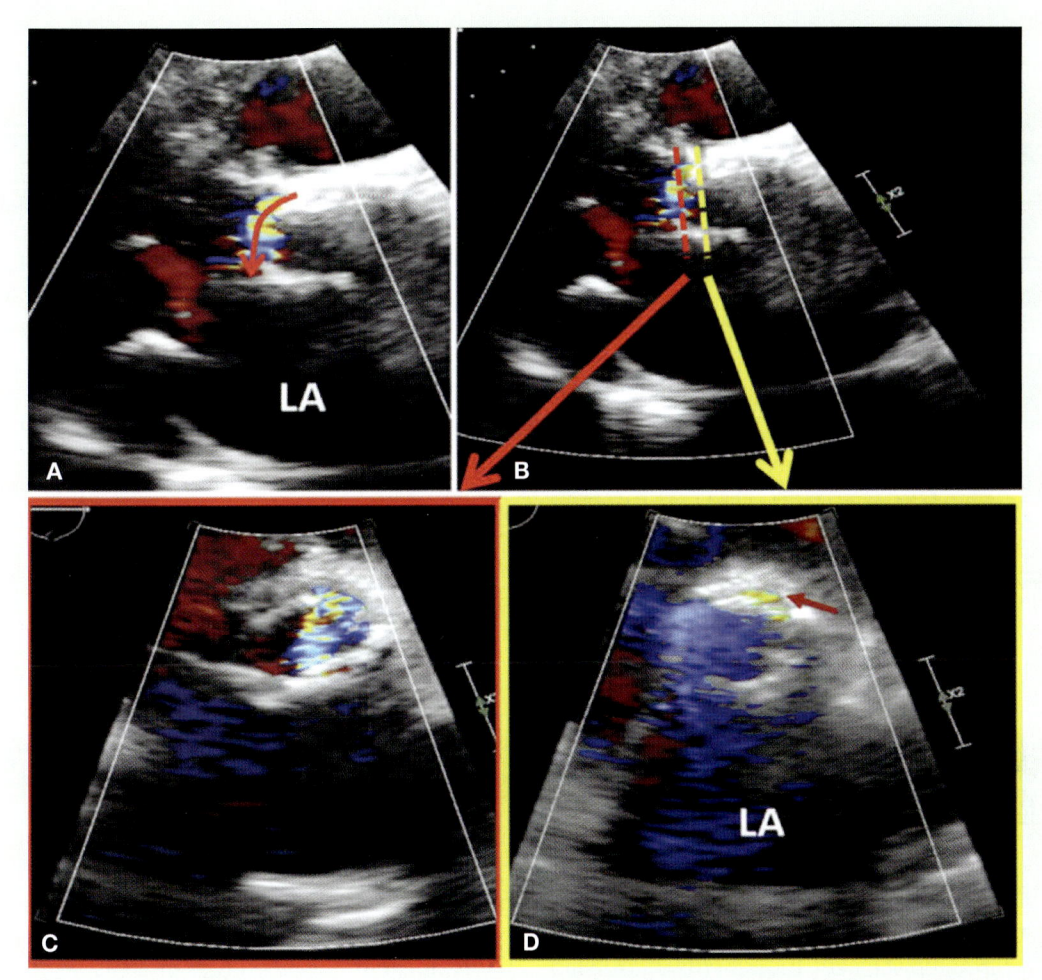

Figure 22.14. Effect of aortic regurgitation eccentricity on color Doppler jet recording when assessing paravalvular regurgitant jet severity after transcatheter aortic valve replacement. In case of an eccentric jet in the left ventricular outflow tract (LVOT) (**A:** curved arrow), the plane below the valve ring (**B:** dashed red) shows a large color jet as it spreads in the LVOT (**C**), overestimating regurgitant jet severity. By selecting the proper short axis (yellow arrow) at the aortic annulus (dashed yellow line) (**D**), the regurgitant jet is best depicted (small red arrow) more consistent with mild paravalvular regurgitant jet. (Reprinted from Zoghbi WA, Asch FM, Bruce C, et al. Guidelines for the evaluation of valvular regurgitation after percutaneous valve repair or replacement: a report from the American Society of Echocardiography Developed in Collaboration with the Society for Cardiovascular Angiography and Interventions, Japanese Society of Echocardiography, and Society for Cardiovascular Magnetic Resonance. *J Am Soc Echocardiogr.* 2019;32(4):431-475. Copyright © 2019 by the American Society of Echocardiography. With permission.)

in the sinuses from PVL. In contrast to native valve AR, the ratio of jet width to LV outflow tract width or jet cross-sectional area to cross-sectional area of the valve or LV outflow tract should not be used to assess the severity of AR since regurgitant jets are frequently eccentric, constrained by, and entrained within the LVOT, leading to rapid jet broadening (**Figure 22.14**).

3. **Answer: A.** The current ACC/AHA indications for percutaneous PVL repair include patients with prosthetic paravalvular regurgitation and symptomatic heart failure (NYHA functional class III to IV) or persistent hemolytic anemia, who have anatomic features that are suitable for percutaneous closure. Intractable hemolytic anemia was defined as hemolytic anemia with hemoglobin ≤10 gm/dL with elevated LDH and low haptoglobin requiring 2 units of blood transfusion and/or erythropoietin injections within 90 days to maintain Hb ≥ 10 gm/dL with no other source for blood loss identified. Closure of less-severe PVL remains controversial. Percutaneous repair is contraindicated in patients with active endocarditis or significant dehiscence involving more than one-fourth to one-third of the valve ring.

4. **Answer: D.** The assessment of the changes in structure and function of bioprosthetic valves is key to allow early detection of bioprosthetic valve dysfunction. Such assessment requires a comprehensive evaluation. ACC guidelines recommend baseline TTE 30 days postprocedure and routine annual TTE follow-up thereafter or at any time if any new symptoms occur or if complications are suspected.

5. **Answer: D.** In a systematic review by Ribeiro et al, the risk factors for coronary obstruction after TAVI were as follows:
   - A low position of the coronary ostia with respect to aortic annulus. Mean height of the left main

ostium was 10.3 mm in the reported cases of coronary obstruction.
- No cases of coronary obstruction related to the frame of the THV was reported.
- Aortic root diameter = 27.8 ± 2.8 mm. A narrow aortic root with shallow sinuses of Valsalva can limit space for native calcified aortic leaflets after valve deployment.
- 83% of patients were women. It has been shown that women have a smaller aortic root and this together with a lower coronary ostia height might explain the increased incidence of coronary obstruction after TAVI among women.

6. **Answer: C.** Key anatomic inclusion criteria for EVEREST trial included a regurgitant jet origin associated with A2-P2 segments of the mitral valve. For patients with functional MR, coaptation length of at least 2 mm and a coaptation depth of no more than 11 mm were required. For patients with leaflet flail, a flail gap < 10 mm and a flail width of <15 mm were required. Thus, Answer C would be an exclusion.

7. **Answer: A.** There are four major categories of percutaneous mitral valve interventions aimed at reducing mitral regurgitation (MR): mitral valve leaflet repair (TEER, and placement of artificial chords), transcatheter mitral valve replacement, mitral annuloplasty, and catheter-based plugging of paravalvular leaks. Among these, edge-to-edge repair and transcatheter mitral valve replacement for patients with failed surgical bioprosthesis and high surgical risk are the only two catheter-based MV intervention approved by the United States Food and Drug Administration (USFDA) for commercial use. For MV TEER, we have MitraClip and Pascal. MitraClip is approved for both degenerative and functional MR. Pascal was recently approved for degenerative MR and is in trial for functional mitral regurgitation. There are no specific devices that have been designed or approved by the Food and Drug Administration (FDA) for PVL closure.

8. **Answer: D.** The intraprocedural assessment of the mitral valve (MV) immediately after deployment includes: (1) ensure adequate leaflet insertion and a stable tissue bridge, (2) ensure valve geometry is not distorted, (3) measure diastolic transmitral gradients, (4) measure residual MV area preferably by 3D planimetry, (5) residual MR—number and localization of jets—quantify with three-dimensional vena contracta area, if possible, (6) look for complications—pericardial effusion and clip detachment.

9. **Answer: D.** Periprocedural TAVI echo evaluation should include assessment of the prosthetic valve function and complications of procedure. Evaluation of prosthetic valve function includes assessment of prosthetic valve gradients and presence of transvalvular or paravalvular aortic regurgitation. Complications of the procedure include aortic prosthesis misplacement either by embolization or improper deployment toward the aorta or left ventricle (LV), mitral regurgitation (MR) caused by aortic prosthesis impingement on the anterior mitral leaflet, damage or distortion of subvalvular apparatus by the delivery system or LV asynchrony caused by right ventricle (RV) pacing, new LV motion abnormalities caused by acute coronary ostial occlusion, cardiac tamponade caused by perforation of RV, and dissection or rupture of aortic root.

10. **Answer: B.** Preprocedural echocardiography should be focused on confirming the presence of severe mitral stenosis (MS) and the anatomical characteristics that are suitable for the procedure. A mitral valve (MV) area <1.5 cm^2 is considered severe MS. Valve area can be estimated with the use of the continuity equation and by using the pressure half-time method. An additional method for assessing the MV area that is not dependent on hemodynamic parameters is performance of planimetry. Compared with 2D echocardiography, planimetry with 3D echocardiography has a better correlation to the valve area calculated using the Gorlin formula. Valve morphology should be assessed for leaflet thickening, mobility, calcification, and subvalvular involvement. The Wilkins score uses echocardiographic findings to predict a successful procedure; a score <8 is correlated with favorable procedural outcomes, whereas a score >11 has shown to correlate with poor results. A 3D echocardiography scoring has been shown to have added value. Moreover, it is important to confirm a symmetrical commissural involvement, with no severe mitral commissural calcification, and to rule out more than mild to moderate (2+) mitral regurgitation (MR) and LA appendage thrombus. These asymmetric deformations of mitral orifice may increase the risk of MR with balloon valvuloplasty.

11. **Answer: D.** An assessment of changes in both hemodynamics and Doppler echocardiographic parameters is important in the overall evaluation of acute changes in MR severity during mitral valve (MV) repair or replacement. Color Doppler is the initial Doppler parameter used for assessing MR (site, number of jets, flow direction, vena contracta, and flow convergence) prior to and during the procedure, with limitations depending on the type of MV intervention. The pulmonary vein flow pattern is used together with other findings in an integrated fashion to assess residual MR and it should be meticulously interrogated in all patients before and during the procedure. Patients with severe MR have either systolic blunting or systolic flow reversal in one or more pulmonary veins. Normalization of pulmonary vein flow after MV interventions strongly suggests that MR has been reduced to mild, with

normalization of left atrial (LA) pressure. Failure of pulmonary vein velocity pattern to improve suggests insufficient MR reduction. Appearance of spontaneous echogenic contrast (SEC) in the LA after MV intervention also suggests significant reduction in MR severity. This may occur because of relative stagnation created by leaflet apposition. A retrospective study by Sato et. al showed that the occurrence of SEC was a strong predictor of greater long-term survival and a lower risk for heart failure hospitalization. The mitral inflow velocity pattern (decrease in mitral E velocity and velocity time integral [VTI]) may be helpful in assessing reduction of MR, particularly in procedures that do not change actual MV structure (annuloplasty and repair of paravalvular regurgitation). A change from an E wave–dominant to an A wave–dominant pattern suggests mild residual MR. Furthermore, measurement of velocity in the LVOT with TEE from deep transgastric views, while challenging, may be helpful in demonstrating an increase in velocity and thus systemic flow. Lastly, a decline in LV ejection fraction after MV intervention suggests significant MR reduction because of increased afterload.

12. **Answer: A.** The left coronary ostium is frequently in the posterior part of the left sinus, and the right coronary ostium is somewhat anterior and superior in the right sinus. The lower position of the left coronary increases its risk for obstruction by a calcified aortic leaflet.

13. **Answer: D.** Echocardiography plays a pivotal role in the intraprocedural guidance of TEER procedures including determining optimal transseptal site, positioning the guide catheters and device, and ensuring optimal device orientation in relation to the line of coaptation at the site of target pathology.

14. **Answer: A.** Per 2020 ACC AHA guidelines, mitral valve TEER is reasonable in severe symptomatic secondary mitral regurgitation patients who have select anatomy. The COAPT trial for transcatheter treatment of secondary MR demonstrated improvement in survival, hospitalization, symptoms, and quality of life in patients with persistent symptoms despite optimization of guideline-directed medical therapy (GDMT) and randomized to TEER. In contrast, MITRA-FR trial enrolled patients with greater degrees of LV enlargement and less severe MR and reported no difference in the composite end point of death or hospitalization. The enrollment criteria in COAPT trial (LVEF between 20% and 50%, LVESD ≤ 70 mm, pulmonary artery systolic pressure ≤70 mmHg, and persistent symptoms [NYHA class II, III, or IV] while on optimal GDMT) are the current standard selection criteria for TEER for secondary MR.

15. **Answer: D.** The default approach is to measure the LVOT diameter using the outer edge-to-outer edge diameter at the lower (ventricular) end of the valve stent. The pulsed-wave Doppler (PWD) sample volume is placed immediately proximal to the site of flow acceleration at the inlet to the stent. Stroke volume is then calculated as usual, assuming a circular LVOT geometry as 0.785 * diameter^2 * VTI. In instances where a self-expanding valve is placed low in the LV, particularly if the lower end of the stent is not in close proximity to the anterior mitral leaflet and interventricular septum, an alternative approach is to measure the inner edge-to-inner edge diameter of the valve stent immediately proximal to the cusps. The PWD sample volume should be placed just inside the stent but proximal to the site of flow acceleration at the cusps (**Figure 22.15**). With transcatheter valves, there is flow acceleration at the inlet to the stent and again at the cusps.

16. **Answer: D.** The surgical or anatomic view suggested by the American Society of Echocardiography guidelines on 3-dimensional echocardiography places the aortic valve anterior or at 12 o'clock with the LAA lateral and interatrial septum medial (**Figure 22.16**).

17. **Answer: A.** The device arms should also be perpendicular to the MV line of coaptation, which is commonly angled relative to the aorta in the three-dimensional (3D) en face view compared with the line of coaptation at A2-P2 (**Figure 22.17**).

18. **Answer: B.** The exclusion criteria in the EVEREST and COAPT trial were flail gap >10 mm, flail width >15 mm, coaptation depth >11 mm, coaptation length < 2 mm, LV ESD > 70 mm, mitral valve area <4 cm^2, commissural segments, and severe mitral annular calcification. Based on the classic EVEREST and COAPT criteria, patient in Figure A with flail P2 and Figure C with functional mitral regurgitation with LVESD ≤ 70 mm and PA systolic pressure ≤70 mm Hg would be an ideal candidate for MV TEER. Patient is Figure B has elevated gradient and MV area <3.5 cm^2, which would be prohibitive for MV TEER.

Although these criteria have been used in the past, with newer techniques, operator experience and better imaging techniques, US Food and Drug Administration, and under the auspices of the Heart Valve Collaboratory, a working group was formed with their first mandate to develop recommendations as to the types of mitral pathoanatomies and clinical care situations (comorbidities and imaging considerations) that define patients who would be unsuitable for treatment with TEER. Using red-yellow-green traffic light analogy, green were the classic EVEREST and COAPT trial patients, yellow were patients with complex anatomy such as multisegment prolapse, non-A2/P2 lesion/commissural disease, and red were patients with prohibitively complex anatomy. Prohibitively complex anatomy includes anatomies associated with stenosis with TEER, anatomies associated with inadequate MR reduction with TEER, and patient limitations that preclude performance of TEER. Small MV orifice

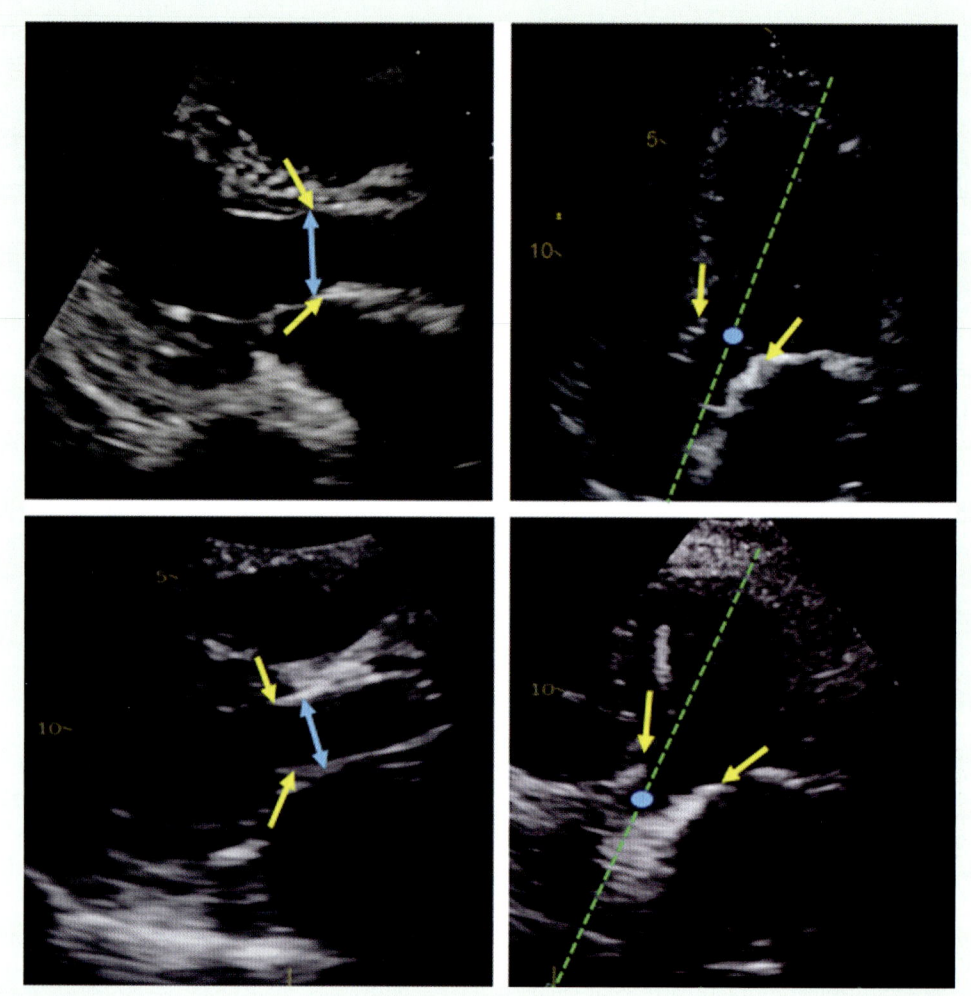

Figure 22.15. Upper panel showing measurement at outer-to-outer edge of the stent (blue) and pulsed-wave (PW) Doppler placed at inlet of the stent. Lower panel shows measurement of left ventricular outflow tract diameter from inner-to-inner edge (blue) in the parasternal long-axis view and PW Doppler placed just inside the stent in the apical 5-chamber view. Yellow arrows point to the lower edge of the stent.

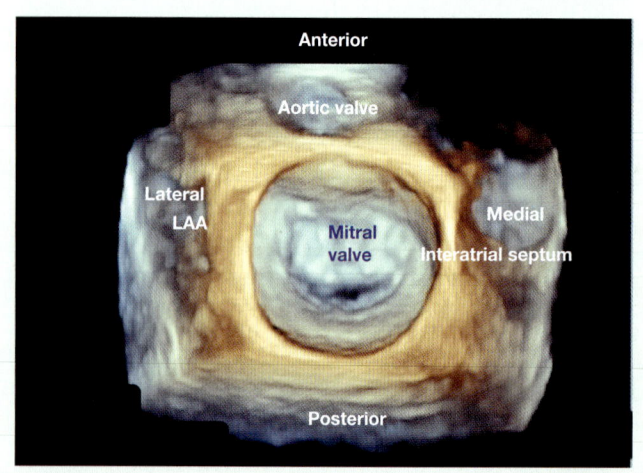

Figure 22.16. Three-dimensional transesophageal echocardiogram view of the mitral valve in the surgical view in systole (LAA: left atrial appendage).

area <3.5 cm² (**Figure 22.18B**) would be prohibitive anatomy.

19. **Answer: B.** Left heart interventional procedures require precise location of the transseptal puncture site to allow a coaxial catheter approach to target structures and provide room within the left atrium for device manipulation. Complementary views when using biplane with TEE are important for optimizing transseptal access. Short-axis views on TEE 30° to 75° provide the anteroposterior and bicaval 90° to 135° provide superior-inferior orientation. For central mitral regurgitation (MR), superior and posterior part of the fossa ovalis would be the ideal location for transseptal puncture (TSP) (**Figure 22.19**). Higher TSP heights are needed for medial jets/medial paravalvular leak (PVL) closure, while a lower site would work for a lateral jet. For percutaneous mitral balloon valvuloplasty and transseptal mitral valve-in-valve implantations, a mid-posterior puncture is adequate.

20. **Answer: B.** Posterior para-aortic regurgitant jets are better imaged on transesophageal echocardiogram (TEE) (Panel A), whereas anterior para-aortic jets are easiest to see on transthoracic imaging. Para-aortic defects are typically smaller than paramitral defects and can usually be closed with a single device as in the example shown. For para-aortic defects, the lower pressure difference between the aorta and

Chapter 22 Interventional Echocardiography: Mitral, Aortic, and Prosthetic Valve Interventions / 471

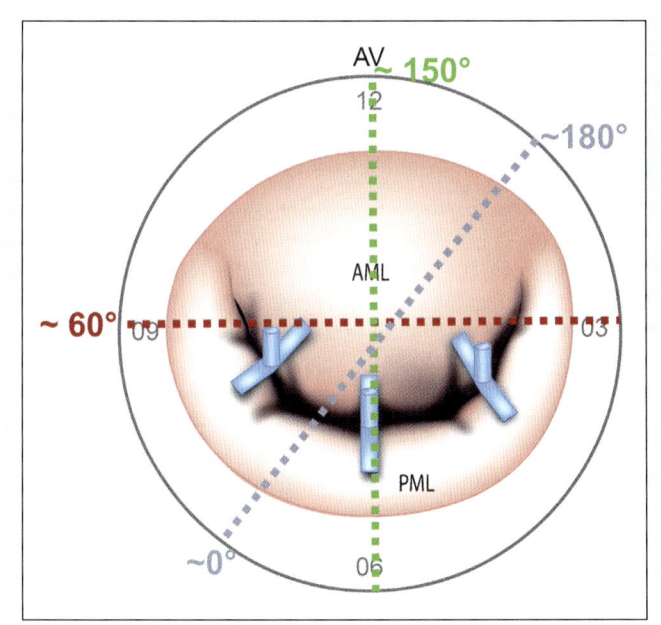

Figure 22.17. Illustration of the MV, surgeon's view in the "clock-face" plane with the aortic valve (AV) at 12 o'clock. For device perpendicularity with the MV leaflet line of coaptation, the arms and paddles are rotated beyond the 12 to 6 o'clock position. In case of a lateral target (A1–P1, left), the device is rotated to a 1 to 7 o'clock or 2 to 8 o'clock orientation. For a medial target (A3–P3, right), the device is rotated counterclockwise to an 11 to 5 o'clock or a 10 to 4 o'clock orientation. Nonconventional TEE imaging planes are often required to confirm leaflet grasping, commonly >150° for a lateral target and <130° for a medial target. The blue, red, and green dashed lines correspond to the ~0°, ~60°, and ~150° mid-esophageal TEE planes. AML, Anterior mitral leaflet; PML, posterior mitral leaflet. (Reprinted from Flint N, Price MJ, Little SH, et al. State of the art: transcatheter edge-to-edge repair for complex mitral regurgitation. *J Am Soc Echocardiogr.* 2021;34(10):1025-1037. Figure 3. Copyright © 2021 by the American Society of Echocardiography. With permission.)

left ventricle compared to the difference between left ventricles and left atrium for paramitral defects makes hemolysis less likely.

21. **Answer: D.** The only class I indication for intervention is symptomatic mitral stenosis with mitral valve area (MVA) ≤ 1.5 cm², and favorable valve morphology in the absence of contraindication. This patient fulfills this criterion. The reference measurement for MVA is 2D echo planimetry since pressure halftime (PHT) methods may not accurately estimate valve area in the setting of acute increase in LA compliance following balloon valvuloplasty. 3D echo has replaced 2D for planimetry of the mitral orifice since it allows an accurate localization of the tips of the leaflets. These compliance changes normalize 24 to 48 hours after the procedure, when pressure halftime can again be used to assess MVA. Procedural success is defined as an increase of ≥50% of MVA or final area of ≥1.5 cm² with no more than one grade increment in mitral regurgitation (MR) severity assessed by echocardiography 24 hours after the procedure. This is usually accompanied by >50% reduction in mean gradient; however, mean gradient change is not typically used as a criterion for success since it is dependent on multiple hemodynamic parameters including heart rate.

22. **Answer: C.** This is the typical appearance of a periaortic hematoma. Compared to intramural hematoma (which is bleeding into the wall of the aorta), periaortic hematoma arises from a microperforation of all three layers of the aorta, and the hematoma that forms appear as a tissue density mass around the outside of the aortic root. This perforation likely occurs after stretching of the aortic wall from displaced bulky calcium during balloon inflation/deployment of the transcatheter heart valve. This process appears to be self-limiting, with the microperforation sealing quickly once the balloon is deflated or the aorta is no longer stretched. Conservative management of the periaortic hematoma (including administration of protamine, continued intubation with restricted

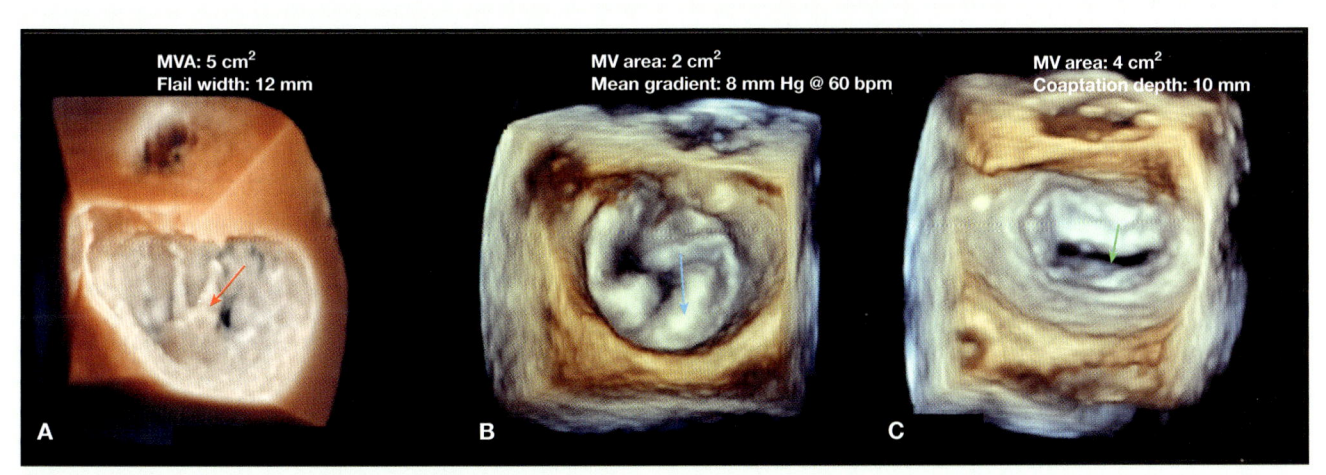

Figure 22.18. Three-dimensional still transesophageal echocardiogram images of the mitral valve in anatomic/surgical view during systole in three different patients presenting for mitral valve (MV) transcatheter edge-to-edge repair. **A:** Classic P2 flail (red arrow). **B:** Severe mitral annular calcification (blue arrow). **C:** Functional mitral regurgitation with coaptation gap (green arrow).

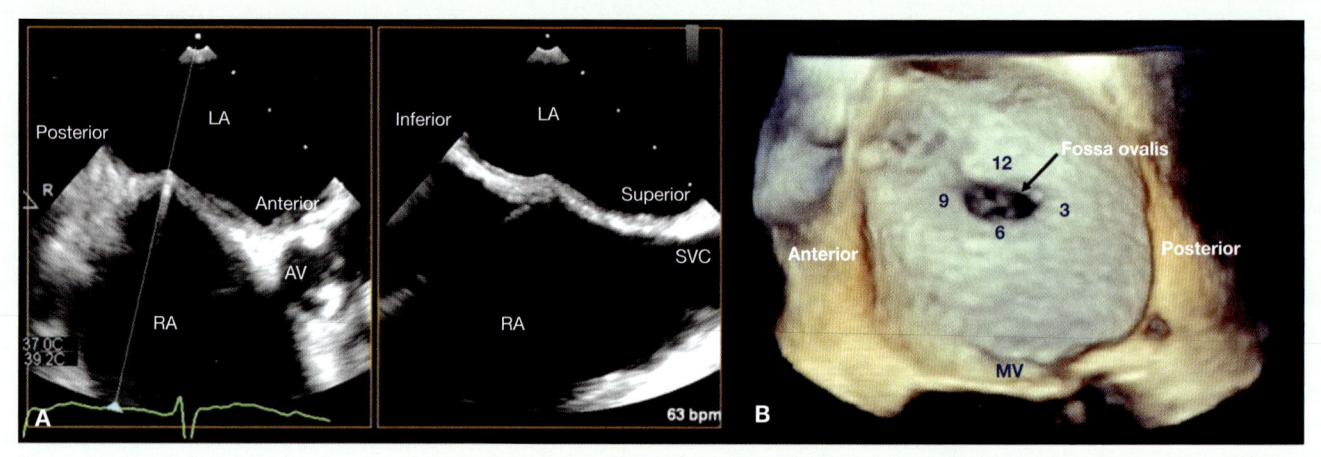

Figure 22.19. A: Two-dimensional transesophageal echocardiogram (TEE) biplane view of the interatrial septum. The anterior-posterior portion of the septum is in the short-axis view on the left and superior-inferior portion of the septum is seen in the orthogonal plane (bicaval view). **B:** 3D TEE still image of the interatrial septum visualized from the left atrial side (MV: mitral valve) with the fossa shown as a clock face. For central MR, the ideal location would be superior and posterior around 1 o'clock.

activity, and meticulous blood pressure control) can result in excellent outcomes and avert open repair. Failure to recognize this complication, however, may result in uncontrolled hypertension, leading to continued bleeding within the wall of the aorta and resulting in an intramural hematoma. Any further balloon dilatation whether direct balloon dilation or valve-in-valve procedure would be contraindicated.

23. **Answer: B.** The patient has degenerative bioprosthetic mitral stenosis with severe reduction in valve area seen in Panel A. A transcatheter valve-in-valve procedure with a balloon expandable valve was performed; the image in Panel B shows a smaller internal diameter of the valve with the edges of the transcatheter valve easily seen. There is no obvious flail leaflet in these images although these are diastolic frames. Thrombus or vegetations on the bioprosthetic valve are not seen on the image provided and the smaller internal diameter on follow-up would not be easily explained by simple lysis of a clot or treatment of vegetation. Transcatheter valve in failed surgical bioprosthesis is an acceptable alternative to surgical reoperation.

24. **Answer: B. Figure 22.20** shows the three-dimensional echocardiographic reconstruction of the left main and left coronary cusp from the coronal plane. D1 is the distance from the annulus to the left coronary ostium and D2 is the distance from the annulus to the tip of the left coronary cusp. Discordance in these measurements with longer cusp than coronary height should trigger an assessment of the risk for coronary occlusion.

25. **Answer: D.** During balloon aortic valvuloplasty imaging, the bulky calcium from the left coronary cusp can be seen on the simultaneous orthogonal view to completely occlude the left main coronary ostium. It is important to remember that during simultaneous multiplane imaging, the orthogonal view is forward rotated 90° and so the left coronary cusp is the cusp closer to the apex of the sector but on the left of the screen. Proceeding directly to transcatheter AVR or placing a left coronary stent prior to deployment would risk complete occlusion of the coronary artery. Because the patient is at a very high surgical risk, she had a wire placed into the left main prior to transcatheter AVR. Following valve deployment, the left main coronary artery became completely occluded. With the wire in the left main, a stent was rapidly deployed with no adverse consequence.

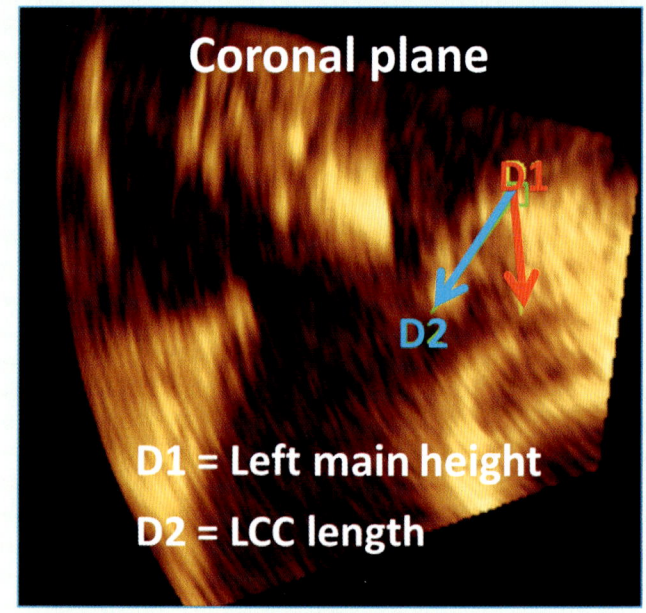

Figure 22.20. Three-dimensional reconstruction preprocedural planning for transcatheter aortic valve implantation.

> **KEY POINTS**
> - Discordance in the measurement of the coronary cusp and coronary height should trigger an assessment of the risk for coronary occlusion.
> - During balloon aortic valvuloplasty imaging, the left main coronary artery orifice can be directly observed for obstruction by displaced calcium on the coronary cusps.
> - Protecting the left main in high-risk patients may then allow rapid response to coronary occlusion following TAVI with placement of stent.

26. **Answer: A.** The surgical anatomic view places the aorta at 12 o'clock, the left atrial appendage (LAA) at 9 o'clock, interatrial septum at 3 o'clock and the posterior annulus at 6 o'clock (**Figure 22.21A**). This is true for both native and prosthetic valves. The anterolateral or lateral defects close to the LAA frequently have a serpiginous superior-to-inferior orientation because of massive left atrial dilation, with the inferior or left ventricular origin of the defect located closer to the valve prostheses. This orientation of the defect may result in tilting of the device after deployment that may not be identified when the device is still attached to the deployment catheter. Once tilted 90° to the annular plane, the device may obstruct normal motion of the anterior tilting disc valve. This device was snared and removed; multiple attempts to close the defect resulted in disc obstruction and the procedure was aborted.

27. **Answer: C.** Tilting disc valves may be obstructed during device deployment which can be recognized immediately by fluoroscopy (if appropriately aligned) and transesophageal echocardiogram (TEE) imaging (**Figure 22.21B**).

> **KEY POINTS**
> - The lateral sewing ring adjacent to the left atrial appendage is a common location for paravalvular regurgitation following surgical mitral valve replacement.
> - Because of the adjacent left atrial appendage and dilatation of the left atrium, the lateral paravalvular defects often have a superior-to-inferior orientation.
> - The orientation of the defect may cause closure devices to tilt such that they seat perpendicular to the plane of the annulus.
> - Any paravalvular closure device, but particularly ones that seat perpendicular to the plane of the annulus, may obstruct the mechanical valve occluders.

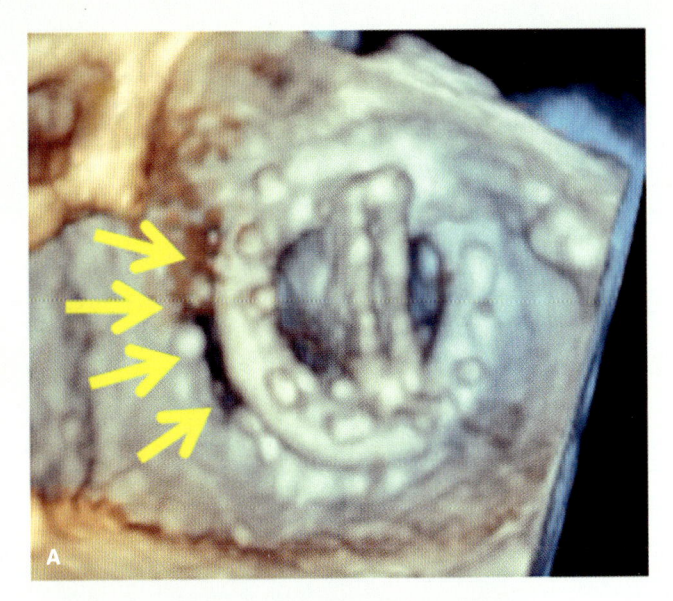

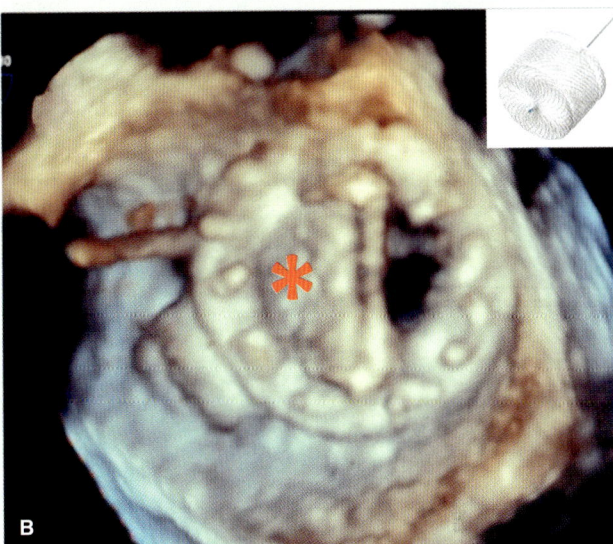

Figure 22.21. A: Surgeon's view of a bileaflet mechanical mitral valve replacement with both discs opening in diastole. The yellow arrows indicate the large region of dehiscence in the lateral sewing ring. **B:** One-disc medial side with normal disc. Mispositioning of the Amplatzer, vascular plug 2 (St. Jude Medical), see inset in **B**, to a vertical position prevents the second disc (red asterisk) from opening. Removing the device prior to deployment or snaring and removing a device after deployment can successfully reverse this complication. Distal embolization is always a risk of this procedure and retrieval of the device can be successfully accomplished by snaring the device or retrieving it with a bioptome. Coronary artery obstruction may occur when para-aortic defects are treated because the device may protrude over the ostia of the coronary arteries. Theoretically, occlusion of the circumflex artery may occur with posterior mitral prosthetic valve devices. If intraprocedural rectification of the complication cannot be accomplished, surgical intervention may be required.

28. **Answer: D.** The current American College of Cardiology (ACC)/American Heart Association (AHA) indications for percutaneous paravalvular leak (PVL) repair include patients with prosthetic valves and symptomatic HF (NYHA functional class III to IV) and persistent hemolytic anemia, who have anatomic features that are suitable for percutaneous surgery

in centers of expertise. Closure of less-severe PVL remains controversial. Percutaneous repair is contraindicated in patients with active endocarditis or significant dehiscence involving more than one-fourth to one-third of the valve ring. Successful PVL closure is defined as reduction of regurgitation to grade ≤1, is achieved in ~70% to 90% of cases, and improves with increasing operator experience. Important procedural complications can include prosthetic leaflet impingement (4%) and device embolization (<1%). Prosthetic leaflet impingement is more common in mechanical and stentless prosthesis and in larger occluder devices with overhang. The anterior-superior defects are also prone to device movement once released. Device embolization can be prevented in most cases by ensuring stability of the device by pushing on it using the sheath/catheter while pulling on the delivery cable before releasing it (tug test). The device can be repositioned or changed for a larger device in case of instability.

29. **Answer: D.** Currently, there are no guidelines on the management of residual iASD closure following transseptal intervention. In the MITHRAS (closure of iatrogenic atrial septal defect following transcatheter mitral valve repair) trial, routine closure of iatrogenic ASD post transcatheter mitral valve repair did not result in improved 6-min walk distance or an improvement in mortality/heart failure hospitalization compared with conservative management despite a normalization in Qp:Qs (baseline Qp:Qs ≥ 1.3). Desaturation on room air due to right-to-left or bidirectional shunting is probably the strongest indication to close iASD during the index procedure. In the case of right-to-left shunt or significant bidirectional shunt in a patient with no hypoxia, iASD closure can be considered if there is severe pulmonary hypertension, right ventricle dysfunction, and significant tricuspid regurgitation. A watchful waiting approach can be used for left-to-right shunt.

For the patient in **Case 3**, given significant hypoxia that did not correct by administration of O_2, iASD was closed with a device (▶ **Video 22.14**).

KEY POINTS
- Consider right-to-left shunting if patients develop hypoxia not corrected by the administration of O_2 intraprocedurally.
- Currently, there are no guidelines for the management of residual iASD closure. iASD closure is strongly indicated in patients with right-to-left or bidirectional shunt with hypoxia on room air.

30. **Answer: A.** Theoretically, planimetry of the mitral orifice has the advantage of being a direct measurement of mitral valve area (MVA) and, unlike other methods, does not involve any hypothesis regarding flow conditions, cardiac chamber compliance, or associated valvular lesions. In practice, planimetry has been shown to have the best correlation with anatomical valve area as assessed on explanted valves. For these reasons, planimetry is considered as the reference measurement of MVA. Planimetry is the method of choice to estimate valve area with the caveat that on-axis imaging of the orifice is required. Three-dimensional echocardiography improves the diagnostic accuracy and reproducibility of this measurement.

However, the gain setting should be just sufficient to visualize the whole contour of the mitral orifice. Excessive gain setting may cause underestimation of valve area, especially when leaflet tips are dense or calcified. The optimal timing of the cardiac cycle to measure planimetry is mid-diastole. Percutaneous mitral balloon valvuloplasty is an option for patients with rheumatic MS given the presence of commissural fusion. It is generally not an option for patients with calcific mitral stenosis without commissural fusion.

31. **Answer: C.** The patient in **Case 5** has acute severe mitral regurgitation (MR) (▶ **Video 22.10**), which is a known infrequent complication of mitral balloon valvuloplasty. This results from disruption of the valve integrity, chordal rupture, or leaflet tearing. Calcified leaflets may be at greater risk of tearing. Nanjappa et al in 2012 looked at patients undergoing PBMV and severe MR—anterior leaflet tear was the cause in 72% of patients (▶ **Video 22.15**). Among 3855 patients, acute severe mitral regurgitation (MR) developed in 1.3% of patients. In this patient, the cause of acute severe MR was anterior leaflet tear with eccentric severe MR jet directed posteriorly. The mitral valve (MV) area improved after MV balloon valvuloplasty. However, the large V wave on hemodynamic tracing and persistent elevated mitral gradient with short PHT should raise a suspicion for significant MR. The acute volume overload on the left ventricle (LV) and left atrium (LA) results in pulmonary congestion and low forward cardiac output. The sudden volume overload increases LA and pulmonary venous pressures, leading to pulmonary congestion and hypoxia, whereas decreased blood delivery to the tissues with a concomitant decrease in LV systolic pressure limits the pressure gradient, driving MR to early systole. Thus, the murmur may be short and unimpressive, as may be the color jet of MR.

The tracings show that the patient became hypotensive with large V wave. Intra-aortic balloon counter pulsation can be helpful to treat acute severe MR. By lowering systolic aortic pressure, intra-aortic balloon counter pulsation decreases LV afterload, increasing forward output while decreasing regurgitant volume. Simultaneously, intra-aortic balloon counter pulsation increases diastolic and mean aortic pressures, thereby supporting the systemic circulation. Prompt mitral valve surgery, preferably mitral repair, if possible, is lifesaving in the symptomatic patient with acute severe primary MR. Most patients with acute severe MR require surgical correction for reestablishment of normal hemodynamics and for relief of symptoms.

KEY POINTS

- The development of MR post PMBV is an infrequent but unpredictable event.
- Wilkins score, although useful for patient selection, has been unable to predict the development of severe MR.
- Suspect severe MR in patients who develop hypotension and hypoxia post PMBV. The only form of definitive therapy in these patients is surgery.

32. **Answer: B.** The small focal protrusions of calcium into the left ventricular outflow tract (**Figure 22.22A**, yellow arrows) are unlikely to result in annular rupture, but more likely to result in paravalvular regurgitation (**Figure 22.22B**, between red arrows) from malapposition of the stent with the wall of the LVOT. Treating with postdilatation is often performed and, in this case, resulted in a significant reduction in paravalvular regurgitation seen in **Figure 22.22C**, red arrow. Annular rupture and paravalvular regurgitation are not typically treated with a second valve (valve-in-valve); however, this may be the treatment of choice for severe central aortic regurgitation.

33. **Answer: A.** Evaluating the extent of calcium is an important task of the preintervention TEE or TTE. Because the valve skirt will land in the LVOT, imaging of this part of the landing zone is essential. Given the focal calcium seen in the LVOT (**Figure 22.22A**, yellow arrows), the patient would be at some risk for paravalvular regurgitation although the severity should be mild.

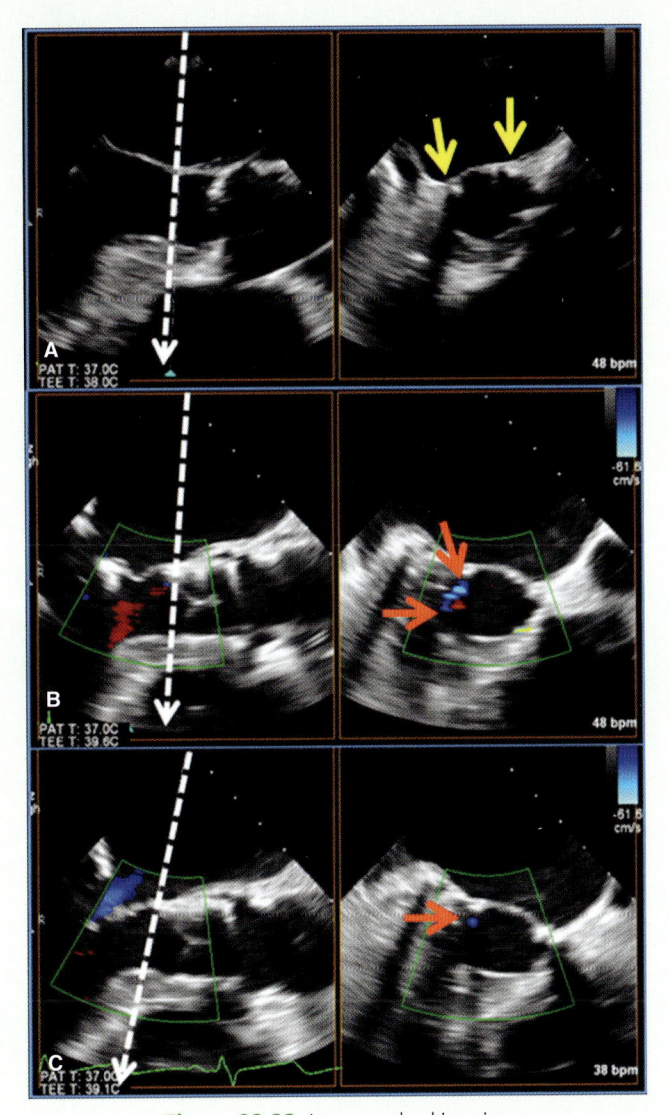

Figure 22.22. Intraprocedural imaging.

KEY POINTS

- Calcification in the LVOT may predict post-TAVI paravalvular regurgitation.
- Imaging the severity of paravalvular regurgitation should be performed below the lowest border of the transcatheter valve (ie, below the skirt of the stented valve) typically in the left ventricular outflow tract and not at the level of the sinuses of Valsalva.
- Although some spontaneous regression may be seen, typically more with the self-expanding valve than the balloon expandable valve, ≥mild regurgitation can be treated with postdilatation.

SUGGESTED READINGS

Alkhouli M, Rihal CS, Holmes DR Jr. Transseptal techniques for emerging structural heart interventions. *JACC Cardiovasc Interv.* 2016;9(24):2465-2480.

American College of Cardiology. *Transcatheter Management of Paravalvular Leaks.* American College of Cardiology; 2017. Accessed October 31, 2019. https://www.acc.org/latest-in-cardiology/articles/2017/02/02/08/25/transcatheter-management-of-paravalvular-leaks

Flint N, Price MJ, Little SH, et al. State of the art: transcatheter edge-to-edge repair for complex mitral regurgitation. *J Am Soc Echocardiogr.* 2021;34(10):1025-1037.

Hahn RT, Kodali SK. State-of-the-art intra-procedural imaging for the mitral and tricuspid PASCAL Repair System. *Eur Heart J Cardiovasc Imaging.* 2022;23(3):e94-e110.

Hahn RT, Kodali S, Tuzcu EM, et al. Echocardiographic imaging of procedural complications during balloon-expandable transcatheter aortic valve replacement. *JACC Cardiovasc Imaging.* 2015;8(3):288-318.

Hahn RT, Nicoara A, Kapadia S, Svensson L, Martin R. Echocardiographic imaging for transcatheter aortic valve replacement. *J Am Soc Echocardiogr.* 2018;31(4):405-433.

Lim DS, Herrmann HC, Grayburn P, et al. Consensus document on non-suitability for transcatheter mitral valve repair by edge-to-edge therapy. *Structural Heart.* 2021;5(3):227-233.

Lurz P, Unterhuber M, Rommel KP, et al. Closure of iatrogenic atrial septal defect after transcatheter mitral valve repair: the randomized MITHRAS trial. *Circulation.* 2021;143(3):292-294.

Otto CM, Nishimura RA, Bonow RO, et al. 2020 ACC/AHA guideline for the management of patients with valvular heart disease: a report of the American College of Cardiology/American Heart Association Joint Committee on clinical practice guidelines [published correction appears in Circulation. 2021 Feb 2;143(5):e229]. *Circulation.* 2021;143(5):e72-e227.

Pibarot P, Herrmann HC, Wu C, et al. Standardized definitions for bioprosthetic valve dysfunction following aortic or mitral valve replacement: JACC state-of-the-art review. *J Am Coll Cardiol.* 2022;80(5):545-561.

Ribeiro HB, Nombela-Franco L, Urena M, et al. Coronary obstruction following transcatheter aortic valve implantation: a systematic review. *JACC Cardiovasc Interv.* 2013;6(5):452-461.

Zoghbi WA, Asch FM, Bruce C, et al. Guidelines for the evaluation of valvular regurgitation after percutaneous valve repair or replacement: a report from the American Society of Echocardiography developed in collaboration with the Society for Cardiovascular angiography and interventions, Japanese Society of Echocardiography, and Society for Cardiovascular Magnetic Resonance [published correction appears in J Am Soc Echocardiogr. 2019 Jul;32(7):914-917]. *J Am Soc Echocardiogr.* 2019;32(4):431-475.

CHAPTER 23

Interventional Echocardiography: Tricuspid Valve, Septum, Left Atrial Appendage, and Hypertrophic Cardiomyopathy

Nishath Quader

QUESTIONS

1. Which of the following is an exclusion for left atrial appendage (LAA) occlusion?
   A. Contraindication for oral anticoagulant therapy.
   B. Valvular atrial fibrillation (AF).
   C. Nonvalvular AF.
   D. $CHA_2DS_2\text{-}VAS_C \geq 1$.

2. Which of the following statements about the $CHA_2DS_2\text{-}VAS_C$ score is **TRUE**?
   A. The $CHA_2DS_2\text{-}VAS_C$ score is a clinical prediction score for estimating the risk of stroke in valvular AF.
   B. The C in $CHA_2DS_2\text{-}VAS_C$ stands for Coumadin.
   C. The S_2 in $CHA_2DS_2\text{-}VAS_C$ stands for prior stroke and high systolic blood pressure.
   D. $CHA_2DS_2\text{-}VAS_C$ score of 2 or greater warrants anticoagulation with either warfarin or a novel oral anticoagulant (NOAC).

3. Which of the following is the most common potential complication of percutaneous LAA occlusion device?
   A. Major bleeding.
   B. Device embolization.
   C. Serious pericardial effusion.
   D. Ischemic stroke.

4. In obstructive hypertrophic cardiomyopathy (HCM), the LVOT gradient influences treatment decisions. Which of the following statements is **TRUE** regarding the LVOT gradient?
   A. LVOT obstruction refers to a mean LV outflow gradient of ≥30 mm Hg.
   B. LVOT obstruction refers to a peak instantaneous LV outflow gradient of ≥30 mm Hg.
   C. Dobutamine may be used to provoke a higher LVOT gradient.
   D. Only symptomatic patients with resting (not provocable) LVOT gradients of ≥50 mm Hg are candidates for intervention.

5. Alcohol septal ablation (ASA) is an alternative to surgery when medical therapy is unsuccessful. Which of the following statements regarding ASA is **TRUE**?
   A. ASA should be considered in symptomatic patients with very severe hypertrophy (septal thickness >30 mm).
   B. Successful ASA is defined by a reduction of the LVOT gradient by at least 30%.
   C. Myocardial contrast echocardiography improves the likelihood of a successful ASA.
   D. Following injection of alcohol, the septum thickens but has reduced excursion.

478 / Clinical Echocardiography Review

6. Which of the following is **NOT** a complication of ASA?
   A. Ventricular septal defect.
   B. Atrial arrhythmia.
   C. Complete heart block.
   D. Death.

7. It is clinically important to distinguish between the obstructive and nonobstructive forms of HCM because management strategies are largely dependent on the presence or absence of symptoms caused by obstruction. Which of the following images in **Figure 23.1** represents flow across the LVOT of a patient with dynamic outflow obstruction?
   A. A.
   B. B.
   C. C.
   D. D.

8. Dilute myocardial contrast is injected into the target septal perforator of four different patients with hypertrophic obstructive cardiomyopathy. Which of the following contrast images in **Figure 23.2** would be consistent with a post-alcohol ablation, large troponin leak, and development of a bundle branch block?
   A. A.
   B. B.
   C. C.
   D. D.

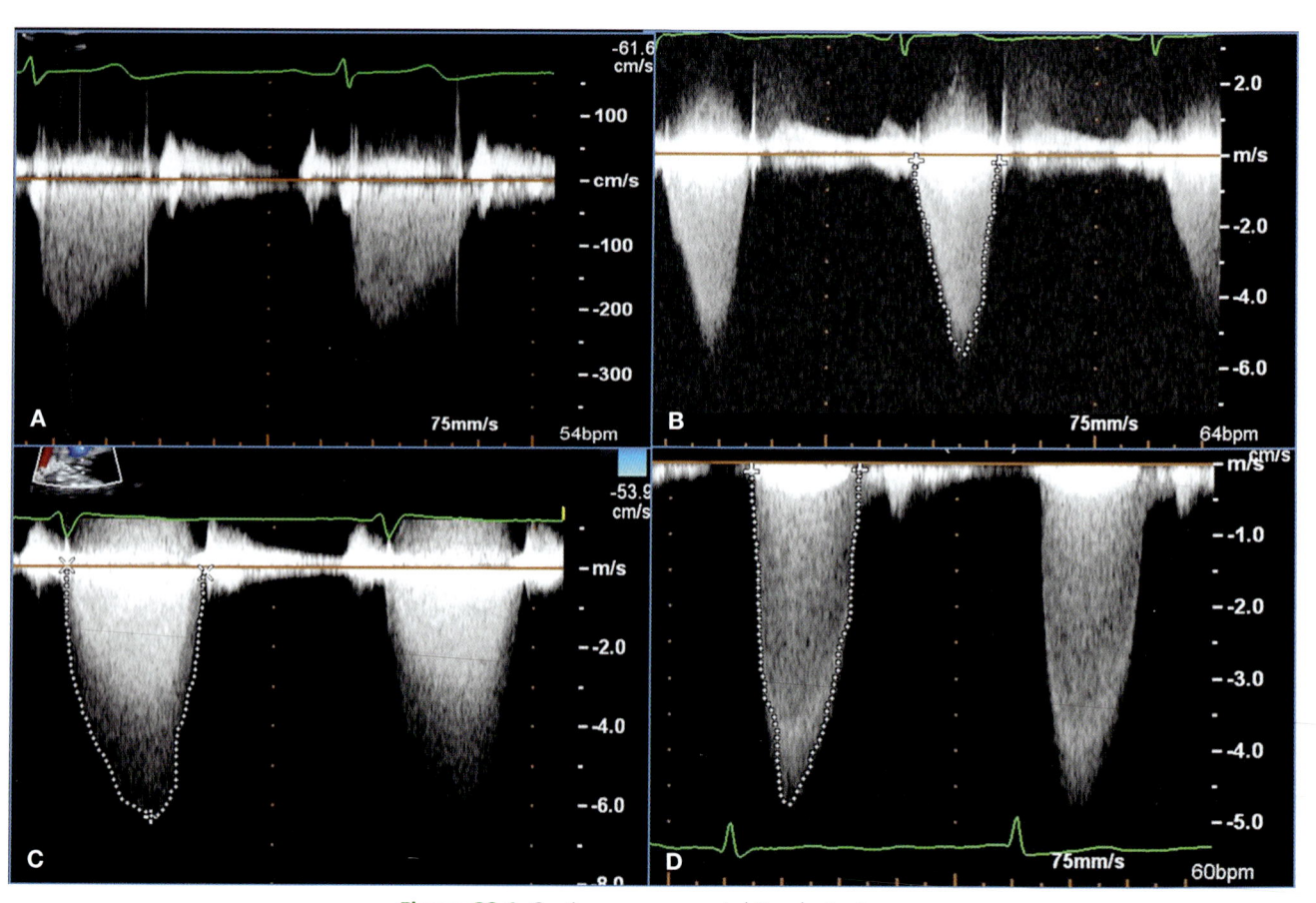

Figure 23.1. Continuous-wave spectral Doppler tracings.

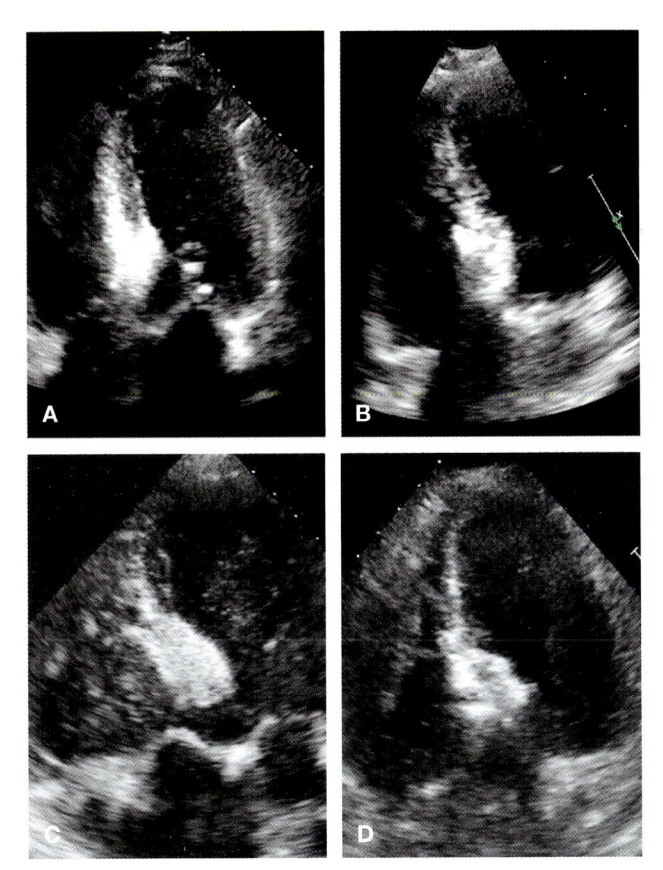

Figure 23.2. Four cases of hypertrophic cardiomyopathy are shown with intraprocedural transthoracic echocardiographic imaging following contrast injection into the septal perforator artery.

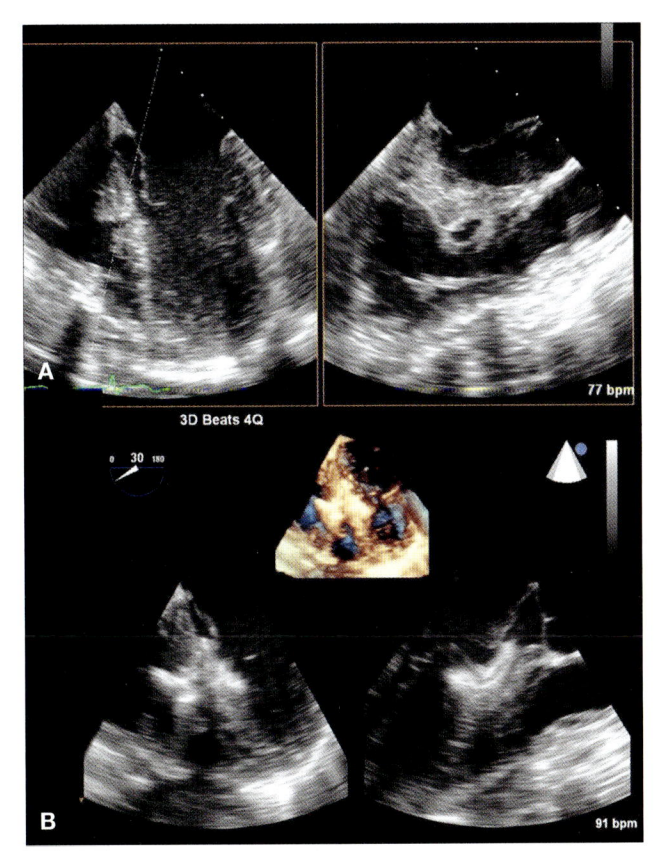

Figure 23.3. Simultaneous multiplane imaging performed at baseline (**A**) and following an emergency procedure (**B**).

9. A 17-year-old boy with no significant medical history was stabbed in the chest and abdomen and underwent left thoracotomy with decompression of the pericardium and repair of a 1-cm right ventricular laceration. The patient continued to have evidence of heart failure and was transferred to your hospital where an emergent TEE revealed the image in **Figure 23.3A**. A procedure was subsequently performed, shown in **Figure 23.3B**. What was missed at the outside hospital (**Figure 23.3A**) and what procedure was performed (**Figure 23.3B**)?
   A. Congenital anomaly of the atrial septum; atrial septal defect closure device placed.
   B. Acute myocardial infarction from transection of the right coronary artery (RCA); RCA stent placed.
   C. Traumatic ventricular septal defect (VSD); VSD closure device placed.
   D. Severe myxomatous mitral valve disease; MitraClip placed.

CASE 1

*A 76-year-old patient with a history of prior stroke, congestive heart failure, hypertension, and diabetes presented with atrial fibrillation on warfarin and a recent gastrointestinal bleed requiring transfusion with 2 units of packed red blood cells. An intracardiac LAA closure was performed (**Figure 23.4**; ▶ Videos 23.1 and 23.2).*

10. Given the initial transseptal catheter shown in **Case 1** (**Figure 23.4A**, ▶ Video 23.1), what is the likely position of the intracardiac LAA occlusion device (in this instance, a Watchman device)?
    A. The LAA closure device will be anterosuperiorly directed.
    B. The LAA closure device will be anteroinferiorly directed.
    C. The LAA closure device will be posteroinferiorly directed.
    D. The LAA closure device will be properly directed along the long axis of the appendage.

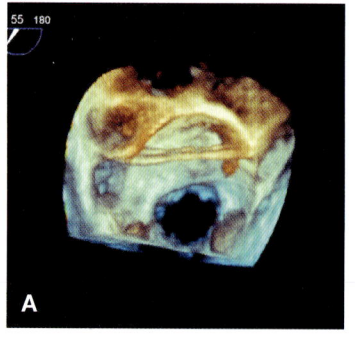

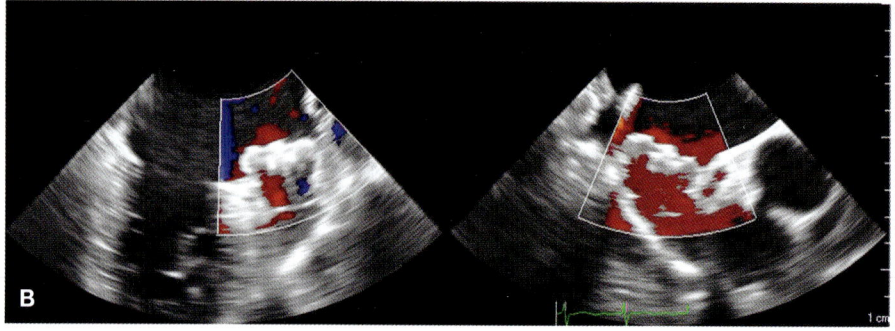

Figure 23.4. Three-dimensional image of the transseptal puncture performed for the LAA closure device (**A**, ▶ Video 23.1) and the 45-day postprocedural follow-up TEE image (**B**, ▶ Video 23.2).

11. Given the 45-day follow-up study of the LAA closure device from the patient in **Case 1** (**Figure 23.4B**, ▶ **Video 23.2**), what would you recommend?
    A. Discontinue warfarin and repeat study at 6-month follow-up.
    B. Discontinue warfarin and begin aspirin and Plavix.
    C. Begin a novel oral anticoagulant.
    D. Continue Coumadin.

12. An 89-year-old woman with atrial fibrillation presents to valve clinic for increasing shortness of breath, fatigue, LE edema, and abdominal bloating. Her TTE reveals severe TR along with a flail leaflet (**Figure 23.5**; ▶ **Video 23.3**):
    Which of the leaflets as indicated by the red arrow is involved?
    A. Anterior.
    B. Posterior.
    C. Septal.
    D. Central.

13. Which of the following is **NOT TRUE** regarding TEE imaging of the tricuspid valve?
    A. Tricuspid valve leaflets are thinner than mitral valve leaflets.
    B. Deep esophageal and gastric views of the tricuspid valve are equivalent to mid-esophageal views.
    C. Because of the location of the tricuspid valve, lateral resolution is essential to imaging.
    D. The larger annular size of the tricuspid valve makes imaging from a mid-esophageal view challenging.

14. Which of the following leaflets noted by the *red arrow* is demonstrated in the following TTE images (**Figure 23.6** and ▶ **Video 23.4**)?
    A. Anterior.
    B. Septal.
    C. Posterior.
    D. Atrial.

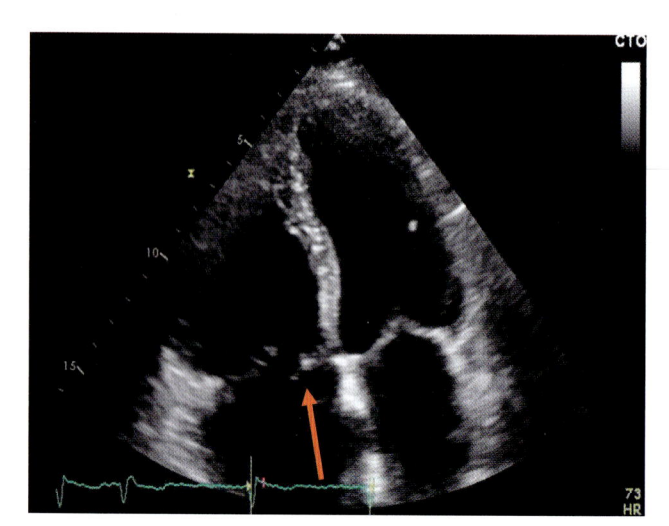

Figure 23.5

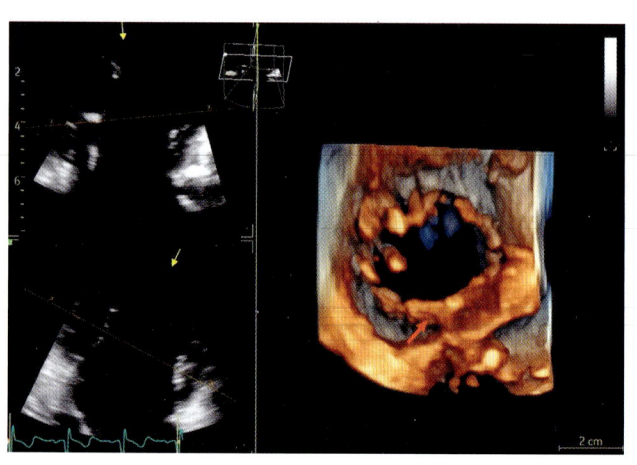

Figure 23.6

Chapter 23 Interventional Echocardiography: Tricuspid Valve, Septum, LAA, and HCM / 481

15. Which tricuspid valve leaflets denoted by an *arrow* is demonstrated in the deep esophageal views (**Figure 23.7** and ▶ **Video 23.5**)?
    A. Septal.
    B. Anterior.
    C. Posterior.
    D. Aortic.

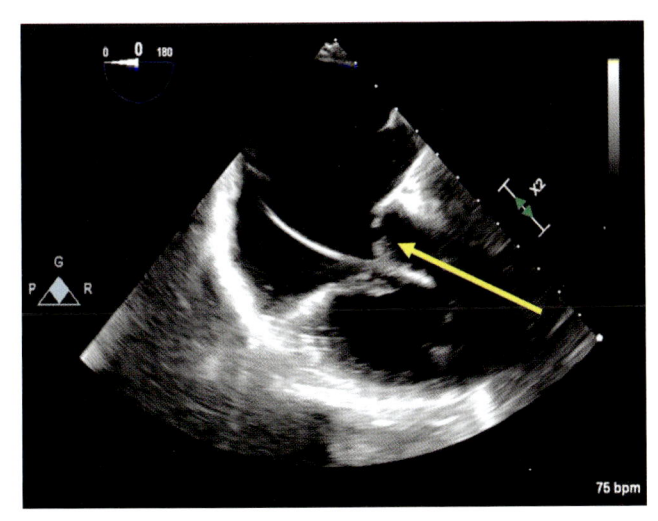

Figure 23.7

16. A 60-year-old woman presents to her cardiologist for evaluation of dyspnea, abdominal bloating, and lower extremity edema. Her echocardiograms reveal severe TR; further imaging with TEE reveals thickening of valve leaflets and commissural shortening/thickening and fusion of chordae tendineae. What is the etiology of this patient's tricuspid regurgitation?
    A. Rheumatic disease.
    B. Carcinoid.
    C. Infective endocarditis.
    D. Congenital disease.

17. A 70-year-old man presents with tricuspid regurgitation where his tricuspid regurgitation is quantified as having an EROA of 50 mm² with vena contracta of 10 mm. How would the severity of his tricuspid regurgitation be graded?
    A. Moderate.
    B. Severe.
    C. Massive.
    D. Torrential.

18. Which of the tricuspid valve leaflets is noted by the arrow in this transesophageal echocardiography view (**Figure 23.8** and ▶ **Video 23.6**)?
    A. Anterior.
    B. Septal.
    C. Posterior.

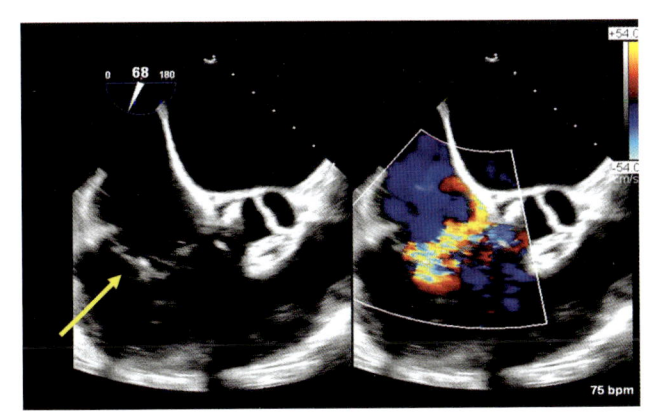

Figure 23.8

19. Which of the following is not a TEE multiplane angle utilized when assessing patients for percutaneous left atrial appendage occlusion devices?
    A. 0°.
    B. 90°.
    C. 60°.
    D. 135°.

20. Which of the following LAA morphologies is represented in the following (**Figure 23.9**)?
    A. Windsock.
    B. Chicken wing.
    C. Broccoli.
    D. Cactus.

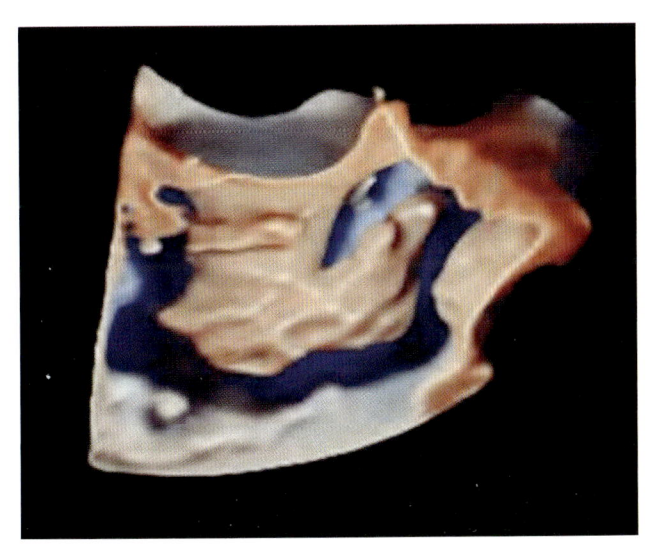

Figure 23.9

21. A 50-year-old obese man undergoes a TEE prior to cardioversion for atrial fibrillation. What is the structure labeled in the ▶ **Video 23.7** and **Figure 23.10** most commonly known as?
A. Atrial myxoma.
B. Lipomatous hypertrophy.
C. Atrial septal closure device.
D. Rhabdomyoma.

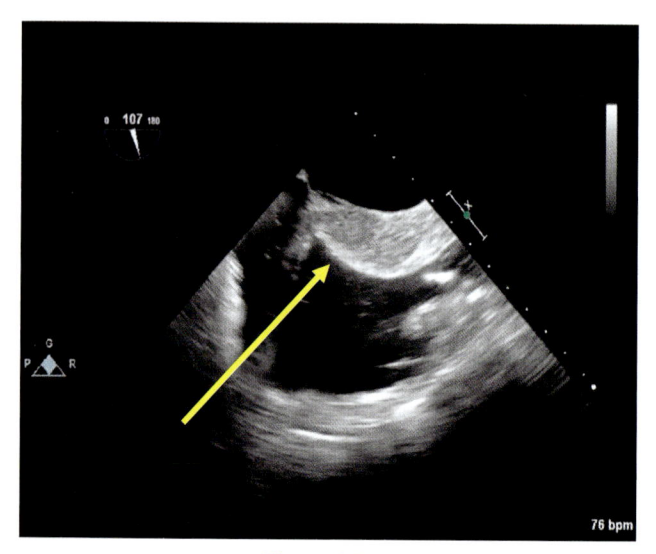

Figure 23.10

22. A 21-year-old man presents with migraine. His transthoracic echocardiogram demonstrates a positive agitated saline study consistent with a patent foramen ovale. He then undergoes a TEE. Name the mobile structure in the RA (arrow) in the following figure/video (**Figure 23.11**; ▶ **Video 23.8**):
A. Bacterial vegetation
B. Thrombus
C. Chiari network
D. Lambl excrescence

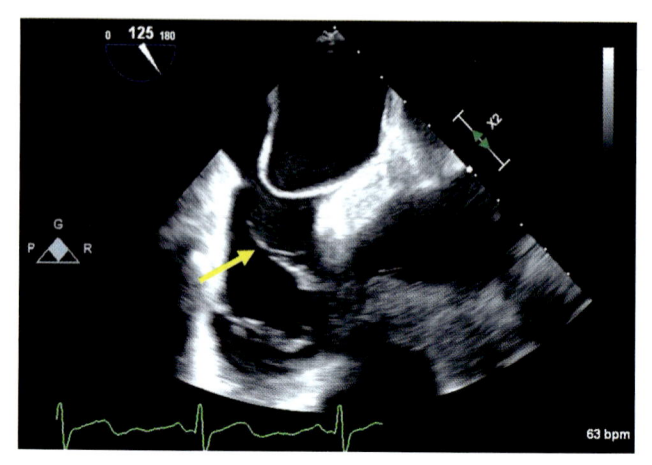

Figure 23.11

23. A 19-year-old woman presents to her cardiologist for evaluation of shortness of breath. Transthoracic echocardiogram reveals right ventricular enlargement. A TEE reveals an atrial septal defect. Which of these atrial septal defects can be successfully closed percutaneously?
A. Primum ASD.
B. Secundum ASD.
C. AV canal defect.
D. Fenestrated septal defect.

24. A 56-year-old woman presents to her cardiologist with chest pain. Her transthoracic echocardiogram reveals RV enlargement. An agitated saline study demonstrates right-to-left shunting with Valsalva. Her TEE reveals the following as indicated by the yellow arrow (**Figure 23.12** and ▶ **Video 23.9**). Select the **BEST** term that describes the finding.
A. Primum ASD.
B. Secundum ASD.
C. AV canal defect.
D. Patent foramen ovale.

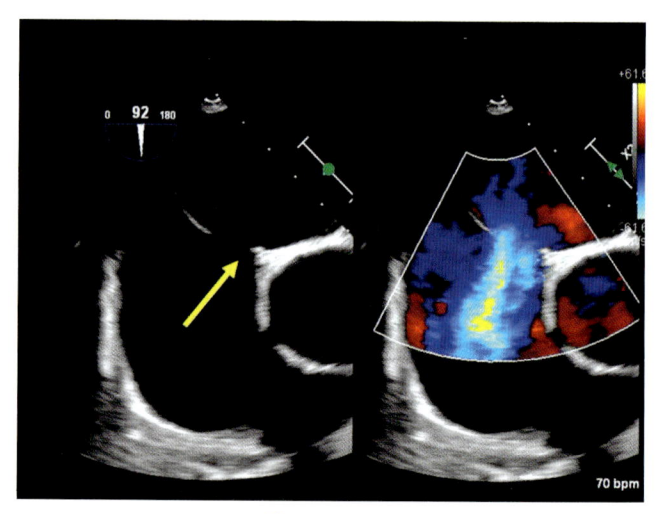

Figure 23.12

25. Which of the following would be an indication to close a secundum ASD percutaneously?
A. Shunt study with Q_p/Q_s of 1.2.
B. Right ventricular enlargement.
C. Anterior rim of 4 mm.
D. Severe irreversible pulmonary hypertension.

26. Which of the following is most likely **NOT** associated with the abnormality seen in the following video (**Figure 23.13**; ▶ Video 23.10)?
    A. RV enlargement.
    B. Anomalous pulmonary vein.
    C. Sinus venosus defect.
    D. Secundum atrial septal defect.

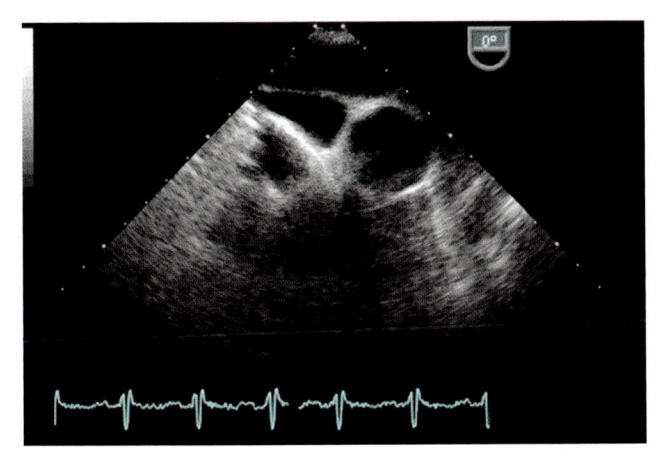

Figure 23.13

27. A 50-year-old man presents with progressive shortness of breath. His cardiac auscultation reveals a loud systolic murmur. He undergoes a TTE and eventually a TEE. Which of the following is represented in the accompanying M-mode image (**Figure 23.14**)?
    A. Aortic stenosis.
    B. Mitral valve prolapse.
    C. Systolic anterior motion of mitral valve.
    D. Mid-systolic closure of the aortic valve.

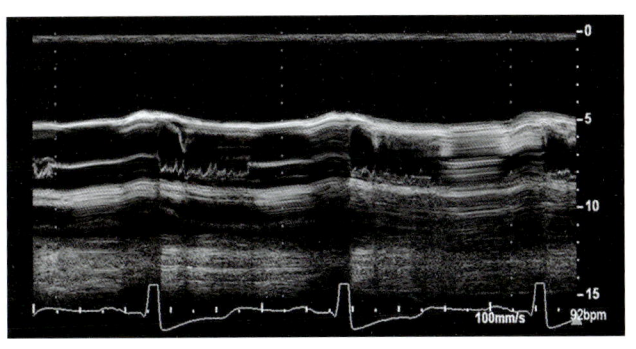

Figure 23.14

28. Based on the findings in **Question 27**, what is the most likely diagnosis?
    A. Aortic stenosis.
    B. Barlow mitral valve.
    C. Hypertrophic cardiomyopathy.
    D. Aortic regurgitation.

29. A 50-year-old man presents to the emergency department with chest pain. His ECG reveals the following (**Figure 23.15**):
    His troponin is mildly elevated. His transthoracic echocardiography reveals the following (**Figure 23.16**; ▶ Video 23.11):
    What is the likely diagnosis?
    A. Apical hypertrophy cardiomyopathy.
    B. Takotsubo cardiomyopathy.
    C. Eosinophilic cardiomyopathy.
    D. Coronary disease and ischemia.

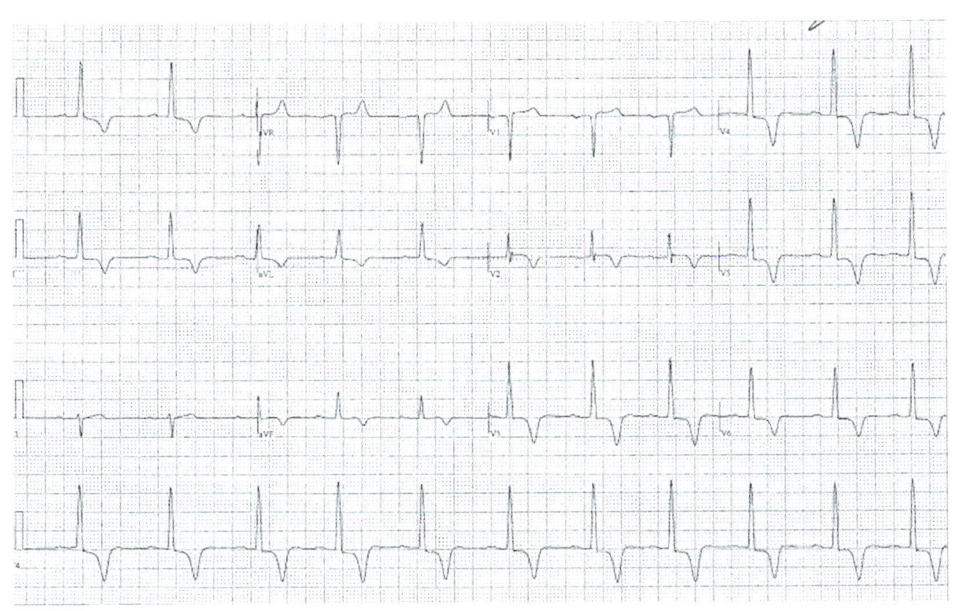

Figure 23.15

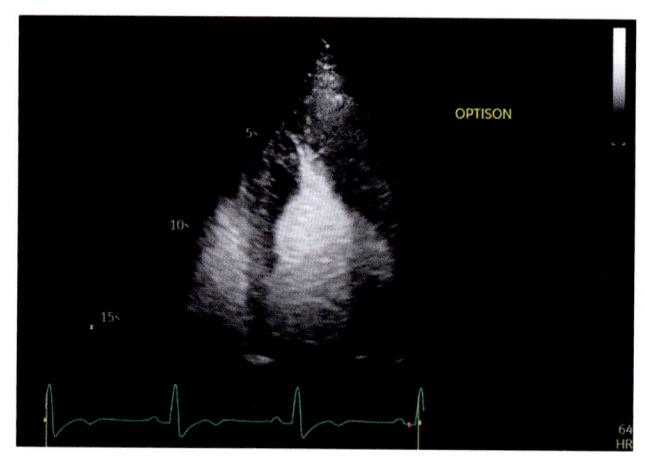

Figure 23.16

30. Which of the following is **NOT TRUE** about atrial septal aneurysms (ASA)?
    A. ASA have been associated with PFOs.
    B. ASA is defined as an excursion of 15 mm from the plane of the atrial septum into the RA or LA.
    C. ASA is defined as a combined total excursion right and left of 15 mm.
    D. ASA has been associated with multiple septal fenestrations.

31. An 89-year-old man with a history of DM, TIA, and atrial fibrillation is undergoing percutaneous LAA occlusion evaluation. Which of the statements is **TRUE** regarding sizing of the left atrial appendage to assess for occlusion devices?
    A. Computed tomography is exclusively utilized for sizing of the LAA.
    B. 2D TEE sizing is comparable to CT sizing.
    C. 3D TEE sizing generally is larger than 2D sizing.
    D. Intracardiac echo is frequently utilized in sizing the LAA.

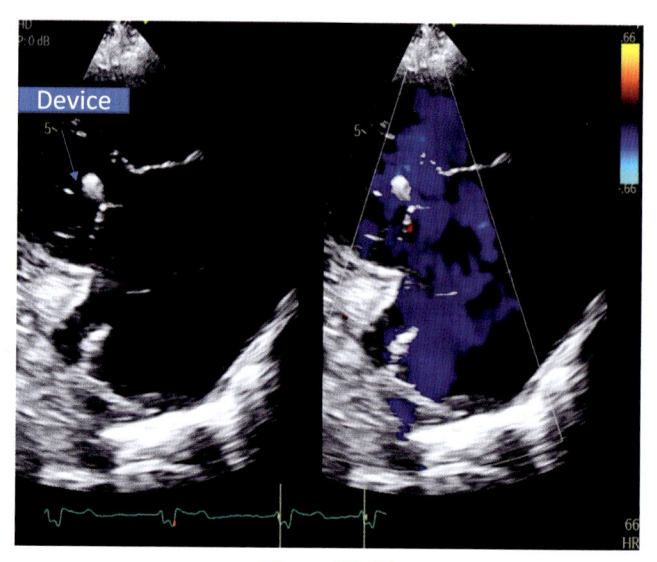

Figure 23.17

32. An 89-year-old man undergoes transcatheter edge-to-edge repair of the tricuspid valve resulting in reduction of tricuspid regurgitation from torrential to severe. His postoperative TTE images are demonstrated in **Figure 23.17** and ▶ **Video 23.12**.
    Which of the tricuspid valve leaflets is freely mobile?
    A. Anterior.
    B. Septal.
    C. Posterior.
    D. Difficult to ascertain from the image provided.

33. Which of the following is not a complication of percutaneous membranous VSD closure?
    A. Tricuspid regurgitation.
    B. Aortic regurgitation.
    C. Mitral regurgitation.
    D. Complete heart block.

34. A 74-year-old man presents for evaluation of his tricuspid regurgitation (**Figure 23.18**, ▶ Video **23.13**). Which of the following is **NOT TRUE** regarding cardiac implantable electronic device (CIED)-induced tricuspid regurgitation?
   A. In CIED-induced TR, the TR color Doppler jet is higher than the coaptation point of the TV leaflets.
   B. The CIED appears to move with or attached to the leaflet.
   C. Both 2D and 3D views are needed to localize which leaflet is affected by the CIED.
   D. In the parasternal short, if a single leaflet is visualized being impinged by the CIED, it is likely the posterior leaflet.

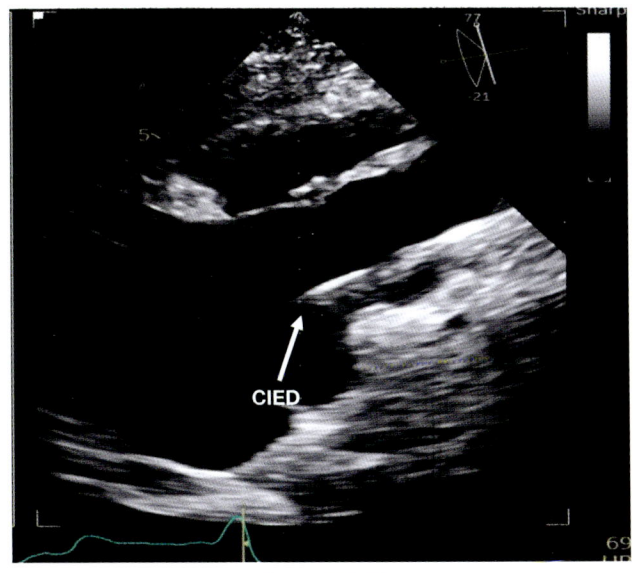

Figure 23.18

ANSWERS

1. **Answer: B.** To date no studies have examined LAA closure in valvular AF and therefore this is not an indication. See the answer to Question 2 for a definition of the CHA$_2$DS$_2$VAS$_c$ score.

2. **Answer: D.** The CHA$_2$DS$_2$-VAS$_c$ score is a clinical prediction rule for estimating the risk of stroke in patients with nonvalvular atrial fibrillation with the acronym standing for C: congestive heart failure (1 point); H: hypertension (1 point); A: age > 75 (2 points); D: diabetes (1 point); S: stroke (2 points); V: vascular disease (1 point); A: age 65 to 74 (1 point); S$_c$: sex category—female (1 point).
   Oral anticoagulation is recommended for CHA$_2$DS$_2$-VAS$_c$ score of 2 or greater.

3. **Answer: C.** In the PROTECT AF trial, 707 patients were randomized to LAA closure with the Watchman device and subsequent discontinuation of warfarin, or warfarin standard therapy. The most frequent primary safety event in the intervention group was serious pericardial effusion (defined as the need for percutaneous or surgical drainage), which occurred in 22 (4.8%) patients. Fifteen of these patients were treated with pericardiocentesis and seven underwent surgical intervention. Other complications included major bleeding in 3.5%, procedure-related ischemic stroke in 1.1%, and device embolization in 0.6%.

4. **Answer: B.** The definition of LVOT obstruction refers to a peak instantaneous LV outflow gradient of ≥30 mm Hg. LVOT gradients of ≥50 mm Hg, either at rest or with provocation, meet the conventional threshold for surgical or percutaneous intervention assuming symptoms cannot be controlled with medications. If the resting outflow gradient is <50 mm Hg, provocative measures may be used to elicit higher gradients. However, dobutamine is no longer recommended as a provocative test as per the ACCF/AHA guidelines. Provocation of a higher gradient may be accomplished with exercise, the strain phase of the Valsalva maneuver and isoproterenol in the cardiac catheterization laboratory.

5. **Answer: C.** The effectiveness of ASA is uncertain with marked HCM (>30 mm) and is generally discouraged in these patients. Successful ASA is defined by a reduction of the LVOT gradient by at least 50%. Myocardial contrast echocardiography has become an important addition to the ASA procedure to identify the vascular distribution of the individual perforator branches, shorten intervention time, reduce infarct size, reduce the likelihood of heart block, and improve the likelihood of success. Following injection of alcohol, the septum thins and has reduced excursion.

6. **Answer: B.** Excluding high-grade atrioventricular block, nonfatal complications occur in 2% to 3% of cases (in experienced centers). Ventricular septal defect is more likely with a septal thickness of <15 mm. Approximately 5% of patients have sustained ventricular tachyarrhythmias during hospitalization for septal ablation with an inhospital mortality rate of up to 2%. Transient heart block occurs in approximately half of patients undergoing alcohol septal ablation. Persistent complete heart block prompting implantation of a permanent pacemaker occurs in 10% to 20% depending on baseline conduction. Although atrial arrhythmias are common with obstructive HCM, they are not a result of ASA.

7. **Answer: B.** Panel A is a continuous-wave Doppler across the tricuspid valve. Panel C is the continuous-wave Doppler across the mitral valve of a patient with obstructive HCM; note the relatively delayed systolic flow pattern since regurgitation occurs secondary to malcoaptation of the leaflets with systolic anterior motion. Panel D is the continuous-wave Doppler across the aortic valve in the setting of a valvular aortic stenosis with rapid generation of a pressure gradient. The concave-to-the-left contour of panel B is the key to making the diagnosis of a dynamic outflow obstruction.

8. **Answer: C.** Contrast injection is used to identify the myocardium supplied by the septal perforator. The larger the volume of muscle supplied, the larger the controlled infarction. **Figure 23.2C** shows the largest region of myocardium supplied by the septal perforator and thus the greatest myocardium at risk for infarction following alcohol injection; this patient also developed a bundle branch block during the procedure. It is important to document the absence of perfusion of myocardial segments remote from the targeted areas for ablation, including the left ventricular anterior wall, right ventricular (RV) free wall, and papillary muscles. Perfusion of these regions may result in cessation of the procedure.

9. **Answer: C.** The *red arrows* **Figure 23.19** point to the knife blade–shaped defect in the muscular ventricular septum that was missed during the initial open heart repair of the right ventricular free wall laceration. Because of extensive blood loss and unstable clinical condition, a transcatheter VSD device was placed under echocardiographic guidance. Imaging is essential for the following reasons: facilitates device selection by allowing accurate assessment of morphology of frequently irregularly shaped defects; allows precise anatomic localization of thin wires and enhances device visualization during positioning and deployment; and allows assessment of potential complications such as device malpositioning, residual shunt, and impingement on surrounding structure (valves).

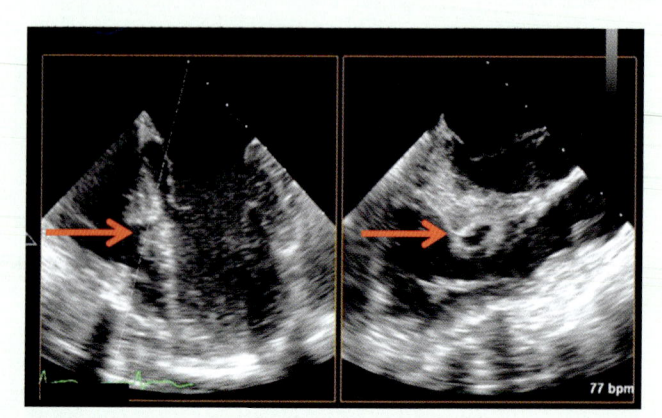

Figure 23.19. The knife blade–shaped defect in the muscular ventricular septum (red arrows).

10. **Answer: A.** The LAA orifice or os typically faces posterior and inferior with the body of the appendage directed anterior, lateral, and superior. Transseptal punctures for the LAA closure device thus should be inferior and posterior in the fossa ovalis, to direct the catheter anterior, lateral, and superior, thus aligning the device with the long axis of the LAA. This transseptal puncture was too anterior and superior. Thus the device will point superior to the LAA orifice. With correct sizing and position, the Watchman device surface should sit at the plane of the LAA orifice as in **Figure 23.20** (▶ **Video 23.14**).

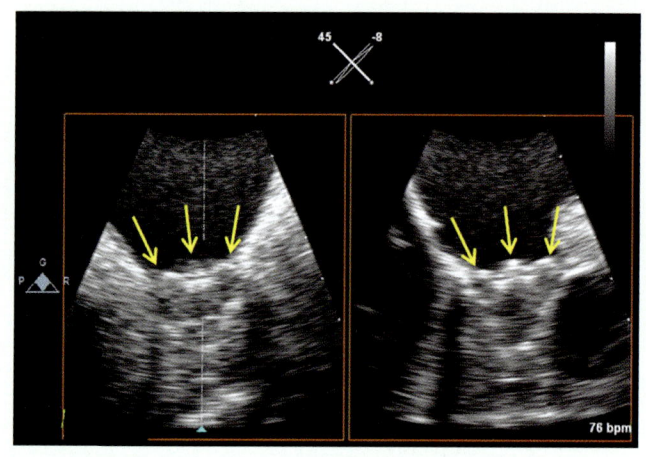

Figure 23.20. Well-positioned Watchman device with surface of the device at the LAA orifice (yellow arrows) (▶ **Video 23.14**).

11. **Answer: D.** The patient has multiple small residual peri-device leaks (**Figure 23.21**, *yellow arrows*) and the inferior edge of the permeable polyester fabric cover sits above the LAA orifice with residual flow into the LAA and underneath the device. Thrombus has developed under the Watchman device in the setting of malpositioning (anterosuperiorly directed). This is an unusual complication of a malpositioned device and the best course would be to continue warfarin and repeat the TEE in 6 months to assess for endothelialization and resolution of the peri-device leaks. Novel oral anticoagulants have an unclear role in patients already with an LAA device.

> **KEY POINTS**
> - For LAA closure, the location of septal puncture is important for optimal positioning of the device.
> - Suboptimal positioning of a LAA closure may contribute to peri-device leak.

12. **Answer: C.** The accompanying image (**Figure 23.22A,B**) shows a transthoracic echocardiogram (TTE) and an apical 4-chamber view. The *red arrow* in **Figure 23.5** indicates the septal leaflet. In **Figure 23.22A,B**, one can visualize the septal leaflet (yellow). The opposing leaflet could be anterior or posterior (red leaflet).

Chapter 23 Interventional Echocardiography: Tricuspid Valve, Septum, LAA, and HCM / **487**

Figure 23.21. The 45-day follow-up study of the LAA closure device with peri-device leak seen (*yellow arrows*).

However, angulation of the probe so that the LVOT is visualized can bring in the anterior leaflet (blue leaflet, **Figure 23.22C**). Angulation of the probe toward the coronary sinus can bring in the posterior leaflet (green leaflet, **Figure 23.22D**). The image provided demonstrates a flail septal leaflet. In the apical 4-chamber view, the septal leaflet is closest to the septum. Angulation of the probe is then needed to determine anterior and posterior leaflets, which are located on the RV free wall.

13. **Answer: B.** Deep esophageal views of the tricuspid valve are not equivalent to mid-esophageal views. The TV is positioned immediately superior to the diaphragm and is very close to the TEE probe in the deep esophageal and transgastric views. Thus, these views can provide superior visualization of the TV compared to the mid-esophageal views. The other choices are all true; the TV leaflets are thinner than the mitral leaflets. This makes imaging these leaflets more challenging. In addition, because the annular plane cannot be aligned perpendicular to the ultrasound beam, there is increased reliance on lateral resolution to image the TV. The tricuspid valve annulus is also 20% larger and less symmetric than the mitral valve.

14. **Answer: B.** 3D imaging of the TV using TTE demonstrates that the septal leaflet is adjacent the interatrial septum and the mitral valve. When viewing the TV from the right ventricular aspect, the anterior leaflet is adjacent to the aortic valve and the posterior leaflet that is positioned close to the free wall. The anterior tricuspid leaflet is located by the aortic valve. The septal leaflet is closer to the septum/mitral valve (see **Figure 23.23A** and **B**).

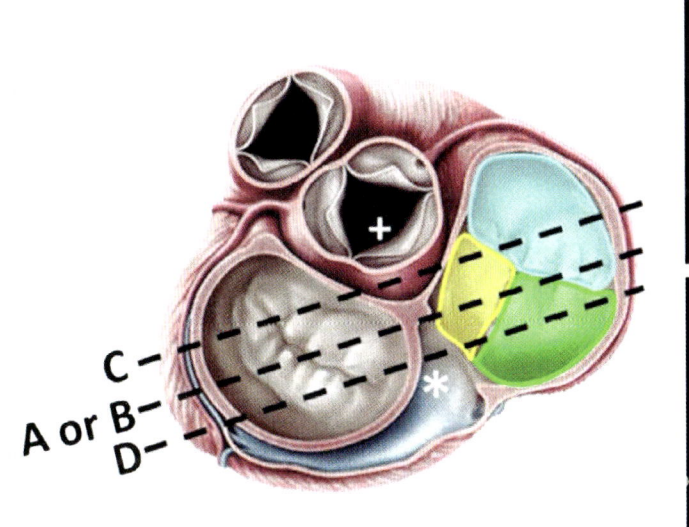

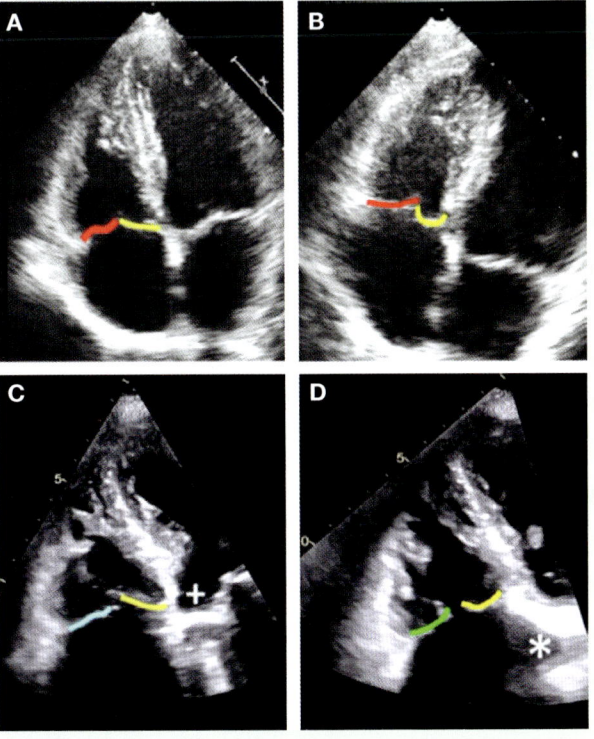

Figure 23.22. +, left ventricular outflow tract; *, coronary sinus. (Reprinted with permission from Hahn RT. State-of-the-art review of echocardiographic imaging in the evaluation and treatment of functional tricuspid regurgitation. *Circ Cardiovasc Imaging*. 2016;9(12):e005332. Figure 3. Copyright © 2016 American Heart Association, Inc.)

488 / Clinical Echocardiography Review

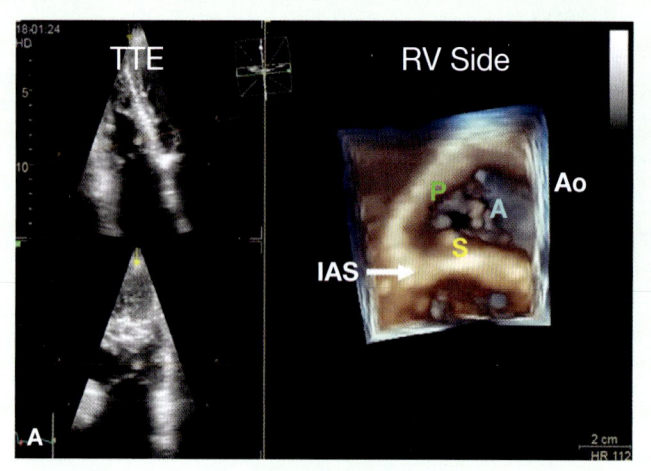

Figure 23.23A

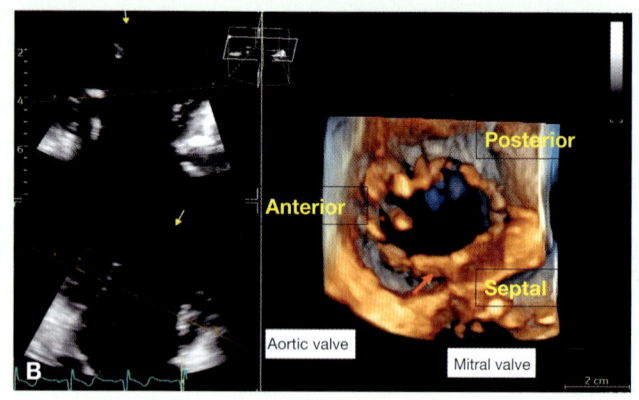

Figure 23.23B

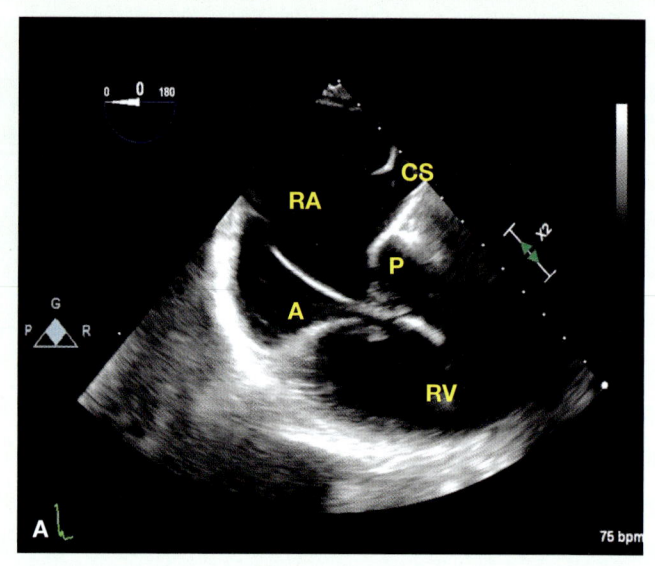

Figure 23.24A

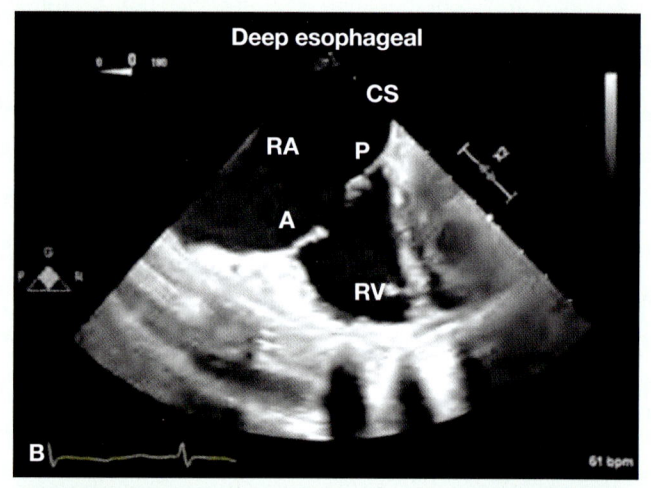

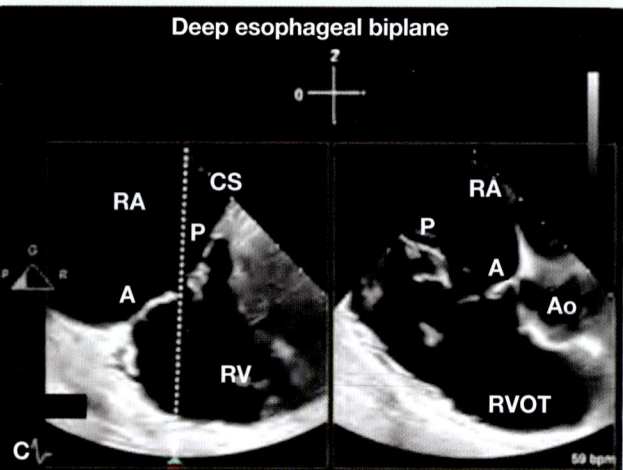

Figure 23.24B,C. Reprinted from Hahn RT, Saric M, Faletra FF, et al. Recommended standards for the performance of transesophageal echocardiographic screening for structural heart intervention: from the American Society of Echocardiography. *J Am Soc Echocardiogr*. 2022;35(1):1-76. Copyright © 2021 by the American Society of Echocardiography. With permission.

15. **Answer: C.** From the deep esophageal views (**Figure 23.24A**), which are closer to the diaphragm, imaging of the tricuspid valve can provide superior views of the leaflets. In this view, with the coronary sinus (CS) visualized, one can assess the posterior leaflet (P) closer to the CS and the anterior leaflet (A) closer to the right ventricular (RV) free wall. Also visualized is a pacemaker wire in the right atrium (RA) and RV. **Figure 23.24B** and **C** again demonstrates the posterior tricuspid leaflet visualized close to the coronary sinus and the anterior leaflet closer to the RV free wall. In TEE imaging, deep esophageal views showing the coronary sinus provide visualization of the posterior tricuspid leaflet.

16. **Answer: A.** Rheumatic involvement of the TV is like what occurs with rheumatic involvement of the mitral valve. There is fibrous thickening of the valve leaflets with fusion of the commissures and thickening, shortening, and fusion of the chordae tendinae. Involvement of the tricuspid valve occurs mostly with involvement of the mitral valve. In carcinoid involvement of the TV, there is deposition of fibrous tissue on the endocardial surface leading to

thickening and retraction of the leaflets and subvalvular apparatus. The leaflets then become fixed in a semiopen position leading to stenosis and regurgitation. Carcinoid disease can involve the mitral valve, but it predominantly affects the tricuspid valve.

17. **Answer: B.** The ASE valve regurgitation guidelines outline several qualitative, semiquantitative, and quantitative ways to grade the severity of TR (**Table 23.1**). These grades can further be broken down into various categories including the term massive and torrential (**Figure 23.25**). Based on the two tables, a vena contracta of 10 mm and EROA of 50 mm² would fall under the severe category.

18. **Answer: C.** Imaging of the tricuspid valve at the 50° to 80° view with the aortic valve visualized demonstrates the anterior leaflet close to the aortic valve and the posterior leaflet closer to the RV free wall (**Figure 23.26**). Biplane imaging shows the septal leaflet; when the biplane cursor is placed on the anterior leaflet, the septal and anterior leaflet is visualized. When the cursor is moved to the posterior leaflet, the septal and posterior leaflets are visualized.

Table 23.1. Summary of the American Society of Echocardiography Recommendations for Grading Severity of TR

TR Severity	Mild	Moderate	Severe
Structural	Bolded signs are considered specific for their TR grade		
TV morphology	Normal or mildly abnormal leaflets	Moderately abnormal leaflets	Severe valve lesions (eg, flail leaflet, severe retraction, large perforation)
RV and RA size	Usually normal	Normal or mild dilation	Usually dilated[a]
Inferior vena cava diameter	Normal <2 cm	Normal or mildly dilated 2.1-2.5 cm	Dilated >2.5 cm
Qualitative Doppler	Bolded signs are considered specific for their TR grade		
Color flow jet area[b]	Small, narrow, central	Moderate central	Large central jet or eccentric wall–impinging jet of variable size
Flow convergence zone	Not visible, transient or small	Intermediate in size and duration	Large throughout systole
CWD jet	Faint/partial/parabolic	Dense, parabolic, or triangular	Dense, often triangular
Semiquantitative	Bolded signs are considered specific for their TR grade		
Color flow jet area (cm²)[b]	Not defined	Not defined	>10
VCW (cm)[b]	<0.3	0.3-0.69	>0.7
PISA radius (cm)[c]	<0.5	0.6-0.9	>0.9
Hepatic vein flow[d]	Systolic dominance	Systolic blunting	Systolic flow reversal
Tricuspid inflow[d]	A-wave dominant	Variable	E-wave >1.0 m/s
Quantitative			
EROA (cm²)	<0.20	0.20-0.39[e]	>0.40
RVOT (mL/beat)	<30	30-44[e]	>45

CWD, continuous-wave Doppler; EROA, effective regurgitant orifice area; PISA, proximal isovelocity surface area; RA, right atrial; RV, right ventricular; RVOT, right ventricular outflow tract; TR, tricuspid regurgitation; TV, tricuspid valve; VCW, vena contracta width
Reprinted from Zoghbi WA, Adams D, Bonow RO, et al. Recommendations for noninvasive evaluation of native valvular regurgitation: a report from the American Society of Echocardiography developed in collaboration with the Society for Cardiovascular Magnetic Resonance. *J Am Soc Echocardiogr*. 2017;30(4):303-371. Copyright © 2017 by the American Society of Echocardiography. With permission.
[a]RV and RA size can be within the "normal" range in patients with acute severe TR.
[b]With Nyquist limit >50 to 70 cm/s.
[c]With baseline Nyquist limit shift of 28 cm/s.
[d]Signs are nonspecific and are influenced by many other factors (RV diastolic function, atrial fibrillation, RA pressure).
[e]There are little data to support further separation of these values.

Parameters	Mild	Moderate	Severe	Massive	Torrential
Vena contracta width (biplane average)	<3 mm	3-6.9 mm	7 mm - 13 mm	14-20 mm	≥21 mm
EROA by PISA	<20 mm^2	20-39 mm^2	40-59 mm^2	60-79 mm^2	≥80 mm^2
3D vena contracta area or quantitative Doppler EROA	-	-	75-94 mm^2	95-114 mm^2	≥115 mm^2
Example:					

Figure 23.25. Reprinted from Hahn RT, Thomas JD, Khalique OK, Cavalcante JL, Praz F, Zoghbi WA. Imaging assessment of tricuspid regurgitation severity. *JACC Cardiovasc Imaging.* 2019;12(3):469-490. Copyright © 2019 by the American College of Cardiology Foundation. With permission; and from Hahn RT, Zamorano JL. The need for a new tricuspid regurgitation grading scheme. *Eur Heart J Cardiovasc Imaging.* 2017;18(12):1342-1343. Reproduced by permission of The European Society of Cardiology.

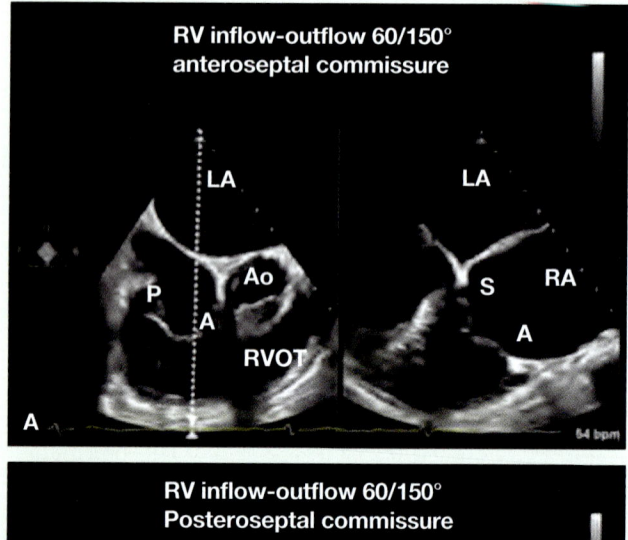

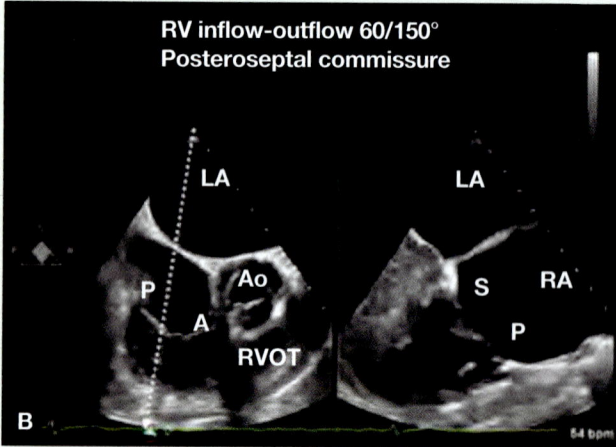

Figure 23.26. Reprinted from Hahn RT, Saric M, Faletra FF, et al. Recommended standards for the performance of transesophageal echocardiographic screening for structural heart intervention: from the American Society of Echocardiography. *J Am Soc Echocardiogr.* 2022;35(1):1-76. Copyright © 2021 by the American Society of Echocardiography. With permission.

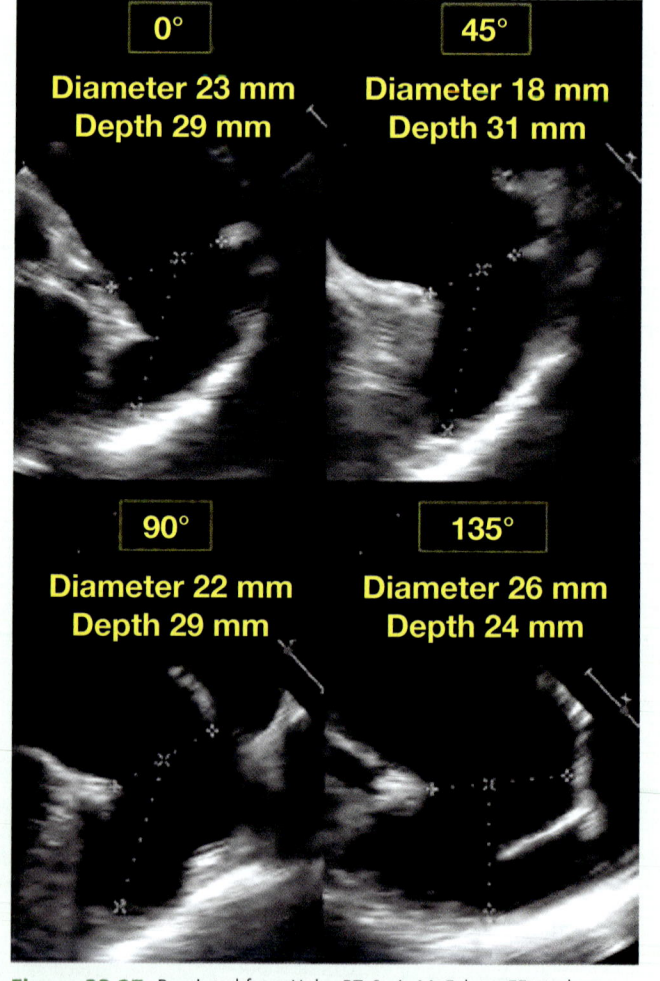

Figure 23.27. Reprinted from Hahn RT, Saric M, Faletra FF, et al. Recommended standards for the performance of transesophageal echocardiographic screening for structural heart intervention: from the American Society of Echocardiography. *J Am Soc Echocardiogr.* 2022;35(1):1-76. Copyright © 2021 by the American Society of Echocardiography. With permission.

Chapter 23 Interventional Echocardiography: Tricuspid Valve, Septum, LAA, and HCM / 491

| Windsock | Chicken wing | Broccoli | Cactus |

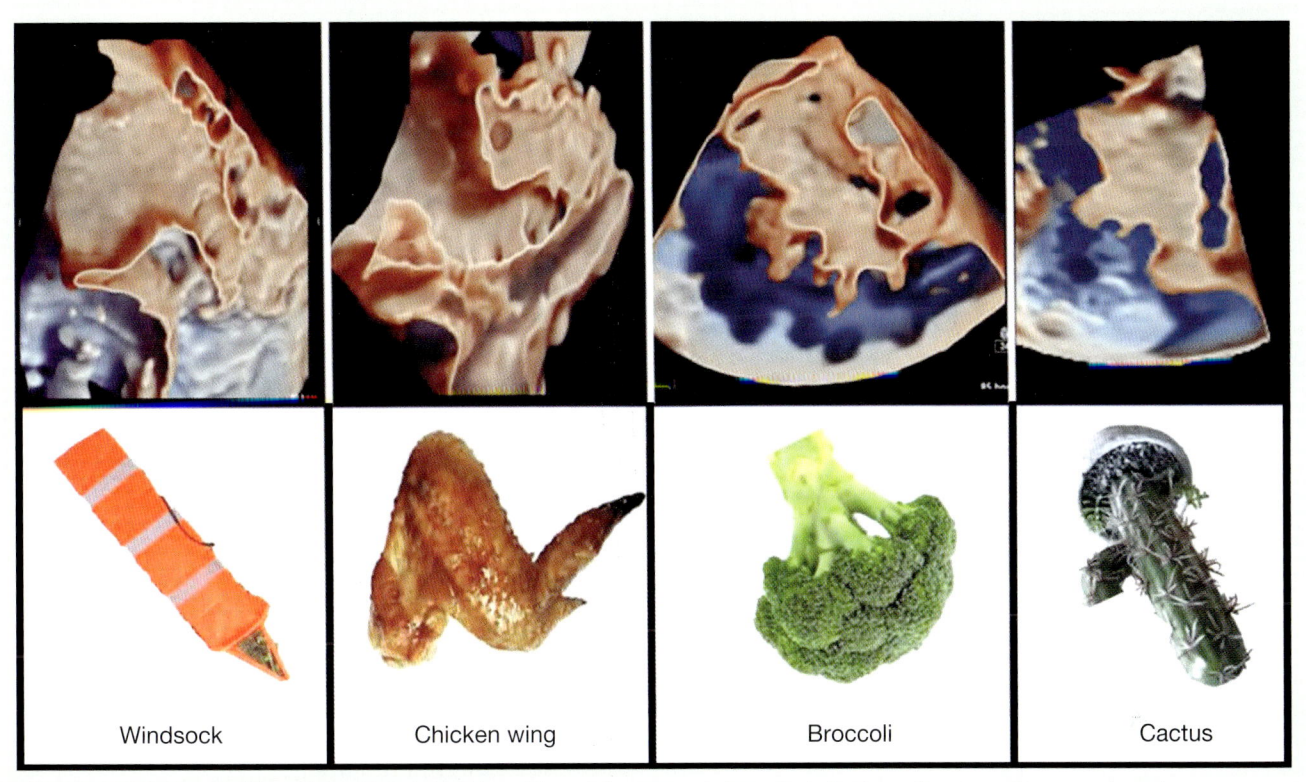

Figure 23.28. Reprinted from Hahn RT, Saric M, Faletra FF, et al. Recommended standards for the performance of transesophageal echocardiographic screening for structural heart intervention: from the American Society of Echocardiography. *J Am Soc Echocardiogr.* 2022;35(1):1-76. Figure 26. Copyright © 2021 by the American Society of Echocardiography. With permission.

19. **Answer: C.** When evaluating patients for percutaneous left atrial appendage occlusion devices, the TEE angles that are necessary are 0°, 45°, 90°, and 135° (**Figure 23.27**). At each of these views, one must measure the maximum depth and diameter of the left atrial appendage.

20. **Answer: B.** The morphology of the left atrial appendage can be broadly classified into four major groups: chicken wing, broccoli, windsock, and cactus (**Figure 23.28**). It is important to note these morphologies, since the risk of embolic events increases with the number of lobes. Also, the more the number of lobes and accessory lobes present, the higher the risk of an unsuccessful percutaneous left atrial appendage closure.

21. **Answer: B.** This entity is characterized by fatty infiltration of the interatrial septum, which can sometimes be confused with a cardiac tumor. The differential for atrial masses includes atrial myxoma. However, atrial myxomas usually arise from the interatrial septum close to the foramen ovale. In lipomatous hypertrophy of the interatrial septum (LHIS), the foramen ovale is preserved. LHIS is also common in obese adults. Rhabdomyomas usually occur in infants and children. LHIS can result in atrial arrhythmias. This is incidentally noted on TTE or TEE.

22. **Answer: C.** The Chiari network is encountered in the right atrium and is a fenestrated, embryonic remnant of the valves of sinus venosus. It lies near the inferior vena cava and the coronary sinus. It is usually of no clinical significance; however, it can sometimes pose diagnostic dilemmas being confused with thrombus and infective endocarditis and can pose challenges to catheter-based procedures. It is also associated with an interatrial septal aneurysm as is seen in the **Figure 23.11** and an interatrial communication.

23. **Answer: B.** Secundum ASDs can be single or multiple defects (the latter may be seen with fenestrated atrial septum). The defects are surrounded by a rim of tissue and hence these can be closed percutaneously. A secundum ASD with a maximal diameter below 38 mm and circumferential rim length over 5 mm is suitable for percutaneously closure. The rims allow the atrial septal closure device to be anchored securely. A primum ASD is an endocardial cushion defect and results in abnormal atrioventricular valve morphology. The primum ASD is bound anteriorly by the AV valve annulus and is therefore not amenable to percutaneous closure. Sinus venosus defect is absence of the sinus venosus septum and thus not a true defect of the atrial septum.

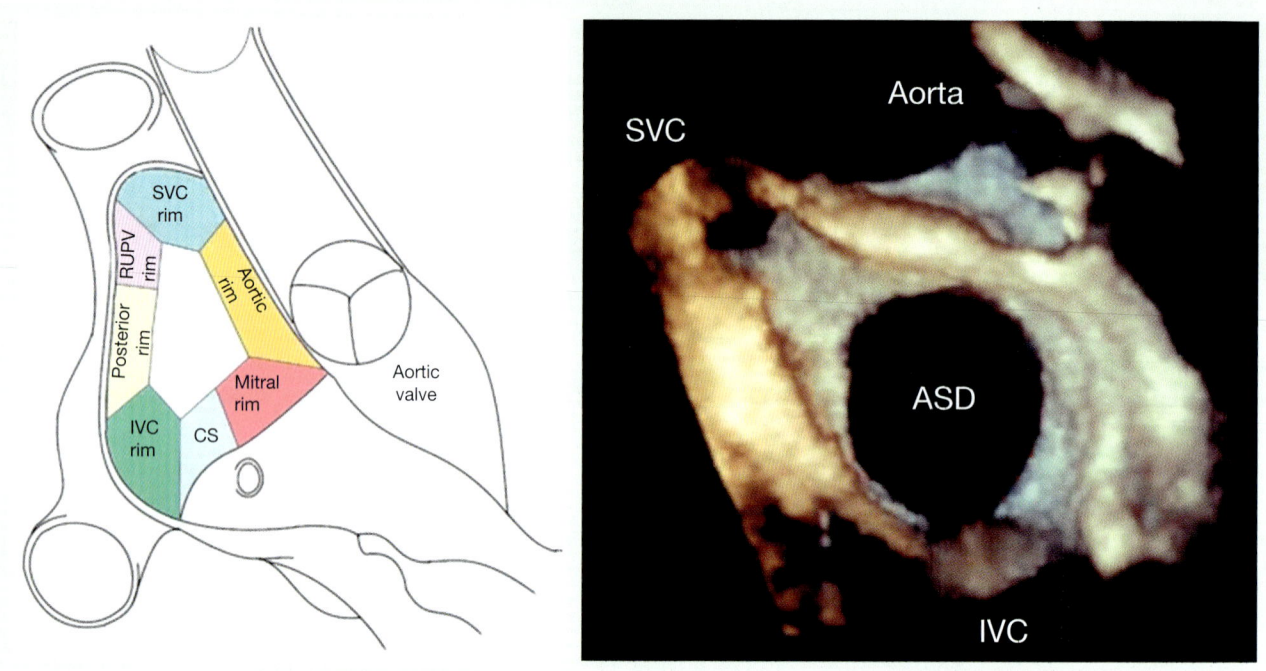

Figure 23.29. Left: From Pillai AA, Balasubramanian V. Transcatheter closure of complex and large ASDs. In: Pillai AA, Balasubramanian V, eds. *Atrial Septal Defects: Diagnosis and Management.* CRC Press; 2021:82. Figure 11.1. Copyright © 2021 by Taylor & Francis Group, LLC. Reproduced by permission of Taylor and Francis Group, LLC, a division of Informa plc. Right: Reprinted from Hahn RT, Abraham T, Adams MS et al. Guidelines for performing a comprehensive transesophageal echocardiographic examination: recommendations from American Society of Echo and the Society of Cardiovascular Anesthesiologists. *J Am Soc Echocardiogr.* 2013;26(9):921-964. Copyright © 2013 by the American Society of Echocardiography. With permission.

Fenestrated septum, although may be closed percutaneously, represents a challenge due to multiple defects present. Generally percutaneous closure is not considered first-line therapy.

24. **Answer: B. Figure 23.12** shows a large defect across the interatrial septum and a small anterior rim. This is representative of a secundum ASD. A primum ASD and an AV canal defect are associated with abnormalities of the AV canal where the AV valves make up part of the rim. This does not represent a patent foramen ovale since it is too large to be a PFO and these usually occur at the fossa ovalis. **Figure 23.29** demonstrates the rims of an atrial septal defect that must be assessed to determine eligibility for percutaneous closure.

25. **Answer: B.** Indications to close a secundum ASD are right heart dilation, ratio of pulmonary flow to systemic flow >1.5, absence of cyanosis, and absence of irreversible or severe pulmonary hypertension. Deficiency of <5 mm of specific rims may exclude someone from percutaneous closure of a secundum ASD.

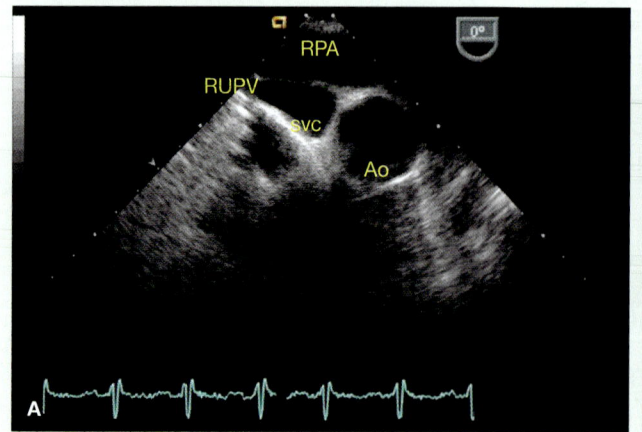

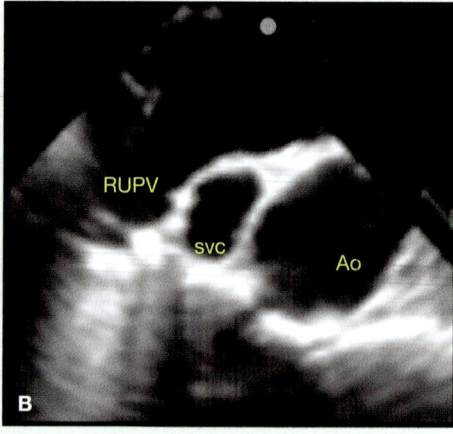

Figure 23.30

26. **Answer: D.** **Figure 23.13** is a high esophageal view showing the superior vena cava (SVC) and aorta (Ao). In **Figure 23.13**, the SVC, which normally is a rounded structure, appears to be a classic "tear drop SVC." This is indicative of anomalous right upper pulmonary venous (RUPV) return into the SVC. These can be associated with sinus venosus defects and right ventricular dilation. Secundum ASDs are usually not associated with anomalous pulmonary venous drainage (see **Figure 23.30A**). The other part of this image is what a normal high esophageal view looks like with a more rounded SVC and clear separation of the RUPV from the SVC (see **Figure 23.30B**).

27. **Answer: D.** In this case, the patient had hypertrophic cardiomyopathy and mid-systolic left ventricular outflow tract obstruction resulting in mid-systolic closure of the aortic valve. ▶ **Video 23.15** demonstrates a long-axis TEE view with severe mitral regurgitation along with systolic anterior motion of the mitral valve along with septal hypertrophy.

    Figure 23.31A-C show the M-mode of aortic stenosis, mitral valve prolapse, and systolic anterior motion of mitral valve.

28. **Answer: C.** Since **Figure 23.14** demonstrates mid systolic closure of the aortic valve, the diagnosis for this patient is hypertrophic cardiomyopathy.

29. **Answer: A.** The ECG with deep T-wave inversions along with the echo findings of apical hypertrophy along with a small apical aneurysm is classis for apical hypertrophic cardiomyopathy. This would not be takotsubo cardiomyopathy since this presents with apical ballooning which is not shown in the video. Eosinophilic cardiomyopathy does not present with an apical aneurysm or the ECG findings of deep T-wave inversions. Patients may present may chest pain along with the ECG and echo findings and may be mislabeled as having CAD and coronary ischemia. Thus, care should be taken to distinguish apical hypertrophic cardiomyopathy with an apical aneurysm from CAD and ischemia.

30. **Answer: B.** Atrial septal aneurysm (ASA) is most often diagnosed on TEE, where a distinction is made between a mobile or redundant atrial septum and an aneurysmal septum. The prevalence is estimated as 1% to 3% of the general population. The most widely accepted criterion for ASA is a >10-mm protrusion (usually in the region of the fossa ovalis) beyond the plane of the atrial septum, into the right or left atrium, or a total combined excursion into the right and left atrium >15 mm. Other criteria have suggested that the base of the protrusion should have a base width of ≥15 mm. The significance of ASA is that there is a high association with atrial septal shunting

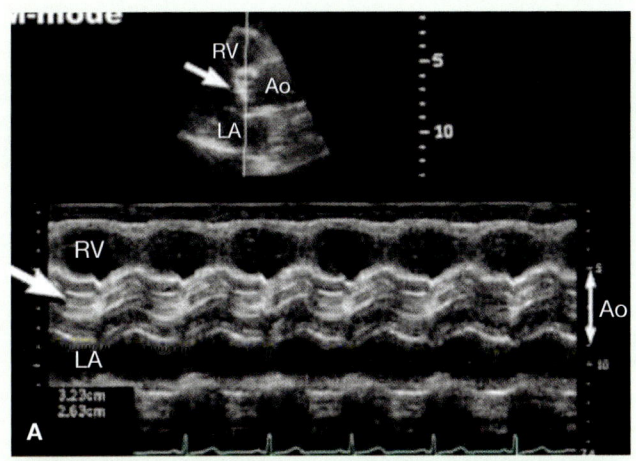

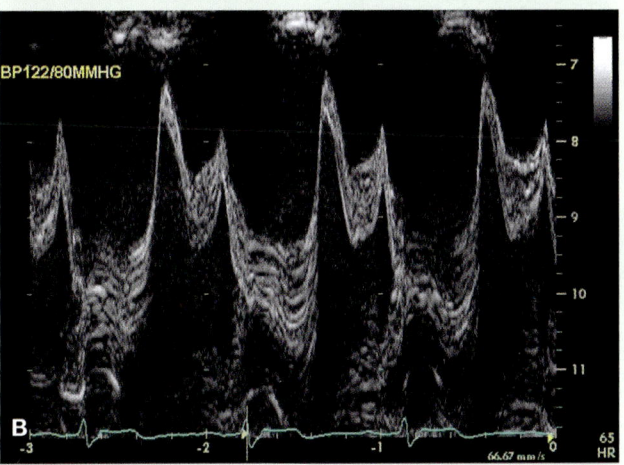

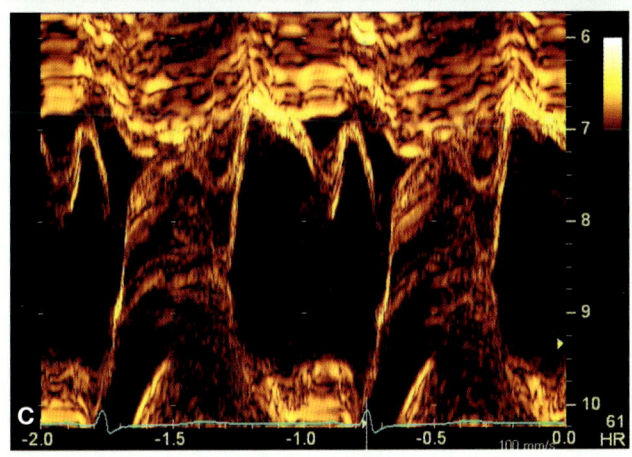

Figure 23.31. A: Aortic stenosis M-mode. (Reprinted by permission from Springer: Bermudez EA. Echocardiographic assessment of aortic stenosis. In: Solomon SD, Bulwer B, eds. *Essential Echocardiography. Contemporary Cardiology.* Humana Press; 2007:214. Copyright © 2007 Humana Press Inc., Totowa, NJ.). **B:** MV prolapse M-mode. **C:** Systolic anterior motion MV M-mode.

including PFO (up to 50% in one study), ASDs, or a fenestrated atrial septum. Therefore, ASA may be associated with cardioembolic risk with an increased occurrence in patients with cryptogenic stroke.

31. **Answer: C.** 3D TEE sizing generally is larger than 2D sizing. Both TEE and CT are used to size the LAA. Both technologies have disadvantages and advantages, and patient characteristics and risk factors need to be taken into consideration when deciding which imaging modality to utilize. 2D TEE sizing consistently provides smaller measurements than CT and 3D TEE sizing. Although there is increasing interest in using ICE for structural heart disease procedures, it is not used for preprocedural planning or for sizing. There are certain advantages of using ICE and the use of ICE intraprocedurally for percutaneous LAA occlusion will likely increase in the near future.

32. **Answer: A.** In the RV inflow view, one can visualize the freely mobile leaflet and the other leaflet within the clip device. The freely mobile leaflet is the anterior leaflet. The other leaflet is likely the septal leaflet since the coronary sinus ostium is visualized. In the four-chamber view, one can see the septal leaflet closer to the interventricular septum. The other leaflet is then the posterior leaflet (**Figure 23.32**).

33. **Answer: C.** A perimembranous VSD is anatomically close to the bundle of His, aortic valve and tricuspid valve. Percutaneous perimembranous VSD closure can cause heart block, aortic regurgitation, and tricuspid regurgitation because of the proximity of these structures to any device used for closure.

34. **Answer: D.** On TTE and TEE, one can follow the trajectory of the device lead into the RV to establish the relationship between CIED and tricuspid valve. There is extreme variability in the size of tricuspid valve leaflets and the number of leaflets. Even though conventionally three tricuspid valve leaflets are described, this may not always be the case. Usually more than one view is needed to localize which tricuspid valve leaflet is affected. In addition, both 2D and 3D imaging may be needed.

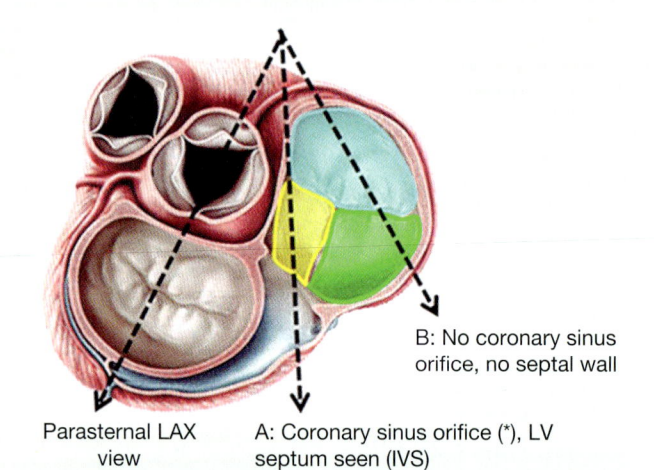

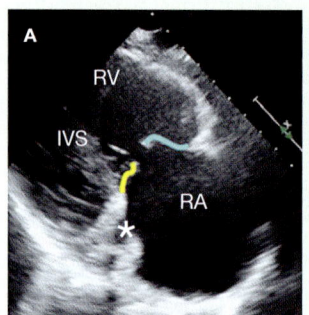

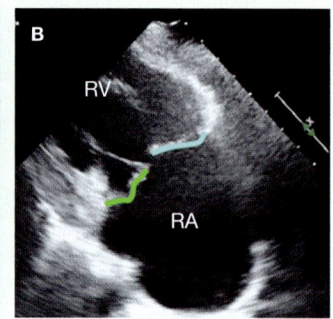

Figure 23.32. In the RV inflow view with the coronary sinus visualized, the anterior leaflet (blue) and septal leaflet (yellow) are visualized. A slight tilt of the probe away from the ostium of the coronary sinus then shows the posterior leaflet (green). (Reprinted with permission from Hahn RT. State-of-the-art review of echocardiographic imaging in the evaluation and treatment of functional tricuspid regurgitation. *Circ Cardiovasc Imaging*. 2016;9(12):e005332. Figures 1 and 3. Copyright © 2016 American Heart Association, Inc.)

SUGGESTED READINGS

Alkhouli M, Holmes DR. Incomplete transcatheter left atrial appendage occlusion: no longer benign. *JACC Cardiovasc Interv*. 2022;15(21):2139-2142.

Hahn RT, Abraham T, Adams MS, et al; American Society of Echocardiography, Society of Cardiovascular Anesthesiologists. Guidelines for performing a comprehensive transesophageal echocardiographic examination: recommendations from the American Society of Echocardiography and the Society of Cardiovascular Anesthesiologists. *Anesth Analg*. 2014;118(1):921-968.

Hahn RT, Thomas JD, Khalique OK, Cavalcante JL, Praz F, Zoghbi WA. Imaging assessment of tricuspid regurgitation severity. *JACC Cardiovasc Imaging*. 2019;12(3):469-490.

Hahn RT, Saric M, Faletra FF, et al. Recommended standards for the performance of transesophageal echocardiographic screening for structural heart intervention: from the American Society of Echocardiography. *J Am Soc Echocardiogr*. 2022;35(1):1-76.

Hahn RT. State-of-the-art review of echocardiographic imaging in the evaluation and treatment of functional tricuspid regurgitation. *Circ Cardiovasc Imaging*. 2016;9(12):e005332.

Hughes RK, Knott KD, Malcolmson J, et al. Apical hypertrophic cardiomyopathy: the variant less known. *J Am Heart Assoc*. 2020;9(5):e015294.

Isakadze N, Lovell J, Shapiro EP, Choi CW, Williams MS, Mukherjee M. Large atrial septal aneurysm associated with secundum atrial septal defect. *CASE (Phila)*. 2022;6(4):187-190.

Mugge A, Daniel WG, Angermann C, et al. Atrial septal aneurysm in adult patients. A multicenter study using transthoracic and transesophageal echocardiography. *Circulation*. 1995;91(11):2785-2792.

Nucifora G, Faletra FF, Regoli F, et al. Evaluation of the left atrial appendage with real-time 3-dimensional transesophageal echocardiography: implications for catheter-based left atrial appendage closure. *Circ Cardiovasc Imaging*. 2011;4(5):514-523.

Schneider B, Hofmann T, Justen MH, Meinertz T. Chiari's network: normal anatomic variant or risk factor for arterial embolic events? *J Am Coll Cardiol*. 1995;26(1):203-210.

Wang DD, Eng M, Kupsky D, et al. Application of 3-dimensional computed tomographic image guidance to WATCHMAN implantation and impact on early operator learning curve: single-center experience. *JACC Cardiovasc Interv*. 2016;9(22):2329-2340.

Yavar Z, Gilge JL, Patel PJ, et al. Lipomatous hypertrophy of the interatrial septum manifesting as third degree atrioventricular block. *JACC Case Rep*. 2020;2(14):2235-2239.

Zoghbi WA, Adams D, Bonow RO, et al. Recommendations for noninvasive evaluation of native valvular regurgitation: a Report from the American Society of Echocardiography developed in collaboration with the Society for Cardiovascular Magnetic Resonance. *J Am Soc Echocardiogr*. 2017;30(4):303-371.

CHAPTER 24

Cardiomyopathies

Antonio Lewis-Camarago and Craig R. Asher

QUESTIONS

1. In which of the following conditions is a normal or mildly increased left ventricular wall thickness a typical cardiac phenotypic presentation by echocardiography?
   A. Diabetes.
   B. Primary restrictive cardiomyopathy.
   C. Systemic sclerosis.
   D. Radiation heart disease.
   E. All of the above.

2. A 48-year-old woman presents to the emergency room (ER) complaining of shortness of breath and new-onset palpitations. The initial electrocardiogram (EKG) shows atrial flutter at a rate of 150 bpm with 2:1 atrioventricular (AV) conduction. A transthoracic echocardiogram (TTE) is performed, and it reveals 4-chamber dilatation with severe biventricular systolic dysfunction. Which of the following statements regarding this patient's cardiomyopathy is **CORRECT**?
   A. It is most likely irreversible.
   B. Successful cardioversion to sinus rhythm will usually improve LV systolic function to normal in days.
   C. The presence of moderate to severe mitral regurgitation suggests that the cardiomyopathy is due to valvular heart disease.
   D. If recovery of LV function occurs after successful cardioversion, a recurrent episode of atrial flutter will likely not be well tolerated.

3. Which of the following statements about peripartum cardiomyopathy is **CORRECT**?
   A. If the LV ejection fraction (EF) normalizes after the initial cardiomyopathy episode, it is unlikely that there will be a recurrence of LV systolic dysfunction in subsequent pregnancies.
   B. Up to 25% of patients have marked improvement in LV systolic function and clinical symptoms after the initial episode.
   C. Most women present with symptoms and echocardiographic abnormalities between months 3 and 6 postpartum.
   D. Normal inotropic response measured during dobutamine stress echocardiography may serve as a predictor of the likelihood of recurrence of LV systolic dysfunction with subsequent pregnancy.

4. A 49-year-old man with a history of pulmonary sarcoidosis is seen in clinic for evaluation of syncopal episodes. As part of the evaluation, he had a 12-lead EKG that revealed complete AV block. Which of the following findings on TTE is most specific for the diagnosis of cardiac involvement?
   A. Severely increased wall thickness.
   B. Grade 2 or 3 diastolic dysfunction.
   C. Thinning of the basal anterior septal wall.
   D. Pulmonary hypertension.
   E. Pericardial effusion.

5. A 52-year-old man presents for a 3-month follow-up echocardiogram after chemotherapy for lymphoma with an anthracycline-based regimen. He is asymptomatic and clinically appears well. At baseline, his LVEF was 68% with a peak global longitudinal strain (GLS) of −25%. On follow-up echocardiogram, his LVEF is 58% and GLS is −22.5%. Which of the following statements is **CORRECT**?
   A. There is evidence of cardiotoxicity based on a reduction in LVEF.
   B. There is no evidence of cardiotoxicity.
   C. There is evidence of cardiotoxicity based on reduction in GLS.
   D. It is uncertain whether there is cardiotoxicity, and a repeat echocardiogram should be done in 3 months.

6. Which echocardiographic parameter is consistent with hypertensive left ventricular hypertrophy (LVH) rather than physiologic hypertrophy of athlete's heart when evaluating an echocardiogram of an Olympic marathon runner?
   A. Relative wall thickness (RWT) >0.42.
   B. RV dilation.
   C. Increased left atrial (LA) volume.
   D. Increased LV mass.
   E. None of the above.

7. A 47-year-old woman underwent chemotherapy and radiation for Hodgkin lymphoma 20 years previously. Which of the following echocardiographic findings are most specific for radiation heart disease?
   A. Aorto-mitral curtain thickening or calcification.
   B. Pericardial thickening/pericardial effusion.
   C. Severe aortic regurgitation.
   D. Ascending aorta calcification.
   E. None of the above.

8. Which of the following statements regarding the prediction of sudden cardiac death (SCD) in patients with hypertrophic cardiomyopathy (HCM) is **CORRECT**?
   A. Older patients with HCM have a higher risk than younger patients.
   B. Nonobstructive forms are associated with higher risk than obstructive forms.
   C. Apical aneurysms are associated with higher risk.
   D. Increased wall thickness, only if LV wall thickness is >3 cm is associated with higher risk.
   E. LV dysfunction with LVEF <60% is associated with higher risk.

9. Which of the following statements best describes the most typical echocardiographic appearance of cardiac hemochromatosis?
   A. Nondilated LV cavity with severe increased wall thickness.
   B. Restrictive diastolic filling pattern with normal LV wall thickness.
   C. Mildly dilated LV cavity with global LV dysfunction and normal or mildly increased LV wall thickness.
   D. Severely dilated LV cavity with regional LV dysfunction and severely increased LV wall thickness.
   E. None of the above.

10. Based on echocardiographic criteria, which asymptomatic athlete should be allowed to participate in competitive sports without further testing?
    A. A 20-year-old male American football player with an LVEF = 65%, $LVID_d$ = 5.3 cm, septal wall thickness 1.6 cm, posterior wall thickness 1.2 cm, and lateral mitral annular e′ 6 cm/s.
    B. A 21-year-old male basketball player with $LVID_d$ = 5.9 cm, $LVIS_d$ = 3.6 cm, LVEF = 60%, septal wall thickness 1.3 cm, posterior wall thickness 1.3 cm, left atrial volume 37 mL/m², and lateral mitral annular e′ 18 cm/s.
    C. A 26-year-old male soccer player with LVEF = 55%, $LVID_d$ = 5.2 cm, and proximal right ventricular outflow tract measurement (parasternal short-axis) in diastole 3.8 cm.
    D. A 24-year-old male basketball player with LVEF = 60%, $LVID_d$ = 5.3 cm, mitral valve prolapse with moderate MR, aortic diameter at the sinuses of Valsalva 4.3 cm, at the ST junction 4.1 cm, and mid-ascending aorta 3.8 cm.
    E. None of the above.

11. A 28-year-old asymptomatic woman is diagnosed with apical HCM after workup of an abnormal EKG. Genetic testing does not reveal a pathogenic mutation. Which of the following statements regarding family screening for her 30-year-old brother is **CORRECT**?
    A. A normal EKG and echocardiogram excludes the diagnosis of HCM and no further testing is required.
    B. A normal EKG and echocardiogram and a negative genetic test excludes the diagnosis of HCM and no further testing is required.
    C. If EKG and echocardiogram are normal, repeat studies should be performed in 1 to 2 years.
    D. If EKG and echocardiogram are normal, repeat studies should be performed in 3 to 5 years.
    E. None of the above.

12. A 32-year-old man presents to the ER with angina and an abnormal EKG. Pertinent findings on physical examination include an S4 gallop. As part of his cardiac evaluation, a TTE is performed. It shows an apical LV thickness of 19 mm, interventricular septal thickness of 11 mm, and posterior wall thickness of 10 mm. Which of the following associated findings is most likely to be found in this patient?
    A. Normal left atrial volume.
    B. Left ventricular outflow tract (LVOT) peak velocity by continuous-wave Doppler of 3 m/s after amyl nitrite administration.
    C. Systolic anterior motion of the mitral valve.
    D. Normal LV cavity linear dimension in diastole.
    E. All of the above.

13. Which of the following echocardiographic findings are consistent with LV noncompaction/excessive trabeculation phenotype?
    A. Three layers of myocardium should be identifiable (endocardial, myocardial, and epicardial).
    B. The ratio of the noncompacted to compacted layers should be >1.5:1.
    C. Deep recesses filled with blood from the LV cavity should be seen by contrast echocardiography or color Doppler.
    D. The most commonly affected regions are the midventricular anterior, inferoseptum, and apex.
    E. All of the above.

14. Which of the following measures of diastolic function is most likely found in a patient with restrictive cardiomyopathy?
    A. Color M-mode propagation velocity (V_p) = 70 cm/s.
    B. Peak mitral inflow early diastolic filling velocity = 120 cm/s; tissue Doppler e′ lateral velocity = 6 cm/s.
    C. Mitral inflow E deceleration time = 165 ms.
    D. Pulmonary vein Doppler systolic velocity = 40 cm/s; diastolic velocity = 50 cm/s.
    E. None of the above.

15. Which of the following findings is most specific for the diagnosis of cardiac amyloidosis?
    A. Average apical segments longitudinal strain (LS)/average combined basal + mid LS >1.0.
    B. Granular sparkling pattern of LV myocardium.
    C. Tissue Doppler mitral annular e′ velocity, a′ velocity, and S velocity <8 cm/s.
    D. Grade 3 diastolic dysfunction.
    E. None of the above.

16. A 45-year-old man with recurrent diastolic heart failure and systemic symptoms including fever and night sweats underwent a TTE. Based on **Figure 24.1**, which of the following statements about this patient's condition is **CORRECT**?
    A. RV involvement is common.
    B. Mitral regurgitation is uncommon.
    C. Left atrial pressure is usually normal.
    D. LV thrombus is uncommon.

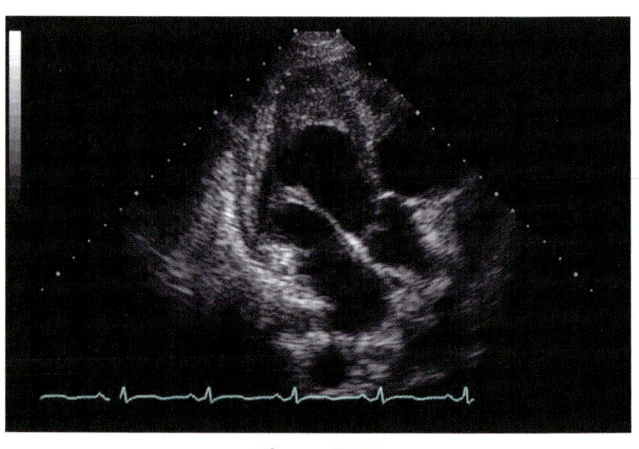

Figure 24.1

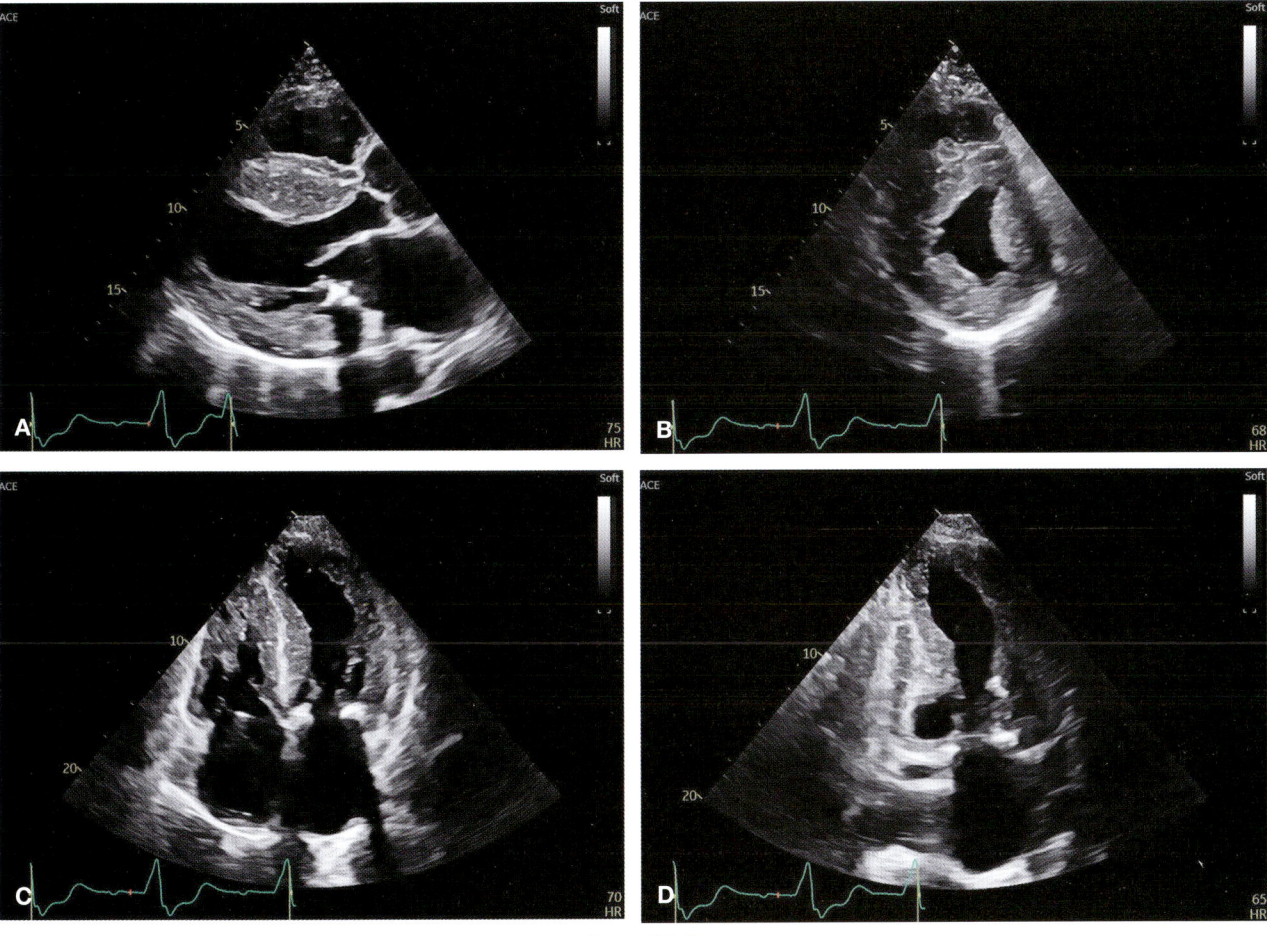

Figure 24.2

17. A 44-year-old man presents for evaluation of worsening dyspnea and palpitations. He has a family history of sudden cardiac death. A resting echocardiogram is performed and is shown in **Figure 24.2A-D**. LVEF is 65%.

    Which of the following parameters would suggest that enzyme replacement therapy may be beneficial in this patient?
    A. Exercise-induced LVOT obstruction.
    B. Severe asymmetric septal wall thickness.
    C. Grade 2 diastolic dysfunction.
    D. Thinning of the basal inferolateral wall.
    E. None of the above.

18. A 27-year-old man presents to clinic for a cardiac evaluation due to a family history of cardiomyopathy (CM). He is asymptomatic and EKG is normal. An outside echocardiogram was done and reported as normal. Findings include an interventricular and posterior wall thickness, both of 1.0 cm; $LVID_d$ = 5.0 cm and normal diastolic function.

    Figure 24.3 is obtained from the study. Which of the following conclusions can be made?
    A. Findings rule out HCM.
    B. Findings are suggestive of HCM.
    C. Data are insufficient to make conclusions.

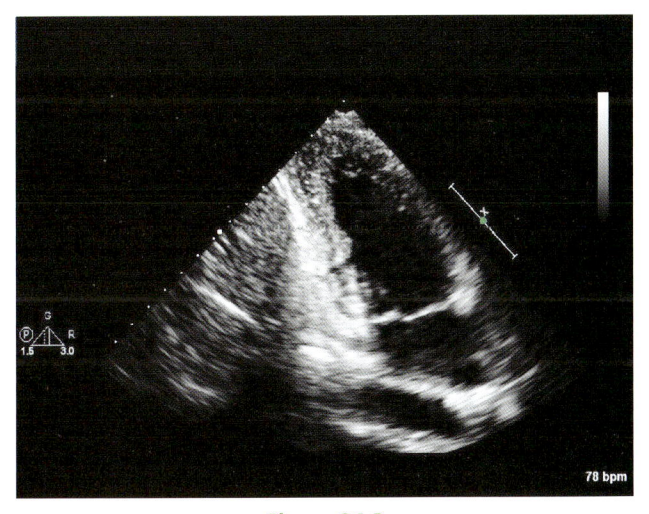

Figure 24.3

500 / Clinical Echocardiography Review

19. A 38-year-old man presents to the ER following an episode of syncope preceded by palpitations. The patient denies chest pain or previous syncopal episodes. Telemetry monitoring reveals frequent premature ventricular contractions, but no arrhythmias. EKG reveals T-wave inversion in V2 and V3. A TTE is performed. **Figure 24.4A,B** are obtained.
 Which of the following statements about this patient's condition is **CORRECT**?
 A. Associated LV dilated cardiomyopathy is common.
 B. Isolated RVOT dilation is a diagnostic feature.
 C. Pulmonary hypertension is common.
 D. Right atrial dilation is a diagnostic feature.
 E. All of the above.

20. A 61-year-old woman presents to the ER with findings consistent with heart failure. She is in pulmonary edema and a poor historian. An echocardiogram is done in the ER and the cardiology consultation team is at the bedside. Laboratory testing is pending. **Figure 24.5A-D** shows pertinent images from the study.
 What is the most likely underlying etiology of the patient's valvular heart disease?
 A. Rheumatic heart disease.
 B. End-stage renal disease.
 C. Homozygous familial hypercholesterolemia.
 D. Radiation heart disease.
 E. None of the above.

21. A 45-year-old man from Colombia presents with a 2-month history of exertional dyspnea, orthopnea, and lower extremity edema. He moved to the United States 6-months prior for employment. A 12-lead EKG shows frequent PVCs and a RBBB. His TTE is shown in **Figure 24.6A-C** and **Video 24.1**.
 Besides ventricular systolic dysfunction, what other echocardiographic findings would be most suggestive of Chagas cardiomyopathy?
 A. Increased biventricular wall thickness with normal LV systolic function.
 B. Presence of increased trabeculations in noncompacted myocardium.
 C. Moderate functional mitral regurgitation due to leaflet tethering.
 D. Regional wall motion abnormalities in noncoronary territories.
 E. None of the above.

22. A 61-year-old man is admitted to the cardiology service from the ER with symptoms and signs consistent with heart failure with preserved ejection fraction (HFpEF). An echocardiogram is done in the ER and shows LVEF = 55%, LVH, and abnormal diastolic function. Which of the following GLS patterns is least suggestive of a myopathic disease (**Figure 24.7**)?
 A. GLS pattern A.
 B. GLS pattern B.
 C. GLS pattern C.
 D. GLS pattern D.
 E. GLS pattern E.

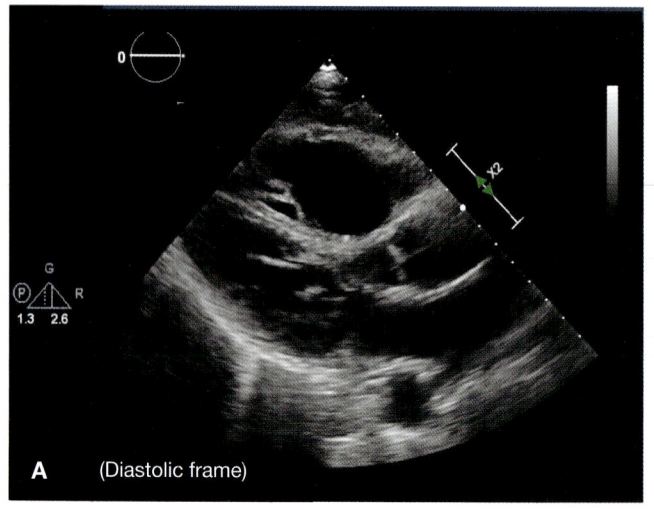

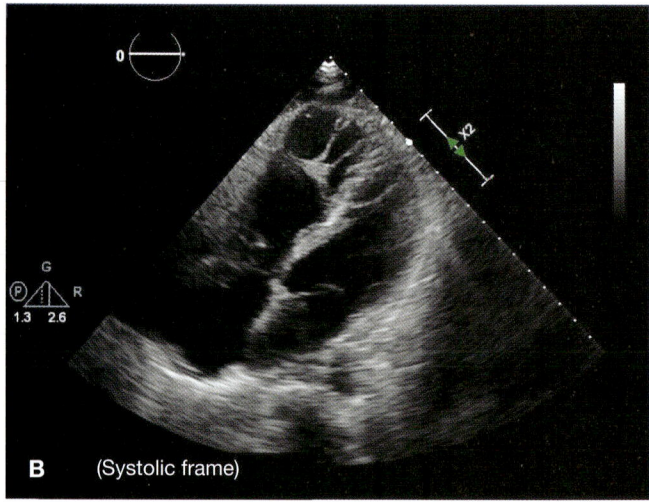

A (Diastolic frame) B (Systolic frame)

Figure 24.4

Chapter 24 Cardiomyopathies / 501

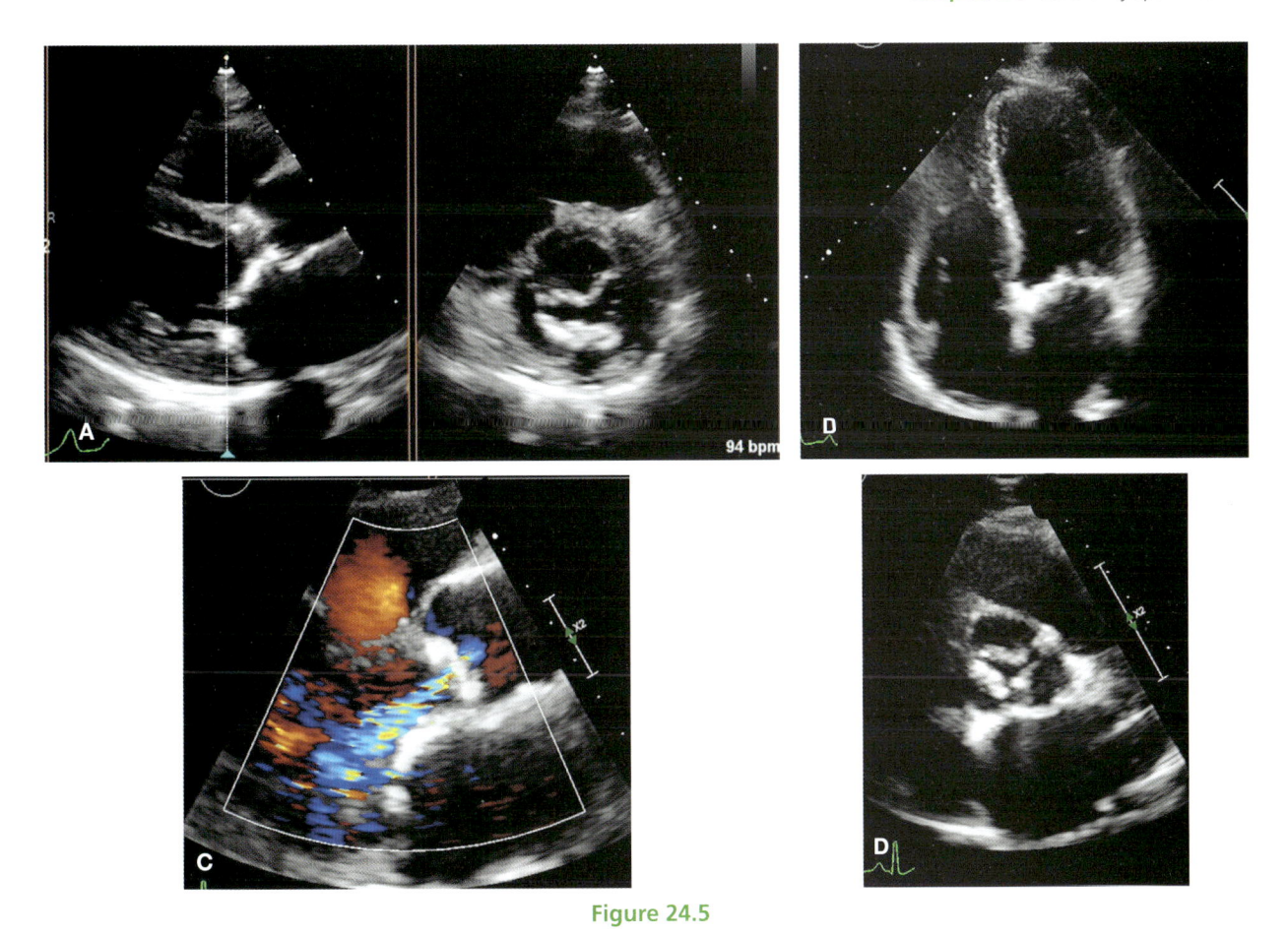

Figure 24.5

23. A 74-year-old man presents with dyspnea on exertion and presyncope. Which of the following diagnoses is most likely based on **Figure 24.8A** (pulsed-wave Doppler) and **Figure 24.8B** (speckle tracking GLS polar plot)?
  A. Subaortic membrane and LV hypertrophy.
  B. Cardiac amyloidosis with LVOT obstruction.
  C. Hypertrophic cardiomyopathy with LVOT obstruction.
  D. Hypertrophic cardiomyopathy without LVOT obstruction.
  E. None of the above.

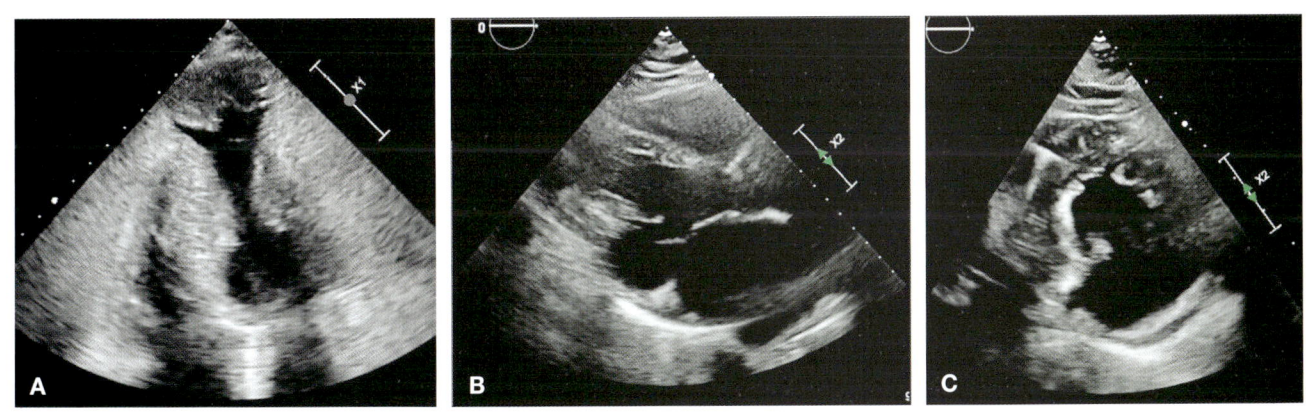

Figure 24.6. Courtesy of Dr. Julian Gelves, Fundación Cardioinfantil – Instituto de Cardiología, Bogotá, Colombia.

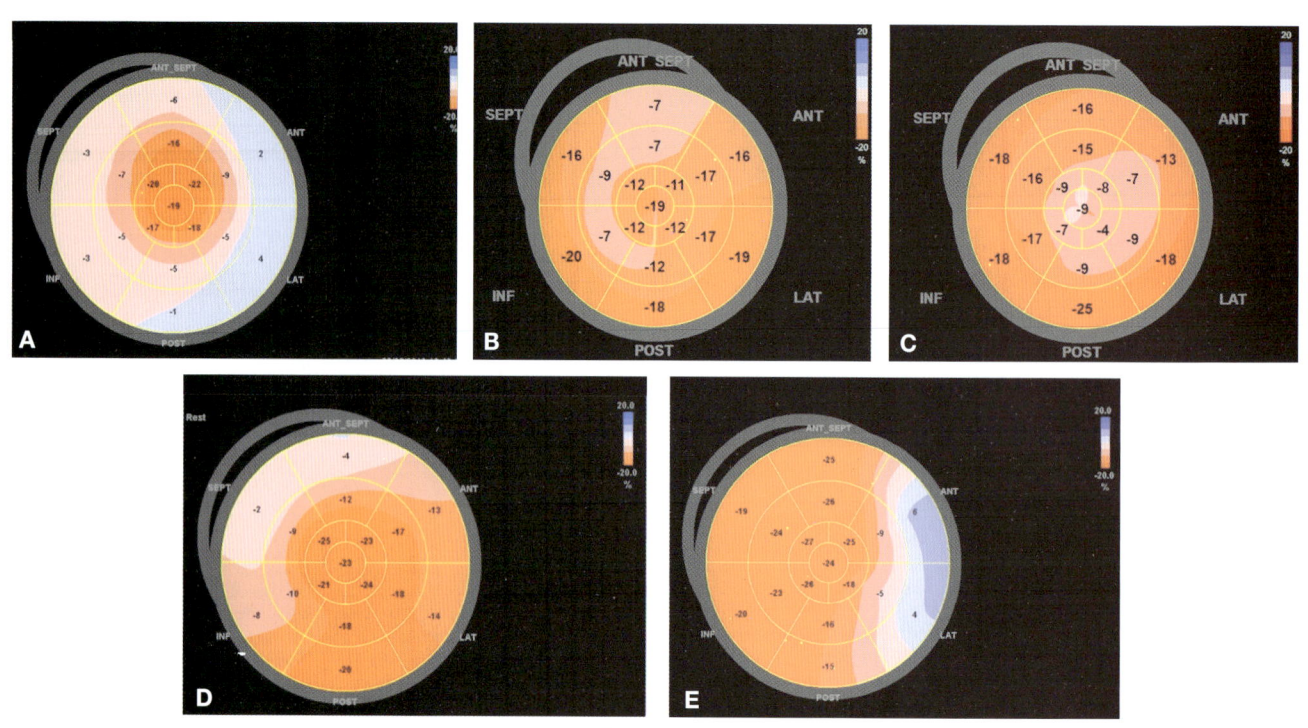

Figure 24.7

24. A 54-year-old woman with shortness of breath of unknown etiology presents for a TTE. Which of the following statements regarding the images (apical 4-chamber, apical 2-chamber, reverse 4-chamber view, and GLS polar plot) are most accurate (**Figure 24.9**)?
   A. Findings are suggestive of cardiac involvement in muscular dystrophy.
   B. Findings are suggestive of cardiac involvement in Fabry disease.
   C. Findings are suggestive of cardiac involvement in sarcoidosis.
   D. Findings are suggestive of Chagas disease.
   E. None of the above.

25. Which of the following statements regarding the images shown in **Figure 24.10A,B** of a patient with HCM is **CORRECT**?
   A. The patient is most likely sarcomere mutation negative.
   B. The patient is most likely over 50 years of age.
   C. The patient most likely has right ventricular hypertrophy.
   D. The risk of SCD is low.
   E. None of the above.

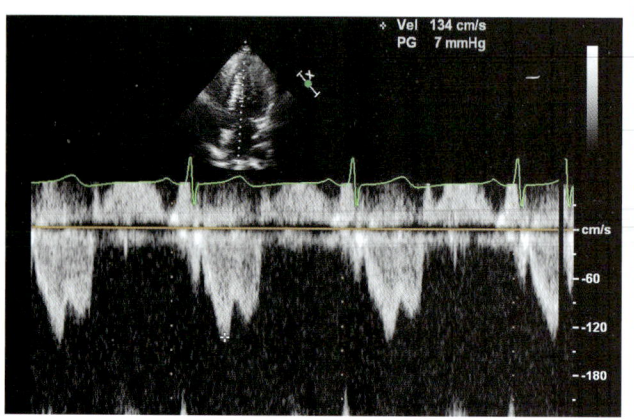

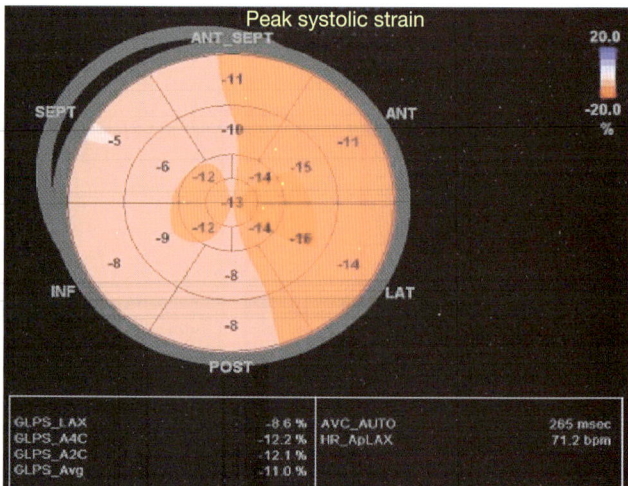

Figure 24.8

Chapter 24 Cardiomyopathies / 503

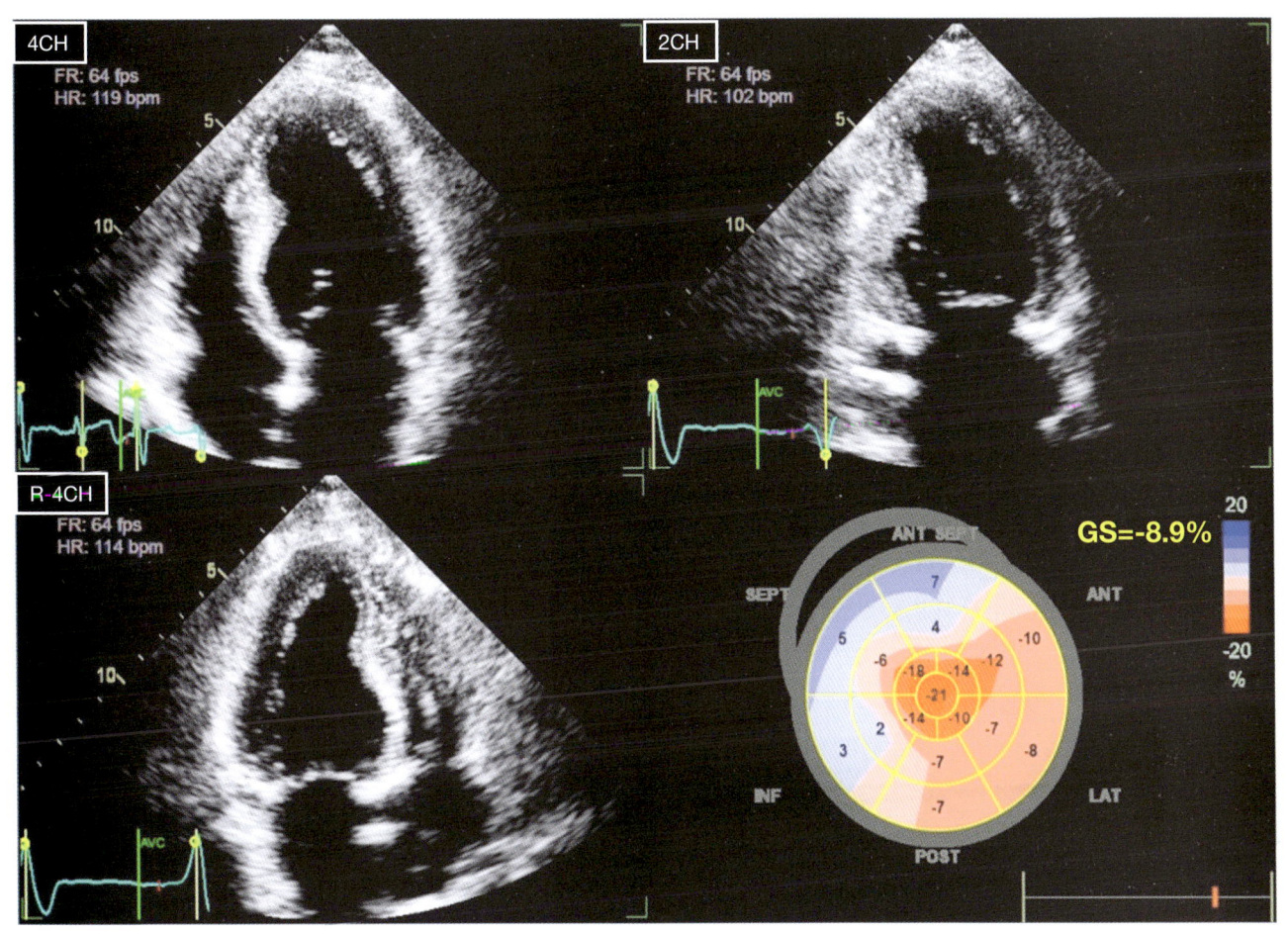

Figure 24.9

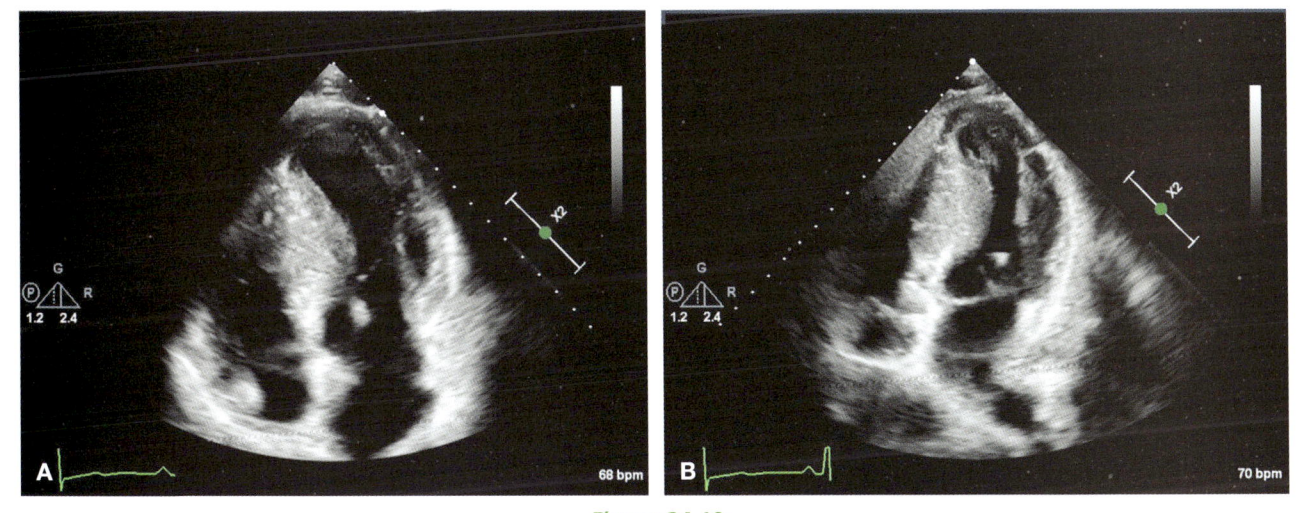

Figure 24.10

26. A 14-year-old boy presents to the ER with symptoms and signs of congestive heart failure. He has a history of intellectual disability and muscular weakness. On presentation, laboratory testing is notable for an elevated CPK. His EKG show sinus rhythm with a short PR interval and delta wave consistent with a left-sided preexcitation pattern. A TTE is done and echo images are shown in **Figure 24.11A-C**.

Which of the following clinical impressions is most likely?
A. A sarcomeric gene mutation is present.
B. A dystrophin gene mutation is present.
C. A LAMP-2 gene mutation is present.
D. A mutation in the GLA gene coding for alpha-galactosidase A is present.
E. None of the above.

27. A 52-year-old woman with midcavitary HCM presents for an annual echocardiogram. She is asymptomatic and participates in recreational running. The sonographer performing the study notices an unusual continuous-wave Doppler pattern and presents it to the interpreting cardiologist (**Figure 24.12**).

What is the significance of this tracing?
A. It likely represents an artifact and has no significance.
B. It demonstrates intracavitary obliteration, which has no significant clinical importance.
C. It demonstrates intracavitary obliteration and an apical abnormality that is clinically important.
D. It demonstrates a mitral regurgitant jet that is not significant because it is not severe regurgitation.
E. None of the above.

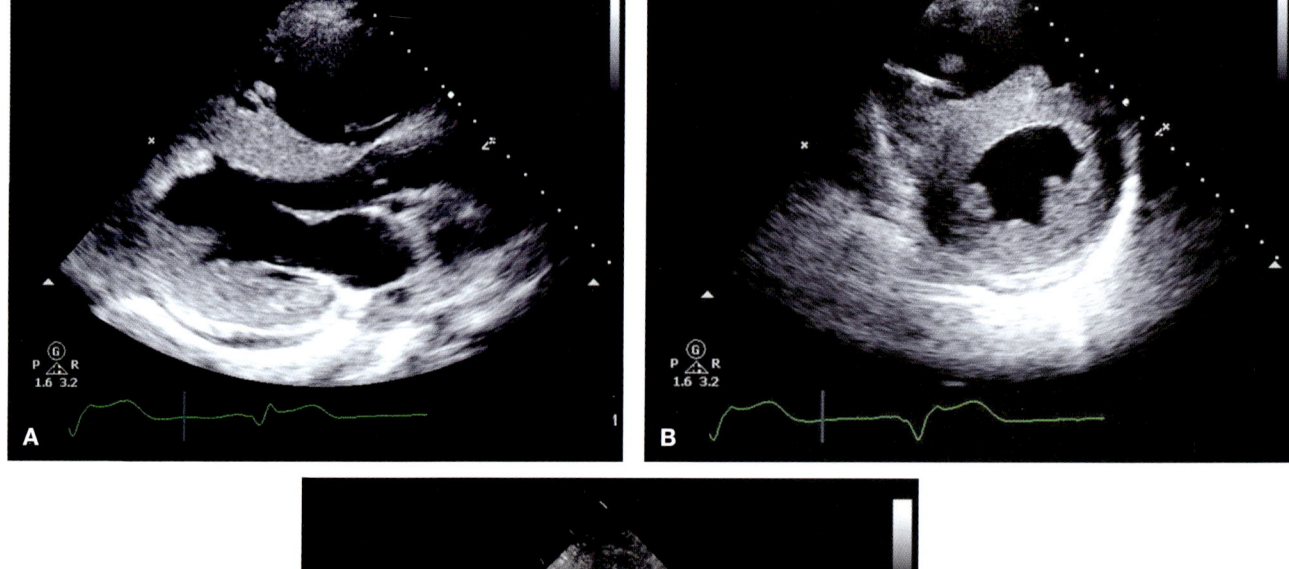

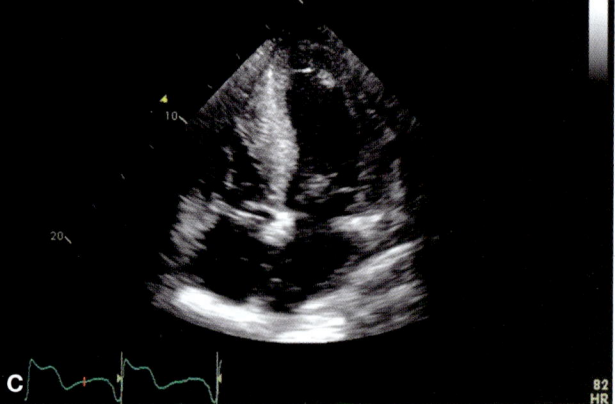

Figure 24.11

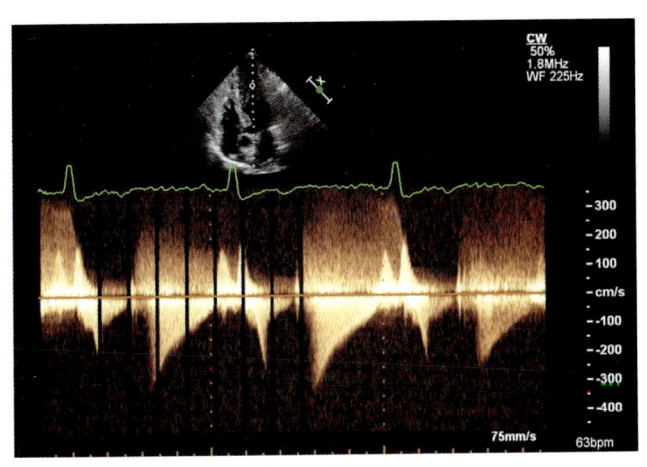

Figure 24.12

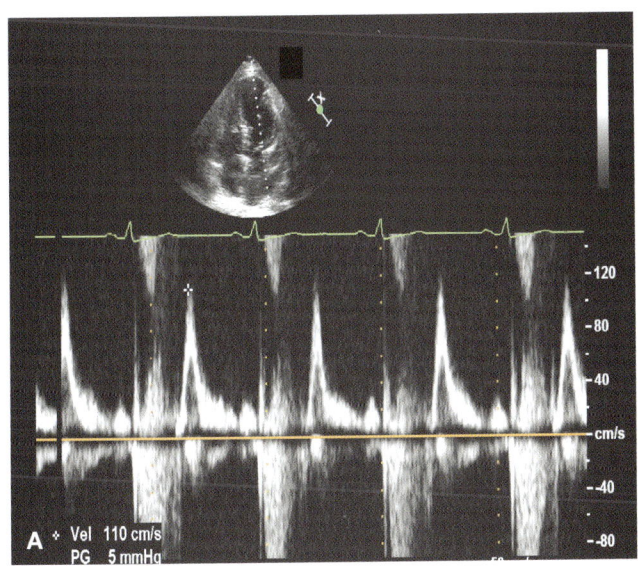

Figure 24.13A

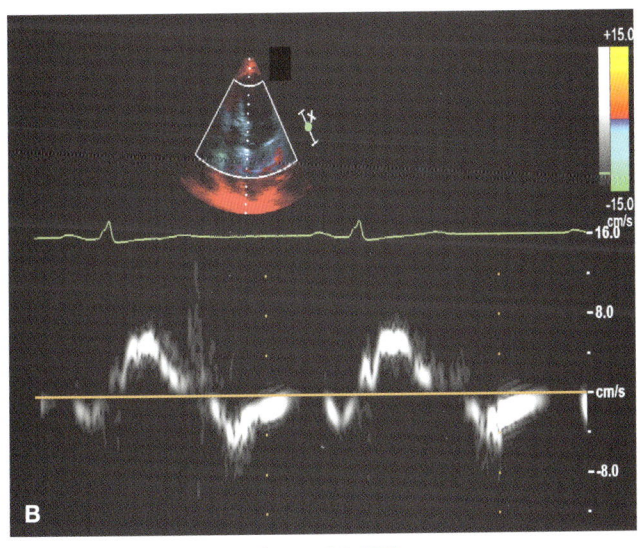

Figure 24.13B

28. A 26-year-old woman presents to the office for evaluation of dyspnea on exertion and lower extremity edema. The rhythm is sinus. On echocardiogram (**Figure 24.13A** and **B**), the following findings are seen: $LVID_d$ = 4.4 cm; $LVID_s$ = 2.9 cm; LVEF = 60%; IVS = 1.1 cm; and PW = 1.1 cm.
    Which of the following diagnoses is the most likely for this patient?
    A. Primary restrictive cardiomyopathy.
    B. Noncardiac etiology for her symptoms.
    C. Constrictive pericarditis.
    D. Early-stage HCM.
    E. None of the above.

29. A 36-year-old woman underwent a gynecologic surgery. Immediately after waking up from surgery, she developed pelvic pain and subsequently chest pain and hypotension. A loud systolic ejection murmur was heard. An EKG showed sinus rhythm at 84 bpm and diffuse ST depressions with T-wave inversions. She was thought to be experiencing an analphylactic reaction to one of the anesthetic agents. Phenylephrine was initiated and the murmur resolved. A stat echocardiogram was done. Apical 4-chamber images in diastole (**Figure 24.14A**) and systole (**Figure 24.14B**) are shown with contrast enhancement.
    What is the most likely cause of the systolic murmur?
    A. Ventricular septal defect.
    B. Left ventricular outflow tract obstruction.
    C. Mitral regurgitation.
    D. Aortic stenosis.
    E. None of the above.

30. A 67-year-old man with a history of atrio-ventricular (AV) and biventricular pacing for severe LV dysfunction associated with prior myocardial infarctions presents with recurrent CHF (**Figure 24.15A-C**)
    Which of the following management options do you recommend?
    A. Consideration for mitral valve repair or replacement.
    B. Diuresis only.
    C. Diuresis and shortening the AV delay.
    D. Diuresis and lengthening of the AV delay.
    E. None of the above.

506 / Clinical Echocardiography Review

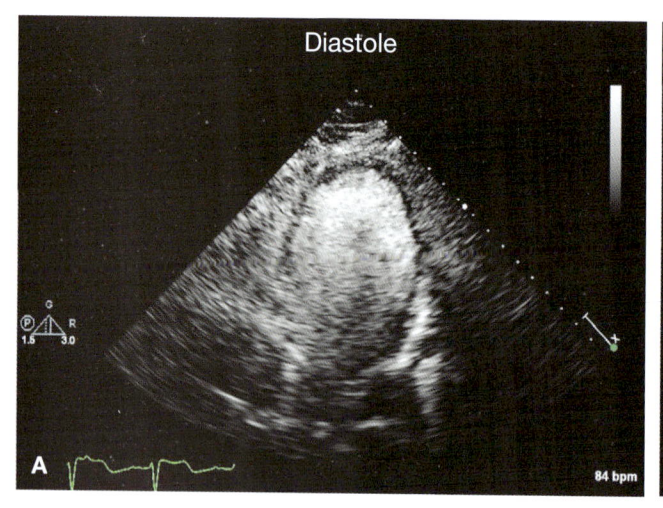

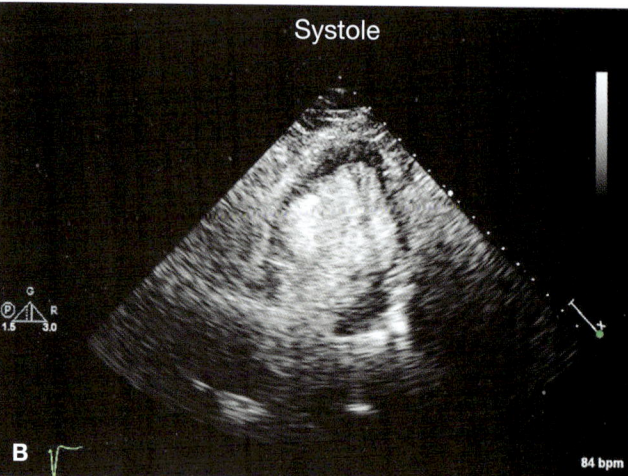

Figure 24.14

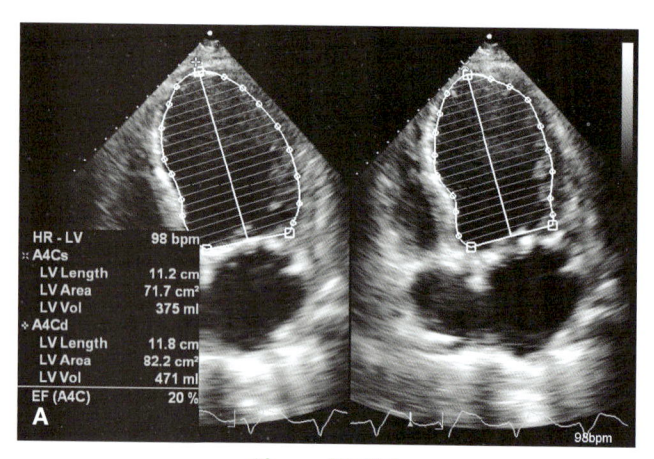

Figure 24.15A

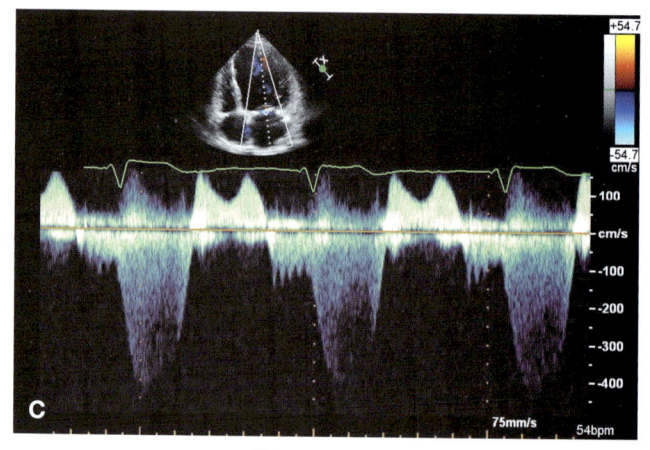

Figure 24.15C

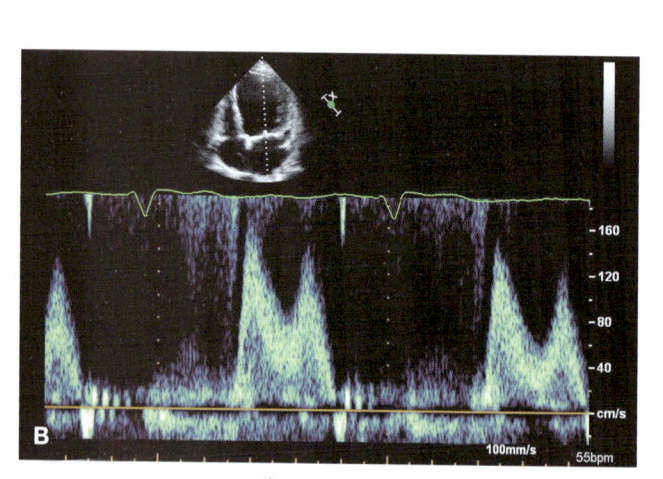

Figure 24.15B

A. Asymmetric septal hypertrophy with resting LVOT gradient >30 mm Hg, LVEDP >20 mm Hg.
B. Asymmetric septal hypertrophy with rest LVOT gradient >30 mm Hg, LVEDP <20 mm Hg.
C. Asymmetric septal hypertrophy with provocable LVOT gradients >30 mm Hg, LVEDP >20 mm Hg.
D. Symmetric septal hypertrophy with LVOT gradients >30 mm Hg, LVEDP >20 mm Hg.
E. None of the above.

31. A 27-year-old man with HCM undergoes his annual echocardiogram. The following M-mode images are available for review. Which statements BEST characterize the echocardiographic findings in **Figure 24.16A-B**?

Chapter 24 Cardiomyopathies / 507

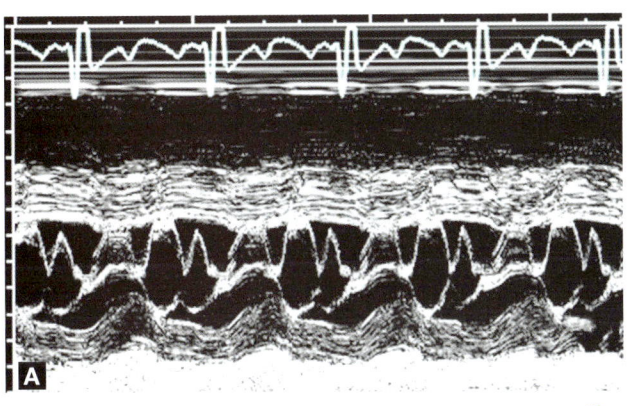

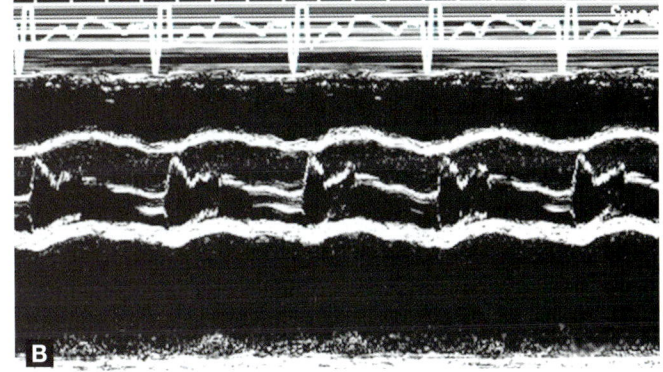

Figure 24.16

32. A 74-year-old man with HCM undergoes a routine follow-up echocardiogram. **Figure 24.17** shows the MR jet continuous-wave Doppler tracing from the apical 4-chamber view.

    The BP is 149/74 mm Hg at the time of the study. Of note, the patient appears euvolemic. Which of the following estimates of the LVOT gradient is most accurate?
    A. LVOT gradient is ~80 mm Hg.
    B. LVOT gradient cannot be determined with the available information.
    C. LVOT gradient is ~60 mm Hg.
    D. All of the above.

33. Based on the information presented in **Case 1** and the GLS seen in **Figure 24.18A** and **B**, which of the following interpretations is **CORRECT**?
    A. There is normal GLS, with normal regional variability.
    B. There is near-field clutter leading to apical artifact.
    C. There is regional and global reduction in longitudinal strain.
    D. A and C.
    E. None of the above.

34. To confirm the patient in **Case 1** has an abnormality, which of the following should be performed next?
    A. Dobutamine echocardiogram.
    B. Contrast for LV opacification.
    C. Cardiac catheterization.
    D. Cardiac magnetic resonance imaging.
    E. None of the above.

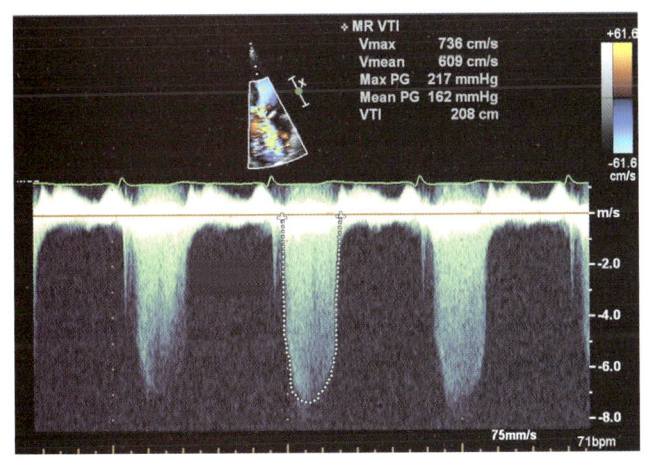

Figure 24.17

CASE 1

An 80-year-old woman is referred for a dobutamine echocardiogram due to dyspnea on exertion and edema. The baseline two-dimensional echocardiogram is interpreted as normal LV size and function, normal wall thickness, no regional wall motion abnormalities, grade I diastolic dysfunction, and no significant valvular abnormalities.

CASE 2

A 21-year-old male rookie professional football player presents for preparticipation screening prior to the start of the season. The evaluation takes place in a busy scouting combine within a gymnasium. He is asymptomatic. He has no personal or family history of heart disease. He is 6'4" and 210 lb. His physical examination is unremarkable. However, his EKG is interpreted as borderline abnormal due to a rightward axis. There is no LVH, Q waves, or T-wave abnormalities. Therefore, a limited echocardiogram is performed (**Figure 24.19A-H**, ▶ Video 24.2A-C) with a portable echocardiography machine.

Echocardiographic measurements:
LVIDd = 5.8 cm; IVS = 1.2 cm; PW = 1.2 cm; LV mass index = 131 g/m^2; RWT = 0.41.

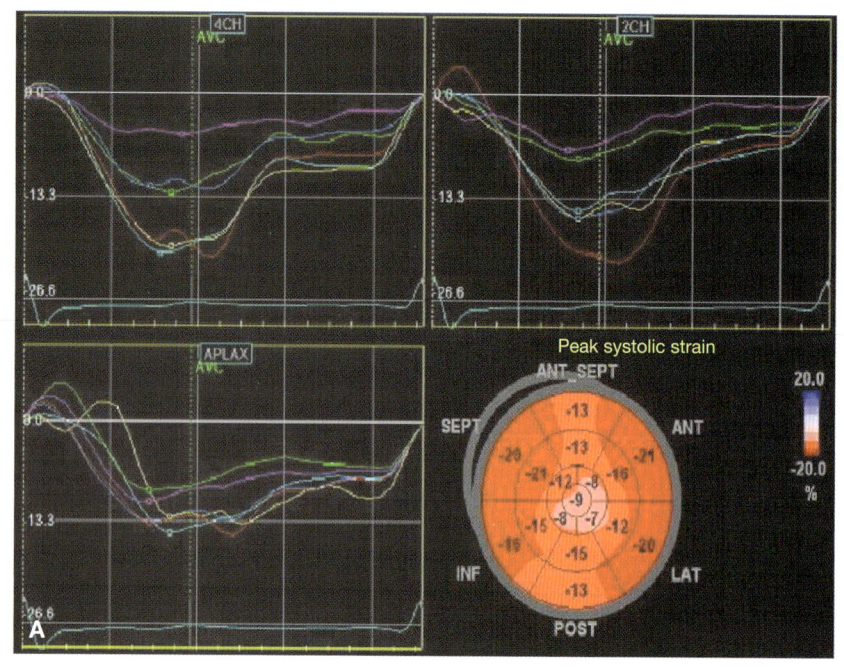

Figure 24.18A

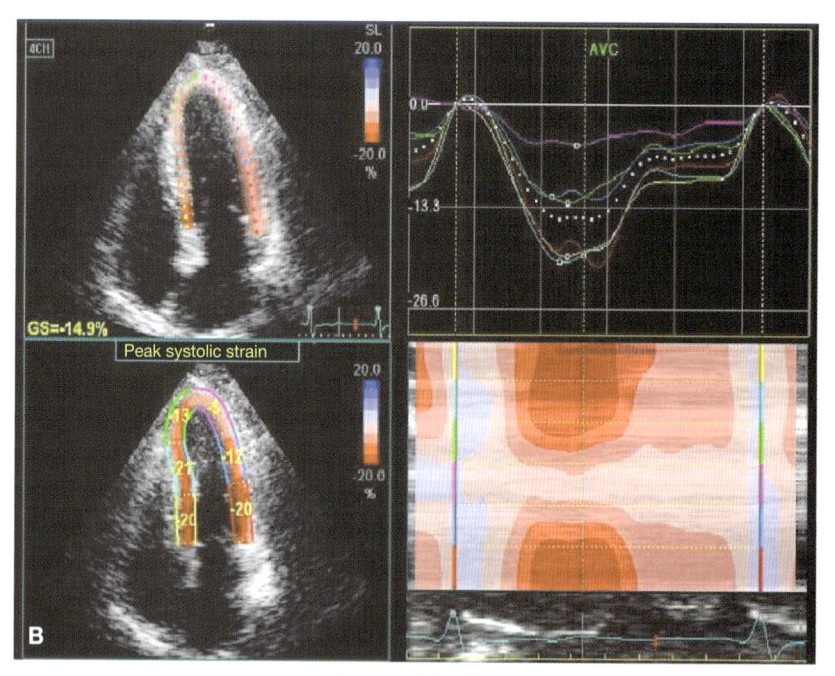

Figure 24.18B

35. Based on the clinical and echocardiographic data provided in **Case 2**, which of the following statements is **CORRECT**?
    A. The athlete should be cleared to play with no further testing required.
    B. Findings are concerning for an early form of HCM and therefore he should not be cleared to play until further testing is performed.
    C. The athlete should be cleared to play, although yearly testing should be performed due to concern for early manifestation of HCM.

Chapter 24 Cardiomyopathies / 509

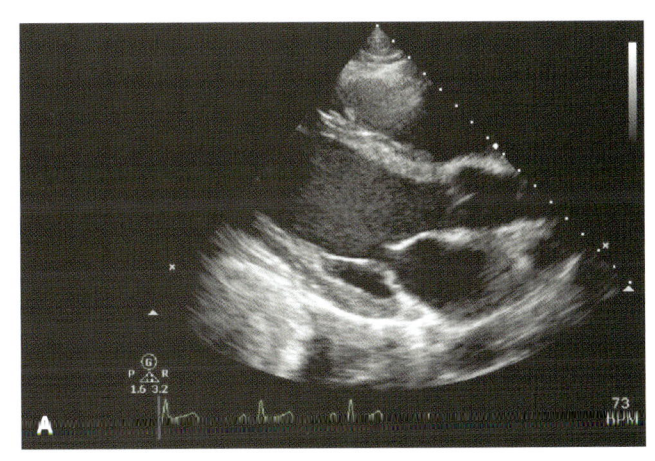

Figure 24.19A

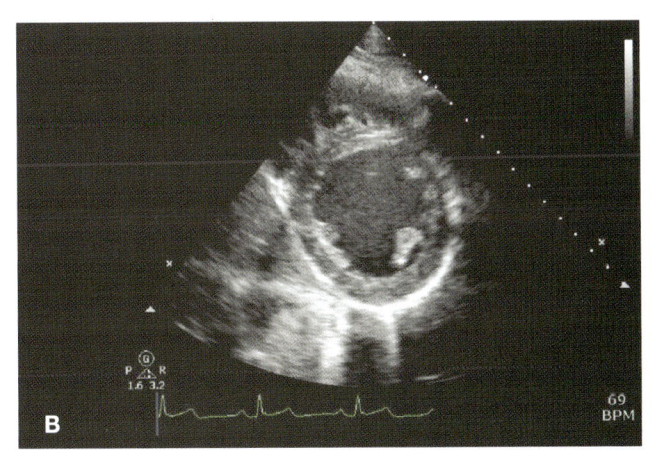

Figure 24.19B

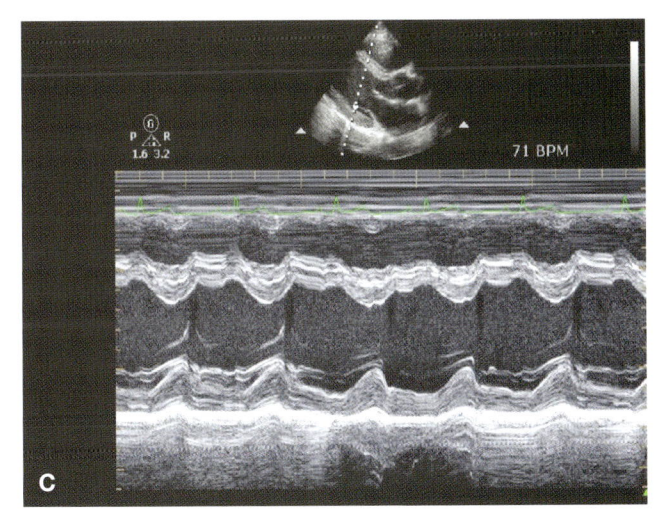

Figure 24.19C

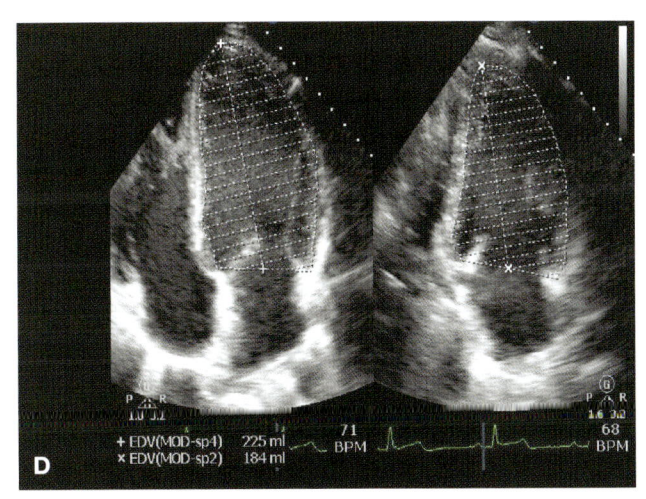

Figure 24.19D

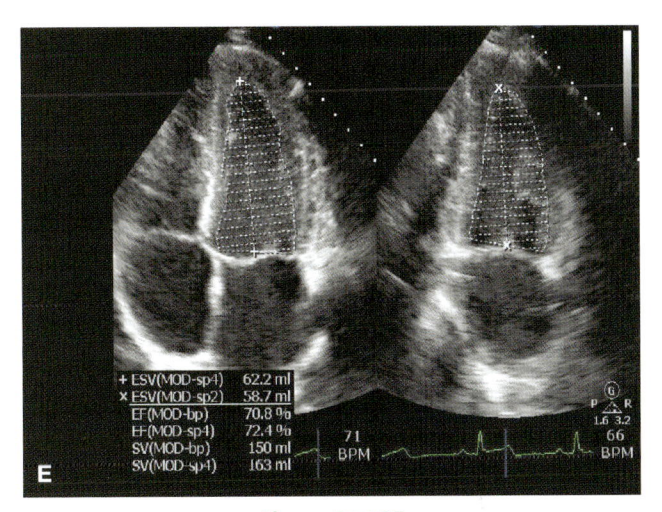

Figure 24.19E

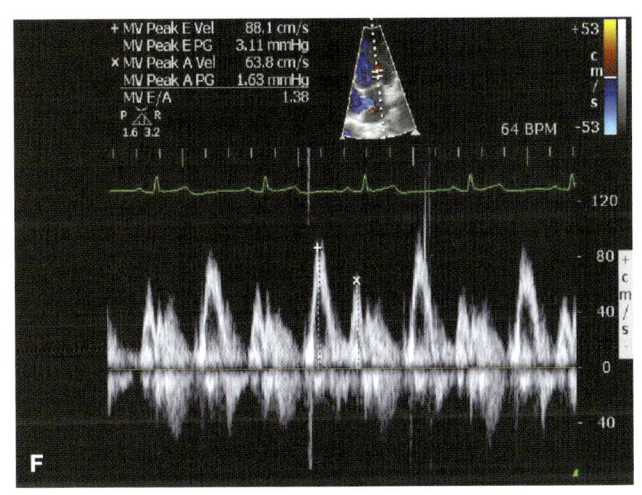

Figure 24.19F

36. Which of the following criteria has been found to be the most helpful for discriminating athlete's heart from HCM in individuals within the "gray zone" of LVH?
   A. Septal e′ >9 cm/s.
   B. Left atrial size (>34 mL/m^2).
   C. Longitudinal strain <15% (in absolute terms).
   D. Relative wall thickness (RWT) (<0.5-0.6).
   E. None of the above.

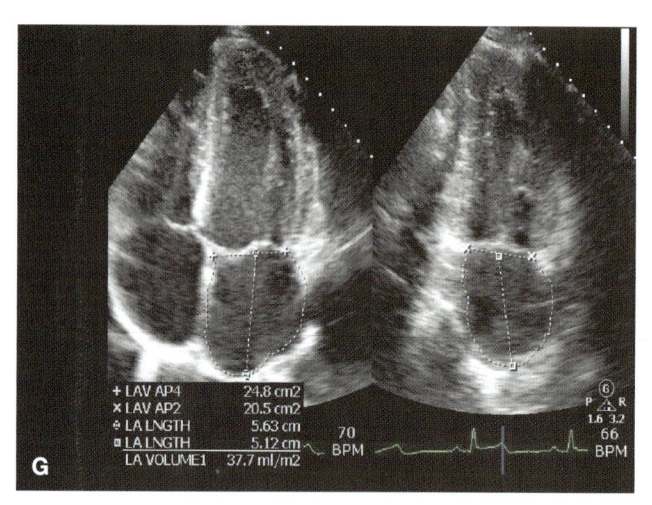

Figure 24.19G

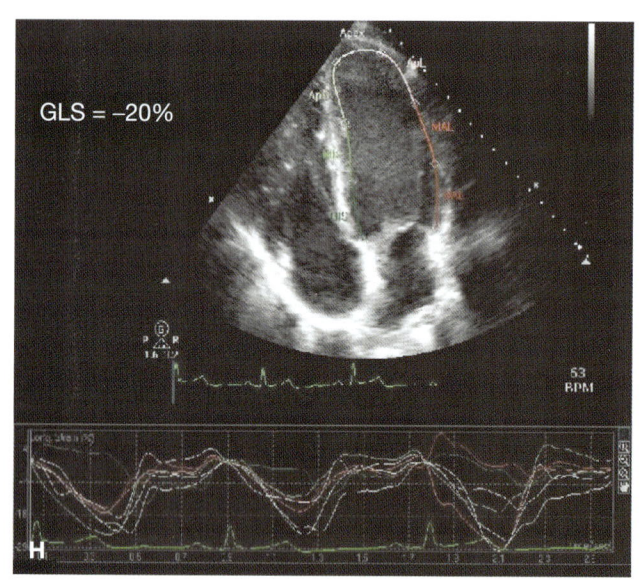

Figure 24.19H

CASE 3

A 77-year-old black man is admitted to the hospital with decompensated heart failure. He has poorly controlled hypertension with two prior admissions for diastolic heart failure, end-stage renal disease on dialysis, and coronary artery disease with prior stents. His medications on admission include carvedilol, isosorbide dinitrate, clonidine, hydralazine, and bumetanide. His physical examination was consistent with CHF. An EKG on admission is shown (**Figure 24.20A**).

Additional echocardiographic images are shown (**Figure 24.20B-J**, ▶ **Video 24.3A-C**).

37. Based on the available information from **Case 3**, which of the following diagnoses is likely?
   A. Hypertrophic cardiomyopathy.
   B. Hypertensive heart disease.
   C. Cardiac amyloidosis.
   D. All are possible.
   E. None of the above.

38. What information do you recommend next to clarify the diagnosis in the patient from **Case 3**?
   A. Cardiac MRI.
   B. Endocardial biopsy.
   C. Genetic testing for HCM.
   D. Strain imaging.
   E. None of the above.

CASE 4

A 67-year-old man is referred for consideration for myectomy. He was diagnosed with HCM 2 years previously and has had two hospitalizations for severe dyspnea and heart failure. Other PMH included sick sinus syndrome with a permanent pacemaker and COPD. His family history is notable for a brother who died suddenly at the age of 54. Medications are furosemide and metoprolol.

On examination, JVP is 10 cm H_2O, there are bibasilar crackles in the lung fields, and the cardiac examination is notable for an S3 gallop and a medium-pitched systolic ejection murmur at the LUSB that increases with the strain phase of Valsalva. There is pitting edema bilaterally.

Labs include a Cr = 0.9 and NT-BNP = 3330. EKG was sinus rhythm (not pacing). CXR shows pulmonary edema (see **Figure 24.21A-E**, ▶ **Video 24.4A-D**).

Echo data: $LVID_d/LVID_s$ = 3.6 cm/2.0 cm, proximal septum = 2.0 cm, LV diastolic volume = 86 mL, LV systolic volume = 43, LVEF = 50%, LAVi = 52 mL/m^2, and PASP = 40 mm Hg.

39. The findings in **Case 4** are consistent with what grade of diastolic dysfunction?
   A. Grade I.
   B. Grade II.
   C. Grade III.
   D. Cannot be determined.

40. What recommendation is most appropriate for the patient in **Case 4**?
   A. Alcohol septal ablation.
   B. Myectomy.
   C. Optimize pacing with short AV delay.
   D. Other.
   E. A and C.

Figure 24.20

512 / Clinical Echocardiography Review

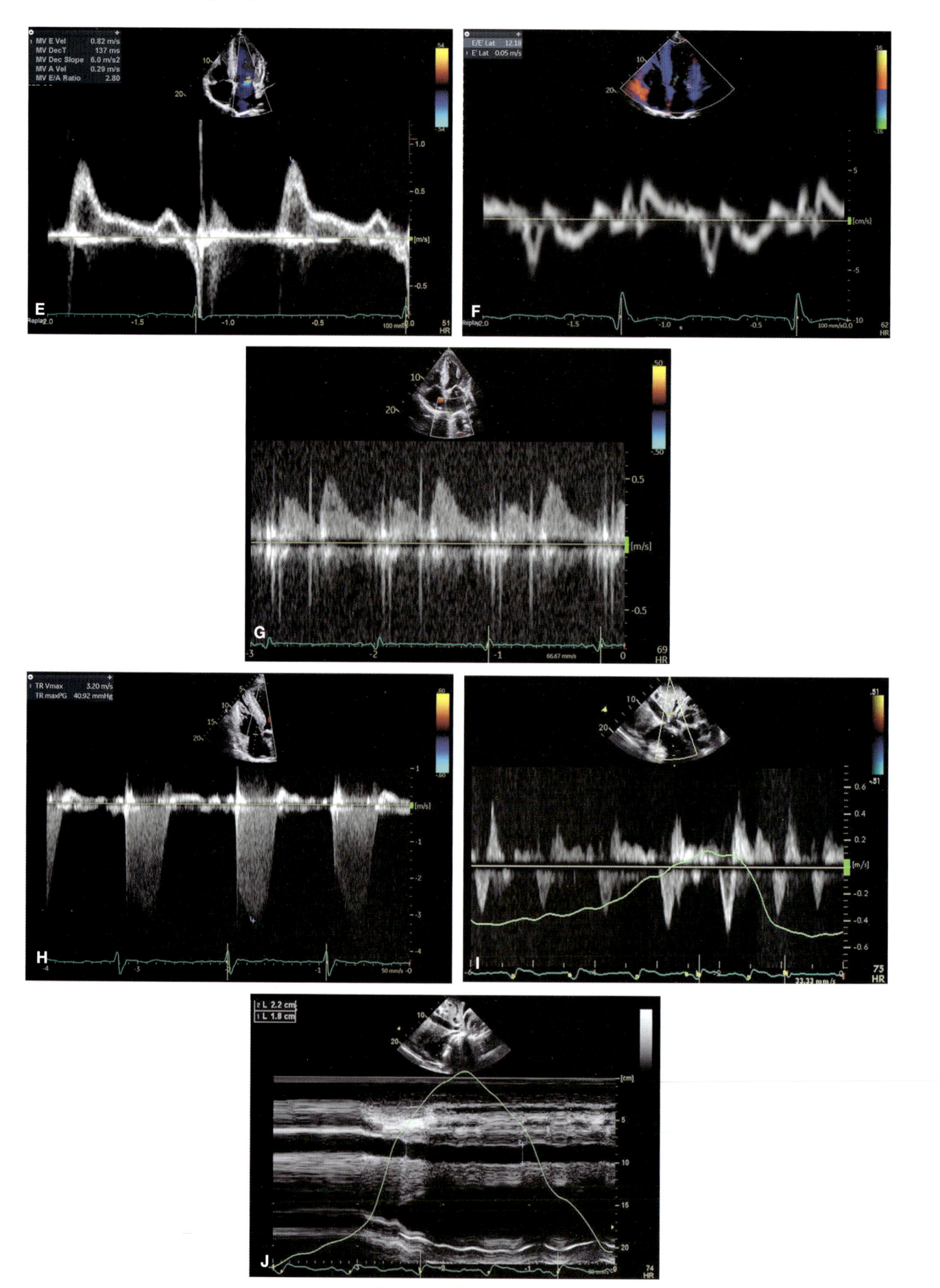

Figure 24.20. *Continued*

Chapter 24 Cardiomyopathies / 513

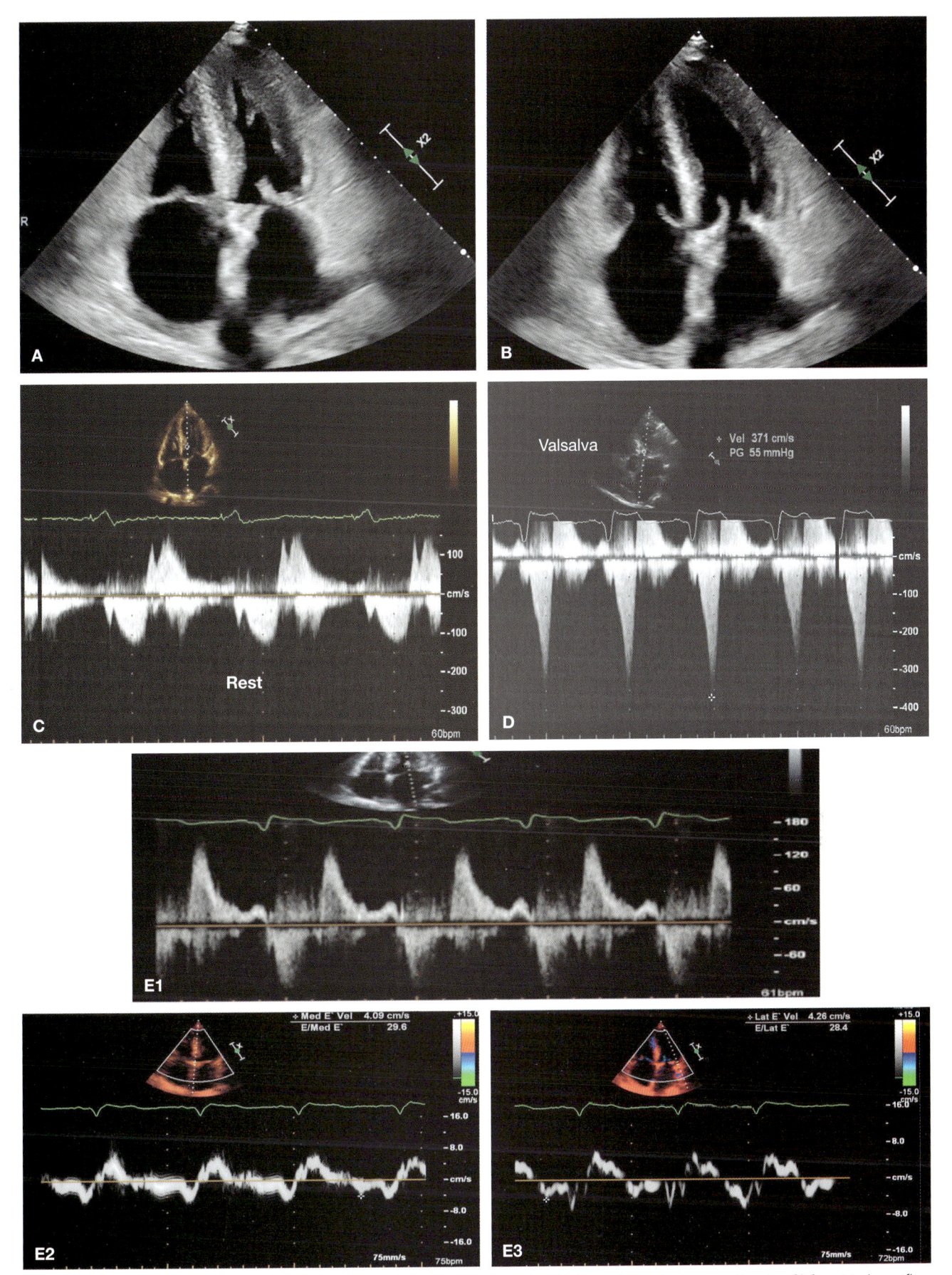

Figure 24.21. A: Apical 4-chamber view systolic frame. **B:** Apical 4-chamber view diastolic frame. **C:** Continuous wave Doppler of left ventricular outflow (LVOT) at rest. **D:** Continuous wave Doppler of LVOT with Valsalva. E: Mitral inflow (top panel), medial annular tissue Doppler (middle panel), lateral annular tissue Doppler (bottom panel). **E:** Mitral inflow (**E1**, top panel), medial tissue Doppler (**E2**, left panel), lateral tissue Doppler (**E3**, right panel).

ANSWERS

1. **Answer: E.** Increased left ventricular (LV) wall thickness is a common phenotypic appearance of many types of cardiomyopathies. When increased LV wall thickness is not due to a readily identifiable cardiac or systemic etiology like hypertension, obesity, or an aortic valve disorder that contributes to pressure and or volume overload, an explanation should be sought. Often times, the initial suspicion for cardiomyopathies such as hypertrophic cardiomyopathy or cardiac amyloidosis is based on an echocardiographic finding of increased LV wall thickness. Mechanisms for increased wall thickness include increased mass of muscle (physiologic or pathologic hypertrophy) or nonmuscle endocardial/myocardial infiltration, inflammation, fibrosis, or storage of cellular or extracellular materials. Cardiac amyloidosis is an example of an extracellular infiltrative process, while Fabry disease causes an intracellular storage of substance, both contributing to significantly increased LV wall thickness. However, some forms of cardiomyopathies (such as listed in the answers) especially of interstitial or fibrotic nature more often have normal or only mildly increased myocardial thickness. Importantly, ancillary findings such as atrial size and function, diastolic function, right and left heart filling pressures and pulmonary pressures, tissue Doppler annular velocities, and strain appearance may be the clues to a myopathic process (**Figure 24.22**).

2. **Answer: D.** The patient has "arrhythmia-induced cardiomyopathy." It is a reversible form of cardiomyopathy that occurs secondary to abnormal heart rhythms, including SVT, AF, and PVCs. It should be diagnosed only when other forms of structural heart disease are excluded. The main echocardiographic features are LV systolic dysfunction and dilatation with increased left and right heart pressures. Dilatation tends to be biventricular with mild thinning and no associated hypertrophy. The presence of moderate to severe mitral regurgitation without structural abnormalities of the mitral valve does not support a valvular cardiomyopathy, but rather is likely functional due to LV dilation. The prognosis for arrhythmia-induced cardiomyopathy related to tachyarrhythmias is generally good with most patients recovering normal function over time with correction of the underlying arrhythmia. However, the time course of recovery may be unpredictable, often taking months to years and usually largely dependent on duration of the arrhythmia. Among patients who have recovered normal function after restoration of a normal rhythm, a recurrent arrhythmia has been reported to cause rapid decline in LV function. This is thought to be due to persistence of structural and electrical abnormalities of the LV.

3. **Answer: D.** Peripartum cardiomyopathy is characterized by the development of heart failure symptoms (with an LVEF <45%) during the last month of pregnancy or during the first 5 months postpartum, in the absence of any other identifiable cause of heart failure. In addition to systolic dysfunction, echocardiography may demonstrate LV and RV dilation, functional mitral and tricuspid regurgitation, pulmonary hypertension, and biatrial enlargement. Importantly, intracardiac LV thrombus may occur and lead to thrombotic complications due to the hypercoagulable state of pregnancy. Most studies have found that >50% of patients fully recover with normalization of LVEF and resolution of symptoms. For woman having a recurrent pregnancy despite

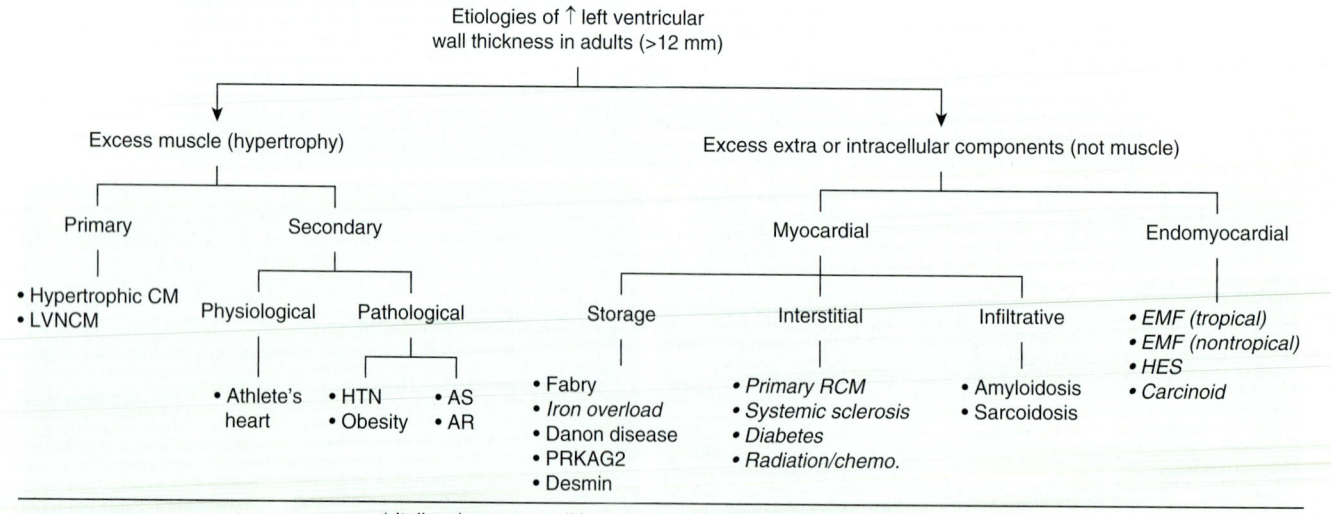

Italics denotes conditions that may have normal wall thickness

Figure 24.22. Etiologies of increased left ventricular wall thickness in adults (>12 mm). AR, aortic regurgitation; AS, aortic stenosis; EMF, endomyocardial fibrosis; HES, hypereosinophilic syndrome; HTN, hypertension; LVNCM, left ventricular noncompaction cardiomyopathy; RCM, restrictive cardiomyopathy.

persistent cardiomyopathy, the risks of heart failure and mortality is high. There is also a significant risk of relapse in women with normalization of LVEF. The most important predictor of adverse events and long-term recovery is the LVEF at the time of diagnosis, with additional predictors of worse outcomes including LV dilatation, LV thrombus, and RV dysfunction. In a small series of patients who had recovered from peripartum cardiomyopathy, dobutamine stress echocardiography was demonstrated to be a useful tool to predict the safety of a recurrent pregnancy. Those women who had recovery of LVEF to normal and maintain normal contractile function with dobutamine have a lower risk of recurrence of peripartum cardiomyopathy.

4. **Answer: C.** Histologic and clinical criteria for the diagnosis of cardiac sarcoidosis are available from the Japanese Circulation Society 2016 Guideline on Diagnosis and Treatment of Cardiac Sarcoidosis. Among the major clinical criteria are thinning of the basal ventricular septum (**Figure 24.23A** and **B**, white arrow) or abnormal ventricular wall anatomy (including aneurysms, regional wall thickening, thinning of the middle ventricular septal wall) and LVEF <50% or focal ventricular wall asynergy. Although commonly present, diastolic dysfunction, pulmonary hypertension, and the presence of pericardial effusion are nonspecific findings. Severely increased LV wall thickness is a rare finding. In the setting of a dilated cardiomyopathy with noncoronary territory wall motion abnormalities or aneurysms involving the inferior lateral basal wall and apex, cardiac sarcoid should be suspected. Reduced global longitudinal strain with regional abnormalities particularly in the septum may also be present (see **Table 24.1**).

5. **Answer: B.** Anthracycline-based chemotherapeutic agents are used to treat several forms of malignancy, but are associated with acute and chronic cardiotoxicity. The current criteria for cardiotoxicity (or CTRCD, cancer therapy-related cardiac dysfunction) proposed by the 2022 European Society of Cardiology guidelines in the absence of HF symptoms are: (1) any new reduction in LVEF below 40%; (2) a new reduction in >10 percentage points to a LVEF 40% to 49%; (3) a new reduction in <10 percentage points to an LVEF 40% to 49% and either a relative decrease in GLS by >15% from baseline or a new rise in cardiac biomarkers; or (4) an LVEF >50% and a relative decrease in GLS by >15% from baseline and/or a new rise in cardiac biomarkers.

Table 24.1. Echocardiographic Findings Suggestive of Cardiac Sarcoidosis

Most specific

- Thinning of the basal septum (anterior/inferior)
- Abnormal ventricular wall anatomy:
  - Ventricular aneurysms (RV apex, LV apex or inferolateral wall)
  - Regional ventricular wall thickening
  - Thinning of midventricular septal wall
- Regional wall motion abnormalities LV (noncoronary distribution)

Nonspecific

- LV dysfunction (LVEF <50%) or LV dilatation
- RV dysfunction/dilatation (rare mimic of RV cardiomyopathy)
- Diastolic dysfunction
- Pericardial effusion
- Papillary muscle dysfunction
- Severe increased LV wall thickness (rare mimic of HCM)
- Pulmonary hypertension
- Reduced GLS or regional (noncoronary distribution) LS

GLS, global longitudinal strain; HCM, hypertrophic cardiomyopathy; LS, longitudinal strain; LV, left ventricular; LVEF, left ventricular ejection fraction; RV, right ventricular.

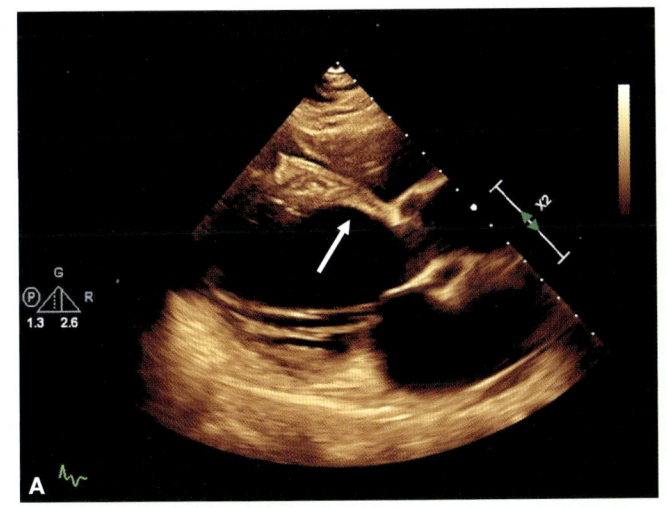

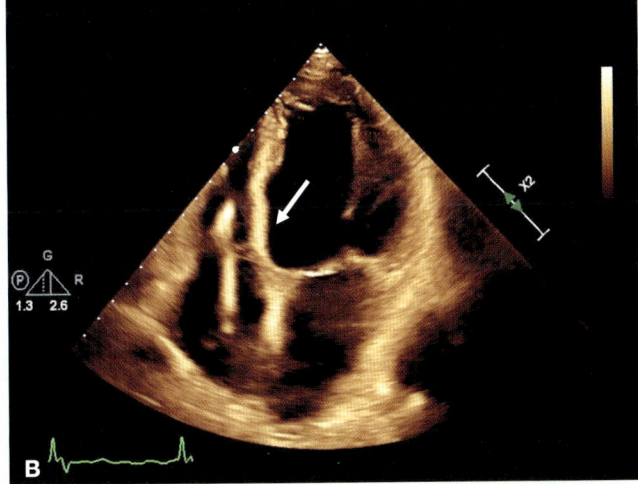

Figure 24.23

Baseline LVEF and GLS are recommended in all patients before cardiotoxic cancer treatment initiation to stratify risk and identify significant changes during treatment. The prognosis of patients who develop doxorubicin cardiotoxicity is generally poor and usually irreversible; therefore, there have been efforts to predict which patients are at risk. Global longitudinal strain (GLS) measured by speckle tracking echocardiography has been found to be the most sensitive predictor of subclinical LV dysfunction. A cutoff value of >15% relative reduction in GLS is considered abnormal and thus the 10% drop (−25% to −22.5%) in this patient would not be consistent with cardiotoxicity. However, if cardiac biomarkers were available and abnormal, criteria for cardiotoxicity would be met.

6. **Answer: A.** RWT is determined as 2× the posterior wall thickness/left ventricular internal dimension in diastole. A RWT > 0.42 indicates concentric remodeling or concentric hypertrophy depending on whether LV mass is normal or increased, respectively. Exercise-induced cardiac remodeling, often called "athletes' heart," is an adaptive increase in cardiac chamber size and/or wall thickness promoted by the volume and pressure loads of exercise. Notably, athletes who perform endurance exercise are more prone to adaptations that lead to larger cardiac chamber size, whereas resistance training leads to changes where hypertrophy predominates. Therefore, RWT might be increased in isometric activity only in athletes (such as powerlifters) but is a less common presentation of athlete's heart and would not be expected in an Olympic marathon runner. For an endurance athlete, there is balanced chamber dilatation and hypertrophy and therefore an RWT < 0.42 with increased LV mass results in a pattern of eccentric hypertrophy See **Figure 24.24**. An increase in LA volume and LV mass may occur with both athlete's heart and hypertensive LVH. RV dilation is usually not present with hypertensive LVH but is common with athlete's heart. Several other parameters of systolic and diastolic function may help to differentiate these conditions including tissue Doppler and strain. All these variables should be normal in athlete's heart but may be abnormal with pathologic forms of LVH.

7. **Answer: A.** Radiation-associated heart disease is a consequence of radiation treatment for various mediastinal or thoracic cancers, most commonly breast cancer and lymphoma. It appears years to decades following treatment. Cardiac involvement includes coronary artery stenosis, valvular, myocardial, pericardial, aortic, and conduction disease. Since it involves the myocardium, it is often considered a form of acquired endomyocardial restrictive cardiomyopathy. With radiation, valve cusps and leaflets undergo fibrotic changes with thickening and restriction with or without calcification, leading to regurgitation or stenosis. Valve regurgitation is more commonly found than stenosis. Aortic insufficiency is the most common pathology followed by aortic stenosis, probably due to the fact the aortic valve is usually closest to the radiation field. Aorto-mitral curtain thickening or calcification (junction between the base of the anterior mitral leaflet and the aortic root) is a specific finding suggesting radiation-associated disease. Calcification of the mitral annulus and subvalvular apparatus is also common. The aorto-mitral curtain is typically spared from most degenerative or acquired conditions, with the exception of endocarditis, aortitis, or advanced calcific conditions such as end-stage renal disease. When thickening or calcification of the aorto-mitral curtain is seen in conjunction with aortic or mitral valve disease, as well as myocardial disease, it is highly suggestive of radiation-associated disease (**Table 24.2**).

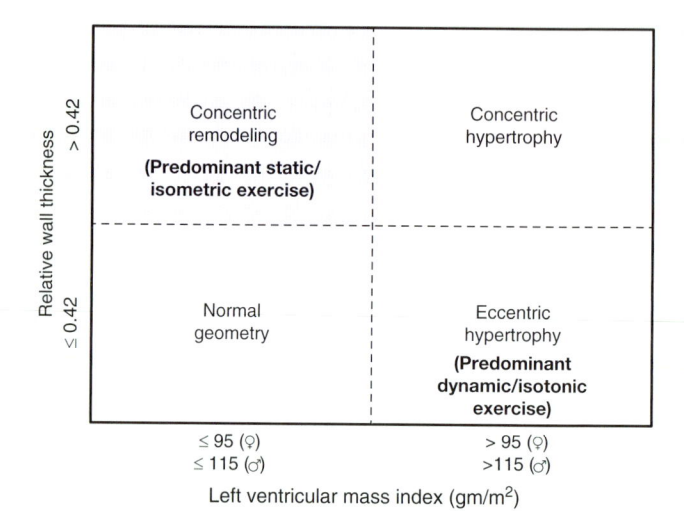

Figure 24.24. Reprinted from Lang RM, Badano LP, Mor-Avi V, et al. Recommendations for cardiac chamber quantification by echocardiography in adults: an update from the American Society of Echocardiography and the European Association of Cardiovascular Imaging. *J Am Soc Echocardiogr.* 2015;28(1):1-39.e14. Copyright © 2015 by the American Society of Echocardiography. With permission.

8. **Answer: C.** Several structural and functional features of HCM are associated with an increased risk of SCD (see **Table 24.3**). Structural features include the degree of LV wall thickness, left atrial size, presence of an apical aneurysm, and progression to the dilated-hypokinetic cardiomyopathy (end-stage or burned-out stage of HCM) with reduced LVEF <50%. Although an LV wall thickness in any segment of >28 to 30 mm is considered an indication for an implantable cardiac defibrillator, increasing LV wall thickness appears to be associated with a continuous increase in risk. Functional features of HCM associated with risk of SCD include the degree of LVOT obstruction. Comparative studies by Maron et al demonstrated that LVOT obstruction (>30 mm Hg) was associated with a higher incidence of SCD,

Table 24.2. Echocardiographic Findings Suggestive of Radiation Heart Disease

Myocardial involvement

- Normal LV wall thickness and nondilated cavity
- Normal LV function (with HFpEF/restrictive CM)
- Ischemic CM with LV dysfunction < nonischemic CM/preserved LV function
- Regional wall motion abnormalities/scar (coronary or noncoronary territory)
- Reduced global/regional GLS (even with preserved LV function)
- Biatrial enlargement/reduced atrial function/atrial strain
- Reduced DTI (e′, s′)
- Reduced stroke volume with preserved LV function
- Advanced diastolic dysfunction with ↑ LAP (usually grade II, III)
- RV dysfunction and pulmonary HTN

Pericardial involvement

- Pericardial thickening/calcification
- Pericardial effusion (usually small, may have effusive constrictive pericarditis)
- Constrictive pericarditis (with associated findings)
- Regional GLS reduced (strain reversus)

Valve involvement

- Valve leaflet thickening, calcification and restriction
- Aorto-mitral curtain thickening/calcification (specific hallmark)
- Mitral annular and leaflet calcification (spares tips and commissures)
- Aortic stenosis > mitral stenosis
- Mitral, aortic, tricuspid, and pulmonic (regurgitation > stenosis; left > right-sided)
- Mixed regurgitation/stenosis

Aortic involvement

- Ascending aortic/aortic arch calcification (porcelain aorta)
- Aortic annulus calcification
- Aortic root calcification

CM, cardiomyopathy; DTI, doppler tissue imaging; GLS, global longitudinal strain; HFpEF, heart failure with preserved ejection fraction; HTN, hypertension; LAP, left atrial pressure; LV, left ventricular; RV, right ventricular.

Table 24.3. Echocardiographic Features of HCM Associated With Increased Risk of Sudden Cardiac Death

- Massive LVH (>28-30 mm) in any segment
- LV systolic dysfunction, LVEF < 50% (burned-out phase)
- LV apical aneurysm (independent of size)
- LA size (per ESC criteria, measured in mm)
- LVOT gradient (per ESC criteria, measured as continuous variable)

ESC, European Society of Cardiology; HCM, hypertrophic cardiomyopathy; LA, left atrial; LV, left ventricular; LVEF, left ventricular ejection fraction; LVH, left ventricular hypertrophy; LVOT, left ventricular outflow tract.

---

compared to nonobstructors. In addition, patients who have undergone myectomy appear to have a reduction in SCD risk and likelihood of appropriate ICD shocks, though these data are based on nonrandomized comparisons and do not negate guideline-based indications for ICD.

9. **Answer: C.** Cardiac involvement in hemochromatosis is a form of iron storage disease with deposition in various organs including the myocardial cells of the heart (iron overload cardiomyopathy). It may be a hereditary (primary) or acquired condition. Aside from myocardial storage, there is also interstitial inflammation contributing to myocardial damage. Therefore, whereas many forms of myocardial storage disorders have increased LV wall thickness, iron overload cardiomyopathies usually do not. By the American Heart Association (AHA) classification of cardiomyopathies, it is characterized as a secondary cardiomyopathy since it is part of a systemic disease. In addition to LV involvement, conduction abnormalities and supraventricular arrhythmias are common manifestations. Cardiac involvement in iron overload cardiomyopathy evolves through a progression of structural and functional abnormalities. In the early stages, diastolic dysfunction, including tissue Doppler abnormalities may be the first manifestation, despite normal LV size, wall thickness, and systolic function. Some patients may progress to advanced diastolic dysfunction (restrictive phenotype), but this is a less common presentation. For others, as the disease progresses, there is a decrease in LV systolic function, LV cavity dilation, and biatrial enlargement (dilated phenotype). LV wall thickness is usually normal or mildly increased even in the later stages. Identification of iron overload cardiomyopathy is important since treatment with chelating agents or phlebotomy may improve cardiac function. Cardiac MRI is the gold standard diagnostic test for cardiac iron overload cardiomyopathy.

10. **Answer: B.** All of the features noted are echocardiographic findings that are consistent with athlete's heart (see **Table 24.4**). In athlete's heart, there may be an increase in LV cavity size (uncommonly beyond 6.0 cm), and in a small group of athletes, there may be a symmetric increase in LV wall thickness (between 1.3 and 1.5 cm—"the gray zone"). There is normal LV systolic and diastolic function. Four-chamber enlargement may be seen. Answer A is consistent with HCM with a septal

Table 24.4. Typical Echocardiographic Features of Athlete's Heart vs Hypertrophic Cardiomyopathy

	Athlete's Heart	HCM
$LVID_d$	Normal or ↑ (<6.0 cm)	↓ or normal
LV wall thickness	Normal or ↑ (≤15 mm)	↑ (often IVS/PW ≥1.3)
RWT	<0.5-0.6	≥0.5-0.6
LVEF	Normal or low normal (LVEF ≥50%)	Normal or ↑
$RVID_d$	Normal or ↑	Normal
RV wall thickness	Normal	Normal or ↑
LA volume index	Normal or ↑	Normal or ↑
RA volume index	Normal or ↑	Normal
Aorta	Normal or ↑ (<4.2 cm)	Normal
Diastolic function	Normal	Abnormal
e' (TDI)	>9 cm/s	<9 cm/s
Longitudinal strain[a]	>15%	<15%

HCM, hypertrophic cardiomyopathy; IVS, interventricular septum; LA, left atrial; LV, left ventricle; LVEF, left ventricular ejection fraction; $LVID_d$, left ventricular internal dimension in diastole; PW, posterior wall; RA, right atrial; RV, right ventricle; $RVID_d$, right ventricular internal dimension in diastole; RWT, relative wall thickness; TDI, tissue Doppler imaging. Cutoff values may depend on age, race, size, and type of sport played. Different cutoff values are seen in female athletes.
[a]Expressed in absolute terms.

wall thickness outside of the gray zone, asymmetric hypertrophy, and normal LV cavity size with a reduced tissue Doppler annular velocity. Answer C is suggestive of arrhythmogenic RV dysplasia due to RVOT dilation (normal size proximal RVOT in the parasternal short-axis view is <3.6 cm) and unbalanced RV dilation, with normal LV chamber size. Answer D is suggestive of Marfan syndrome due to the presence of aortic root dilation and mitral valve prolapse.

11. **Answer: D.** The ACC/AHA 2020 guidelines for the diagnosis and treatment of patients with HCM has a class I recommendation for performing both clinical screening (EKG/echocardiogram) and cascade genetic testing (when a pathogenic variant has been identified in the index family member) in first-degree relatives at risk. A pathogenic variant was not identified in the index patient in this question; therefore, there is no indication to do cascade genetic testing in family members. Electrocardiography and echocardiography monitoring is recommended at 3 to 5 year intervals starting in adulthood, and more frequently in children and adolescence. Screening intervals of at-risk family members who are phenotype and genotype negative can be tailored to more frequent intervals when there are: (1) symptoms suggestive of HCM; (2) they are involved in activities or occupations associated with higher risk, such as competitive sports; or (3) the index family member has had a more malignant course or an earlier age of onset of HCM. There are not data to determine when screening of asymptomatic family members can be discontinued, though current guidelines recommend to screen at least to age 50s.

12. **Answer: D.** The patient presents with features consistent with apical HCM. Apical HCM is typically characterized as an LV apex >15 mm, with apical to posterior wall thickness ratio >1.5, although a lower threshold has been suggested of >13 mm, or a relative increase of apex to base thickness in early stages (often with associated EKG findings). Apical HCM can be either isolated (normal wall thickness except the apex) or mixed (increased LV wall thickness of nonapical segments, especially the septum). In isolated apical HCM, systolic anterior motion of the mitral valve or LV outflow obstruction either at rest or after provocative maneuvers does not occur. Left ventricular cavity linear dimension in diastole is usually normal although LV cavity volume may be reduced, with associated reduced stroke volume. LV systolic function is usually normal or increased. LA volume is typically increased and diastolic function is abnormal. Apical outpouchings or apical aneurysms may occur in patients with apical HCM especially with midcavitary obliteration. Since apical aneurysms in HCM are associated with VT, SCD, HF, LV dysfunction, LV thrombus, and embolic events, they should be sought after. Apical abnormalities may only be seen if contrast echocardiography is performed. Other clues to apical aneurysms include pooling of blood or contrast at the apex, midventricular gradients and hypertrophy, and paradoxical diastolic flow within the LV cavity. **Figure 24.25** shows the progression of apical HCM to an apical aneurysm.

13. **Answer: C.** Various echocardiographic criteria have been proposed to describe LV noncompaction/excessive LV trabeculation phenotype. These include: (1) a two-layer myocardium with a thin compacted epicardial layer and thick noncompacted endocardial layer; (2) a ratio of noncompacted to compacted myocardium of >2.1 measured in end-systole in the short-axis view; (3) deep intertrabecular recesses with continuity to the LV cavity; (4) prominent trabeculations; and (5) predominant localization to the midlateral, midinferior, and apical regions.

Historically, left ventricular noncompaction cardiomyopathy (LVNCM) had been classified as a

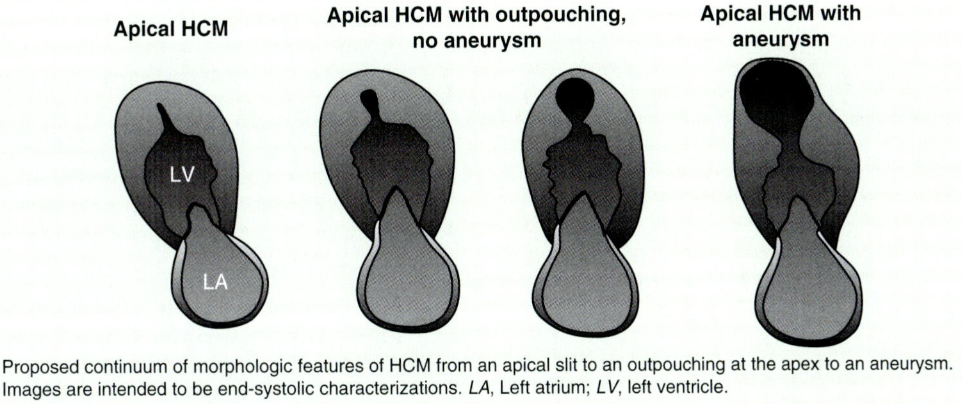

Figure 24.25. Reprinted from Binder J, Attenhofer Jost CH, Klarich KW, et al. Apical hypertrophic cardiomyopathy: prevalence and correlates of apical outpouching. *J Am Soc Echocardiogr.* 2011;24(7):775-781. Copyright © 2011 American Society of Echocardiography. With permission.

Proposed continuum of morphologic features of HCM from an apical slit to an outpouching at the apex to an aneurysm. Images are intended to be end-systolic characterizations. *LA*, Left atrium; *LV*, left ventricle.

primary genetic cardiomyopathy according to the AHA proposed classification scheme. As an isolated cardiomyopathy, LVNCM is rare. However, noncompacted left ventricular (LV) myocardium (or excessive trabeculations of the LV) may occur in association with other genetic, chromosomal, neuromuscular, or congenital syndromes or cardiac abnormalities. It has also been reported to occur as a physiologic adaptive response to many conditions such as athletic training, pregnancy, or hematologic disorders. Therefore, it may range from a genetic cardiomyopathy associated with serious cardiovascular morbidity and mortality to a pathologic response to pressure and volume overload, to a normal process of cardiac remodeling that may be dynamic and reversible over time, with prognosis dependent on associated clinical presentation or ventricular remodeling such as LV dilatation, dysfunction, or hypertrophy. In view of this diverse presentation, recent 2023 European Society of Cardiology Cardiomyopathy Guidelines and an expert panel paper recommend that noncompaction be considered as a phenotype of excessive LV trabeculations with deep intertrabecular recesses and should not be considered as a distinct cardiomyopathy.

14. **Answer: B.** In restrictive cardiomyopathy, diastolic dysfunction is usually advanced. The left atrial or left ventricular end-diastolic pressure is usually elevated. LV size and systolic function are often normal. Answer B describes a patient with a high mitral E-wave velocity, a decreased mitral annular tissue Doppler e′ lateral velocity, and an E/e′ ratio of 20 suggestive of elevated LV filling pressure. In restrictive cardiomyopathy, color M-mode velocities would be expected to be delayed (propagation velocity, V_p < 50 cm/s), with pulmonary vein systolic to diastolic velocity ratio of <0.5 and a mitral deceleration time <160 ms. Other expected findings include LA volume index >34 mL/m^2, and E/A ratio >2, elevated pulmonary artery and right atrial pressure, and abnormal left ventricular and left atrial strain.

15. **Answer: A.** Cardiac amyloidosis is an infiltrative cardiomyopathy due to deposition of amyoid fibrils originating from either bone marrow cells (AL) or liver cells (ATTR), wild-type or hereditary. Both types of amyloid have similar appearances on echocardiography and several structural and functional features on 2-dimensional echocardiography and Doppler and strain may raise suspicion. Many of these features are nonspecific such as increased LV wall thickness, granular sparkling pattern, low TDI velocities, and advanced diastolic dysfunction. However, regional GLS patterns are among the most specific features of cardiac amyloidosis with an apical sparing pattern aiding to differentiate from other etiologies of increased LV wall thickness such as aortic stenosis, hypertensive heart disease, and hypertrophic cardiomyopathy. Since visual diagnosis of an apical sparing pattern is subjective, it is important to be familiar with the quantitative equivalent, which is determined as an average apical segment LS/average combined basal + mid LS >1.0. See **Table 24.5** for common echocardiographic features of cardiac amyloidosis.

16. **Answer: A.** The patient has Loeffler endocarditis, a disorders associated with variable degrees of eosinophilia or evidence of eosinophil-mediated organ involvement. It may be a primary myeloproliferative disorder or secondary to infections, allergic conditions, or tumors. Loeffler endocarditis differs from endomyocardial fibrosis, which is seen in endemic tropical areas. Some consider Loeffler endocarditis an earlier stage of endomyocardial fibrosis. These are forms of restrictive cardiomyopathy with similar echocardiographic features. There are three stages of disease due to eosinophil-mediated toxic endomyocardial damage: (1) necrotic, (2) thrombotic, and (3) fibrotic. If treated prior to the fibrotic stage, reversibility may occur. Echocardiographic findings are listed in **Table 24.6**. Signature findings of cardiac involvement in EMF and Loeffler endocarditis include Merlon sign, which describes

Table 24.5. Echocardiographic Findings Suggestive of Cardiac Amyloidosis

Two-dimensional echo

- ↑ LV wall thickness (symmetric most common but asymmetric, sigmoid septum, reversed septal contour possible)
- ↑ RV wall thickness
- "Granular sparkling pattern" of LV myocardium
- Biatrial enlargement with abnormal LA/RA strain
- Thickened valves and atrial septum
- Pericardial and pleural effusions
- Dilated IVC and hepatic veins
- SAM (uncommon)

Doppler

- ↓ LV stroke volume (low output) with preserved LV function
- Advanced diastolic dysfunction (usually grade II or III) with ↑ LAP
- Pulmonary HTN
- Blunted PV and HV S wave consistent with ↑ LAP/RAP
- Loss of PV AR
- ↓ mitral annular velocities ("5, 5, 5" sign—s', e', a' DTI velocities <5 cm/s)
- Aortic stenosis (most often paradoxical low-flow low-gradient AS)
- LVOT obstruction (uncommon)

Strain

- Reduced global and regional LV GLS
- Apical sparing pattern or relative regional strain ratio (RRSR or RELAPS)—average apical LS/average combined base + mid LS >1.0
- Septal apical-base ratio (SAB) >2.9
- EF strain ratio >4.1

AR, atrial reversal; AS, aortic stenosis; DTI, Doppler tissue imaging; EF, ejection fraction; GLS, global longitudinal strain; HTN, hypertension; HV, hepatic vein; IVC, inferior vena cava; LA, left atrial; LAP, left atrial pressure; LS, longitudinal strain; LV, left ventricular; LVOT, left ventricular outflow tract; PV, pulmonary vein; RA, right atrial; RAP, right atrial pressure; RV, right ventricular; S, systolic; SAM, systolic anterior motion.

---

a hypercontractile basal ventricle opposing an obliterated apex which is hypo/akinetic and a "square root sign" seen on M-mode echocardiography of the basal LV cavity showing exaggerated early rapid diastolic septal and posterior wall motion after exaggerated systolic motion. A classification of endomyocardial fibrosis distribution has been proposed by Shaper et al (**Figure 24.26B**) and includes RV involvement as seen in **Figure 24.26A**.

17. **Answer: D.** This echocardiogram is from a patient diagnosed with Fabry cardiomyopathy (CM). Fabry disease is an X-linked lysosomal storage disease due to an enzyme deficiency of alpha-galactosidase A, which results in progressive intracellular glycosphingolipid accumulation affecting several organs including the heart. Fabry CM can be misdiagnosed as HCM. Characteristic features of cardiac involvement include increased LV wall thickness, preserved LV systolic function, normal LV dimensions, and impaired diastolic function. Although asymmetric increased wall thickness may occur, Fabry CM generally has a symmetric pattern. Systolic anterior motion of the mitral valve (SAM) and LVOT obstruction may occur, but are not common. Specific features of Fabry CM not typical of HCM are lacking. A "binary appearance" of the layers of LV septal wall was described as a specific feature of Fabry CM, although subsequent studies did not confirm this finding. There is a predilection for involvement of the basal inferolateral wall resulting in hypokinesis, akinesis, fibrosis, and subsequent thinning. **Figure 24.2D** (apical 2-chamber view) shows a thinned/akinetic/aneurysmal basal inferior wall (though more typically inferolateral wall) in a patient with Fabry disease. This can be detected as reduced GLS in the region. This is a later sign by echocardiography and is more likely to be detected on cardiac MRI with delayed enhancement. Diagnosis of Fabry CM is very important since enzyme replacement therapy or chaperone therapy, if initiated early enough in the disease course, has proven to improve cardiac function and reduce wall thickness. See **Table 24.7**.

18. **Answer: B.** There is a crypt in the basal segment of the inferior wall. Although there is not full agreement on a definition, crypts are usually characterized as blood-filled "V-" or "U"-shaped invaginations in the myocardium, perpendicular to the endocardium, extending at least 50% toward the epicardium as seen in end-diastole. Crypts are most often located in the basal/mid septum or inferior wall. They may be single or multiple in number and disappear during systole. They are important since they have been reported to be present in genotype (+), phenotype (−) individuals with HCM. However, crypts are also seen in patients without HCM, particularly in those with hypertension. Therefore, given the clinical history of a family member with CM, it is likely that this patient would test positive for HCM. Notably, crypts have been observed to disappear when hypertrophy develops. While echocardiography can be useful at detecting crypts, cardiac MRI has been the test of choice to evaluate for subclinical HCM findings. **Table 24.8** illustrates other associated echocardiographic features suggesting early expression of HCM. In **Figure 24.27**, the arrow points to the crypt.

19. **Answer: B.** The clinical and echocardiographic findings are consistent with RV cardiomyopathy (or ARVC), which is a myocardial disease characterized by fibrofatty ventricular replacement, ventricular arrhythmias, and the risk of SCD. Diagnostic findings of RV cardiomyopathy seen on echocardiography are noted in **Table 24.9**. Modified task force criteria for the diagnosis of RV cardiomyopathy

Table 24.6. Echocardiographic Findings Suggestive of Cardiac Endomyocardial Fibrosis/Loeffler Disease

- Endomyocardial thickening with obliteration of LV/RV apex with fibrosis/thrombus
- Hypoechogenic wall thickening (thrombotic)
- Hyperechogenic wall thickening (fibrotic)
- Scattered patches of hyperechogenic fibrosis (apex, free wall, papillary muscles, septum)
- Small LV/RV cavity size
- LV/RV function preserved (normal myocardial motion, restricted endomyocardium)
- Biatrial enlargement
- Mitral regurgitation due to fibrous or thrombotic retraction of posterior papillary muscles, subvalvular apparatus
- Tricuspid regurgitation due to fibrous retraction TV
- Pericardial effusion
- Advanced grade diastolic dysfunction (restrictive pattern with high left- and right-sided filling pressures) typical of restrictive cardiomyopathy
- Merlon sign (hyperkinetic basal segments with hypo/akinetic apex)
- Exaggerated M-mode LV base showing early rapid diastolic septal and posterior wall motion "square root sign".

LV, left ventricular; RV, right ventricular; TV, tricuspid valve.

were proposed in 2010. Major criteria applicable to echocardiography include: (1) RV akinesia, dyskinesis, or aneurysm; (2) parasternal long-axis or short-axis severe RVOT dilatation; or (3) reduced RV fractional area change (≤33%). Minor criteria include: (1) RV akinesis or dyskinesis, (2) parasternal long-axis or short-axis RVOT nonsevere dilatation, and (3) reduced RV fractional area change (>33% to ≤40%). RV cardiomyopathy presenting as a dilated LV cardiomyopathy is well-described, but not common. **Figure 24.4A** shows parasternal long-axis image in diastole with RVOT dilatation. **Figure 24.4B** shows apical 4-chamber image in systole with prominence of the moderator band, RV dilatation, and an RV apical aneurysm in the region of the "triangle of dysplasia."

20. **Answer: D.** As reviewed in the answer to question 7, aorto-mitral curtain thickening or calcification (junction between the base of the anterior mitral leaflet and the aortic root) is a specific finding suggesting radiation-associated disease. This is well demonstrated in the images shown in **Figure 24.5A,B** and **C**. In addition, there is aortic stenosis, aortic regurgitation, and mitral stenosis present. Mitral and aortic stenosis are present with mitral annular, leaflet, and cusp calcification but without commissural fusion of the aortic and mitral valves. Commissural fusion is an expected finding with rheumatic heart disease,

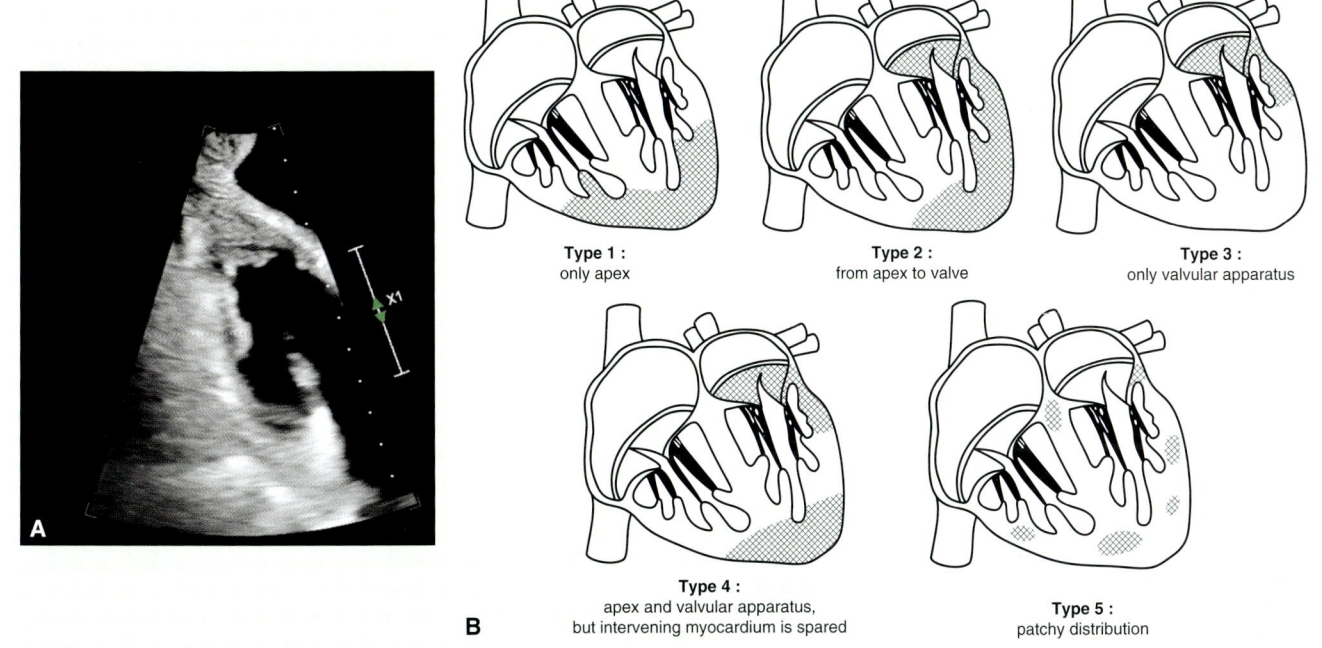

Figure 24.26. A: Focused right ventricular (RV) view showing RV infiltration of endomyocardial fibrosis. **B:** Reprinted from Polito MV, Hagendorff A, Citro R, et al. Loeffler's endocarditis: an integrated multimodality approach. *J Am Soc Echocardiogr.* 2020;33(12):1427-1441. Copyright © 2020 by the American Society of Echocardiography. With permission.

Table 24.7. Echocardiographic Findings Suggestive of Fabry Disease

- Symmetric > asymmetric ↑ LV wall thickness (mimics HCM)
- Nonobstructive > obstructive physiology (SAM/LVOT obstruction less common)
- Inferolateral basal wall hypokinesis/akinesis/thinning
- ↓ basal inferolateral GLS (early finding) or global reduced GLS (with normal LVEF)
- Papillary muscle hypertrophy and hyperechogenicity (disproportionate to LVH)
- Diastolic dysfunction and left atrial enlargement (and impaired atrial strain)
- RV ↑ wall thickness
- "Binary appearance" LV septum or hyperechogenic endocardium (nonspecific)
- Aortic root dilatation

GLS, global longitudinal strain; HCM, hypertrophic cardiomyopathy; LV, left ventricular; LVEF, left ventricular ejection fraction; LVH, left ventricular hypertrophy; LVOT, left ventricular outflow tract; RV, right ventricular; SAM, systolic anterior motion.

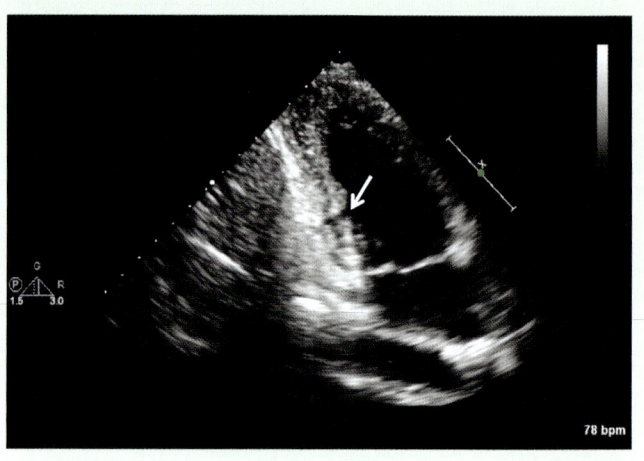

Figure 24.27

both for the mitral and aortic valve. In addition to rheumatic heart disease, end-stage renal disease and homozygous familial hypercholesterolemia may cause valvular calcification and stenosis but do not typically involve the aorto-mitral curtain, especially to the extent seen in these images (Answers A-C are incorrect).

Table 24.8. Echocardiographic Features Suggestive of Early Phenotypic Hypertrophic Cardiomyopathy

- Myocardial crypts (most often basal inferoseptum/inferior wall)
- Regional or global abnormalities of LV GLS
- Elongated mitral leaflets with chordal slack
- Hypermobile, hypertrophied, multiheaded papillary muscles
- Apical and anterior displacement of papillary muscles
- Atypical insertion of chordae or papillary muscle (LVOT, anterior leaflet)
- Chordal SAM
- Reduced TDI mitral annular e' or s'
- Abnormal diastolic function (mitral inflow or pulmonary veins)
- Mild LVH with concentric remodeling or hypertrophy (↑ RWT)

GLS, global longitudinal strain; LV, left ventricular; LVH, left ventricular hypertrophy; LVOT, left ventricular outflow; RWT, relative wall thickness; SAM, systolic anterior motion; TDI, tissue doppler imaging.

21. **Answer: D.** Chagas cardiomyopathy is a vector-borne zoonotic disease endemic to the Americas, caused by infection of the parasite *Trypanosoma cruzi*. The cardiac manifestations include an acute and chronic form of myocarditis. In most cases, the acute infection is unrecognized and the chronic condition appears years to decades later. The pathophysiology of chronic myocardial damage is likely a result of persistent immune-mediated inflammation, necrosis, and fibrosis, which commonly affects small arterioles, leading to myocardial damage and predisposing to arrhythmias. Due to this vasculitis-like inflammation, regional wall motion abnormalities in a noncoronary distribution are common at any stage of the disease. These are located mainly at the LV apex and inferior and inferolateral walls (**Figure 24.6A-C**). The microvascular inflammation can be so severe that thinning of the myocardial segments can lead to formation of aneurysms, which are prone to thrombus formation (seen on **Figure 24.6A**). The use of ultrasonic enhancing agents for LV opacification and wall motion evaluation is recommended. Typical electrocardiographic findings in Chagas myocarditis include right bundle branch block, left anterior hemiblock, AV block, and multifocal premature beats. **Table 24.10** summarizes common features of Chagas cardiomyopathy. Increased biventricular wall thickness is more suspicious of an infiltrative cardiomyopathy, mitral regurgitation due to leaflet tethering is a common association with ischemic and DCM, and noncompacted myocardium is not a major manifestation of Chagas disease.

22. **Answer: E.** Global longitudinal strain (GLS) patterns displayed in bull's eye plots derived from 2-dimensional speckle tracking imaging provide a visual overview of myocardial regional and global function. These patterns, while not always specific, may suggest etiologies of myocardial or pericardial disorders. GLS pattern A is a classic example of apical sparing, often a signature finding of cardiac amyloidosis.

Table 24.9. Echocardiographic Features of Right Ventricular Cardiomyopathy

- RV cavity dilation (rest or stress)
- RV outflow tract dilation (in isolation or associated with cavity dilation)
- RV dysfunction (rest or stress)
- RV regional abnormalities
- Reduced RV regional GLS
- Prominent trabeculations/moderator band
- Aneurysms (systolic) in the "triangle of dysplasia"
- Sacculations (diastolic outpouchings) in the "triangle of dysplasia"
- Dilated LV cardiomyopathy

GLS, global longitudinal strain; LV, left ventricular; RV, right ventricular.
"Triangle of dysplasia" consists of the basal right ventricular inflow, right ventricular outflow, and apex.

GLS pattern B shows predominantly reduced basal anteroseptal strain from a patient with cardiac sarcoidosis. GLS pattern C shows predominantly reduced apical strain seen in a patient with apical hypertrophic cardiomyopathy. This can be referred to as "blueberry-on-top" strain pattern GLS pattern D shows predominantly reduced septal strain from a patient with an asymmetric septal hypertrophy pattern of hypertrophic cardiomyopathy. GLS pattern E shows a preserved septal strain > lateral strain, due to tethering of the myocardium, in a patient with constrictive pericarditis. This is an example of "strain reversus," which is the strain equivalent to "annulus reversus" where the tissue Doppler annular e' medial

Table 24.10. Echocardiographic Findings Suggestive of Chagas Cardiomyopathy

Acute
- Global LV dilatation and dysfunction (myocarditis)
- Pericardial effusion

Chronic
- Biventricular dilatation and dysfunction
- Regional abnormalities of noncoronary territory (most common apical, inferior, inferolateral wall, usually basal)
- Aneurysm (LV apex, inferior, inferolateral; RV uncommon)
- Thrombus (in aneurysmal segments)
- Functional MR and TR
- Dilated LA and abnormal diastolic function
- ↓ Global and regional GLS
- Pericardial effusion

GLS, global longitudinal strain; LA, left atrium; LV, left ventricular; MR, mitral regurgitation; RV, right ventricular; TR, tricuspid regurgitation.

velocity is higher than the e' lateral velocity (opposite of normal), a characteristic finding in constrictive pericarditis. Although GLS pattern E is similar to what may be seen with cardiomyopathies that have a predilection for involvement in the inferolateral basal region such as Fabry disease, sarcoidosis, Chagas disease, or muscular dystrophy, extension to the anterolateral wall is less typical with these conditions.

23. **Answer: C.** The patient has asymmetric septal hypertrophy with dynamic LVOT obstruction. The pulsed-wave Doppler pattern shows the "lobster claw pattern" with a mid-systolic dip in velocity as depicted by the white arrow (**Figure 24.28**). The sample volume is placed just apical to the point of LVOT obstruction due to systolic anterior motion (SAM) of the mitral valve. There is an initial high velocity followed by a mid-systolic drop in velocity during SAM-septal contact when afterload exceeds the LV contractility. This finding is consistent with LVOT obstruction usually with peak gradients >60 mm Hg. The speckle tracking peak longitudinal strain polar plot shown in **Figure 24.8B** shows a regional, predominantly septal reduction in GLS. This pattern is consistent with asymmetric septal hypertrophy due to HCM. It is not consistent with cardiac amyloidosis, which has a characteristic apical sparing strain pattern.

24. **Answer: C.** The images show relative thinning of the basal anteroseptal and basal inferoseptal walls with normal mid-anteroseptal and mid-inferoseptal thickness. This is not a typical pattern of coronary artery disease. Thinning of the basal anteroseptal wall is characteristic and relatively specific for cardiac sarcoidosis with granulomatous infiltration and scarring. The basal anteroseptal wall can also be preferentially affected by a few other conditions including myocarditis. Basal inferolateral wall thinning occurs with several types of myocardial diseases including muscular dystrophies, Fabry disease, and Chagas disease. Cardiac sarcoidosis can

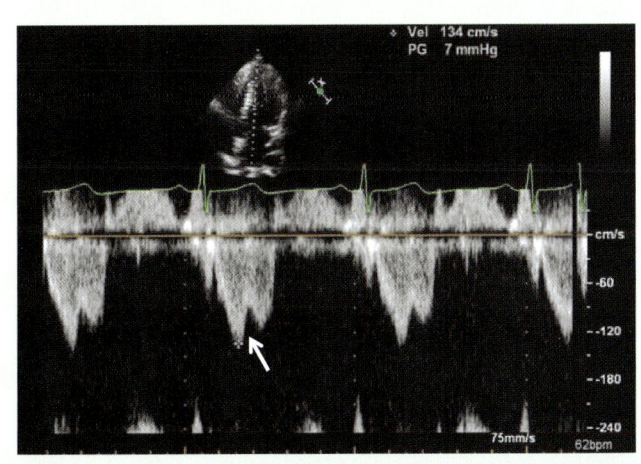

Figure 24.28

also involve the inferolateral region, although this is a less common finding. Furthermore, there is an appearance of an apical sparing pattern, though in this context with regional wall abnormalities, cardiac amyloidosis is not likely. See **Figure 24.23A** and **B** showing PLAX and apical 4-chamber views in a patient with known sarcoidosis, ventricular tachycardia, and ICD. Arrows point to the thinning of the antero- and inferoseptum. **Table 24.1** lists echocardiographic findings suggesting cardiac sarcoidosis.

25. **Answer: C. Figure 24.10A,B** shows hypertrophy with reverse septal curvature. Reversed septal curvature means that the shape of the LV cavity is crescent-shaped with the hypertrophy convex toward the left side. There are age-related differences seen in patients with HCM. Younger patients typically have asymmetric hypertrophy involving the septum with reversed septal curvature and right ventricular hypertrophy. Elderly patients more often have a localized proximal septal hypertrophy (septal bulge) that is due in part to geometric changes in the heart with aging. The LV cavity shape and septal curvature are normal (concave toward the left side, with ovoid-shaped LV cavity) and right ventricular hypertrophy is not present. The elderly form of HCM is associated with sarcomeric mutations in 8% of patients, whereas the reversed septal curvature shape is associated with sarcomeric mutations in 79% of patients. Most patients with this elderly form of HCM present with symptoms due to LVOT obstruction, though sudden cardiac death is uncommon. **Figure 24.29** demonstrates the various LV and RV cavity shapes associated with HCM.

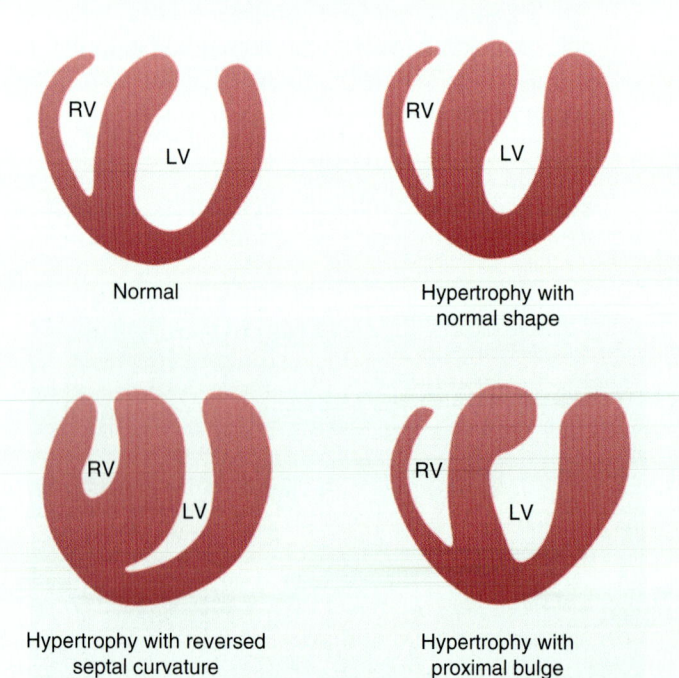

Figure 24.29. Reprinted with permission from Lever HM, Karam RF, Currie PJ, Healy BP. Hypertrophic cardiomyopathy in the elderly. Distinctions from the young based on cardiac shape. *Circulation*. 1989;79(3):580-589. Copyright © 1989 by American Heart Association.

26. **Answer: C.** The echocardiographic images show severe symmetric increased LV wall thickness. Clinical history, EKG, and echocardiographic findings together can be highly suggestive of the underlying cause of specific cardiomyopathies. When increased LV wall thickness is seen along with a preexcitation pattern on EKG, the differential diagnosis should include (1) Fabry disease; (2) Danon disease; and (3) PRKAG2 mutation. Danon disease is a X-linked storage disease (lysosomal and glycogen) associated with intellectual disability, skeletal myopathy, and cardiac dysfunction most often presenting as a severe cardiomyopathy with heart failure. Danon disease is caused by a defect in the *LAMP2* gene. Sarcomeric gene mutations are the primary cause of HCM, though HCM does not present with systemic symptoms. Dystrophin gene mutations contribute to the development of muscular dystrophies that may cause cardiomyopathy and skeletal myopathy, but are not usually associated with preexcitation. A mutation in the *GLA* gene causes a deficiency in alpha-galactosidase A, which is the cause of Fabry disease. However, Fabry disease is not typically associated with advanced skeletal myopathy. PRKAG2 cardiomyopathy is a rare infiltrative glycogen storage disease this is also associated with increased LV wall thickness, preexcitation, conduction disease, and an unusual "stripes" pattern of bull's eye GLS.

27. **Answer: C.** The continuous-wave Doppler tracing is called the "mid-systolic signal void." This finding is seen with HCM and midcavity obliteration. It suggests an apical akinetic aneurysm. See **Figure 24.30**, the first flow (white arrow) is early systolic LV cavity ejected flow before cavity obliteration. The "mid-systolic signal void" occurs because there is cessation of flow with midcavity obliteration (white dashed arrow) for the remainder of systole. The second flow is a low velocity paradoxical diastolic flow (yellow arrow) from blood trapped in the apex toward the basal cavity. This occurs because of the presence of the apical abnormality. The apical pressure remains higher than in the basal/mid cavity resulting in a paradoxical flow towards the base during early diastole. Since apical abnormalities are not always well recognized especially if contrast is not given, this Doppler pattern should alert the interpreting physician to further investigate. HCM with apical aneurysms are associated with ventricular tachycardia, sudden cardiac death, congestive heart failure, and left ventricular apical thrombus. ▶ **Video 24.5AB** shows the same patient with midcavity hypertrophy, cavity obliteration, and apical aneurysm.

28. **Answer: A.** Primary restrictive cardiomyopathy is a rare form of cardiomyopathy associated with heart failure that usually presents at an early age in adulthood. It is usually a diagnosis of exclusion after other etiologies for restrictive cardiomyopathy and

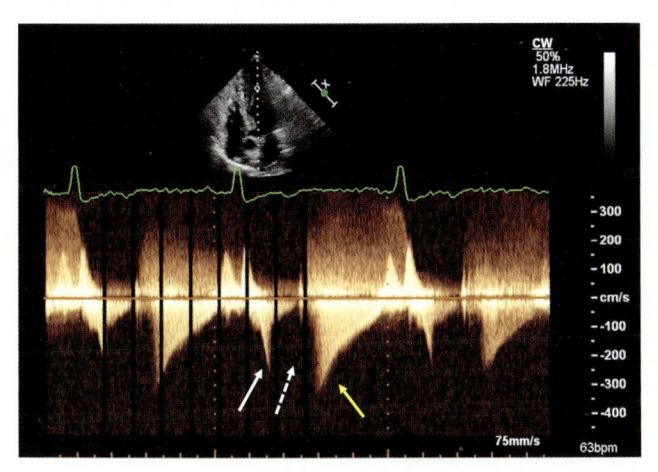

Figure 24.30

Table 24.11. Causes of Systolic Anterior Motion (SAM) of the Mitral Valve and Left Ventricular Outflow Obstruction

- Hypertrophic cardiomyopathy
- Proximal septal bulge of the elderly
- Stress cardiomyopathy
- Other cardiomyopathies (Fabry, amyloid—uncommon)
- Anterior MI (with preserved basal septal function)
- Post aortic valve replacement
- Post mitral valve repair
- Aberrant/anomalies of mitral valve leaflets/apparatus
- Dobutamine echo (hyperdynamic state)
- Extreme reductions preload, afterload, contractility
- Cardiac compression (effusions, ascites, etc.)

MI, myocardial infarction.

pericardial disease are excluded. The hallmark of all restrictive cardiomyopathies is advanced diastolic dysfunction. In this patient, the e' annular velocity is ~4 cm/s and the mitral inflow pattern is restrictive with a short deceleration time, E/A ratio >2, and an E/e' ratio near 25 consistent with high left-sided filling pressures. Other echocardiographic features of primary restrictive cardiomyopathy include normal LV size and systolic function, biatrial enlargement, and pulmonary hypertension. However, the wall thickness in this form of cardiomyopathy is usually normal or mildly increased consistent with the histologic finding of marked interstitial fibrosis. See **Figure 24.22** for causes of increased LV wall thickness.

29. **Answer: B.** The clinical history and echocardiographic images are most consistent with Takotsubo (stress cardiomyopathy). Several variants of stress cardiomyopathy have been described including (1) classical apical ballooning (apical akinesis) variant with proximal to mid-hyperkinesis; (2) midventricular ballooning; (3) basal or reverse variant with hypokinesis of the basal segment and apical hyperkinesis; and (4) focal variant. Right ventricular apical involvement may also occur. The classical apical variant remains the most common, typically presenting in postmenopausal women after a physical or emotional trigger. However, women and men of all ages may experience any of the variants. **Figure 24.14B** shows basal and apical wall thickening with absence of thickening in the midcavity, consistent with midventricular ballooning, in this case a manifestation of anaphylaxis. Left ventricular obstruction due to systolic anterior motion of the mitral valve is a well-recognized consequence of the classical apical variant and may contribute to hypotension. Although not described with the midventricular variant, reduction in the murmur with phenylephrine, an alpha 1 agonist suggests obstruction. Often SAM of the mitral valve is thought to be pathognomonic of hypertrophic cardiomyopathy but is actually seen with many other conditions. **Table 24.11** reviews causes of SAM.

30. **Answer: C.** The patient has severe LV cavity dilation (end-diastolic volume 471 mL) and severe LV dysfunction (LVEF = 20% by the method of discs). On continuous-wave Doppler (**Figure 24.31**, white arrow), diastolic mitral regurgitation (MR) is seen. Diastolic MR may occur during AV pacing when the AV delay is too long. Atrial contraction is completed before the onset of ventricular contraction and therefore the mitral valve remains open but with a left ventricular pressure that is higher than the left atrial pressure. Diastolic MR contributes to symptoms, which may improve with shortening the AV delay.

31. **Answer: A.** Classic M-mode tracings for HCM are shown. **Figure 24.32A** (left panel) shows asymmetric septal hypertrophy with prolonged SAM septal contact in systole (yellow arrow). Prior to use of continuous-wave Doppler ultrasound to determine LVOT gradients, M-mode echocardiographic estimates of obstruction were utilized. A prolonged SAM-septal contact of >30% of systole generally correlated with a resting LVOT gradient >30 mmHg. Similarly, M-mode tracings

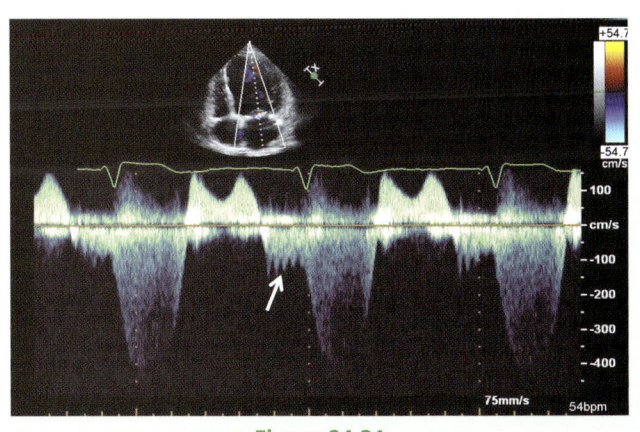

Figure 24.31

526 / Clinical Echocardiography Review

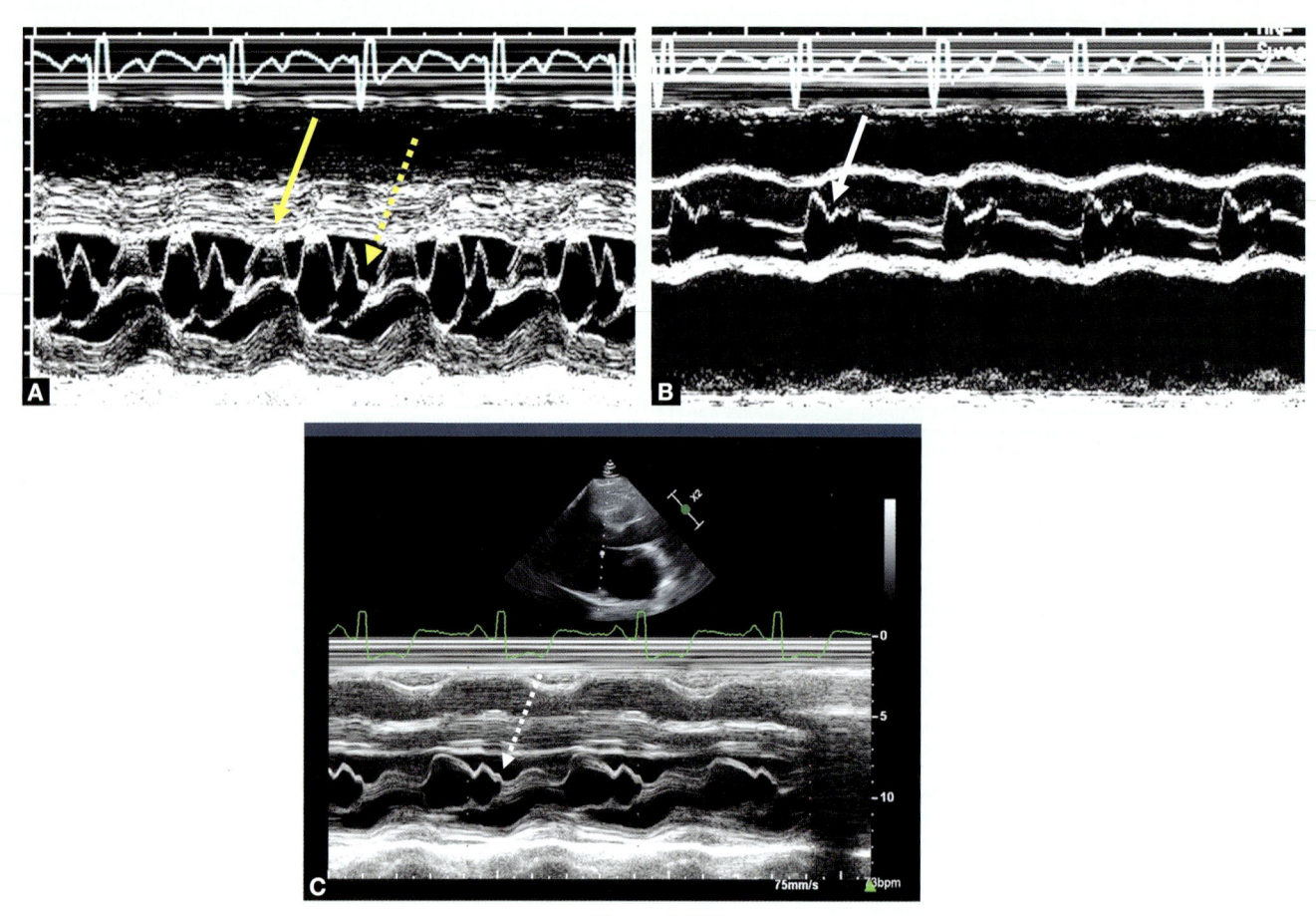

Figure 24.32

of the aortic valve are shown; **Figure 24.32B** (right panel) shows aortic notching and fluttering (white arrow) consistent with LVOT obstruction. Finally, a B-bump is seen on M-mode (**Figure 24.32A**, left panel, dashed yellow arrow), with a second example of a B-bump better seen with increased sweep speed on **Figure 24.32C** (dashed white arrow), which is consistent with a significantly elevated LVEDP, usually >20 mm Hg.

32. **Answer: A.** The LVOT gradient can be estimated from the MR jet, especially if the left atrial pressure (LAP) is expected to be low. In this circumstance, the MR jet will represent the pressure gradient between the left ventricular systolic pressure (LVSP) and the left atrial pressure (LAP)—217 mm Hg—or pressure difference = $4v^2$ MR jet, where v = 7.36 m/s or 217 mm Hg. If we assume the LAP is 10 mm Hg, the LVSP = 217 + 10 = 227 mm Hg. Then, the LVSP—the systolic blood pressure (SBP) = the LVOT gradient, 227—149 = 78 mm Hg. **Figure 24.33** shows the LVOT gradient from the same patient.

33. **Answer: C.** The GLS is −14.9%, which is abnormal (normal is −18% to −20%). In addition, there is regional variability with reduction of longitudinal strain at the apex, particularly toward the lateral wall. In normal individuals, apical longitudinal strain is generally higher than the mid and basal segments. Although the history suggests that the LV wall thickness and wall motion are normal, strain can detect regional abnormalities due to disease states not evident with conventional two-dimensional echocardiography.

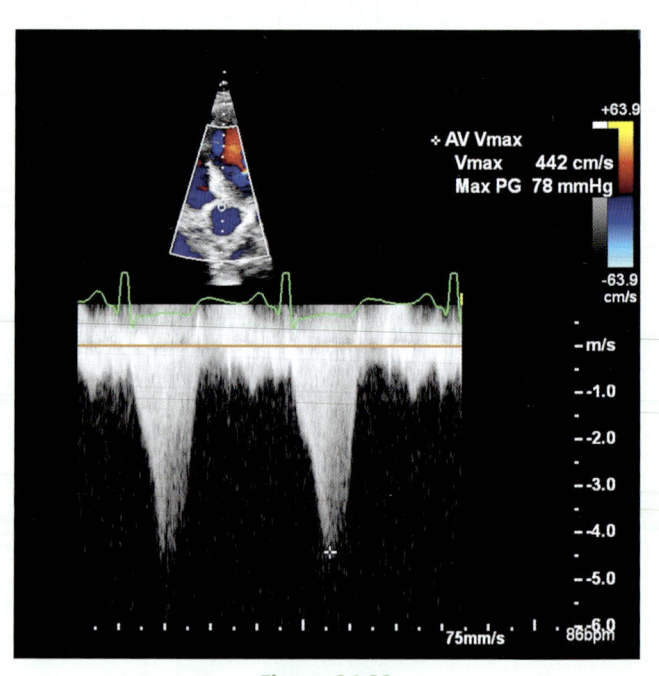

Figure 24.33

34. **Answer: B.** The patient has a mild form of apical HCM that was not evident on the two-dimensional echocardiogram. An apical wall motion abnormality or infarct could also explain the regional variability in strain. Contrast was given and demonstrated a small area of apical hypertrophy (see **Figure 24.34**, white arrow points to apical hypertrophy in the apical 4-chamber view). In addition, not stated in the history was that the EKG (**Figure 24.35**) showed LVH with repolarization abnormalities and T-wave inversions consistent with the diagnosis of apical HCM.

> **KEY POINTS**
> - Regional GLS may provide clues to CAD or myocardial diseases not readily evident on 2-dimensional echocardiographic imaging.
> - Correlation of EKG findings, 2D echocardiography with contrast, and GLS is helpful in the diagnosis of apical HCM.

35. **Answer: A.** The clinical and echocardiographic findings are all consistent with athlete's heart. The echocardiographic findings include a dilated LV cavity with normal systolic function, mild LVH with relative wall thickness (RWT) consistent with eccentric hypertrophy, and an increased LV mass index (**Figure 24.24**). Diastolic function is normal and LA volume index is increased. The longitudinal peak systolic strain is normal at −20%. All of these findings are consistent with athlete's heart. Although there is mild LVH and an increase in LV mass index, the degree of hypertrophy falls in the "gray zone" of hypertrophy (13-15 mm), which, with concomitant LV dilation, is generally associated with physiologic, not pathologic, hypertrophy. Therefore, there are no findings concerning for HCM that require additional testing (**Table 24.4**).

36. **Answer: D.** Numerous echocardiographic variables have been used to distinguish LVH related to athlete's heart from HCM, particularly when LVH falls within the "gray zone" (**Table 24.4**). Although, the approach for distinguishing physiologic from pathologic hypertrophy should include clinical information, EKG, echocardiography, and sometimes cardiac MRI, usually echocardiographic data are sufficient. Since most athletes' hearts that fall within the "gray zone" also have associated LV dilation, RWT serves as an important criterion to distinguish these conditions. RWT = $2PW/LVID_d$ and an RWT <0.6 (or <0.5 in some studies) is generally consistent with athlete's heart, and an RWT above these values is more likely to be HCM. Athlete's heart would be expected to have a longitudinal strain >15%, not <15% in absolute terms.

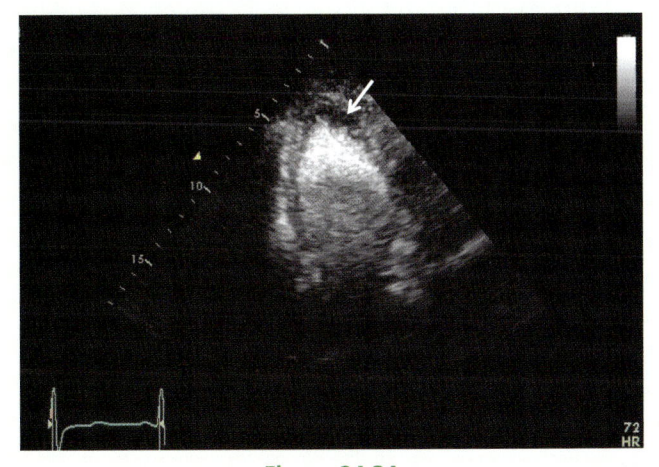

Figure 24.34

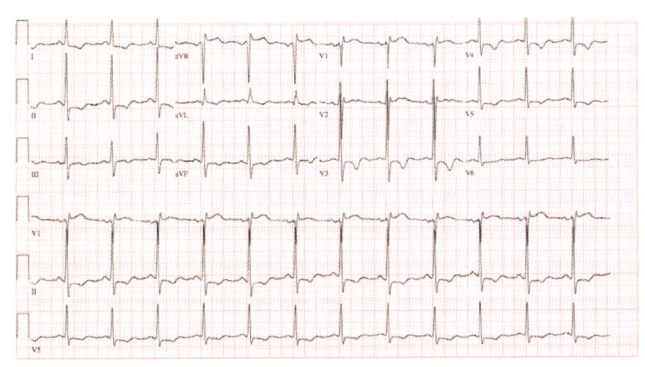

Figure 24.35

> **KEY POINTS**
> - Clinical, EKG, and echocardiographic information should be used to distinguish athlete's heart from HCM.
> - Multiple echocardiographic criteria should be assessed to make this distinction (see **Table 24.4**).
> - RWT is a useful criterion to distinguish athlete's heart from HCM, since the LV cavity is usually dilated with athlete's heart.

37. **Answer: D.** The available clinical, EKG, and echocardiographic information do not allow for a confident diagnosis of either HCM, hypertensive heart disease, or cardiac amyloidosis. The clinical information suggests that hypertensive heart disease is a possibility given the requirement for multiple antihypertensive agents with end-stage renal disease and LVH on EKG. Nonobstructive HCM is also a possibility given the severe degree of increased LV wall thickness. Although, by definition, HCM is usually only diagnosed when other reasons for LVH are excluded, there are some patients that have a form of "hypertensive hypertrophic cardiomyopathy" where the degree of hypertrophy may be

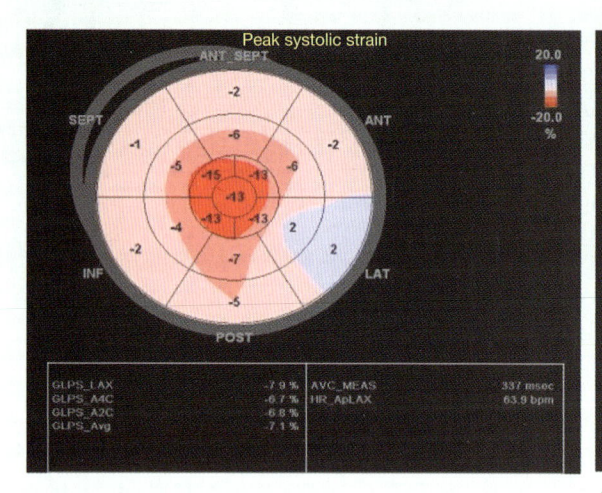

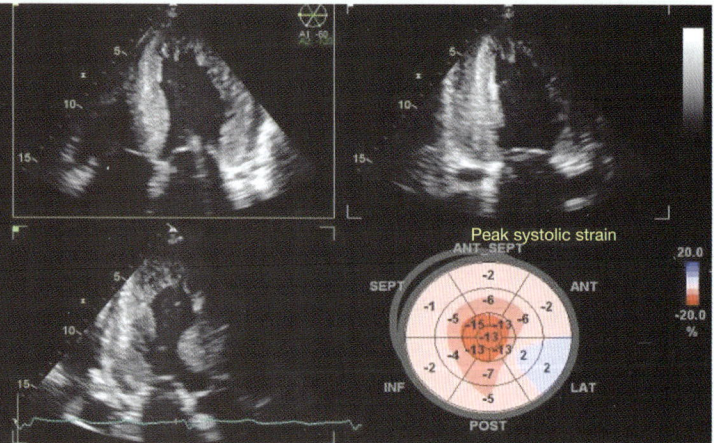

Figure 24.36

considered out of proportion to the degree of HTN. The more likely diagnosis is cardiac amyloidosis given the findings of severe symmetric increased LV wall thickness, restrictive diastolic filling pattern with high LAP, elevated RAP and pulmonary HTN, and a pericardial effusion. The presence of ESRD on dialysis further complicates the diagnosis and can by itself explain the high filling pressure and pericardial effusion. **Figure 24.22** classifies different etiologies of increased LV wall thickness in adults.

38. **Answer: D.** Speckle tracking strain imaging has been found to be very helpful to distinguish etiologies of increased LV wall thickness. The apical sparing pattern seen with cardiac amyloidosis is distinct from other causes of LVH such as HTN, HCM, or aortic stenosis. However, as of yet, AL and ATTR (wild-type or mutant) amyloid cannot be distinguished using strain data. The patient had ATTR wild-type amyloidosis, which had been overlooked because he was hypertensive and thought to have hypertensive heart disease and diastolic heart failure. **Figure 24.36** shows the strain images from this patient demonstrating apical sparing pattern.

KEY POINTS

- Clinical data, EKG and standard echocardiography may not be adequate to distinguish causes of increased LV wall thickness.
- Speckle tracking longitudinal strain provides additional information to make these distinctions.

39. **Answer: C.** The diastolic function assessment is consistent with a restrictive diastolic filling pattern (grade III). The E/a ratio is >2, the mitral deceleration time is 150 ms, the E/e' ratio is near 30, and the LAVi is 52 mL/m^2, all findings consistent with a high left-sided filling pressure, also consistent with the clinical history and physical examination, CXR with pulmonary edema, and elevated BNP level.

40. **Answer: D.** The patient from **Case 4** has cardiac amyloidosis, not HCM, and therefore the treatment options offered are not appropriate. Although increased LV wall thickness and SAM suggest HCM, the echocardiographic clue to an alternative diagnosis is the presence of a restrictive diastolic filling pattern. A restrictive phenotype of HCM (associated with specific genetic mutations) is reported to occur in only ~2% of patients. Although SAM of the mitral valve is often considered to be a relatively specific sign of HCM, it is well described in several other conditions including cardiac amyloidosis (**Table 24.11**). An additional clue to an alternative diagnosis from HCM is the presence of CHF with pulmonary edema. Unless there is LV dysfunction, AF, or primary causes of severe MR, most patients with HCM do not develop severe signs of CHF and pulmonary edema.

KEY POINTS

- A restrictive filling pattern is present in approximately 2% of patients with HCM.
- SAM of the mitral valve may occur in patients with cardiac amyloidosis.
- Clinical signs of CHF with overt pulmonary edema is uncommon due to LVOT obstruction alone in HCM, and usually does not occur unless there is LV dysfunction, AF, or severe MR from primary causes.

SUGGESTED READINGS

Binder J, Attenhofer Jost CH, Klarich KW, et al. Apical hypertrophic cardiomyopathy: prevalence and correlates of apical outpouching. *J Am Soc Echocardiogr*. 2011;24(7):775-781.

Gebhard C, Stahli B, Greutmann M, Biaggi P, Jenni R, Tanner FC. Reduced left ventricular compacta thickness: a novel echocardiographic criterion for non-compaction cardiomyopathy. *J Am Soc Echocardiogr*. 2012;25(10):1050-1057.

Kansal MM, Lester S, Surapaneni P, et al. Usefulness of two-dimensional and speckle tracking echocardiography in "gray-zone" left ventricular hypertrophy to differentiate professional football player's heart from hypertrophic cardiomyopathy. *Am J Cardiol*. 2011;108(9):1322-1326.

Lang RM, Badano LP, Mor-Avi V, et al. Recommendations for cardiac chamber quantification by echocardiography in adults: an update from the American Society of Echocardiography and the European Association of Cardiovascular Imaging. *J Am Soc Echocardiogr*. 2015;16(3):233-270.

Lever HM, Karam RF, Currie PJ, Healy BP. Hypertrophic cardiomyopathy in the elderly. Distinctions from the young based on cardiac shape. *Circulation*. 1989;79(3):580-589.

Lyon AR, Lopez-Fernandez T, Couch L, et al; ESC Scientific Document Group. 2022 ESC guidelines on cardio-oncology developed in collaboration with the European hematology association (EHA), the European Society for therapeutic Radiology and Oncology (ESTRO) and the International Cardio-Oncology Society (IC-OS). *Eur Heart J*. 2022;43(41):4229-4361.

Nagueh SF, Phelan D, Abraham T, et al. Recommendations for multimodality cardiovascular imaging of patients with hypertrophic cardiomyopathy: an update from the American Society of echocardiography, in collaboration with the American Society of Nuclear Cardiology, the Society for cardiovascular magnetic resonance, and the Society of cardiovascular Computed tomography. *J Am Soc Echocardiogr*. 2022;35(6):533-569.

Oh JK, Tajik AJ, Edwards WD, Bresnahan JF, Kyle RA. Dynamic left ventricular outflow tract obstruction in cardiac amyloidosis detected by continuous-wave Doppler echocardiography. *Am J Cardiol*. 1987;59(9):1008-1010.

Olson LJ, Baldus WP, Tajik AJ. Echocardiographic features of idiopathic hemochromatosis. *Am J Cardiol*. 1987;60(10):885-889.

Ommen SR, Mital S, Burke MA, et al. 2020 AHA/ACC guideline for the diagnosis and treatment of patients with hypertrophic cardiomyopathy: executive summary—a report of the American College of Cardiology/American heart Association Joint Committee on clinical practice guidelines. *Circulation*. 2020;142(25):e533-e557.

Petersen SE, Jensen B, Aung N, et al. Excessive trabeculation of the left ventricle: JACC—cardiovascular imaging expert panel paper. *J Am Coll Cardiol Img*. 2023;16(3):408-425.

Rapezzi C, Aimo A, Barison A, et al. Restrictive cardiomyopathy: definition and diagnosis. *Eur Heart J*. 2022;43(45):4679-4693.

Shaper AG. Cardiovascular disease in the tropics. II. Endomyocardial fibrosis. *Br Med J*. 1972;3(5829):743-746.

Tabira A, Misumi I, Sato K, et al. Mid-ventricular obstructive cardiomyopathy after Takotsubo cardiomyopathy: a case report. *Intern Med*. 2023;62(16):2365-2373.

CHAPTER 25

Durable and Temporary Left Ventricular Mechanical Circulatory Support Devices and Orthotopic Heart Transplantation

Basant Arya and Raymond F. Stainback

QUESTIONS

1. Which of the following are considered important aspects of the preoperative transesophageal echocardiogram (TEE) in patients awaiting left ventricular assist device (LVAD) implantation?
   A. Evaluating degree of aortic regurgitation (AR).
   B. Determining presence of a cardiac-level shunt.
   C. Identification of intracardiac thrombi.
   D. Assessing right ventricular (RV) function.
   E. All of the above.

2. Which of the following is an absolute contraindication to LVAD implantation?
   A. Small left ventricular (LV) cavity.
   B. LV apical thrombus.
   C. Acute bacterial endocarditis.
   D. Severe mitral regurgitation (MR).
   E. None of the above.

3. Which valvular lesions must be corrected prior to or at the time of LVAD implantation?
   A. Severe mitral stenosis (MS).
   B. Severe aortic stenosis (AS).
   C. Moderate AR.
   D. Severe mitral MR.
   E. Choices A and C.

4. The following approaches are acceptable for treating greater than mild AR prior to LVAD implantation **EXCEPT**:
   A. Aortic valve replacement with a bioprosthesis.
   B. Completely oversewing the valve (by suturing along all coaptation zones).
   C. Performing a central coaptation (Park) stitch.
   D. Aortic valve replacement with a mechanical valve.
   E. Choices A and C.

5. Why is secondary mitral regurgitation (MR) expected to improve after LVAD implantation?
   A. Reduced LV size.
   B. Reduced filling pressures.
   C. Improved coaptation of the mitral valve leaflets.
   D. All of the above.
   E. Choices A and C.

6. Which of the statements below are included in the definition of severe right heart failure (RVF) post-LVAD implantation?
   A. Requirement of a RV assist device.
   B. >14 consecutive days of intravenous (IV) inotropic support.
   C. Right ventricular basal diameter greater than 4.8 cm.
   D. Development of severe TR.
   E. A and B.

7. Which of the following echocardiographic parameters are least reliable in assessing AR post-LVAD implantation?
   A. Vena contracta.
   B. Pressure half-time.
   C. LV outflow tract (LVOT) AR jet height.
   D. Pulsed Doppler evaluation of aortic diastolic flow reversal.
   E. B and D.

8. A patient with dilated cardiomyopathy is undergoing evaluation for LVAD. A high-quality IV saline contrast study at rest is negative for patent foramen ovale (PFO) or intracardiac shunting. Does this finding definitively exclude the presence of a PFO?
   A. Yes.
   B. No.
   C. Yes, if RA pressure is normal.
   D. Yes, if no significant MR.
   E. None of the above.

9. What is the **BEST** approach to a PFO prior to LVAD implantation?
   A. No intervention is necessary; a PFO is not hemodynamically significant enough to cause clinical issues post-LVAD implantation.
   B. Percutaneous closure.
   C. Surgical closure at the time of device implantation.

10. A patient is undergoing surgical LVAD implantation. Intraoperative TEE shows normal RV size and function soon after LVAD activation. Shortly thereafter, the RV suddenly becomes dilated with reduced systolic function and increased TR severity. What is the most likely culprit?
    A. Right ventricular failure due to prolonged cardiopulmonary bypass.
    B. Air emboli from the LV cavity into the right coronary artery (RCA).
    C. Typical RV response to surgical manipulation of the heart.
    D. Acute pulmonary embolism.
    E. None of the above.

11. If initiation of LVAD support results in a sudden decrease in arterial oxygen saturation, the clinician performing the intraoperative TEE should be alerted to the possibility of which cardiac pathology?
    A. Right-to-left shunt.
    B. Severe AS.
    C. Severe AR.
    D. Cardiac tamponade.
    E. None of the above.

12. Assuming there is no significant valve regurgitation or shunting, calculate the cardiac output given the parameters. Right ventricular outflow tract
    - RVOT TVI: 12 cm
    - RVOT diameter: 2.5 cm
    - LVOT diameter: 2.0 cm
    - Heart rate: 70 bpm
    A. 3.9 L/min.
    B. 4.1 L/min.
    C. 4.5 L/min.
    D. 6.1 L/min.
    E. Unable to calculate; more information needed.

13. A 56-year-old man with ischemic cardiomyopathy underwent HeartMate II LVAD implantation. His postoperative course was uneventful. His LVAD speed is set at 9200 rpm. Predischarge echocardiogram shows a left ventricular internal diameter diastole (LVID$_d$) of 5.3 cm, normal RV size and function, mild MR, mild TR, and intermittent aortic valve opening. He is discharged on warfarin, carvedilol, lisinopril, and furosemide. Two weeks later, he presents to the emergency room complaining of dyspnea, lower extremity edema, and dark urine. He also reports multiple LVAD alarms in the past 48 hours. Interrogation of the LVAD controller confirms both low flow and high power alarms. LVAD speed is 9200 rpm. Labs reveal LDH of 1032 U/L and INR 1.3. Bedside echocardiography reveals LVID$_d$ of 6.6 cm, moderate to severe MR, aortic valve opening with every cardiac cycle, and nonuniform inflow cannula velocities.
    What is the most likely cause of the patient's symptoms and echocardiographic findings?
    A. Inadequate LV unloading due to low LVAD speed.
    B. Right ventricular failure.
    C. Hypovolemia secondary to gastrointestinal bleed.
    D. LVAD pump thrombosis.
    E. None of the above.

14. An LVAD patient is undergoing a TTE for evaluation of palpitations and low flow alarms. The sonographer calls to inform you the LVID$_d$ is 3.1 cm and the interventricular septum is shifted to the left, nearly abutting the inflow cannula. What is your initial assessment and plan of action?
    A. The LV is appropriately decompressed; make no changes to the LVAD setting.
    B. The patient is hypovolemic; give a fluid bolus and make no changes to the LVAD setting.
    C. The patient is having a suction event; decrease the LVAD speed.
    D. The patient has RV failure; consider right ventricular assist device (RVAD) placement.
    E. None of the above.

15. When evaluating an LVAD patient with suspected RV dysfunction, which group of echocardiographic parameters would be most diagnostic?
    A. RV size and function, AR severity, inferior vena cava (IVC) size, TR severity.
    B. RV size and function, interventricular septal position, IVC size and collapsibility, TR severity, pericardial assessment.
    C. RV size and function, severity of MR, IVC size and collapsibility, pulmonary artery pressure, TR severity, LV ejection fraction.
    D. RV size and function, severity of AR, interventricular septal position, severity of TR, systolic PA pressure.
    E. None of the above.

16. A 25-year-old woman with nonischemic cardiomyopathy underwent HeartMate II placement. Her early postoperative course was complicated by mild RV dysfunction. Predischarge echocardiogram during LVAD pump speed = 8800 rpm showed improved RV function, LVID$_d$ of 5.1 cm, and a continuously closed aortic valve. Her discharge medical therapy included carvedilol, lisinopril, and warfarin. She now returns to clinic for routine follow-up. Physical examination is notable for palpable radial pulses. LVAD controller shows power of 10.5 W and pulsatility index (PI) of 5.6. Labs are pending. Scheduled surveillance LVAD optimization echocardiography is performed at speeds of 8400 rpm, 8800 rpm, and 9200 rpm. The echocardiography technician notifies you that the LVID$_d$ is >6 cm at all speeds assessed. The aortic valve now opens with every beat, and the outflow cannula velocities change minimally with speed change. What is the most likely explanation for the echo findings?
    A. The patient has recurrent RV failure and the LVAD speed should be decreased.
    B. There is severe AR and she should be referred for a TEE.
    C. There is LVAD impeller thrombosis and the patient should be admitted for further treatment.
    D. The patient is not adequately unloaded and the LVAD speed should be increased.
    E. None of the above.

17. Which choice describes the **CORRECT** method of obtaining blood pressure (BP) in a nonpulsatile LVAD patient?
    A. The BP cuff is inflated with a handheld audible Doppler evaluation of the brachial or radial artery. The pressure at which there is an audible Doppler signal as the cuff is deflated is considered the mean arterial BP.
    B. The BP cuff is inflated with a handheld audible Doppler evaluation of the brachial or radial artery. The pressure at which there is an audible Doppler signal as the cuff is deflated is considered the systolic BP. The diastolic BP is the pressure at which the audible signal disappears.
    C. The BP cuff is inflated as usual to obtain systolic and diastolic BP.
    D. There is no way to assess the BP noninvasively. You must place a radial arterial line for an accurate BP in this type of patient.
    E. None of the above.

18. High estimated LVAD flow with normal power can signify which of the following?
    A. Moderate to severe AR.
    B. Incomplete aortic valve opening.
    C. Pericardial tamponade.
    D. Right ventricular failure.
    E. Moderate to severe MR.

19. Which of the following echocardiographic sign(s) characterize a suction event?
    A. Small LV chamber size.
    B. Interventricular septal shift toward the LV.
    C. Small RV chamber size.
    D. Severe MR.
    E. A and B.

20. What are the recommended methods to assess LV size and function post-LVAD implantation?
   A. LV size: LVID$_d$ from two-dimensional parasternal long-axis image.
   LV function: LVEDv: biplane method of disks, modified Simpson rule.
   B. LV size: LVID$_d$ from two-dimensional parasternal long-axis image.
   LV function: LVOT stroke volume.
   C. LV size: biplane method of disks, modified Simpson rule.
   LV function: LVEF biplane method of disks, modified Simpson rule.
   D. LV size: biplane method of disks, modified Simpson rule.
   LV function: RVOT stroke volume.
   E. None of the above.

21. Which is most appropriate for determining LV filling pressures (diastolic function) post-LVAD implantation?
   A. Mitral E velocity.
   B. Left atrial volume.
   C. Pulmonary vein inflow.
   D. Interpretation of diastolic dysfunction is not appropriate.
   E. B and C.

22. When performing an LVAD speed change echocardiogram, which of the following should be assessed with each incremental adjustment to the LVAD speed?
   A. LVID$_d$.
   B. Interventricular septum position.
   C. Aortic valve opening frequency/duration.
   D. MR severity, TR severity, and peak TR velocity.
   E. All of the above.

23. Which of the following are reasons to terminate a speed change echocardiogram?
   A. Suction event.
   B. Patient symptoms including palpitations, dizziness, chest pain, shortness of breath, or headache.
   C. Inflow or outflow cannula flow reversal.
   D. Hypertension (MAP > 100 mm Hg).
   E. All of the above.

CASE 1

A 65-year-old woman with a history of nonischemic cardiomyopathy 6 months post HVAD LVAD implantation presents to clinic with complaints of dyspnea on exertion, orthopnea, and mild lower extremity edema. Her HVAD speed is 2400 rpm, and medications since hospital discharge include lisinopril, carvedilol, spironolactone, and bumetanide. LVAD interrogation reveals no device alarms. A TTE was performed to further evaluate her symptoms, shown in **Figure 25.1** *(A, B—parasternal long-axis; C, D—apical views).*

24. Based on **Case 1** (and **Figure 25.1**), which of the following statements is **CORRECT**?
   A. There is a large thrombus in the LV apex.
   B. The patient has severe MR.
   C. The HVAD cannula is in the appropriate location.
   D. There is evidence of a subacute suction event and the HVAD rpm should be decreased.
   E. None of the above.

CASE 2

A 75-year-old man underwent HeartMate II LVAD placement as destination therapy for ischemic cardiomyopathy. His preoperative TTE showed trivial AR. A repeat study prior to discharge was notable for LVID$_d$ 5.3 cm, mild MR, and trace AR at LVAD speed 8600 rpm. The patient now presents to clinic with complaint of lower extremity edema, dyspnea, and fatigue. There are no LVAD device alarms. A speed change echocardiogram is performed with images shown in **Figure 25.2**. *You note the LVID$_d$ increases with increasing LVAD speed.*

25. What is the most likely explanation for the findings in **Case 2** (**Figure 25.2**)?
   A. LVAD inflow cannula obstruction.
   B. Development of significant, continuous AR.
   C. Development of moderate MR.
   D. All of the above.
   E. B and C.

534 / Clinical Echocardiography Review

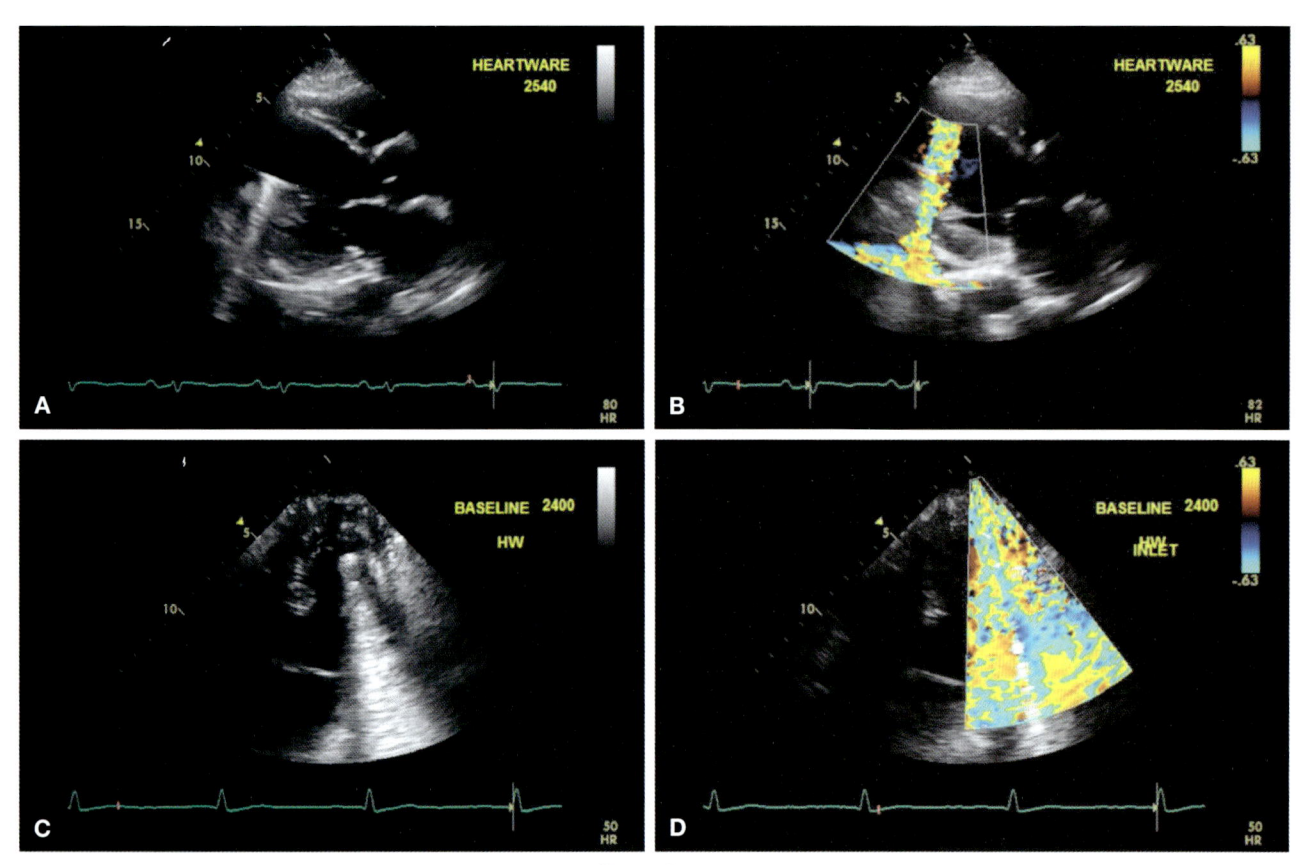

Figure 25.1

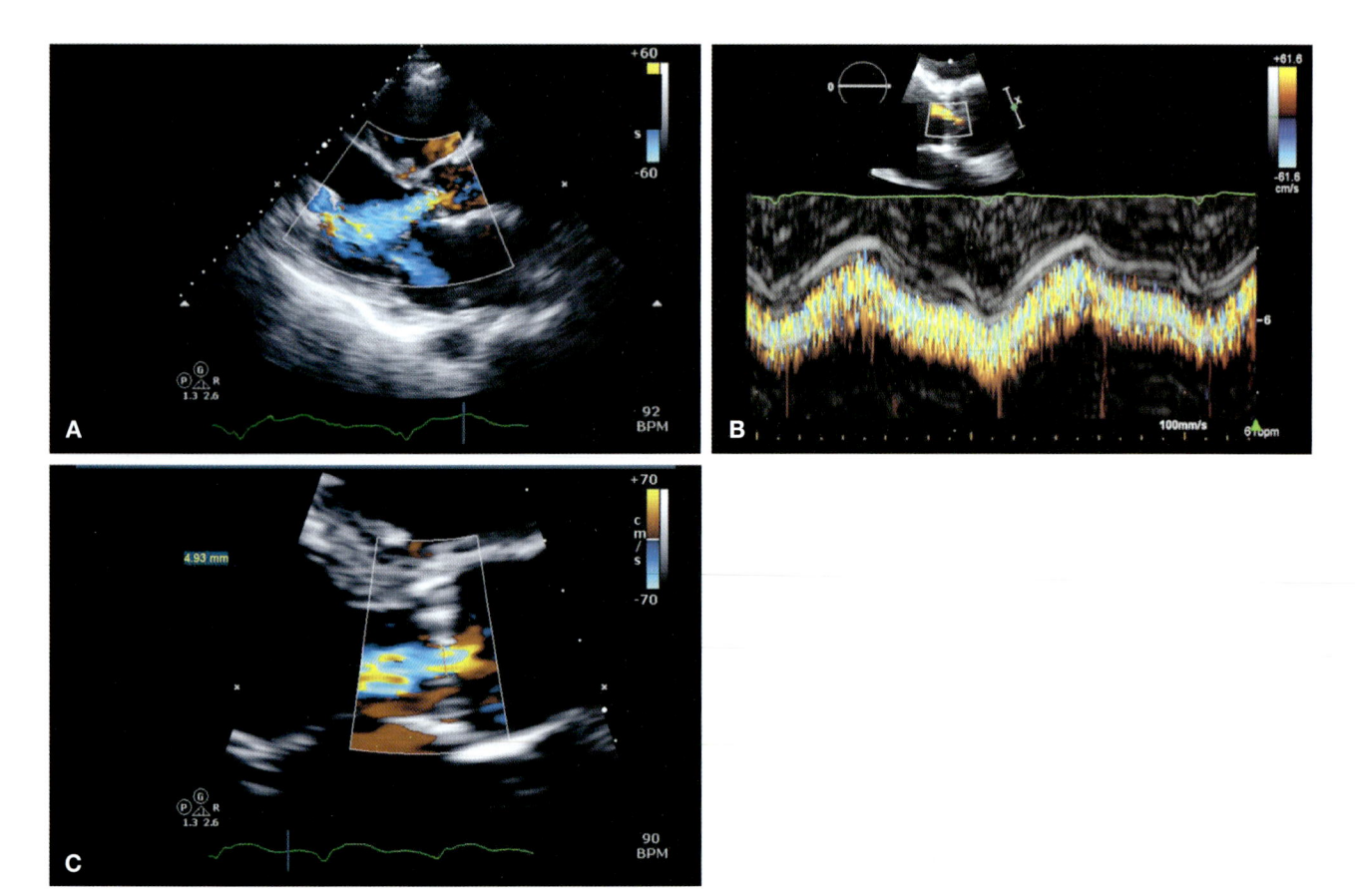

Figure 25.2. A: Parasternal long-axis with color Doppler. **B:** M-mode with superimposed color Doppler. **C:** Parasternal long-axis with color Doppler and zoom.

26. **Figure 25.3** shows various images of LVAD inflow cannula orientation in the same patient by TTE and TEE.

    In general, which is the **BEST** standard imaging view for LVAD inflow cannula spectral Doppler interrogation?
    A. Parasternal long-axis.
    B. Apical 4-chamber.
    C. Parasternal short-axis.
    D. TEE 4-chamber.
    E. No best view.

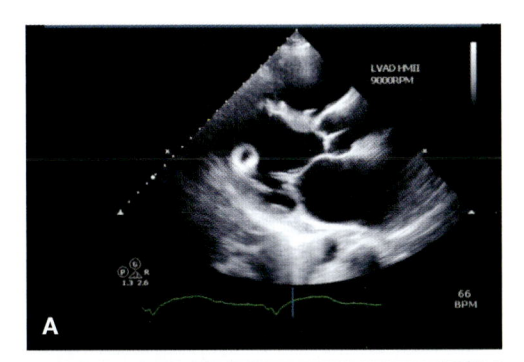

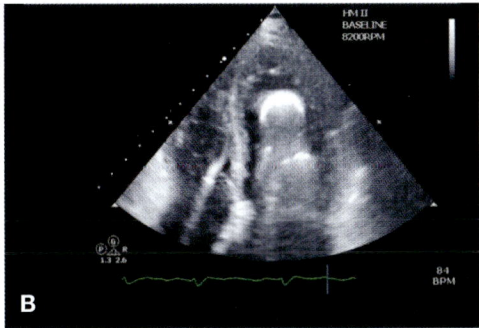

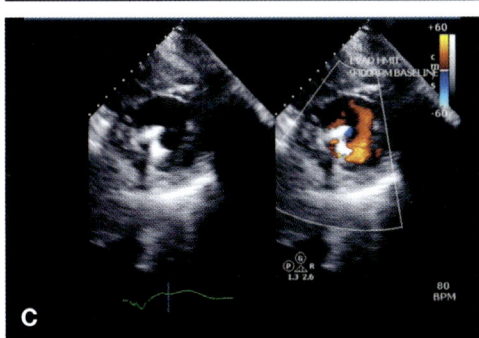

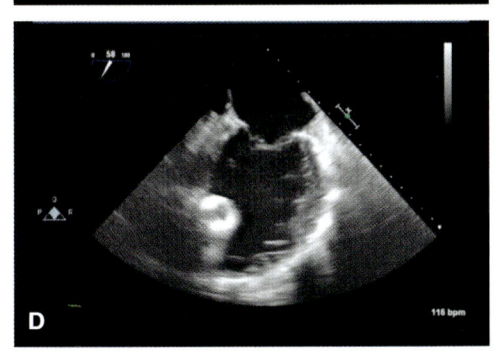

Figure 25.3

CASE 3

*A 55-year-old woman with a history of non-Hodgkin lymphoma complicated by chemotherapy-induced cardiomyopathy underwent HVAD implantation as a bridge-to-transplant (BTT). The patient subsequently underwent a successful orthotopic heart transplant (OHT), complicated by postoperative Staphylococcus aureus bacteremia. The patient is referred for TEE to evaluate for endocarditis (*Figure 25.4*).*

27. Which statement **CORRECTLY** describes the structure seen adjacent to the right atrium (*denoted by the arrow*) in the bicaval view from the patient in **Case 3** (and **Figure 25.4**)?
    A. There is a residual continuous flow LVAD outflow graft material anterior to the right atrium.
    B. There is a Swan-Ganz catheter in the right pulmonary artery.
    C. There is a loculated pericardial effusion around the right atrium.
    D. There is an enlarged coronary sinus in the transplanted heart.

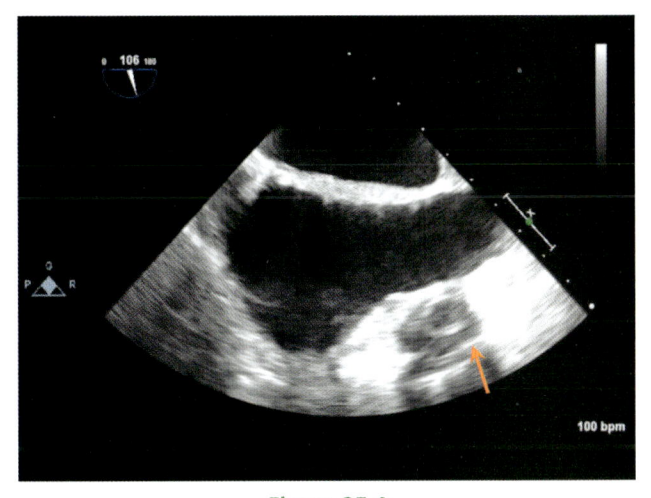

Figure 25.4

CASE 4

A 62-year-old man with a history of coronary artery disease and ischemic cardiomyopathy underwent HeartMate II LVAD implantation. The LVAD is currently at 9400 rpm. On examination, the mean arterial pressure is 90 mm Hg and there is no palpable pulse. TTE is performed, which includes M-mode through the aortic valve, seen in **Figure 25.5A,B**.

536 / Clinical Echocardiography Review

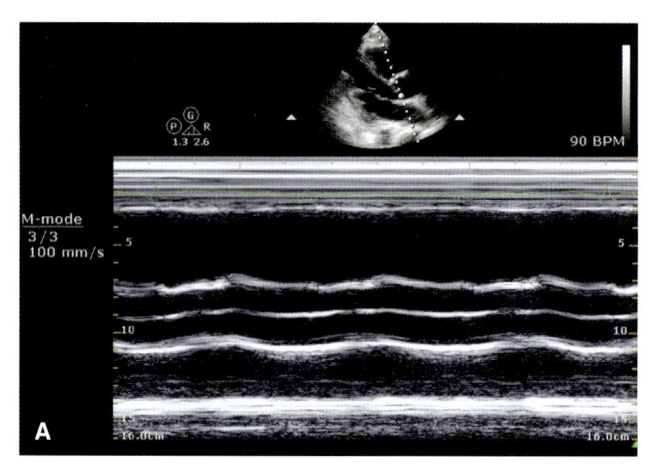

Figure 25.5A

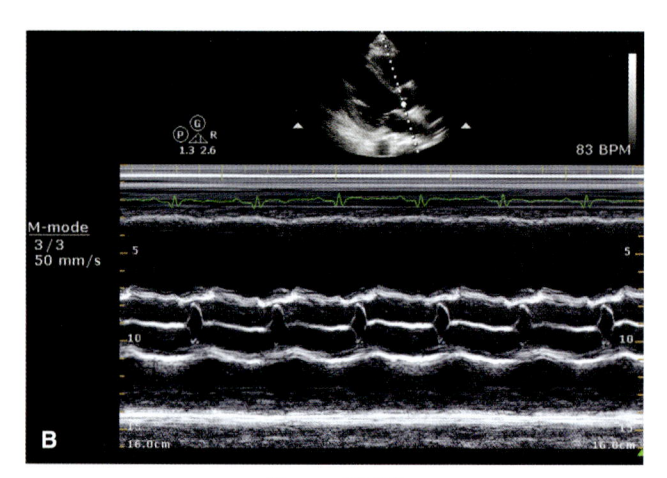

Figure 25.5B

28. What change most likely occurred to account for the change in aortic valve M-mode between **Figure 25.5A** and **Figure 25.5B** in the patient from **Case 4**?
A. Increased LVAD speed.
B. Increased LVAD power.
C. Decreased LVAD pulsatility index.
D. Decreased LVAD speed.
E. B and C.

CASE 5

A 43-year-old woman with history of dilated cardiomyopathy underwent HeartMate II LVAD implantation. Her postoperative course was complicated by recurrent gastrointestinal bleeding. A TTE was performed prior to discharge, and is seen in **Figure 25.6A**. *The patient was ultimately discharged with an LVAD speed of 9200 rpm, off warfarin. The patient now presents to LVAD clinic for routine follow-up and scheduled LVAD optimization echocardiogram with speed change. Follow-up images are shown in* **Figure 25.6B-D**.

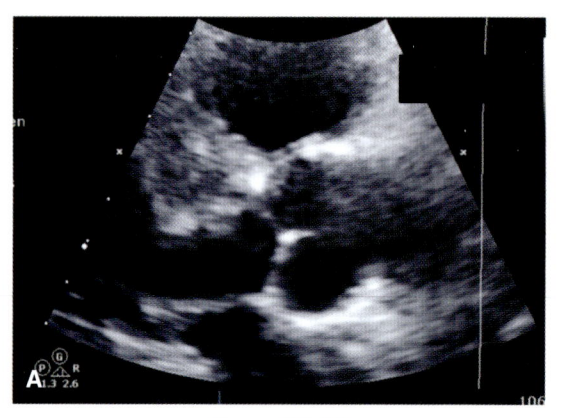

Figure 25.6A

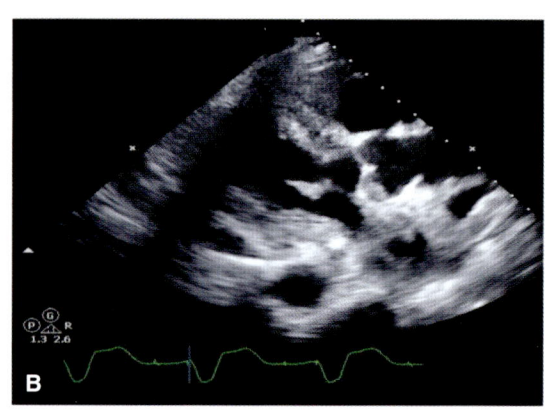

Figure 25.6B

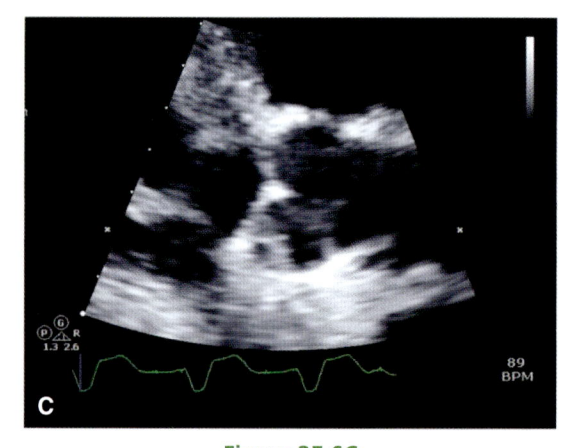

Figure 25.6C

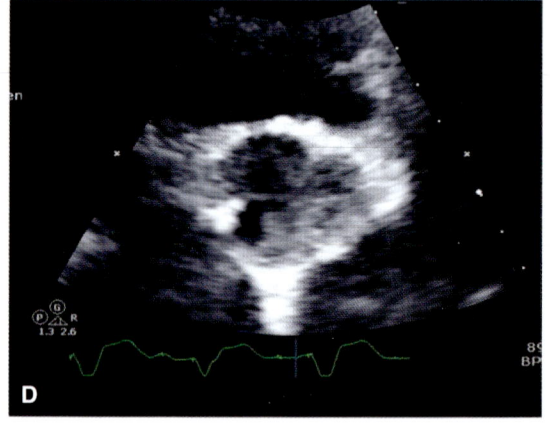

Figure 25.6D

29. What do you recommend for the patient in **Case 5**?
    A. Proceed with study as ordered at speeds of 8800, 9000, and 9400 rpm.
    B. Check blood cultures and start empiric antibiotics.
    C. Image at baseline speed only and notify managing physician.
    D. Obtain immediate surgical consultation.
    E. B and C.

30. In which clinical scenario do you see the above HeartMate II outflow graft velocities (**Figure 25.7**)?
    A. Normal LVAD function.
    B. LVAD power spike.
    C. LVAD suction event.
    D. Unable to interpret due to inappropriate cannula velocity interrogation.

CASE 6

A 34-year-old man underwent HeartMate II LVAD implantation for nonischemic cardiomyopathy. The LVAD speed is set at 8200 rpm. On postoperative day 7, he undergoes routine TTE. Four standard TTE images are shown in **Figure 25.8**.

31. What do you recommend for the patient in **Case 6**?
    A. Decrease the LVAD speed to allow aortic valve opening.
    B. Consider mitral valve replacement for severe MR.
    C. Normal postoperative LVAD study; continue current care.
    D. Increase the LVAD speed to optimize unloading of the LV.
    E. A and B.

CASE 7

A 20-year-old man with a remote history of cardiac transplantation for hypoplastic left heart presents to clinic for routine follow-up. He is currently taking tacrolimus and prednisone for immunosuppression and has had no episodes of rejection. Physical examination reveals normal heart sounds, a 2/6 systolic murmur at the left sternal border, clear lung sounds, and no edema. Laboratory testing reveals a tacrolimus level of 6. A surveillance echocardiogram is performed.

32. Based on the scenario presented in **Case 7**, what is shown in **Figure 25.9**?
    A. Cor triatriatum.
    B. Pericardial effusion adjacent to the left atrium.
    C. Typical posttransplant appearance.
    D. Pericardial cyst.
    E. Moderate mitral annular calcification.

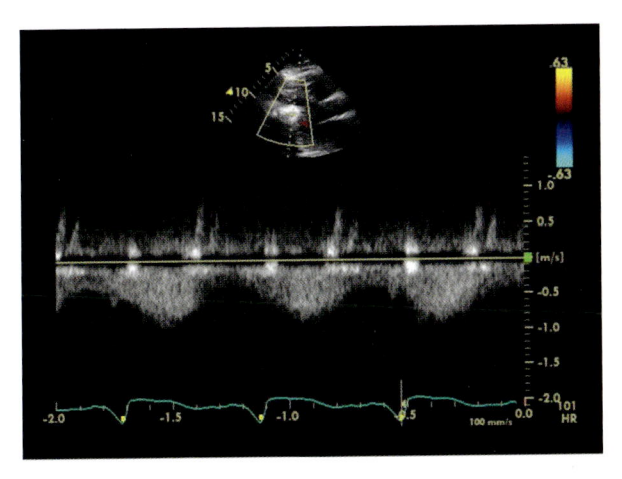

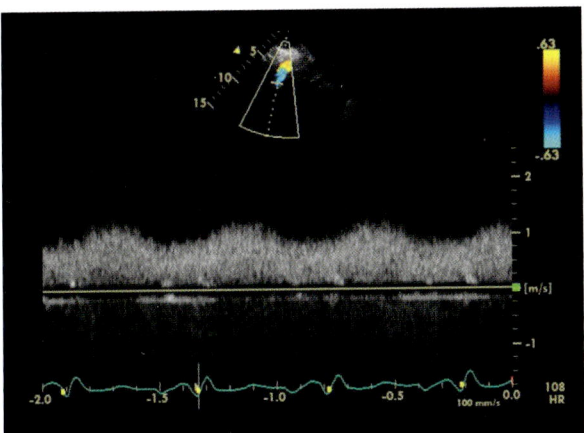

Figure 25.7

538 / Clinical Echocardiography Review

A Parasternal long axis

B Apical 4-chamber

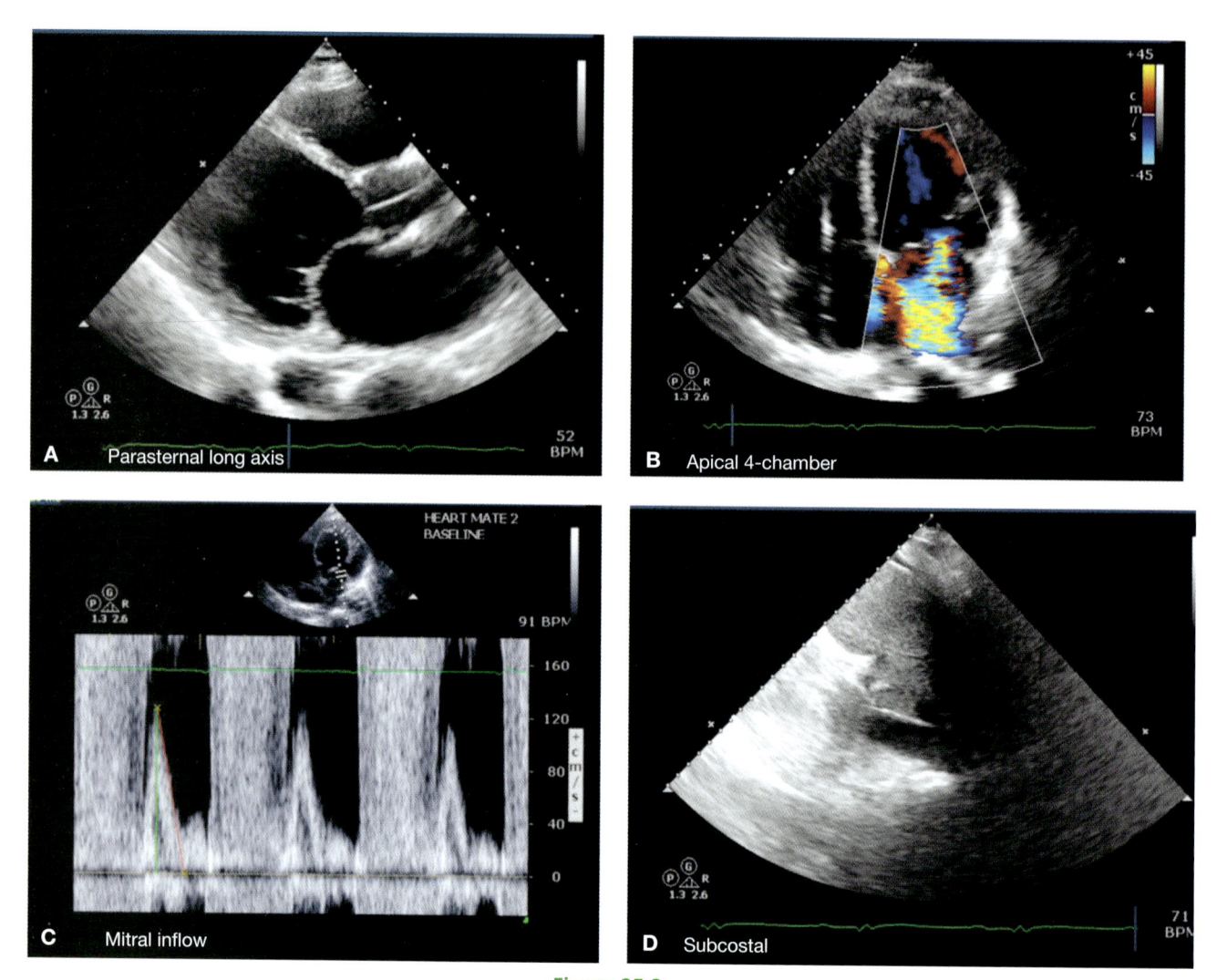

C Mitral inflow

D Subcostal

Figure 25.8

CASE 8

*A LVAD patient is undergoing TTE for evaluation of palpitations and low flow alarms. The parasternal long-axis images (**Figure 25.10**, ▶ **Videos 25.1** and **25.2**) with CW Doppler interrogation of the LVAD inflow cannula are obtained.*

---

33. For the patient in **Case 8**, based on findings (**Figure 25.10**, ▶ **Videos 25.1** and **25.2**), what is your initial assessment and plan of action?
   A. The LV is appropriately decompressed; make no changes to the LVAD setting.
   B. The patient is hypovolemic; give a fluid bolus and make no changes to the LVAD setting.
   C. The patient is having a suction event; decrease the LVAD speed.
   D. The patient has RV failure; consider RVAD placement.

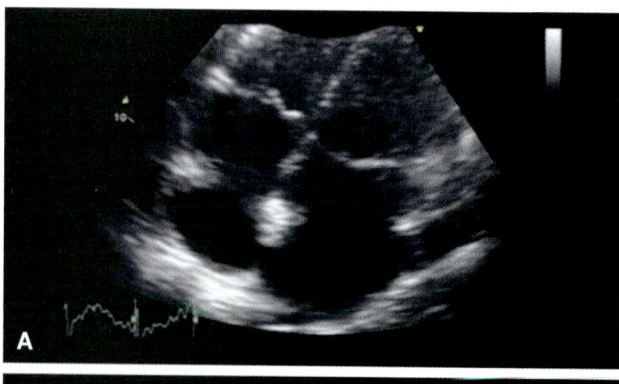

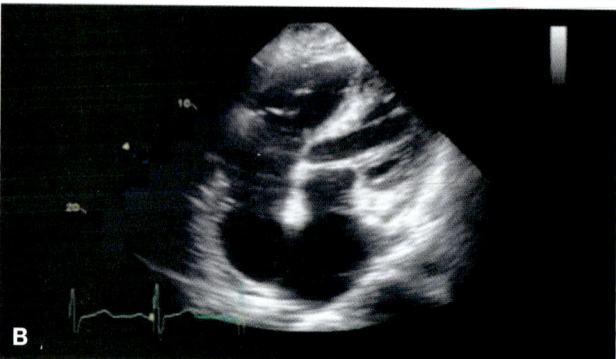

Figure 25.9. **A** and **B:** Apical 4-chamber views.

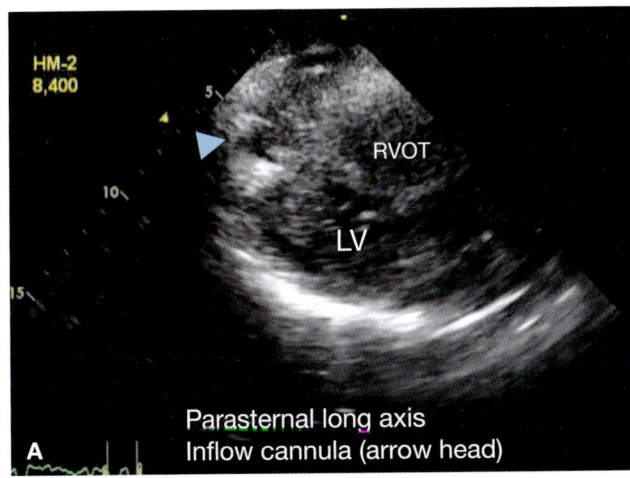

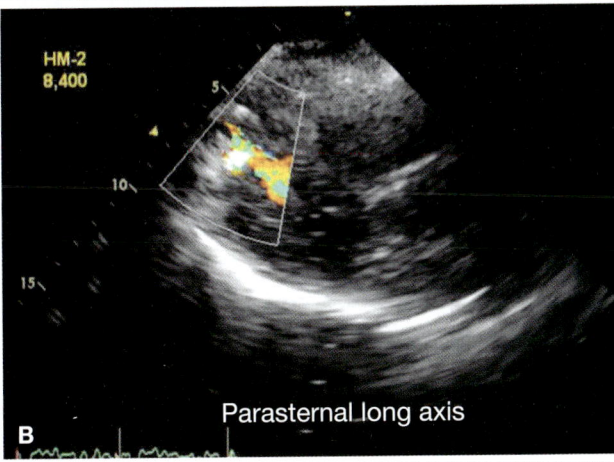

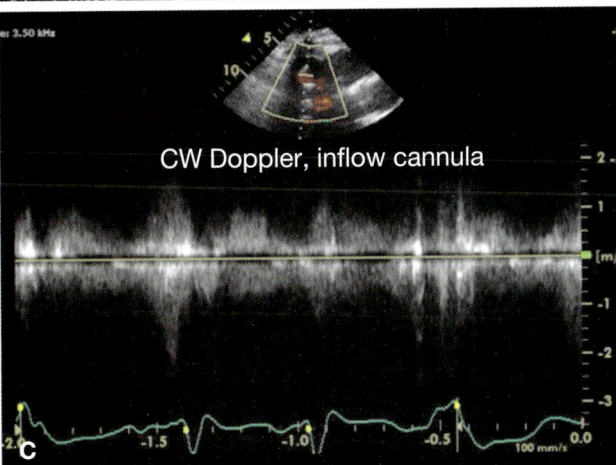

Chapter 25 Durable and Temporary LV Mechanical Circulatory Support Devices and Orthotopic Heart Transplantation / 539

Figure 25.10

CASE 9

A 45-year-old woman with end-stage renal disease, COPD, and nonischemic cardiomyopathy undergoes LVAD implantation. Postoperatively she remains hypotensive, requiring multiple inotropes, and chest films show worsening pulmonary edema at a low HM II pump speed of 7800 rpm. A TTE is ordered. The parasternal short-axis, RV inflow, and apical 4-chamber views are shown in **Figure 25.11A-C** *respectively and* ▶ **Videos 25.3** *to* **25.5**.

34. What is the likely cause of the patient's deteriorating clinical status in **Case 9** (see **also Figure 25.11** and ▶ **Videos 25.3 to 25.5**)?
    A. There is a thrombus at the LVAD inflow cannula.
    B. The patient has RV failure and should be considered for an RVAD.
    C. The LVAD speed is too low and should be increased to optimize RV unloading.
    D. There is a large pericardial effusion compressing the LV and causing tamponade.

35. A 68-year-old man with ischemic cardiomyopathy, diabetes, and hypertension is now 7 years status post orthotropic heart transplantation. Surveillance left heart catheterization with coronary angiography cardiac allograft vasculopathy (CAV) screening was deferred due to worsening renal dysfunction and poor vascular access. A dobutamine stress echo was ordered instead, and this test appeared to be clearly normal. Which is the **CORRECT** statement for stress echo in OHT patients?
    A. Stress echo is not recommended due to rapid resting HR related to OHT cardiac denervation.
    B. Dobutamine stress echo has high sensitivity and high specificity for CAV detection and may replace coronary angiography for CAV screening when readily available.
    C. Dobutamine stress echo has low sensitivity and should be considered only when coronary angiography is contraindicated.
    D. Treadmill stress echo is better than pharmacologic stress since exercise capacity assessment is a valuable component.
    E. None of the above.

36. In which clinical scenario do you see the above HeartMate 3 outflow graft velocities (**Figure 25.12**)?
    A. Normal LVAD function.
    B. LVAD power spike.
    C. LVAD suction event.
    D. Unable to interpret due to inappropriate cannula velocity interrogation.

540 / Clinical Echocardiography Review

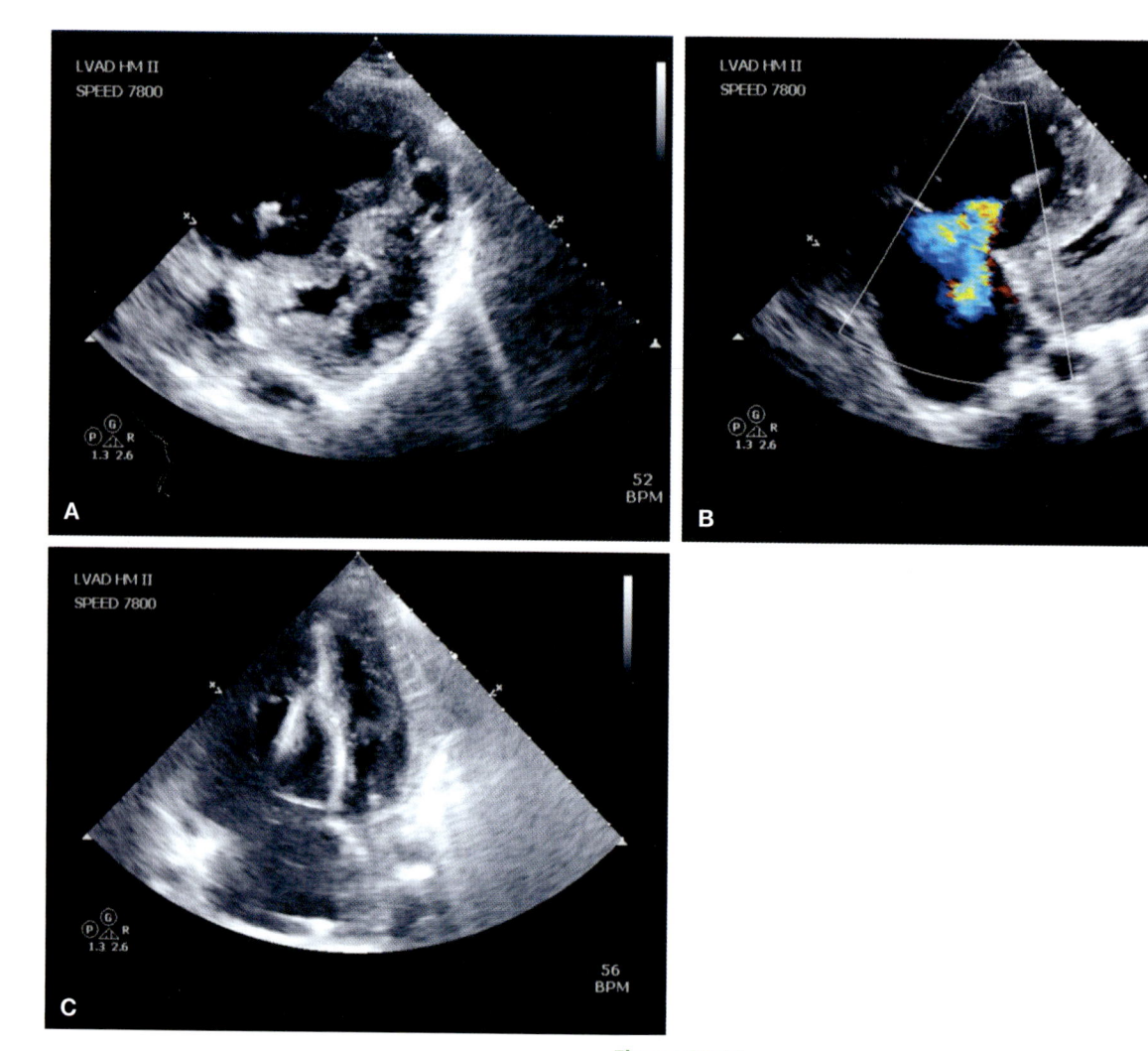

Figure 25.11

CASE 10

A 69-year-old man with end-stage renal disease, type 2 diabetes, hypertension, dyslipidemia, coronary artery disease, and congestive heart failure (EF 35%-39%) is scheduled to undergo multivessel PCI to the LAD and RCA. An Impella CP percutaneous left ventricular assist device was inserted under fluoroscopic guidance in the catheterization lab prior to coronary interventions. After successful PCIs, transthoracic images were obtained (**Figure 25.13** and ▶ **Video 25.6A,B**) in the CCU to evaluate the Impella CP catheter position.

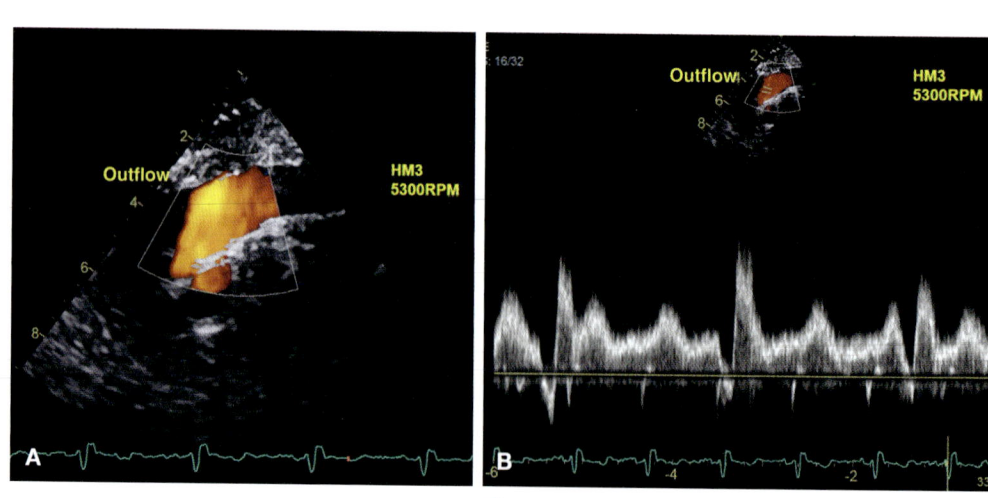

Figure 25.12

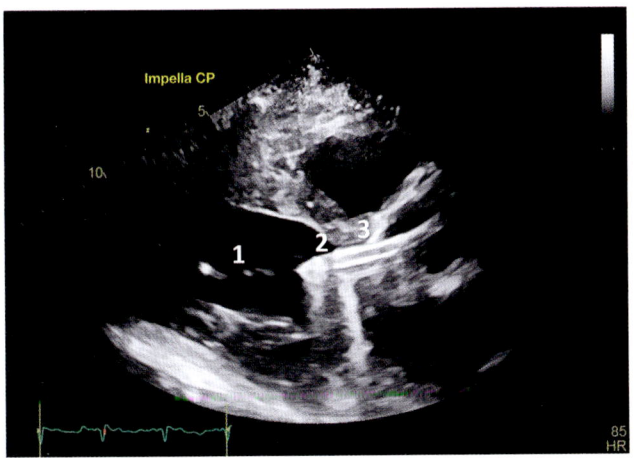

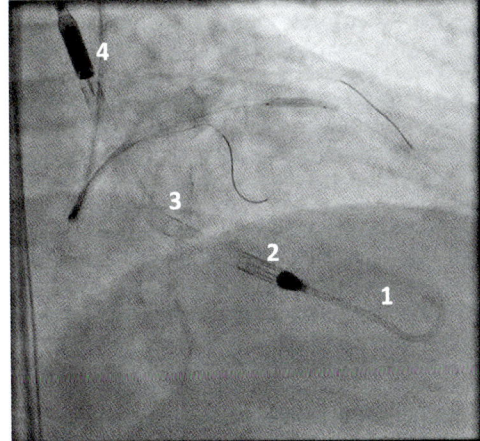

Chapter 25 Durable and Temporary LV Mechanical Circulatory Support Devices and Orthotopic Heart Transplantation / 541

Figure 25.13

37. Regarding the patient in **Case 10** (**Figure 25.13** and ▶ **Video 25.6**), which is most **CORRECT**?
    A. Impella CP components include 1. pigtail catheter, 2. inlet cage, 3. cannula, and 4. outlet area and power motor.
    B. Impella CP catheter 1. pigtail catheter, 2. outlet area and power motor, 3. cannula, and 4. inlet cage.
    C. Optimal Impella CP position as measured by TTE is about 3.5 cm from the mid-inlet cage (LV) to the aortic annulus.
    D. Optimal Impella CP position as measured by TTE is about 3.5 cm from the mid-outlet area to the aortic annulus.
    E. A and C.

CASE 11

A 58-year-old man is seen in the heart transplant clinic for post-hospital discharge follow-up including echocardiography. Three weeks ago, he had an orthotopic heart transplantation for nonischemic cardiomyopathy. Postoperative course was uncomplicated and a predischarge echocardiogram showed normal LV and RV function and no significant pericardial effusion.

His follow-up outpatient clinic visit echo is shown in **Figure 25.14** (▶ **Video 25.7A,B**).

38. Based on **Case 11** (as well as **Figure 25.14** and ▶ **Video 25.7A,B**), which of the following are echocardiographic features of early/acute allograft rejection?
    A. Reduction in left ventricular systolic function.
    B. Increase in left ventricular mass and wall thickness.
    C. New pericardial effusion.
    D. Choices A and B are correct.
    E. Choices A, B, and C are correct.

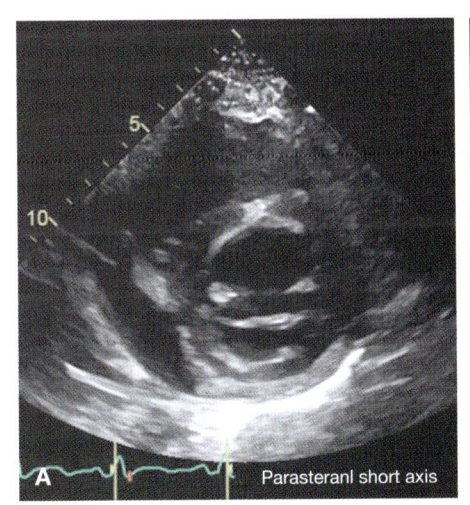

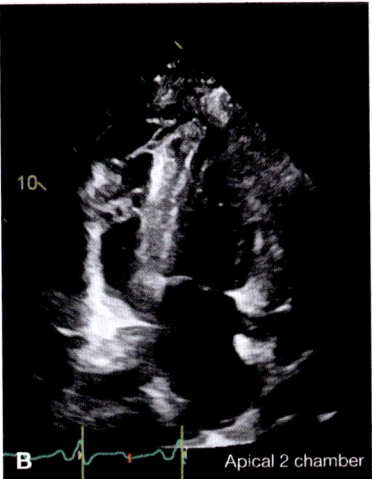

Figure 25.14

ANSWERS

1. **Answer: E.** Among the most important aspects of preimplantation TEE are reevaluation of the degree of AR, determination of the presence or absence of a cardiac-level shunt, identification of intracardiac thrombi, assessment of RV function, and evaluation of the degree of TR. These conditions may have been undiagnosed or underappreciated on previous imaging examinations or may have progressed in the intervening time. Their presence may alter the surgical plan or influence the decision for biventricular support.

2. **Answer: C.** While the LV diastolic dimension and LV end-diastolic volume are moderately or severely increased in most patients considered for a LVAD, limited data suggest that a smaller LV cavity (defined by a LV diastolic dimension of <6.3 cm) is associated with increased 30-day morbidity and mortality after LVAD implantation. A normal or small LV cavity size is certainly a *red flag* finding, but not an absolute contraindication to LVAD implantation. This finding should be clearly communicated to the heart failure team. An intracardiac thrombus is not an absolute contraindication for LVAD implantation but may increase the risk of stroke during the LV cannulation portion of the procedure. Acute endocarditis (or any other active infection) *is* an absolute contraindication to device implantation because of the risk of bacterial seeding of a newly implanted LVAD. Mitral regurgitation typically improves after LVAD implantation and thus is not considered a contraindication, although some recent data suggest that failure of MR to improve following LVAD implantation may be an indication for more frequent follow-up and careful clinical management.

3. **Answer: E.** Moderate or severe MS can prevent adequate LVAD cannula inflow and must be corrected before LVAD implantation. In contrast, AS of any severity may be present without affecting LVAD function, because LVADs completely bypass the native LV outflow tract. Significant AR enables a blind loop of flow in which blood enters the LVAD from the left ventricle, is pumped into the ascending aorta, but then flows back into the LV through the aortic valve, and thus must be addressed prior to LVAD implantation. Surgical treatment options for significant native valve AR include replacement with a bioprosthesis, completely oversewing the valve (by suturing along all coaptation zones) or by performing a central coaptation (Park) stitch. It is important to note that patients with significant AS or who undergo surgical aortic valve closure to correct AR will have minimal to zero forward flow in the event of LVAD failure. Mitral regurgitation that is significant preoperatively is often markedly improved after initiation of LVAD support because of reduced LV size, reduced filling pressures, and improved coaptation of the mitral valve leaflets after LVAD implantation. For this reason, any degree of MR is acceptable in LVAD candidates.

4. **Answer: D.** When present at LVAD implantation, significant AR enables a blind loop of flow in which blood enters the LVAD from the LV, is pumped into the ascending aorta, but then flows back into the LV through the regurgitant aortic valve. The presence of more-than-mild AR should be communicated to the implanting surgeon, because recent guidelines advise confirmation by perioperative TEE and surgical correction of AR before LVAD implantation. Surgical treatment options for significant native valve AR include replacement with a bioprosthesis, completely oversewing the valve (by suturing along all coaptation zones) or by performing a central coaptation (Park) stitch. Completely oversewing the aortic valve cusps effectively eliminates AR, but leaves the patient with no means of LV ejection in the event of LVAD failure. When the aortic cusp integrity is good, a central coaptation (Park) stitch technique can treat central AR while allowing aortic forward flow through the residual commissural zones during reduced LVAD support or in the event of LVAD pump failure. Aortic valve replacement with a mechanical valve is discouraged due to the prohibitively high risk of valve thrombus formation.

5. **Answer: D.** MR that is significant preoperatively is often markedly improved after initiation of LVAD support because of reduced filling pressures, reduced LV size, and improved coaptation of the mitral valve leaflets. For this reason, any degree of MR is acceptable in LVAD candidates.

6. **Answer: E.** The Interagency Registry for Mechanically Assisted Circulatory Support (INTERMACS) defines right heart failure (RHF) after LVAD implantation as "signs and symptoms of persistent right ventricular (RV) dysfunction," which can include echo parameters such as "C" and "D." There currently are no accepted criteria for mild versus moderate post-LVAD RVF, which may be transient. However, the designation of *severe* RVF additionally requires the need for a mechanical RV assist device or >14 days consecutive IV inotropic support. Right heart failure following LVAD can be problematic to predict, occurs in approximately 20% of patients, and is associated with significantly increased morbidity and mortality.

7. **Answer: E.** More-than-mild AR detection on a preoperative exam is a red flag finding. For many reasons, AR severity may be underestimated in cardiogenic shock patients. The preoperative AR assessment should include analysis of vena contracta width and LVOT jet height, integrated with other evidence of hemodynamically significant AR to guide the need for possible surgical intervention on the aortic valve. After LVAD implantation, AR severity assessment can be difficult in part due to variability of the aortic valve

opening and closure duration. With high levels of LV support, the aortic valve opening may completely cease, leading to continuous (pan systolic and pan diastolic) AR such that even a small aortic regurgitant orifice can produce a high regurgitant volume, and this is further affected by afterload conditions. AR severity assessment by pressure half-time and pulsed Doppler has not been validated in the setting of LVAD support and is presumed unreliable due to the continuous nature of LV unloading in addition to the turbulent and continuous outflow into the proximal aorta. There is consensus that either an AR vena contracta ≥0.3 cm (A) or AR (LVOT) jet height (>46%) can frequently be reliably measured and can also indicate clinically significant AR after LVAD implantation.

8. **Answer: B.** In evaluating patients with advanced heart failure for atrial septal defects and PFOs, the use of IV agitated saline exam combined with an appropriately performed Valsalva maneuver is necessary (but also often also insufficient) because elevated left and/or right atrial pressures may reduce interatrial pressure gradients and preclude detectable right-to-left atrial level shunting. When the LA pressure is not too high, the RA pressure can transiently exceed the LA pressure immediately following Valsalva maneuver release. If this pressure differential occurs during RA IV saline opacification, the transient shunt can be visibly detected by 2D echo. However, even with a Valsalva maneuver, the false-negative rate can be high when the LA pressure is very high (frequent with advanced HF) or in the presence of competitive inferior vena cava negative contrast. Additional perioperative TEE with the use of color Doppler (to detect an incompetent PFO tunnel flow, left-to-right flow) and immediate post-LVAD activation is also needed to definitively exclude a PFO, which would shunt avidly after LVAD activation.

9. **Answer: C.** A PFO, present in up to 30% of the general population, increases the risk of hypoxemia and paradoxical embolization in patients receiving LVAD support. Patent foramen ovale or any other interatrial communication should be closed at the time of device implantation.

10. **Answer: B.** Durable surgically implanted LVADs require coring in the region of the LV apex for inflow cannula insertion. This part of the procedure is inevitably accompanied by some degree of entrained air on the left side of the heart. Subsequent deairing maneuvers require continuous TEE guidance. The ostium of the RCA is situated anteriorly in the aortic root and is a common destination for air ejected from the left ventricle. Acute RV dysfunction or dilatation and/or an increase in the severity of TR suggest the possibility of air embolization to the RCA. This complication may resolve with watchful waiting. Post cardiopulmonary bypass RV failure (A) would not be preceded by a period of relatively normal RV function. Although acute pulmonary embolism could present with these findings, it is less likely in this setting while the patient is on cardiopulmonary bypass and fully heparinized.

11. **Answer: A.** After initiation of LVAD support, early imaging of the interatrial septum with color Doppler and with IV injection of agitated saline contrast to confirm the absence of an atrial septal communication is recommended. This is particularly important if initiation of LVAD support results in a sudden decrease in arterial oxygen saturation, the hallmark of an unmasked PFO or other right-to-left shunt.

12. **Answer: B.** In the absence of significant pulmonary valve regurgitation, the net cardiac output (combined native LV outflow and LVAD conduit flow) is the same as the right-sided cardiac output. The right-sided output is calculated by using the following commonly applied equation: RVOT cardiac output = RVOT pulsed Doppler TVI × [3.14 × (RVOT diameter/2)^2 × HR] or RVOT TVI × 0.785 × (RVOT diameter)^2 × HR. When the aortic valve does not open, and there is no significant AR, the RVOT-derived cardiac output is the same as the LVAD cardiac output. When the AV opens significantly and an adequate LVOT TVI can be measured with pulsed Doppler (and in the absence of significant AR), the LVAD cardiac output should equal the RVOT-derived cardiac output minus the LVOT cardiac output.

13. **Answer: D.** Clinical features associated with pump thrombosis include hemolysis, which is characterized by hemoglobinuria along with elevated lactate dehydrogenase, total bilirubin, and plasma-free hemoglobin levels. On echocardiography, primary pump dysfunction secondary to thrombosis may manifest as signs of reduced LV unloading in comparison with the previous surveillance examination. Echocardiographic signs of impaired pump performance (reduced LV unloading) include an increased $LVID_d$, worsened MR, septal shift toward the RV, and increased aortic valve opening duration or frequency in comparison to the prior echocardiogram. Although this LVAD (and the HVAD) is no longer implanted, a legacy patient population remains and this complication can occur in currently approved devices.

14. **Answer: C.** During suction events, the LVAD decompresses the LV chamber to an abnormally small size, leading to a right-to-left interventricular septal shift. Interventricular septal contact with the LVAD inflow cannula can induce ventricular arrhythmias and trigger LVAD alarms. Monitoring for possible suction events is an important component of a speed change echocardiogram. The treatment recommendation for a suction event is typically twofold: (1) decrease the pump speed and (2) identify and treat the underlying cause of the event. Hypovolemia and/or acute RV failure can precipitate suction events, but not enough information is provided to suggest the underlying cause.

15. **Answer: B.** After LVAD implantation, the RV begins to receive a significantly increased stroke volume. In some cases, the RV cannot accommodate this sudden increase in flow and, as a result, fails. If RVF is severe, LV preload (from the RV) can be inadequate, leading to a small LV (and possible suction event) if the pump speed is too high for prevailing conditions. Clinicians must maintain a high index of suspicion for RV dysfunction post-LVAD implantation and have a low threshold to perform an echocardiographic examination. Findings concerning for RV failure post-LVAD include RV enlargement, reduced RV function, interventricular septal position continuous shift toward the LV, dilated IVC, and worsening TR. Although the systolic PA pressure may be elevated, its estimation using the simplified Bernoulli equation method is unreliable with very severe TR. Because post-LVAD tamponade can clinically resemble RVF, a careful evaluation for significant pericardial effusion/hematoma is required. These are critical changes to recognize and diagnose promptly as they will greatly affect patient management.

16. **Answer: C.** Echocardiographic features associated with impeller thrombosis include reduced LV unloading in comparison with prior examinations. Specifically, these patients have increased $LVID_d$ despite increasing LVAD speed, worsening MR, and increased aortic valve opening and rightward shift of the ventricular septum (inadequate LV unloading). LVAD controller alarms indicating high power and elevated pulsatility index (PI) are also markers of LVAD dysfunction, especially impeller thrombosis.

17. **Answer: A.** The arterial blood pressure during examination is required for echocardiography interpretation, particularly when it comes to comparison with prior exams. A Doppler ultrasound blood pressure is defined as the cuff pressure at which a Doppler signal is obtained at the brachial or radial artery. In nonpulsatile LVAD patients, it is only appropriate to measure/document a mean arterial pressure. The sonographer may record current measurements from an invasive arterial blood pressure monitoring system that is already in place (eg, in an ICU).

18. **Answer: A.** Significant AR may be associated with a high estimated LVAD flow but with normal power. Aortic regurgitant volume can lead to an increased LV preload, which may result in increased native LVOT output and AV opening, with intermittent AR on color Doppler. Alternatively, the AR may be continuous if the LV systolic contractile force is not sufficient to interrupt the regurgitant aortic flow. With severe AR, spectral Doppler interrotation of the inflow cannula or outflow graft typically demonstrates augmented diastolic flow velocity (nadir diastolic flow velocity) and relatively reduced peak systolic flow velocity.

19. **Answer: E.** LVAD suction events relate to contact of the inflow cannula and the LV endocardium, which results in reduced inflow cannula flow. During suction events, the LVAD decompresses the LV chamber to an abnormally small size, resulting in a right-to-left ventricular septal shift. Patients with a malpositioned inflow cannula may be predisposed to the development of intermittent inflow cannula obstruction. Hemodynamic compromise can occur even if the inflow cannula is not physically obstructed, but LV preload falls to an unsustainable level from overpumping.

20. **Answer: A.** The $LVID_d$ from the two-dimensional parasternal long-axis image is considered the most *reproducible* measure of LV size after LVAD implantation. LV volumes determined by the Simpson's biplane or single-plane method better reflect the LV size than do linear measurements and should be used when technically feasible (usually in stable outpatients); Simpson method–derived volumes can be more difficult to obtain after LVAD implantation in the early phase due to wounds, suboptimal patient position, or shadowing associated with the inflow cannula. The LV size can be an important baseline metric for tracking response to therapy and device function, but it may change minimally during centrifugal pump ramp studies, depending upon afterload conditions. Systolic function is difficult to evaluate in the setting of continuous LVAD unloading, and the LVEF is a poor proxy and seldom relevant except in the setting of the infrequently used formal LVAD weaning protocol.

21. **Answer: A.** It may be assumed that LVAD patients have markedly abnormal baseline diastolic function. Many of the standard LV diastolic function parameters can be measured after LVAD implantation. However, they have not been validated in this specific population. Left atrial volume (Choice B) is typically increased in patients with dilated cardiomyopathy. A large left atrium post LVAD would not be unusual or reflect LA pressure in the setting of continuous LV unloading by the LVAD. Pulmonary vein inflow patterns are not routinely included in diastolic function in non-LVAD (or LVAD) patients although they could provide supplemental information in many situations. However, the mitral E velocity and estimated systolic PA pressure can be important variables for serial echo evaluations or during ramp studies since both will increase in the setting of inadequate LV unloading and may improve/normalize with pump speed and/or medical therapy adjustments.

22. **Answer: E.** LVAD optimization echocardiography consists of routine comprehensive TTE (or modified exam, depending on indication) at the baseline speed setting, followed by stepwise incremental adjustments to the LVAD speed, with collection of prespecified echocardiographic parameters at

each new speed that reflect LVAD and/or native LV function (eg, LVID$_d$, interventricular septal position, aortic valve opening frequency/duration, RVOT VTI, outflow graft Doppler, TR and/or MR severity). The sonographer should make appropriate notation of the LVAD speed assessed to help the interpreting clinician. There may be confusion with regard to the terms LVAD "speed change" or "ramp" echo protocols due to lack of consensus. "Ramp" protocol is likely the more appropriate name for a study performed with systematic changes in the pump speed and variable reassessment at each speed. An "optimization" ramp protocol would be used for surveillance where no problem is suspected, but device settings are sought, which are not too close to the upper or lower boundaries of safe pump operation. A ramp protocol could also be used to assess a suspected problem, which may or may not be due to an inappropriate speed setting.

23. **Answer: E.** Speed change echo testing is typically performed only if a patient is therapeutically anticoagulated. Risks include embolic events associated with sudden aortic valve opening (return to pulsatile flow) in the event of undiagnosed aortic root thrombus or the potential liberation of peripheral or internal pump thrombi, particularly at lower pump speeds. Reasons to stop a speed change test include (1) completion of the test; (2) a suction event (at higher speeds); (3) new symptoms, which may be related to hypoperfusion or hypotension; (4) hypertension; (5) and cannula flow reversal.

24. **Answer: C.** The pericardial location of the HVAD impeller results in a prominent, characteristic color and a spectral Doppler artifact, unique to this device, that generally precludes Doppler interrogation of the inflow cannula. The HVAD spectral and color Doppler artifacts occur only when the inflow cannula appears within the imaging sector. Therefore, successful color and spectral Doppler interrogation of other cardiac structures is possible whenever the imaging plane excludes the HVAD inflow cannula.

> **KEY POINTS**
> - The HVAD intrapericardial impeller results in a characteristic two-dimensional and color Doppler artifact.
> - The artifact is only present in the imaging sector of the impeller device.
> - This artifact precludes proper interrogation of the LV inflow.

25. **Answer: B.** New-onset ("de novo") AR occurs (often gradually) after LVAD implantation, more frequently in patients with no aortic valve opening (approximately 30% of LVAD patients). Significant AR is a key finding, given its known adverse effects on LVAD performance, morbidity, and mortality. Note in this patient with continuous aortic insufficiency, the vena contracta width is >4 mm.

> **KEY POINTS**
> - "De novo" AR is more common in LVAD patients with no aortic valve opening and detection of its development/progression is an important component of surveillance echocardiography.
> - Post-LVAD AR should be suspected with failure to unload the LV.

26. **Answer: E.** Ideally, the inflow cannula will have been inserted near the LV apex and aligned with the LV major axis, pointing toward the mitral valve. For technical reasons related to patient morphology, surgical access, and device characteristics, the ideal cannula position cannot be achieved, even though the LVAD may be functioning normally. In this example, the inflow cannula orientation is clearly NOT toward the mitral valve. The inflow zone appears unobstructed by best views. Inflow cannula Doppler interrogation might be best achieved using the parasternal long-axis view (**Figure 25.3A**), although this is not certain. There is no one best inflow cannula Doppler view for all LVAD patients, and the sonographer should investigate multiple windows to find the best view, using color and spectral Doppler to screen for inflow obstruction (not possible for HVAD devices, however).

> **KEY POINTS**
> - The LV inflow cannula is ideally apically placed and oriented toward the mitral valve in alignment with the LV major axis, but this may not be the case.
> - Sonographers should image the inflow cannula in multiple views to determine its orientation and the best view for spectral Doppler interrogation.

27. **Answer: A.** In HeartMate II, HVAD, and HeartMate 3 LVADs, the outflow graft follows a course anterior to the right atrium on its way to the proximal ascending aorta. In certain cases, such as in this patient who underwent OHT with biatrial technique, or in rare cases of successful LVAD explantation (without OHT), a portion of the outflow graft remains and might be seen in the bicaval view as in this TEE.

546 / Clinical Echocardiography Review

> **KEY POINTS**
> - A portion of the LVAD outflow graft may be seen as it courses anterior to the right atrium on its way to the proximal ascending aorta.

28. **Answer: D.** The aortic valve opening frequency and duration are most accurately assessed by recording multiple cardiac cycles at a slow M-mode sweep speed. The valve should be characterized as either opening with every cardiac cycle, opening intermittently, or remaining closed. At higher LVAD speeds, the LV is decompressed and aortic valve opening may be only intermittent or none at all (image A). Decreasing the LVAD speed (as seen in this example) reduces LV unloading and pump-generated LV afterload enabling aortic valve opening through native LV contraction. It is important to note that continuously closed aortic cusps have been associated with the development of aortic root thrombus, which may be transient or associated with commissural fusion. In many LVAD patients, aortic valve opening cannot be achieved at therapeutic pump speeds. Pump speed changes that might lead to new aortic valve opening should be made after exclusion of aortic root thrombus and verification of therapeutic anticoagulation.

    LVAD power is a direct measurement of pump motor voltage and current and generally varies directly with speed. It is measured continuously and displayed on the controller panel as an average over time in watts (a typical value is <10 W). Flow (L/min) is an estimated value that is directly related to the selected speed and power. Pulsatility denotes the difference between the minimum and maximum flows calculated by the device. Speed is the only parameter on both the HeartMate II and HeartWare HVAD that can be manually changed using the device controller. The other parameters vary according to the LVAD operating speed.

> **KEY POINTS**
> - M-mode aids in determining the frequency and duration of aortic valve opening in LVAD patients.
> - A decrease in LVAD speed reduces LV unloading through the pump and promotes aortic valve opening.

29. **Answer: C.** These images demonstrate the development of an aortic root thrombus in the setting of a continuously closed aortic valve. Speed change testing is typically performed only if a patient is receiving therapeutic doses of warfarin or parenteral anticoagulation therapy. Risks of performing speed changes include embolic events associated with sudden aortic valve opening in the event of undiagnosed aortic root thrombus or the potential liberation of peripheral or internal pump thrombi, particularly at lower pump speeds. In general, strong consideration should be given to deferring speed change examinations if baseline imaging shows a possible intracardiac or aortic root thrombus.

> **KEY POINTS**
> - Aortic root thrombus may occur as a complication of a continuously closed aortic valve in patients on a LVAD.
> - Evaluation for aortic root thrombus should be performed prior to speed change examinations due to the potential for liberation with sudden aortic valve opening.

30. **Answer: A.** Color and spectral Doppler interrogation of a properly aligned HeartMate II and HVAD outflow graft should reveal laminar, unidirectional flow. Due to native LV contractility, outflow graft flow remains pulsatile to some degree even when the aortic valve does not open. In general, outflow graft peak systolic flow velocities should be <1.5 to 2.0 m/s (usually in the range of 1.0 m/s). Higher velocities suggest possible localized obstructions (graft kinks or outflow graft-to-aorta anastomosis obstructions). Outflow graft velocities >2 m/s warrant further evaluation, although such speeds have been observed in normally functioning HVAD devices. Absent or minimal nadir diastolic flow (lowest diastolic velocity) suggests device internal thrombosis or obstruction. "High" nadir diastolic flows approaching peak systolic flow velocities suggest nearly complete LVAD support and/or severe aortic regurgitation. Note: CW Doppler is used to screen for inflow cannula obstruction for HM II and HM III devices, characterized by "spiky" irregular peak systolic velocities >2 m/s. Spectral Doppler of the HVAD cannula is not possible due to characteristic artifact.

    Note that the forward outflow graft flow–velocity profile will appear either above or below the baseline in the spectral Doppler display, depending upon the sonographer's positioning of the sample volume within the graft. There is no standard recommendation for a positive versus negative outflow graft display other than to provide the most coaxial alignment and to ensure that the flow direction is apparent.

> **KEY POINTS**
> - Inflow and outflow cannula flows should be interrogated by pulsed, continuous, and color Doppler. However, HVAD inflow velocities cannot be measured due to device Doppler artifact.
> - HeartMate II inflow cannula velocities are typically <1.5 m/s, with higher velocities suggesting obstruction.
> - Outflow graft velocities >2 m/s at any speed may be abnormal and warrant further evaluation.

31. **Answer: D.** The images above at LVAD speed 8200 rpm demonstrate a dilated LV with increased LV diastolic dimension, significant MR, elevated early mitral inflow velocities with rapid deceleration, and a dilated IVC. Persistence of significant MR after initiation of LVAD support may indicate inadequate LV unloading, as LV unloading generally leads to reduced mitral valve annular dilatation, improved leaflet coaptation, and reduced MR severity. Mitral inflow velocities can also be helpful in determining adequacy of LV unloading. In this patient, increasing the LVAD speed will allow the LV to decompress and reduce the MR.

> **KEY POINTS**
> - Findings consistent with inadequate LV unloading include a dilated LV, significant MR, elevated early mitral inflow velocities with rapid deceleration, and a dilated IVC.
> - An increase in LVAD speed may aid to optimize LV unloading.

32. **Answer: C.** These images represent the typical biatrial appearance seen in some patients following orthotopic heart transplant (OHT) with biatrial anastomosis. The suture line appears as thickened hyperechoic tissue in the mid-atrial septum and mid-atrial walls, separating donor atrial tissue from recipient atrial tissue. Note: this also represents an atrial electrical barrier resulting in asynchronous donor and recipient atrial contractility, hampering the interpretation of certain Doppler assessments (eg, unpredictable pulmonary vein flow velocity patterns). This appearance is less common today, as an increasing number of patients undergo OHT with bicaval anastomosis.

> **KEY POINTS**
> - Orthotopic heart transplant with biatrial anastomosis results in a typical appearance on echocardiography of biatrial enlargement/elongation.
> - Most heart transplants are currently done with bicaval anastomosis and so this is now a less common finding.

33. **Answer: C.** LVAD suction events relate to contact of the inflow cannula and the LV endocardium, which results in reduced inflow cannula flow and can be associated with a change in clinical status (eg, presyncope and/or palpitations from ventricular arrhythmias) and/or LVAD function. Any condition that produces LV underfilling places a patient at risk for LVAD suction events. These events can result from hypovolemia, RV failure, cardiac tamponade, and/or pump speed settings that are too high for the prevailing hemodynamic conditions. During suction events, the LVAD "sucks down" the LV chamber to an abnormally small size, leading to a right-to-left ventricular septal shift. Patients with a malpositioned inflow cannula may be predisposed to the development of intermittent inflow cannula obstruction and/or ventricular arrhythmias from mechanical contact with adjacent (usually septal) endocardium. Note: Although the HVAD inflow cannula cannot be directly interrogated by Doppler, the intermittent irregular inflow cannula obstruction usually produces blunted irregular outflow graft flow velocity pattern. Internal impeller or graft thrombosis does not cause irregular flow patterns such as this.

> **KEY POINTS**
> - LV suction events are manifested as a small LV cavity with right-to-left ventricular septal shift.
> - They result from inflow cannula contact with the LV endocardium.
> - LV suction events may lead to symptoms, arrhythmias, or hemodynamic effects.

34. **Answer: B.** This patient may have had some degree of preoperative RV failure unmasked by LVAD activation or de novo postoperative RVF, which can be difficult to predict. LVAD unloading of the LV exposes the RV to near-normal left-sided cardiac output, which can overload a weak RV, leading to acute RV failure in predisposed patients. This patient has an enlarged RV with significant interventricular septal shift to the left, a small LV cavity, and severe TR consistent with LVAD-associated acute RV failure. It is important to note that the current LVAD speed of 7800 rpm is very low and cannot be reduced further and increasing the speed would exacerbate the situation. Temporary RVAD support may enable RV recovery or bridge to transplant, assuming OHT candidacy.

> **KEY POINTS**
> - RV dysfunction post-LVAD initiation may be unmasked.
> - With unloading of the LV after LVAD initiation, the RV is suddenly exposed to near-normal cardiac output, which may lead to RV failure.

548 / Clinical Echocardiography Review

35. **Answer: C.** Coronary artery graft vasculopathy (CAV) remains prevalent after OHT and is the leading cause of death in OHT patients surviving >1 year. Coronary angiography using the ISHLT CAV classification system is the gold standard for early detection and follow-up, typically performed every 1 to 2 years. Dobutamine or treadmill stress echo received a class IIb recommendation for CAV screening in adult OHT patients in the updated 2022 ISHLT HT management guidelines. This guarded recommendation is due to *low test sensitivity* (high rates of false-negative tests) of stress echo for CAV detection, which may be related to the diffuse nature of CAV. Stress echo may be used cautiously in this patient population when invasive coronary angiography is contraindicated.

36. **Answer: A.** This is a normal HeartMate 3 (HM 3) outflow graft pulsed Doppler image. All of the comments relating to the HM II and the HVAD outflow graft Doppler noted in the **Questions 25 to 30** discussion also apply to the HM 3. What is different about the spectral Doppler pattern in this normally functioning HM 3 outflow Doppler image? The outflow graft flow velocity pattern contains a distinct, brief (0.35 sec) periodic (every 2 seconds) biphasic velocity shift cycle superimposed upon the familiar continuous flow pattern with systolic flow augmentation from the native heart. This new superimposed pattern is caused by a programmed impeller pump speed shift of (−) 2000 rpm immediately followed by (+) 2000 rpm relative to the baseline fixed pump speed. This creates an "artificial pulse" designed to minimize flow stasis within the system.

    Note: The HM II is no longer FDA approved due to superior third-generation devices and the HVAD device was recalled from the market in June of 2021. However, echocardiographers must remain familiar with these legacy devices, which remain implanted and normally functioning in a significant number of patients as of this publication. At this time, the HM 3 is the only durable surgical device with FDA approval (2018 approval for destination therapy).

37. **Answer: E.** The Impella CP is a percutaneous LVAD, which is FDA approved for use in high-risk percutaneous coronary interventions. It is also approved in the treatment of acute left ventricular failure not responsive to optimal medical management.

    The Impella CP catheter (as well as the larger surgically placed similar Impella 5.0) consists of four major components (**Figure 25.15A**: (1) a distal flexible pigtail, (2) an inlet cage, (3), the conduit cannula, and (4) an outlet area which is just proximal to the adjacent micro-impeller axial flow pump.

    Echocardiography is frequently used to confirm optimal catheter position since the device can become displaced after patient movement (including CPR) or transfers even after initial confirmation of adequate placement by fluoroscopic and/or TEE guidance.

    The parasternal long-axis view on TTE and the mid-esophageal long-axis view on TEE are the best

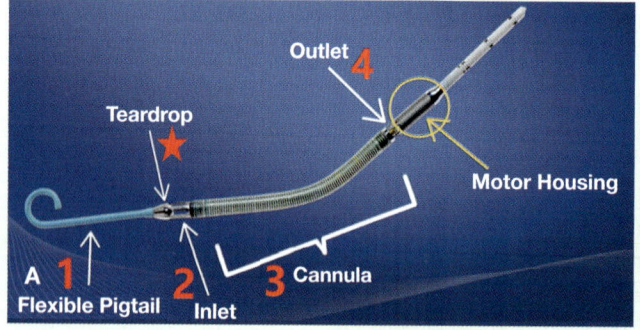

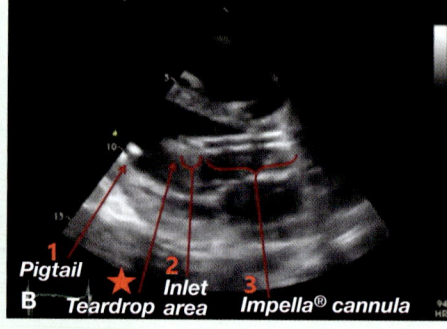

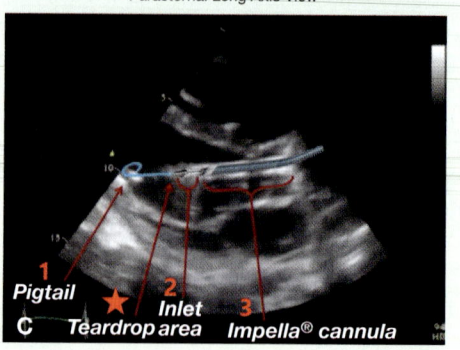

Figure 25.15. Impella® is a trademark of Abiomed, Inc. Used with permission. From Assessing Impella® Heart Pump Position with Echocardiography. https://www.heartrecovery.com

views to identify accurate placement of the Impella catheter.

As shown in **Figures 25.15B** and **25.15C**, the thin distal pigtail (1) is mounted upon a brightly hyperechoic distal "teardrop" structure (*). The inlet area (2) is the blood inflow zone and appears as an hypoechoic (dark) "gap" between the distal teardrop (*) and the cannula (3). Ideally, the mid-inflow area to aortic annuls distance should be in the range of 3.5 cm and this can be easily determined using the echo device electronic calipers.

Note: in **Figure 25.13**, the distance between the inflow area (2) and the aortic annulus is obviously much less than 3.5 cm, and the device should be advanced so that the inflow area is safe within the LV and not so close to the aortic valve. Care is taken to direct the pigtail catheter away from the submitral apparatus when possible, with the inflow area away from the mitral leaflets, which could become entrained by device suction or otherwise distorted. The outflow area and pump motor (4) are positioned well above the aortic annulus and in the ascending aorta (seen on the fluoroscopic images but frequently not visible on TTE or TEE images).

Echocardiography also helps identify several important conditions that may be contraindications to Impella CP placement including presence of LV thrombus, mechanical aortic valve, moderate or severe aortic regurgitation, severe aortic stenosis/calcification (equivalent to an orifice area <0.6 cm^2), postinfarct VSD, or significant right heart failure.

Supplementary information: temporary LVAD Impella 5.5. In contrast to the Impella CP (and the Impella 5.0), the surgically placed Impella 5.5 LVAD (▶ **Video 25.8**) provides greater LV unloading and can be used for longer duration. The catheter system is devoid of the distal pigtail component, making it more apt to become inadvertently completely expelled from the LV. The Impella 5.5 mid-inflow zone–to–aortic annulus distance should be approximately 5.0 cm for this device (as opposed to 3.5 cm for the pigtailed Impella devices). Acquired images should include a device-type annotation.

38. **Answer: E.** While reduction in LV systolic function early after transplantation warrants endomyocardial biopsy to exclude acute rejection, the degree of LV systolic dysfunction may not correlate with the severity of rejection on the biopsy. Other echocardiographic features with lower sensitivity and specificity include increase in the LV mass/wall thickness and appearance of pericardial effusion. While patients undergoing orthotropic heart transplantation are at risk for development of pericardial effusion due to the usual causes after cardiac surgery (including postpericardiotomy syndrome and pericardial hemorrhage), there are also several unique risk factors associated with development of pericardial effusions in this population including acute allograft rejection, use of sirolimus, and right ventricular perforation during endomyocardial biopsies. A temporal relation between development of moderate or large pericardial effusions and allograft rejection that may involve the pericardium has been reported.

In our patient, the echocardiogram shows normal LV and RV function and moderate pericardial effusion around the inferior LV and RV with fibrinous strands. No echocardiographic or clinical signs of increased intrapericardial pressure were noted. Following the echo, the patient was admitted and underwent an endomyocardial biopsy, which showed grade 2 rejection. He was treated with high-dose IV steroids. Repeat echocardiogram in 4 weeks' time showed complete resolution of the pericardial effusion. A new pericardial effusion is a critical finding in an OHT patient either before or after endomyocardial biopsy.

SUGGESTED READINGS

Assessing Impella Heart Pump Position with Echocardiography. Abiomed. Heartrecovery.com.

Bennett MK, Roberts CA, Dordunoo D, Shah A, Russell SD. Ideal methodology to assess systemic blood pressure in patients with continuous-flow left ventricular assist devices. *J Heart Lung Transplant*. 2010;29(5):593-594.

Estep JD, Stainback RF, Little SH, Torre G, Zoghbi WA. The role of echocardiography and other imaging modalities in patients with left ventricular assist devices. *JACC Cardiovasc Imaging*. 2010;3:1049-1064.

Estep JD, Vivo RP, Krim SR, et al. Echocardiographic evaluation of hemodynamics in patients with systolic heart failure supported by a continuous-flow LVAD. *J Am Coll Cardiol*. 2014;64(12):1231-1241.

Masarone D, Kittleson M, Gravino R, Valente F, Petraio A, Pacileo G. The role of echocardiography in the management of heart transplant recipients. *Diagnostics (Basel)*. 2021;11(12):2338.

Shah NR, Cevik C, Hernandez A, Gregoric ID, Frazier OH, Stainback RF. Transthoracic echocardiography of the HeartWare left ventricular assist device. *J Card Fail*. 2012;18(9):745-748.

Stainback RF, Estep JD, Agler DA, et al. Echocardiography in the management of patients with left ventricular assist devices: recommendations from the American Society of Echocardiography. *J Am Soc Echocardiogr*. 2015;28(8):853-909.

Velleca A, Shullo MA, Dhital K, et al. The International Society for Heart and Lung Transplantation (ISHLT) guidelines for the care of heart transplant recipients. *J Heart Lung Transplant*. 202342(5):e1-e141.

CHAPTER 26

Systemic Disease

Daniel Sykora and Sunil Mankad

QUESTIONS

1. A 56-year-old homeless man with a body mass index of 17 kg/m² and recently diagnosed cardiomyopathy undergoes echocardiography. The following Doppler variables are obtained. Left ventricular outflow tract time-velocity integral (LVOT TVI) = 36 cm; aortic valve TVI = 40 cm; LVOT diameter = 2.2 cm; heart rate = 86 bpm; and body surface area = 1.9 m². No significant valvular heart disease is identified. Which nutritional deficiency is most likely?
   A. Selenium deficiency.
   B. Thiamine deficiency.
   C. Carnitine deficiency.
   D. Folate deficiency.
   E. Vitamin B$_{12}$ deficiency.

2. A 60-year-old male farmer presents with 1 month of progressive exertional dyspnea, lower extremity edema, skin pigmentation changes, and palpitations. He is highly physically active, at a normal weight, but was recently diagnosed with type 2 diabetes mellitus by his primary care provider. His echocardiogram is shown in **Figure 26.1** and ▶ **Video 26.1**. What is the most likely cardiac diagnosis?
   A. Dilated left ventricle and systolic dysfunction secondary to hemochromatosis.
   B. Heart failure with preserved ejection fraction secondary to diabetes mellitus type 2.
   C. Ischemic cardiomyopathy.
   D. Right ventricular heart failure from pulmonary hypertension.
   E. Large pericardial effusion.

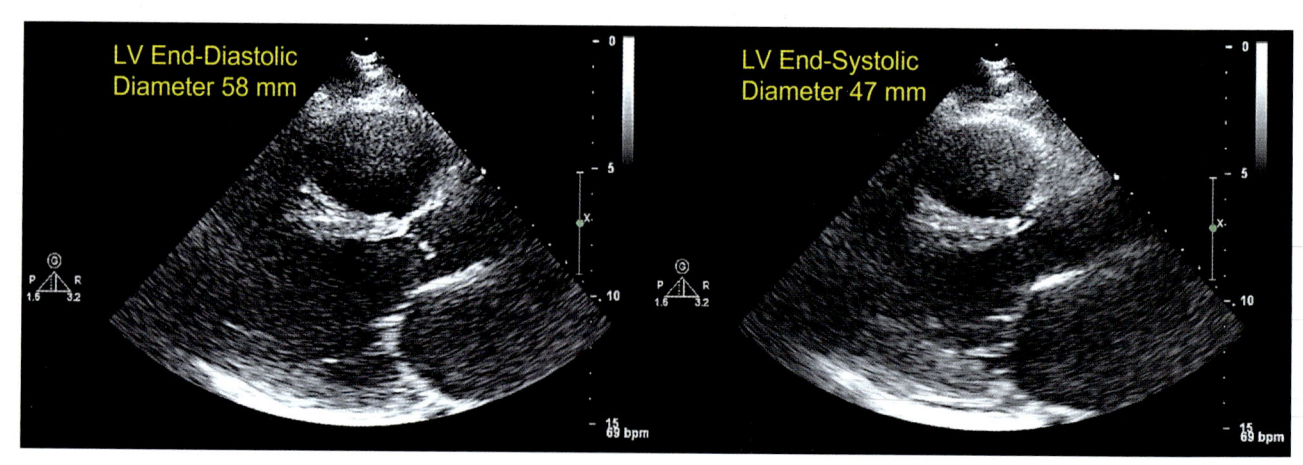

Figure 26.1

3. A 62-year-old woman with a long-standing history of systemic lupus erythematosus presents to the emergency department with subacutely worsening fatigue, weight gain, and orthopnea. She has not visited the rheumatologist in a decade but states her lupus has been well controlled with hydroxychloroquine. Electrocardiogram reveals second degree Mobitz II atrioventricular block. Echocardiography reveals reduced LV ejection fraction of 40% and the findings in **Figure 26.2**. The most likely diagnosis is:
   A. Pulmonary arterial hypertension.
   B. Alcoholic cardiomyopathy.
   C. Cardiac manifestation of systemic lupus erythematosus.
   D. Hydroxychloroquine cardiotoxicity.
   E. None of the above.

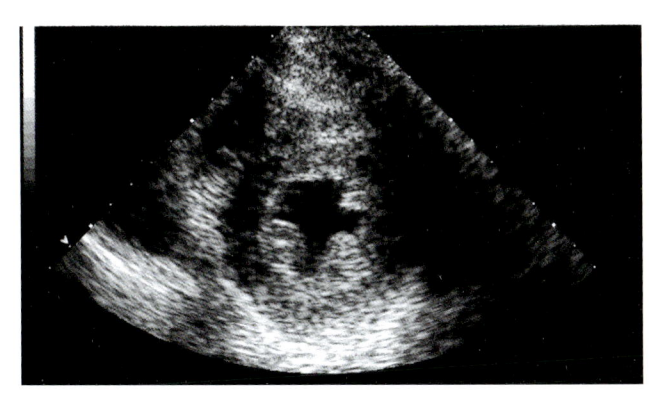

Figure 26.2

4. A 58-year-old woman presents to her primary care provider with complaints of weight loss, tremor, insomnia, palpitations, and orthopnea for 3 weeks. Physical exam reveals irregular tachycardia and subsequent electrocardiogram reveals atrial fibrillation with a rapid ventricular response. An echocardiogram will most likely reveal:
   A. Increased concentric left ventricular wall thickness.
   B. Sclerotic aortic valve.
   C. Dilated left ventricle with cardiomyopathy.
   D. Regional wall motion abnormalities.
   E. None of the above.

5. A 22-year-old man presents with 1 week of increasing shortness of breath associated with bilateral lower extremity swelling. Three months ago, he underwent the treatment of Hodgkin lymphoma. The mitral inflow peak E wave and mitral annular e′ velocities are 110 and 3 cm/s, respectively. There are no significant valvular abnormalities. A small circumferential pericardial effusion is present. The most likely explanation for these findings is:
   A. Noncardiac etiology.
   B. Severe anemia.
   C. Early doxorubicin cardiotoxicity.
   D. Radiation-induced heart disease.
   E. None of the above.

6. A 19-year-old man with severe ataxia and cerebellar dysarthria is referred for an echocardiogram. Echocardiographic findings are shown in **Figure 26.3** (parasternal short-axis view), ▶ **Video 26.2**, and ▶ **Video 26.3** (parasternal long-axis and short-axis views, respectively). The most likely diagnosis is:
   A. HIV cardiomyopathy.
   B. Friedreich ataxia.
   C. Hypertrophic obstructive cardiomyopathy.
   D. Arrhythmogenic right ventricular cardiomyopathy.
   E. None of the above.

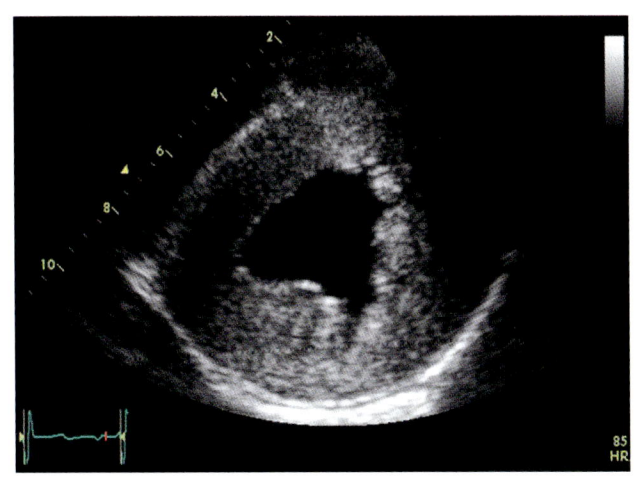

Figure 26.3

7. A patient with long-standing poorly controlled hypertension and chronic renal failure on maintenance hemodialysis undergoes an echocardiogram. LV size and systolic function are normal. There is increased concentric wall thickening. There is severe left atrial enlargement. The E/A ratio is 2.0, and the E/e′ ratio is 25. The aortic and mitral valves are thickened and calcified and associated with moderate aortic, mitral, and tricuspid regurgitation. There is severe mitral annular calcification. The right ventricular (RV) systolic pressure is 60 mm Hg. A small pericardial effusion is present. Which of the following tests should be reviewed at the time of the echocardiogram to help evaluate for cardiac involvement with amyloid?
   A. Complete blood cell count.
   B. Serum creatinine level.
   C. Serum brain natriuretic peptide.
   D. Chest x-ray.
   E. Electrocardiogram (ECG).

8. A 68-year-old woman presents with 1 month of epistaxis, purpuric rash, and shortness of breath. Broad laboratory evaluation reveals elevated erythrocyte sedimentation rate and Proteinase 3-ANCA. Which of the following echocardiographic findings is most likely in this patient?
   A. Regional wall motion abnormalities not confined to a specific coronary artery territory.
   B. Concentric increased wall thickness and restrictive physiology consistent with an infiltrative cardiomyopathy.
   C. Aortic cusp perforation with severe aortic regurgitation.
   D. Large pericardial effusion with cardiac tamponade.
   E. None of the above.

9. A 46-year-old man with dyspnea undergoes a transthoracic echocardiogram, which demonstrates reduced systolic function with normal LV dimension. Which of the following conditions that can cause reduction in ejection fraction is most often associated with normal LV cavity dimension?
   A. Amyloidosis.
   B. Sarcoidosis.
   C. Hemochromatosis.
   D. Human immunodeficiency virus (HIV).
   E. Excess alcohol.

10. A 32-year-old man with no prior cardiac history is undergoing evaluation for presumed cardiogenic syncope and subacute exertional dyspnea with orthopnea. Chest x-ray is shown in **Figure 26.4**. Twelve lead EKG is shown in **Figure 26.5**. Holter monitoring reveals frequent non-sustained ventricular tachycardia. His echocardiogram is shown in ▶ **Video 26.4** and ▶ **Video 26.5**. What is the most likely diagnosis?
    A. Takotsubo cardiomyopathy.
    B. Cardiac sarcoidosis.
    C. Hypertrophic obstructive cardiomyopathy.
    D. Arrhythmogenic right ventricular cardiomyopathy.
    E. None of the above.

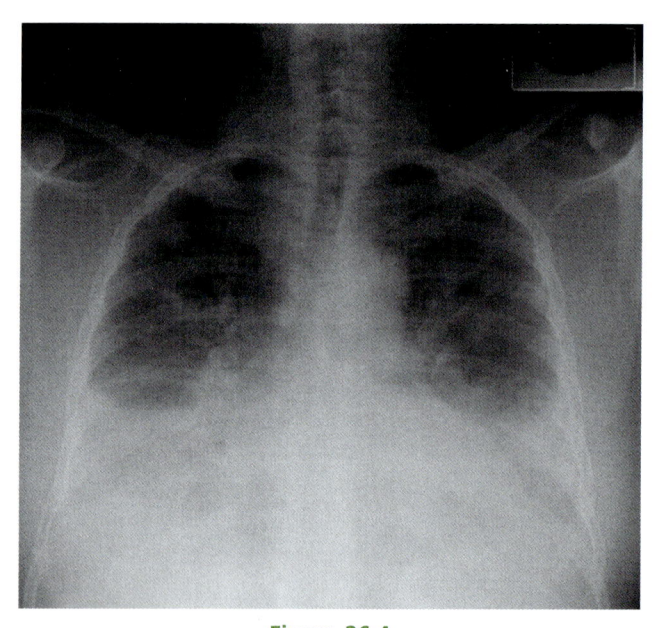

Figure 26.4

Chapter 26 Systemic Disease / 553

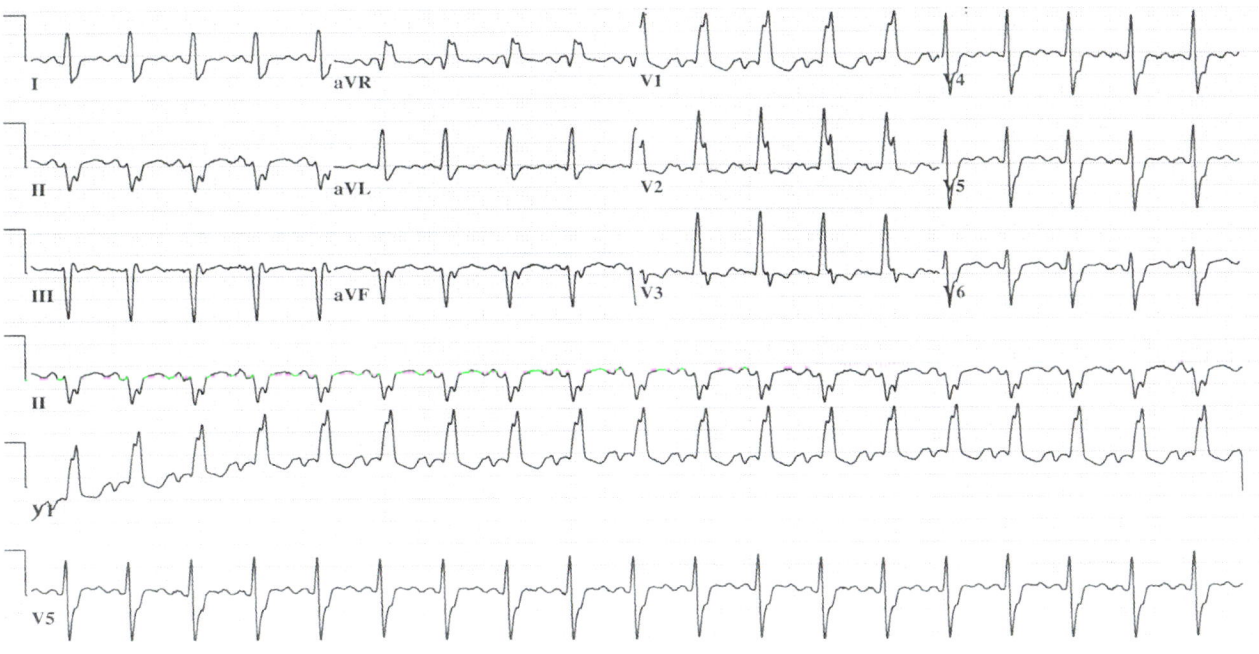

Figure 26.5

11. A 43-year-old Caucasian male presents with findings of progressive fatigue, dyspnea, and pedal edema over a 6-month period. After an episode of atypical chest pain during which he had a flat serial pattern but elevated troponin T, he underwent coronary artery angiography which demonstrated normal epicardial coronary arteries. An echocardiogram was performed and representative images are shown **Figures 26.6-26.9** and ▶ **Videos 26.6-26.9**. Serum light chains are elevated and demonstrate an abnormal pattern. Which of the Bullseye global longitudinal LV strain patterns would typically be seen in this condition?
   A. Figure 26.6
   B. Figure 26.7
   C. Figure 26.8
   D. Figure 26.9
   E. None of the above.

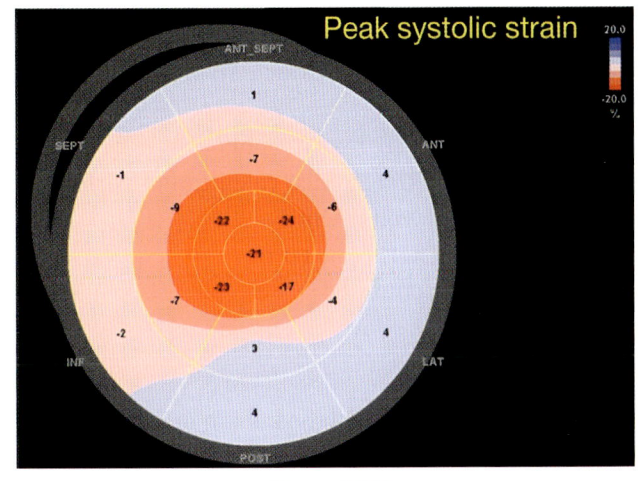

Figure 26.7

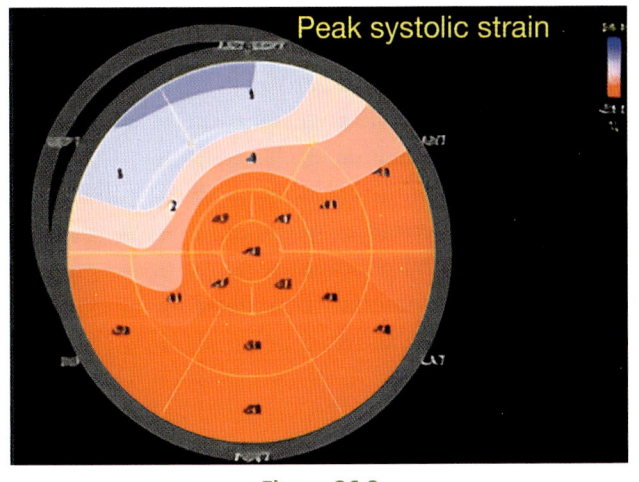

Figure 26.8

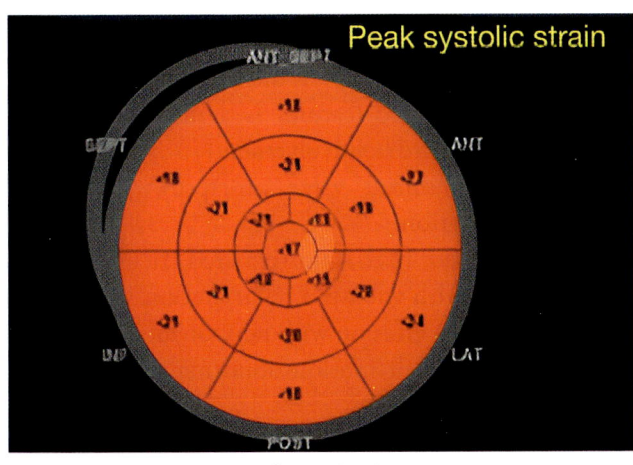

Figure 26.6

Figure 26.9

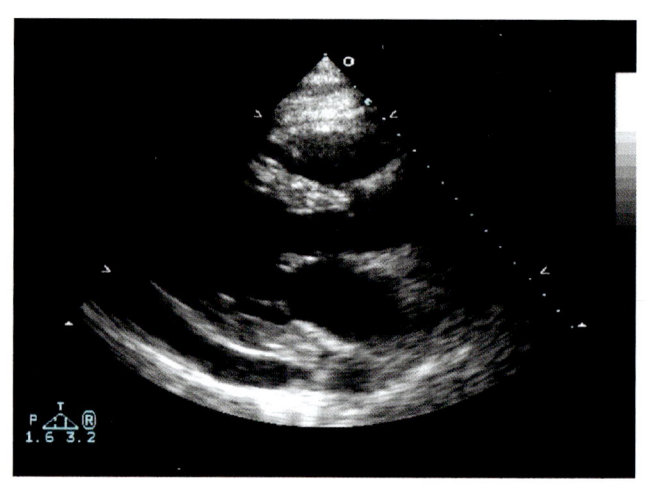

Figure 26.10

12. A 45-year-old woman presents with dyspnea. She has a remote history of Hodgkin lymphoma and received mantle radiation many years ago. An echocardiogram is requested. Which of the following echocardiographic findings would suggest radiation-related cardiovascular disease in this patient?
    A. Left ventricular hypertrophy.
    B. Anterior mitral annular calcification with multivalvular involvement.
    C. Ascending aortic dilatation.
    D. Pericardial effusion.
    E. None of the above.

13. A 28-year-old man with no known medical comorbidities is hospitalized for 6 weeks of progressive exertional dyspnea and dysphagia. Investigation of his dysphagia reveals esophageal candidiasis and very low CD4 cell count. Echocardiogram is performed to investigate his dyspnea and findings are shown in **Figure 26.10** and ▶ **Video 26.10**. What is the most likely diagnosis?
    A. Kaposi sarcoma of the heart.
    B. Human immunodeficiency virus with symptomatic pericardial effusion.
    C. Typical viral pericarditis.
    D. Primary pulmonary hypertension.
    E. None of the above.

14. A 60-year-old woman has a history of labile hypertension. She complains of a severe headache, diaphoresis, central chest pain, and profound shortness of breath, lasting 20 minutes, shortly after total abdominal hysterectomy. The blood pressure is 130/85 mm Hg in the right arm and 140/90 mm Hg in the left arm. Additional findings are a fourth heart sound and bibasilar crackles. The chest x-ray demonstrates pulmonary edema. The ECG demonstrates sinus tachycardia, LV hypertrophy, and widespread ST segment depression. An echocardiogram demonstrates akinesis of the mid and apical LV segments. The LV ejection fraction is 25%. A coronary angiography is performed and demonstrates normal epicardial coronary arteries. The most likely explanation for these findings is:
    A. Coronary artery vasospasm.
    B. Coronary artery thromboembolism.
    C. Pheochromocytoma.
    D. Cushing syndrome.
    E. None of the above.

15. A 61-year-old woman has long-standing rheumatoid arthritis and is referred for an echocardiogram to evaluate dyspnea. Which of the following echocardiographic features is a manifestation of rheumatoid cardiac involvement?
    A. Bileaflet mitral valve prolapse with mitral regurgitation.
    B. Thickened, fixed, and retracted tricuspid valve leaflets with tricuspid regurgitation.
    C. Pericardial effusion with tamponade physiology.
    D. Regional wall motion abnormalities and diastolic dysfunction.
    E. None of the above.

16. A 67-year-old woman with no prior history of cardiac disease presents with severe chest pain and dyspnea over the past 24 hours. Initial ECG demonstrates ST elevation in the anterior precordial leads and she is immediately taken to the cardiac catheterization laboratory. Coronary angiography demonstrates only mild epicardial coronary artery disease. Echocardiography is performed and representative end-diastolic and end-systolic 4-chamber images are shown in **Figures 26.11** and **26.12**. The apical 4 chamber video is shown in ▶ Video 26.11. Which of the following may be present in this patient?
    A. Persistent LV systolic dysfunction at 1 year.
    B. Dynamic LV outflow tract obstruction.
    C. Markedly increased cardiac troponin T.
    D. Increased urinary 5-hydroxyindole acetic acid.
    E. None of the above.

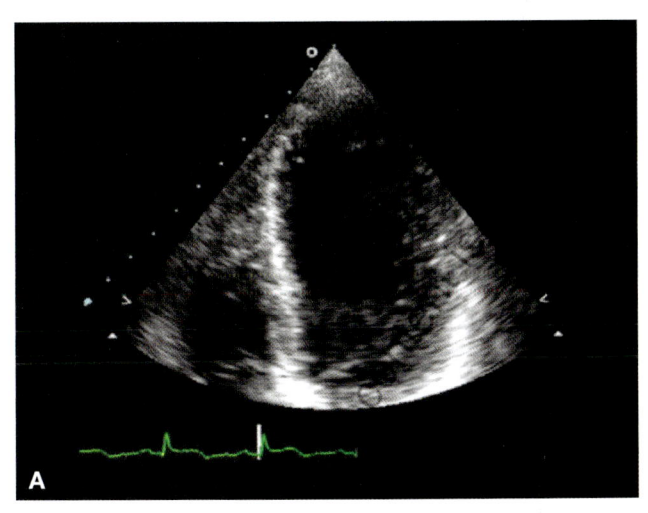

Figure 26.11. End diastole.

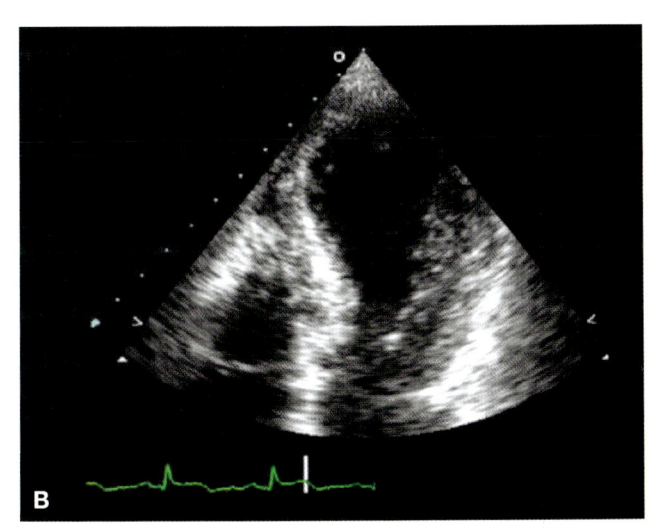

Figure 26.12. End systole.

17. A 66-year-old woman who appears younger than her stated age presents with complaints of dyspnea, arthralgias, and swelling of her hands and feet. Echocardiography is performed and a short-axis view is provided in **Figure 26.13**. What is the most likely diagnosis?
    A. Cardiac amyloidosis.
    B. Scleroderma.
    C. Hemochromatosis.
    D. Rheumatoid arthritis.
    E. None of the above.

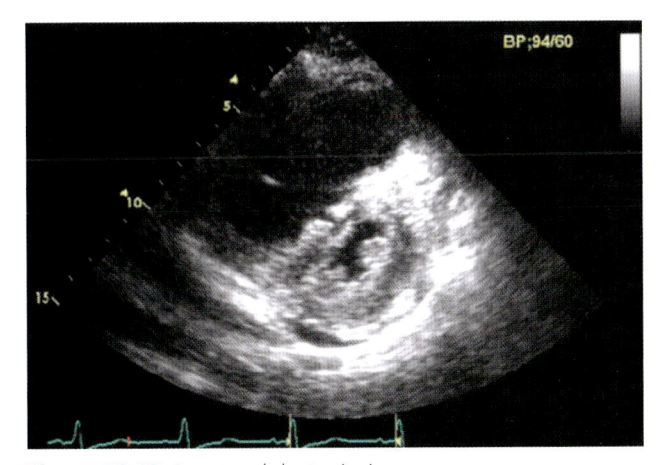

Figure 26.13. Parasternal short-axis view.

18. A transesophageal echocardiogram (TEE) is obtained in a 29-year-old woman who presents with symptoms of arthralgias, low-grade fever, chest pain, skin rash, and photosensitivity. There is no history of illicit drug use. Chest x-ray demonstrates small bilateral pleural effusions. Initial laboratory tests demonstrate a mildly elevated white blood cell count, elevated creatinine level of 1.5 mg/dL, and an elevated erythrocyte sedimentation rate of 45 mm/h. Based on the TEE image (120°) shown in **Figure 26.14** and in ▶ **Videos 26.12** and **26.13**. What is the most likely diagnosis?
    A. Ergot-alkaloid use.
    B. Infective endocarditis.
    C. Libman-Sacks endocarditis.
    D. Rheumatic mitral valve disease.
    E. None of the above.

556 / Clinical Echocardiography Review

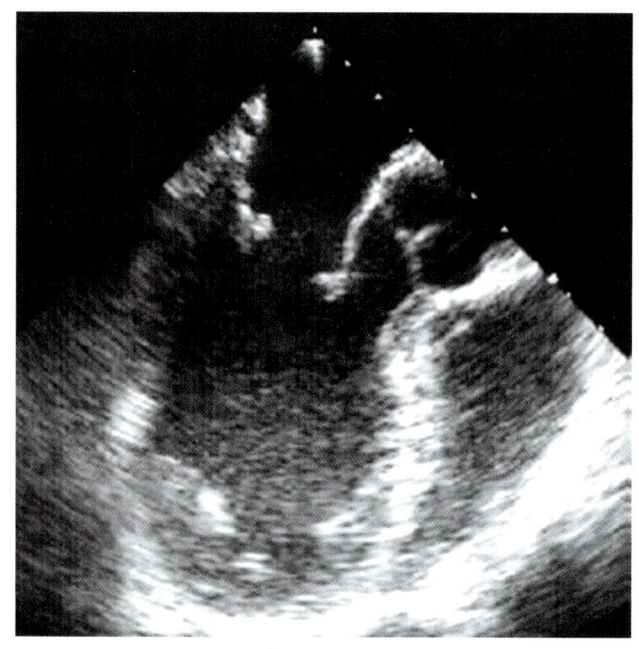

Figure 26.14

19. A 20-year-old man is being evaluated for palpitations. The physical examination is unremarkable except for red skin lesions involving the groin. The ECG demonstrates LV hypertrophy and the echocardiogram demonstrates increased concentric wall thickness measuring 18 mm. The skin lesions are shown in **Figure 26.15**. Which of the following conditions most likely accounts for the echocardiographic findings in this patient?
A. Acromegaly.
B. Amyloid.
C. Fabry disease.
D. Hypertrophic cardiomyopathy.
E. None of the above.

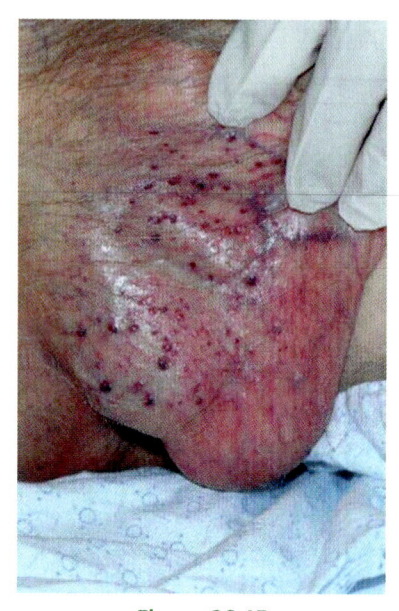

Figure 26.15

20. A 1-year-old boy has a history of seizures. His mother remembers that a prenatal echocardiogram was abnormal, but she was reassured and told that follow-up echocardiography was all that was needed. He is an active child and has no cardiovascular symptoms. The physical examination is unremarkable except for the skin lesion shown (**Figure 26.16**). A transthoracic echocardiogram is obtained (**Figure 26.17**). Which statement below describes the **BEST** course of management for this patient?
A. Reassurance and follow-up echocardiography is recommended in 1 year.
B. Whole-body computed tomography is indicated to identify the primary tumor.
C. Prognosis is poor and thus surgical resection is not recommended.
D. Surgical resection is indicated now to prevent further growth and potential damage to sensitive cardiac structures.
E. None of the above.

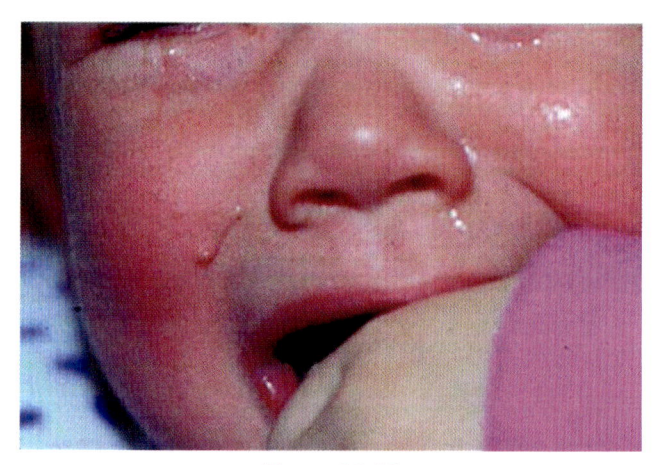

Figure 26.16

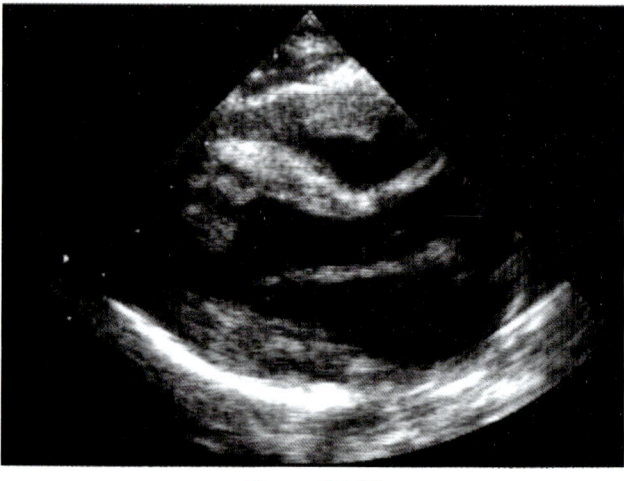

Figure 26.17

21. A 23-year-old man is sent for an echocardiogram because of a widened mediastinum appreciated on chest x-ray performed during a routine preemployment physical examination. He has a history of lens dislocation as a child. His grandfather died suddenly of an unknown cause. The pertinent echocardiographic images are shown in the high parasternal long-axis view shown in **Figure 26.18**. Which of the following is the **BEST** course of action?
   A. TEE to better evaluate the aorta and aortic valve.
   B. Cardiac surgical consultation for elective aortic root replacement.
   C. Treatment with beta-blockers, avoid heavy lifting, and reassessment in 6 months.
   D. Treatment with losartan, avoid heavy lifting, and reassessment in 1 year.
   E. None of the above.

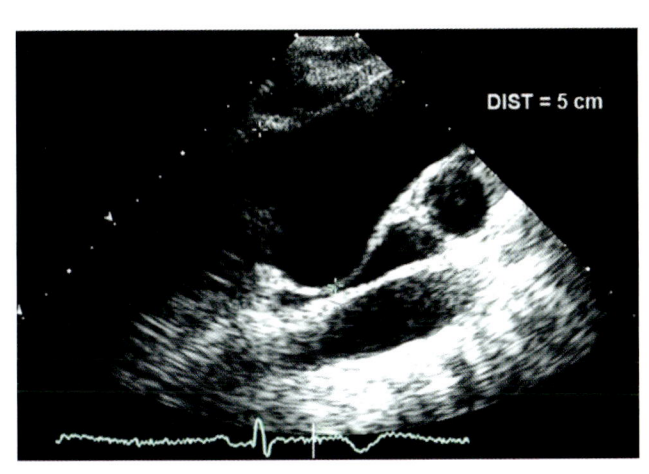

Figure 26.18

22. A 29-year-old Asian woman is referred to echocardiography for the assessment of fatigue and a murmur noted on physical examination. Pertinent features on physical examination include inability to measure a blood pressure in the left arm, a left carotid and subclavian bruit, and a long decrescendo diastolic murmur. An abdominal bruit is also noted. Laboratory testing is remarkable for mild normocytic anemia and increased erythrocyte sedimentation rate and C-reactive protein. An echocardiogram is obtained. The ascending aorta is dilated measuring 45 mm at the mid ascending level; the sinus dimension is normal. Other pertinent images are demonstrated in **Figures 26.19-26.21**. Which of the following diagnoses is most likely in this patient?
   A. Marfan syndrome.
   B. Takayasu arteritis.
   C. Familial thoracic aortic aneurysmal disease.
   D. Ankylosing spondylitis.
   E. None of the above.

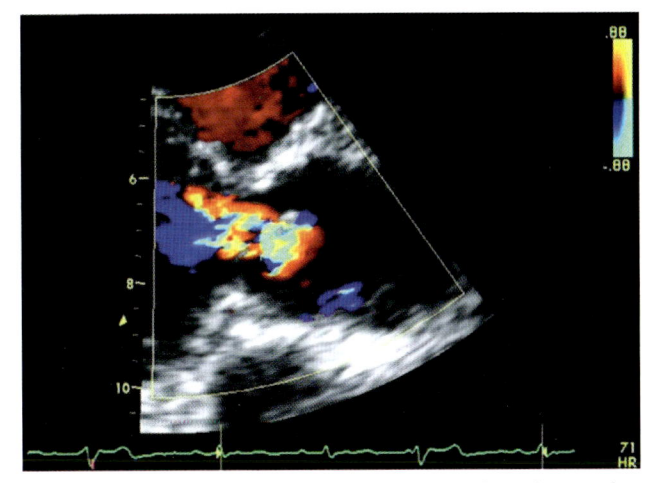

Figure 26.19. Parasternal long-axis with color-Doppler and zoom of the aortic valve.

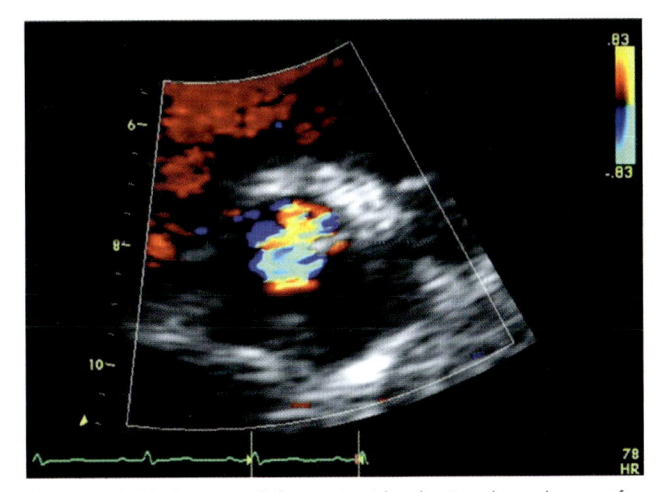

Figure 26.20. Parasternal short-axis with color Doppler and zoom of the aortic valve.

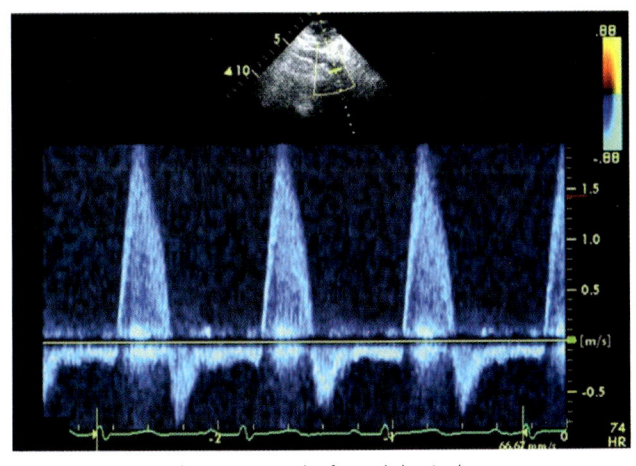

Figure 26.21. Pulse wave Doppler from abdominal aorta.

558 / Clinical Echocardiography Review

23. A patient with a diagnosis of metastatic carcinoid presents to the echocardiographic laboratory for evaluation. She has features of right heart enlargement with associated dysfunction and severe tricuspid valve regurgitation. Additional echo-Doppler images are obtained. What do the echo-Doppler images of the RV outflow tract in **Figures 26.22-26.24** demonstrate?
  A. Severe pulmonary valve regurgitation.
  B. Severe pulmonary valve stenosis.
  C. Severe pulmonary hypertension.
  D. Patent ductus arteriosus.
  E. None of the above.

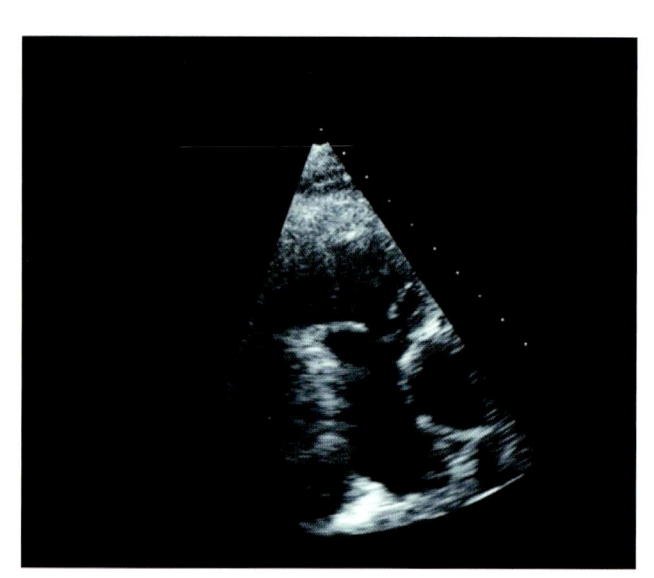

Figure 26.22

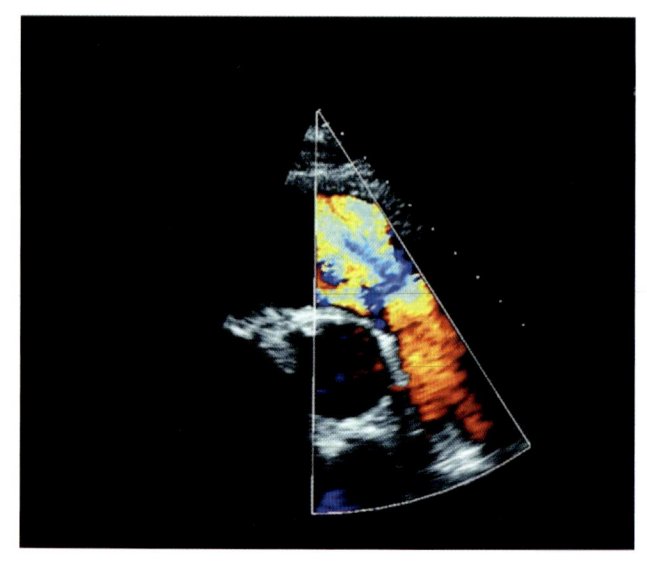

Figure 26.23

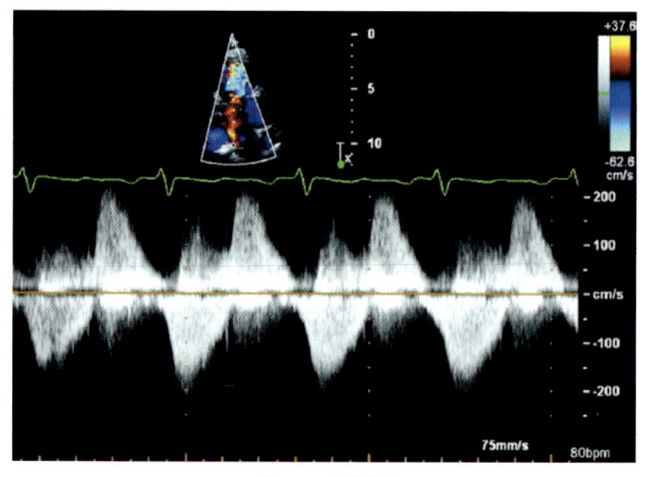

Figure 26.24

24. A patient with a history of flushing, diarrhea, and weight loss presents for echocardiographic evaluation. The finding in **Figure 26.25** and in **Videos 26.14** and **26.15** is noted. What is the most likely cause of the finding?
  A. Extra-adrenal catecholamine-secreting paraganglioma (extra-adrenal pheochromocytoma).
  B. Thrombus.
  C. Metastatic carcinoid tumor.
  D. Coronary artery aneurysm.
  E. None of the above.

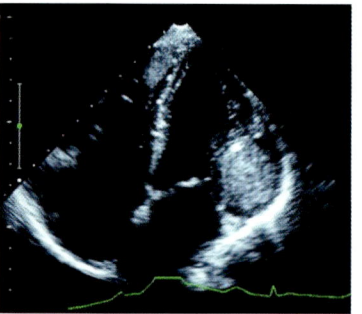

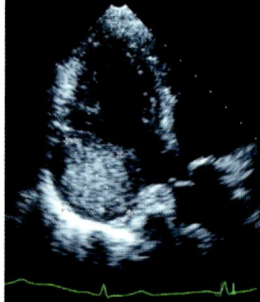

Figure 26.25

25. The LV M-mode, mitral inflow pulsed-wave (PW) Doppler, mitral annulus tissue Doppler, and hepatic vein Doppler in **Figures 26.26-26.29** were obtained in a 56-year-old man with prior history of non-Hodgkin disease and radiation therapy. What radiation-associated complication is present?
  A. Pericardial effusion.
  B. Constrictive pericarditis.
  C. LV hypertrophy.
  D. Restrictive cardiomyopathy.
  E. None of the above.

Figure 26.26. M-mode of the left ventricle with respirometer.

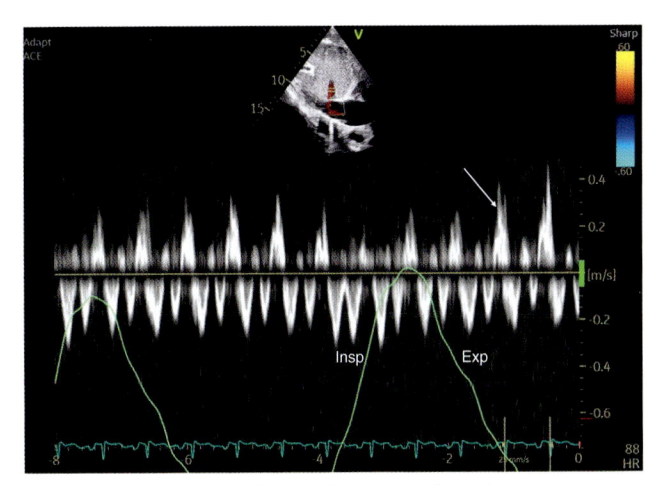

Figure 26.29. Hepatic vein pulsed wave Doppler with respirometer. Arrow points to expiratory diastolic reversal.

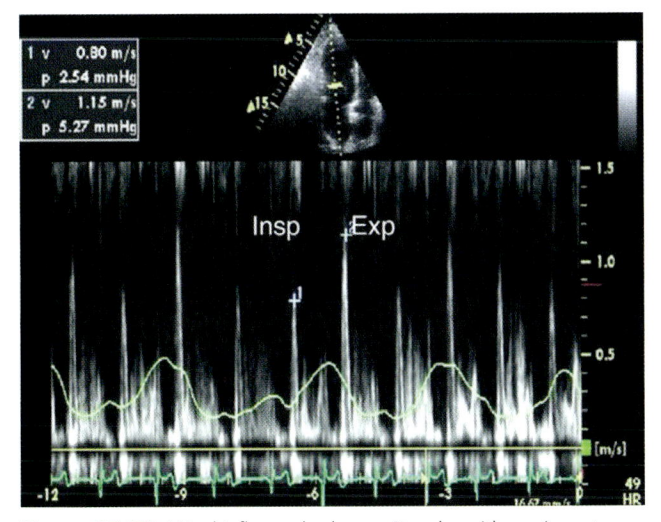

Figure 26.27. Mitral inflow pulsed-wave Doppler with respirometer.

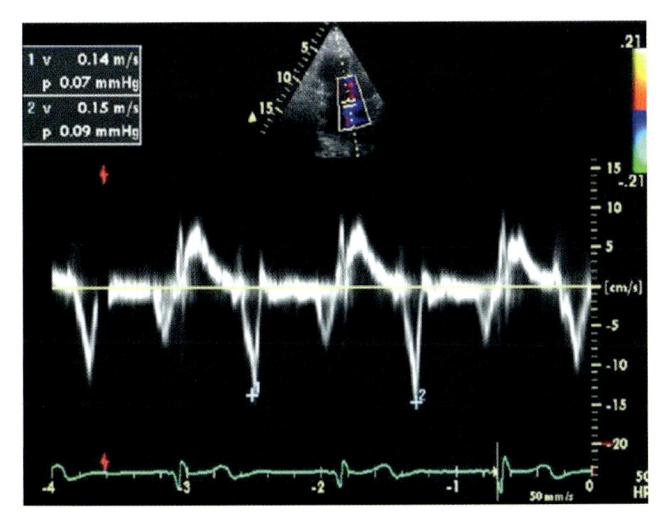

Figure 26.28. Mitral medial annulus tissue Doppler.

CASE 1

A 54-year-old man presents with progressive dyspnea. Physical examination is consistent with congestive heart failure and also reveals an apical III/VI holosystolic murmur. ECG demonstrates sinus tachycardia and no other abnormalities. Echocardiography is performed without and with the aid of contrast ▶ Video 26.16 and ▶ Video 26.17 of the 4-chamber view without and with contrast and Figure 26.30 of the mitral inflow PW Doppler.

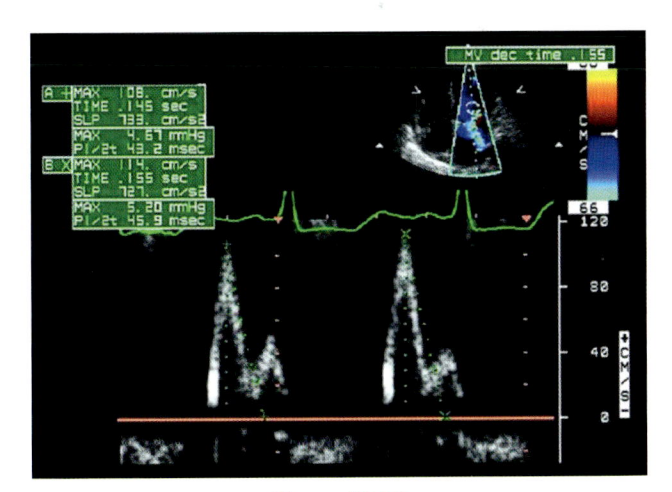

Figure 26.30

26. What is the most likely diagnosis of the patient in **Case 1**?
    A. Apical hypertrophic cardiomyopathy.
    B. Gaucher disease.
    C. Fabry disease.
    D. Eosinophilic endomyocardial disease.
    E. None of the above.

27. Which of the following is typically associated with the condition of the patient in **Case 1**?
   A. Aortic regurgitation.
   B. Isolated LV involvement.
   C. LVOT obstruction.
   D. Restrictive cardiomyopathy.
   E. None of the above.

CASE 2

A 72-year-old woman with chest pain and ST elevation on ECG undergoes coronary angiography that demonstrates minimal coronary atherosclerosis. Left ventriculography is performed and an end-systolic frame is shown in **Figure 26.31**:

The patient is transferred to the ICU where she becomes hypotensive and develops a systolic heart murmur. Urgent echocardiography is performed.

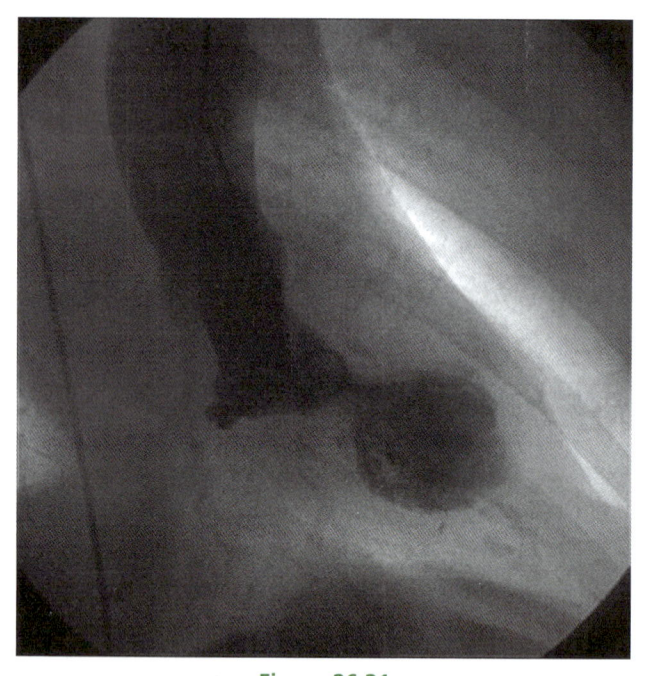

Figure 26.31

28. Based on the echocardiographic images in ▶ **Video 26.18 and** ▶ **Video 26.19**, the cause of hypotension for the patient in **Case 2** is:
   A. Papillary muscle rupture.
   B. LVOT obstruction.
   C. Ventricular septal defect.
   D. Acute severe aortic regurgitation.
   E. None of the above.

29. What is the most appropriate course of action for the patient in **Case 2**?
   A. Dobutamine.
   B. Phenylephrine, cautious beta-blockade, and fluid administration.
   C. Urgent surgery for papillary muscle repair.
   D. Percutaneous closure with an Amplatzer occluder device.
   E. None of the above.

CASE 3

A 68-year-old man who is an ex-competitive cyclist presents with gradually progressive dyspnea and lightheadedness. ECG demonstrates small Q waves in the inferior leads and normal voltages. Initial laboratory evaluations, including blood count and serum chemistries, are normal. 2D echocardiography is performed (▶ **Video 26.20** *and* ▶ **Video 26.21**), *as well as transmitral pulsed-wave and mitral annular tissue Doppler are performed (***Figure 26.32** *and* **Figure 26.33***).*

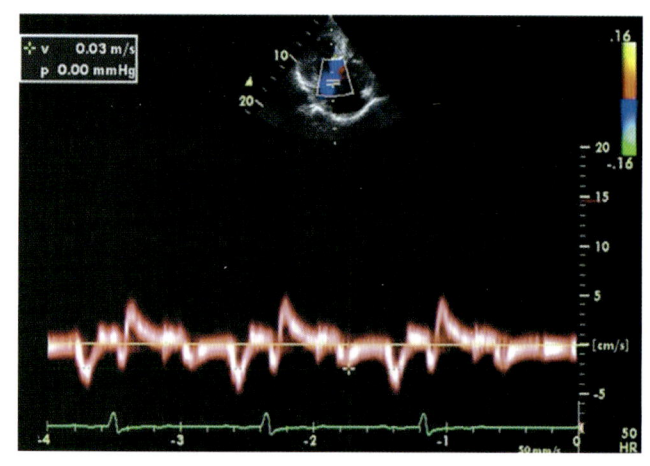

Figure 26.32. Mitral medial annulus tissue Doppler.

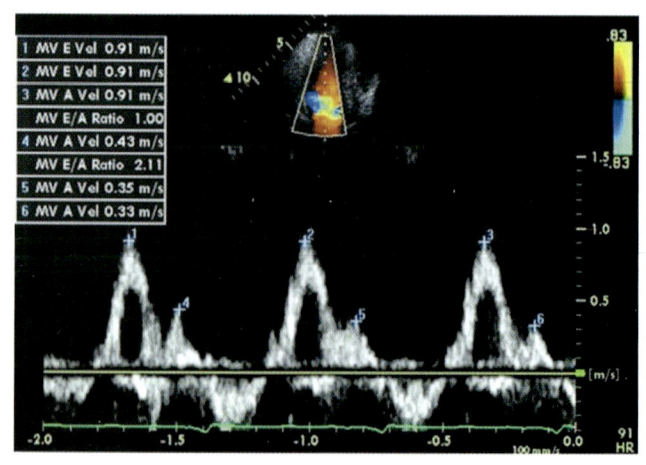

Figure 26.33. Mitral inflow pulsed-wave Doppler.

Chapter 26 Systemic Disease / 561

30. What is the most likely diagnosis for the patient in **Case 3**?
    A. Cardiac amyloidosis.
    B. Hypertrophic cardiomyopathy.
    C. Athlete's heart.
    D. Hypertensive heart disease.
    E. Hemochromatosis.

31. Which of the following is most helpful in distinguishing this diagnosis from other causes of increased LV wall thickness for the patient from **Case 3**?
    A. Restrictive filling physiology.
    B. Systolic anterior motion of the mitral apparatus.
    C. Normal e' velocity.
    D. Inverse relationship between LV mass and ECG voltage.
    E. None of the above.

CASE 4

A 46-year-old woman presents to her physician with lightheadedness and presyncope for 2 days with a background of increasing shortness of breath with exertion for 1 month. The examination is notable for jugular venous distention, soft heart sounds, and bilateral non-pitting pedal edema. The ECG demonstrates sinus bradycardia and low-voltage QRS complexes.

An echocardiogram is obtained and the pertinent 2D images are shown in ▶ Video 26.22, ▶ Video 26.23, and ▶ Video 26.24. The mitral annular e' velocity is 8 cm/s.

32. The most likely explanation for the constellation of findings in the patient from **Case 4** is:
    A. Breast cancer.
    B. Cardiac amyloid.
    C. Hypothyroidism.
    D. Renal failure.
    E. Systemic lupus erythematosus (SLE).

33. The next best course of action for the patient in **Case 4** is:
    A. Observation until a specific etiology is identified and treat the underlying disorder.
    B. Nonsteroidal anti-inflammatories.
    C. High-dose oral steroids.
    D. Echocardiography-guided pericardiocentesis.
    E. None of the above.

34. With appropriate therapy, which of the following echocardiographic parameters would most likely decrease for the patient in **Case 4**?
    A. Isovolumic contraction interval.
    B. LVOT time-velocity integral.
    C. Mitral annular diastolic velocity.
    D. Mitral annular systolic velocity.
    E. None of the above.

CASE 5

A 33-year-old woman with systemic lupus erythematosus, negative blood cultures, and a history of recent stroke now presents with a recurrent transient ischemic attack. A transesophageal echocardiogram is performed with an abnormality noted on the aortic valve shown in long-axis and short-axis views. She has no symptoms of heart failure and her left ventricular size and ejection fraction are normal (▶ Video 26.25 and ▶ Video 26.26).

35. What additional test would be of most value in identifying the etiology of the aortic valve abnormality for the patient in **Case 5**?
    A. Erythrocyte sedimentation rate.
    B. Antiphospholipid antibody blood test.
    C. Cardiac MRI.
    D. CT Pet Scan.
    E. None of the above.

36. The best treatment for the condition of the patient in **Case 5** is:
    A. Aspirin.
    B. Novel oral anticoagulant.
    C. Immediate aortic valve replacement.
    D. Warfarin anticoagulation or heparin.
    E. None of the above.

CASE 6

A 25-year-old woman with a history of bilateral adrenalectomy for Cushing syndrome undergoes a transthoracic echocardiogram for palpitations and shortness of breath. The physical examination is unremarkable except for pigmented lip lesions. The lip lesions are shown in **Figure 26.34**, *and representative echocardiographic images are shown in ▶ Video 26.27 and ▶ Video 26.28.*

562 / Clinical Echocardiography Review

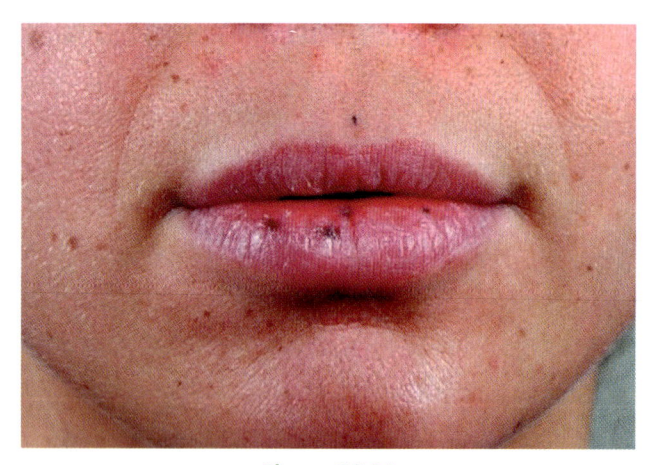

Figure 26.34

37. The most likely diagnosis of the abnormality seen on the echocardiogram (▶ Videos 26.27 and 26.28) for the patient in **Case 6** is:
    A. Angiosarcoma.
    B. Fungal endocarditis.
    C. Myxoma.
    D. Renal cell carcinoma.
    E. Thrombus.

38. The patient undergoes surgical exploration and removal of the mass. The postoperative course is uneventful and the patient is asymptomatic. An echocardiogram is performed 3 months postoperatively; 4-chamber and RV images are demonstrated in ▶ **Video 26.29A,B**. The most likely explanation for the finding shown in the follow-up echocardiogram is:
    A. CAT (calcified amorphous tumor).
    B. Metastatic disease.
    C. Recurrent thrombus.
    D. Synchronous lesion missed at the time of the first surgery.
    E. None of the above.

CASE 7

A 52-year-old woman is referred to the echocardiographic laboratory for further evaluation of symptoms of fatigue, exertional dyspnea, and lower extremity edema.

She had her appendix removed many years ago and was told that there was a tumor in the appendix. No additional information is available.

39. Based on the echocardiographic images in **Figure 26.35**, ▶ **Video 26.30,** and ▶ **Video 26.31** what is the cause of this patient's symptoms from **Case 7**?
    A. Carcinoid heart disease.
    B. Arrhythmogenic RV dysplasia.
    C. Drug-related valve disease.
    D. Ebstein anomaly.
    E. None of the above.

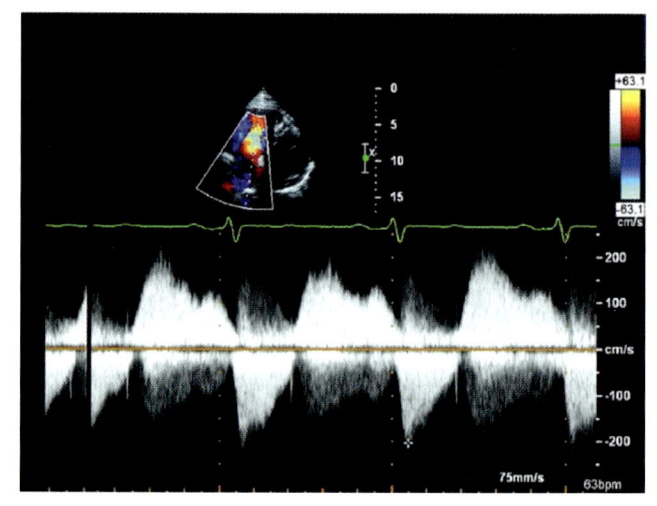

Figure 26.35. Tricuspid valve continous wave Doppler signal.

40. Which of the following tests would help confirm the suspected clinical diagnosis for the patient in **Case 7**?
    A. Serum angiotensin-converting enzyme (ACE) level.
    B. Subcutaneous fat aspirate.
    C. Complete blood cell count with differential white blood cell count and smear.
    D. Urinary 5-hydroxyindole acetic acid
    E. None of the above.

CASE 8

A 35-year-old Caucasian woman with no history of rheumatic fever and a long-standing history of migraine headaches now presents with multiple murmurs and dyspnea. An echocardiogram is performed (▶ Video 26.32).

41. Based on the clinical and echocardiographic features shown in ▶ **Video 26.32** of the patient from **Case 8**, which of the following is the most likely diagnosis?
  A. Ergot-associated valvular disease.
  B. Aortic and mitral valve endocarditis.
  C. Anterior mitral valve leaflet prolapse.
  D. Radiation-induced valvular heart disease.
  E. None of the above.

42. Which of the following is **CORRECT** in regard to the "reverse-dagger" shape of the tricuspid regurgitation velocity shown in the patient from **Case 8** (▶ **Video 26.32**)?
  A. The shape is due to high right atrial pressure.
  B. The shape is characteristic for all tricuspid regurgitation velocities.
  C. The shape is due to rapid rise of right atrial pressure.
  D. The shape is due to pulmonary hypertension.
  E. None of the above.

ANSWERS

1. **Answer: B.** Selenium, thiamine, and carnitine deficiencies are all associated with the development of a reversible cardiomyopathy that responds to the repletion of the deficient vitamin/mineral. Folate and B_{12} deficiency are not usually associated with a cardiomyopathy. Thiamine deficiency or beriberi is usually seen in alcoholic patients with poor nutrition and produces a clinical syndrome that is characterized by high-output cardiac failure. Selenium deficiency, also called Keshan disease, is usually seen in patients undergoing total parenteral nutrition or in patients from areas where food is grown in selenium-deficient soil and results in cardiac enlargement and systolic heart failure. Carnitine deficiency may be primarily due to a genetic defect or secondary because of total parenteral nutrition deficiency or liver or renal disease. Carnitine is required for normal energy metabolism and contractile function in the heart and its deficiency can result in systolic impairment.

    The description of a homeless man with a low body mass index and cardiomyopathy is suspicious for nutritional deficiency as a potential etiology. The Doppler variables shown in this question can be used to calculate the cardiac output and index. Cardiac output = stroke volume (cross-sectional area × left ventricular outflow tract time-velocity integral [LVOT TVI]) × heart rate = 3.14 × (LVOT diameter)²/4 × 36 × 86 = 11.8 L/min. Cardiac index = cardiac output/body surface area = 6.2 L/min/m². Although selenium and carnitine deficiency can also cause cardiomyopathy, only thiamine deficiency causes high cardiac output failure. The correct answer is therefore (B) thiamine deficiency.

2. **Answer: A.** Hereditary hemochromatosis is an autosomal recessive iron-storage disease associated with mutations in the HLA-linked *HFE* gene and is seen almost entirely in people of northern European descent. There is accumulation of iron in the heart, liver, endocrine organs (eg, pancreas and pituitary gland), skin (leading to characteristic bronze hyperpigmentation), and gonads. When cardiac involvement is present, the disease is usually in the advanced stage with multiorgan involvement (diabetes, cirrhosis, arthritis, and impotence). The severity of myocardial dysfunction is proportional to the extent of myocardial iron deposition as intracellular iron is directly cytotoxic to myocytes. Cardiac manifestations include congestive heart failure, arrhythmias, conduction abnormalities, and rarely sudden cardiac arrest.

    Echocardiographic findings usually consist of mild LV dilatation, LV systolic dysfunction, normal or mildly increased wall thickness, relatively normal cardiac valves, and biatrial enlargement. **Figure 26.1** demonstrates a mildly dilated LV with an end-diastolic diameter of 58 mm and an LV end-systolic diameter of 47 mm (LV EF by linear method 34%). The LV diastolic filling pattern is usually restrictive and morphologic two-dimensional echocardiographic features are essentially those of dilated cardiomyopathy. Untreated hereditary hemochromatosis is fatal, but appropriate phlebotomy treatment can improve some complications of iron overload, including cardiomyopathy.

    The correct answer is (A) dilated left ventricle and systolic dysfunction. LV wall thickness may be mildly increased but is frequently normal. In the figure and video shown, the LV wall thickness is normal. Regional wall motion abnormalities are not typically present as would be present in the case of an ischemic cardiomyopathy. Although secondary pulmonary hypertension and RV dysfunction may be present due to restrictive LV physiology, this is not a prominent finding. Pericardial effusion is not typical and is not seen in the figure or video. The diagnosis of hemochromatosis is now often made

564 / Clinical Echocardiography Review

by cardiac magnetic resonance imaging utilizing T2 relaxation time.

3. **Answer: D.** This patient presents with newly diagnosed cardiomyopathy with increased wall thickness and conduction abnormality in the setting of chronic hydroxychloroquine therapy without regular monitoring. The most likely diagnosis is hydroxychloroquine cardiotoxicity, a rare but severe adverse effect of chronic hydroxychloroquine therapy. Typical manifestations include restrictive or hypertrophic cardiomyopathy with diastolic dysfunction and biatrial enlargement. Electrophysiologic abnormalities including atrioventricular blocks or bundle branch blocks are also common. Endomyocardial biopsy is the gold standard diagnostic methodology and prognosis is highly variable.

   Pulmonary arterial hypertension would primarily manifest with right ventricular enlargement and dysfunction. She has no noted history of alcohol misuse or echocardiographic evidence of dilated cardiomyopathy. Systemic lupus erythematosus has many cardiac manifestations, but most commonly causes pericarditis or pericardial effusion (not present on **Figure 26.2**), myocarditis, coronary arteritis, marantic endocarditis, or conduction disease.

4. **Answer: C.** This patient most likely has hyperthyroidism with secondary tachycardia-induced cardiomyopathy (T-CMP). T-CMP is a cardiomyopathy associated primarily with prolonged supraventricular arrhythmias or frequent ectopic beats. It is typically reversible with correction of the underlying tachycardia.

   Evaluation of T-CMP using echocardiography usually reveals dilated cardiomyopathy. Differentiation from idiopathic dilated cardiomyopathy can be challenging in the absence of well-documented chronic tachycardia, but echocardiographically, LV dimension and mass index are typically lower in T-CMP with more frequent post-extra systolic potentiation of LV wall motion.

   T-CMP characteristically features preserved LV wall thickness and absence of hypertrophy. The patient's clinical history is less consistent with symptomatic aortic stenosis or ischemic cardiomyopathy. Shown in ▶ **Video 26.33** are apical 4 and 2 chamber views demonstrating the dilated cardiomyopathy. **Figure 26.36** demonstrates the chest X-ray before treatment with a dilated cardiac silhouette (**Figure 26.36A**, left) which normalized 6 months after treatment (**Figure 26.36B**, right).

5. **Answer: C.** In this patient, the E/e' ratio is 37, which is consistent with marked elevation in LV filling pressures. This observation points to either anthracycline cardiotoxicity or radiation-induced myocardial disease since both conditions can be associated with severe diastolic dysfunction. Manifestations of radiation-induced heart disease usually occur years after therapy. Thus, the most likely explanation for these findings is early doxorubicin toxicity. In view of the severe diastolic dysfunction, a cardiac explanation for this patient's symptoms is most likely. The mitral annular velocity should not be affected by anemia per se, although anemia in addition to diastolic dysfunction in this patient is a possibility. Anemia causes the mitral inflow velocity to increase secondary to a generalized high-flow state.

   Doxorubicin is an anthracycline, and the incidence of cardiotoxicity is related to the cumulative dose administered. The risk is increased in patients with underlying heart disease, when anthracyclines are used concurrently with other cardiotoxic agents or radiation and in patients undergoing subsequent hematopoietic cell transplantation. Cardiotoxicity may occur early (usually around 3 months after

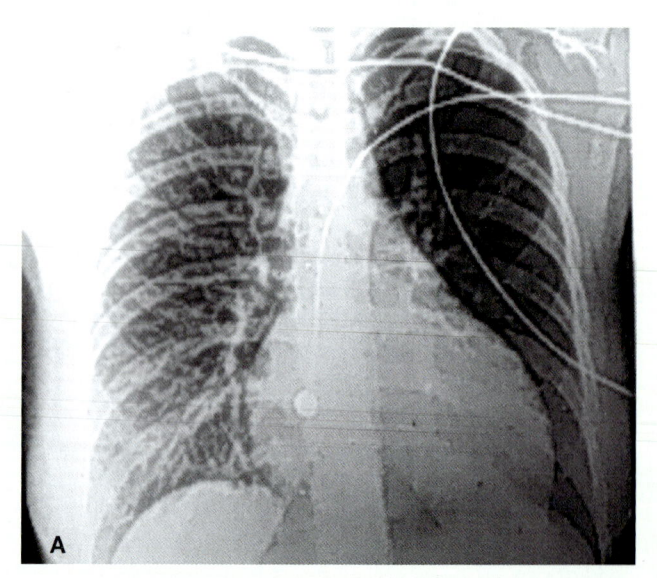

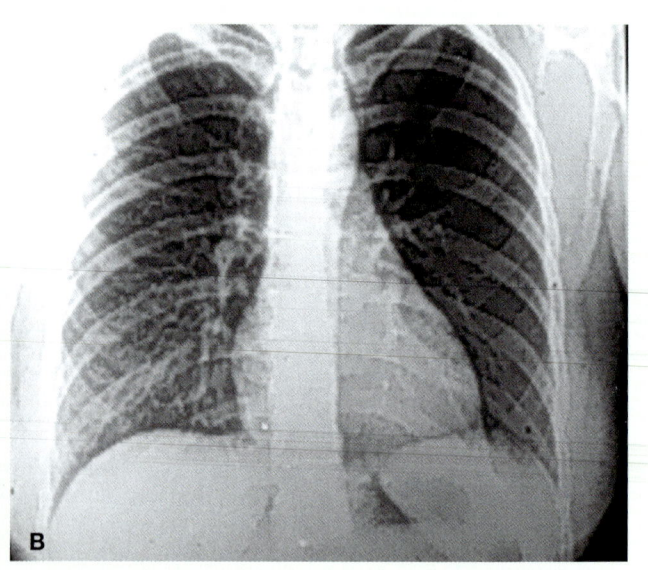

Figure 26.36

treatment) or may occur late (sometimes decades after treatment is completed) presenting as a non-ischemic dilated cardiomyopathy.

6. **Answer: B.** Friedreich ataxia, an autosomal recessive degenerative disorder, is the most common hereditary ataxia and manifests clinically with neurologic dysfunction (ataxia, cerebellar dysarthria, and areflexia), cardiomyopathy, and diabetes mellitus. Echocardiographic abnormalities are common, reported in 86% of patients, and are useful in confirming a diagnosis of Friedreich ataxia since cardiac involvement is not present in other ataxic disorders. **Figure 26.3** reveals concentric left ventricular cardiomyopathy, which is the most common echocardiographic manifestation of Friedreich ataxia. Other findings include globally decreased LV function, decreased LV end-diastolic diameter, and prominent papillary muscles (shown in ▶ **Video 26.2** and ▶ **Video 26.3**).

HIV myocarditis or cardiomyopathy most often presents with pericardial effusion and diastolic dysfunction, or more rarely dilated cardiomyopathy and systolic dysfunction in advanced disease. Echocardiographic findings of Friedreich ataxia occasionally mimic hypertrophic cardiomyopathy, but the absence of systolic anterior motion of the mitral valve, dynamic LV outflow tract obstruction, and careful clinical correlation with presenting neurologic symptoms allow for accurate diagnosis. While arrhythmogenic right ventricular cardiomyopathy (ARVC) can involve the left ventricle, it would not cause the presenting neurologic symptoms. Left ventricular abnormalities in ARVC may be fully evaluated by cardiac CT or magnetic resonance imaging techniques.

7. **Answer: E.** This patient has many of the typical cardiac manifestations of chronic renal failure. These include significant diastolic dysfunction (manifested by left atrial enlargement and restrictive filling Doppler hemodynamics), generalized valve thickening, and pericardial effusion, which are usually of no hemodynamic significance if unrelated to acute uremic pericarditis. Calcification of the valves results in both regurgitant and stenotic lesions. Mitral annular calcification is also common and is caused by derangements in calcium and phosphorous metabolism (see **Tables 26.1** and **26.2**). Other findings that may be seen include regional wall motion abnormalities secondary to underlying coronary artery disease. Concentric wall thickening is often seen in patients with chronic renal failure and is usually secondary to long-standing hypertension; however, another important complication of long-standing renal failure is amyloidosis. An important distinguishing feature between wall thickening secondary to hypertension versus amyloid is the low or inappropriately normal voltage seen on the ECG in amyloid. Thus, it is important to review the ECG when concentric wall thickening is appreciated in this clinical setting. However, the absence of ECG low voltage does not exclude cardiac amyloidosis, nor is this finding diagnostic of amyloidosis. If there is high clinical suspicion for amyloidosis, the next most appropriate step after appropriate blood and urine testing would be either cardiac MRI or ^{99m}Tc-pyrophosphate scintigraphy.

Table 26.1. Echocardiographically Detected Aortic Valve Abnormalities Associated With Systemic Disease

Cusp Abnormality
Thickening
Postinflammatory
Rheumatic heart disease
SLE
Antiphospholipid syndrome
Rheumatoid arthritis
Seronegative spondyloarthropathy
Radiation
Infiltrative
Amyloid
Mucopolysaccharidosis[a]
Sarcoid
Calcification
Renal disease
Hyperparathyroidism
Other
Carcinoid
Drug-induced
Discrete mass
Vegetation
Infective endocarditis
Noninfective endocarditis (Libman-Sacks)
Antiphospholipid syndrome
SLE
Sjögren syndrome
ANCA-associated vasculitis
Aortic Valve Abnormalities Associated with Ascending Aortic Disorders
Inherited connective tissue disorders
Marfan
Loeys Dietz
Ehlers Danlos
Osteogenesis imperfecta
Pseudoxanthoma elasticum
Inflammatory
Giant cell arteritis
Takayasu
Behçet
Hypertension

ANCA, anti-neutrophil cytoplasmic antibody; SLE, systemic lupus erythematosus.
[a]Mitral more commonly affected than aortic.

Table 26.2. Echocardiographically Detected Mitral Valve Abnormalities Associated With Systemic Disease

Leaflet Abnormality

Thickening
  Postinflammatory
    Rheumatic heart disease
    Systemic lupus erythematosus
    Antiphospholipid antibody syndrome
    Rheumatoid arthritis
    ANCA-associated vasculitis
  Infiltrative
    Amyloid
  Other
    Carcinoid
    Drug-induced
    Radiation

Discrete mass
  Vegetation
    Infective endocarditis
    Noninfective endocarditis (Libman-Sacks)
    Systemic lupus erythematosus
    Antiphospholipid antibody syndrome
    ANCA-associated vasculitis
    Sjögren syndrome
    Malignancy

Mitral valve prolapse
  Inherited disorders
    Marfan
    Loeys Dietz
    Ehlers Danlos
    Osteogenesis imperfecta
    Pseudoxanthoma elasticum
    Fabry disease

Mitral Annulus

Calcification
  Renal failure

Subvalvular Apparatus

Postinflammatory
  Rheumatic heart disease

Other
  Carcinoid
  Drug-induced
  Radiation

Endocardium

Infiltrative
  Sarcoid
  Hypereosinophilia
  Amyloid
  Inflammatory
  Myocarditis

ANCA, anti-neutrophil cytoplasmic antibody.

8. **Answer: A.** Granulomatosis with polyangiitis is a systemic necrotizing small vessel vasculitis characterized by granulomatous lesions with predilection for pulmonary and renal involvement. Recent research has identified a high frequency of echocardiographic abnormalities that appear related to granulomatosis with polyangiitis and are associated with increased mortality even though cardiac involvement is often clinically silent. Regional wall motion abnormalities that are not confined to a typical coronary artery distribution are a typical finding seen in infiltrative disorders, such as granulomatosis with polyangiitis, sarcoidosis, and cardiac amyloid. When present in younger patients with a low cardiovascular risk profile, granulomatosis with polyangiitis and sarcoid should be considered. In patients with granulomatosis having polyangiitis, the granulomatous inflammation may resolve with treatment including resolution of the regional wall motion abnormalities. Although pericardial effusions are common, they are usually small and hemodynamically insignificant. The aortic and mitral valves may be involved but valvular regurgitation is seldom severe (see **Tables 26.1** and **26.2**). Granulomatosis with polyangiitis may manifest as a cardiomyopathy but this is usually an isolated dilated cardiomyopathy.

9. **Answer: A.** Amyloid cardiac disease is caused by extracellular deposition of proteins in the myocardium. Characteristic echocardiographic features of amyloid include LV wall thickening with evidence of diastolic dysfunction. In advanced disease, wall thickening progresses resulting in a restrictive cardiomyopathy with a nondilated or small LV cavity.

    Sarcoidosis is a noncaseating granulomatous disorder. Granulomatous infiltration of the myocardium can cause both systolic and diastolic dysfunction. Cardiac sarcoidosis may present as a dilated cardiomyopathy. Hemochromatosis can lead to a dilated cardiomyopathy characterized by heart failure and conduction disturbances due to excess deposition of iron within the myocardium. Cardiac involvement in hemochromatosis can be diagnosed on the basis of clinical evaluation, specialized laboratory testing, and cardiac imaging. HIV causes dilated cardiomyopathy in approximately 1%–3% of patients with acquired immunodeficiency virus. The causes of cardiac damage include drug toxicity, secondary infection, myocardial damage by HIV, and an autoimmune process induced by HIV or other cardiotropic viruses, such as coxsackie virus, cytomegalovirus, or Epstein-Barr virus. Excessive alcohol consumption can lead to myocardial dysfunction. Alcohol is believed to be toxic to cardiac myocytes via oxygen-free radical damage and abnormal cardiac protein synthesis. Abstinence can lead to a dramatic improvement in cardiac function if the disease is diagnosed early.

10. **Answer: B.** The clinical presentation of this relatively young man with ventricular arrhythmia, heart failure, and bilateral hilar pulmonary infiltrates is concerning for sarcoidosis. Patients with sarcoid cardiac disease may have a known history of sarcoidosis or cardiac involvement may be the first identification of the disease. The characteristic echocardiographic features seen in sarcoid heart disease include LV systolic dysfunction with regional wall motion abnormalities that do not follow a usual coronary artery distribution. Additional findings in sarcoid heart disease include atrioventricular block, ventricular arrhythmias, abnormal wall thickness, and perfusion defects affecting the anteroseptal and apical regions. Also shown in the images is the important finding of a basal inferior wall aneurysm, this finding is not in a typical distribution of prior coronary artery disease-related myocardial infarction and is typical of cardiac sarcoidosis.

LV dysfunction with apical dyskinesis and preserved basal cardiac function suggests stress-induced cardiomyopathy. In this disorder, typically the contractile function of the mid and apical segments of the left ventricle are depressed, and there is compensatory hyperkinesis of the basal walls, producing ballooning of the apex with systole. Stress-induced cardiomyopathy (Takotsubo syndrome) is much more common in women than in men and is frequently, but not always triggered by an acute illness or by emotional and/or physical stress. Normal LV cavity size with increased LV wall thickness and LVOT obstruction suggests hypertrophic cardiomyopathy. Hypertrophic cardiomyopathy has an autosomal-dominant pattern of inheritance, characterized by hypertrophy of the left ventricle, with variable clinical manifestations and morphologic and hemodynamic abnormalities. In a subset of patients, the site and extent of cardiac hypertrophy results in obstruction to LV outflow. Less commonly, LV outflow obstruction can be seen with infiltrative cardiomyopathy such as amyloid. Right atrial and ventricular enlargement with reduced systolic function as an isolated finding would be uncommon in patients with sarcoidosis. This finding would suggest a left-to-right shunt at the atrial or pulmonary vein level. Alternatively, this could be seen in patients with arrhythmogenic RV cardiomyopathy.

11. **Answer: B.** This patient presents with a clinical picture and echocardiographic features of cardiac amyloidosis. The patients echocardiogram demonstrates increased LV wall thickness (concentric) as shown in ▶ **Video 26.6,** ▶ **Video 26.7,** ▶ **Video 26.8,** and ▶ **Video 26.9**. His EKG demonstrates relatively low voltage in the limb leads for the degree of increased wall thickness (**Figure 26.37**) and although this is consistent with and may be an important reason to pursue additional testing, it is not always present in cardiac amyloidosis. Amyloidosis involves the extracellular deposit of insoluble amyloid proteins into multiple organs including the kidney, heart, liver, gastrointestinal tract, and tongue. If the heart is involved, this leads initially to diastolic heart failure but may progress to systolic heart failure later in the course. There is valvular thickening, increased thickening of the atrial septum, and a typical speckled appearance on echocardiography although this finding is less specific in the era of harmonic imaging and with newer ultrasound platforms with increased resolution/frame rate. Importantly, there is regional variability in LV systolic function, which can be best identified with global longitudinal strain. Global longitudinal strain is often reduced but typically there is "apical sparing" noted in cardiac amyloidosis, which can be visualized as a "cherry on top" appearance on Bullseye imaging. ▶ **Video 26.6** and ▶ **Video 26.7** demonstrates increased LV wall thickness with preserved shortening fraction, a small pericardial effusion, a left pleural effusion, and thickening of the valves that are typically seen in patients with amyloidosis who present with an elevated troponin or heart failure. ▶ **Video 26.8** and ▶ **Video 26.9** confirm those findings but also better demonstrate the valve thickening, apical sparing nature of this disease, and the increased thickness of the atrial septum. **Figure 26.38** summarizes the regional pattern variation in global LV longitudinal strain due to increased wall thickness from various etiologies.

12. **Answer: B.** Chest radiation can cause late cardiovascular disease, which can manifest as dyspnea. Possible causes include conduction system disease, coronary artery disease, pericardial constriction, and myocardial disease, which manifest as restrictive cardiomyopathy or endocardial disease. The endocardial disease causes valve thickening, typically affecting the aortic-mitral intervalvular fibrosa

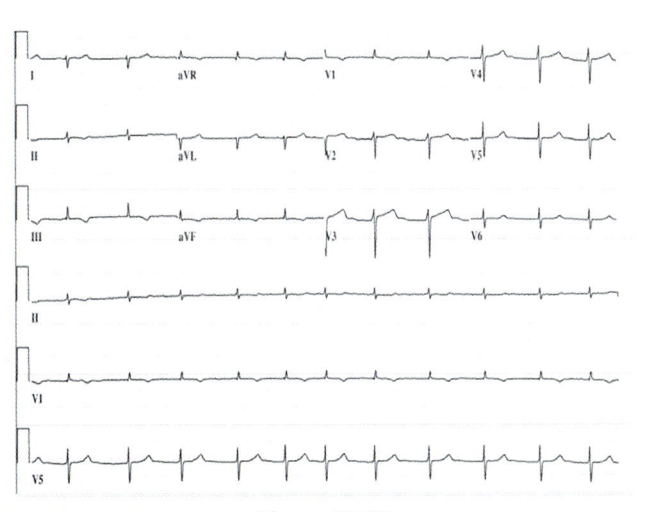

Figure 26.37

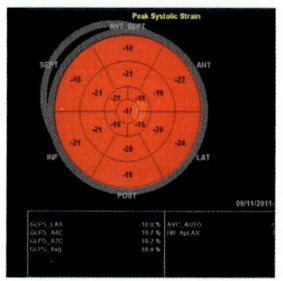

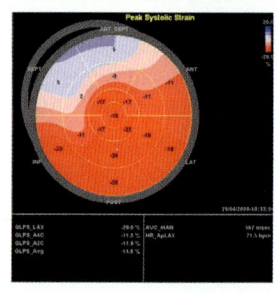

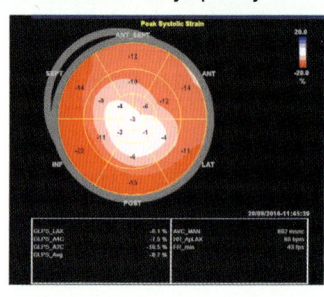

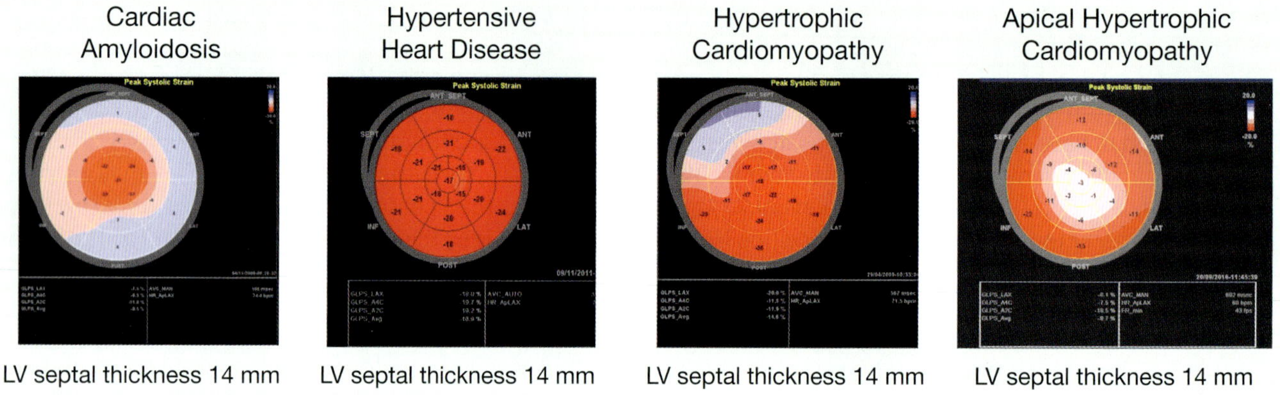

Cardiac Amyloidosis	Hypertensive Heart Disease	Hypertrophic Cardiomyopathy	Apical Hypertrophic Cardiomyopathy
LV septal thickness 14 mm	LV septal thickness 14 mm	LV septal thickness 14 mm	LV septal thickness 14 mm

Figure 26.38

with calcification and associated valve dysfunction (see **Figure 26.39** and **Tables 26.1** and **26.2**). The right-sided valves are less commonly affected. A comprehensive echo-Doppler examination is an excellent test to determine whether there is a structural cardiac cause of dyspnea in a patient with prior radiation.

LV hypertrophy would not be expected after cardiac radiation. This finding would suggest systemic hypertension or outflow tract obstruction. Ascending aortic dilatation is not noted in patients with radiation-induced heart disease. Pericardial effusion can occur during chest radiation or early after completion but would not be expected as a late complication of chest irradiation.

13. **Answer: B.** This young male patient presents with new cellular immunodeficiency and a new opportunistic infection, greatly raising a concern for HIV infection and acquired immunodeficiency syndrome (AIDS). A variety of cardiac abnormalities have been associated with HIV infection, including pericardial effusion, dilated cardiomyopathy, primary pulmonary hypertension, and Kaposi sarcoma of the heart. The cardiac manifestations of HIV disease have been greatly altered by the introduction of highly active antiretroviral therapy (ART). As overall survival has improved and HIV has become a chronic infection, coronary artery disease has become the most important cardiovascular complication and attention has focused on aggressive risk factor modification.

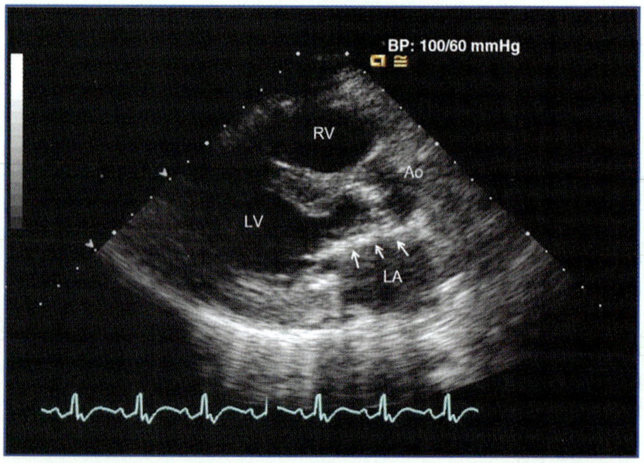

The most common clinical manifestation of HIV disease in the pre-ART era was pericardial effusion, seen in approximately 20% to 40% of patients. This remains the case in the developing world and in resource-limited settings where access to ART is limited. Pericardial effusions are typically asymptomatic but serve as a marker of advanced disease and worse prognosis. It is much less common in the ART era.

Kaposi sarcoma involving the heart is very rare and usually diagnosed as an incidental finding at autopsy. When present, it is typically found in subepicardial adipose tissue. Typical acute pericarditis could present with pericardial effusion but would not explain this patient's profound immunosuppression and opportunistic infection. Primary pulmonary hypertension has been reported in HIV but is a rare finding seen in less than 0.5% of AIDS patients and would not explain his pericardial effusion.

14. **Answer: C.** Coronary vasospasm and atherosclerotic coronary artery disease are unlikely to cause the distribution of regional wall motion abnormalities seen in this patient. Takotsubo cardiomyopathy, subarachnoid hemorrhage, and pheochromocytoma result in catecholamine-mediated severe subendocardial myocardial ischemia that can occur in the absence of epicardial coronary artery disease. The clue to the diagnosis in this patient is the prior history of labile hypertension and acute chest pain episode associated with severe headache occurring shortly after abdominal surgery. Pheochromocytoma typically presents with paroxysms of severe hypertension with associated headache, diaphoresis, and chest pain sometimes precipitated by abdominal surgery or even tumor palpation. Cardiac manifestations of pheochromocytoma include hypertensive

Figure 26.39. Parasternal long-axis view demonstrating anterior mitral annular and aortic-mitral intervalvular fibrosa calcification. AO, Aorta; LV, left ventricle; RV, right ventricle; LA, left atrium.

heart disease, reversible regional wall motion abnormalities, and a dilated cardiomyopathy. The diagnosis is confirmed by measuring plasma and urinary catecholamines or 24-hour urine metanephrines as well as computed tomography identification of the adrenal tumor. Rarely, an extra-adrenal cardiac pheochromocytoma may present as a cardiac mass characteristically located in the atrioventricular groove. Cushing syndrome is due to excess glucocorticoid. The cardiac manifestations include moderate chronic diastolic hypertension rather than paroxysms of systolic hypertension and acute symptoms around the time of stress.

15. **Answer: D.** Rheumatoid arthritis may involve the heart in many ways. Coronary artery disease as well as diastolic heart failure is commonly seen in patients with rheumatoid arthritis. Antimalarial therapy used in the treatment may result in reversible cardiomyopathy.

    Despite small pericardial effusions being common, acute pericarditis and large pericardial effusions with tamponade are rare. Nevertheless, occult constrictive pericarditis may occur and if unrecognized, can result in significant morbidity and mortality. Rheumatic nodules may involve all cardiac structures including valves but infrequently result in significant valve dysfunction. Mitral valve prolapse is not generally associated with rheumatoid arthritis. Thickened, fixed, and retracted tricuspid valve leaflets with tricuspid regurgitation would be expected in patients with carcinoid and drug-related valve disease (see **Tables 26.1** and **26.2**).

16. **Answer: B.** The echocardiogram demonstrates significant apical and midventricular akinesis (**Figure 26.11** and **Figure 26.12**). The patient is a postmenopausal woman with a presentation that simulates acute myocardial infarction. These features are all consistent with Takotsubo cardiomyopathy.

    Takotsubo cardiomyopathy (also known as stress cardiomyopathy or apical ballooning syndrome) is a reversible cardiomyopathy triggered by profound psychological or physical stress and has a clinical presentation that is similar to acute myocardial infarction. Most patients are postmenopausal women. Proposed criteria for the diagnosis of Takotsubo cardiomyopathy require all four of the following characteristics: (1) electrocardiographic abnormalities (usually ST elevations followed by T wave inversion), (2) transient apical, mid-wall, or basal wall motion abnormalities, (3) absence of obstructive coronary artery disease or acute plaque rupture, and (4) absence of other conditions, such as significant head trauma, intracranial hemorrhage, pheochromocytoma, or another etiology of myocardial dysfunction. Catecholamine-induced microvascular dysfunction is currently postulated as a likely mechanism. According to recent reports, RV apical dysfunction may be present in 30% to 40% of cases. Improvement/resolution of LV systolic dysfunction normally occurs between 1 and 4 weeks as demonstrated in ▶ **Video 26.34**. Dynamic LVOT obstruction, which is due to basal hyperkinesis, is a well-described complication of Takotsubo cardiomyopathy and may result in hypotension. Persistent LV systolic dysfunction is not an expected complication in Takotsubo cardiomyopathy. Although cardiac troponin T is always elevated, the elevation is usually mild and disproportionate to the degree of cardiac compromise. Increased urinary 5-hydroxyindole acetic acid is seen in carcinoid patients.

    It is important to remember that Takotsubo cardiomyopathy is a diagnosis of exclusion and can only be diagnosed once obstructive coronary disease and acute plaque rupture have been excluded. Similar wall motion abnormalities can also result from myocardial infarction due to the occlusion of a large wraparound left anterior descending artery. Hence, coronary angiography is required for the diagnosis even in the setting of typical regional wall motion abnormalities.

17. **Answer: B.** The two-dimensional echocardiographic findings of a pericardial effusion and an enlarged right ventricle with a D-shaped LV cavity due to pulmonary hypertension are suspicious for scleroderma. The clinical presentation of a patient who appears younger than her stated age, likely due to taut facial skin, dyspnea, arthralgias, and swelling of the hands and feet is also consistent with a diagnosis of scleroderma. Pulmonary hypertension is present in 8% to 12% of scleroderma patients and even in a higher frequency in patients with CREST syndrome. Pulmonary hypertension accounts for 30% of deaths and screening for pulmonary hypertension and prompt initiation of treatment is recommended.

    RV dysfunction, reduced cardiac index, and pericardial effusion are markers of poor prognosis in PH. Please see **Figure 26.13** (parasternal short-axis view), ▶ **Video 26.35** (parasternal long-axis view), and ▶ **Video 26.36** (parasternal short-axis view) which demonstrate the flattening of the interventricular septum from the right ventricle toward the left ventricle during both systole and diastole, consistent with right ventricular pressure overload. **Figure 26.40** demonstrates the elevated tricuspid regurgitation spectral Doppler velocity consistent with pulmonary hypertension.

    The most common primary cardiac abnormality associated with scleroderma is a pericardial effusion, often small. The myocardium may be involved with fibrosis or sclerosis and systolic and diastolic dysfunction may be present. Systemic and pulmonary hypertension are prominent secondary complications of scleroderma.

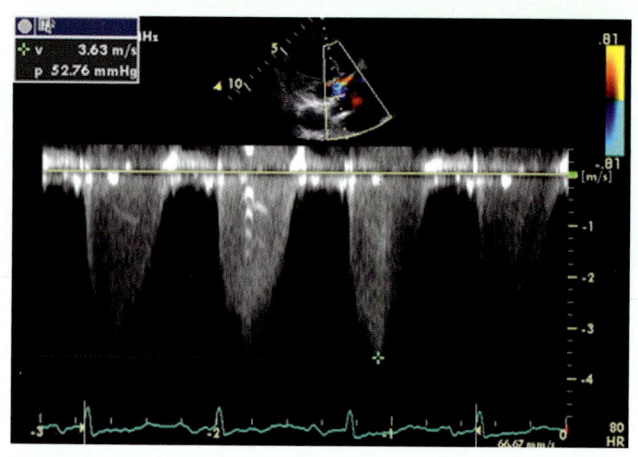

Figure 26.40. Spectral Doppler of tricuspid regurgitation signal.

Cardiac amyloidosis is an infiltrative cardiomyopathy that results in a restrictive disease and is characterized by increased biventricular wall thickness. Hemochromatosis can lead to a dilated cardiomyopathy due to excess deposition of iron within the myocardium. Finally, cardiac manifestations of rheumatoid arthritis include pericarditis and less commonly dilated cardiomyopathy with congestive heart failure.

18. **Answer: C.** The TEE images (**Figure 26.14**, **Video 26.12**, and **Video 26.13**) demonstrate small verrucous valvular lesions on the tips of the mitral valve leaflets. In the clinical setting of a young woman with arthralgias, low-grade fever, skin rash, photosensitivity, elevated white blood cell count, pleural effusion, and no history of illicit drug use, the most likely diagnosis is SLE with Libman-Sacks endocarditis.

Libman-Sacks endocarditis (also known as nonbacterial thrombotic endocarditis or marantic endocarditis) refers to a characteristic verrucous valvular lesion that usually affects the mitral valve in patients with SLE. The lesion can present on the atrial or ventricular aspects of the mitral leaflets and may extend to the chordal and papillary structures. The aortic valve is the second most affected valve, but whether the ventricular or vessel sides of the aortic leaflets are more commonly affected is not yet well-defined. Libman-Sacks lesions rarely lead to significant valve dysfunction but carry a considerable risk of embolization (14%-91%).

Ergot-alkaloid use is associated with valvulopathy and valvular regurgitation usually affecting the aortic and mitral valves. Echocardiographic features of infective endocarditis are an oscillating intracardiac mass on a valve or other cardiac structure, abscesses, and dehiscence of a prosthetic valve. The vegetations are typically on the "upstream" surface of the regurgitant jet of the affected valve, that is, on the atrial aspect of atrioventricular valves and on the ventricular aspect of the aortic valve. Rheumatic mitral valve disease is associated with thickened and calcified mitral leaflets and subvalvular apparatus, "hockey-stick" deformity of the anterior leaflet and relative immobility of the posterior leaflet, and associated stenosis or regurgitation (see **Tables 26.1** and **26.2**).

19. **Answer: C.** The clue to the correct diagnosis in this case lies in the dermatologic findings. The skin lesions are angiokeratomas, which occur commonly in the groin, hip, and periumbilical areas. They are characteristically seen in patients with Fabry disease. Fabry disease is a rare X-linked inborn error of the glycosphingolipid metabolic pathway that results in the accumulation of globotriaosylceramide in several organs, including the skin, kidney, nervous system, cornea, and the heart, leading to the clinical manifestations that usually begin in childhood or adolescence. The prominent features include severe neuropathic pain, telangiectasias and angiokeratomas, heat and exercise intolerance, and gastrointestinal symptoms, such as abdominal pain and diarrhea. Renal manifestations include proteinuria and renal failure. Cardiac involvement is usually manifested by concentric LV hypertrophy, myocardial dysfunction, aortic and mitral valve abnormalities (see **Tables 26.1** and **26.2**), and conduction abnormalities. In some patients, LV hypertrophy may be the only overt manifestation of the disease. Fabry disease may be present in about 1% of patients suspected to have hypertrophic cardiomyopathy. Thus, in patients presenting with unexplained LV hypertrophy, Fabry disease should be included in the differential diagnosis. The diagnosis is usually confirmed by demonstrating decreased leukocyte or plasma alpha-Gal A activity but can also be made histologically on endomyocardial biopsy.

Acromegaly, cardiac amyloid, and Fabry disease can all result in increased LV wall thickness, and rarely asymmetric wall involvement that can mimic hypertrophic cardiomyopathy. Moreover, dynamic LVOT obstruction, typically seen in hypertrophic obstructive cardiomyopathy with systolic anterior motion of the anterior mitral leaflet may be present. In cardiac amyloid, the ECG voltage would be expected to be normal or even reduced and is thus an unlikely diagnosis in this case. This case illustrates the importance of integrating the clinical and echocardiographic findings to make an accurate diagnosis. A binary appearance of the myocardium on echocardiography with a bright endocardium and epicardium and less bright mid-myocardium has been described in Fabry disease **Video 26.37**.

20. **Answer: A.** The skin lesion is an angiofibroma, which is a typical skin lesion seen in patients with tuberous sclerosis. Tuberous sclerosis is an inherited autosomal-dominant neurocutaneous disorder that is characterized by multiorgan system involvement, including multiple benign hamartomas of the brain,

eyes, heart, lung, liver, kidney, as well as skin. The diagnosis of tuberous sclerosis is made clinically. The characteristic cardiac feature of tuberous sclerosis is a rhabdomyoma, the most frequent cardiac neoplasm of childhood representing 60% of pediatric cardiac tumors. Rhabdomyomas are benign tumors that almost always present as multiple lesions. Although they are often associated with tuberous sclerosis, they can occur as an isolated finding. They typically develop in utero and are often detected on prenatal ultrasound. They occur with equal frequency in both ventricles growing in the ventricular walls or on the atrioventricular valves. They vary in size from a few millimeters to a few centimeters and may be pedunculated often obstructing ventricular inflow or outflow. The morbidity and mortality associated with these tumors reflect the potential for flow abnormalities if they grow to sufficient size to restrict blood flow. Although many are asymptomatic, some present with heart failure, a cardiac murmur, or arrhythmia. A unique and peculiar feature of cardiac rhabdomyomas is that they usually undergo spontaneous regression in the first few years of life. There is no evidence that these tumors undergo malignant transformation, and no treatment is necessary for asymptomatic tumors. Thus, the most appropriate management strategy in this patient is reassurance with follow-up echocardiography in 1 year as well as family screening for affected siblings.

21. **Answer: B.** This young man has Marfan syndrome. The characteristic pear-shaped dilatation of the aortic root (aortic sinuses) is characteristic and a major diagnostic criterion of this autosomal-dominant inherited condition usually resulting from a fibrillin 1 gene mutation (see **Table 26.1**). An additional major Ghent diagnostic criterion is the history of lens dislocation. Since there is an increased risk of aortic dissection or rupture when the aortic caliber reaches a dimension of 50 mm, elective aortic root replacement is indicated as first-line therapy.

    A TEE is not indicated at this time since the patient is asymptomatic and there is no suspicion of a dissection flap on the image shown. Although beta-blockers or angiotensin receptor blockers are both used in patients with Marfan syndrome to delay the progression of aortic root dilatation, this patient should preferentially undergo aortic surgery in the near future due to the size of the aorta and family history of sudden death, presumed to be related to aortic dissection.

22. **Answer: B.** Takayasu arteritis is a chronic vasculitis of unknown etiology affecting primarily the aorta and its primary branches. **Figure 26.19** and **Figure 26.20** document aortic regurgitation. **Figure 26.21** demonstrates pulsed-wave Doppler of the abdominal aorta documenting diastolic flow reversals consistent with severe aortic regurgitation. The inflammation may be localized or may involve the entire vessel. The initial vascular lesions frequently occur in the middle or proximal subclavian artery. As the disease progresses, the carotids, vertebrals, brachiocephalic, right middle or proximal subclavian artery, and aorta may also be affected. The abdominal aorta and pulmonary arteries are involved in approximately 50% of patients. The inflammatory process causes thickening of the walls of the affected arteries or involved segment of the aorta. The proximal aorta may become dilated secondary to inflammatory injury. Aortic valve regurgitation may be present and is usually caused by the dilatation of the proximal ascending aorta (see **Table 26.1**).

    Marfan syndrome is associated with aortic root enlargement, with or without aortic regurgitation, but is not associated with carotid, subclavian, or abdominal bruits and loss of pulses in the absence of dissection. Isolated mid ascending aortic enlargement is not typically seen in patients with Marfan disease. Abnormal acute-phase reactants would also not be expected. Familial thoracic aortic aneurysmal disease is an aneurysmal disorder that occurs in the absence of syndromic features. It is inherited in an autosomal-dominant manner with decreased penetrance and variable expression. Aneurysms can affect the ascending or descending thoracic or abdominal aorta and also the intracranial vascular system. Ankylosing spondylitis is a chronic inflammatory disease of the axial skeleton manifested by back pain and progressive stiffness of the spine. Asymptomatic cardiovascular disease secondary to ankylosing spondylitis is not uncommon, especially aortic regurgitation. This is caused by scar tissues in the aortic valve cusps and neighboring aorta.

23. **Answer: A.** The echocardiographic images of the RV outflow tract demonstrate thickening of the pulmonary valve cusps (**Figure 26.22**), and the color-flow images demonstrate a broad-based regurgitant jet of pulmonary regurgitation (**Figure 26.23**). The continuous-wave Doppler signal (**Figure 26.24**) is dense and demonstrates a diastolic signal that decelerates rapidly to baseline. All of these features are consistent with severe pulmonary valve regurgitation related to carcinoid involvement of the pulmonary valve. The characteristic features of carcinoid heart disease include thickening and reduced mobility of the tricuspid valve leaflets with associated tricuspid valve regurgitation. Pulmonary valve involvement occurs in two-thirds of patients and is shown in the RV outflow tract parasternal view in ▶ **Video 26.38**. The pulmonary valve leaflets are thickened and retracted with limited mobility leading to complete failure of coaptation best seen in the parasternal short-axis view of the pulmonary valve shown in ▶ **Video 26.39**. Left-sided valve

disease is recognized in about 10% of patients with carcinoid syndrome and right-sided carcinoid heart disease usually due to the presence of an intracardiac right to left shunt, ovarian carcinoid, or pulmonary carcinoid.

Severe pulmonary valve stenosis is characterized by a high systolic antegrade signal across the pulmonary valve, and systolic doming of the pulmonary valve cusps is usually also noted. Carcinoid heart disease can occasionally cause severe pulmonary valve stenosis, but pulmonary regurgitation is more common. The antegrade signal across the pulmonary valve in this patient is of low velocity (<2 m/s), which is not consistent with severe pulmonary valve stenosis.

Severe pulmonary hypertension is characterized by a low-antegrade systolic continuous-wave Doppler signal across the pulmonary valve. However, in severe pulmonary hypertension, the diastolic Doppler signal is of high velocity. An estimate of the pulmonary artery end-diastolic pressure can be made by measuring an elevated pulmonary regurgitant end-diastolic velocity. Patent ductus arteriosus is a communication between the main pulmonary artery and the descending thoracic aorta, which persists from fetal life. Color-flow Doppler echocardiography will demonstrate continuous flow from the descending thoracic aorta to the pulmonary artery, in the absence of severe pulmonary hypertension. This signal originates in the region of the proximal left pulmonary artery. The continuous-wave Doppler profile will demonstrate a high systolic signal with persistent flow throughout the cardiac cycle in the absence of pulmonary hypertension.

24. **Answer: C.** Metastatic carcinoid to the heart affects less than 5% of patients with metastatic carcinoid disease. This usually occurs in conjunction with carcinoid valve disease, more often right-sided than left-sided (see **Tables 26.1** and **26.2**). The echocardiographic appearance of a metastatic carcinoid tumor is not diagnostic but generally appears as a homogeneous, circumscribed, noninfiltrating mass, which can affect the left or right ventricular myocardium. The history of flushing, diarrhea, and weight loss are consistent with the clinical features of carcinoid syndrome. The mass in **Figure 26.25**, ▶ **Video 26.14**, and ▶ **Video 26.15** is located in the basal lateral intramyocardial wall and measures 3.5 × 4.5 cm.

Extra-adrenal catecholamine-secreting paraganglioma (extra-adrenal pheochromocytoma) should be suspected when the patient presents with a clinical triad of headache, sweating, and tachycardia. The diagnosis can be confirmed biochemically by measuring 24-hour urinary fractionated metanephrines and catecholamines. Radiologic evaluation is performed to locate the tumor after biochemical confirmation. About 10% of the tumors are extra-adrenal. Thrombus would not be expected in the right atrioventricular groove. Thrombus usually occurs in the left atrium in patients with atrial fibrillation or mitral stenosis, in the left ventricle in the setting of a myocardial infarction with resultant regional wall motion abnormality or in the right heart chambers in patients with atrial fibrillation, or a venous thrombosis in transit. Coronary artery aneurysm can be seen in the right atrioventricular groove. Commonly, there is flow noted in an atrioventricular groove aneurysm by echocardiography, differentiating it from solid masses.

25. **Answer: B.** The M-mode demonstrates prominent inspiratory leftward motion of the ventricular septum. The mitral inflow pulsed-wave (PW) Doppler demonstrates significant (>25%) respiratory variation with increased expiratory E velocity and decreased inspiratory E velocity. The mitral annulus tissue Doppler demonstrates a normal e' of > 8 cm/s (14 cm/s). Finally, the hepatic vein Doppler demonstrates expiratory diastolic reversals. These findings are consistent with a diagnosis of constrictive pericarditis. A history of radiation therapy is the third most common cause of constrictive pericarditis, after idiopathic causes and prior cardiac surgery.

Radiation therapy may also result in restrictive cardiomyopathy. Mitral annulus e' velocity is especially helpful in distinguishing between restrictive cardiomyopathy and constrictive pericarditis. A value >8 cm/s (this patient had e' of 14 cm/s) strongly favors constrictive pericarditis. Although hepatic vein diastolic reversals may be seen with restrictive cardiomyopathy, these are typically inspiratory rather than expiratory. Finally, respiratory variation in mitral inflow and ventricular septal shift would not be expected with restrictive cardiomyopathy. A pericardial effusion can occur during or early after the completion of chest radiation but would not be expected as a late complication. LV hypertrophy would not be expected as a complication of radiation therapy. The M-mode does not show evidence of pericardial effusion or LV hypertrophy.

26. **Answer: D.** The echocardiogram demonstrates LV apical thickening and obliteration and biatrial enlargement, which is suspicious for either apical hypertrophic cardiomyopathy or eosinophilic endomyocardial disease. Contrast images demonstrate a layer of nonperfusing thrombus in the apex, consistent with eosinophilic endomyocardial disease. Mitral inflow PW Doppler demonstrates restrictive filling physiology, which is also consistent with eosinophilic endomyocardial disease.

Cardiac involvement occurs in most patients with the hypereosinophilic syndrome defined as unexplained eosinophilia with >1500 eosinophils per cubic mm for more than 6 months, associated with organ involvement. Cardiac manifestations include biventricular apical thrombotic-fibrotic endocardial obliteration, limited motion of the posterior mitral leaflet with mitral regurgitation due to thickening of the inferobasal wall (see **Table 26.2**), and restrictive ventricular diastolic filling physiology.

Apical hypertrophic cardiomyopathy can be differentiated from eosinophilic endomyocardial disease by the use of myocardial contrast, which demonstrates apical perfusion with a slit-like cavity within the hyperdynamic myocardium. It is typically associated with giant T wave inversions on ECG. Gaucher disease is a lysosomal storage disease and cardiac manifestations include LV thickening, left-sided valvular thickening, diastolic dysfunction, and pericardial effusion. Fabry disease is a glycosphingolipid-storage disease and cardiac manifestations include LV thickening, left-sided valvular thickening, mitral regurgitation, and myocardial dysfunction.

27. **Answer: D.** Mitral rather than aortic regurgitation and biventricular involvement are typically seen in patients with eosinophilic endomyocardial disease (see **Table 26.2** and ▶ **Video 26.40**). This is usually the result of fibrosis extending up the lateral LV wall and restricting posterior leaflet mobility. LVOT obstruction is not associated with this condition. Both RV and LV involvement may be present in this form of restrictive cardiomyopathy.

KEY POINTS

- Cardiac involvement occurs in most patients with hypereosinophilic syndrome.
- Eosinophilic endomyocardial disease is characterized by biventricular apical thrombotic-fibrotic obliteration, mitral regurgitation due to the restriction of posterior mitral leaflet motion from inferobasal endocardial thickening, and restrictive physiology.
- Myocardial contrast is helpful in distinguishing eosinophilic endomyocardial disease from apical hypertrophic cardiomyopathy.
- Mitral regurgitation can develop due to fibrosis extending into the basal posterior mitral valve leaflet and restricting leaflet excursion.

28. **Answer: B.** The clinical presentation and left ventriculogram are consistent with Takotsubo cardiomyopathy The echocardiogram demonstrates apical and midventricular akinesis and basal hyperkinesis with dynamic outflow tract obstruction, systolic anterior motion of the mitral leaflets, and associated posteriorly directed mitral regurgitation. LVOT obstruction is an important complication of Takotsubo cardiomyopathy and may result in clinically significant hypotension. Mitral regurgitation, either in association with mitral systolic anterior motion or due to papillary muscle displacement/dysfunction has also been described as a potential complication of Takotsubo cardiomyopathy.

Papillary muscle rupture, ventricular septal defect, and severe aortic regurgitation are not common complications of Takotsubo cardiomyopathy and are not present in this case.

29. **Answer: B.** The dynamic LVOT obstruction with associated mitral systolic anterior motion and mitral regurgitation is the result of basal LV hyperkinesis. The most appropriate remedy is to increase LV afterload with phenylephrine and to reduce basal hyperkinesis with gradual initiation of beta-blockade. Cautious fluid administration may also be helpful, unless significant mitral regurgitation is present. Dobutamine would exacerbate the dynamic outflow tract obstruction. Percutaneous or surgical management is not indicated.

KEY POINTS

- Ten percent of Takotsubo cardiomyopathy patients have hemodynamic instability. This may be due to LV systolic dysfunction but dynamic LVOT obstruction is also a possible complication of this syndrome and may result in clinically significant hypotension/shock. It is the result of basal LV hyperkinesis and mitral valve systolic anterior motion with resultant dynamic LVOT obstruction.
- Other possible causes of shock in patients with Takotsubo cardiomyopathy include profound LV systolic dysfunction and severe mitral regurgitation, either in association with mitral systolic anterior motion or due to displacement/dysfunction of the papillary muscles.

30. **Answer: A.** The echocardiogram demonstrates severe concentric thickening of the left ventricle (not left ventricular hypertrophy), a granular myocardial echotexture, and biatrial enlargement and thickened cardiac valves (see **Tables 26.1** and **26.2**). The subcostal view also shows a thickened RV free wall (10 mm) and a small posterior pericardial effusion. These two-dimensional features are highly suggestive of cardiac amyloidosis. Mitral inflow PW Doppler demonstrates a restrictive filling pattern (E/A ratio of 3 and deceleration time of <160 ms) and tissue Doppler demonstrates severely reduced annular e' velocity of 3 cm/s. The mitral E/e' ratio is 30, which is consistent with severely increased LV filling pressures.

The ECG findings of normal voltages despite severely increased wall thickness and pseudo-infarction are also consistent with amyloidosis. Overall, the two-dimensional and Doppler features are classic for cardiac amyloidosis.

Hypertrophic cardiomyopathy is less likely given the diffuse nature of increased LV thickness (although this can sometimes be present), increased RV thickness, valvular thickening, and pericardial effusion as well as ECG findings. Athlete's heart may be associated with increased LV thickness and enters the differential because of the history of the patient being an ex-competitive cyclist but notably this entity is associated with a normal mitral e' velocity. Hypertensive heart disease may be associated with increased LV thickness, reduced mitral e' velocity, and increased mitral E/e' velocity but would not be associated with the other abnormalities described. Finally, echocardiographic findings of hemochromatosis are those of a dilated cardiomyopathy with normal or mildly increased LV wall thickness.

31. **Answer: D.** Cardiac amyloidosis is associated with an inverse relationship between LV mass and ECG voltage since the increased wall thickness is due to interstitial amyloid fibril deposition rather than LV hypertrophy. ECG features may include low limb lead (<5 mm) or precordial lead (<10 mm) voltages and a pseudoinfarct pattern. Fairly good sensitivity and specificity for the diagnosis of cardiac amyloidosis have been described using various combinations of increased LV wall thickness and low ECG voltages or LV mass/ECG voltage ratios. In contrast, hypertensive heart disease, hypertrophic cardiomyopathy, and athlete's heart—where wall thickness is increased due to LV hypertrophy—are associated with a proportional relationship between LV mass and ECG voltage. Restrictive filling physiology is not unique to cardiac amyloidosis and may also be seen in other conditions where LV wall thickness is increased such as hypertrophic cardiomyopathy or hypertension. Systolic anterior motion of the mitral apparatus is a typical feature of obstructive hypertrophic cardiomyopathy but can also be seen in other conditions such as hypertensive heart disease in the elderly (when sigmoid basal septal hypertrophy is present) or occasionally in cardiac amyloidosis. A normal e' velocity helps to distinguish athlete's heart from pathologic causes of increased LV wall thickness (such as hypertensive heart disease, cardiac amyloidosis, or hypertrophic cardiomyopathy). In addition, the value of parametric or "bull's eye" LV longitudinal strain pattern can be valuable in determining the etiology of increased LV wall thickness (please see answer explanation to question 11).

> **KEY POINTS**
> - Cardiac amyloidosis is an infiltrative cardiomyopathy.
> - Echocardiographic findings include increased biventricular and atrial wall thickness, valvular thickening, panvalvular regurgitation, pericardial effusion, and restrictive physiology.
> - Cardiac amyloidosis is associated with an inverse relationship between LV mass and ECG voltage.

32. **Answer: C.** This patient has hypothyroidism. Although the echocardiogram demonstrates a large pericardial effusion with RV collapse suggesting cardiac tamponade, a definitive etiology cannot be made on the basis of the echocardiogram alone. In this case, all of the conditions above can result in a pericardial effusion and should be included in the differential diagnosis.

Cardiac tamponade is an unlikely consequence in patients with cardiac amyloid, renal failure, SLE, as well as hypothyroidism. Nevertheless, cardiac tamponade can rarely occur in all of these conditions. The clue to the correct answer lies in the physical examination that reveals non-pitting pedal edema (pretibial myxedema secondary to interstitial accumulation of glycosaminoglycans) and bradycardia in the setting of cardiac tamponade making hypothyroidism the most likely explanation for the clinical and echocardiographic findings in this patient.

The low voltage on the ECG is unhelpful to distinguish a cause since the findings may reflect attenuation of the ECG signal by the large pericardial effusion. Furthermore, although we would expect a higher mitral annular velocity in a middle-aged woman, diastolic dysfunction can be present in all of these conditions except in a patient with breast cancer who otherwise has no cardiac disease. The incidence of pericardial effusion in hypothyroidism varies depending on the severity of the disease and occurs in 30% to 80% of patients with severe disease.

33. **Answer: D.** Since the patient is symptomatic, experiencing lightheadedness and presyncope, and there is evidence of collapse of the right-sided chambers, therapeutic echocardiographic-guided pericardiocentesis is indicated at this time. Had the effusion been smaller and without associated hemodynamic compromise, it would have been reasonable to reevaluate the effusion after confirming the diagnosis and restoring a euthyroid state.

34. **Answer: A.** Overt hypothyroidism can result in impaired ventricular systolic and diastolic performance manifested by the prolongation of the isovolumic contraction and relaxation intervals as well

as a frank dilated cardiomyopathy and congestive heart failure. Thus, in this patient with hypothyroidism, the only echocardiographic parameter that would be expected to decrease with thyroid supplementation is the isovolumic contraction interval since this is a measure of cardiac contractility—the shorter the interval, the better the myocardial contractility. Both systolic and diastolic mitral annular velocities are likely to increase as systolic and diastolic function improves and the LVOT time-velocity integral will also increase since the cardiac output will likely increase with treatment. Apart from pericardial effusion and reduced cardiac output (related to a reduction in heart rate and contractility) and diastolic function, other cardiac manifestations of hypothyroidism include increased LV mass and LV wall thickness, which may rarely be asymmetric.

KEY POINTS
- Pericardial effusion is a common cardiac manifestation of severe hypothyroidism.
- Reversible systolic and diastolic dysfunction can occur in patients with hypothyroidism.

35. **Answer: B.** Transesophageal echocardiography (TEE) demonstrates globular vegetations on the aortic valve. In a patient with systemic lupus erythematosus (SLE) and negative blood cultures, the diagnosis of nonbacterial thrombotic endocarditis (NBTE) is most likely. This is also most prevalent in the presence of a positive antiphospholipid antibody (Answer B) or anti-cardiolipin antibody test. In patients with SLE, observational studies using TTE have reported prevalence rates of 6% to 11%, with higher rates (43%) observed when the more sensitive TEE is performed. A high index of clinical suspicion is critical for the diagnosis of NBTE. The definitive diagnosis can be made pathologically by the demonstration of thrombi on autopsy or surgical specimens. However, the routine acquisition of the valvular tissue is not practical such that clinicians are reliant upon a constellation of clinical, echocardiographic, and absence of microbiologic findings for the diagnosis of NBTE. Typically, the demonstration of valvular vegetations on echocardiography in the absence of systemic infection in patients who are at high risk of NBTE provide strong evidence to support the diagnosis. Computed tomography of the brain or magnetic resonance imaging may be performed in those with suspected cerebral embolization due to NBTE, but cardiac MRI or CT PET imaging is unlikely to be of benefit.

36. **Answer: D.** Oral anticoagulation with warfarin or treatment with heparin is the treatment of choice to reduce the risk of embolic events and NBTE, in general, does respond to this treatment with surgical treatment reserved for those patients with refractory symptoms, severe valvular regurgitation, or heart failure due to valvular dysfunction. Immediate aortic valve replacement would not be the initial treatment. Novel oral anticoagulants have not been demonstrated to be effective in NBTE.

KEY POINTS
- NBTE is a rare condition and has been reported in every age group, most commonly affecting patients with advanced malignancy and those with SLE or antiphospholipid antibody positive status.
- NBTE, also called marantic endocarditis, Libman-Sacks endocarditis, or verrucous endocarditis is a form of noninfectious endocarditis, that is characterized by the deposition of thrombi on heart valves (mostly aortic and mitral).
- TEE is more sensitive than TTE for the detection of vegetations, particularly for small lesions (<5 mm)
- Treatment of NBTE usually consists of systemic anticoagulation and therapy directed at treating the underlying malignancy or associated condition. Surgery is performed in selected cases that do not have an advanced malignancy. In patients with NBTE, treatment with therapeutic dose low molecular weight heparin or unfractionated heparin or warfarin (but not novel oral anticoagulants or aspirin) is continued indefinitely.
- Despite therapy, the prognosis from NBTE is generally poor.

37. **Answer: C.** This patient has Carney syndrome. The Carney complex is an inherited, autosomal dominant disorder characterized by multiple tumors, including atrial and extracardiac myxomas, schwannomas, and various endocrine tumors. The cardiac myxomas generally are diagnosed at an earlier age than sporadic myxomas and have a higher tendency to recur. In addition, patients have a variety of pigmentation abnormalities, including pigmented lentigines and blue nevi on the face, neck, and trunk. The skin lesions present in this young woman are lentigines, which are characteristically seen in patients with Carney syndrome. This finding, combined with the history of adrenal tumors, makes it the most likely diagnosis. Therefore, the mass seen in the right atrium is most likely a myxoma (Answer C). Even though myxomas (the most common benign primary cardiac tumor) typically arise in the left atrium and are most often attached to the fossa ovalis membrane by a thin stalk, the "atypical" location is characteristic of this syndrome. Angiosarcoma is a malignant tumor with a dismal

prognosis (rarely exceeding 6 months) and often presents as a broad-based right atrial mass near the inferior vena cava. Epicardial, endocardial, and intracavitary extensions are common. They may be associated with a pericardial effusion, presenting with cardiac tamponade. Fungal endocarditis may mimic a right-sided mass lesion when tricuspid valve involvement is present, even resulting in tricuspid valve obstruction. The clinical setting is usually intravenous drug abuse or indwelling intravenous infusion catheter in patients with renal failure or undergoing chemotherapy. Valve destruction is usually present with valvular regurgitation. Renal cell carcinoma, which characteristically metastasizes to the right-sided cardiac chambers as a tumor/thrombus via the inferior vena cava as well as thrombi in transit from the deep venous system may also present as right-sided masses and therefore should be included in the differential diagnosis.

38. **Answer: D.** It is imperative that careful scrutiny for other lesions is undertaken since multiple synchronous lesions are commonly present. In this instance, the RV lesion was missed during the initial assessment (Answer D). A CAT is an acronym describing a calcified amorphous tumor that probably represents a calcified thrombus. This is a benign finding and would not be expected in this patient. These tumors are benign but recurrent tumors can occur mandating careful lifelong echocardiographic follow-up.

> **KEY POINTS**
> - It is important to integrate the history and physical examination findings when making an echocardiographic diagnosis.
> - When atrial myxomas arise in unusual locations and multiple tumors are present, think of Carney syndrome.
> - Do not focus on one abnormality at the exclusion of other synchronous lesions or abnormalities!

39. **Answer: A.** The patient presents with symptoms of right heart failure and the echocardiographic images demonstrate thickening and malcoaptation of the tricuspid valve leaflets with severe tricuspid regurgitation. The tricuspid valve leaflets are thickened, fixed, and often retracted in a semi-open position. There is a laminar jet of tricuspid regurgitation noted in the right atrium, and the continuous-wave Doppler signal demonstrates a dense systolic signal with a cutoff sign consistent with rapid equalization of pressures between the right atrium and right ventricle. The characteristic echocardiographic features of carcinoid heart disease include progressive thickening and reduced mobility of the tricuspid valve leaflets with associated tricuspid valve regurgitation. Rarely, tricuspid inflow obstruction is noted; when present, it is always associated with tricuspid valve regurgitation. An example of a 3D TTE image of a patient with tricuspid carcinoid valve disease demonstrating the thickened, fixed, and immobile tricuspid valve leaflets "en-face" from the right ventricular perspective is shown in ▶ **Video 26.41**. The pulmonary valve thickening and reduced mobility eventually occurs in two-thirds of patients with carcinoid heart disease and primarily causes pulmonary valve regurgitation. Occasionally pulmonary valve cusp thickening and annulus narrowing cause right ventricular outflow tract obstruction. Left-sided carcinoid valve disease is rare, occurring in about 10% of patients with carcinoid valve disease. Left-sided carcinoid valve disease is characterized by thickening and reduced mobility of the mitral valve leaflets and/or aortic valve cusps. Left-sided valve disease occurs most commonly in patients with a patent foramen ovale that allows some of the serotonin-rich blood to traverse into the left-heart chambers without being filtered by the lungs. Left-sided valve disease is also found in patients with very active carcinoid syndrome and high levels of circulating serotonin.

Arrhythmogenic RV dysplasia is characterized by ventricular arrhythmias and fatty replacement of the RV free wall. The fibrofatty replacement of the RV myocardium initially produces regional wall motion abnormalities and eventual RV dilation. Drug-related valve disease has been reported to occur with ergot alkaloid derivatives, anorexigens, and pergolide (see **Tables 26.1** and **26.2**). These agents cause primarily left-sided valve disease but tricuspid valve disease can also occur. The echocardiographic appearance of drug-related valve disease includes thickening of the valve leaflets or cusps with reduced mobility. Echocardiographic images are similar to those seen in carcinoid valve disease. However, the patient history is consistent with carcinoid rather than drug-related valve disease. Ebstein anomaly is a congenital cardiac disorder, which involves apical displacement of the septal and posterior tricuspid leaflets and variable tethering of the anterior leaflet. Tricuspid regurgitation is a common finding in patients with Ebstein anomaly. Additional echocardiographic features include right heart enlargement with dysfunction and atrial septal defect or patent foramen ovale.

40. **Answer: D.** Urinary 5-hydroxyindole acetic acid is a breakdown product of serotonin and is measured using a 24-hour urine collection. Patients with carcinoid heart disease have increased levels of circulating serotonin related to metastatic disease. Serotonin is produced by the primary tumor and metastases. Increased serotonin levels have been demonstrated to cause tricuspid and pulmonary

valve thickening and associated regurgitation. The mechanism is thought to be the activation of the 5HT 2B receptors on the valves. The diagnosis of carcinoid can be confirmed by pathologic examination of the primary tumor or metastases, increased 24-hour urine 5-hydroxyindole acetic acid, and/or by octreoscan.

Serum angiotensin-converting enzyme (ACE) level is often elevated in patients with sarcoidosis. Subcutaneous fat aspirate is used to help confirm suspected primary amyloid. Complete blood cell count with differential white blood cell count and smear is performed when hypereosinophilic syndrome is suspected. Eosinophilic endomyocardial disease affects primarily the endocardium and valves.

> **KEY POINTS**
> - Patients with carcinoid syndrome usually present with flushing and diarrhea.
> - Carcinoid heart disease is characterized by thickening and regurgitation of the right-sided cardiac valves.
> - Serotonin is responsible for the valve damage that occurs in patients with carcinoid syndrome.

41. **Answer A.** The Ergot derivatives ergotamine and methysergide were previously used widely for the prophylaxis and treatment of migraines but are used less frequently due to available alternatives with better adverse risk profiles. Their notable cardiac toxicity is the induction of valvular abnormalities similar to those seen with carcinoid syndrome. The echocardiographic and pathologic features of the valve disease seen in patients with drug-induced valvular disease are similar to those occurring in carcinoid heart valve disease. But unlike carcinoid valvular disease in which right heart valve involvement occurs to a far greater extent than left-sided valve disease, ergotamine associated valve disease effects both right and left-sided heart valves. Other agents linked with similar valvular findings include the appetite suppressant combination of fenfluramine and dexfenfluramine ('Fen-Phen') and the dopamine agonists, pergolide and cabergoline, used for the treatment of Parkinson disease. The link between these agents and disease states appears to be the stimulation of the serotonin 2B receptors which in turn stimulates fibroblast proliferation and valvular thickening (via the 5-HT 2B receptor). Fenfluramine and dexfenfluramine augment serotonergic activity, while phentermine may contribute to the fenfluramine valvulopathy by interfering with the pulmonary clearance of serotonin. In severe cases, valve leaflets become retracted and progressive immobile with significant valvular regurgitation. There is some anterior leaflet override but no anterior mitral valve leaflet prolapse is seen. No intracardiac vegetations are seen and the clinical history does not suggest endocarditis.

42. **Answer: C.** Typically the shape of the tricuspid regurgitant jet is a symmetrical parabolic curve. However, in the setting of torrential tricuspid valve regurgitation, the large volume of blood re-entering the right atrium during systole causes a rapid rise in right atrial pressure, which equilibrates with the right ventricular pressure and terminates the regurgitant waveform to be more triangular. This pattern does not indicate pulmonary hypertension (nor does it exclude this). This pattern usually does not occur with less than severe tricuspid regurgitation and does not mean that right atrial pressure is elevated.

> **KEY POINTS**
> - Echocardiography to assess valve morphology and regurgitation is indicated in patients with a history of use of any drug associated with valvular heart disease who have a heart murmur, symptoms of valvular heart disease, or a technically inadequate auscultatory examination.
> - Echocardiographic features of drug-induced valvular heart disease may mimic other disorders such as rheumatic valvular heart disease and carcinoid valvular heart disease. A comprehensive history is crucial.
> - Drugs implicated to cause valve damage via the serotonin (5-HT) pathway include ergot derivatives ergotamine and methysergide, ergot-derived dopamine agonists pergolide and cabergoline, 3,4-methylenedioxymethamphetamine (MDMA; known as ecstasy), fenfluramine, dexfenfluramine, and benfluorex. Phentermine, an appetite suppressant, has not as of yet been implicated.

SUGGESTED READINGS

Alzubaidee MJS, Dwarampudi RS, Mathew S, et al. A systematic review exploring the effect of human immunodeficiency virus on cardiac diseases. *Cureus.* 2022;14(9):e28960.

Arany Z, Elkayam U. Peripartum cardiomyopathy. *Circulation.* 2016;133(14):1397-1409.

Bhattacharyya S, Schapira AH, Mikhailidis DP, Davar J. Drug-induced fibrotic valvular heart disease. *Lancet.* 2009;374(9689):577-585.

Borowski A, Ghodsizad A, Cohnen M, Gams E. Recurrent embolism in the course of marantic endocarditis. *Ann Thorac Surg.* 2005;79(6):2145-2147.

Correa R, Salpea P, Stratakis CA. Carney complex: an update. *Eur J Endocrinol*. 2015;173(4):M85-M97.

Kittleson MM, Maurer MS, Ambardekar AV, et al. Cardiac amyloidosis: evolving diagnosis and management—a scientific statement from the American Heart Association. *Circulation*. 2020;142(1):e7-e22.

Kouranos V, Sharma R. Cardiac sarcoidosis: state-of-the-art review. *Heart*. 2021;107(19):1591-1599.

Martin CA, Lambiase PD. Pathophysiology, diagnosis and treatment of tachycardiomyopathy. *Heart*. 2017;103(19):1543-1552.

Oliveira GH, Seward JB, Tsang TS, Specks U. Echocardiographic findings in patients with Wegener granulomatosis. *Mayo Clin Proc*. 2005;80(11):1435-1440.

Phelan D, Collier P, Thavendiranathan P, et al. Relative apical sparing of longitudinal strain using two-dimensional speckle-tracking echocardiography is both sensitive and specific for the diagnosis of cardiac amyloidosis. *Heart*. 2012;98(19):1442-1448.

Ram P, Penalver JL, Lo KBU, Rangaswami J, Pressman GS. Carcinoid heart disease: review of current knowledge. *Tex Heart Inst J*. 2019;46(1):21-27.

Roldan CA, Shively BK, Crawford MH. An echocardiographic study of valvular heart disease associated with systemic lupus erythematosus. *N Engl J Med*. 1996;335(19):1424-1430.

Tanaka H. Efficacy of echocardiography for differential diagnosis of left ventricular hypertrophy: special focus on speckle-tracking longitudinal strain. *J Echocardiogr*. 2021;19(2):71-79.

Templin C, Ghadri JR, Diekmann J, et al. Clinical features and outcomes of Takotsubo (stress) cardiomyopathy. *N Engl J Med*. 2015;373(10):929-938.

CHAPTER 27

Pericardial Diseases

Terrence D. Welch

QUESTIONS

1. According to the 2015 European Society of Cardiology Guidelines for the diagnosis and management of pericardial diseases, in which of the following clinical situations would an echocardiogram be LEAST appropriate?
   A. Suspected acute pericarditis.
   B. Routine follow-up of a known, small pericardial effusion in a clinically stable patient.
   C. Suspected effusive-constrictive pericarditis.
   D. Computed tomographic imaging demonstrating a new, moderate-sized pericardial effusion.

2. Which of the following findings argues most strongly against hemodynamically significant pericardial disease?
   A. Right atrial collapse.
   B. Right ventricular free wall inversion.
   C. Exaggerated trans-mitral flow velocity variation with respiration.
   D. Normal inferior vena cava size and >50% collapse with "sniff" maneuver.

3. Two-dimensional (2D) echocardiographic features of congenital absence of the pericardium resemble those found in which of the following conditions?
   A. Mitral regurgitation.
   B. Aortic stenosis.
   C. Ventricular septal defect.
   D. Atrial septal defect.

4. Which of the following features can be found in both pericardial constriction and cardiac tamponade?
   A. Right ventricular diastolic collapse.
   B. Right atrial diastolic collapse.
   C. Prominent increase in trans-tricuspid valve and decrease in trans-mitral valve Doppler velocities with inspiration.
   D. Reversal of diastolic flow in the hepatic vein during inspiration.

5. In the presence of a dilated inferior vena cava (IVC), which of the following echocardiographic findings would yield the highest sensitivity and specificity in diagnosing constrictive pericarditis (CP)?
   A. Interventricular septal shift with inspiration.
   B. A septal e′ velocity ≥9 cm/s.
   C. Hepatic vein expiratory diastolic flow reversal.
   D. Interventricular septal shift with inspiration and either a septal e′ velocity ≥9 cm/s or hepatic vein expiratory diastolic flow reversal.

6. Which of the following echocardiographic techniques is best for evaluating pericardial thickness?
   A. M-mode transthoracic echocardiography.
   B. Speckle-tracking echocardiography.
   C. Tissue Doppler echocardiography.
   D. Trans-esophageal echocardiography.

7. Which of the following may prevent right ventricular free wall diastolic collapse in a patient with cardiac tamponade?
   A. Rapid collection of the pericardial fluid.
   B. Aortic stenosis.
   C. Pulmonary hypertension in cor pulmonale.
   D. Atrial fibrillation.

8. Which of the following conditions is characterized by diastolic flow reversal in the hepatic veins that is most prominent in expiration as compared with inspiration?
   A. Constrictive pericarditis (CP).
   B. Restrictive cardiomyopathy.
   C. Congenital absence of the pericardium.
   D. Severe tricuspid regurgitation.

9. Which of the following is most correct regarding the use of medial mitral annular tissue Doppler velocities to differentiate CP from RCM?
   A. ≥9 cm/s favors CP.
   B. <15 cm/s favors CP.
   C. ≥4 cm/s favors CP.
   D. <12 cm/s favors CP.

10. Which of the following best explains the enhanced respiratory variation in ventricular filling in constrictive pericarditis?
    A. Dissociation of intrathoracic and intracardiac pressures.
    B. Decreased ventricular interdependence.
    C. Equalization of intrathoracic and extrathoracic pressures.
    D. Intrathoracic and extrathoracic dissociation.

11. Which of the following is frequently seen in CP but is not necessarily a specific sign for constriction?
    A. B bump.
    B. Abnormal interventricular septal motion.
    C. Pulmonary hypertension.
    D. Dilated coronary sinus.

12. Demonstration of which of the following is obligatory for the diagnosis of CP?
    A. Abnormal hemodynamics.
    B. Pericardial thickening/calcification.
    C. Pulmonary hypertension.
    D. Biatrial enlargement.

13. Which of the following statements is most accurate regarding the differentiation of CP from COPD using echocardiography?
    A. In COPD, the mitral inflow pattern is restrictive.
    B. In COPD, the highest mitral E velocity occurs toward the beginning of inspiration, whereas in CP it occurs immediately after the onset of expiration.
    C. In CP, the superior vena cava flow velocities do not change significantly with respiration.
    D. In CP, respirophasic ventricular septal shift is observed.

14. Which of the following is the most common primary neoplasm of the heart associated with a pericardial effusion?
    A. Myxoma.
    B. Hemangioma.
    C. Angiosarcoma.
    D. Rhabdomyoma.

15. Which of the following is an echocardiographic feature of a pericardial cyst?
    A. It is commonly located behind the atrium.
    B. It is usually located at the cardiophrenic angle.
    C. It is usually located near the left ventricular (LV) apex.
    D. It is usually located near the transverse sinus.

16. Which of the following statements is correct regarding pericardial disease?
    A. Loculated pericardial effusions can cause significant hemodynamic compromise.
    B. Features of pericardial constriction are always persistent.
    C. Cardiac tamponade does not occur with small pericardial effusions.
    D. Chronic calcific CP is never associated with myocardial disease.

17. A 43-year-old patient presented to the emergency department with chest pain. The unusual two-dimensional echocardiographic images, shown in **Figure 27.1A,B** are consistent with:
    A. CP.
    B. Acute pericarditis.
    C. Absent pericardium.
    D. Pericardial cyst.

Chapter 27 Pericardial Diseases / 581

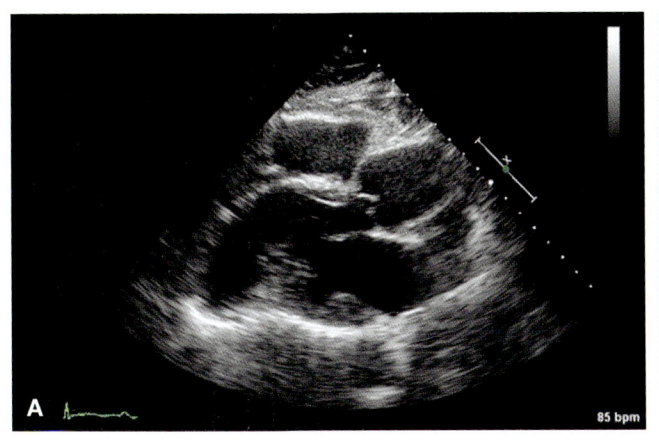

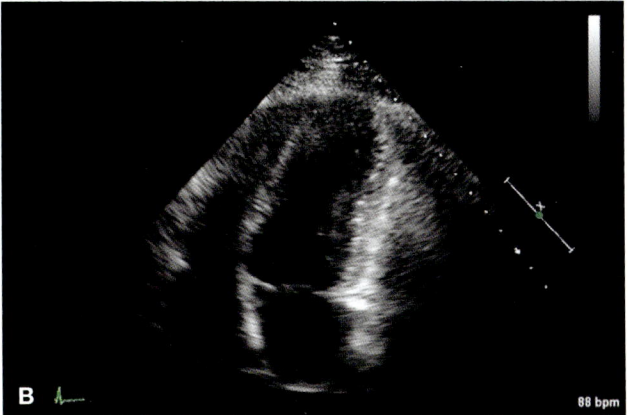

Figure 27.1

18. The labeled portion (white arrow) of the two-dimensional echocardiographic image in **Figure 27.2** is consistent with:
    A. Pleural effusion.
    B. Pericardial effusion.
    C. Pericardial cyst.
    D. Mediastinal cyst.

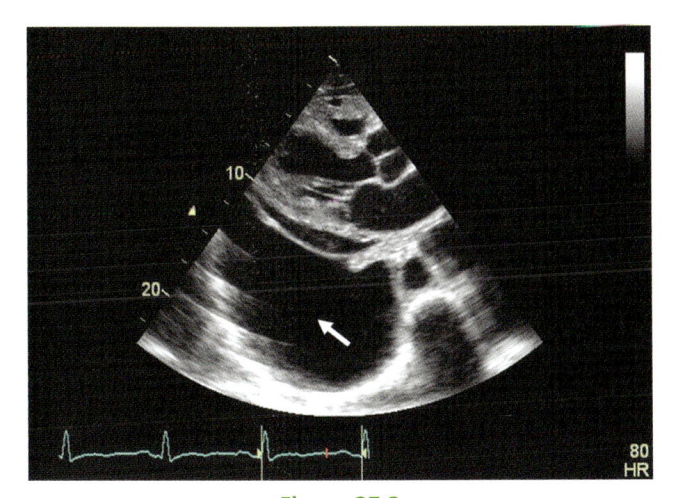

Figure 27.2

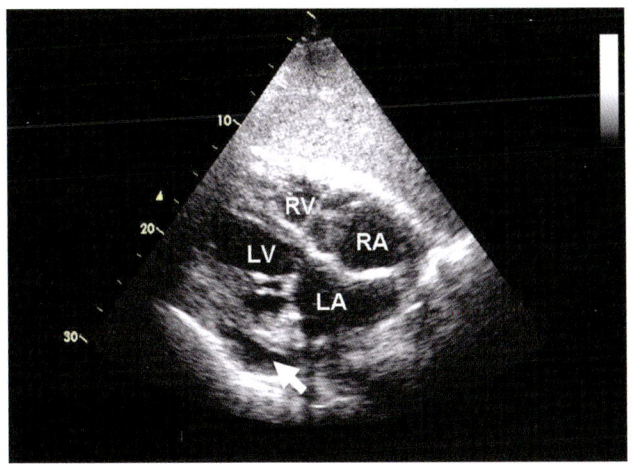

Figure 27.3

20. The labeled portion (white arrow) of the two-dimensional echocardiographic image in **Figure 27.4** is consistent with:
    A. Epicardial fat.
    B. Mediastinal hemorrhage.
    C. Pericardial effusion.
    D. Pleural effusion.

19. The labeled portion (white arrow) of the two-dimensional echocardiographic image in **Figure 27.3** is consistent with:
    A. Pericardial cyst.
    B. Loculated pericardial effusion.
    C. Pericardial metastasis.
    D. CP.

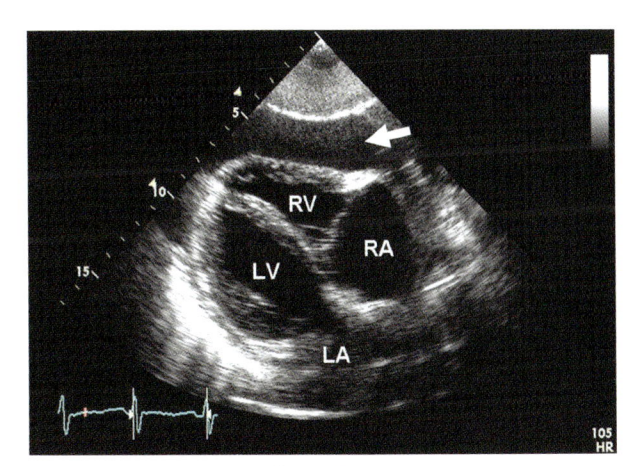

Figure 27.4

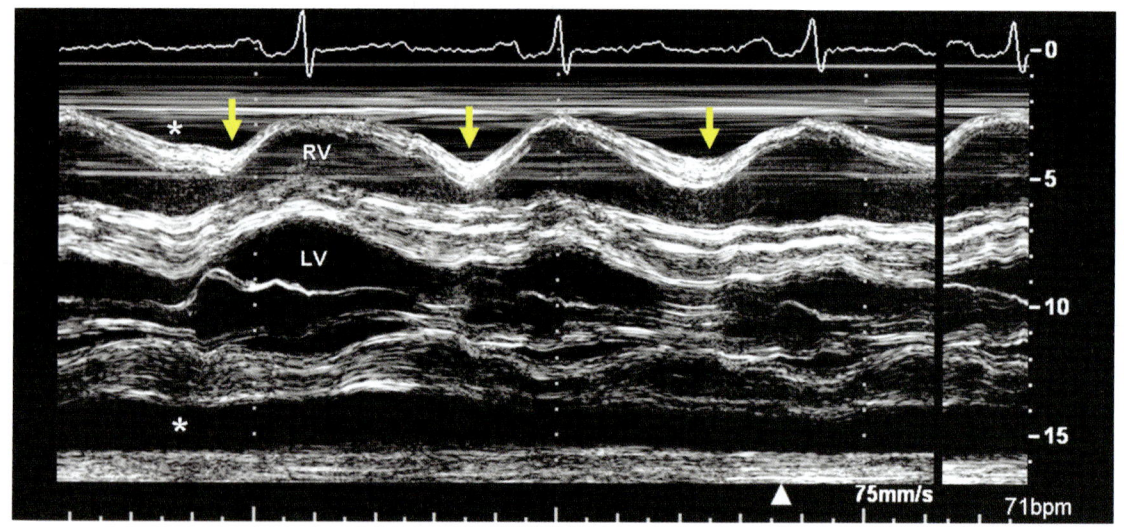

Figure 27.5

21. The M-mode echocardiographic features shown in **Figure 27.5** are suggestive of:
    A. Pleural effusion.
    B. CP.
    C. Pulmonary hypertension.
    D. Cardiac tamponade.

22. The transmitral and transtricuspid flow profiles shown in **Figure 27.6** in a patient with a large pericardial effusion are most consistent with:
    A. Cardiac tamponade.
    B. Constrictive pericarditis.
    C. A normal pattern.
    D. Pulmonary hypertension.

23. The M-mode echocardiogram shown in **Figure 27.7** refers to the early diastolic motion of the interventricular septum (arrow 1) and LV posterior wall (arrow 2). This unique motion pattern is seen in which of the following pericardial diseases?
    A. Cardiac tamponade.
    B. Absent pericardium.
    C. Chronic CP.
    D. Chronic pericardial effusion.

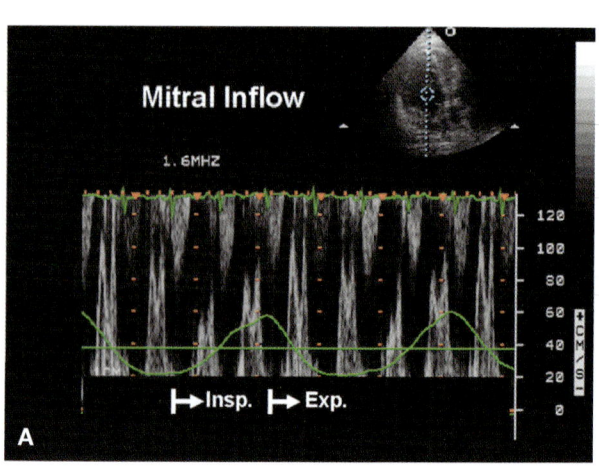

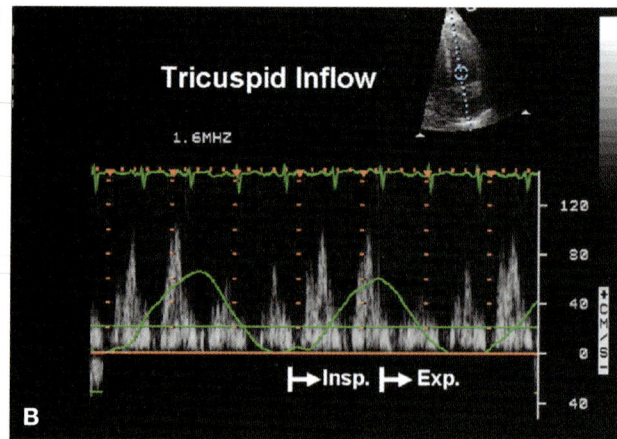

Figure 27.6

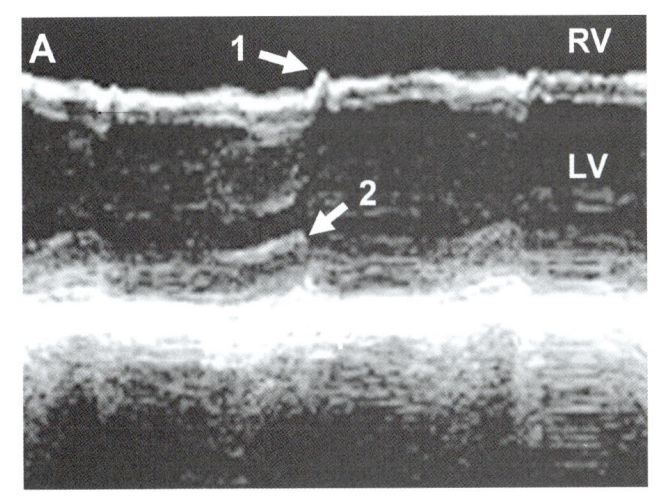

Figure 27.7

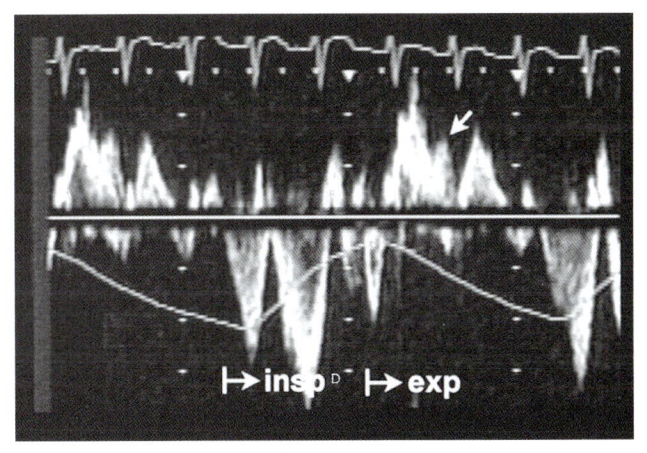

Figure 27.9

24. Figure 27.8 shows velocities from the medial mitral annulus in a patient with CP. What relationship would be expected to be seen between pulmonary capillary wedge pressure (PCWP) and the E/e′ ratio?
A. E/e′ varies directly proportional to the PCWP.
B. E/e′ varies inversely proportional to the PCWP.
C. No relationship exists between E/e′ and the PCWP.
D. E/e′ varies exponentially with PCWP.

26. The two-dimensional echocardiogram for an 82-year-old patient in Figure 27.10 (with white arrow pointing to a key finding) is consistent with which of the following diagnoses?
A. Acute pericarditis.
B. Pericardial metastasis.
C. Pericardial cyst.
D. Pleural effusion.

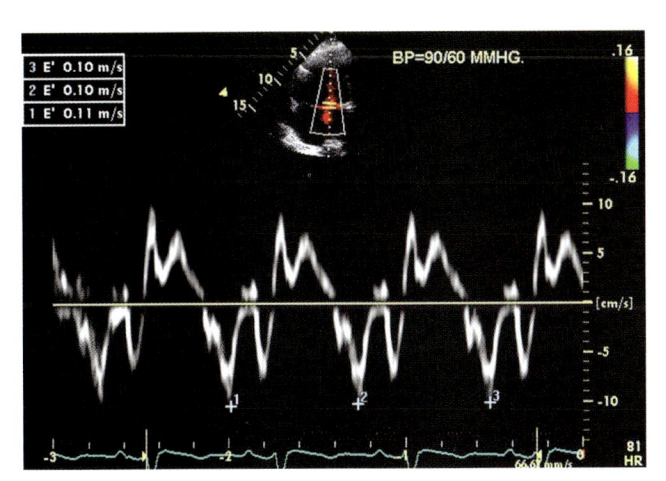

Figure 27.8

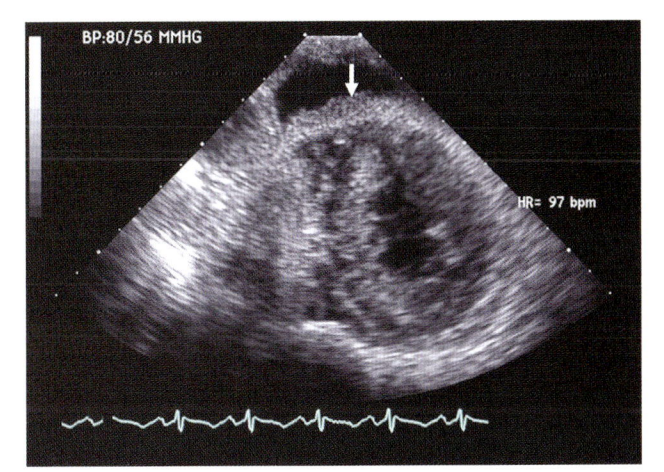

Figure 27.10

25. Figure 27.9 shows hepatic vein pulsed wave Doppler. The features are consistent with:
A. Inspiratory diastolic flow reversals seen in CP.
B. Inspiratory systolic flow reversals seen in CP.
C. Expiratory diastolic flow reversals seen in CP.
D. Expiratory systolic flow augmentation seen in CP.

27. Which of the following best characterizes the respiration-related ventricular septal shift that is expected in CP?
A. The septum shifts to the right with inspiration.
B. The septum shifts to the left with inspiration.
C. The septum shifts to the left with expiration.
D. The septum is shifted to the left in both inspiration and expiration.

28. In conducting a tissue Doppler assessment to differentiate CP from restrictive cardiomyopathy (RCM), what does the finding of mitral *annulus reversus* signify?
   A. An inverse relationship between E/e′ and left atrial pressure in patients with CP.
   B. In contrast to what happens in RCM, mitral annular velocities are increased in patients with CP.
   C. The relationship between the septal and lateral mitral annular velocities is reversed in patients with CP, with the septal e′ commonly being higher than the lateral e′.
   D. In contrast to what happens in RCM, mitral annular velocities are decreased in patients with CP.

CASE 1

A 70-year-old patient was initially admitted with a febrile illness, a small left-sided pleural effusion, and a small pericardial effusion without signs of tamponade on echocardiographic examination. A comprehensive noninvasive workup did not yield evidence for infection or another etiology for the illness. The patient became asymptomatic and afebrile and was discharged several days later. One week later, the patient was readmitted for progressive dyspnea and edema. The patient was afebrile with a heart rate of 100 bpm, blood pressure of 118/80 mm Hg, and an oxygen saturation level of 92%. Auscultation did not reveal any murmurs or a friction rub. The jugular venous pressure was noted to be elevated and there was edema in both legs. Chest radiography demonstrated cardiomegaly and enlarged bilateral pleural effusions. Thoracentesis drained a serous fluid with transudative characteristics. An echocardiogram was performed again; the transmitral and hepatic vein Doppler recordings are shown in **Figure 27.11**. *Cardiac magnetic resonance imaging confirmed significant pericardial thickening with diffuse late-gadolinium enhancement; the pericardial effusion remained small.*

29. What is the **BEST** next step at this time for the patient in **Case 1**?
   A. Anti-inflammatory drugs and diuretics.
   B. Pericardiectomy.
   C. Pericardial biopsy.
   D. Pericardiocentesis.

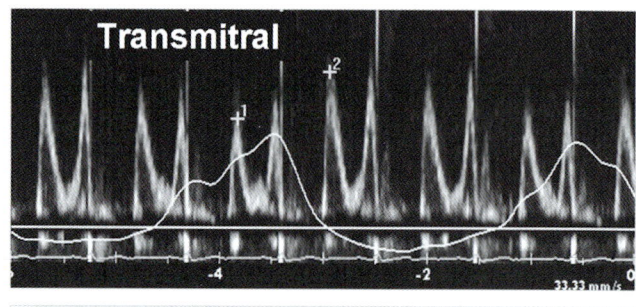

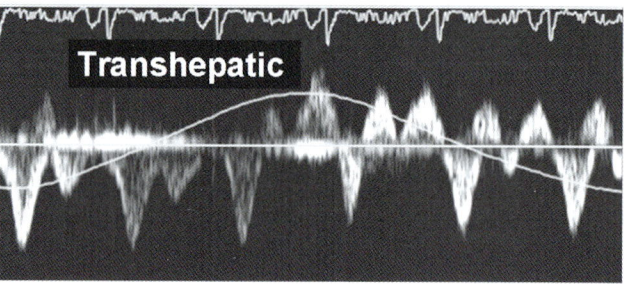

Figure 27.11

30. In the following weeks, the patient from **Case 1** recovered significantly; the edema and the pleural effusions subsided progressively and ultimately resolved. A CT scan performed 5 weeks later showed that the pericardial thickness had decreased and that there was no pleural or pericardial effusion. Follow-up echocardiographic examination showed no evidence for ventricular interdependence or dissociation of intrathoracic and intracardiac pressures. The patient's diagnosis is therefore most consistent with:
   A. Chronic Constrictive Pericarditis.
   B. Transient Constrictive Pericarditis.
   C. Myocarditis.
   D. Familial Mediterranean fever.

CASE 2

A 53-year-old patient with previous coronary artery bypass grafting was admitted for chest discomfort and shoulder pain, both of which worsened with inspiration. The patient was also short of breath. Clinical examination showed normal vital signs and jugular venous pressure. CT in the emergency department ruled out pulmonary embolism and showed a potential pericardial effusion. Echocardiographic images are shown in **Figure 27.12** *and* ▶ **Video 27.1A and B**.

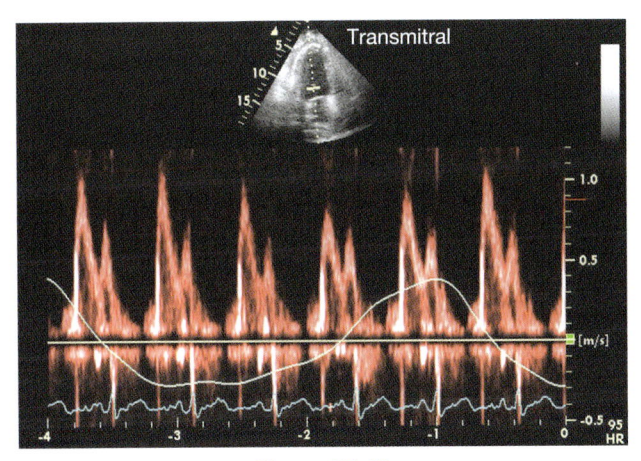

Figure 27.12

31. For the patient in **Case 2,** which of the following diagnoses is most consistent with his presentation?
  A. Occult CP.
  B. Occult effusive CP.
  C. Loculated pericardial effusion.
  D. Pericardial neoplasm.

32. The patient in **Case 2** underwent cardiac catheterization for hemodynamic assessment. If filling pressures are confirmed to be normal at rest, which of the following maneuvers would be most indicated to allow the diagnosis to be made?
  A. Volume loading.
  B. Amyl nitrite challenge.
  C. Hand grip maneuver.
  D. Nitric oxide challenge.

CASE 3

A 35-year-old patient presented with shortness of breath for 1 week. Chest x-ray showed cardiomegaly and a left-sided pleural effusion. The echocardiogram revealed a large pericardial effusion.

33. Which of the following echocardiographic findings would signify the least hemodynamic compromise from the effusion for the patient in **Case 3**?
  A. Early-diastolic collapse of the right ventricle.
  B. Late-diastolic collapse of the right atrium.
  C. No chamber collapse.
  D. Late-diastolic collapse of the left atrium.

34. The patient in **Case 3** underwent an echo-guided pericardiocentesis. Part of the procedure is shown in ▶ **Video 27.2**. Which of the following **BEST** describes what the echocardiogram is showing?
  A. Identification of blood coagulum in the pericardial cavity.
  B. Spontaneous echo contrast in the pericardial cavity.
  C. Stranding within the pericardial space.
  D. Injection of agitated saline contrast.

CASE 4

A 38-year-old patient presented with a 1-year history of bilateral leg edema and shortness of breath. The review of systems was positive for significant weight gain over the last month. The patient's medical history was unremarkable other than a documented episode of viral pericarditis 4 years prior that resolved with nonsteroidal anti-inflammatory medication. The evaluation showed no hepatic or kidney disease. An echocardiogram was performed. The transhepatic and transmitral flow tracings are shown in **Figure 27.13**.

35. Which of the following maneuvers would be most likely to cause the transmitral flow tracing to show more prominent changes with respiration for the patient in **Case 4**?
  A. Trendelenburg position (head down).
  B. Leg raising.
  C. Head up tilt.
  D. Administration of intravenous fluid.

36. Which of the following additional echocardiographic findings would be most likely for the patient in **Case 4**?
  A. Mitral medial e′ of 4 cm/s and lateral e′ of 6 cm/s.
  B. Mitral medial e′ of 10 cm/s and lateral e′ of 9 cm/s.
  C. Ventricular septum that is flat and shifted to the left throughout the respiratory cycle.
  D. Small IVC that collapses with sniff maneuver.

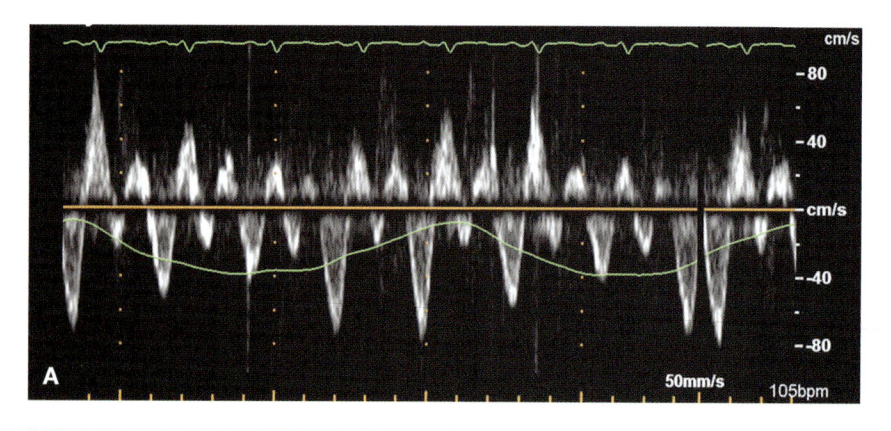

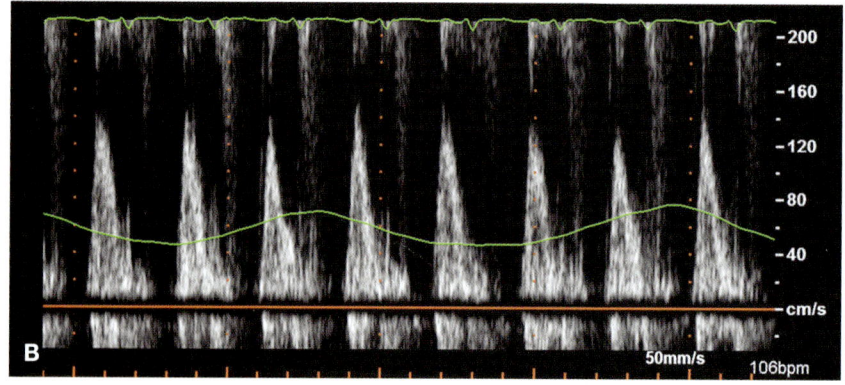

Figure 27.13. **A:** Transhepatic. **B:** Transmitral.

CASE 5

A 46-year-old patient with a history of Hodgkin lymphoma requiring radiation therapy as a child presented with congestive heart failure. This was presumed to be secondary to mitral and tricuspid valve insufficiency. The patient underwent a mitral valve replacement with a St. Jude mechanical valve and a tricuspid valve repair, and was readmitted a few months later with bilateral pleural effusions requiring thoracentesis. The patient was also noted to have abdominal ascites. A diagnosis of CP was made by echocardiogram. To differentiate the extent of pericardial versus myocardial disease related to radiation, myocardial function was analyzed by speckle-tracking strain echocardiography (▶ Video 27.3A,B of speckle tracking strain imaging performed in apical 4-chamber and parasternal short-axis views).

37. Which of the following would be most consistent with radiation-induced CP (without significant myocardial involvement)?

A. Reduced longitudinal and circumferential strains.
B. Relatively normal longitudinal strain and reduced circumferential strain.
C. Reduced longitudinal and normal circumferential strain.
D. Normal longitudinal and circumferential strains.

38. Which of the following is true about left ventricular mechanics in a patient with CP?
A. Longitudinal strain values are similar in CP and RCM.
B. LV rotation is not changed compared to normal controls.
C. Circumferential strain is significantly increased compared to normal controls.
D. Longitudinal strain has an additive value to early diastolic mitral annular velocity (e′) in differentiating between CP and RCM.

ANSWERS

1. **Answer: B.** The 2015 European Society of Cardiology Guidelines for the diagnosis and management of pericardial diseases (available at https://www.escardio.org/Guidelines/Clinical-Practice-Guidelines) provide a class I recommendation for echocardiography as the first-line imaging modality for all cases of suspected pericardial disease or bleeding within the pericardial space. Decisions regarding follow-up echocardiographic imaging should be individualized based on the patient's diagnosis and clinical course. According to these guidelines, a known, small effusion in a stable patient does not necessarily require routine echocardiographic follow-up and would therefore provide the weakest justification for echocardiography of the options presented. Moderate or large effusions, or those for which intervention has been performed, would generally justify surveillance imaging as would the diagnosis of constrictive pericarditis.

2. **Answer: D.** In the absence of positive pressure ventilation, a plethoric inferior vena cava (diameter >21 mm and/or <50% collapse with "sniff") suggests increased central venous pressure and is therefore an expected finding with hemodynamically significant pericardial disease (tamponade and constriction). Although there are exceptions (eg, after significant diuresis or with severe dehydration), the absence of inferior vena cava plethora makes the diagnosis of hemodynamically significant pericardial disease unlikely. The other answer choices represent abnormal findings found in cardiac tamponade.

3. **Answer: D.** With congenital absence of the pericardium, the heart acquires an unusual "teardrop" appearance, with elongated atria and bulbous ventricles, and the position of the heart shifts to the left. The right ventricle may appear enlarged, there is excessive mobility of the posterior left ventricular wall, and septal motion may become paradoxical. The right ventricle becomes abnormally prominent by echocardiography, and the constellation of findings may mimic those found with an atrial septal defect causing right ventricular volume overload. The other answer choices would not be expected to cause the right ventricle to become enlarged or prominent by echocardiography.

4. **Answer: C.** Prominent increase in trans-tricuspid valve and decrease in trans-mitral valve Doppler velocities on inspiration occur in both constrictive pericarditis and tamponade. With both of these diagnoses, the cardiac chambers operate in a fixed and noncompliant volume, leading to ventricular interdependence (ie, the ventricles compete with each other for space). The abnormal pericardium and/or pericardial contents are also thought to "insulate" the intracardiac chambers from the intrathoracic respiratory pressure changes in both disorders. As the pressure in the extrapericardial pulmonary veins decreases normally with inspiration, a reduced pulmonary venous-to-left atrial gradient contributes to the inspiratory decrease in LV filling. Opposite changes in the filling of the two ventricles are seen on expiration, with left-sided cardiac filling occurring at the expense of right-sided cardiac filling. The reduction in right heart filling during expiration may also be manifested as blunting or reversal of diastolic flow in the hepatic veins. Diastolic collapse of the right-sided cardiac chambers occurs only in tamponade. Features of cardiac tamponade are shown in **Table 27.1**, and some of the most prominent differences between cardiac tamponade and constriction are summarized in **Table 27.2**.

Table 27.1. Features of Cardiac Tamponade

Clinical	Imaging
• Beck's triad: hypotension, distended neck veins, and muffled heart sounds • Absent Y-descent in jugular venous pulse • Paradoxical pulse (>10 mm Hg fall in systolic blood pressure with inspiration)	• Large effusion (might occur with small effusion if rapidly collecting) • Reduced LV size • Dilated IVC and hepatic veins • Right atrial and ventricular diastolic collapse • Respiratory variation in ventricular sizes (variation in position of interventricular septum) • Exaggerated respiratory variations in mitral and tricuspid flow (↑ tricuspid, ↓ mitral, and ↓ aortic with inspiration) • Low hepatic vein velocities, decreased forward diastolic hepatic vein velocities with prominent reversals in expiration

IVC, inferior vena cava; LV, left ventricular.

5. **Answer: D.** The assessment for constrictive pericarditis should include a comprehensive, pericardial-protocol echocardiogram. Based on work from authors at the Mayo Clinic, three echocardiographic features that are independently associated with the diagnosis of constriction are (1) the presence of respiration-related ventricular septal shift, (2) preserved or increased medial mitral annular e' velocity (typically ≥9 cm/s), and (3) prominent hepatic vein expiratory diastolic flow reversal. Inferior vena cava plethora (maximum diameter ≥21 mm and/or degree of inspiratory collapse <50%) is nearly

Table 27.2. Similarities and Differences Between Constrictive Pericarditis (CP) and Cardiac Tamponade

	Tamponade	CP
Fixed cardiac volume limiting cardiac filling ↑ respiratory variation of ventricular filling	Present	Present
Ventricular interdependence and dissociation of intracardiac and intrathoracic pressures (respirophasic septal shift and variation in mitral and hepatic vein Doppler profiles)	Present	Present
Equal left- and right-sided diastolic pressures	Present	Present
Dilated noncollapsing IVC	Present	Present
Exaggerated (>10 mm Hg) fall in systolic blood pressure with inspiration (Paradoxical pulse)	Common	Uncommon
Systemic venous wave morphology	Absent Y descent	Steep and deep Y-descent
Inspiratory change in systemic venous pressure	Decrease (normal)	Increase or no change (Kussmaul sign)
Square root sign in ventricular pressure	Absent	Present

IVC, inferior vena cava.

always present in constriction and should be considered a prerequisite (rare exception: in the setting of relative hypovolemia, in which constriction can become "occult"). The combination of ventricular septal shift and either medial e' velocity ≥9 cm/s or hepatic vein expiratory diastolic flow reversal ratio ≥0.79 corresponded to the highest combination of sensitivity (87%) and specificity (91%) in the Mayo Clinic study. See **Table 27.3** for a summary of echocardiographic features of CP and **Figure 27.14** for a suggested algorithm for the echocardiographic diagnosis of CP based on the Mayo Clinic criteria.

6. **Answer: D.** Transesophageal echocardiography offers superior resolution and allows for more accurate assessment of pericardial thickness when compared to transthoracic echocardiography. Pericardial thickness of ≥3 mm on transesophageal echocardiography has been reported to be 95% sensitive and 86% specific for the detection of a thickened pericardium (confirmed by computed tomography). **Figure 27.15** shows a transesophageal echocardiogram (4-chamber transverse plane view) and the corresponding transaxial computed tomographic image from a patient with a markedly thickened pericardium (up to 18 mm) over the right side of the heart (reproduced from http://circ.ahajournals.org). White arrows point to the thickened pericardium (P).

Table 27.3. Principal Echocardiographic Findings in Constrictive Pericarditis

Finding	Comment
Ventricular septal shift with respiration	2D and M-mode; septum shifts toward LV during inspiration and toward RV during expiration
Variation in mitral inflow pulsed-wave Doppler velocities with respiration	Reduced velocity during inspiration; variation will typically be 15%-35%
Preserved or increased mitral annular tissue Doppler velocities	Medial e' typically ≥9 cm/s; medial e' will often be higher than lateral e'; note that tissue Doppler will be less reliable in the setting of concomitant myocardial disease
Hepatic vein expiratory diastolic flow reversals (pulsed-wave Doppler)	May be technically challenging to perform
IVC plethora	Typically >21 mm diameter and/or <50% collapse with "sniff"
Unique myocardial strain profile	Typically preserved global longitudinal strain with reduced lateral wall compared to septal; reduced circumferential strain

IVC, inferior vena cava; LV, left ventricular; RV, right ventricular.

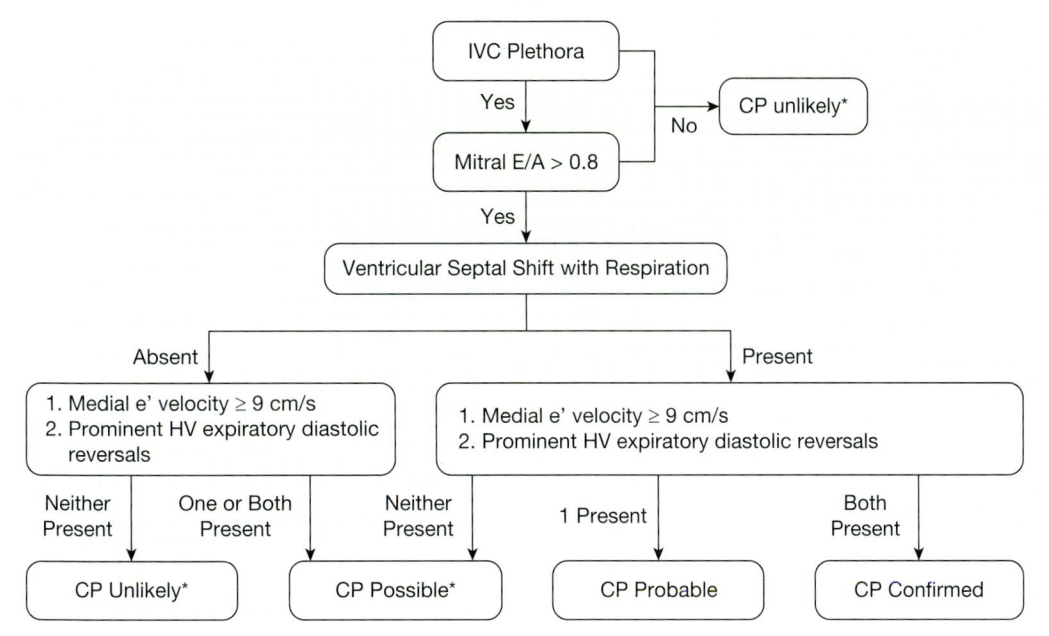

Chapter 27 Pericardial Diseases / 589

Figure 27.14. Suggested algorithm for the echocardiographic diagnosis of constrictive pericarditis (CP), based on the Mayo Clinic criteria. HV, hepatic vein; IVC, inferior vena cava. (Adapted by permission from Nature: Syed FF, Schaff HV, Oh JK. Constrictive pericarditis–a curable diastolic heart failure. *Nat Rev Cardiol.* 2014;11(9):530-544. Copyright © 2014 Springer Nature.)

7. **Answer: C.** One of the features of a hemodynamically significant pericardial effusion is right ventricular early diastolic collapse and/or right atrial late diastolic (often extending into systole) collapse. This 2D echocardiographic sign usually reflects that pericardial fluid has accumulated to the elastic limit of the pericardial sac, causing a significant increase in pericardial pressure. Increasing the pressure beyond this point will be at the expense of the cardiac chambers with the lowest pressures and will typically be reflected as indentation of right-sided chambers during diastole. However, when right-sided pressures are abnormally high, as in severe pulmonary hypertension, pressures of the RV and RA may be elevated to levels equal to or even higher than that of the pericardial pressure, thus preventing right-sided diastolic collapse. In this case, the first chamber to exhibit diastolic collapse may be the left atrium. The other answer choices would not prevent RV diastolic collapse in tamponade. Refer to **Table 27.1** for a summary of the clinical features of tamponade.

8. **Answer: A.** Hepatic vein diastolic flow reversal during expiration is a classic feature of constrictive pericarditis (CP). During expiration, left-sided cardiac filling is favored, as the pulmonary-venous-to-left-atrium gradient is restored (after being reduced during inspiration; see also the answer explanation for Question 4). The increased left-sided filling can only be accommodated by a shift in the position of the interventricular septum toward the right. This creates a relatively smaller and less-compliant right ventricle and is manifested in the hepatic vein as a reversal of flow in late-diastole. In contrast, reversal of hepatic vein flow occurs most prominently during inspiration in restrictive cardiomyopathy. Severe

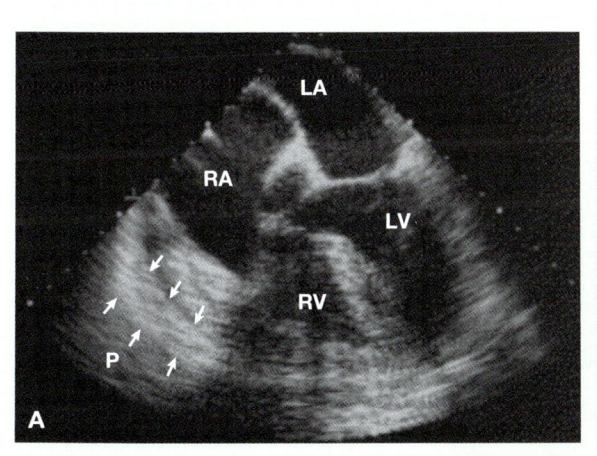

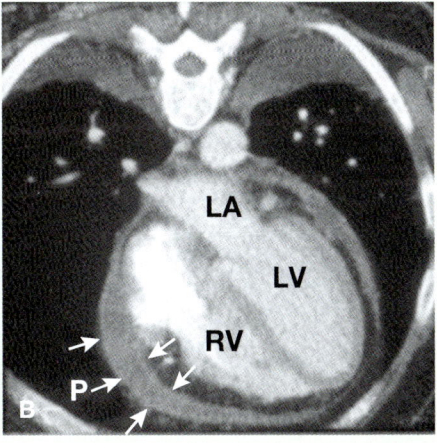

Figure 27.15

tricuspid regurgitation would typically correspond to the reversal of systolic flow in the hepatic veins, which is most prominent during inspiration.

9. **Answer: A.** A preserved or increased medial e' velocity is an important clue that suggests constriction in a patient with a heart failure syndrome. In a large study evaluating patients with constriction vs those with restriction or severe tricuspid regurgitation, a cut point of medial e' ≥9 cm/s was found to be best for identifying constriction. It should be noted that patients with radiation-induced CP may be exceptions to this "rule" as concomitant myocardial disease may decrease the e' velocity. The relationship between the medial and lateral e' values should also be assessed when evaluating for CP. In patients who do not have CP, mitral lateral e' velocity is higher than the medial e' velocity. In CP, the medial e' velocity often exceeds the lateral, which has been termed *annulus reversus*. This finding is likely due to the tethering of the lateral wall by the diseased pericardium.

10. **Answer: A.** There are two fundamental pathophysiologic mechanisms that underlie many of the echocardiographic findings in CP: (1) dissociation of intrathoracic and intracardiac pressures and (2) ventricular interdependence (also termed "enhanced ventricular interaction"). In patients with CP, the pulmonary venous pressure is influenced by the inspiratory fall in thoracic pressure, whereas the LV pressure is shielded from respiratory pressure variations in the diseased pericardium. Thus, inspiration lowers the pulmonary venous, but not left-sided intracardiac pressures (at least to the same degree), thereby decreasing the pressure gradient for ventricular filling. The less favorable filling pressure gradient during inspiration reduces LV filling and is evident in the decreased transmitral filling velocities (E velocities). The reduced LV filling leads to shift in the ventricular septum to the left and helps allow for augmented RV filling. These changes are all reversed during expiration: left-sided cardiac filling is restored, the ventricular septum shifts to the right, and RV filling decreases. Answer B is incorrect because ventricular interdependence is increased in CP. Answers C and D refer to the relationship between intrathoracic and extrathoracic pressures, which would not be expected to cause ventricular filling variation in CP.

11. **Answer: B.** Abnormal ventricular septal motion, in general, may be seen in a variety of clinical situations, including after cardiac surgery, with left bundle branch block or pacing, with right ventricular pressure and/or volume overload states, and in CP. There is, however, a distinctive type of abnormal ventricular septal motion, termed "respirophasic septal shift," that is more specific for CP. In CP, total cardiac volume is fixed by the noncompliant pericardium. The ventricles fill at the expense of each other, and shifting of the ventricular septum allows this to happen. During inspiration, right ventricular filling is favored, and the septum shifts to the left (**Figure 27.16**, arrow 1); the opposite occurs during expiration. Refer to the answers to questions 4 and 10 for additional details about the mechanism for this phasic alteration in filling of the ventricles. Note that the respirophasic septal shift is distinct from the beat-to-beat "bounce" or "shudder" (**Figure 27.16**, arrow 2) that can also be seen in CP. The beat-to-beat movement is probably due to ventricular interdependence on a millisecond timescale based

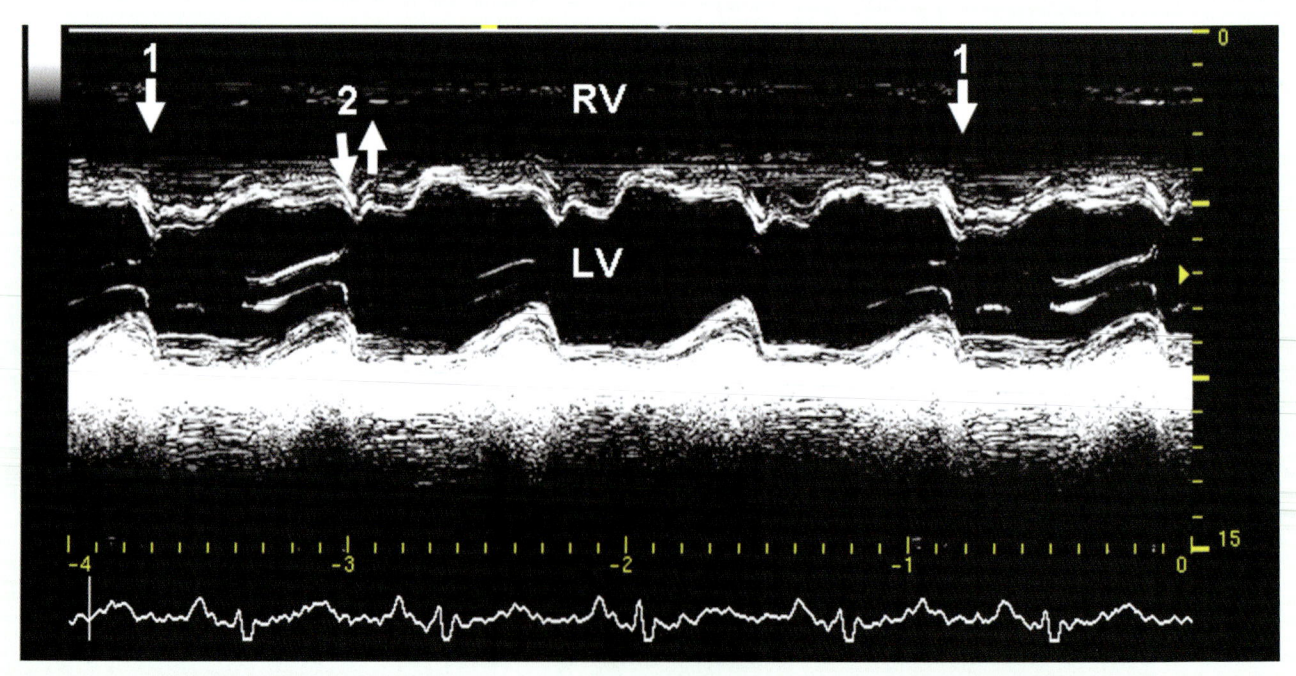

Figure 27.16

on hemodynamic work published from the Mayo Clinic but is deemed a less reliable clinical sign of CP because it is hard to differentiate from other types of abnormal septal motion (such as with conduction abnormalities, etc.). A B-bump is an M-mode sign of diastolic dysfunction, and neither this, nor the other choices, would be expected in CP.

12. **Answer: A.** Demonstration of constrictive physiology (ventricular interdependence) and elevated filling pressures (in the absence of hypovolemia) are key requisites for the diagnosis of CP and can occur in the absence of a thickened pericardium. Significant pulmonary hypertension and more than mild atrial enlargement are not typical features of CP.

13. **Answer: C.** Severe COPD or asthma can sometimes be accompanied by marked intrathoracic pressure swings that impact right and left ventricular filling and create the appearance of constriction in the absence of any pericardial pathology. Assessment of the SVC Doppler profile is a helpful means for distinguishing CP from obstructive pulmonary disease in these situations. Patients with obstructive pulmonary disease have a marked increase in inspiratory superior vena cava systolic flow velocity (**Figure 27.17A**, arrows), which is not seen in those with CP (**Figure 27.17B**). Prominent respiratory variation in mitral E velocity, with the highest mitral E velocity after the onset of expiration, can be present in patients with CP and COPD. The same is true for a respirophasic ventricular septal shift, which occurs in CP but can also appear in COPD when intrathoracic pressure swings are marked. The transmitral inflow pattern is more likely to be restrictive (E/A ≥ 2) in CP than in COPD.

14. **Answer: C.** The most common primary neoplasm of the heart associated with pericardial effusion is angiosarcoma. The majority of cardiac angiosarcomas arise as mural masses in the right atrium. Typically, they completely replace the atrial wall and fill the entire cardiac chamber. They may invade adjacent structures (eg, vena cava, tricuspid valve). These tumors are typically both symptomatic and rapidly fatal. Extensive pericardial spread and encasement of the heart often occur. Note, however, that the most common tumors to affect the pericardium and cause effusion are metastatic.

15. **Answer: B.** The most common location of a pericardial cyst is in the right cardiophrenic angle. A pericardial cyst appears as a round fluid-filled density, usually 2 to 4 cm in diameter, although sometimes larger.

16. **Answer: A.** Loculated pericardial effusions can cause significant hemodynamic compromise, depending on location and size, and may be most likely to occur after cardiac surgery. Features of pericardial constriction can be transient and may resolve with the use of anti-inflammatory drugs. Features of cardiac tamponade are not entirely dependent upon the volume of pericardial fluid collection; the rate of fluid collection is very important, and rapidly accumulated small effusions can still cause tamponade. Longstanding chronic CP may be associated with concomitant myocardial diseases (particularly in patients who have received chest radiation therapy) or lead to epicardial fibrosis and myocardial atrophy.

17. **Answer: C.** Absence of the pericardium is associated with the enlargement of the right ventricle and shift of the heart to the left, resulting in more of the right ventricle being seen on the routine left parasternal echocardiogram. Unusual windows for obtaining traditional-appearing images of the left ventricle are often needed. Acute pericarditis may be associated with pericardial thickening or effusion, but often there are no diagnostic echocardiographic findings. CP has typical hemodynamic features that cannot be identified on still-frame 2D echocardiographic images. A pericardial cyst is a round fluid-filled structure, most commonly located at the right cardiophrenic angle.

18. **Answer: A.** Left pleural effusions can present as large echo-free spaces that resemble pericardial effusions. These can be recognized because they appear as very large posterior spaces without any anterior

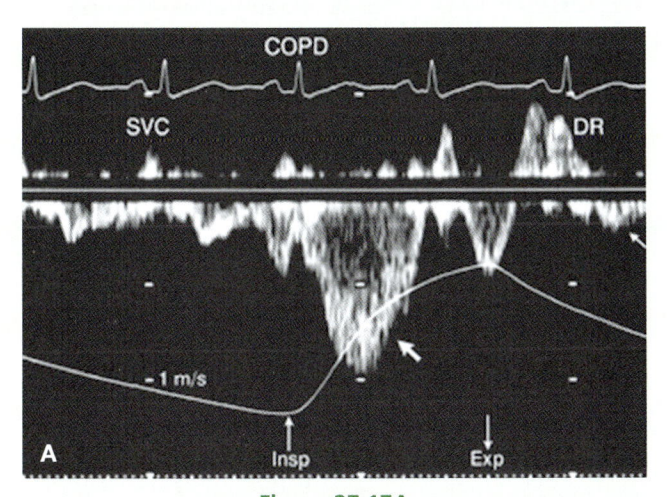

Figure 27.17A

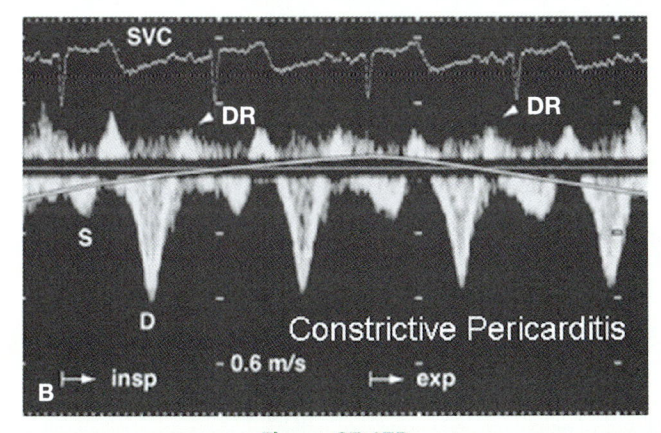

Figure 27.17B

component. Generally, in the parasternal long-axis view, pleural effusions are located posterior to the descending aorta, whereas pericardial effusions are located anterior to the aorta.

19. **Answer: B.** Pericardial fluid can become loculated or compartmentalized, and in this example, it is located adjacent to the left heart in the subcostal image shown. Loculated fluid in the pericardium under pressure may produce severe hemodynamic instability. Small effusions are generally confined to the region behind the left ventricle when the patient is in a supine position and may appear to vanish when the patient sits up, as they drain to the apical region.

20. **Answer: C.** This patient has a large loculated anterior pericardial effusion. Pericardial fluid typically appears as an echo-free space on two-dimensional imaging. Pericardial fat usually can be distinguished from fluid because of the characteristic subtle echotexture of the adipose tissue. In addition, pericardial fat remains constant in size throughout the cardiac cycle. A pleural effusion will be seen outside of the parietal pericardium.

21. **Answer: D.** **Figure 27.5** shows M-mode features of early diastolic collapse of the right ventricular free wall in cardiac tamponade. The yellow arrows point to right ventricular diastolic collapse. The * denotes the pericardial effusion. The primary abnormality is compression of all cardiac chambers due to increased pericardial pressure. The pericardium has some degree of elasticity; but once the elastic limit is reached, the ventricles must compete with each other for the fixed volume determined by the increased intrapericardial pressure. Ultimately, pericardial pressure rises to the point that chamber collapse occurs and cardiac filling and output fall. The other answer choices would not lead to right ventricular diastolic collapse.

22. **Answer: A.** The respiratory variation of mitral and tricuspid flow velocities in cardiac tamponade is greatly increased and out of phase, reflecting the increased ventricular interdependence in which the hemodynamics of the left and right heart chambers are directly influenced by each other to a much greater degree than normal. The pathophysiology of tamponade relates to the effect of the excessive pericardial fluid limiting cardiac filling as the cardiac chambers compete with the pericardial fluid in the "fixed" and noncompliant space. Ventricular diastolic filling is reduced because of reduced inflow pressure gradients. Inspiration increases venous return to the right heart, with a simultaneous decrease in left heart filling, while expiration increases left heart filling with decrease in right heart filling. This explains the opposite respiratory variation of mitral and tricuspid inflow by Doppler echocardiography. For peak mitral E inflow velocity, the maximal drop occurs with the first beat of inspiration, and there is typically >30% variation when compared with the first beat of expiration. The formal calculation of this would entail the following: [(expiratory velocity – inspiratory velocity)/expiratory velocity × 100]. For peak tricuspid E inflow velocity, the maximal drop is on the first beat of expiration, and there is typically >60% variation when compared with the first beat of inspiration. Significant respiratory variation of the mitral and tricuspid inflows should not be used as a stand-alone criterion for tamponade; the presence of chamber collapse increases specificity for tamponade significantly. Finding abnormal venous flow in the hepatic vein or superior vena cava is also helpful in the diagnosis of tamponade. Expected findings include marked systolic over diastolic component, expiratory accentuation of this difference, and expiratory reversal of diastolic flow. See **Table 27.4** for a summary of the reported test performance characteristics for the principal echocardiographic features of tamponade. With CP, the pattern of mitral and tricuspid flow variation with respiration is comparable to that observed in cardiac tamponade, but typically less exaggerated (**Table 27.2**). In the case presented, the marked variation in Doppler flows and large effusion are

Table 27.4. Test Performance Characteristics for Echocardiographic Findings in Tamponade

	Sensitivity (%)	Specificity (%)
Any Collapse	90	65
RA Collapse	68	66
RV Collapse	60	90
RA + RV Collapse	45	92
Abnormal Venous Flow[a]	75	91
Abnormal Venous Flow + 1 Collapse	67	91
Abnormal Venous Flow + 2 Collapses	37	98

Adapted from Merce J, Sagrista-Sauleda J, Permanyer-Miralda G, Evangelista A, Soler-Soler J. Correlation between clinical and Doppler echocardiographic findings in patients with moderate and large pericardial effusion: implications for the diagnosis of cardiac tamponade. *Am Heart J*. 1999;138(4 pt 1):759-764. Copyright © 1999 Elsevier. With permission.
[a]Abnormal venous (hepatic vein or superior vena cava) defined as marked systolic over diastolic component, expiratory accentuation of this difference, and expiratory reversal of diastolic flow.

most consistent with tamponade, and would not be seen as a normal pattern or with pulmonary hypertension.

23. **Answer: C.** In CP, the diseased and inelastic pericardium restricts total cardiac volume, which can cause abnormalities of LV wall motion during diastole. With its high temporal resolution, M-mode provides an important opportunity to evaluate such wall motion. The first arrow notes the abnormal early diastolic oscillatory motion of the interventricular septum, which might be best termed a "shudder." This appears to be related to ventricular interdependence on a millisecond timescale. The second arrow denotes the steep movement of the left ventricular inferolateral wall in early diastole before it meets the limit imposed by the constrictive pericardium and abruptly "flattens." An effusion is not shown in the M-mode recording. Congenitally absent pericardium would not be expected to have these signature M-mode findings and is better diagnosed with 2D echocardiography.

24. **Answer: B.** In contrast to the direct correlation between E/e′ and PCWP in patients with myocardial disease, an inverse relationship is generally seen in patients with CP (**Figure 27.18**), in a phenomenon termed *annulus paradoxus*. In contrast to other forms of heart failure, in which reduction in mitral annular velocities (both medial and lateral) is expected, constriction is typically associated with normal to exaggerated mitral annular velocities, particularly at the medial annulus (given that the lateral annulus is likely to be able to move less due to the overlying diseased pericardium). As the constriction becomes more severe, it is postulated that the medial mitral e′ becomes more exaggerated. Therefore, the E/e′ ratio may actually decrease progressively, even as filling pressures are increasing. Note that a study from the Cleveland Clinic cast some doubt as to the reliability of this finding; this may have been due to the heterogeneity of patients with constriction in the study, but regardless, *annulus paradoxus* should not be considered a key criterion for the diagnosis of constriction

25. **Answer: C.** Hepatic vein diastolic flow reversal with expiration suggests CP, even when the transmitral flow velocity pattern may not be diagnostic. Hepatic vein flow reversal that increases with expiration reflects enhanced ventricular interaction (also termed ventricular interdependence) and dissociation of intracardiac and intrathoracic pressures. During expiration, left ventricular filling is favored and the ventricular septum shifts toward the right, ultimately leading to the reversal of flow in the hepatic vein. The white arrow in **Figure 27.9** refers to hepatic vein diastolic reversal. Forward flow augmentation in the hepatic veins is most evident during inspiration and not expiration. Inspiratory diastolic flow reversals are characteristic of RCM, and inspiratory systolic flow reversals are characteristic of severe tricuspid regurgitation.

26. **Answer: B.** The irregular echodensity attached to the pericardium most likely represents metastatic disease, of the answer choices provided. Acute pericarditis may not cause discernible changes on a transthoracic echocardiogram or may be associated with pericardial thickening or a new pericardial effusion (typically an echo-free space); sometimes the pericardial effusion may contain inflammatory material such as fibrinous strands, but a mass like the one shown would not be expected. A pericardial cyst is a round, fluid-filled (echo-free space) structure, most common at the right cardiophrenic angle. A pleural effusion usually manifests as an echo-free space within the pleural cavity. Metastatic lesions are the most common neoplasms to affect the heart and to cause pericardial disease.

27. **Answer: B.** CP is typically marked by unique respiration-related shifting of the interventricular septum; this is considered one of the more sensitive findings for CP. The respiration-related septal shift in CP is caused by the dissociation of intrathoracic and intracardiac pressures and ventricular interdependence described in the answers to Questions 4, 10, and 11. During inspiration, left-heart filling decreases and right-heart filling is favored, with a shift in the septum toward the left. During expiration, left-heart filling increases at the expense of right-heart filling and the septum shifts back to the right. Identifying this finding typically requires extended 2D and M-mode clips of the septum in multiple views. See **Figure 27.19** and accompanying Video 27.4 for examples. Answers A and C describe the opposite of what would be expected. Answer D describes the persistent septal flattening toward the left that can be seen with severe right-heart pressure overload.

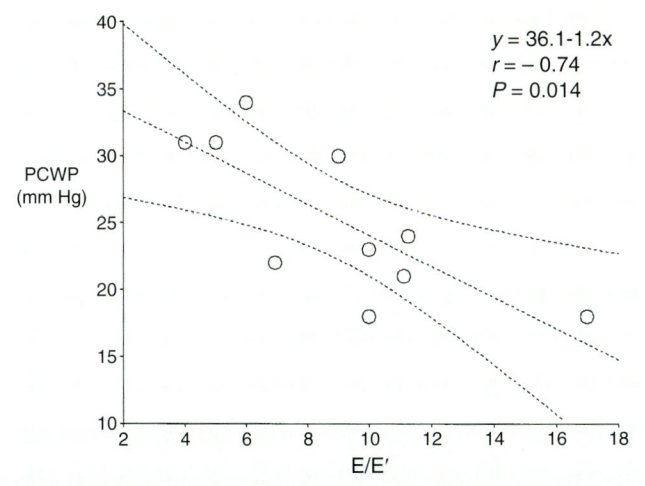

Figure 27.18. Reprinted with permission from Ha JW, Oh JK, Ling LH, Nishimura RA, Seward JB, Tajik AJ. Annulus paradoxus: transmitral flow velocity to mitral annular velocity ratio is inversely proportional to pulmonary capillary wedge pressure in patients with constrictive pericarditis. *Circulation*. 2001;104(9):976-978.

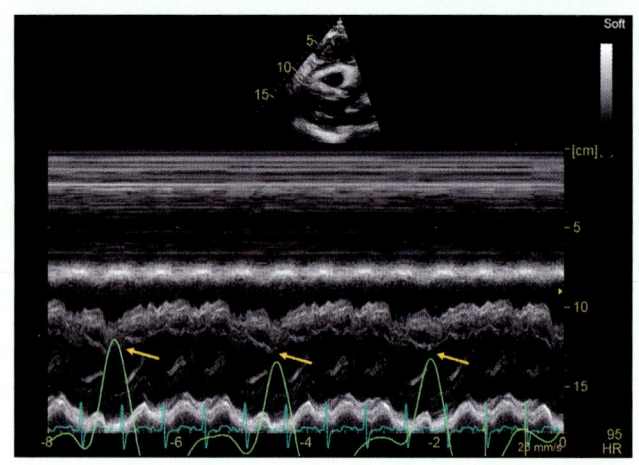

Figure 27.19. Respiration-related ventricular septal shift in constrictive pericarditis. M-mode recording through the ventricular septum in the parasternal long-axis view. The orange arrows mark the shift of the interventricular septum toward the left during inspiration.

28. **Answer: C.** The term *annulus reversus* refers to the reversed relationship of the medial and lateral e′ velocities in patients with CP as compared to most normal patients and those with RCM or other forms of heart failure. In patients without CP, the lateral mitral annular velocity will typically be higher than the medial mitral annular velocity. In CP, the lateral annulus is thought to be tethered by the adherent pericardium, which reduces the lateral e′ velocity; the medial annulus, on the other hand, is not tethered, and medial e′ velocities can become higher than the lateral e′ velocities. But even more important than *annulus reversus* is the concept that in CP, mitral annular velocities tend to be normal or even supranormal, which stands in contrast to RCM and essentially all other forms of heart failure, which nearly always are characterized by low e′ velocities. A reversed relation between E/e′ and left atrial pressure is called *annulus paradoxus*; as previously described in question 24, this phenomenon occurs because the accentuated e′ velocities decrease the E/e′ ratio in CP, despite high filling pressures.

29. **Answer: A. Figure 27.11** shows significant respiratory variations in mitral E velocity (lower velocity during inspiration and higher during expiration) and a hepatic vein Doppler pattern (reversal of flow in late diastole during expiration) that are consistent with the diagnostic criteria for CP by Doppler echocardiography. Also expected would be a respiration-related ventricular septal shift and preserved or increased mitral annular e′ velocities (typically with the medial being greater than the lateral). These clinical and echocardiographic features, coupled with the MRI findings (delayed gadolinium enhancement of the pericardium signifies inflammation) are consistent with acute inflammatory pericarditis with constriction. CP in such a situation may resolve spontaneously, but should generally be managed with anti-inflammatory therapy in the hope of faster recovery and a lower likelihood of progression to chronic constriction. The typical first-line therapy would include a nonsteroidal anti-inflammatory agent plus colchicine for two to 3 months or longer; for those with contraindications to this therapy, or for those whose syndromes remain refractory, glucocorticoid therapy is typically employed. Interleukin-1 inhibitor therapy could also be considered as an alternative to glucocorticoid therapy, although it has not been specifically studied in inflammatory constrictive pericarditis without pericardial pain. Diuretics can be used to improve symptoms related to congestion. Pericardiocentesis would not be the next best step, given the small size of the effusion, absence of tamponade features, and lack of any evidence for infection. Pericardial biopsy is not the next best step and is not commonly employed, but could be considered if there is no response to treatment over the next several weeks. Pericardiectomy is generally reserved for patients whose inflammatory constriction has transitioned into chronic fibrotic constriction despite maximal medical therapies.

30. **Answer: B.** The resolution of edema and pleural effusion with documentation of reduction in pericardial thickening on the computed tomography scan is consistent with the diagnosis of transient pericardial constriction. In some cases, inflammatory constriction may transition into chronic fibrotic CP, which would be characterized by continued clinical and imaging findings of CP. The presentation and course are not suggestive of myocarditis or familial Mediterranean fever.

> **KEY POINT**
> - In the absence of symptoms that suggest chronicity of disease (eg, cachexia, atrial fibrillation, hepatic dysfunction, or pericardial calcification), patients with newly diagnosed CP who are hemodynamically stable and have some evidence of inflammation using biomarkers (CRP and ESR) or imaging (late gadolinium enhancement of the pericardium on cardiac MRI) may be given a trial of medical therapy (anti-inflammatory) for 3 to 6 months before pericardiectomy is recommended.

31. **Answer: B.** Apical 2-chamber and short-axis views of the left ventricle in ▶ **Video 27.1A,B** show marked thickening of the parietal and visceral pericardium with a small loculated pericardial effusion. **Figure 27.12** shows increased respiratory variation of transmitral flow. Both these features, and the apparent absence of any elevation in venous pressure, suggest the presence of occult effusive CP (relatively rare presentation, most likely in a hypovolemic patient). The presence of the pericardial effusion and constrictive

hemodynamics makes effusive CP, rather than CP or a simple loculated effusion, the best answer. There is no evidence for a pericardial neoplasm.

32. **Answer: A.** Significant pericardial disease can exist without overt manifestations. Occult constrictive pericardial disease is identified by normal baseline hemodynamics and normal LV systolic function with a characteristic response to rapid volume infusion. Following the intravenous administration of 1000 mL of normal saline over 6 to 8 minutes, striking elevations of filling pressures are seen during cardiac catheterization along with more marked manifestation of ventricular interdependence on simultaneous right and left ventricular pressure tracings. The remainder of the answers would predominantly affect afterload and preload and would not be expected to help demonstrate constrictive physiology.

> **KEY POINT**
> - In some patients, physical and hemodynamic features of constriction are not apparent in their baseline state; but when rapidly fluid challenged, they will present a typical hemodynamic CP pattern. This subtype is called occult CP (or occult effusive CP, if a pericardial effusion is present).

33. **Answer: C.** The absence of any chamber collapse signifies less hemodynamic effect from the effusion, and therefore makes clinical tamponade much less likely. Cardiac tamponade is a situation in which abnormal pericardial fluid contents raise the pericardial pressure and impair the ability of the cardiac chambers to fill. When the pericardial pressure exceeds the cardiac chamber pressure, collapse of that chamber on the echocardiogram will be noted, and this is considered a hallmark sign of tamponade. Right-sided chamber collapse is most likely as those chambers typically have lower diastolic pressure than the left-sided chambers. Right atrial collapse occurs the earliest and has the best specificity for tamponade when it persists for 1/3 or more of the cardiac cycle. Tamponade is also typically associated with marked variation in mitral E velocities and blunted or reversed diastolic flow in the hepatic veins during expiration. ▶ **Video 27.5** shows an example of chamber collapse in tamponade.

34. **Answer: D.** The echocardiographic clip shows the pericardial space containing a cloud of echogenic bubbles after the injection of agitated saline via the pericardiocentesis needle. Although pericardiocentesis has been shown to be a relatively safe procedure, there are hazards, with one of the most feared being myocardial perforation. Having the opportunity to clearly outline the space from which the fluid is withdrawn is therefore of particular interest in maximizing the safety of the procedure. A current technique of echocardiography with saline contrast enhancement involves the injection of a few milliliters of agitated saline solution. In the pericardium, contrast movement is slow and swirling and has a longer half-life. Performing this procedure helps in ensuring that the catheter is within the pericardial cavity and not within the cardiac chambers. Stranding within the pericardial space is seen most often in inflammatory pericarditis and appears as linear attachments across the pericardial space from the parietal to the visceral pericardium. Blood coagulum would typically appear as a semi-organized echodensity within the pericardial space and be less free-flowing than the agitated saline bubbles. Spontaneous echo contrast is typically seen at sites of blood stasis as in the left atrium in some patients with atrial fibrillation.

> **KEY POINT**
> - Tamponade requires the removal of fluid from the pericardium to restore normal cardiac filling and output. Agitated saline contrast echocardiography is a simple, effective technique that aids the localization of needle position during pericardiocentesis.

35. **Answer: C.** The upper panel in **Figure 27.13** shows respiratory changes in the hepatic vein flow Doppler velocity profile. The presence of exaggerated diastolic flow reversals suggests CP. The lower panel in **Figure 27.13** shows relatively minor respiratory changes in transmitral flow velocities. Sometimes, in the setting of markedly high cardiac filling pressures, the expected respiratory changes in transmitral filling velocities can be muted. To bring out these changes, repeat transmitral Doppler evaluation with the patient in a head up tilt, or while seated or post-diuresis, should be considered. These maneuvers reduce preload and may accentuate the dissociation of intrathoracic and intracardiac pressures; this leads to the augmentation of the corresponding respiratory changes in transmitral filling velocities. The other answer choices would augment preload.

36. **Answer: B.** CP would be suggested by a preserved mitral medial e′ (typically ≥9 cm/s), and particularly one that exceeds the lateral e′, as previously discussed in Question 28. The tissue Doppler velocities in answer A would be more likely in a patient with restrictive cardiomyopathy. A consistently flattened ventricular septum would be most suggestive of severe pulmonary hypertension. A small and collapsing IVC would suggest normal venous pressure, which would be unusual in CP (see rare exception in "occult" CP as in questions 31 and 32).

KEY POINT

- A lack of typical respiratory transmitral flow velocity changes should not exclude the diagnosis of CP, particularly if other findings for CP are present; Some patients may have high enough filling pressures that mitral inflow variation becomes muted; imaging in the head up tilt or seated position will decrease preload and may help to bring out variation in transmitral velocities in these patients. While mitral inflow variation should be assessed as part of the CP workup, it is not one of the three (respiratory ventricular septal shift, mitral medial e' ≥9 cm/s, and hepatic vein expiratory diastolic flow reversals) most important diagnostic echo criteria for CP.

Table 27.5. Myocardial Mechanics in Constrictive Pericarditis (CP) and Restrictive Cardiomyopathy (RCM)

Deformation Parameter	CP	RCM
Longitudinal strain	Normal	Decreased
Longitudinal early diastolic velocity (e')	Normal or increased	Decreased
Regional longitudinal systolic strain ratio (lateral LV to septal LV)	Decreased	Normal
Circumferential strain	Decreased	Normal
Apical untwisting velocity	Decreased	Normal

37. **Answer: B.** Video 27.3A shows the apical 4-chamber view of the left ventricle longitudinal strain values obtained by speckle tracking imaging. With pericardial restraint and potential epicardial involvement, LV expansion in CP is limited in the circumferential rather than in the longitudinal direction. Accordingly, patients with CP typically have preserved longitudinal strain values but have reduced circumferential strain values. Note, however, that longitudinal strain values may be regionally affected by the adherent pericardium, with the antero-lateral LV and RV free walls being most likely to have reduced longitudinal strain values compared to the septum. See **Figure 27.20** for an example of longitudinal systolic strain values in CP, presented in a "bullseye" format. Also note that patients with radiation-induced CP may also have radiation-induced myocardial disease; in that case, global longitudinal strain may be reduced along with circumferential strain.

38. **Answer: D.** The relationship between different principal strains and myocardial rotation are presented in **Table 27.5**. It has been shown that the global longitudinal strain, whether measured by 2D speckle tracking echocardiography or feature tracking cardiac magnetic resonance, is of additive value to early diastolic mitral annular velocities (e') in differentiating CP from restrictive cardiomyopathy (RCM). Because longitudinal fibers are relatively spared in CP and are greatly affected in RCM, global longitudinal strain is significantly lower in patients with RCM compared to patients with CP. Patients with CP, on the other hand, usually have depressed LV rotation and circumferential strains compared to normal.

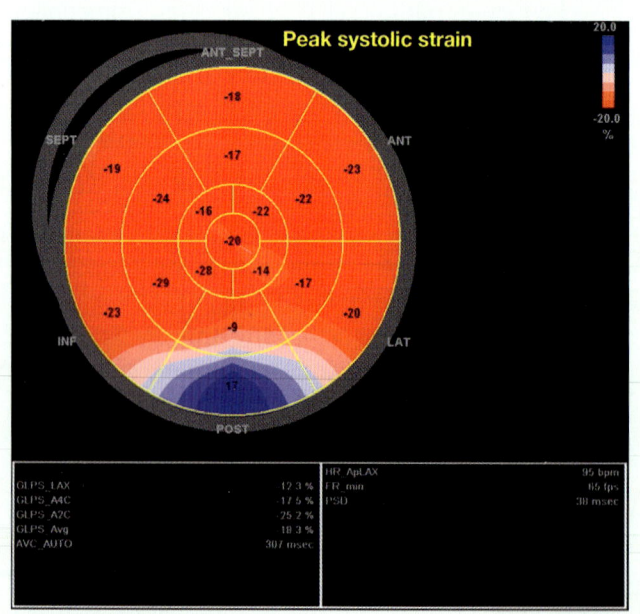

Figure 27.20. Strain imaging in constrictive pericarditis. Longitudinal systolic strain presented in a bullseye map demonstrates the overall preserved longitudinal systolic strain (average −19.1%). Inferolateral strain is prominently reduced compared to septal strain because of the tethering effects of the adherent, diseased pericardium. After pericardiectomy, the regional strain pattern normalizes (strain reversus)

KEY POINT

- Pericardial tethering in constriction limits rotational and circumferential mechanics of the left ventricle, whereas the longitudinal mechanics are relatively normal. Regional longitudinal mechanics may be depressed in CP in the anterolateral and RV free walls. These findings differ from those expected in RCM and make the assessment of myocardial strain a helpful part of the echocardiographic assessment.

SUGGESTED READINGS

Adler Y, Charron P, Imazio M, et al. 2015 ESC guidelines for the diagnosis and management of pericardial diseases: the Task Force for the diagnosis and management of pericardial diseases of the European Society of Cardiology (ESC)endorsed by—the European Association for Cardio-Thoracic Surgery (EACTS). *Eur Heart J*. 2015;36(42):2921-2964.

Alajaji W, Xu B, Sripariwuth A, et al. Noninvasive multimodality imaging for the diagnosis of constrictive pericarditis. *Circ Cardiovasc Imaging*. 2018;11(11):e007878.

Cosyns B, Plein S, Nihoyanopoulos P, et al. European Association of Cardiovascular Imaging (EACVI) position paper: multimodality imaging in pericardial disease. *Eur Heart J Cardiovasc Imaging*. 2015;16(1):12-31.

Hoit BD. Pericardial effusion and cardiac tamponade in the new millennium. *Curr Cardiol Rep*. 2017;19(7):57.

Klein AL, Abbara S, Agler DA, et al. American Society of Echocardiography clinical recommendations for multimodality cardiovascular imaging of patients with pericardial disease: endorsed by the Society for Cardiovascular magnetic resonance and Society of Cardiovascular computed tomography. *J Am Soc Echocardiogr*. 2013;26(9):965-1012.e15.

Klein A, Wang T, Cremer P, et al. Pericardial diseases: international position statement on new concepts and advances in multimodality cardiac imaging. *J Am Coll Cardiol Img*. 2024;8:937-988.

Kusunose K, Dahiya A, Popović ZB, et al. Biventricular mechanics in constrictive pericarditis comparison with restrictive cardiomyopathy and impact of pericardiectomy. *Circ Cardiovasc Imaging*. 2013;6(3):399-406.

Merce J, Sagrista-Sauleda J, Permanyer-Miralda G, Evangelista A, Soler-Soler J. Correlation between clinical and Doppler echocardiographic findings in patients with moderate and large pericardial effusion: implications for the diagnosis of cardiac tamponade. *Am Heart J*. 1999;138(4 pt 1):759-764.

Sengupta PP, Krishnamoorthy VK, Abhayaratna WP, et al. Disparate patterns of left ventricular mechanics differentiate constrictive pericarditis from restrictive cardiomyopathy. *JACC Cardiovasc Imaging*. 2008;1:29-38.

Spodick DH. Acute cardiac tamponade. *N Engl J Med*. 2003;349(7):684-690.

Syed FF, Schaff HV, Oh JK. Constrictive pericarditis—a curable diastolic heart failure. *Nat Rev Cardiol*. 2014;11(9):530-544.

Welch TD, Ling LH, Espinosa RE, et al. Echocardiographic diagnosis of constrictive pericarditis Mayo Clinic criteria. *Circ Cardiovasc Imaging*. 2014;7(3):526-534.

CHAPTER 28

Aortic Diseases

Alejandro Sanchez-Nadales, Craig R. Asher, and Gian M. Novaro

QUESTIONS

1. Which of the following statements is **CORRECT** regarding measurement of the ascending aorta by transthoracic echocardiography (TTE) in adults?
   A. The diameter should be measured during end systole.
   B. The size of the aorta should be interpreted in view of an individual's height.
   C. The tubular ascending aorta cannot be adequately visualized.
   D. The size of the aorta should be measured preferably by M-mode.

2. Which of the following statements is **CORRECT** regarding measurement of the ascending aorta by TTE in pediatric populations?
   A. The aorta should be measured in systole.
   B. The aorta should be measured by M-mode.
   C. The aorta should be measured using a leading edge–to–leading edge convention.
   D. The aortic size measurement in pediatric populations is no different than in adults.

3. Which of the following statements regarding aortic anomalies is **CORRECT**?
   A. A bovine aorta is defined as the left subclavian artery arising from the innominate artery.
   B. A bovine aortic branching pattern is present in 1% of individuals.
   C. A bovine aorta is readily detectable from a standard parasternal long-axis image.
   D. A bovine aorta is defined as the left common carotid artery arising from a common origin with the innominate artery.

4. In which of the following locations are complex aortic atheroma most likely to occur?
   A. Ascending aorta.
   B. Aortic arch.
   C. Innominate artery.
   D. Descending aorta.

5. The so-called "blind spot" which occurs when imaging the distal ascending aorta by transesophageal echocardiography (TEE) is most commonly created by acoustic interference from which structure?
   A. Sliding hiatal hernia.
   B. Transverse sinus.
   C. Trachea or bronchus.
   D. Azygos vein.

6. Which of the following statements is **CORRECT** regarding the findings on TEE in patients with a traumatic thoracic aortic deceleration injury?
   A. The most common finding is a type B dissection extending from above to below the diaphragm.
   B. The most common finding is a type B intramural hematoma extending from above to below the diaphragm.
   C. The most common finding is a type A dissection.
   D. The most common finding is a localized thick flap in the region of the aortic isthmus.

7. Which of the following statements is **CORRECT** regarding distinguishing the true lumen from the false lumen in a patient with an aortic dissection?
   A. The true lumen is usually bigger in size than the false lumen.
   B. The true lumen has delayed, slow flow with thrombosis.
   C. There is systolic expansion in the true lumen.
   D. The true lumen has predominantly retrograde flow.

8. An aneurysm of the ascending aorta is best characterized by which of the following definitions?
   A. Aortic dilatation to at least 2.0 times the expected normal diameter.
   B. Aortic dilatation to at least 1.5 times the size of the descending aorta.
   C. Aortic dilatation of ≥4.5 cm in an adult.
   D. Aortic dilatation of ≥4.0 cm in an adult.

9. Which of the following statements is **CORRECT** regarding Marfan syndrome–related aortic disease?
   A. Aortic aneurysms are primarily in the region above the aortic root.
   B. A descending aortic aneurysm without an ascending aortic aneurysm is rare.
   C. Isolated abdominal aortic aneurysms are common.
   D. An "onion bulb" appearance with dilatation of the aortic root with sinotubular effacement and a relatively normal size ascending aorta may be seen.

10. Which of the following statements regarding a right-sided aortic arch is **CORRECT**?
    A. The nonmirror image type may result in compression of the esophagus by an aberrant right subclavian artery.
    B. A diverticulum of Kommerell may be associated with an aberrant left subclavian artery and the nonmirror image type.
    C. The nonmirror image type is usually associated with congenital cardiac anomalies.
    D. The mirror image type often occurs with no other cardiac abnormalities.

11. Which of the following series of aortic dimensions would most likely be considered pathologic for a 30-year-old woman undergoing a TTE for chest pain?
    A. Annulus—2.2 cm; sinus—3.2 cm; ST junction—3.5 cm; tubular—3.6 cm.
    B. Annulus—2.0 cm; sinus—3.6 cm; ST junction—3.4 cm; tubular—3.4 cm.
    C. Annulus—2.3 cm; sinus—3.6 cm; ST junction—3.3 cm; tubular—3.4 cm.
    D. Annulus—1.9 cm; sinus—3.7 cm; ST junction—3.4 cm; tubular—3.6 cm.

12. Which of the following pairings of aortic abnormalities and disease states or syndromes is **BEST** described?
    A. Supravalvular aortic stenosis–Turner syndrome.
    B. Aortic coarctation–Shone complex.
    C. Aortic coarctation–Noonan syndrome.
    D. Supravalvular aortic stenosis–Down syndrome.

13. Which of the following anatomic abnormalities of the aorta is most likely to be associated with cyanotic heart disease requiring corrective surgery during infancy?
    A. An overriding aorta, malalignment VSD and minimal pulmonary stenosis.
    B. An aorta that is anterior to the pulmonary artery associated with atrioventricular discordance and ventricular-arterial discordance.
    C. An aorta that is anterior to the pulmonary artery associated with atrioventricular concordance and ventricular-arterial discordance.
    D. A periductal aorta–pulmonary connection with normal pulmonary pressure.

14. Which of the following statements regarding bicuspid aortic valve–associated aortic abnormalities is **CORRECT**?
    A. The tubular ascending aorta is usually the region with the greatest degree of dilatation.
    B. The aortopathy of bicuspid aortic valves rarely involves the aortic arch.
    C. Most patients with bicuspid aortic valves have predominant enlargement of the aortic sinuses.
    D. Approximately 20% of patients with a bicuspid aortic valve have coarctation of the aorta.

600 / Clinical Echocardiography Review

15. A 68-year-old man undergoes a cardiac catheterization which demonstrates no significant obstructive coronary artery disease. Within 1 hour after the catheterization, he complains of severe chest pain. The electrocardiogram is normal. An aortic dissection is diagnosed by a TEE. A cardiac surgeon is called. The cardiologist tells the surgeon that the dissection should be classified as a DeBakey type 2/Stanford A with a variant form limited, iatrogenic hematoma. Which of the following statements is **CORRECT**?
   A. There is an intramural aortic hematoma localized to the aortic arch.
   B. There is an intramural hematoma distal to the left subclavian artery.
   C. There is an intramural hematoma extending from the ascending aorta to the femoral artery.
   D. There is an intramural aortic hematoma in the ascending aorta.

16. A 67-year-old woman is admitted to the hospital with a 2-day history of hemianopsia. A head computed tomography scan reveals multiple ischemic infarcts suggestive of emboli and a TEE is performed to evaluate a source of embolism. Based on **Figure 28.1** showing the distal aortic arch, which of the following statements **BEST** describes the finding?
   A. There is a large vegetation.
   B. There is a large protruding atheromatous plaque.
   C. There is a localized intramural hematoma.
   D. There is a large aortic thrombus.

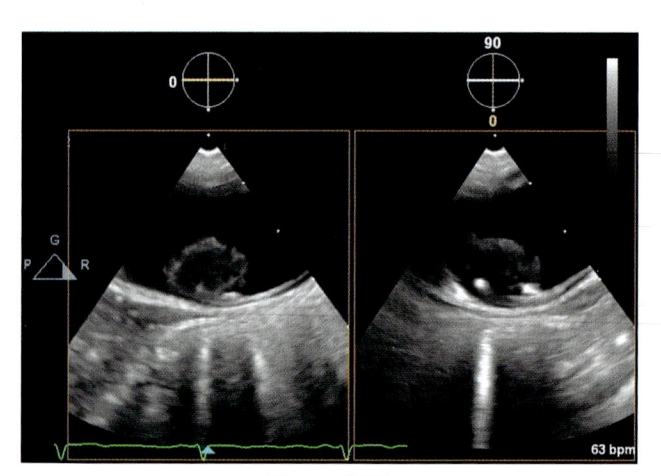

Figure 28.1

17. A 78-year-old man underwent a TEE for atrial fibrillation prior to cardioversion. Which of the following statements regarding the image of the upper descending thoracic aorta shown in **Figure 28.2** is **CORRECT**?
   A. There is grade 1 atheroma.
   B. There is grade 2 atheroma.
   C. There is grade 3 atheroma.
   D. There is grade 4 atheroma.

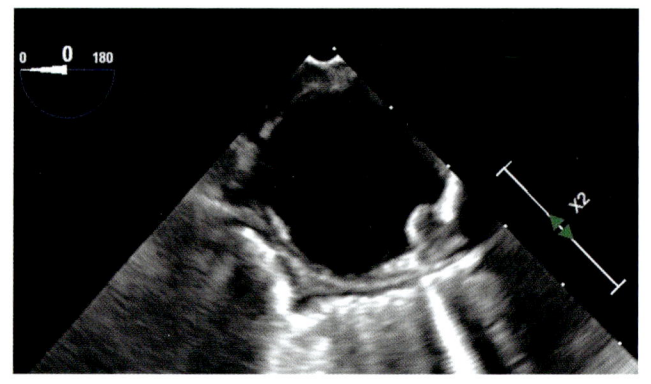

Figure 28.2

18. A 42-year-old woman underwent a TTE due to an episode of congestive heart failure. The aortic valve was found to be bicuspid. Which of the following statements is **CORRECT** regarding the two-dimensional echocardiographic, color Doppler, and continuous-wave Doppler tracing obtained from the suprasternal notch (**Figure 28.3** and Video 28.1)?
   A. The peak pressure gradient obtained by the simplified Bernoulli equation will equal the pressure gradient obtained at cardiac catheterization.
   B. The peak pressure gradient obtained by the simplified Bernoulli equation will be less than obtained at cardiac catheterization.
   C. The peak pressure gradient obtained by the simplified Bernoulli equation will be greater than obtained at cardiac catheterization.
   D. None of the above.

Chapter 28 Aortic Diseases / 601

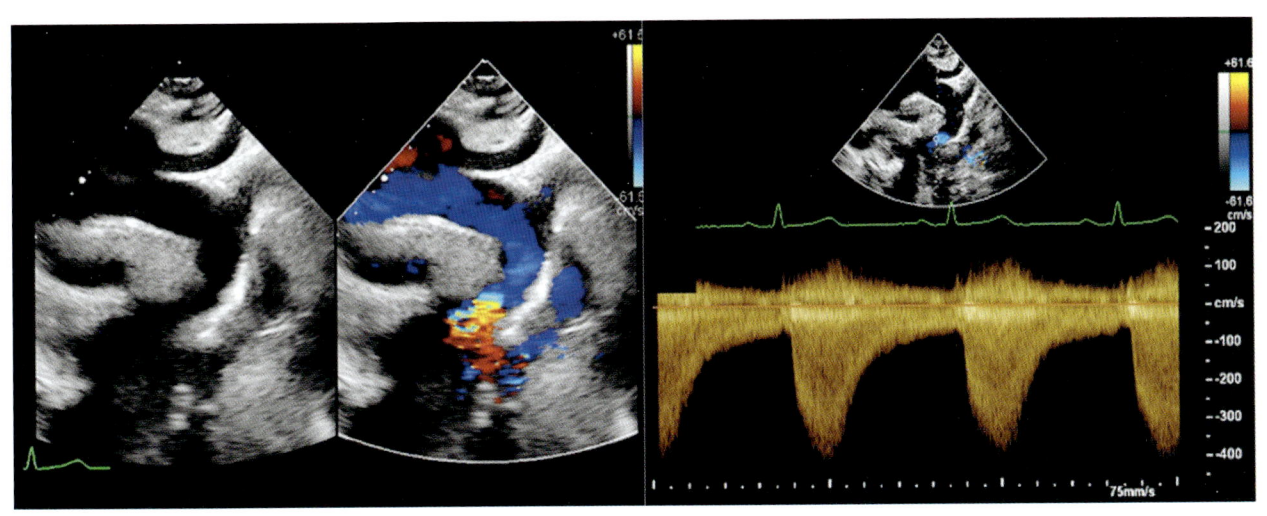

Figure 28.3

19. Match the numbers with the anatomic structure based on this TTE suprasternal notch image (**Figure 28.4**)?
  A. 1—right pulmonary artery; 2—left atrium; 3—transverse sinus; 4—innominate artery; 5—innominate vein.
  B. 1—left atrium; 2—transverse sinus; 3—right pulmonary artery; 4—innominate vein; 5—innominate artery.
  C. 1—left atrium; 2—right pulmonary artery; 3—transverse sinus; 4—innominate vein; 5—innominate artery.
  D. 1—right pulmonary artery; 2—left atrium; 3—transverse sinus; 4—innominate artery; 5—innominate vein.

20. A 47-year-old-woman presents with chest pain following a motor vehicle accident (MVA). She experienced blunt trauma hitting the steering wheel with no deployment of the airbags. Upon arrival to the ER, her vital signs are normal and physical examination is notable for absence of a heart murmur and equal pulses. An EKG is normal. A bedside echocardiogram is performed by the cardiology fellow in the ER and an abnormal aortic root image is seen in **Figure 28.5**.
Which of the following statements is most consistent with the clinical history and image shown?
  A. There is a localized aortic dissection.
  B. There is an aortic transection.
  C. There is a coronary anomaly.
  D. There is aortic calcification.

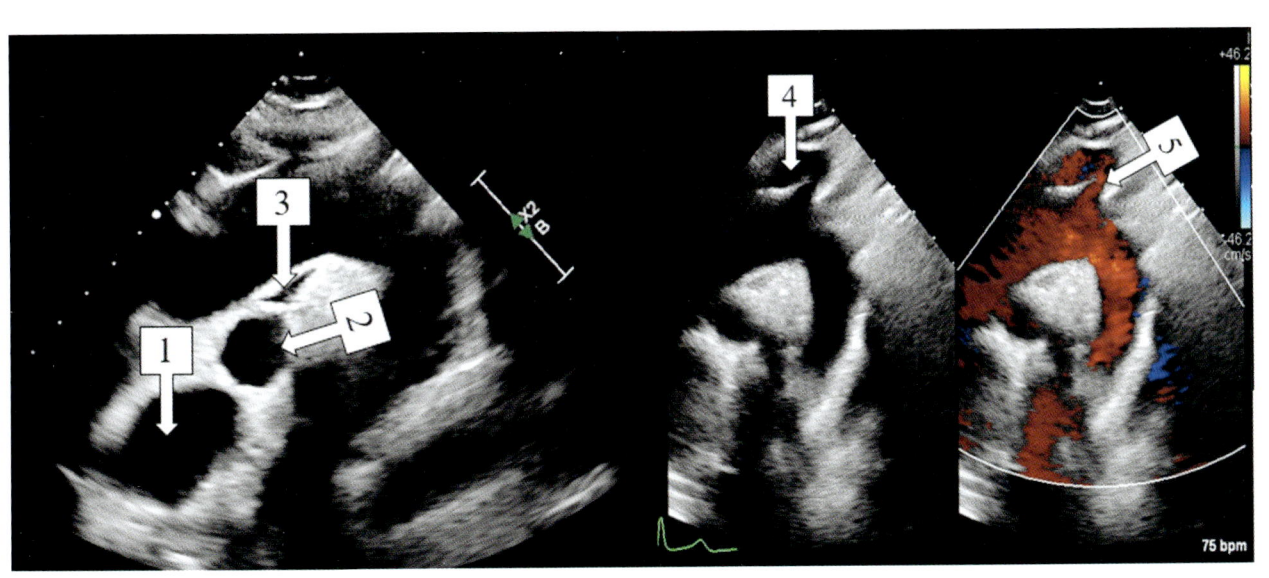

Figure 28.4

602 / Clinical Echocardiography Review

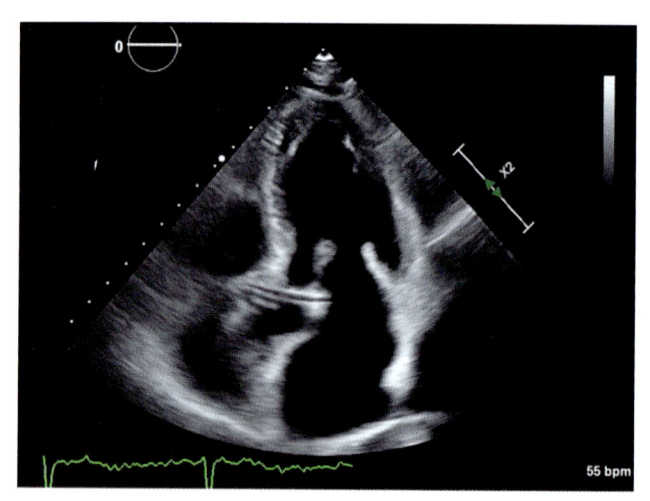

Figure 28.5

21. A 44-year-old man underwent TEE prior to cardioversion for atrial fibrillation. Based on the image in **Figure 28.6** and ▶ **Video 28.2** of the aortic valve, which of the following statements is **CORRECT** regarding associated findings?
  A. Aortic regurgitation is common but aortic aneurysms or dissections are not.
  B. Aortic root aneurysms are commonly associated.
  C. Aortic coarctation is commonly associated.
  D. Aortic dissection or rupture may occur without aortic dilatation.

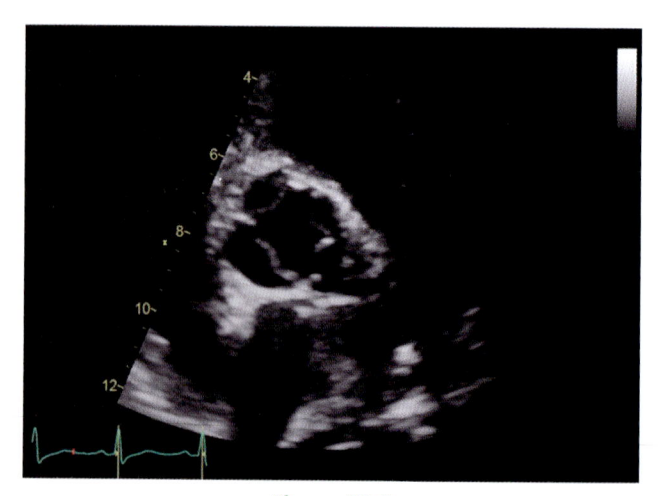

Figure 28.6

22. A 38-year-old man with bicuspid aortic valve disease and moderate aortic regurgitation is found to have an aortic aneurysm with the following dimensions (sinus of Valsalva—4.8 cm; sinotubular junction—4.7 cm; tubular ascending aorta—5.0 cm). Which of the following statements regarding the aorta in this patient is most accurate (**Figure 28.7**)?

  A. The aortic arch is not likely to be enlarged.
  B. The aortic arch is likely to be enlarged.
  C. The descending aorta is likely to be enlarged.
  D. A coarctation of the aorta is likely to be found.

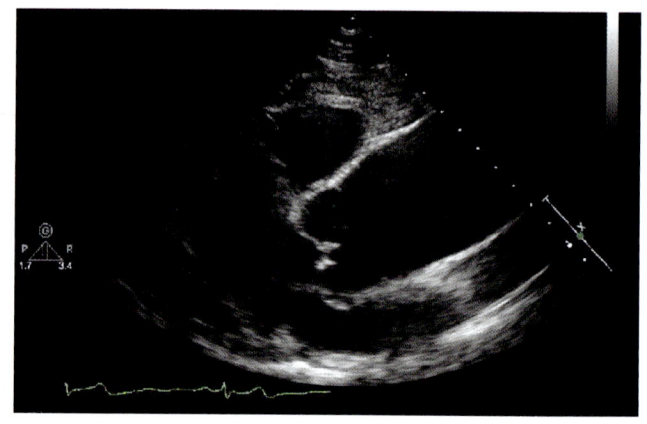

Figure 28.7

23. Which of the following statements is **CORRECT** regarding the TTE image, **Figure 28.8** of the ascending aorta?
  A. The image was most likely obtained from the suprasternal notch window.
  B. The image was most likely obtained from a standard parasternal window.
  C. The image was most likely obtained from a nonstandard parasternal window with lateral and inferior movement of the transducer.
  D. The image was most likely obtained from a nonstandard parasternal window with medial and superior movement of the transducer.

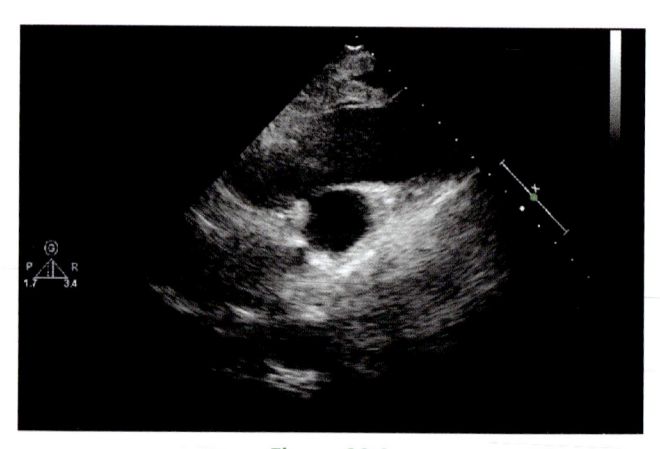

Figure 28.8

24. A 37-year-old man underwent a routine outpatient TTE because of palpitations. His physical examination is unremarkable. An abnormality is noted, which prompts a TEE. From the long-axis view in **Figure 28.9**, which of the following statements is **CORRECT** about the abnormality shown (see *arrow*)?
    A. It involves the left coronary cusp.
    B. It is usually a congenital anomaly.
    C. Rupture would likely be fatal due to cardiac tamponade.
    D. Rupture would likely be fatal due to aortic dissection.

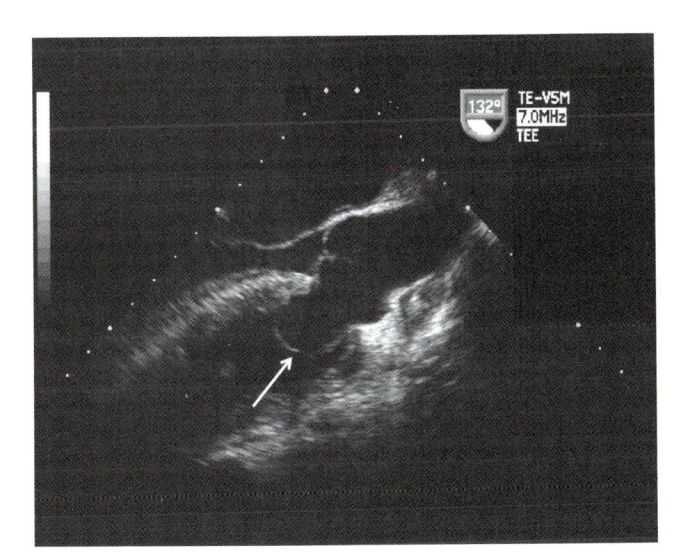

Figure 28.9

25. A 50-year-old woman underwent a TTE due to shortness of breath and a heart murmur. The image, **Figure 28.10** is obtained from the suprasternal notch (▶ **Video 28.3** parasternal short-axis view). Which of the following additional findings on this study would be most influential regarding determining the need for intervention?
    A. $Q_p/Q_s = 1.7$.
    B. Dilated left ventricle.
    C. Dilated right ventricle.
    D. Dilated right atrium.

26. A 73-year-old man with a history of hypertension and chronic kidney disease presented with the acute onset of chest pain radiating to his upper back. TEE was performed to rule out an acute aortic dissection. Based on **Figure 28.11**, which of the following statements is **CORRECT**?

A. A descending thoracic aortic pseudoaneurysm is present.
B. There is evidence of a type B aortic dissection.
C. A congenital vascular anomaly is detected.
D. Portion of a left pleural effusion can be seen.

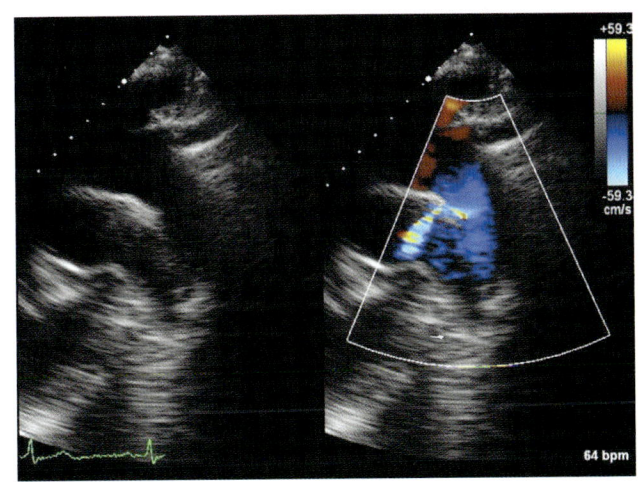

Figure 28.10

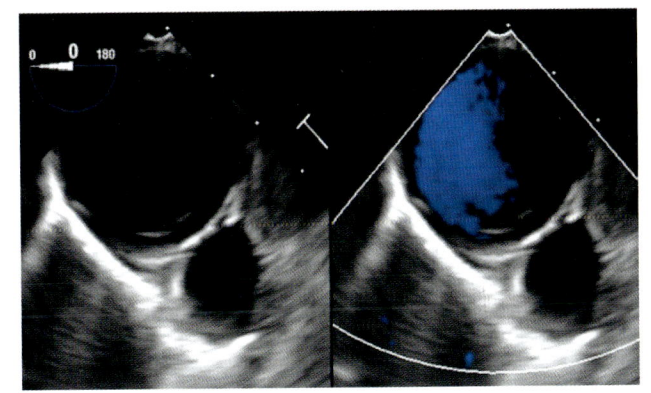

Figure 28.11

27. A 21-year-old woman with Turner syndrome underwent a surgical coarctation of the aorta repair as a child. She was lost to follow-up but now presents with poorly controlled blood pressure and claudication. Which of the following statements is **CORRECT** regarding the Doppler image obtained from the abdominal aorta shown in **Figure 28.12**?
    A. The Doppler pattern is diagnostic of coarctation of the aorta.
    B. The Doppler pattern cannot be interpreted without additional Doppler images proximal to the coarctation site.
    C. The Doppler pattern cannot be interpreted due to a suboptimal angle between the aorta and the ultrasound beam.
    D. None of the above.

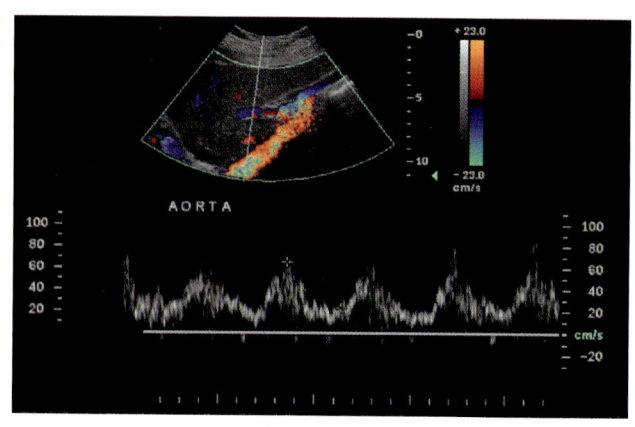

Figure 28.12

28. An 88-year-old man is diagnosed with a type A aortic dissection. He is being considered for a research protocol for thoracic endovascular aortic repair (TEVAR) of the ascending aorta. In order to qualify for the procedure, the surgeon requires information on specific characteristics of the dissection flap. TEE images are shown in (**Figure 28.13**; ▶ Video 28.4A and B). Which of the following statements is **CORRECT** based on these images?
    A. The true lumen is the larger lumen and it has no significant flow.
    B. The true lumen is the smaller lumen and it is patent.
    C. The false lumen is the smaller lumen and it has normal flow.
    D. None of the above.

29. A 72-year-old hypertensive man underwent a TEE due to severe back pain. **Figure 28.14** was obtained at the level of the upper descending thoracic aorta. Which of the following statements is **CORRECT** regarding this image?
    A. There is an intramural hematoma with the arrow pointing to a penetrating ulcer.
    B. There is a complex atheromatous plaque.
    C. The thickening of the aorta is due to aortitis.
    D. There is an intramural hematoma with the arrow pointing to displaced intimal calcium.

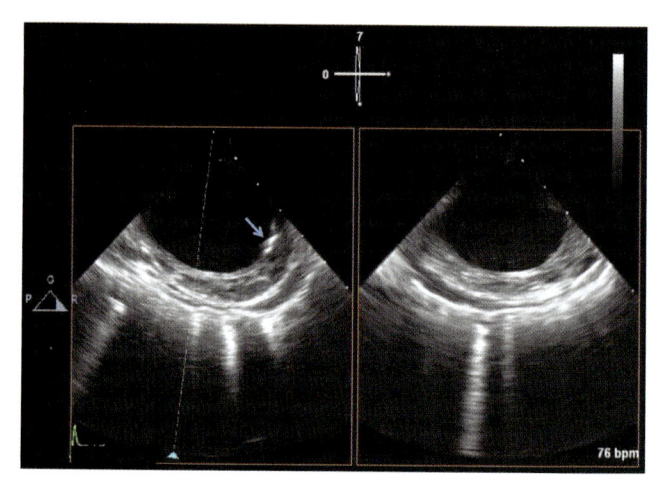

Figure 28.14

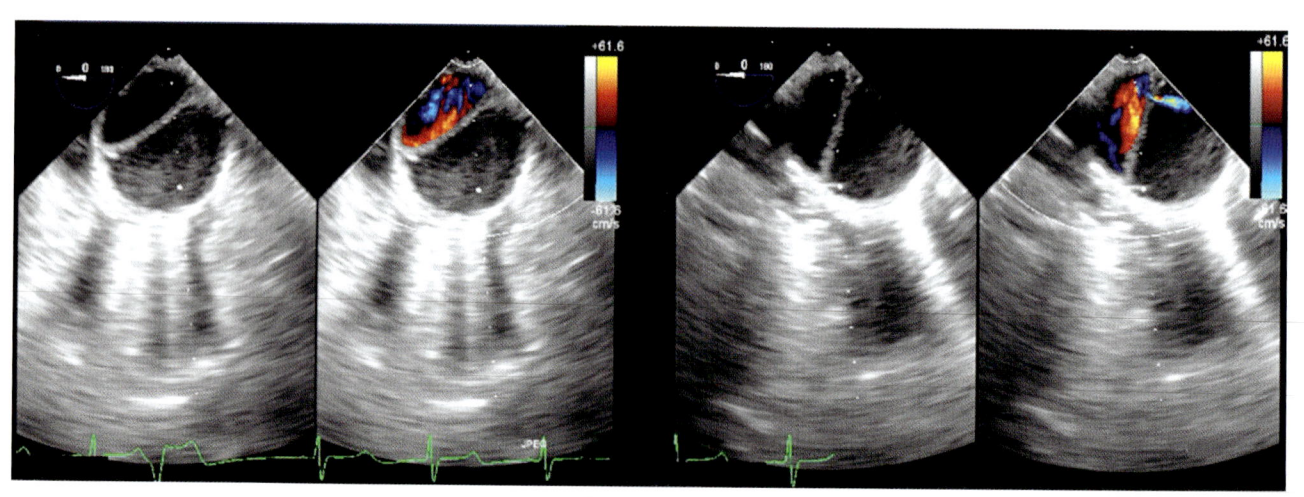

Figure 28.13

CASE 1

A 67-year-old male smoker presents to the ER with ongoing chest and back pain. A computed tomography of the chest shows no evidence of acute aortic dissection or intramural hematoma. He is then taken to the cardiac catheterization laboratory and angiography shows nonobstructive coronary artery disease. He continues to have ongoing chest and back pain. A TEE is performed for further evaluation.

30. Which of the following statements is most accurate regarding the images shown (**Figure 28.15**) of the patient from **Case 1**?
   A. The findings are consistent with a saccular aneurysm of the aortic arch.
   B. The findings are consistent with an intramural hematoma.
   C. The findings are consistent with aortic endarteritis.
   D. The findings are consistent with a penetrating aortic ulcer.

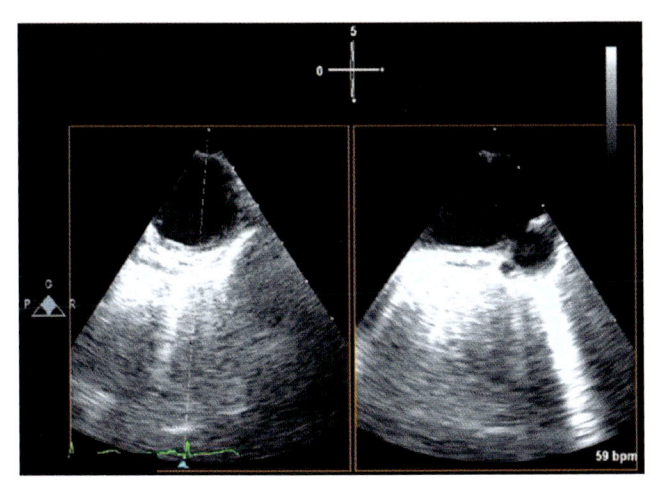

Figure 28.15

CASE 2

A 47-year-old man presents with intermittent substernal chest pain during the preceding week. His past medical history is significant for arthritis for the past 15 years. On presentation, he is afebrile and nontoxic appearing, but his WBC is 20,000. Cardiovascular examination is notable for a grade 2/6 early peaking systolic ejection murmur at the base and a grade 1/4 decrescendo diastolic murmur radiating to the left lower sternal border. A TEE is performed to assess for endocarditis (**Figure 28.16**, see arrowhead).

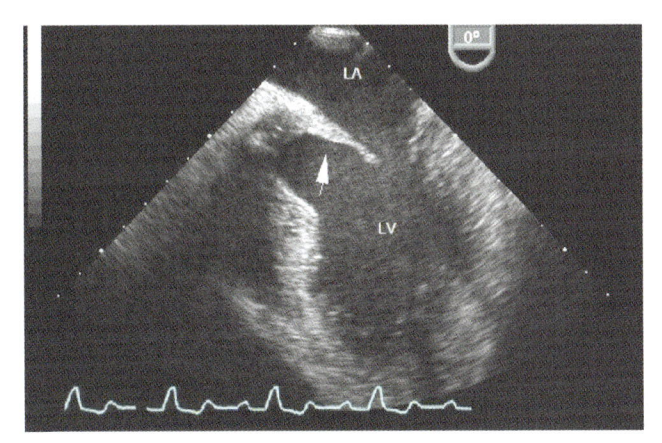

Figure 28.16

31. Which of the following statements about the abnormality shown in the patient from **Case 2** is **CORRECT**?
   A. Associated findings may include an aortic intramural hematoma.
   B. Associated findings may include a localized intimal dissection flap.
   C. Associated findings may include proximal aortitis.
   D. Associated findings may include mitral valve endocarditis.

CASE 3

A 48-year-old man with history of hypertension was transferred from a cruise ship after lifting weights with severe chest pain radiating down to his left shoulder and arm. Cardiovascular examination is notable for a BP—170/96 mm Hg (right arm). The heart sounds are notable for a reduced intensity S1, a soft systolic ejection murmur, and a 3/4 decrescendo diastolic murmur at the right upper sternal border. An electrocardiogram shows inferior ST depressions. A TEE is done to rule out aortic dissection (**Figure 28.17**; ▶ **Video 28.5**).

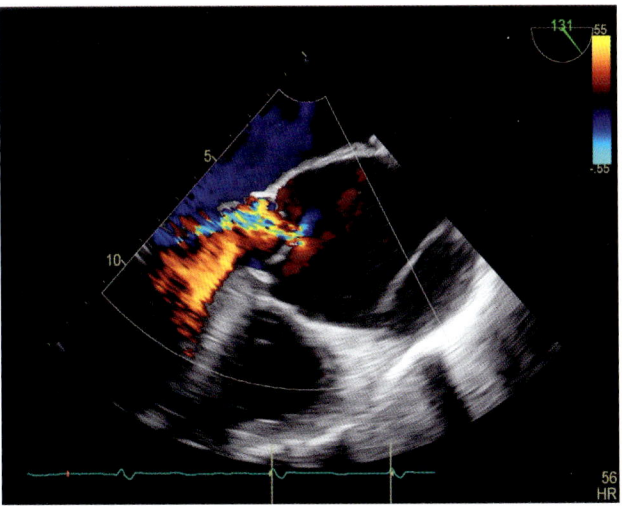

Figure 28.17

32. The patient from **Case 3** is taken for emergency heart surgery. Which of the following statements is most accurate?
    A. Aortic valve replacement should be performed.
    B. Aortic valve repair should be considered based on the mechanism of aortic regurgitation.
    C. Aortic valve repair or replacement will not likely be required if the ascending aorta is replaced.
    D. None of the above.

CASE 4

A 44-year-old woman with a history of severe aortic regurgitation underwent aortic valve replacement surgery with an aortic homograft. The postpump intraoperative TEE confirmed a normal functioning aortic homograft and an intact ascending aorta. Her postoperative course was uneventful. One month later, a baseline postoperative echocardiogram showed an abnormality of the homograft. She denied fevers, night sweats, or chest pain.

33. For the patient in **Case 4**, based on the ▶ **Video 28.6A–C**, which of the following statements is most accurate?

    A. Typical postoperative changes post homograft are present.
    B. A postoperative periaortic root hematoma is present.
    C. A postoperative periaortic root abscess is present.
    D. None of the above.

CASE 5

*A 62-year-old man presents with complaints of chest and back pain, orthopnea, and syncope. His medical history is remarkable for longstanding hypertension. On presentation, his blood pressure is 90/64 mm Hg and heart rate is 110 bpm in sinus rhythm. He is found to have cardiomegaly and pulmonary edema by chest radiograph. A bedside TEE is performed (▶ **Video 28.7A, B**).*

34. Which of the following therapies is most appropriate in this patient's management?
    A. Emergent surgical repair.
    B. Urgent pericardiocentesis.
    C. High-dose intravenous hydrocortisone.
    D. Intravenous beta-blocker therapy.

ANSWERS

1. **Answer: B.** The size of the ascending aorta correlates with several anthropometric measures. Aortic size correlates most closely with height, body surface area, gender, and increasing age (**Table 28.1**). Aortic size correlates less well with body weight as an isolated factor. In a majority of individuals, the aortic root and proximal and mid portion of the tubular ascending aorta can be adequately imaged from the transthoracic left parasternal window from various intercostal spaces. The right parasternal view can be helpful when visualization is inadequate in the left parasternal views. Correlation between computed tomography or magnetic resonance angiography of the ascending aorta at the aortic root and proximal and mid ascending aorta is good when TTE image quality is adequate. Because it is subject to pulsatile blood flow, the aortic

Table 28.1. Aortic Root Dimensions in Normal Adults

Aortic Root	Absolute Values (cm)		Indexed Values (cm/m²)	
	Men	**Women**	**Men**	**Women**
Annulus	2.6 ± 0.3	2.3 ± 0.2	1.3 ± 0.1	1.3 ± 0.1
Sinuses of Valsalva	3.4 ± 0.3	3.0 ± 0.3	1.7 ± 0.2	1.8 ± 0.2
Sinotubular junction	2.9 ± 0.3	2.6 ± 0.3	1.5 ± 0.2	1.5 ± 0.2
Proximal ascending aorta	3.0 ± 0.4	2.7 ± 0.4	1.5 ± 0.2	1.6 ± 0.3

Adapted from Roman et al. and Hiratzka et al.
From Lang RM, Badano LP, Mor-Avi V, et al. Recommendations for cardiac chamber quantification by echocardiography in adults: an update from the American Society of Echocardiography and the European Association of Cardiovascular Imaging. *Eur Heart J Cardiovasc Imaging*. 2015;16(3):233–270.

size varies between systole and diastole. However, the aorta should be imaged ideally during end diastole in a perpendicular plane to the long axis of the aorta using the leading edge–to–leading edge technique (**Figure 28.18**). M-mode is used primarily for assessing the size of the aortic root, whereas two-dimensional echocardiography can be used to visualize the aortic root and tubular ascending aorta.

2. **Answer: A.** The American Society of Echocardiography (ASE) Pediatric Guidelines recommend measuring the aorta by two-dimensional imaging in systole during maximum expansion using an inner edge–to–inner edge convention. This convention, which is in contrast to the leading edge–to–leading edge end-diastolic measurement recommended in adults, was chosen since it is believed to correlate best with prognosis especially in disease states such as Marfan syndrome. In systole, the aorta is exposed to the highest wall stress and therefore systolic measurements may be more predictive of aortic complications such as aortic dissection. There are separate guidelines from the ASE pertaining to adults that recommend measurements be made in end diastole not in systole. Since these guidelines are not aligned, it is important to recognize that measurement differences may occur when individuals transition from pediatric to adult echocardiography laboratories. In general, measurements made in systole may be 1 to 2 mm greater than those made in diastole for younger individuals with compliant aortas.

3. **Answer: D.** The term "bovine aortic arch" refers to a common anatomic variant pattern of the aortic arch. Although a common misnomer (the human bovine aortic arch variant does not resemble the aortic arch pattern found in cattle), it remains a widely used descriptive term in the medical literature. Two different configurations typically occur, the most common being when the innominate artery and the left common carotid artery have a common origin, and the second when the left common carotid artery arises directly from the innominate artery (**Figure 28.19**).

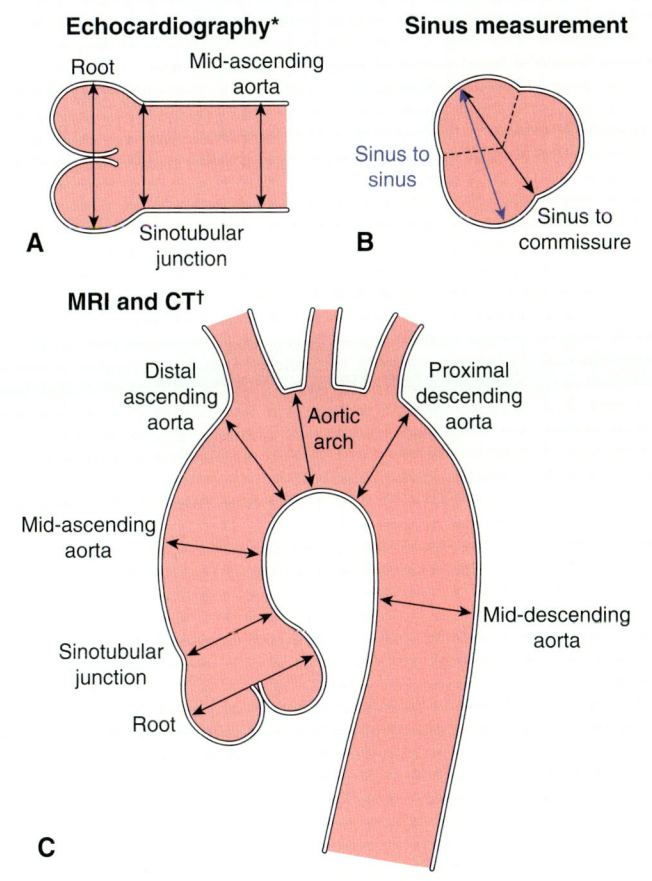

Figure 28.18. **A:** Schematic shows the leading edge–to–leading edge measurement technique used in echocardiography, from left to right: measurement of the aortic root (sinuses of Valsalva), sinotubular junction, and proximal tubular ascending aorta. **B:** Inner wall–to–inner wall measurements of the aortic root used in MRI and CT. In addition, a consistent approach to measuring all three sinuses with MRI and CT is necessary. The sinus-to-commissure and sinus-to-sinus measurements can both be used, but consistency is necessary for interval surveillance. **C:** Standard measurement locations for MRI and CT with the inner wall–to–inner wall technique. CT, computed tomography; MRI, magnetic resonance imaging. *Leading edge–to–leading edge. †Inner wall–to–inner wall. (Reprinted from Writing Committee Members, Isselbacher EM, Preventza O, et al. 2022 ACC/AHA guideline for the diagnosis and management of aortic disease: a report of the American Heart Association/American College of Cardiology Joint Committee on Clinical Practice Guidelines. *J Am Coll Cardiol.* 2022;80(24):e223-e393. Copyright © 2022 by the American College of Cardiology Foundation and the American Heart Association, Inc. Adapted from Borger MA, Fedak PWM, Stephens EH, et al. The American Association for Thoracic Surgery consensus guidelines on bicuspid aortic valve-related aortopathy: full online-only version. *J Thorac Cardiovasc Surg.* 2018;156:e41-e74. Copyright © 2018 by The American Association for Thoracic Surgery. With permission.)

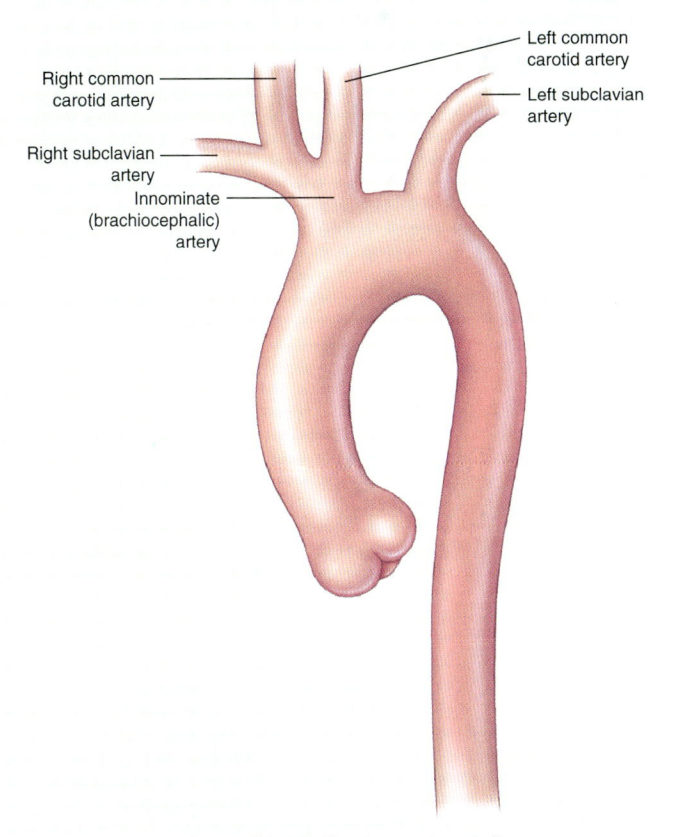

Figure 28.19. "Bovine aortic arch."

These aortic configurations occur in about 22% of individuals. Recent data suggest that a bovine arch may be a risk marker of thoracic aortic aneurysm and imaging to assess for aneurysm may be reasonable. The aortic arch and great vessels are not visualized from the standard parasternal window but can be best imaged from the suprasternal notch.

4. **Answer: D.** Complex aortic atheromas are usually defined as ≥4 to 6 mm thickness or mobile. These characteristics are most strongly associated with embolic risk including stroke and peripheral embolization and can be defined by TEE. Complex aortic atheromas are most often seen in the descending aorta followed by the aortic arch and ascending aorta in decreasing prevalence. TEE is not adequate to visualize the innominate artery although complex atheromas are infrequent in this region.

5. **Answer: C.** A potential limitation of TEE for the evaluation of the thoracic aorta is the so-called "blind spot." This area encompasses an approximately 3 cm portion of the distal ascending aorta up to and including the proximal arch. The "blind spot" is caused by the interposition of air most commonly from the trachea or bronchus causing acoustic interference between the transducer and the aorta. The "blind spot" is not caused by interference from the transverse sinus or azygos vein. Although a hiatal hernia may interfere with cardiac imaging from the mid to lower TEE windows, it is not the cause of the aortic "blind spot." Despite the potential for the "blind spot" to interfere with aortic imaging, the diffuse processes of the aorta infrequently render it a significant limitation. During cardiac surgery, the "blind spot" can be overcome by epiaortic imaging, using a stand-off to enhance ultrasound transmission to the aorta or by a deep transgastric view at 0°, which may visualize the entire ascending aorta (**Figure 28.20**).

6. **Answer: D.** TEE may provide a rapid and accurate diagnosis of traumatic aortic injury. Most traumatic aortic injuries are the result of abrupt deceleration resulting in shearing of the aorta in the region of the isthmus. The aortic isthmus is the region between the left subclavian artery and the first intercostal arteries where the aorta is fixed to the thoracic cage by the ligamentum arteriosum and intercostal arteries. Although many patients experience complete transection of the aorta after motor vehicle accidents and do not survive, some with less severe injuries may be rapidly diagnosed and undergo life-saving surgery.

   Figure 28.21 shows the three types of blunt aortic trauma (BAT) classification with characterization by TEE images at the level of the isthmus. BAT type I—intimal tears; type II—intramural hematoma; type III—pseudoaneurysm; and type IV—rupture. Type I intimal tears may have associated mural thrombus. Type II are localized intramural hematomas. Type III results in aortic subadventitial disruption and pseudoaneurysm or contained rupture. This may manifest as a thick medial flap that unlike a spontaneous aortic dissection flap runs near perpendicular to the aortic wall in long-axis view with similar color Doppler flow in each side of the flap and associated hemomediastinum. Type IV ruptures do not typically survive to be imaged.

7. **Answer: C.** Distinguishing the true from the false lumen in patients with aortic dissection has important

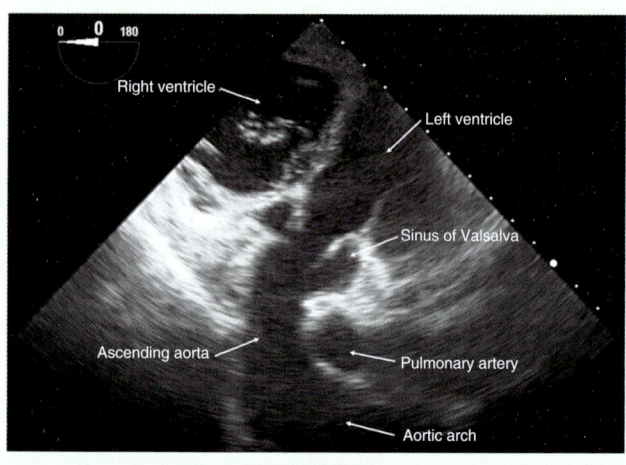

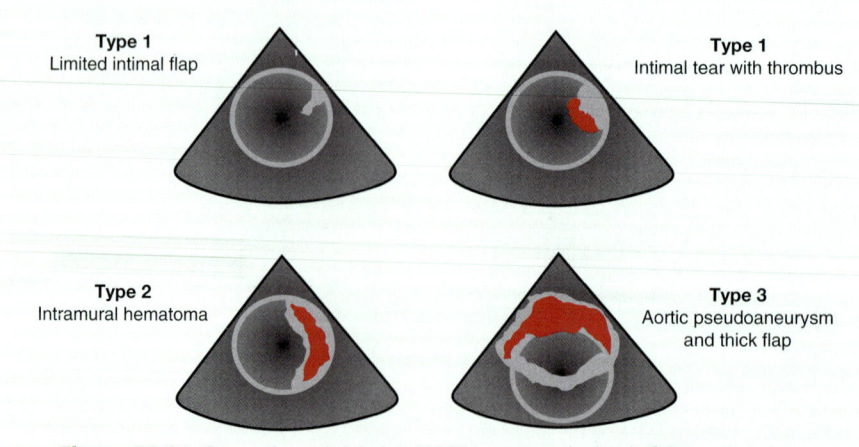

Figure 28.20

Figure 28.21. Traumatic aortic injuries, 0° TEE images at the level of the aortic isthmus.

Table 28.2. Echocardiographic Differentiation Between True and False Lumens

	True Lumen	False Lumen
Lumen Size	True < False	False > True
Pulsation	Systolic expansion/Diastolic collapse	Diastolic expansion/Systolic compression
Flow Direction	Systolic antegrade flow	Systolic antegrade flow reduced or absent or retrograde flow
Flow Communication	From true to false lumen in systole	
Spontaneous echo contrast	Absent or low intensity	Common ± pronounced
Thrombus	Minimal or none	Complete or partial

From Anderson B, Park MM, eds. *Basic to Advanced Clinical Echocardiography: A Self-Assessment Tool for the Cardiac Sonographer.* Wolters Kluwer; 2021. Adapted with permission from Evangelista A, Flachskampf FA, Erbel R, et al. Echocardiography in aortic diseases: EAE recommendations for clinical practice. *Eur J Echocardiogr.* 2010;11(8):645-658.

surgical and prognostic implications. With TEE, it may be possible to determine if the false lumen provides flow to aortic arch vessels, thus compromising flow. The true lumen is generally the smaller lumen that receives brisk systolic antegrade flow and expands during systole. Flow communication into the false lumen may occur. In contrast, the false lumen is generally the larger lumen but is compressed during systole and receives reduced systolic antegrade flow, which is delayed and lower in velocity. Thrombosis of the false lumen, not the true lumen, may occur and may be complete or partial (**Table 28.2**).

8. **Answer: C.** Aneurysmal dilatation of an artery such as the aorta is usually defined as a localized or diffuse increase in diameter to at least 1.5 times greater than the normal expected size. That is, if the artery is normally 3.0 cm in diameter for a given patient based on age, gender, and body surface area, an aortic aneurysm would be present if the maximal diameter was equal to or greater than 4.5 cm or at least 50% greater than the expected size. However, this characterization is unsatisfactory when defining aneurysms of the ascending aorta. The more important factor in defining an aneurysm of the ascending portion is its natural history. Studies have shown that populations at risk of aortic events are those with an ascending aortic diameter of ≥4.0 cm and at even greater risk with a diameter of ≥4.5 cm. As such, it is suggested by the ACC/AHA 2022 Guideline for the Diagnosis and Management of Aortic Disease that ascending aortas be defined as dilated when 4.0 to 4.4 cm and as an aneurysm when ≥4.5 cm. Also, because of confusion and misuse with the term ectasia, it is preferred that the term dilation be used when referring to mild aortic enlargement.

9. **Answer: D.** Marfan syndrome is a systemic disorder of connective tissue characterized primarily by aortic aneurysms and other cardiovascular, skeletal, and ocular abnormalities. The condition is caused by a genetic mutation in the *FBN1* gene. A principal manifestation (major criteria) for diagnosis of Marfan syndrome is dilatation/aneurysms of the ascending aorta involving the sinuses of Valsalva. This is the most common site for aneurysm formation. Dilatation/aneurysms of the aortic arch and descending thoracic and thoracoabdominal aorta are also common and can develop in the absence of coexisting ascending aortic aneurysms. Isolated abdominal aortic aneurysms are, however, relatively rare.

10. **Answer: B.** Right aortic arch is defined as descent of the aorta at the level of the transverse arch to the right of the trachea. The two most common types of right-sided aortic arches are mirror image and nonmirror image (aberrant left subclavian artery). Mirror image type is commonly associated with congenital heart disease (most often tetralogy of Fallot), whereas nonmirror image type is infrequently associated with other congenital cardiac malformations. In mirror-image right aortic arch, the left innominate artery originates as the first branch (from patient left to right), followed by right carotid artery and right subclavian artery (**Figure 28.22A**). In nonmirror image right aortic arch, the sequence of branching (from patient left to right) is left carotid artery, right carotid artery, right subclavian artery, and then left subclavian artery (**Figure 28.22B**). The left (aberrant) subclavian artery originates from the proximal descending aorta often with a prominent diverticulum (diverticulum of Kommerell) at its origin. A diverticulum of Kommerell is associated with risk of rupture and dissection. The left subclavian artery courses behind the esophagus and trachea and can produce a vascular ring with esophageal compression.

11. **Answer: A.** The normal shape of the aorta is well established and characterized by sinus of Valsalva diameter > sinotubular junction diameter, and sinus

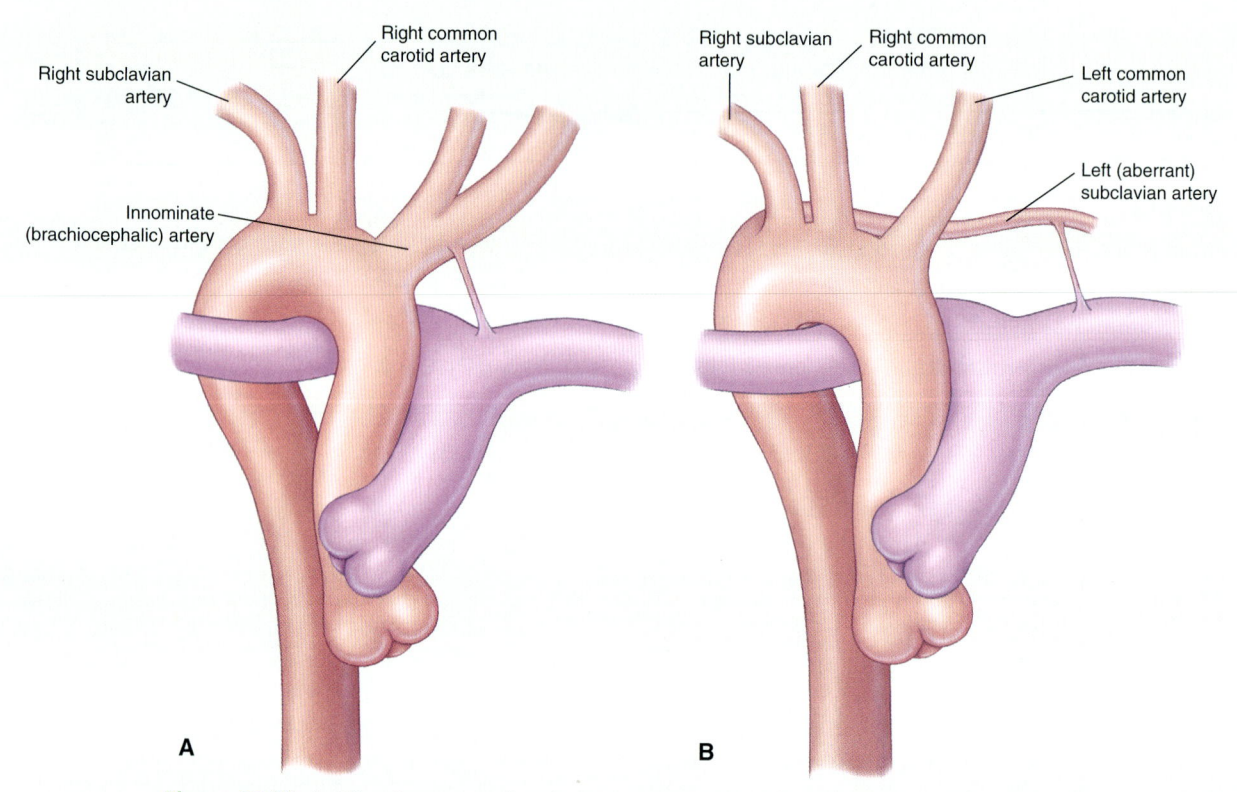

Figure 28.22. A: Mirror image type of a right aortic arch. **B:** Nonmirror image type of a right aortic arch.

of Valsalva diameter > tubular ascending aortic diameter. In general, the diameter at the sinus of Valsalva is approximately 0.3 cm in men and 0.2 cm in women greater in size than the tubular ascending aortic diameter. Thus, the presence of a tubular ascending aorta of greater size than the sinus of Valsalva size is the most likely choice to represent a pathologic process despite normal overall dimensions.

12. **Answer: B.** Shone complex is a rare congenital heart disease comprised typically of four obstructive left heart lesions: supravalvular mitral ring, parachute-like mitral valve (commonly associated with mitral stenosis), subaortic stenosis, and aortic coarctation. Valvular aortic stenosis with a bicuspid aortic valve may also occur. Turner syndrome has commonly recognized cardiac malformations. The most common cardiac defects are coarctation of the aorta and a bicuspid aortic valve. Other abnormalities associated with Turner syndrome can include aortic aneurysms and dissection. Noonan syndrome is a genetic disease typified by facial anomalies, short stature, webbed neck, undescended testes, and congenital heart defects. The classic cardiac malformations reported in Noonan syndrome are pulmonary stenosis and hypertrophic cardiomyopathy. Down syndrome (or trisomy 21) is frequently associated with congenital heart defects, the most common of which are atrioventricular septal defects.

13. **Answer: C.** An aorta that is anterior to the pulmonary artery associated with atrioventricular concordance and ventricular-arterial discordance refers to the anatomic configuration of D-transposition of the great arteries (**Figure 28.23**). D-transposition (complete or uncorrected transposition) is a cyanotic congenital heart defect in which the aorta is anterior and to the right of the pulmonary artery. It is characterized by the aorta arising from the morphologic right ventricle and the pulmonary artery arising from the morphologic left ventricle resulting in two separate circulatory systems. The condition is often diagnosed in utero by ultrasound, but if not, cyanosis upon birth will immediately lead to the diagnosis.

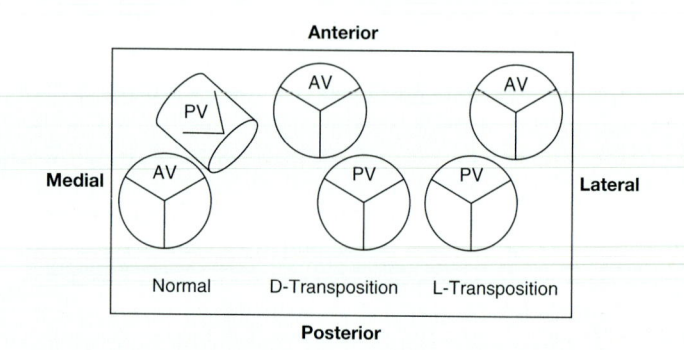

Figure 28.23. The aorta is in front of the pulmonary artery in transposition of the great arteries and is either to the right (D) or to the left (L) of the pulmonary artery. (Adapted from Klein AL, Asher CR. *Clinical Echocardiography Review: A Self-Assessment Tool.* Wolters Kluwer Health/Lippincott Williams & Wilkins; 2011. Fig 23-17.)

An aorta that is anterior to the pulmonary artery associated with atrioventricular discordance and ventricular-arterial discordance refers to L-transposition or congenitally corrected transposition. L-transposition is an acyanotic congenital heart defect in which the aorta is anterior and to the left of the pulmonary artery. It is characterized by double discordance (a "double switch") where the atrial and ventricular connections are discordant and the ventricular to great artery connections are discordant. Blood flow is from the right atrium into the right-sided morphologic left ventricle through the pulmonary artery to the lungs. From the lungs, blood flow returns from the pulmonary veins into the left atrium, to the left-sided morphologic right ventricle and to the aorta. Since circulation is physiologically corrected, patients survive into adulthood.

An aorta overriding the ventricular septum with a malalignment ventricular septal defect describes tetralogy of Fallot. This cyanotic heart defect is classically described by four malformations: a ventricular septal defect, pulmonary stenosis, an overriding aorta, and right ventricular hypertrophy. The degree of pulmonary stenosis varies and is the main determinant of disease severity and degree of cyanosis. This condition is often diagnosed at birth or during the first year of life depending on cyanosis severity. A periductal aorta–pulmonary connection with normal pulmonary pressure refers to a patent ductus arteriosus. When a patent ductus remains untreated, depending on its size, pulmonary hypertension and heart failure can develop. In the absence of pulmonary hypertension, the condition is well tolerated and can persist into adulthood.

14. **Answer: A.** Bicuspid aortic valves are associated with ascending aortic dilatation with a prevalence of approximately 50%. The tubular ascending aorta is usually the region with the greatest degree of dilatation. The underlying predisposition is likely related to genetic abnormalities of connective tissue along with flow-related stress, which render the aorta susceptible to dilatation, aneurysm, and aortic dissection. The ACC/AHA guidelines recommendations for aortic replacement in bicuspid aortic valve aortopathy are listed in **Table 28.3**.

Patterns and classifications of ascending aortic dilatation in patients with bicuspid aortic valves have been proposed. **Figure 28.24** demonstrates some of the more common variations. **Figure 28.24A** shows an aortic root predominant pattern, which is in fact relatively uncommon. **Figure 28.24B** shows a pattern of relative sparing of the aortic root with tubular ascending aortic predominance and aortic arch sparing. **Figure 28.24C** shows a pattern of diffuse involvement of the aortic root, tubular ascending aorta, and aortic arch. Other patterns are possible with aortic arch dilatation common but usually not to the degree that requires surgical intervention.

Coarctation of the aorta is a commonly associated congenital malformation, which develops in patients with bicuspid aortic valves. It occurs in ~5% of all bicuspid aortic valve patients. Conversely, in those patients with coarctation of the aorta, a bicuspid aortic valve is present >50% of the time.

15. **Answer: D.** Several classification systems have been developed to describe aortic dissection involving the thoracic aorta. There are three classifications commonly in use and are based either on the location/extent of the dissection or on the underlying pathophysiology. The DeBakey classification has types I, II, IIIa, and IIIb and is based on the location/extent of aortic dissection. The Stanford classification has types A and B and is based on whether the dissection is in the proximal or distal aorta. The Svensson classification has classes 1 to 5 and is based on the pathophysiology of aortic syndrome.

The patient described has a DeBakey type 2/Stanford A with a variant form limited, iatrogenic

Table 28.3. Recommendations for Aortic Replacement in Bicuspid Aortic Valve Aortopathy

An ascending aorta or aortic root diameter of ≥5.5 cm
A cross-sectional ascending aortic or root area (cm) to height (m) ratio of ≥10 cm²/m
An ascending aorta or root diameter of 5.0-5.4 cm, and a risk factor: • Family history of aortic dissection • Aortic growth rate ≥0.3 cm/y • Coarctation of the aorta • Root phenotype aortic aneurysm
In those undergoing aortic valve surgery, an ascending aorta or root diameter of ≥4.5 cm
Consider an ascending aorta or root diameter of 5.0-5.4 cm, if low surgical risk

Derived from Writing Committee Members, Isselbacher EM, Preventza O, et al. 2022 ACC/AHA guideline for the diagnosis and management of aortic disease: a report of the American Heart Association/American College of Cardiology Joint Committee on Clinical Practice Guidelines. *J Am Coll Cardiol.* 2022;80(24):e223-e393.

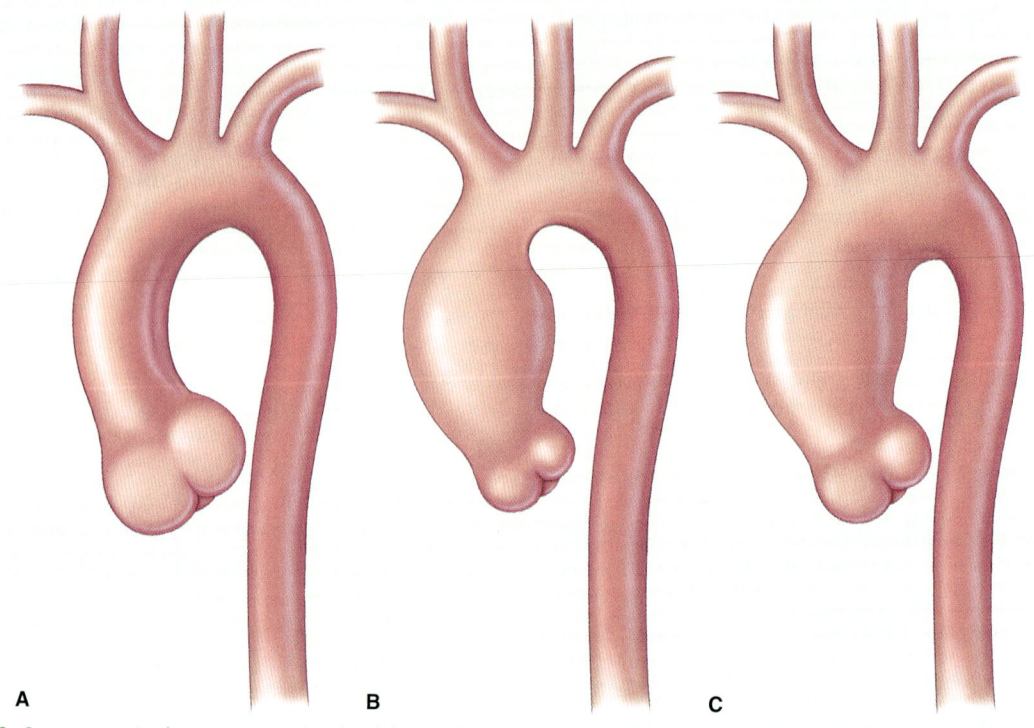

Figure 28.24. Common aortic phenotypes associated with bicuspid aortic valves. **A:** Aortic root predominant. **B:** Aortic root–sparing tubular ascending aorta predominant. **C:** Diffuse involvement including aortic root, tubular ascending aorta, and aortic arch.

hematoma. DeBakey type 2 refers to the ascending aortic location, Stanford A similarly locates the dissection in the ascending aorta or arch, and by Svensson classification, there is a class 5 iatrogenic intramural hematoma (**Table 28.4**).

16. **Answer: D.** The TEE image depicts a large pedunculated aortic thrombus in the distal aortic arch/proximal descending thoracic aorta. Although most sources of emboli from the aorta are related to complex atherosclerotic plaques, large aortic thrombi may also occur. A majority of these thrombi develop in areas of diffuse atheromatous disease, but they may also occur in regions with minimal or no apparent atherosclerosis. An alternative etiology of aortic thrombus is an underlying hypercoagulable state such as antiphospholipid antibody syndrome or malignancy. Treatment for aortic thrombi has not been well established although anticoagulant therapy is supported by some studies. If recurrent embolic events occur, surgical removal of the aortic thrombi may be necessary.

Aortic thrombi do not predispose to aortic dissection although they may be seen at the site of traumatic aortic disruption. Aortic aneurysms may be a site for aortic thrombus formation but usually they appear as mural and layered and not pedunculated. Bacteremia may lead to mycotic aneurysms or atheromatous plaques with superimposed infection but not usually isolated infective masses.

Table 28.4. Classification of Aortic Dissection Involving the Thoracic Aorta

DeBakey Classification	Region of Aorta Involved
Type I	Ascending, arch ± descending
Type II	Ascending only
Type IIIa	Descending (above diaphragm)
Type IIIb	Descending (extends below diaphragm)

Stanford Classification	Region of Aorta Involved
Type A	Ascending ± arch/descending
Type B	Arch/descending, not ascending

Svensson Classification	Type of Aortic Syndrome
Class 1	Classic intimal flap (2 lumens)
Class 2	Intramural hematoma (no intimal flap)
Class 3	Localized intimal flap
Class 4	Penetrating aortic ulcer
Class 5	Iatrogenic/posttraumatic

17. **Answer: D.** The TEE image of the upper descending thoracic aorta depicts severe aortic atheromatous plaque of >0.5 mm, grade 4. There are no apparent mobile or ulcerated components. Plaque size can be graded based on intimal or atheroma thickness. There are a few published grading systems for atheroma with small differences in cutoff ranges for atheroma severity. The grading system endorsed by the 2015 multimodality imaging of thoracic aorta in adults guidelines and standards is shown in **Table 28.5**. Distinguishing intimal thickening from atheroma is not always easily characterized. Intimal thickening is typically diffuse, homogeneous, mild, and without significant calcification.

Table 28.5. Grading System for Severity of Aortic Atherosclerosis

Grade	Severity (Atheroma Thickness)	Description
1	Normal	Intimal thickness <2 mm
2	Mild	Mild intimal thickening (2-3 mm)
3	Moderate	Atheroma >3-5 mm (no mobile/ulcerated components)
4	Severe	Atheroma >5 mm (no mobile/ulcerated components)
5	Complex	Grade 2-4 plus mobile or ulcerated components

Reprinted from Goldstein SA, Evangelista A, Abbara S, et al. Multimodality imaging of diseases of the thoracic aorta in adults: from the American Society of Echocardiography and the European Association of Cardiovascular Imaging—endorsed by the Society of Cardiovascular Computed Tomography and Society for Cardiovascular Magnetic Resonance. *J Am Soc Echocardiogr*. 2015;28:119-182. Copyright © 2015 by the American Society of Echocardiography. With permission.

18. **Answer: C.** The continuous-wave Doppler profile is consistent with coarctation of the aorta with a high-velocity systolic and a diastolic flow (continuous flow, sawtooth pattern). The simplified Bernoulli equation typically overestimates the peak gradient obtained at cardiac catheterization. This occurs because the precoarctation velocity is often elevated due to flow acceleration and bicuspid aortic valve disease. However, using the modified Bernoulli equation, $P = 4(V_2^2 - V_1^2)$, where the proximal velocity V_1 is accounted for results in a good correlation between Doppler echocardiography and cardiac catheterization.

19. **Answer: C.** The suprasternal notch view by TTE provides visualization of the distal ascending aorta, aortic arch and branch vessels, and upper descending aorta. Recognition of normal anatomy in this view is important. The structures labeled are: 1—left atrium; 2—right pulmonary artery; 3—transverse sinus; 4—innominate vein; and 5—innominate artery. The proximal portion of the left subclavian and left carotid artery can be seen in most individuals. The vessel border between the innominate vein and artery may be confused for a dissection flap if normal anatomy is not known. Typically, continuous low-velocity flow is seen in the innominate vein with flow direction opposite to that in the aortic arch.

20. **Answer: C.** There is a coronary anomaly. The double-barreled structure is an anomalous coronary artery, in this case the left circumflex (LCX) arising from the right coronary cusp (RCC) and coursing posteriorly to the aortic root. The coronary artery is superimposed on the aortic root due to a slice thickness artifact. There are several hallmark findings of an anomalous coronary from the RCC. The "crossed aorta sign" describes the tubular structure running perpendicular to the aortic root. This is also referred to as the retroaortic anomalous coronary (RAC sign), where the tubular structure courses from the RCC, posterior to the aorta, to above the mitral annulus and atrioventricular groove, toward the left AV groove. The anterior plane, and smaller size of the vessel, above the AV groove distinguishes the vessel from the posteriorly located coronary sinus. Another sign is the "bleb sign," typically seen best on TEE as a vessel at the junction of the posterior aortic root noncoronary cusp and base of the mitral valve leaflet (**Figure 28.25**, *arrow points to bleb sign*). Additionally, in some individuals, in the short-axis view at the level of the aortic valve (either TTE or TEE), a retroaortic vessel can sometimes be seen.

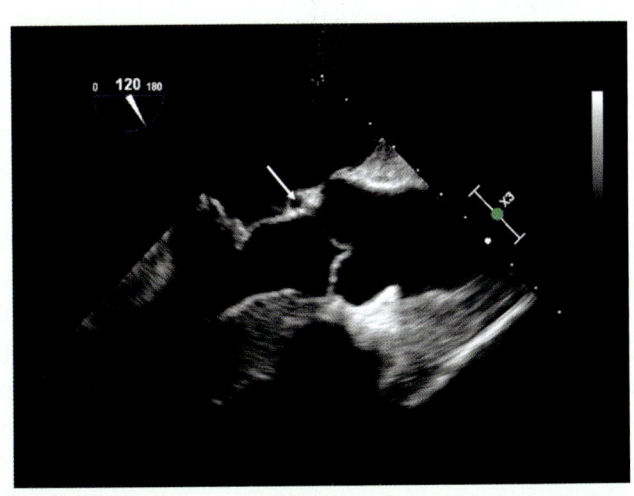

Figure 28.25

614 / Clinical Echocardiography Review

21. **Answer: A.** The TEE image shows a quadricuspid aortic valve. Quadricuspid aortic valves are rare congenital anomalies commonly associated with aortic regurgitation. Although mild to moderate dilatation may occur with quadricuspid aortic valves, associated aortic conditions such as aneurysms, dissection, rupture, and coarctation are uncommon. In contrast, the other rare congenital aortic valve anomaly, unicuspid valves are commonly associated with aortic aneurysms. It is important to note that there are classifications of quadricuspid aortic valves that characterize the relative sizes of each cusp.

22. **Answer: B.** The aortic arch is likely to be enlarged in this patient with a bicuspid aortic valve and a dilated aortic root and ascending aorta. The aortopathy of bicuspid aortic valves is due to both genetic predispositions and hemodynamic flow patterns. Several studies have begun to elucidate the association between bicuspid aortic valve morphology and aortic shapes and dilatation patterns. However, these associations are still under study and not well established. It is recognized that the aortic arch is commonly enlarged in patients with bicuspid aortic valves and particularly in those that have more diffuse dilatation involving the sinus of Valsalva, sinotubular junction, and tubular ascending aorta. The descending aorta is not known to be involved with the aortopathy of bicuspid aortic valves.

23. **Answer: D.** The TTE image of the ascending aorta was obtained from the parasternal window moving up an interspace and medially toward the sternum. This is the most common nonstandard parasternal long-axis transducer orientation to improve the quality of visualization of the ascending aorta. Additionally, the right parasternal or suprasternal notch windows may visualize portions of the ascending aorta. Since the great vessels are not seen in this image, it is not consistent with a suprasternal notch view. The vessel posterior to the ascending aorta is the right pulmonary artery.

24. **Answer: B.** The TEE images of the aortic root demonstrate a right coronary sinus of Valsalva aneurysm. Aortic sinus of Valsalva aneurysms may be congenital (associated with other cardiac abnormalities such as bicuspid aortic valve or ventricular septal defect, or connective tissue disorders such as Marfan syndrome or Ehlers-Danlos syndrome) or acquired secondary to infection or trauma. A male predominance occurs. The right sinus of Valsalva followed by the noncoronary sinus is the most commonly involved site for sinus of Valsalva aneurysms. If rupture occurs, a communication develops into adjacent chambers and rarely extracardiac rupture occurs. With rupture into an adjacent chamber, a continuous high-velocity flow (or murmur) occurs with a high velocity diastolic component. Clinically patients may present with hypotension or shock, not cardiac tamponade. **Figure 28.26A** and **Video 28.8A** show a TEE long-axis view at 120° with and without color Doppler with a ruptured right sinus of Valsalva aneurysm into the right ventricle (arrow points to the site of rupture and color Doppler flow). **Figure 28.26B** shows a schematic of how rupture of each sinus could affect the heart.

25. **Answer: B.** The parasternal short-axis and suprasternal notch views show color Doppler flow from the descending aorta to the pulmonary artery consistent with a patent ductus arteriosus (PDA). A PDA should be considered in any patient with a murmur of unknown cause. Several views can be utilized to detect a PDA including the parasternal short-axis view with orientation toward the pulmonary artery bifurcation as seen in **Figure 28.27**, the high left parasternal view (mostly used in pediatrics), and the suprasternal notch view (most sensitive view in adults). The color Doppler flow is continuous if the pulmonary vascular resistance is less than the systemic vascular resistance. The hemodynamic significance of a PDA depends on the size of the defect and amount of flow into the pulmonary artery. Left-sided volume overload (left atrial or left ventricular dilatation) and pulmonary hypertension occur with hemodynamically significant PDAs. Although Q_p/Q_s is often calculated during TTE when shunts are present, the accuracy may not be optimal due to difficulties measuring the pulmonary

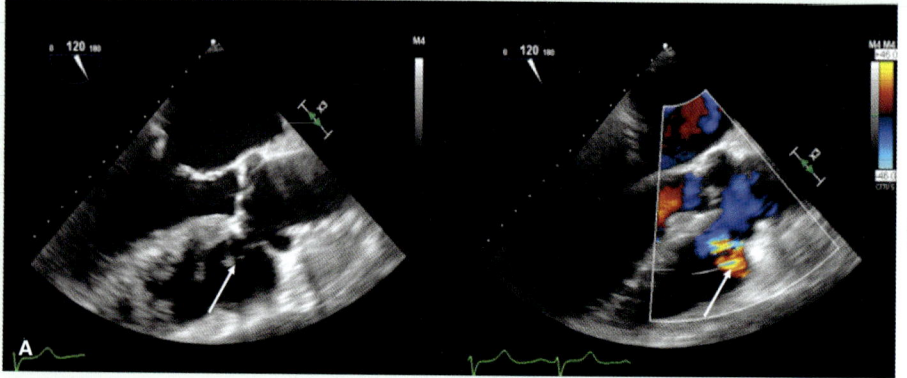

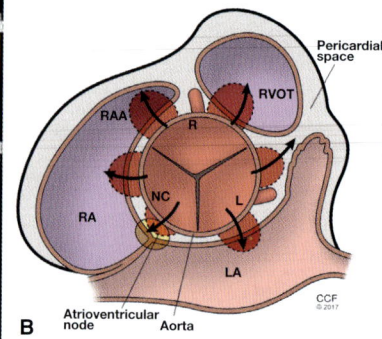

Figure 28.26. **B:** Reprinted with permission, Cleveland Clinic Foundation ©2024. All Rights Reserved.

Chapter 28 Aortic Diseases / 615

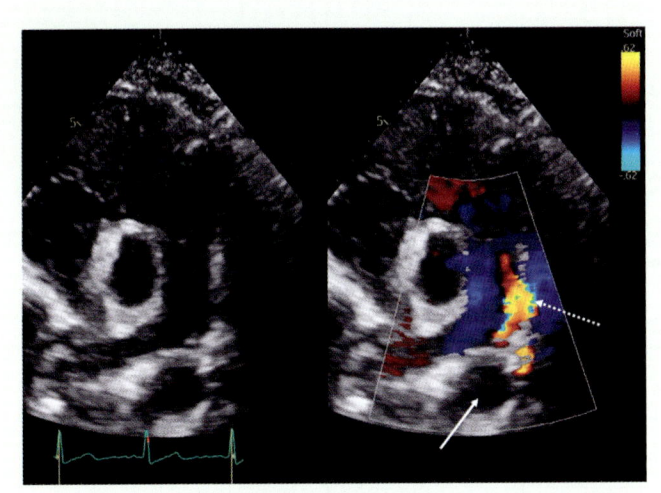

Figure 28.27

valve annulus (see **Figure 28.27** and ▶ **Video 28.3**). (The solid arrow points to the descending aorta and the dashed arrow points to the continuous flow into the left pulmonary artery.)

26. **Answer: C.** The TEE image of the descending thoracic aorta shows a vascular structure distinct from the aorta consistent with the appearance of a persistent left superior vena cava (PLSVC). The course of a PLSVC runs from the left upper thorax in continuation of the left internal jugular and left subclavian veins running lateral to the arch, posterior to the descending aorta, and, most commonly when isolated, into the coronary sinus. **Figure 28.28A** shows a longitudinal view of the PLSVC on its course toward the coronary sinus. **Figure 28.28B** shows a markedly dilated coronary sinus adjacent to the left atrium on a mid-esophageal view. A PLSVC is the most common congenital venous anomaly encountered in the chest, occurring in 0.3% to 0.5% of the population, and drains into the coronary sinus in 90% of cases. Arrows point to PLSVC on multiple views.

27. **Answer: A.** The pulsed Doppler spectral profile taken from the abdominal aorta is consistent with recoarctation of the aorta in this patient with claudication and prior coarctation repair. The findings consistent with coarctation include: (a) low-velocity systolic flow; (b) persistent higher-velocity diastolic forward flow (the "diastolic tail"); (c) low systolic-diastolic flow ratio; (d) decreased pulsatility; and (e) delay in systolic peak velocity. Although the proximal coarctation velocity is unknown in this patient, a very low forward cardiac output would be necessary to have such low systolic velocities. This is not clinically compatible with a hypertensive patient. The angle of insonation of the Doppler beam and the abdominal aorta is not optimal; however, these images were obtained with angle correction as is typically done in the vascular laboratory. A normal pulsed Doppler spectral profile of the abdominal aorta has an early, rapid upstroke and downstroke, a higher systolic to diastolic flow ratio, an early reversal of flow in diastole, and more pronounced pulsatility.

28. **Answer: B.** Differentiation of the true and false lumen can usually be accurately determined with TEE. In this patient, the true lumen is the smaller lumen and it is patent. There is a flow communication seen by color Doppler from the true lumen to the false lumen in the far right panel. The true lumen can be identified by systolic expansion with compression of the false lumen. The flow in systole is typically fast and antegrade. In contrast, the false lumen more often is the larger lumen and has slow or absent flow and may have thrombus (**Table 28.2**). Distinguishing the lumens has implications regarding prognosis and management, particularly if the coronary arteries, great vessels, or peripheral vessels originate from the false lumen.

29. **Answer: D.** The image shows an intramural hematoma with displaced intimal calcification. An aortic intramural hematoma is characterized by TEE as a circumferential or crescent-shaped smooth margined thickening of the aortic wall without an

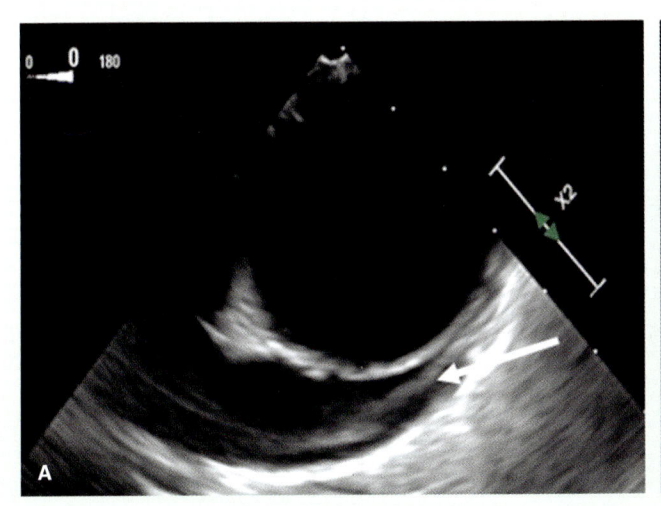

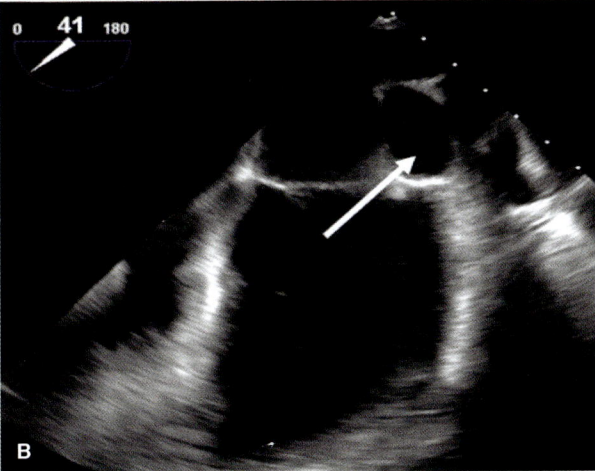

Figure 28.28

Table 28.6. Echocardiographic Features of Aortic Intramural Hematoma

- Circular or crescent-shaped thickening of the aortic wall
- Thickening of the aortic wall >5 mm
- Continuous and smooth margined thickening of the aortic wall
- Absence of intimal flap or communication with the aortic lumen
- Reduction in the size of the aortic lumen due to thickening of the aortic wall
- Echolucent areas within aortic wall
- Displacement of intimal calcium next to aortic lumen

intimal flap. The degree of aortic wall thickening is generally >5 mm. Intimal calcium may be displaced toward the lumen of the vessel by the accumulation of medial hematoma. Echolucent areas in the aortic wall may be seen suggestive of noncommunicating blood in the medial hematoma (**Table 28.6**). An intramural hematoma is generally continuous over a relatively localized or extensive portion of the aorta and sometimes may coexist with regions of the aorta that have an intimal flap.

Severe aortic atheromatous disease or mural thrombus can appear similar to intramural hematoma. Aside from the obvious differences in clinical presentation, echocardiographic features can help differentiate these entities. In contrast to the features described above seen with intramural hematomas, atheroma or mural thrombus is typically discrete, with irregular borders, protruding or mobile components, is not contiguous and has scattered calcifications. Another mimic of intramural hematoma is a thrombosed false lumen. The pathophysiology of an intramural hematoma and an intimal flap with a thrombosed lumen is similar. A penetrating aortic ulcer results in a localized intramural hematoma though the ulcer may be identified as the initiating event. Aortic thickening due to aortitis is usually mild and does not usually present a diagnostic dilemma relative to intramural hematoma.

30. **Answer: D.** The TEE image is consistent with a penetrating aortic ulcer on the upper descending thoracic aorta with a saccular aneurysm. Typical features consistent with a penetrating aortic ulcer include a large calcified atheromatous plaque with a craterlike outpouching of the aortic wall. Histologically, a penetrating ulcer is characterized by a break in the internal elastic lamina with medial hematoma. Consequences of a penetrating ulcer include a saccular aneurysm, pseudoaneurysm, aortic dissection, or aortic rupture. Risk factors for complications include the depth and diameter of the outpouching.

A symptomatic penetrating ulcer is an acute aortic syndrome and surgery should be considered. Thoracic endovascular aortic repair (TEVAR) has become an attractive option for management of penetrating ulcers depending on the site of involvement. Penetrating aortic ulcers are most often seen in the descending thoracic aorta in smokers.

KEY POINTS

- Penetrating aortic ulcer represents a form of acute aortic syndrome.
- Features of penetrating aortic ulcers include: (1) calcified atheromatous plaque; (2) craterlike outpouching; (3) intramural hematoma; and (4) complications including aortic dissection, pseudoaneurysm, saccular aneurysm, or aortic rupture.

31. **Answer: C.** The TEE image shows diffuse thickening of the aortic-mitral curtain extending to the anterior leaflet of the mitral valve in a patient with aortitis. Although this finding may be associated with aortic valve endocarditis with periaortic root abscess, the clinical history is consistent with an inflammatory aortitis. The inflammatory process may involve the ascending aorta extending to the sinuses of Valsalva, aortic leaflets, annulus, and aortic-mitral curtain. Findings most commonly associated with aortitis include aortic aneurysms and aortic regurgitation. **Figure 28.29A** and **B** shows the TEE long-axis (**A**) and descending aorta views (**B**) of the aorta demonstrating diffuse aortic wall thickening due to aortitis.

KEY POINTS

- Thickening of the aortic-mitral curtain may result from aortitis or endocarditis with associated periaortic abscess.
- Aortitis is a well-recognized manifestation of primary and secondary systemic inflammatory conditions or infectious etiologies.
- Aortitis may involve all segments of the aorta and extend to involve the aortic root, leaflets, and annulus.

32. **Answer: B.** The patient has an acute type A aortic dissection with aortic regurgitation. Aortic regurgitation is common in the setting of ascending aortic dissection occurring in over half of patients. Several mechanisms that account for aortic regurgitation have been described: (a) dilated aortic root with tethering of the leaflets and poor coaptation; (b) leaflet prolapse due to asymmetric dissection depressing cusp below annulus; (c) disruption of annular support leading to flail leaflet; (d) large redundant proximal dissection flap with prolapse into the left ventricular outflow

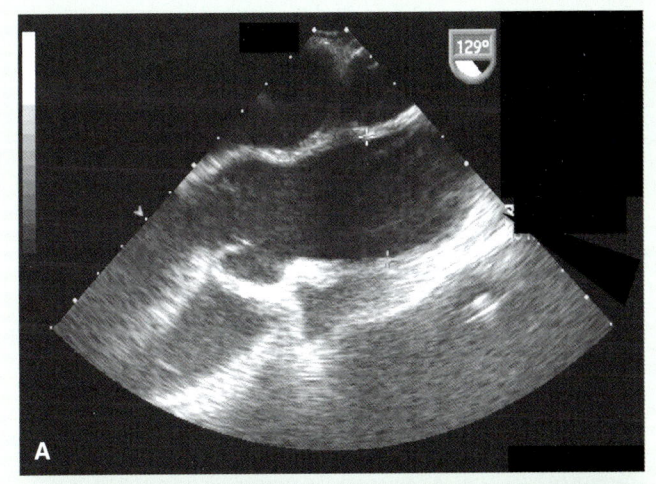

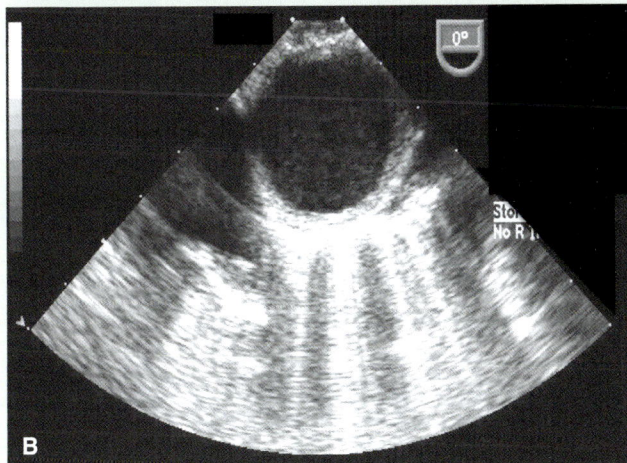

Figure 28.29

tract in diastole causing disruption of coaptation; and (e) associated primary valve abnormalities such as a bicuspid aortic valve. **Figure 28.17** and ▶ **Video 28.5** show an aortic dissection flap in the proximal ascending aorta and moderate aortic regurgitation. TEE can accurately distinguish the mechanism of aortic regurgitation as well as the severity and aid surgeons in determining the feasibility of repair. Numerous aortic valve–sparing procedures have been successfully performed with supracoronary aortic grafting. However, replacement of the aorta alone will not likely resolve aortic regurgitation in this setting.

KEY POINTS
- Aortic regurgitation is common with type A aortic dissection.
- Mechanisms of aortic regurgitation in type A aortic dissection involve disruption of leaflet coaptation, annular or aortic root size or geometry, and underlying abnormal aortic valve disease.
- Aortic valve–sparing procedures are feasible in many patients with type A aortic dissection depending on the mechanism and severity of aortic regurgitation.

33. **Answer: B.** The abnormality seen on this TEE is a large periaortic echodense space with pockets of echolucencies. The aortic homograft appears well seated with mild aortic regurgitation, which is valvular and centrally directed. The appearance of the large periaortic echodense space is most consistent with an organized fluid or blood collection. The differential diagnosis in this patient includes blood/hematoma, purulent fluid/abscess/endocarditis, and massive serous edema. Typical postoperative changes following aortic homograft do include edema and hematoma formation though the size and extent seen here are to a greater extent than usual. Suspected abscess of the aortic root can now be evaluated with PET/CT imaging, which will show uptake of FDG if an infective etiology is present. The fluid collection in this case was periaortic blood/hematoma related to partial suture dehiscence and paravalvular leak at the annulus level. As a result, a fistulous communication developed between the outflow tract and the periaortic space where blood accumulated. With the use of a transcatheter closure device, the paravalvular communication was occluded and the hematoma resolved over time.

KEY POINTS
- Fluid collections in the periaortic root space detected by echocardiography may represent blood/hematoma, edema, or purulent material such as abscess formation.
- Distinguishing between these entities is difficult and should be based on additional echocardiographic features, clinical information, and if necessary PET/CT imaging.

34. **Answer: A.** The TEE images reveal an acute type A aortic dissection presenting with a large pericardial effusion (hemopericardium). The long-axis images show an intimal flap at the level of the aortic root confirming the diagnosis of a proximal dissection. Based on the clinical history and echo images, there is evidence of cardiac tamponade. In this setting, the patient should be taken immediately to the operating room for aortic surgery. Small series have demonstrated concerns regarding pericardiocentesis in patients with cardiac tamponade and aortic dissection. In some cases after the removal of pericardial fluid, rapid decompensation and death has occurred, possibly related to augmented ventricular function and propagation of the dissection. Thus when cardiac tamponade is present along with proximal aortic dissection, immediate surgery should be performed unless a surgical team is not available and the patient is in extremis.

> **KEY POINTS**
> - When cardiac tamponade is present along with proximal aortic dissection, immediate surgery is indicated.
> - Pericardiocentesis should not be performed in unstable patients with cardiac tamponade due to aortic dissection unless surgical support is not readily available.

SUGGESTED READINGS

Goldstein SA, Evangelista A, Abbara S, et al. Multimodality imaging of diseases of the thoracic aorta in adults: from the American Society of echocardiography and the European association of cardiovascular imaging—endorsed by the Society of cardiovascular computed tomography and Society for cardiovascular magnetic resonance. *J Am Soc Echocardiogr*. 2015;28(2):119-182.

Lang RM, Badano LP, Mor-Avi V, et al. Recommendations for cardiac chamber quantification by echocardiography in adults: an update from the American Society of Echocardiography and the European Association of Cardiovascular Imaging. *J Am Soc Echocardiogr*. 2015;16(3):233-270.

Lopez L, Saurers DL, Barker PCA, et al. Guidelines for performing a comprehensive pediatric transthoracic echocardiogram: recommendations from the American Society of Echocardiography. *J Am Soc Echocardiogr*. 2024;37:119-170.

Verma S, Siu SC. Aortic dilatation in patients with bicuspid aortic valve. *N Engl J Med*. 2014;370(20):1920-1929.

Writing Committee Members; Isselbacher EM, Preventza O, Hamilton Black Iii J, et al. 2022 ACC/AHA guideline for the diagnosis and management of aortic disease: a report of the American Heart Association/American College of Cardiology Joint Committee on clinical Practice guidelines. *J Am Coll Cardiol*. 2022;80(24):e223-e393.

CHAPTER 29

Atrial Fibrillation

Maria Fadous and Jordan B. Strom

QUESTIONS

1. A 75-year-old man with a history of hypertension is admitted to the hospital after a transient ischemic attack and is found to be in atrial fibrillation (AF). He is referred for a transesophageal echocardiogram (TEE). Which echo finding is associated with an increased risk of left atrial (LA) thrombus?
   A. Patent foramen ovale.
   B. LA appendage velocities >50 cm/s.
   C. LA volume index of <25 mL/m².
   D. Spontaneous echo contrast (SEC).

2. Which LA measurements best correlates with the maintenance of sinus rhythm after cardioversion?
   A. LA volume index of 30 mL/m² and LA appendage velocity 40 cm/s.
   B. LA volume index of 30 mL/m² and LA appendage velocity 50 cm/s.
   C. LA volume index of 40 mL/m² and LA appendage velocity 40 cm/s.
   D. LA volume index of 40 mL/m² and LA appendage velocity 30 cm/s.

3. Transmitral E/e′ best estimates pulmonary capillary wedge pressure (PCWP) in a patient with which cardiac pathology?
   A. Mitral annuloplasty ring.
   B. Severe mitral annular calcification (MAC).
   C. Atrial fibrillation.
   D. Mechanical mitral valve.

4. Which of the following is most suggestive of increased left ventricular filling pressures in patients with atrial fibrillation?
   A. Isovolumic relaxation time (IVRT) of 80 ms.
   B. Deceleration time (DT) of pulmonary venous diastolic velocity of 250 ms.
   C. Septal E/e′ ratio of 13.
   D. LA volume index of 35 mL/m².

5. In patients with aortic stenosis (AS) and AF, which statement is **CORRECT**?
   A. Doppler mean gradients should be averaged out of three beats.
   B. Doppler mean gradients often overestimate AS severity when obtained in AF compared to sinus rhythm.
   C. Atrial fibrillation is associated with lower forward flow compared to sinus rhythm.
   D. A peak left ventricular outflow tract (LVOT) to aortic velocity ratio (Doppler velocity index or DVI) of 0.3 is suggestive of severe AS.

6. Why are right atrial appendage (RAA) thrombi significantly less frequent then left atrial appendage (LAA) thrombi?
   A. RAA velocities are usually higher than those in the LAA.
   B. LAA neck is larger and "traps" thrombi.
   C. RAA width is larger and lacks anatomic remodeling during AF.
   D. RAA does not fibrillate.

7. Which statement regarding the LAA anatomy is **FALSE**?
   A. The normal diameter of the LAA orifice ranges from 10 to 24 mm.
   B. The orifice of the LAA is typically located posteriorly and laterally.
   C. The ridge between the orifice of the LAA and the pulmonary vein is a fold of LA wall tissue and serous pericardium.
   D. The LAA can have up to five lobes.

8. Assessment of LAA function can provide incremental information about the risk of thrombus formation, embolic events, and success of cardioversion. Which of the following statements is **CORRECT**?
   A. The pulsed Doppler sample volume should be placed as distally as possible in the LAA cavity.
   B. LAA velocities decrease progressively with age.
   C. LAA velocities are typically lower and slower in atrial flutter than in atrial fibrillation.
   D. LAA fractional area change is the preferred method of assessment of LAA function.

9. LAA emptying velocities of <20 cm/s are associated with spontaneous echocardiographic contrast, thrombus formation, and embolic events. Which wave (**Figure 29.1**) represents the late diastolic LAA emptying velocity in sinus rhythm?
   A. Wave 1.
   B. Wave 2.
   C. Wave 3.
   D. Wave 4.

10. In which patient would the development of AF be most hemodynamically compromising?
    A. Hypertrophic cardiomyopathy with a resting LVOT velocity of 4 m/s.
    B. Bicuspid aortic valve with a peak velocity of 3 m/s.
    C. Mitral annular calcification with a mean gradient of 5 mm Hg across the mitral valve.
    D. Mitral regurgitation with a peak velocity of 6 m/s.

11. Possible causes of ongoing thromboembolism in patients with paroxysmal AF but no clinical recurrence of AF include all of the following **EXCEPT**:

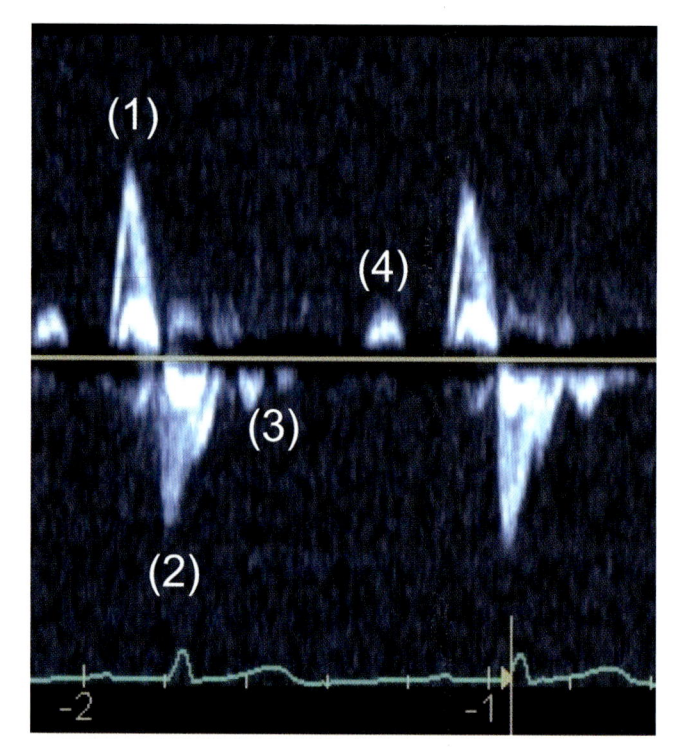

Figure 29.1

   A. Thrombus development during asymptomatic periods of AF.
   B. Transient demand–associated increase in mitral regurgitation.
   C. Mechanical discordance of the LAA and body of the LA.
   D. Coexistent complex aortic plaque.

12. A 78-year-old patient with AF requires assessment of the LAA prior to planned pulmonary vein isolation. He has a proximal esophageal stricture with dysphagia. The best alternative imaging modality to assess the LAA for thrombus would be:
    A. Transthoracic echocardiography (TTE) with harmonic imaging.
    B. TTE with echo contrast.
    C. Cardiac magnetic resonance imaging.
    D. Intracardiac echocardiography (ICE).

13. Recovery of LA mechanical function following cardioversion of AF to sinus rhythm:
    A. Occurs within 24 hours.
    B. Is related to recovery of the electrocardiogram (ECG) P-wave height.
    C. Is inversely related to LA volume.
    D. Is directly related to the duration of AF prior to cardioversion.

14. Left atrial strain is a predictor of atrial fibrillation occurrence and recurrence, and its value seems to be associated with thromboembolic risk. Which of the following phases of the left atrial cycle is indicated by the arrow (**Figure 29.2**)?
   A. Contraction phase.
   B. Reservoir phase.
   C. Conduit phase.
   D. Relaxation phase.

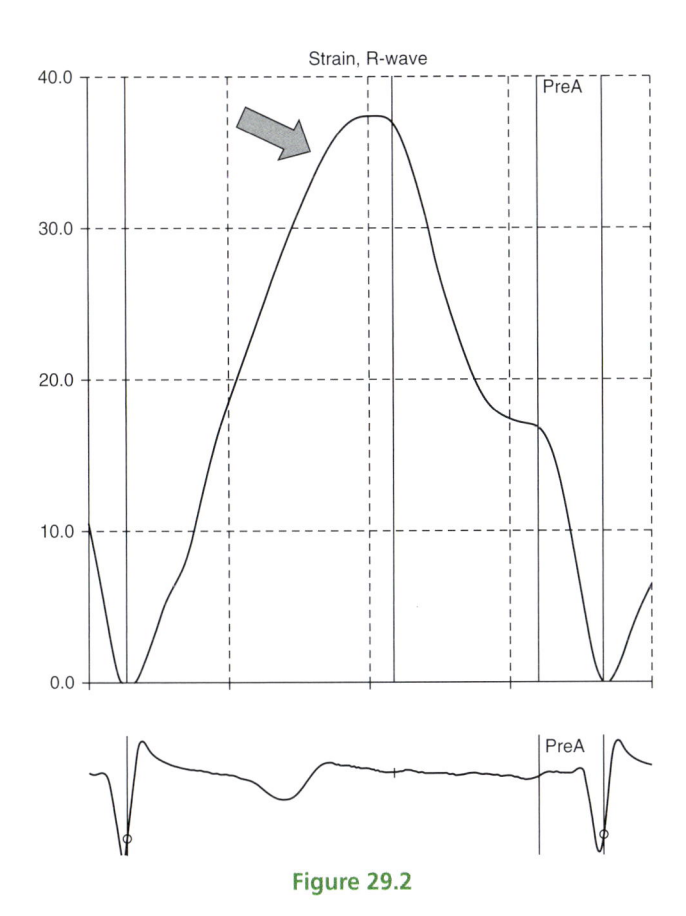

Figure 29.2

15. A 68-year-old woman with AF is referred for TEE due to a transient ischemic attack. Which of the following is **TRUE** about her TEE finding in Video 29.1?
   A. Its prevalence is the same for both AF and atrial flutter.
   B. Mitral regurgitation worsens this finding.
   C. There is an association with LA myxoma.
   D. It is an independent predictor of thromboembolic risk.

16. What can be inferred from these Doppler findings (**Figure 29.3**)?
   A. There is a high probability of maintaining sinus rhythm after cardioversion.
   B. This is associated with an increased risk of thromboembolism.
   C. There is severe pulmonary hypertension.
   D. The patient should be referred for pulmonary vein isolation (PVI).

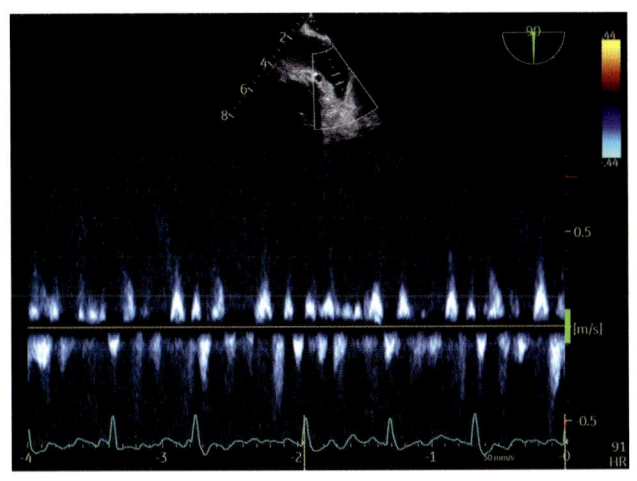

Figure 29.3

17. A 22-year-old man presents with increasing dyspnea and decreased exercise tolerance that has limited his ability to participate in his basketball league. A TTE is performed (**Figure 29.4**). What would confirm the diagnosis?
   A. Increased gradient across the mitral valve.
   B. LAA contiguous with the basal (proximal) chamber.
   C. LAA contiguous with the apical (distal) chamber.
   D. Normal apical 2-chamber view (eg, this is an artifact).

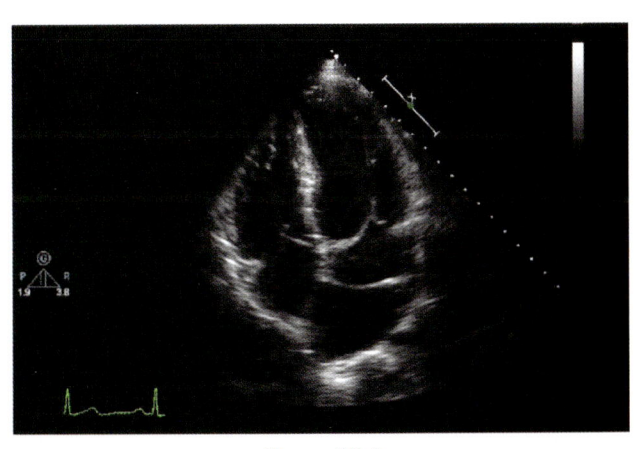

Figure 29.4

622 / Clinical Echocardiography Review

Figure 29.5

18. An 83-year-old man with a history of AF presents with a transient ischemic attack. The patient was therapeutic on warfarin at the time of hospitalization (INR = 2.5). The patient was referred for a TEE for further workup. During TEE inspection of the left atrium, a small patent foramen ovale was observed, but no LA or LAA thrombi were seen. A view of his aortic arch is shown in **Figure 29.5**. Based on these echo findings, what should be recommended?
   A. Percutaneous closure of the patent foramen ovale.
   B. Increase the target INR to 3 to 4.
   C. Add statin therapy.
   D. Confirmation with contrast chest computed tomography (CT).

19. A 64-year-old man with a sternotomy scar is admitted to the hospital with atypical chest pain and new-onset AF. The patient denies neurologic symptoms and is without focal neurologic findings on physical examination. INR on admission is 2.1. The patient's TEE is without evidence of LA or LAA thrombi or valvular thrombus. Coronary angiography was performed the following day. Although there was no significant coronary disease, fluoroscopy of the aortic valve as in ▶ **Video 29.2** was observed. Based on these findings, what would you recommend?
   A. Warfarin therapy with goal INR 2.5.
   B. Warfarin therapy with goal INR 3.0.
   C. Anticoagulation with direct oral anticoagulant (DOAC).
   D. Treatment with low-dose systemic fibrinolytic therapy.

20. A 78-year-old man without prior medical history is admitted with a 1-day history of palpitations and shortness of breath. Based on the M-mode finding in **Figure 29.6**, what would you recommend?
   A. Emergent cardiac surgery.
   B. Thrombolytics.
   C. Check TSH.
   D. Alcohol septal ablation.

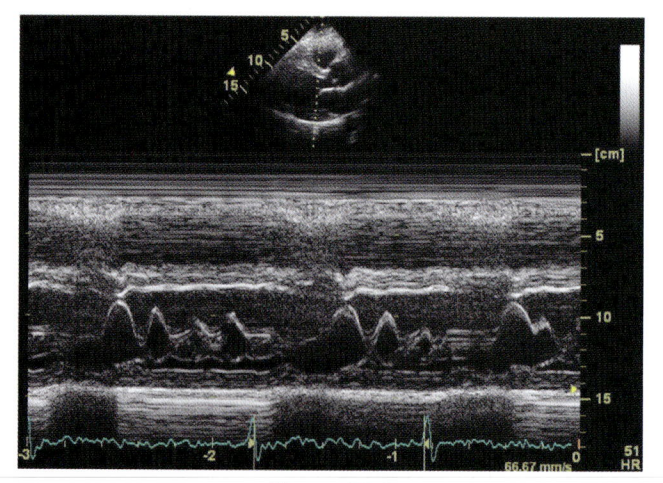

Figure 29.6

21. A 43-year-old woman with a history of paroxysmal AF is referred for an echocardiogram. Based on **Figure 29.7**, which statement is **TRUE**?
   A. Direct current cardioversion is contraindicated.
   B. Emergent cardiac surgery is warranted.
   C. Risk for sudden cardiac death is increased.
   D. This is a normal variant.

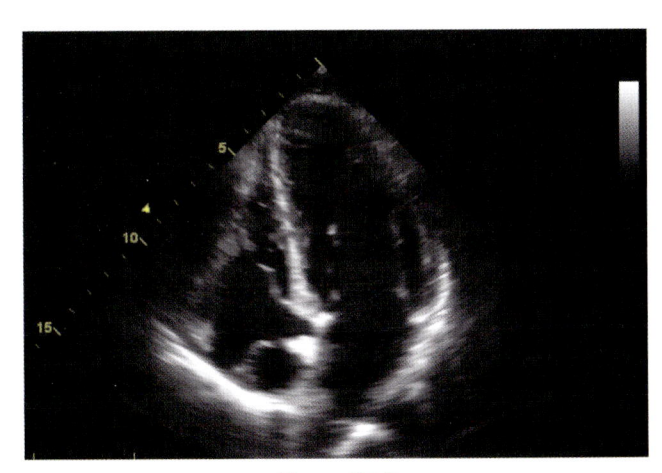

Figure 29.7

22. An 81-year-old man is admitted to the hospital for chest pain and shortness of breath and found to have an acute myocardial infarction. The patient is referred for TEE for a questionable transient ischemic attack on hospital day 2. Based on the Doppler findings in **Figure 29.8**, which of the following statements is **CORRECT**?
   A. The patient's prognosis is worse than if this finding were not seen on Doppler.
   B. This finding occurs in approximately 50% of acute myocardial infarctions.
   C. The patient should be referred for percutaneous closure.
   D. The estimated PCWP is 30 mm Hg.

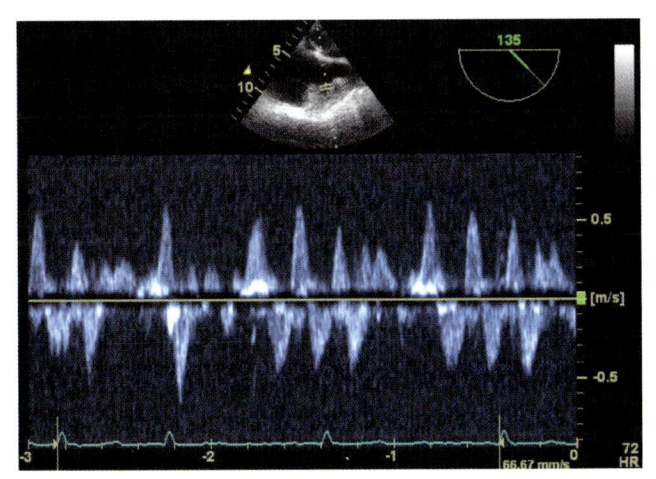

Figure 29.8

23. A 58-year-old man with a history of AF is referred for a TEE prior to cardioversion. Although there was no evidence of LAA thrombus, this image (**Figure 29.9**) was seen. What is a **TRUE** statement regarding this finding?

A. Electrical cardioversion is contraindicated.
B. Emergent surgery is warranted.
C. It is a normal variant.
D. A malignancy workup is needed.

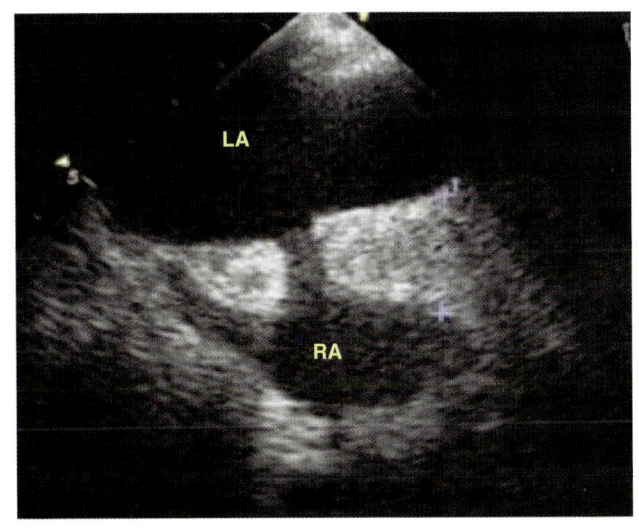

Figure 29.9

24. A 55-year-old man is referred for electrical cardioversion for symptomatic AF/atrial flutter. Based on the Doppler findings in **Figure 29.10**, what would be expected immediately postcardioversion?
   A. Decreased risk of thromboembolism.
   B. Recurrence of AF.
   C. Improvement of LA function.
   D. Decreased velocities in the LAA.

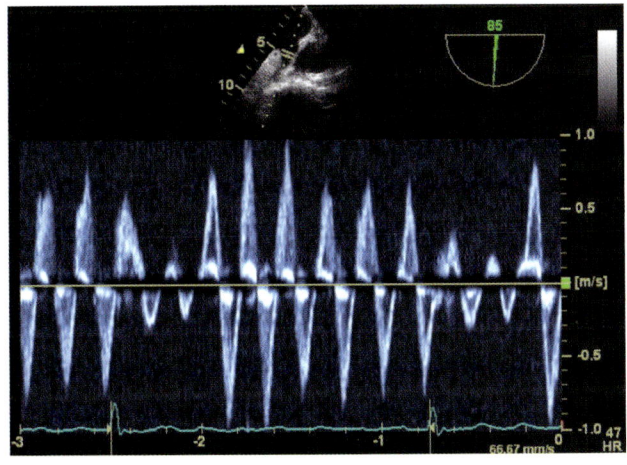

Figure 29.10

25. A 62-year-old woman presents to the hospital with occasional palpitations and is found to be in atrial fibrillation. Her heart rate is 112 bpm and her blood pressure is 130/80 mm Hg. You perform a TEE prior to attempting direct current cardioversion (DCCV). Given the findings shown in ▶ **Video 29.3**, what would you recommend?
A. Proceed with DCCV.
B. Cancel DCCV and recommend chemical cardioversion.
C. Cancel DCCV and recommend rate control.
D. Cancel DCCV and recommend PVI.

26. A 38-year-old man presents with intermittent palpitations that started 48 hours ago. His ECG shows atrial fibrillation. He denies any history of hypertension, diabetes, heart failure, or stroke. During his TTE, he spontaneously converts back to sinus rhythm. Based on the findings in **Figure 29.11**, how would you manage this patient?
A. No anticoagulation.
B. Aspirin.
C. DOAC.
D. Warfarin.

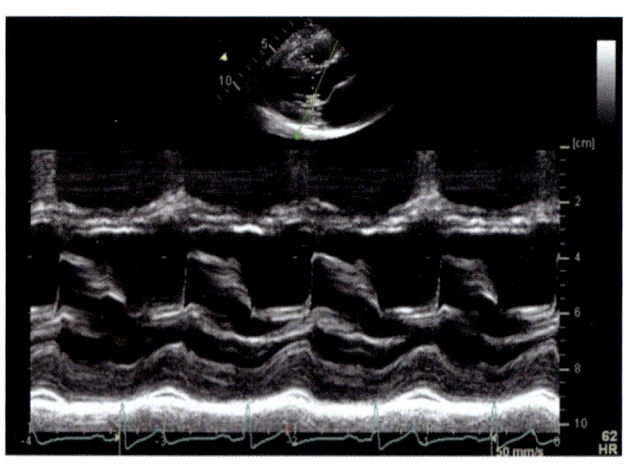

Figure 29.11

27. What is the preferred imaging modality to evaluate for LA thrombi?
A. TTE with IV-administered contrast agent and harmonic imaging.
B. Three-dimensional (3D) TTE.
C. TEE.
D. Pulsed-wave Doppler through the LAA.

CASE 1

A 50-year-old man is referred for PVI for treatment of paroxysmal AF. A TEE is ordered prior to his procedure.

28. What is the specificity of TEE for diagnosing the finding shown in **Case 1** and ▶ **Video 29.4**?
A. 80% to 85%.
B. 85% to 90%.
C. 90% to 95%.
D. >95%.

29. The patient in **Case 1** is started on anticoagulation and he undergoes a successful PVI procedure several months later. Three months post procedure, he develops progressive shortness of breath with exertion. He is referred for TEE which demonstrates the findings in **Figure 29.12**. Based on these Doppler findings, what is the likely etiology of his shortness of breath?
A. Mitral stenosis.
B. AF.
C. Severe mitral regurgitation.
D. Pulmonary vein stenosis.

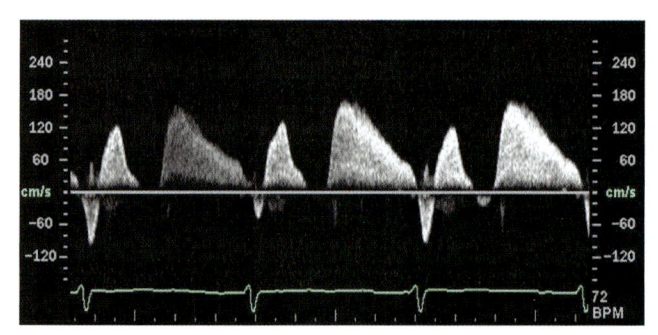

Figure 29.12

CASE 2

A 72-year-old man with paroxysmal AF presents with a transient ischemic attack and is referred for a TEE. The LA is normal in size on the images in Figure 29.13.

30. Based on the findings in **Case 2**, what would you recommend?
A. Start warfarin with a goal INR of 3 to 4 and reimage in 3 weeks.
B. Nothing, this is an artifact.
C. Refer for cardiac surgery.
D. Percutaneous transseptal removal.

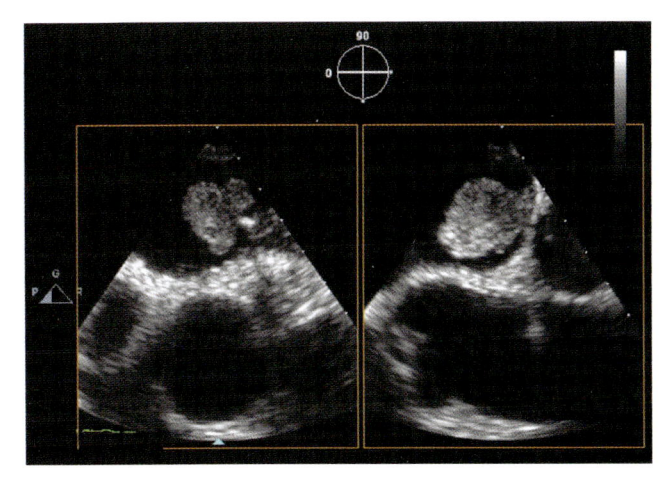

Figure 29.13

31. Which statement is **TRUE** regarding this finding on echocardiogram from **Case 2**?
   A. There is no risk of recurrence after resection.
   B. It is usually malignant.
   C. It is usually attached to the interatrial septum.
   D. It is most commonly found in the right atrium.

32. **Figure 29.13** combined with what other pathology is found in patients with Carney complex?
   A. Schwannomas.
   B. Anomalous pulmonary veins.
   C. Right-sided aorta.
   D. Bicuspid aortic valve.

CASE 3

A 78-year-old man with paroxysmal atrial fibrillation and recurrent gastrointestinal bleeding undergoes percutaneous left atrial appendage occlusion (LAAO). His postoperative course is unremarkable with no recurrent gastrointestinal bleeding. His 45-day follow-up TEE is shown below (**Figure 29.14**).

33. Which of the following statements is **TRUE** regarding the patient in **Case 3**?
   A. Peri-device leak is a common complication following LAAO.
   B. Large leaks are defined as leaks >10 mm.
   C. Device endothelialization usually occurs within 14 days post implantation.
   D. This is unlikely to resolve without treatment.

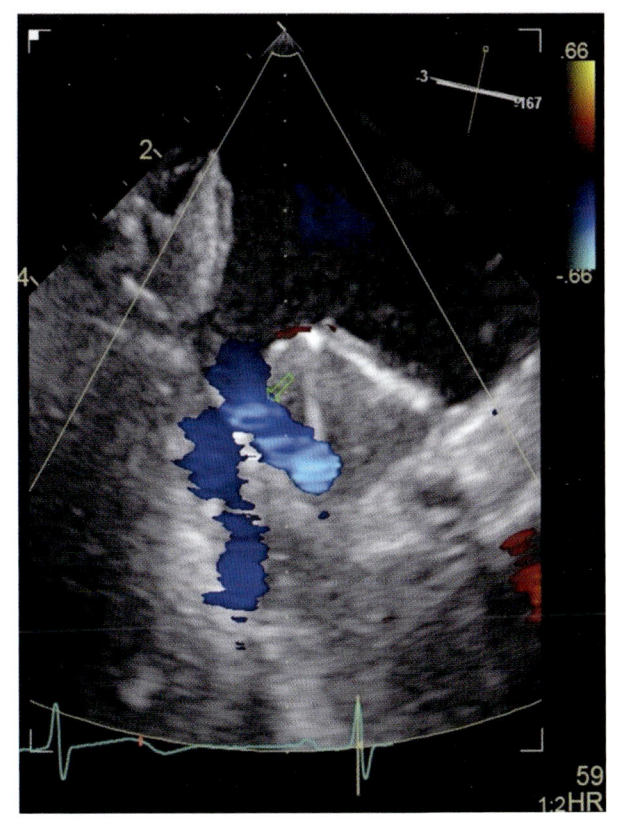

Figure 29.14

34. A routine 1-year surveillance TEE shows the following (**Figure 29.15**). How would you manage this patient?
   A. Repositioning of LAAO device.
   B. Start a DOAC.
   C. Start intravenous antibiotics.
   D. Reassurance.

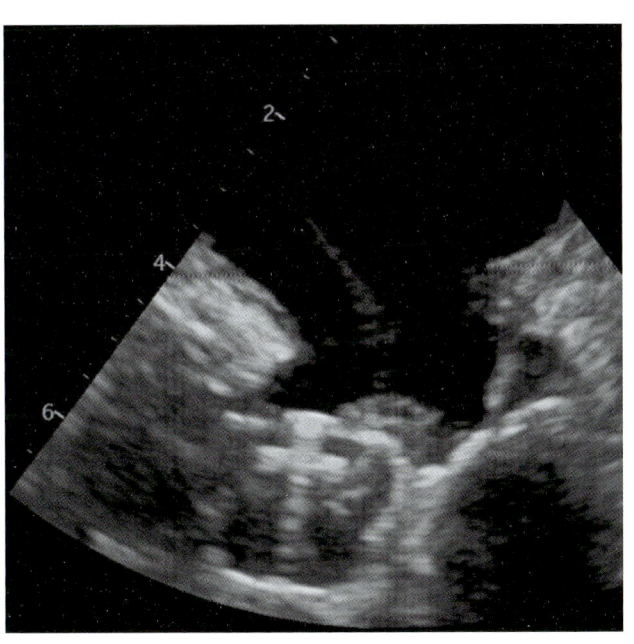

Figure 29.15

ANSWERS

1. **Answer: D.** SEC is present in over 50% of all patients with AF and in over 80% of those with an LAA thrombus or a recent thromboembolic event. Patent foramen ovale is an important contributor to cryptogenic stroke in the young but is unassociated with thromboembolic events in AF. LAA flow velocities >50 cm/s are normal, as is LA volume index of 25 mL/m² (normal ≤34 mL/m²).

2. **Answer: B.** LA size is important prognostically in AF. Progressive enlargement is associated with a decreased probability of maintaining sinus rhythm. Moreover, LA size (in particular, LA minimum size) is associated with incident AF in the general population. LAA velocity is also thought to be a predictor of the likelihood of maintaining sinus rhythm after cardioversion. Answer B has the smallest LA size and highest LAA velocity and is therefore the best option.

3. **Answer: C.** Atrial fibrillation is the best choice among these options. E/e' should not be used to determine PCWP in patients with mitral valve prostheses or severe MAC, as e' velocities may not reflect diastolic relaxation and correlate poorly with PCWP. In the case of moderate or greater MAC, mitral E/A ratio and IVRT may be used to identify those with increased PCWP. E/e' remains an accurate estimate of PCWP in AF. Additionally, while LA reservoir strain has been associated with LA pressure outside of the setting of AF, LA reservoir strain values are depressed regardless of the LA pressure in patients with AF and thus should not be used for estimation of LA pressure in this population.

4. **Answer: C.** In patients with AF, Doppler assessment of LV diastolic function is limited by the variability in cycle length, the absence of organized atrial activity, and the frequent occurrence of LA enlargement regardless of filling pressures. Doppler measurements that may have value in identifying those with increased PCWP in AF include:
   - Peak acceleration rate of mitral E velocity of ≥1900 cm/s²
   - Isovolumic relaxation time (IVRT) of ≤65 ms
   - Deceleration time (DT) of pulmonary venous diastolic velocity of ≤220 ms
   - E/V$_p$ ratio of ≥1.4
   - Septal E/e' ratio of ≥11

5. **Answer: C.** Forward flow is one of the main determinants of mean gradient. As AF is associated with lower forward flow, AS severity may be underestimated by the flow-dependent MG when obtained by echocardiography during AF compared with sinus rhythm. In patients with atrial fibrillation, mean gradient should be calculated as the average of five cycles with the least variation of R-R intervals and as close as possible to normal heart rate. A Doppler velocity index (DVI) < 0.25 is suggestive of severe aortic stenosis.

6. **Answer: C.** The larger RAA width and lack of anatomic remodeling may partially explain the substantially lower prevalence of RAA thrombus found among patients with AF. All the other choices are false statements.

7. **Answer: B.** The LAA is a blind-ending structure with the orifice typically located superiorly and laterally, adjacent to the anterolateral commissure of the mitral valve. The normal diameter of the ostium ranges from 10 to 24 mm. The ridge between the ostium of the LAA and the left superior pulmonary vein is a triangular fold of LA wall tissue and serous pericardium (AKA the left lateral ridge or warfarin ridge due to its frequent confusion for a thrombus). Autopsy studies have shown that the LAA can vary from having one to as many as five lobes (**Figure 29.16**; the arrow points to one of the multiple lobes of the LAA).

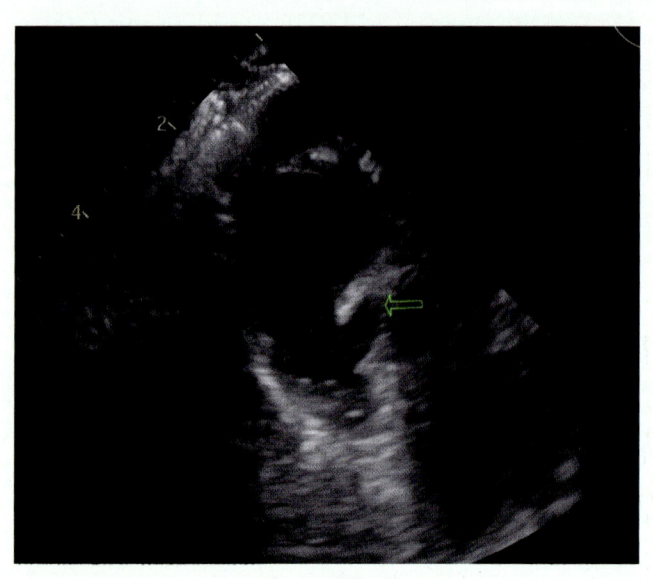

Figure 29.16

8. **Answer: B.** Doppler measurement of LAA flow velocities is currently the preferred method of assessment of LAA function. The pulsed Doppler sample volume is typically placed 1 to 2 cm from the orifice within the chamber. LAA flow velocities progressively decline with age and are typically higher and slower in atrial flutter than in atrial fibrillation.

9. **Answer: A.** In a normal LAA spectral Doppler trace, four waves are seen during sinus rhythm (see **Figure 29.1**):
   1. LAA contraction and emptying during atrial systole, which is seen above the baseline;
   2. LAA filling during early ventricular systole, which is seen below the baseline;
   3. Systolic reflection waves (positive and negative), which represent passive flow during the remainder of systole alternating on both sides of the baseline;
   4. Early diastolic LAA emptying during LV early filling seen above the baseline.

10. **Answer: A.** The patient in Answer A has a resting gradient of 64 mm Hg across the LVOT, which is quite elevated. Patients with hypertrophic cardiomyopathy and LVOT obstruction often have compromised left ventricular (LV) filling due to abnormal relaxation secondary to myofibril disarray. Additionally, systolic anterior motion of the anterior leaflet of the mitral valve, which results in outflow tract obstruction and mitral regurgitation, can severely compromise cardiac output. The development of AF in such a patient would compromise LV filling significantly. Answers B through D are essentially mild forms of their respective pathologies.

11. **Answer: B.** Prolonged rhythm monitoring in patients with AF documents frequent episodes of clinically silent periods of AF. TEE studies suggest that 25% of patients with paroxysmal AF demonstrate periods in which the ECG and body of the LA are in sinus rhythm, while the LAA has a fibrillatory pattern on pulsed-wave Doppler (**Figure 29.17**). Aortic plaque is found in over 50% of patients with AF with nearly 50% of these with complex plaque. Complex plaque is associated with thromboembolism. In the AF population, at least moderate mitral regurgitation has been shown to be associated with a decreased risk of clinical stroke.

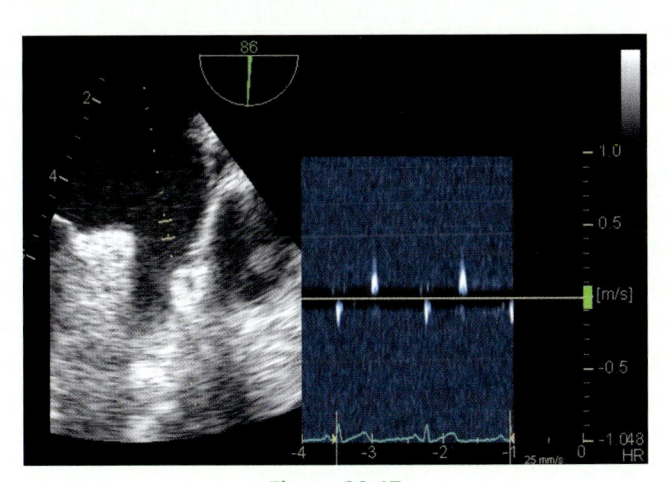

Figure 29.17

12. **Answer: D.** Though TTE with echo contrast improves definition of the LAA, it has not been shown to be as efficacious as TEE for identifying LAA thrombi. Cardiac MRI has an inferior sensitivity and specificity for LAA thrombi, likely due to the irregular rhythm and slow LAA flow leading to stagnant blood flow and false positive interpretation. Gated cardiac computed tomography, when adequate, has comparable performance as TEE for detection of LAA thrombus but is not listed as an answer choice. ICE with the ICE probe advanced into the main pulmonary artery has been shown to be extremely accurate (vs TEE) for identifying thrombus in the LAA. Though expensive, the catheter is the same catheter used in the subsequent pulmonary vein isolation procedures to guide the transseptal puncture.

13. **Answer: D.** Though there may be apparent sinus rhythm with full recovery of atrial waveforms on ECG, atrial mechanical function as assessed by transmitral Doppler may remain depressed for several weeks after successful cardioversion. Recovery of LA mechanical function is related to the duration of AF prior to cardioversion, with full recovery within 24 hours for those with AF of <2 weeks, within a week for those with AF of <4 to 6 weeks, and within a month for those with AF for >2 months.

14. **Answer: B.** LA deformation is a cyclic process, which can be subdivided into three phases (**Figure 29.18**):
    1. the reservoir phase (corresponding to ventricular systole);
    2. the conduit phase (when the mitral valve is open in early ventricular diastole and there is passive LV filling);
    3. the contraction or booster pump phase (in late ventricular diastole occurring with atrial contraction in patients in sinus rhythm).

    While a normal reference range for LA reservoir strain is 39% (95% CI, 38%-41%) and 17% (95% CI, 16%-19%) for contraction strain, a cutoff of LA reservoir strain of less than 18% or contraction strain less than 8% has been associated with increased LA pressure. Abnormal left atrial reservoir and contractile strain have also been associated with a higher risk of incident atrial fibrillation and ischemic stroke, even in those with normal LA size and normal LV function.

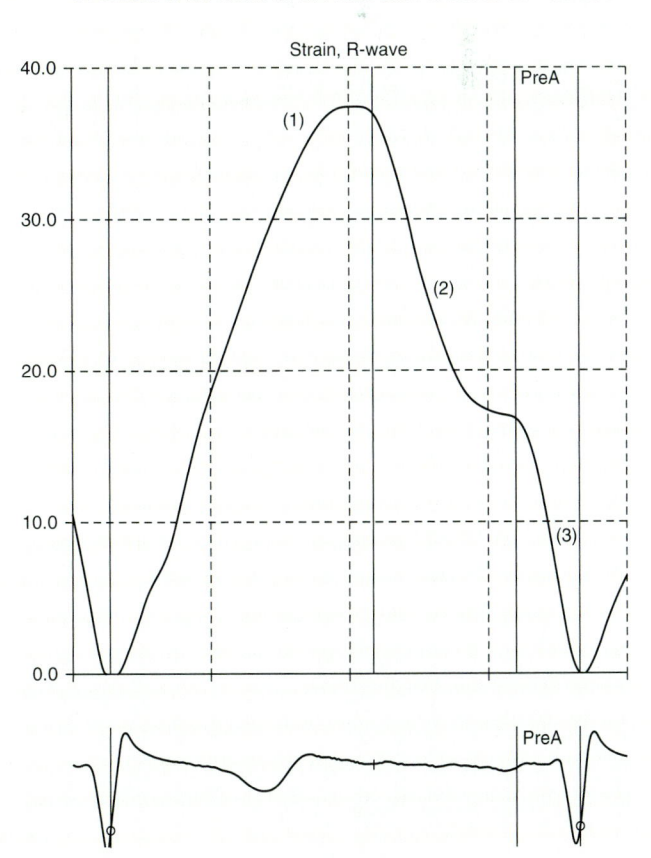

Figure 29.18

15. **Answer: D.** ▶ **Video 29.1** shows prominent spontaneous echo contrast (SEC) in the LAA. SEC is an independent predictor of thromboembolic risk and is associated with an increase in embolic rate in patients with AF. SEC is on a continuum with "sludge" and thrombus. Mitral regurgitation appears to be associated with a lower frequency of SEC. There is a strong association between LA SEC and LA thrombi. The prevalence of SEC occurs more frequently in AF than in atrial flutter. There is no known association between SEC and LA myxoma.

16. **Answer: B.** The risk of stroke is increased with marked reductions in blood flow velocity, particularly in the LAA or posterior LA. A low-appendage ejection flow velocity is associated with the presence of appendage thrombus and with dense SEC. LAA blood flow velocity (>40 cm/s) is thought to be a predictor of the likelihood of maintaining sinus rhythm after cardioversion. There are no definitive findings that suggest that this patient has severe pulmonary hypertension or should be referred for pulmonary vein isolation (PVI) based on atrial appendage velocities.

17. **Answer: C.** Cor triatriatum sinister is differentiated from a supravalvular mitral ring by the position of the LAA (**Figure 29.19**, white arrow). In cor triatriatum sinister, the left appendage is part of the distal (mitral valve) atrial chamber, while the LAA is part of the proximal (pulmonary vein) atrial chamber in patients with a supravalvular ring.

Cor triatriatum may be associated with other congenital abnormalities (atrial septal defect, persistence of left superior vena cava), but is commonly seen in isolation when found in an adult. It may be associated with increased gradients across the membrane, leading to this patient's symptoms. However, this finding lacks specificity and does not confirm a diagnosis.

Given **Figure 29.19** and this patient's symptoms, an artifact cannot be assumed. Such a finding should be further investigated with multiple views, with and without Doppler. If TTE findings are ambiguous, a TEE may be warranted.

18. **Answer: C. Figure 29.5** reveals a complex aortic plaque, which is defined as ≥4-mm-thick, ulcerated or containing mobile thrombi. Patients who experience a cerebral event should be aggressively treated for secondary prevention with aspirin, statins, blood pressure control, smoking cessation, and glycemic control (if diabetic). Patent foramen ovale closure is not warranted given this patient's age and complex aortic atheroma. Although there is controversy with regard to warfarin therapy and aortic arch plaque, this patient is already therapeutic on antithrombotic agents for his AF. There are no data to demonstrate that a goal INR of 3 to 4 will improve the outcome of patients with aortic atheroma. Confirmation by chest CT is not warranted as **Figure 29.5** represents atheroma and not aortic dissection.

19. **Answer: B.** Fluoroscopy reveals that the patient had a mechanical aortic valve replacement (AVR) with normal disc opening. Based on the 2020 ACC/AHA Valvular Heart Disease Guidelines, in patients with a mechanical AVR and additional risk factors for thromboembolism (eg, AF, previous thromboembolism, LV dysfunction, hypercoagulable state) or an older-generation prosthesis (eg, ball-in-cage), anticoagulation with a vitamin K antagonist (VKA) is indicated to achieve an INR of 3.0 (class I). Given that the patient has been newly diagnosed with AF, the target INR should be increased from 2.5 to 3.0. Direct oral anticoagulants (DOAC) are currently contraindicated in patients with mechanical heart valves. Low-dose systemic fibrinolytic therapy is used to treat mechanical valve thrombosis.

20. **Answer: C.** This M-mode reveals that this patient is in coarse AF. In a patient with new-onset AF, reversible causes of AF (eg, hyperthyroidism) should be investigated and treated, if possible. There are no findings on this M-mode that would suggest that cardiac surgery, thrombolytics, or alcohol septal ablation would be appropriate in this patient.

21. **Answer: D.** This 4-chamber TTE demonstrates a prominent Eustachian valve and is a normal variant. The Eustachian valve is a remnant of the embryologic valve responsible for directing inferior vena caval blood across the atrial septum to the LA. It is a rigid and protuberant structure that arises along the posterior margin of the inferior vena cava to the

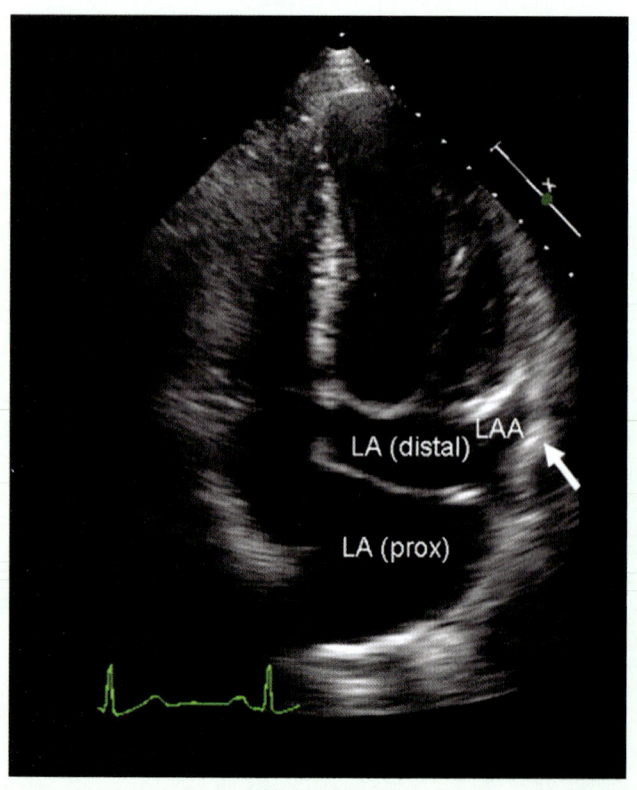

Figure 29.19

border of the fossa ovalis. Although usually immobile, it may occasionally demonstrate independent motion within the RA and can be confused with tumors, vegetations, or thrombi. This should be differentiated from a Chiari network, which is a delicate-appearing, highly mobile, usually fenestrated membranous structure arising near the orifice of the inferior vena cava. Like the Eustachian valve, the Chiari network has little clinical significance but may be confused with pathologic structures, such as vegetations or thrombi.

22. **Answer: A.** This is a pulsed-wave Doppler of the LAA revealing AF/atrial flutter. AF occurs transiently in 6%–10% of patients with an acute myocardial infarction, presumably due to atrial ischemia or atrial stretching secondary to heart failure. These patients have a worse prognosis than those who have acute myocardial infarctions without AF.

23. **Answer: C.** This finding on TEE represents lipomatous hypertrophy of the interatrial septum. In this condition, there is an unencapsulated accumulation of mature adipose tissue in the interatrial septum with sparing of the fossa ovale, which gives it the classic "dumbbell" appearance on both TTE and TEE. It is thought to be a normal variant and is generally considered benign. This finding alone would not be a contraindication for cardioversion.

24. **Answer: D.** Immediately after cardioversion, there is an initial increase in SEC and thus an increased risk of thrombus formation/thromboembolism. This has been described with spontaneous conversion as well as following electrical and pharmacologic cardioversion. These findings are thought to be due to the reduction of LA function ("atrial stunning"), which can last for several weeks after successful cardioversion. Relatively high atrial appendage ejection velocity suggests shorter duration AF, and thus a higher likelihood of long-term maintenance of sinus rhythm. Additionally, there is a reduction in LAA function, demonstrated by decreased velocities through the LAA.

25. **Answer: C.** The TEE shows LAA sludge, a dynamic and gelatinous echodensity without a discrete mass representing a prethrombotic state. In patients with AF, sludge is independently associated with an increased risk for thromboembolism and all-cause mortality. Therefore, electrical or chemical cardioversion should not be attempted and the patient should be treated with anticoagulation and rate control until resolution of the sludge.

26. **Answer: D.** This patient's M-mode tracing demonstrates thickened mitral valve leaflets with a flattened E-F slope, consistent with rheumatic mitral stenosis. In patients with rheumatic mitral stenosis and (1) AF, (2) a prior embolic event, or (3) a LA thrombus, long-term oral anticoagulation with a VKA is indicated independent of CHA2DS2-VASc score. In addition to the much higher risk of embolization with rheumatic valve disease, rheumatic disease may also affect the atrial myocardium, resulting in an increased risk of blood flow stasis and thrombosis in the body of the LA, as well as the LAA for a given severity of mitral stenosis. In the setting of AF and rheumatic heart disease, the use of DOACs may be inferior for stroke prevention when compared to VKA (INVICTUS trial).

27. **Answer: C.** The vast majority of atrial thrombi among patients with AF are located in the LAA. TTE has a reported sensitivity of 39% to 63% in identifying or excluding LAA. Although there is improvement of visualization of the LA and the LAA with IV contrast and harmonic imaging with TTE, TEE still remains the gold standard to evaluate the LA and especially the LAA for thrombi.

28. **Answer: D.** TEE shows a LAA thrombus. TEE has a reported specificity of 99% to 100% for detecting LAA thrombi.

29. **Answer: D.** Pulsed-wave Doppler at the ostium of the pulmonary vein shows elevated velocities and spectral broadening both in systole and diastole, consistent with pulmonary vein stenosis. On TEE, normal right upper pulmonary vein S and D wave velocities are ~50 to 70 cm/s. The mean onset of pulmonary vein stenosis occurs between 2 and 5 months postprocedure.

Pulmonary vein stenosis is one of the potential complications of PVI. Early experience with PVI reported PV stenosis rates of up to 38%. More recent studies report the incidence to be only 1% to 3%. The decline is likely related to a modification of the procedure with ablation now occurring in the body of the LA rather than within the pulmonary vein. A "retrograde" A wave is present confirming sinus rhythm.

KEY POINTS
- TEE has both high sensitivity and specificity for LA thrombi.
- Pulmonary vein stenosis is a potential complication of PVI and should be suspected in those who present with shortness of breath after they have undergone this procedure. Interrogation by pulsed-wave Doppler through the ostia of all four pulmonary veins should be performed to properly evaluate and rule out this condition.

30. **Answer: C.** This is a myxoma that is attached to the left atrial wall via a stalk, which is identified by calcification (the area of increased echogenicity [**Figure 29.20**, white arrow]). Given this patient's history, this myxoma is likely responsible for an embolic phenomenon and should be removed surgically. That it is not an artifact since it can be seen in two different views

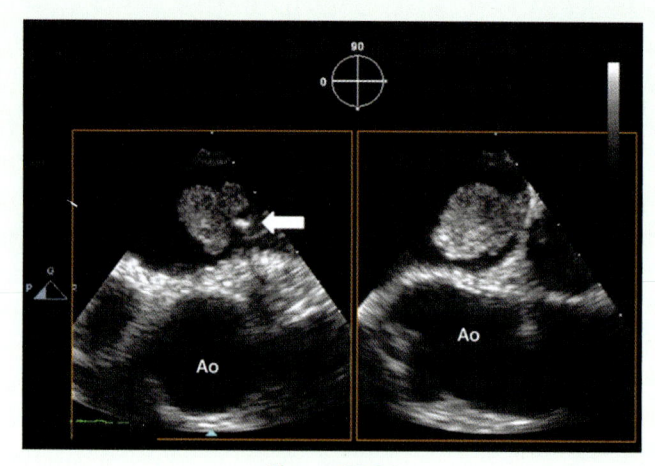

Figure 29.20

(**Figure 29.20**). While it is possible that this may also represent a thrombus, it is unlikely, given the patient's normal-sized LA and clearly demarcated stalk to the left atrial wall. Ao represents Aorta.

31. **Answer: C.** Myxomas are benign tumors and the most common primary cardiac neoplasm. Almost 80% originate in the left atrium. While they commonly are found attached to the interatrial septum, they may be attached anywhere in the heart. Some patients are at risk for recurrence of the myxoma, which may occur in 2% to 5% or the development of additional lesions. Systemic embolization has been reported up to 29%.

32. **Answer: A.** The Carney complex is an inherited, autosomal dominant disorder characterized by multiple tumors. These include atrial and extracardiac myxomas, schwannomas, and various endocrine tumors. Additionally, patients have a variety of pigmentation abnormalities, including pigmented lentigines and blue nevi.

KEY POINTS

- This is not an artifact as it can be seen in two views.
- Myxomas most commonly occur in the left atrium attached to the interatrial septum by a stalk (with calcification at the attachment).
- Myxomas should be removed in the setting of embolic phenomenon.

33. **Answer: A.** Incomplete closure of the LAA resulting in a peridevice leak (PDL) is relatively common after percutaneous left atrial appendage occlusion (LAAO) given the widely variable size, shape, and orientation of the LAA. Large leaks are currently defined as leaks greater than 3 to 5 mm (depending on the study) and are associated with an increased risk of embolic stroke. In patients with PDL (open arrow, **Figure 29.14**), persistent flow around the device may delay or inhibit device endothelialization, which usually occurs within 45 days, and thus render the device susceptible to device-related thrombus formation. Many leaks present at 45 days after the procedure will close on their own over time. Options to close the PDL include methods like embolization coils, plugs, and occluders.

34. **Answer: B.** Formation of a device-related thrombus (DRT) is a potential complication of LAAO, especially early after implant, before endothelization of the device (**Figure 29.21**). DRT occurs in about 3% to 4% of patients post-LAAO and is associated with a significantly increased risk of ischemic events. DRT is managed with oral anticoagulation with either warfarin or DOAC and repeat imaging to ensure resolution.

KEY POINTS

- Percutaneous LAAO is an alternative therapy for stroke prevention in patients with AF who are poor candidates for oral anticoagulants.
- PDLs are common after percutaneous LAAO and often close on their own over time.
- Postprocedural surveillance imaging with TEE is important to detect PDL and DRT.

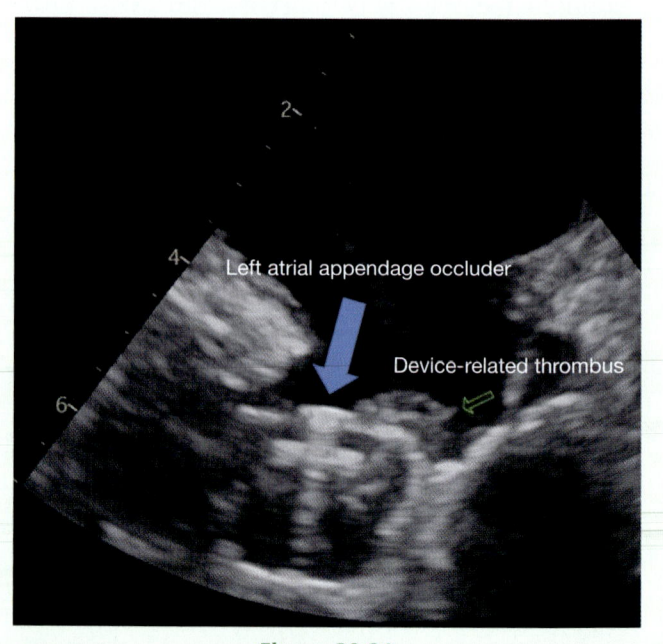

Figure 29.21

SUGGESTED READINGS

Antonielli E, Pizzuti A, Palinkas A, et al. Clinical value of left atrial appendage flow for prediction of long-term sinus rhythm maintenance in patients with nonvalvular atrial fibrillation. *J Am Coll Cardiol*. 2002;39(9):1443-1449.

Inoue K, Khan FH, Remme EW, et al. Determinants of left atrial reservoir and pump strain and use of atrial strain for evaluation of left ventricular filling pressure [published correction appears in *Eur Heart J Cardiovasc Imaging*. 2021. *Eur Heart J Cardiovasc Imaging*. 2021;23(1):61-70.

Klein AL, Grimm RA, Murray RD, et al. Use of transesophageal echocardiography to guide cardioversion in patients with atrial fibrillation. *N Engl J Med*. 2001;344(19):1411-1420.

Lowe BS, Kusunose K, Motoki H, et al. Prognostic significance of left atrial appendage "sludge" in patients with atrial fibrillation: a new transesophageal echocardiographic thromboembolic risk factor. *J Am Soc Echocardiogr*. 2014;27(11):1176-1183.

Manning WJ, Silverman DI, Katz SE, et al. Impaired left atrial mechanical function after cardioversion: relation to the duration of atrial fibrillation. *J Am Coll Cardiol*. 1994;23(7):1535-1540.

Manning WJ, Weintraub RM, Waksmonski CA, et al. Accuracy of transesophageal echocardiography for identifying left atrial thrombi. A prospective, intraoperative study. *Ann Intern Med*. 1995;123(11):817-822.

Writing Committee Members; Otto CM, Nishimura RA, Bonow RO, et al. 2020 ACC/AHA guideline for the management of patients with valvular heart disease: a report of the American College of Cardiology/American Heart Association Joint Committee on clinical practice guidelines. *J Am Coll Cardiol*. 2021;77(4):e25-e197.

Pathan F, D'Elia N, Nolan MT, Marwick TH, Negishi K. Normal ranges of left atrial strain by speckle-tracking echocardiography: a systematic review and meta-analysis. *J Am Soc Echocardiogr*. 2017;30(1):59-70.e8.

Ramchand J, Harb SC, Miyasaka R, Kanj M, Saliba W, Jaber WA. Imaging for percutaneous left atrial appendage closure: a contemporary review. *Structural Heart*. 2019;3(5):364-382.

CHAPTER 30

Right Ventricular Disease and Pulmonary Hypertension

Dimitrios Maragiannis and Sherif F. Nagueh

QUESTIONS

1. Which of the following is **TRUE** about hepatic vein Doppler pattern in patients with severe tricuspid regurgitation?
   A. In severe tricuspid regurgitation during sinus rhythm, hepatic vein Doppler always shows a prominent systolic flow reversal wave.
   B. In severe tricuspid regurgitation during sinus rhythm, systolic flow reversal wave peaks in late systole.
   C. In the absence of severe tricuspid regurgitation, systolic flow reversal may occur in the setting of right ventricular dysfunction.
   D. None of the above.
   E. B and C.

2. Which of the following Doppler parameters can be supportive of tricuspid mechanical valve stenosis?
   A. A prolonged pressure halftime (PHT).
   B. An elevated mean gradient and/or velocity.
   C. $TVI_{prosthesis}/TVI_{LVOT}$ ratio <1.5.
   D. A and B.

3. A patient is reported to have severe right ventricular diastolic dysfunction with a restrictive filling pattern. Which echocardiographic findings support this diagnosis?
   A. A tricuspid E/A ratio <2.1 with a deceleration time >120 ms.
   B. A tricuspid E/A ratio >2.1 with a deceleration time <120 ms.
   C. No diastolic antegrade flow in the pulmonic artery.
   D. None of the above.
   E. All of the above.

4. Which patient has the highest right atrial pressure (RAP)?
   A. IVC maximum diameter at 1.8 cm and minimum diameter with sniffing at 0.8 cm.
   B. IVC maximum diameter at 2.2 cm and minimum diameter with sniffing at 0.9 cm.
   C. IVC maximum diameter at 1.9 cm and minimum diameter with sniffing at 1.3 cm.
   D. IVC maximum diameter at 2.3 cm and minimum diameter with sniffing at 1.3 cm.
   E. IVC maximum diameter at 1.5 cm and minimum diameter with sniffing at 0.7 cm.

5. Which of the following is characteristic of RV structure and function in patients with longstanding arrhythmogenic RV dysplasia (ARVD)?
   A. RV regional dysfunction in RVOT and apical segments.
   B. RV fractional area change of 50%.
   C. Tricuspid regurgitation (TR) jet by continuous-wave Doppler of 3.6 m/s.
   D. Left ventricular (LV) ejection fraction (EF) of 26%.

6. Which of the following tissue Doppler velocities is expected in a 36-year-old patient with primary pulmonary hypertension of 4-year duration?
   A. Septal mitral annulus systolic velocity of 16 cm/s.
   B. Lateral mitral annulus early-diastolic velocity of 14 cm/s.
   C. Septal mitral annulus early-diastolic velocity of 13 cm/s.
   D. Tricuspid annulus systolic velocity of 15 cm/s.
   E. Tricuspid annulus early-diastolic velocity of 13 cm/s.

7. Which of these is an abnormal finding?
   A. Predominant forward hepatic vein diastolic flow in a 25-year-old man.
   B. A hepatic vein atrial reversal velocity of 20 cm/s duration.
   C. A tricuspid E/A ratio of 1.8 in a 34-year-old woman.
   D. A hepatic vein systolic velocity–to–diastolic velocity ratio of 0.3 in a 70-year-old man.
   E. Hepatic vein late-systolic reversal velocity (Vr) of 15 cm/s.

8. In which of the following cases may hepatic venous flow predict RA pressure?
   A. A 55-year-old man with mid-diastolic rumble/holosystolic murmur at the lower left sternal border.
   B. A 61-year-old woman with postoperative dyspnea and paradoxical pulse.
   C. A 65-year-old man with a heart rate of 40 beats/min after bypass surgery and cannon "A" waves in his jugular venous pulse.
   D. A 53-year-old man with low-voltage EKG, postural hypotension, and LV posterior wall thickness of 18 mm.
   E. A 45-year-old man who received a heart transplant 6 months ago.

9. Which of the following is compatible with advanced RV disease in patients with cardiac amyloidosis?
   A. RV free wall thickness of 7 mm.
   B. Deceleration time of tricuspid E velocity of 260 ms.
   C. Tricuspid E/A ratio of 1.
   D. A hepatic venous systolic velocity–to–diastolic velocity ratio of 0.6.
   E. Inspiratory hepatic venous atrial flow reversals.

10. What is the pulmonary artery (PA) systolic pressure in a patient with a peak TR velocity of 3 m/s and a jugular venous pressure of 15 cm?
    A. PA systolic pressure = 51 mm Hg.
    B. PA systolic pressure = 36 mm Hg.
    C. PA systolic pressure = 46 mm Hg.
    D. PA systolic pressure = 40 mm Hg.

11. Which of these patients has the highest pulmonary vascular resistance?
    A. TR jet of 3.6 m/s and time-velocity integral of RVOT systolic flow of 13 cm.
    B. TR jet of 3.3 m/s and time-velocity integral of RVOT systolic flow of 13 cm.
    C. TR jet of 3.6 m/s and time-velocity integral of RVOT systolic flow of 18 cm.
    D. TR jet of 3.5 m/s and time-velocity integral of RVOT systolic flow of 14 cm.

12. What is the mean PA pressure in this patient with TR peak velocity of 3 m/s, pulmonary regurgitation (PR) end-diastolic velocity of 2 m/s, and RA pressure of 10 mm Hg?
    A. Mean PA pressure = 26 mm Hg.
    B. Mean PA pressure = 21 mm Hg.
    C. Mean PA pressure = 33 mm Hg.
    D. Mean PA pressure = 40 mm Hg.

13. What is the PA systolic pressure of this patient with pulmonary stenosis, where peak TR velocity is 4 m/s, peak velocity across pulmonic valve is 3 m/s, and RA pressure is 10 mm Hg?
    A. PA systolic pressure = 46 mm Hg.
    B. PA systolic pressure = 74 mm Hg.
    C. PA systolic pressure = 38 mm Hg.
    D. PA systolic pressure = 50 mm Hg.

14. Which of these statements supports the diagnosis of increased RV systolic pressure?
    A. Acceleration time of 131 ms in systolic flow recorded at RVOT.
    B. Pulmonary regurgitation (PR) peak velocity of 1.5 m/s, and RA pressure of 5 mm Hg.
    C. TR peak velocity of 3.5 m/s.
    D. Flat interventricular septum during diastole only.

15. Which view is the recommended view to measure RV wall thickness?
    A. Modified apical 4-chamber view.
    B. RV inflow view.
    C. Apical 4-chamber view.
    D. RV-focused view.
    E. Subcostal view.

16. Which segment of the RV receives its blood supply from the LAD coronary artery?
  A. Anterior wall.
  B. Inferior wall.
  C. Lateral wall.
  D. Infundibulum.
  E. Moderator band.

17. The myocardial performance index may be spuriously normal in which patient?
  A. Patient with RV systolic dysfunction and right bundle branch block.
  B. Patient with RV systolic dysfunction and left bundle branch block.
  C. Patient with RV systolic dysfunction and restrictive RV filling pattern.
  D. Patient with RV systolic dysfunction and tricuspid E/e' ratio of 3.
  E. Patient with RV systolic dysfunction and IVC diameter of 1.3 cm, and 60% collapse index.

18. Which of these measurements indicates an enlarged RV?
  A. Male subject with RVOT distal diameter of 25 mm.
  B. Female subject with RV basal diameter in the apical 4-chamber view of 3.9 cm.
  C. A 65-year-old male subject with RV end-diastolic volume index by 3D echo of 80 mL/m^2.
  D. Female subject with RV end-diastolic area in apical 4-chamber view of 12.5 cm^2/m^2.
  E. Male subject with RV long-axis dimension of 73 mm.

19. What is the mean PA pressure if PR peak velocity is 3.5 m/s and end-diastolic velocity is 2 m/s with right atrial pressure by central line of 10 mm Hg?
  A. 16 mm Hg.
  B. 26 mm Hg.
  C. 33 mm Hg.
  D. 49 mm Hg.
  E. 59 mm Hg.

20. Which of these measurements by itself indicates the presence of pulmonary hypertension in a patient with heart rate of 66 beats/min?
  A. Peak TR velocity of 2.7 m/s.
  B. Peak PR velocity of 1.9 m/s.
  C. End-diastolic PR velocity of 1.5 m/s.
  D. Isovolumic relaxation time by tissue Doppler of tricuspid valve of 100 ms.
  E. Acceleration time of RVOT flow of 55 ms.

21. Which of these measurements is consistent with increased mean right atrial pressure?
  A. IVC diameter of 2 cm with 80% inspiratory collapse.
  B. Tricuspid E/A ratio of 0.7.
  C. Right atrial end-systolic area of 10 cm^2.
  D. Tricuspid E/e' ratio of 10.
  E. Systolic velocity–to–diastolic velocity ratio of 0.75 in hepatic vein flow.

22. What is dP/dt if the time between TR velocity of 2 m/s and TR velocity of 0.5 m/s is 30 ms?
  A. 200 mm Hg/s.
  B. 300 mm Hg/s.
  C. 400 mm Hg/s.
  D. 500 mm Hg/s.
  E. 600 mm Hg/s.

23. Which of these measurements is consistent with severe TR with aliasing velocity set at 55 cm/s?
  A. Peak TR velocity of 5 m/s.
  B. TR jet area of 7 cm^2.
  C. ERO of 0.2 cm^2.
  D. RV of 38 mL.
  E. VC of 0.8 cm.

24. Which of these conditions is associated with intermittent (not seen in each cardiac cycle) systolic reversal seen in hepatic vein flow?
  A. Pericardial constriction.
  B. Severe tricuspid regurgitation.
  C. Severe tricuspid stenosis.
  D. Junctional rhythm.
  E. Electronic RV pacing.

25. Which of the following is most compatible with the hepatic venous flow in **Figure 30.1**?
   A. A 56-year-old man with systemic hypertension under control with medical therapy.
   B. A 39-year-old woman with hypotension in the setting of acute inferior wall MI.
   C. A 25-year-old man with recurrent septic pulmonary embolism.
   D. A 63-year-old man in atrial fibrillation.

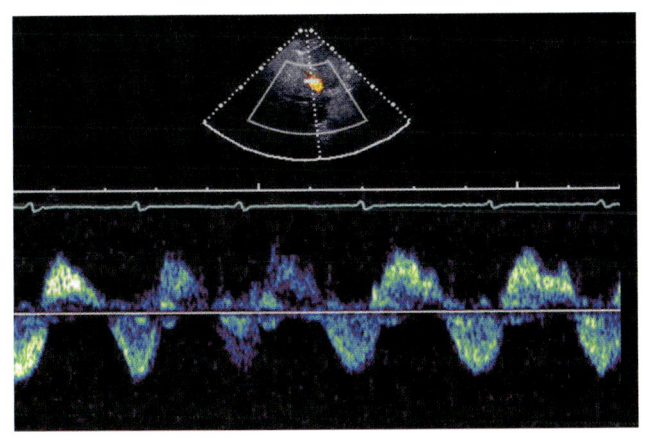

Figure 30.1

26. Which of the following is compatible with the hepatic venous flow in **Figure 30.2**?
   A. A 49-year-old man with dilated cardiomyopathy and systemic and pulmonary congestion.
   B. A 29-year-old woman with pulmonary hypertension and systemic congestion.
   C. A 55-year-old man with cardiac amyloidosis and lower extremity swelling.
   D. A 65-year-old woman with hypertrophic cardiomyopathy and RV hypertrophy.

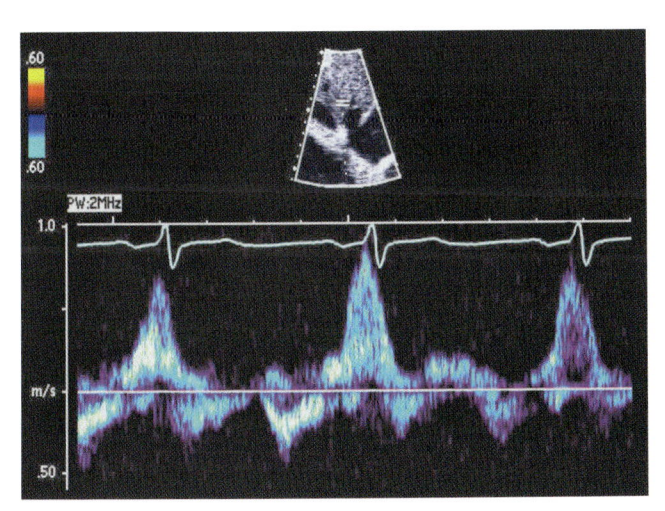

Figure 30.2

27. The following image (**Figure 30.3**) was obtained from an apical 4-chamber view in a 48-year-old man with shortness of breath.
Which of the following conditions is least likely to have caused this finding?
   A. Sinus venosus atrial septal defect.
   B. RV cardiomyopathy.
   C. Severe pulmonary regurgitation.
   D. Patent ductus arteriosus.
   E. Anomalous pulmonary venous return.

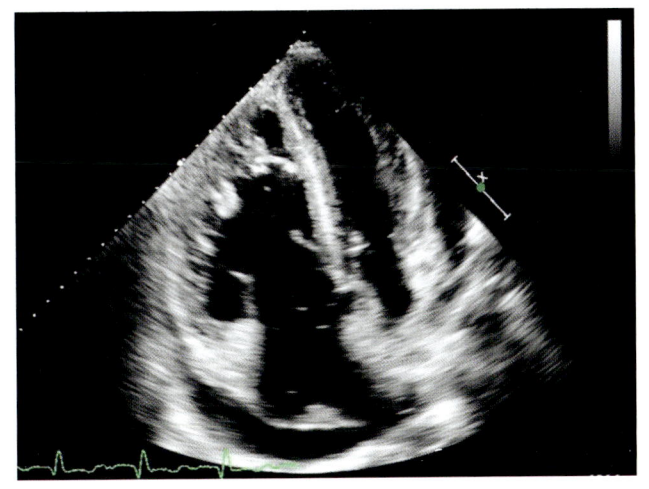

Figure 30.3

28. Tricuspid annular plane systolic excursion (TAPSE) was measured at 6 mm in a 47-year-old patient with cardiac amyloidosis (**Figure 30.4**). Which of the following is **TRUE**?
   A. The lower normal limit for preserved right ventricular function is 17 mm.
   B. TAPSE represents the longitudinal function of the right ventricle.
   C. TAPSE is an accurate assessment of global RV function.
   D. All of the above.
   E. A and B.

A. Mean left atrial pressure is increased.
B. LV relaxation is impaired.
C. Successful treatment with bosentan will lead to an increase in mitral E/A ratio.
D. Left ventricular end-diastolic pressure (LVEDP) is increased.

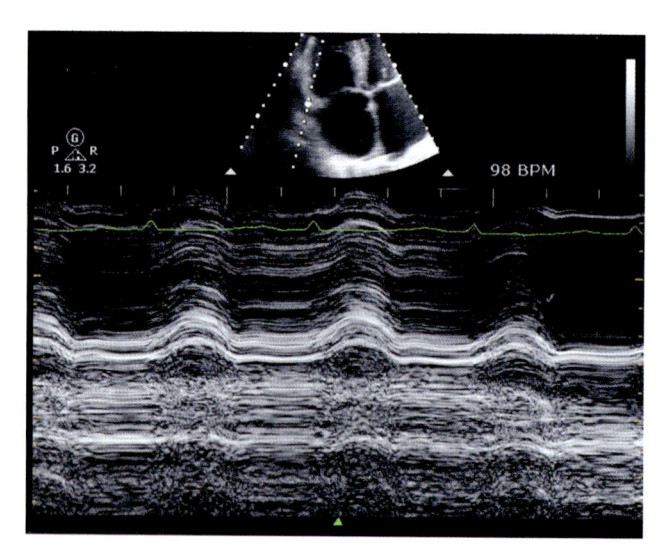

Figure 30.4

29. A 49-year-old woman presents with dyspnea on exertion (▶ **Video 30.1A,B**). What is the diagnosis?
    A. Ebstein anomaly.
    B. Carcinoid heart disease.
    C. Rheumatic valvular disease.
    D. None of the above.

30. Which is **TRUE** about this patient with pulmonary regurgitation (PR) (**Figure 30.5**)?
    A. Right ventricular end-diastolic pressure (RVEDP) is normal.
    B. RV stiffness is increased.
    C. Systolic reversal in the hepatic veins is present.
    D. Tricuspid E/A ratio is 0.6.

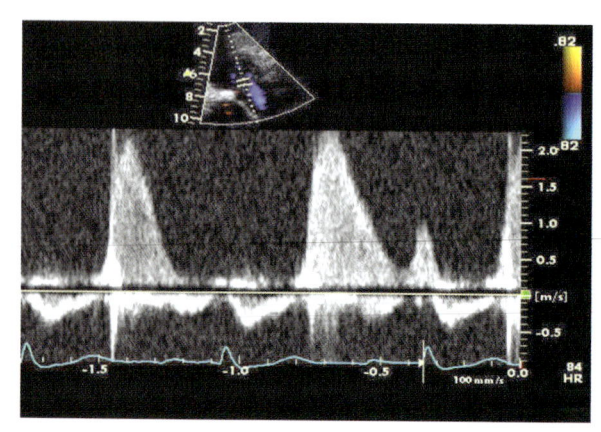

Figure 30.5

31. Choose the **CORRECT** conclusion about LV diastolic function in this patient with pulmonary hypertension (**Figure 30.6**).

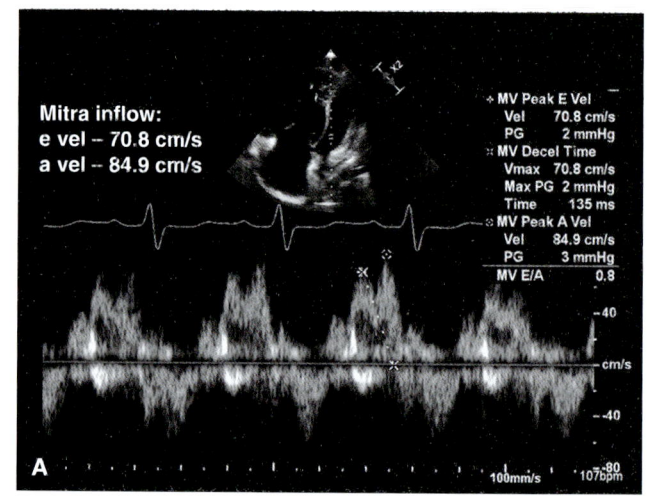

Figure 30.6A

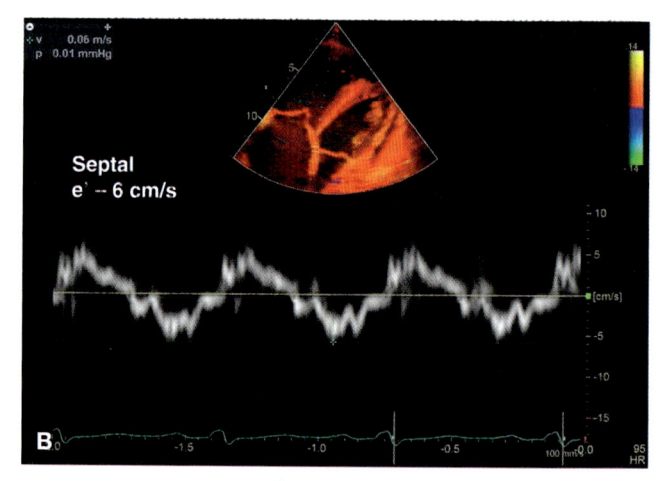

Figure 30.6B

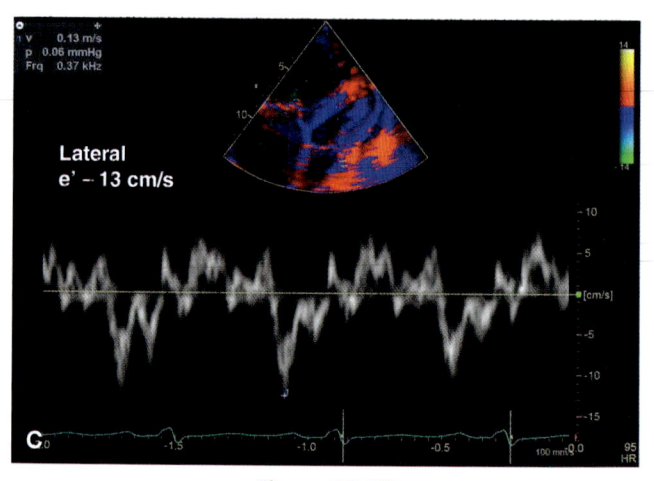

Figure 30.6C

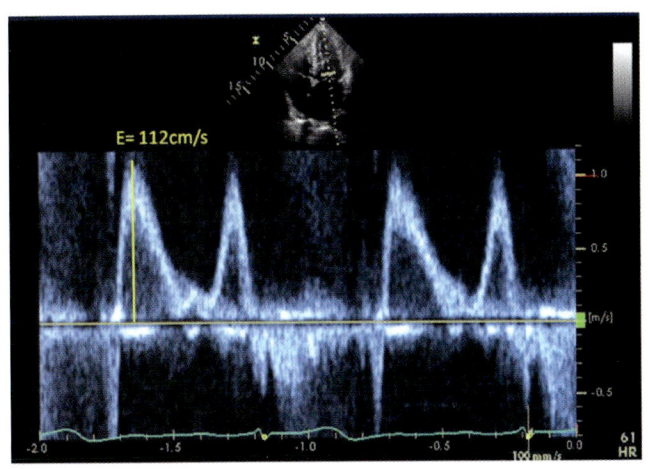

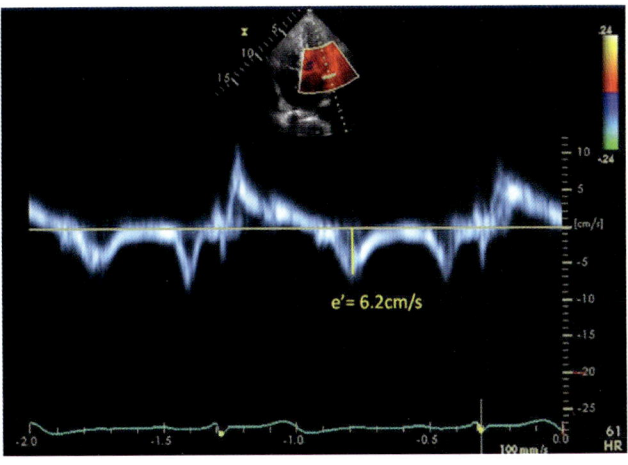

Figure 30.7

32. Choose the **CORRECT** conclusion about LV diastolic function in this patient with pulmonary hypertension (**Figure 30.7**).
    A. Mean left atrial (LA) pressure is normal.
    B. LV relaxation is impaired and LA pressure is increased.
    C. Treatment with diuretics will lead to an increase in mitral E/A ratio.
    D. LVEDP is normal.

33. Choose the **CORRECT** conclusion about LV and RV pressures in this patient with a holosystolic murmur at the left sternal border and a blood pressure of 150/80 mm Hg. The Doppler is obtained from VSD flow at the parasternal short-axis view at the level of the aortic valve (**Figure 30.8**).
    A. RVEDP is higher than left ventricular end-diastolic pressure (LVEDP).
    B. RV systolic pressure is higher than LV systolic pressure.
    C. If the peak velocity is approximately 5.5 m/s, PA systolic pressure is 29 mm Hg in the absence of pulmonary stenosis.
    D. The findings are compatible with a peak TR velocity of 3.5 m/s in the absence of pulmonary stenosis.

34. A 19-year-old man is presenting with shortness of breath. Four-chamber view by transthoracic echocardiography shows a distinct abnormality (▶ **Video 30.2**). Which of the following is **CORRECT**?
    A. Normal wall motion of the RV apex is seen and akinesia of the basal/mid-RV wall.
    B. The findings are suggestive of acute pulmonary embolism.
    C. This pattern can be present only in acute pulmonary embolism.
    D. All of the above.
    E. A and B.

35. What is the PA systolic pressure in this patient, where the TR peak velocity is 2.8 m/s (**Figure 30.9**)? Hepatic venous flow shows an S/D velocity ratio of 0.35.
    A. PA systolic pressure = 31 to 36 mm Hg.
    B. PA systolic pressure = 46 to 51 mm Hg.
    C. PA systolic pressure = 41 to 46 mm Hg.
    D. PA systolic pressure = 36 to 41 mm Hg.

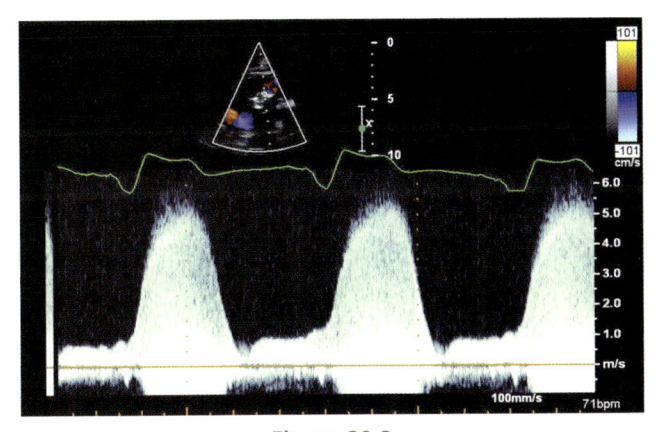

Figure 30.8

Figure 30.9

36. The sonographer is interrogating the hepatic veins flow without a respirometer (**Figure 30.10**).
   A. Inspiration is represented in part I.
   B. Expiration is represented in part I.
   C. Inspiration is represented in part II.
   D. Hepatic vein flow shown was recorded during apnea.

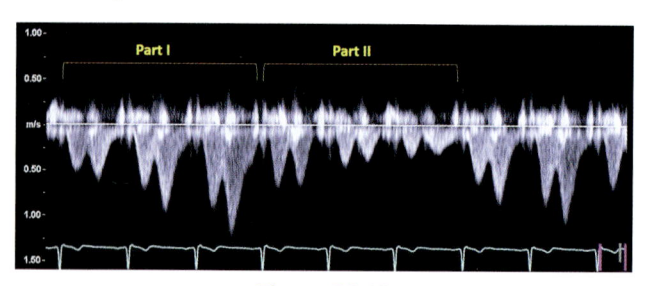

Figure 30.10

37. Which of the following statements are **CORRECT** regarding the RV speckle tracking longitudinal strain image obtained (**Figure 30.11**)?
   A. The view shown is a RV-focused view and RV longitudinal strain should be obtained in the RV-modified view.
   B. RV longitudinal strain should be done as a 6-segment measurement, not a 3-segment measure as seen in this image.
   C. RV longitudinal strain normal valves are not well-established.
   D. RV longitudinal strain has prognostic significance in many disease states.

38. A 57-year-old woman with scleroderma undergoes a baseline echocardiogram to assess for pulmonary hypertension and the pulmonary artery systolic pressure is estimated to be 40 mm Hg. Which of the following statements regarding RV function is **CORRECT** (see **Figure 30.12**)?

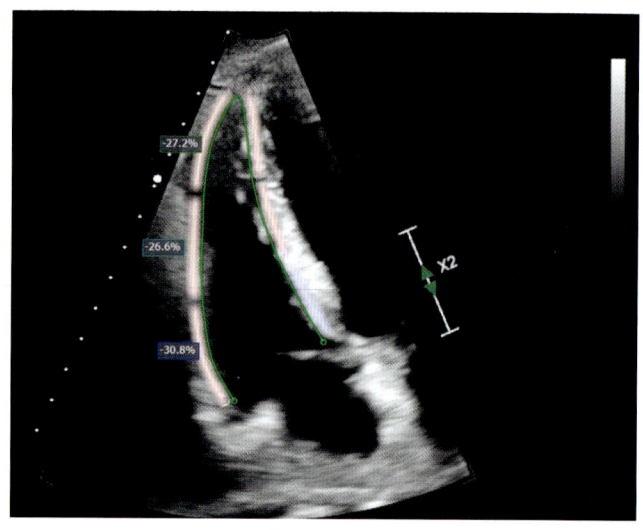

Figure 30.11

   A. 3D RVEF volumes are not useful since they overestimate those from cardiac MRI.
   B. 3D RVEF is an excellent measure of RV contractility.
   C. A normal 3D RVEF is >55% and therefore RVEF of 46.7% is abnormal.
   D. A semiautomated border detection volume technique is recommended for 3D RVEF determination.

39. How much tricuspid regurgitation (TR) is present in **Figure 30.13**?
   A. Cannot be determined as the Nyquist limit is too high.
   B. No TR is present.
   C. Cannot be determined based on the available information.
   D. Severe TR.

CASE 1

An echocardiogram is performed to evaluate hypotension in a patient with CAD after coronary artery bypass surgery. There are limited windows (▶ Video 30.3).

40. Regarding ▶ Video 30.3 in **Case 1**, which of the following is **TRUE**?
   A. RV function is normal.
   B. LV size is normal.
   C. LV stroke volume is reduced.
   D. Patient can benefit from an intra-aortic balloon pump.

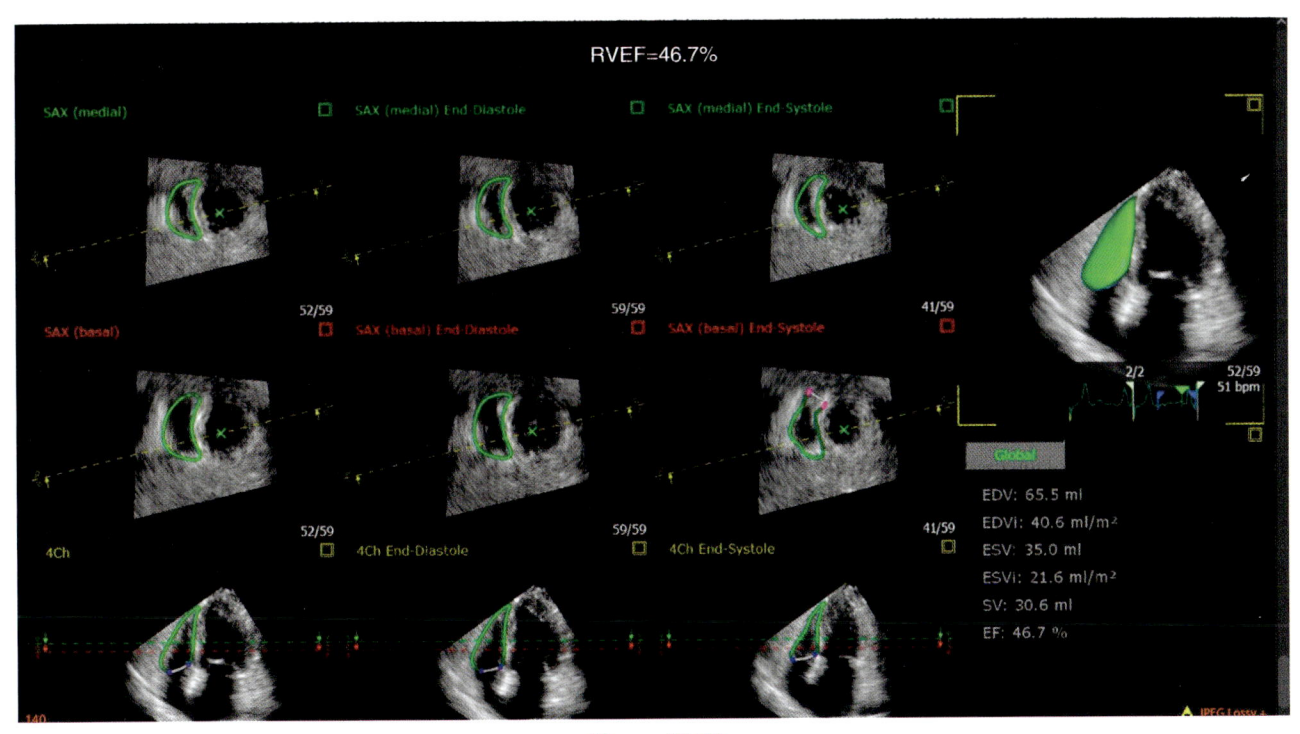

Figure 30.12

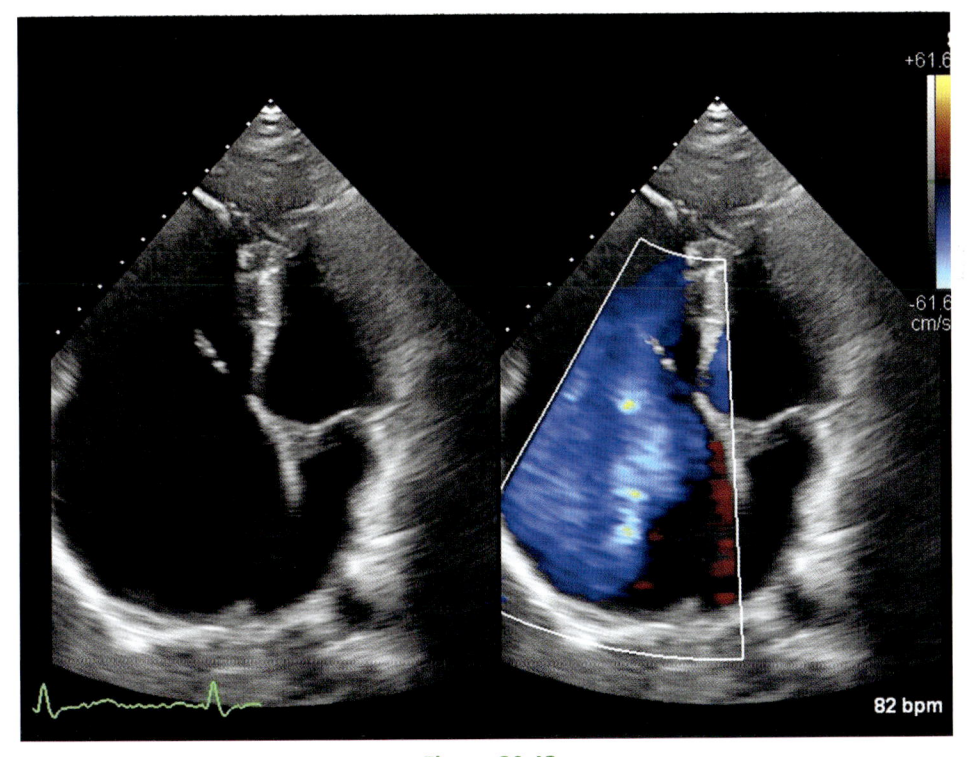

Figure 30.13

41. Concerning **Figure 30.14**, which of the following is **TRUE**?
    A. PA systolic pressure can be reliably estimated based on the TR jet.
    B. Mid-systolic reversal is present in the hepatic veins.
    C. RV systolic pressure is very close to RA "V" wave pressure.
    D. Similar hemodynamic findings are noted in patients with longstanding atrial septal defect (ASD).

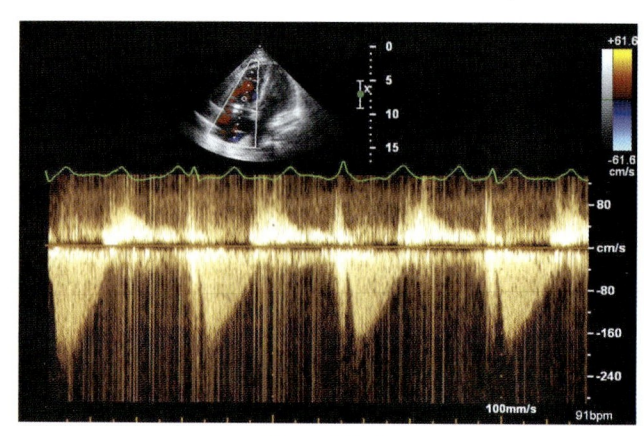

Figure 30.14

A. Echocardiographic contrast agent injection can help determine the underlying etiology.
B. No further evaluation is needed at this time.
C. An increase in LV filling pressures accounts for the exertional hypoxemia.
D. He is likely to have an abnormal brain MRI examination.

CASE 3

The transesophageal view in ▶ Video 30.5 is obtained from a 51-year-old woman in NYHA class IV.

44. Which of the following is **TRUE** regarding **Case 3**, ▶ **Video 30.5**?
    A. The right atrium appears enlarged.
    B. There is predominant left-to-right shunting.
    C. LA pressure is higher than RA pressure.
    D. The lesion is not amenable to percutaneous closure.

CASE 2

The apical views in ▶ Video 30.4A,B were obtained from a 36-year-old man with complaints of recurrent focal weakness of the right upper extremity, and reduced arterial O_2 saturation with exertion.

42. Which of the following is **TRUE** regarding **Case 2**, ▶ **Video 30.4A,B**?
    A. RV size is enlarged.
    B. LVEF appears reduced.
    C. A short-axis view would show a D-shaped septum in systole.
    D. RA "V" wave pressure is increased.

43. Which is **TRUE** regarding the symptoms of the patient in **Case 2**?

45. Which is **TRUE** concerning the TR jet and the pulmonary venous flow signals obtained from the same patient in **Case 3** (**Figure 30.15**)?
    A. Pulmonary vascular resistance is normal.
    B. Septal systolic velocity by tissue Doppler is probably reduced.
    C. Diastolic dysfunction is the etiology of dyspnea.
    D. Mitral regurgitation is the likely etiology of dyspnea.

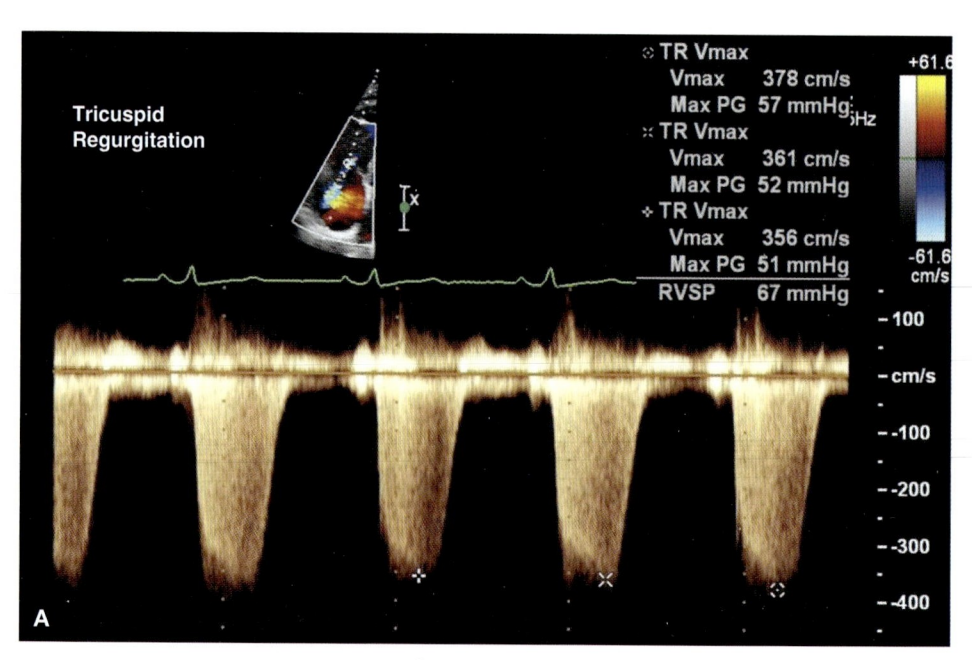

Figure 30.15A

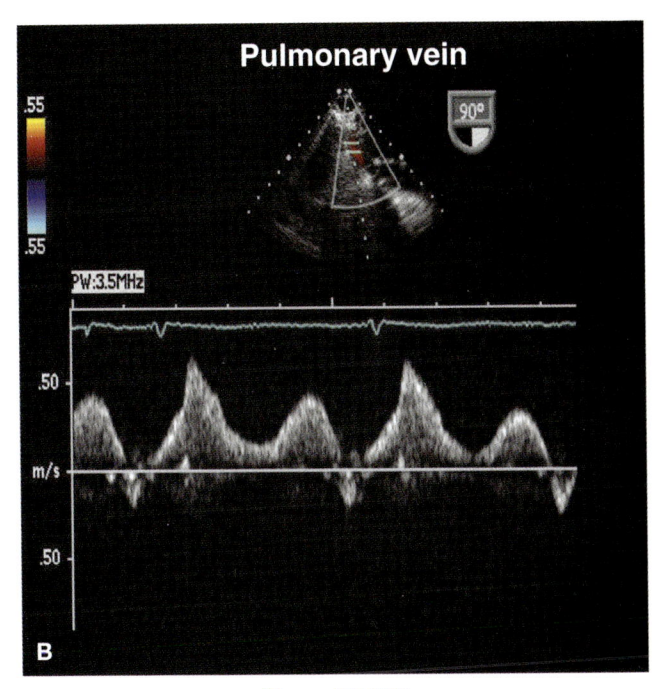

Figure 30.15B

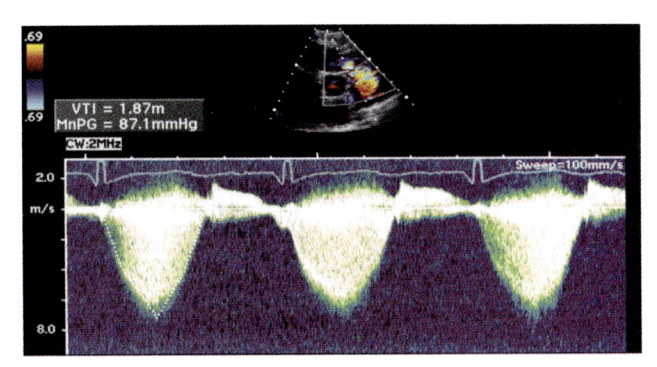

Figure 30.16

C. Hepatic veins will have a prominent atrial reversal signal after RA contraction.
D. The lesion is not amenable to percutaneous intervention.

CASE 4

The parasternal views (▶ Video 30.6A,B) were obtained from a patient with a systolic murmur since birth.

46. Which is **TRUE** regarding **Case 4** and ▶ Video **30.6A,B**?
  A. PA systolic pressure is normal.
  B. RV free wall thickness is likely 4 mm.
  C. LVEF is 50% to 54%.
  D. Color Doppler shows severe PR.

47. Which of the following is **TRUE** about the CW signal recorded at the RVOT obtained from the same patient in **Case 4** (**Figure 30.16**)?
  A. Pulmonary vascular resistance is increased.
  B. Peak TR velocity is likely 4.5 m/s.

CASE 5

The parasternal views in ▶ Video 30.7A,B were obtained from a 36-year-old man with lower extremity swelling.

48. Which is **TRUE** regarding **Case 5** and ▶ Video **30.7A,B**?
  A. RV volumes are normal.
  B. RV systolic pressure is increased.
  C. LVEF is mild to moderately depressed.
  D. There is a positive history of congenital heart disease.

49. Which of the following is **TRUE** about the CW Doppler signal recorded at the RVOT obtained from the same patient in **Case 5** (**Figure 30.17**)?
  A. Pulmonary vascular resistance is increased.
  B. Percutaneous commissurotomy can be considered.
  C. There is an RV septum that is flat in diastole and systole likely present.
  D. There is increased RV diastolic pressures.

642 / Clinical Echocardiography Review

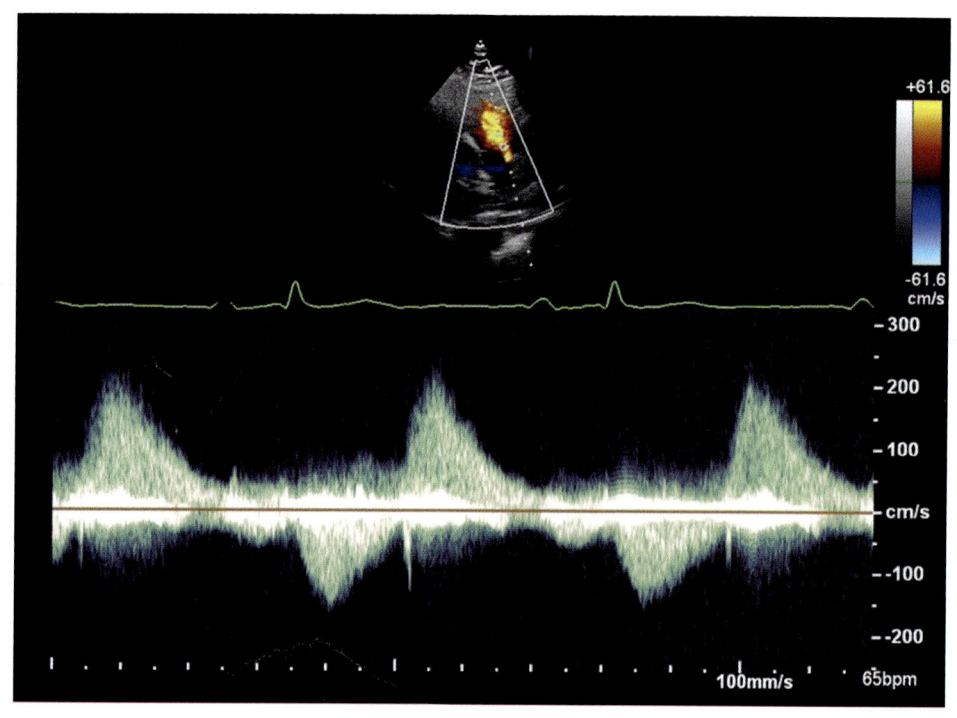

Figure 30.17

ANSWERS

1. **Answer: E.** In severe tricuspid regurgitation during sinus rhythm, hepatic vein Doppler typically shows a prominent, late peaking systolic flow reversal wave. However, systolic flow reversal may also occur in the setting of right ventricular dysfunction. Of note, blunting of the forward flow systolic wave rather than systolic flow reversal may occur in patients with severe TR and a large, compliant right atrium.

2. **Answer: D.** A PHT ≥130 ms can identify a stenotic bileaflet tricuspid mechanical valve. However, rounded spectral Doppler contours are not infrequent and PHT cannot be measured in these cases. In the absence of high-output states (anemia, hyperthyroidism, sepsis) the elevated mean gradient ≥6 mm Hg and/or an elevated velocity ≥1.9 m/s are supportive diagnostic parameters of tricuspid prosthetic valve stenosis. $TVI_{prosthesis}/TVI_{LVOT}$ ≥2.1 suggests mechanical prosthetic stenosis.

3. **Answer: B.** Tricuspid E/A ratio >2.1 with a deceleration time <120 ms are consistent with right ventricular restrictive filling in patients with RV disease. Late-diastolic antegrade flow in the pulmonary artery also suggests increased right ventricular diastolic pressure.

4. **Answer: D.** The normal diameter of IVC is ≤2.1 cm and decreases by at least 50% with inspiration during sniffing. Thus, patients in choices A and E have the lowest RAP (0-5 mm Hg). When the IVC is dilated but collapses by at least 50%, RAP is estimated at 5 to 10 mm Hg. In the presence of a normal diameter but with less than 50% collapse (assuming good effort during sniffing), RAP is usually between 5 and 10 mm Hg. When the IVC is both dilated with less than 50% collapse, RAP is estimated at 15 mm Hg (**Table 30.1**).

5. **Answer: A.** In this cardiomyopathy, there are frequent abnormalities in RV regional and global function. The regional dysfunction is commonly noted in the RVOT, apex, and basal RV free wall in the region of the "triangle of dysplasia." RV dilatation and depressed global systolic function also occur, though not in all patients early on. In one study, dilatation of the RVOT was noted in all patients with ARVD and may occur as an isolated finding. Other abnormalities include abnormally bright moderator band, RV sacculations (or diastolic outpouchings), aneurysm (systolic outpouchings), and trabecular derangements. LVEF is characteristically normal in most patients with ARVD, although infrequently a left-sided cardiomyopathy may occur. Given the presence of RV systolic dysfunction, PA pressures are usually normal and not elevated. Therefore, a peak TR velocity of 3.6 m/s is not consistent with ARVD.

6. **Answer: B.** RV systolic and diastolic functions are depressed in patients with pulmonary hypertension. Because of the RV contribution to septal function, both septal systolic and diastolic mitral annulus tissue Doppler velocities are reduced. Likewise, tricuspid annulus velocities at the lateral side of the tricuspid annulus are reduced in these patients. On the other hand, LV function is preserved, and early-diastolic velocities at the lateral side of the mitral annulus are usually normal.

Table 30.1. Estimation of RA Pressure on the Basis of IVC Diameter and Collapse

Variable	Normal (0-5 [3] mm Hg)	Intermediate (5-10 [8] mm Hg)		High (15 mm Hg)
IVC diameter	≤2.1 cm	≤2.1 cm	>2.1 cm	>2.1 cm
Collapse with sniff	>50%	<50%	>50%	<50%
Secondary indices of elevated RA pressure				• Restrictive filling • Tricuspid E/e' > 6 • Diastolic flow predominance in hepatic veins (systolic filling fraction <55%)

Ranges are provided for low and intermediate categories, but for simplicity, midrange values of 3 mm Hg for normal and 8 mm Hg for intermediate are suggested. Intermediate (8 mm Hg) RA pressures may be downgraded to normal (3 mm Hg) if no secondary indices of elevated RA pressure are present, upgraded to high if minimal collapse with sniff (<35%) and secondary indices of elevated RA pressure are present, or left at 8 mm Hg if uncertain.
IVC, inferior vena cava; RA, right atrial.

7. **Answer: D.** The flow in the hepatic veins is largely determined by RAP during the cardiac cycle (see **Table 30.2**). In normal subjects, antegrade flow from the hepatic veins to the RA occurs in systole (S) and diastole (D). With RA contraction, brief retrograde late-diastolic flow (Ar), as well as late-systolic flow (Vr), occurs into the hepatic veins. It is feasible to record high-quality signals by transthoracic imaging from the subcostal window in most ambulatory patients. Hepatic vein flow velocities can be used to asses RAP. In general, a lower proportion of forward systolic flow is indicative of increased RAP, except in healthy young subjects where this finding is normal. Similar to mitral inflow, young subjects have a tricuspid E/A ratio that is >1 with a short deceleration time (DT), and reduced RA contribution to RV filling.

Table 30.2. Summary of RAP Estimation Using Hepatic Venous Flow

Mean RAP	Hepatic Veins
0-5 mm Hg	$V_S > V_D$
5-10 mm Hg	$V_S = V_D$
10-15 mm Hg	$V_S < V_D$
≥20 mm Hg	Flow only with V_D

RAP, right atrial pressure; V_D, forward diastolic velocity in hepatic venous flow; V_S, forward systolic velocity in hepatic venous flow.

8. **Answer: D.** There are limitations to using hepatic venous flow to predict RAP. These include the presence of tricuspid valve stenosis or regurgitation, pericardial compression syndromes, high-grade AV block, and heart transplants. The presence of a restrictive cardiomyopathy is not a limitation. Option A is consistent with tricuspid stenosis/regurgitation. Option B is consistent with a postoperative pericardial compression syndrome. The patient in option C has high-grade heart block, and option E is a heart transplant. The presentation in D is consistent with amyloid where the patient has cardiac disease and peripheral neuropathy.

9. **Answer: E.** With advanced RV disease in patients with cardiac amyloidosis, RV free wall thickness is >7 mm, and tricuspid inflow shows a restrictive filling pattern. Hepatic venous flow at this stage is characterized by reduced forward systolic flow, increased forward diastolic flow, and inspiratory diastolic atrial flow reversal.

10. **Answer: C.** PA systolic pressure is given by $4(V_{TR})^2$ + RAP. A jugular venous pressure of 15-cm water corresponds to 15 × 0.7 or 10 to 11 mm Hg, since 1-cm water corresponds to 0.7 mm Hg. Accordingly, PA systolic pressure is given by $4(3)^2$ + 10, or 46 mm Hg.

11. **Answer: A.** Pulmonary vascular resistance (PVR) is derived invasively as (mean PA pressure − wedge pressure)/cardiac output. It can be estimated noninvasively by using the ratio between peak velocity of TR jet (as a surrogate of PA pressure) and time-velocity integral of RVOT systolic flow (as a surrogate of cardiac output), using the formula PVR = (TRV_{max}/RVOT TVI) × 10 + 0.16. Options A and C have the highest peak velocity, while option A has the least time-velocity integral of RVOT systolic flow.

12. **Answer: C.** Mean PA pressure is given by PA diastolic pressure +1/3 pulse pressure or (PA systolic pressure + 2 × PA diastolic pressure)/3. This patient has a PA systolic pressure of $4(3)^2$ + 10 or 46 mm Hg. PA diastolic pressure = $4(2)^2$ + 10 or 26 mm Hg. Pulse pressure is given by 46 − 26 or 20 mm Hg. Accordingly, mean PA pressure = 26 + (20/3), or 33 mm Hg. Mean PA pressure can also be estimated using the regression equation: 79 − 0.5 (acceleration time) of the RVOT pulsed Doppler velocity.

Common formulas to estimate mean PA pressure:

- Mean PA pressure = 79 − 0.45 (acceleration time) or 80 − 0.5 (acceleration time)
- Mean PA pressure = 4 (early PR velocity)^2 + estimated RA pressure
- Mean PA pressure = 1/3 (SPAP) + 2/3 (PADP), where SPAP pressure = 4 (TR velocity)^2 + estimated RA pressure and PADP pressure = 4 (late PR velocity)^2 + estimated RA pressure

13. **Answer: C.** RV systolic pressure is given by $4(V_{TR})^2 + RAP$, where V_{TR} is the peak velocity of the TR jet. Therefore, RV systolic pressure = 64 + 10, or 74 mm Hg. The gradient between RV systolic pressure and PA systolic pressure is given by RV systolic pressure − PV systolic pressure = $4(V_{PV})^2$, where V_{PV} is the peak velocity across the pulmonary valve. Therefore, PA systolic pressure = 74 − 36, or 38 mm Hg.

14. **Answer: C.** Mean PA pressure can be estimated using the regression equation: 79 − 0.45 (acceleration time). Therefore, the patient in Option A is predicted to have a mean PA pressure of 20 mm Hg, which is upper limits of normal. Mean PA pressure can also be estimated using the peak velocity of PR to which an estimate of right ventricular end-diastolic pressure (RVEDP), or RAP, is added. Therefore, the mean PA pressure in Option B can be predicted to be: $4(1.5)^2 + 5$ or 14 mm Hg, which is normal. In Option C, the peak systolic pressure is at least: $4(3.5)^2$, or 49 mm Hg, which is consistent with pulmonary hypertension. With increased RV systolic pressure, a D-shaped septum is present in both systole and diastole, and not only during diastole.

15. **Answer: E.** RV free wall thickness is most reliably measured in the subcostal view. In this view, axial resolution results in a more accurate measurement than the other views mentioned in the question in which lateral resolution of the ultrasound beam is relied on. The upper limits of normal RV wall thickness is 5 mm. Epicardial fat pad, trabeculations, and papillary muscles are excluded when performing this measurement.

16. **Answer: E.** The moderator band receives its blood supply from the LAD coronary artery. The acute marginal branch of the RCA provides the blood supply to the anterior and lateral RV walls. The conus artery (usually a branch from the RCA) provides the blood supply to the infundibulum region of the RV. The inferior wall of the RV gets its blood supply from the posterior descending branch of the RCA (see **Figure 30.18** with RV segments with corresponding coronary blood supply).

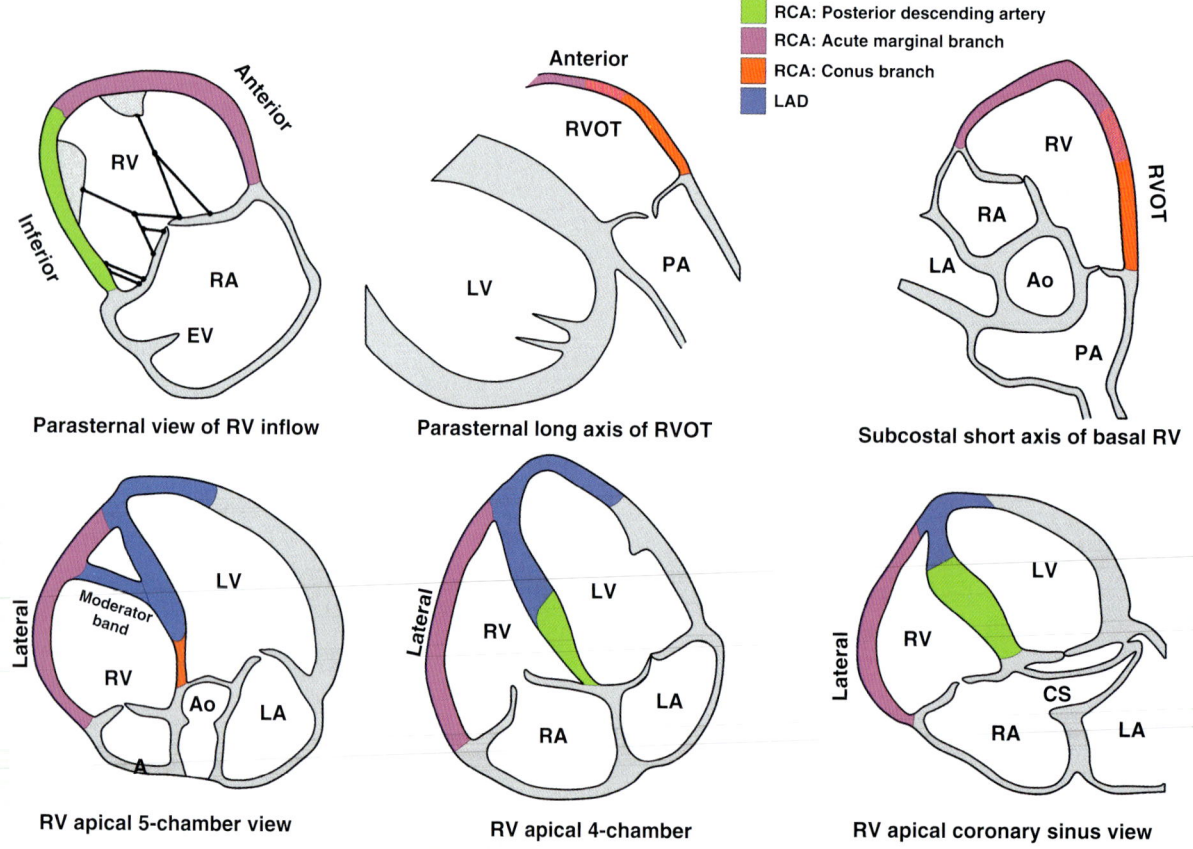

Figure 30.18. Segmental nomenclature of the right ventricular walls, along with their coronary supply. *Ao*, aorta; *CS*, coronary sinus; *LA*, left atrium; *LAD*, left anterior descending artery; *LV*, left ventricle; *PA*, pulmonary artery; *RA*, right atrium; *RCA*, right coronary artery; *RV*, right ventricle; *RVOT*, right ventricular outflow tract. (Reprinted from Rudski LG, Lai WW, Afilalo J, et al. Guidelines for the echocardiographic assessment of the right heart in adults: a report from the American Society of Echocardiography endorsed by the European Association of Echocardiography, a registered branch of the European Society of Cardiology, and the Canadian Society of Echocardiography. *J Am Soc Echocardiogr.* 2010;23(7):685-713; quiz 786-788. Figure 2. Copyright © 2010 by the American Society of Echocardiography. With permission.)

17. **Answer: C.** The myocardial performance index is given by the ratio of the sum of isovolumic contraction time (IVCT) and isovolumic relaxation time (IVRT) divided by ejection time (tissue Doppler MPI > 0.54 is abnormal). It can have a value that falls in the normal range despite RV systolic dysfunction in situations where IVRT is shortened, which happens when RV filling pressures are elevated. The presence of bundle branch block can lead to prolongation of IVCT and thus a higher value and not a lower value of the performance index. Patients in options D and E have a normal mean right atrial pressure, which does not lead to shortening of IVRT. In comparison, the patient in option C with restrictive RV filling pattern has an increased mean RA pressure, which leads to shortened IVRT (see **Figure 30.19** for illustration of RV myocardial performance index).

Table 30.3. Normal Values for RV Chamber Size

Parameter	Normal Range
RV basal diameter (mm)	25-41
RV mid diameter (mm)	19-35
RV longitudinal diameter (mm)	59-83
RVOT PLAX diameter (mm)	20-30
RVOT proximal diameter (mm)	21-35
RVOT distal diameter (mm)	17-27
RV wall thickness (mm)	1-5
RVOT EDA (cm^2)	
Men	10-24
Women	8-20
RV EDA indexed to BSA (cm^2/m^2)	
Men	5-12.6
Women	4.5-11.5
RV ESA (cm^2)	
Men	3-15
Women	3-11
RV ESA indexed to BSA (cm^2/m^2)	
Men	2.0-7.4
Women	1.6-6.4
RV EDV indexed to BSA (mL/m^2)	
Men	35-87
Women	32-74
RV ESV indexed to BSA (mL/m^2)	
Men	10-44
Women	8-36

BSA, body surface area; EDA, end-diastolic area; ESA, end-systolic area; PLAX, parasternal long-axis view; RV, right ventricular; RVOT, RV outflow tract.
Reprinted from Lang RM, Badano LP, Mor-Avi V, et al. Recommendations for cardiac chamber quantification by echocardiography in adults: an update from the American Society of Echocardiography and the European Association of Cardiovascular Imaging. *J Am Soc Echocardiogr.* 2015;28(1):1-39.e14. Copyright © 2015 Elsevier. With permission.

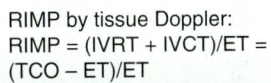

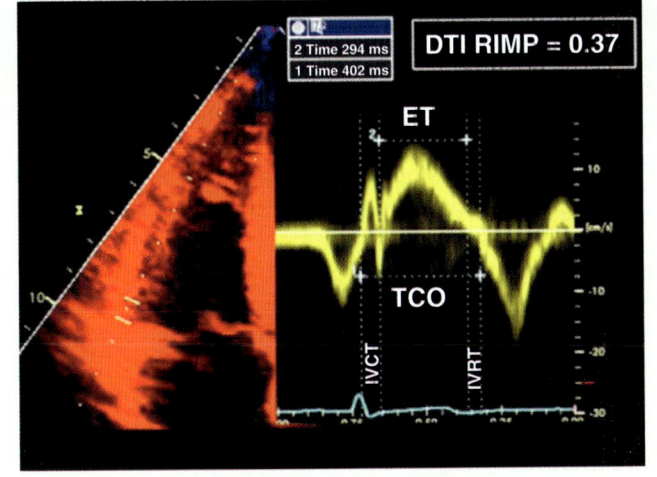

Figure 30.19. Recommendations for the echocardiographic assessment of right ventricular function. DTI, doppler tissue imaging; ET, ejection time; IVCT, isovolumic contraction time; IVRT, isovolumic relaxation time; RIMP, right ventricle myocardial performance index; TCO, tricuspid valve closure to opening time. (Reprinted from Lang RM, Badano LP, Mor-Avi V, et al. Recommendations for cardiac chamber quantification by echocardiography in adults: an update from the American Society of Echocardiography and the European Association of Cardiovascular Imaging. *J Am Soc Echocardiogr.* 2015;28(1):1-39.e14. Copyright © 2015 Elsevier. With permission.)

18. **Answer: D.** The upper limits of normal RVOT distal diameter is 27 mm, and the upper limits of normal basal RV dimension is 4.1 cm. The upper limits of normal value for both measurements is the same for both sexes. The upper limit for RV end-diastolic volume index by 3D echocardiography in males is 86 mL/m^2. For RV end-diastolic area index in females, the upper limits of normal is 11.5 cm^2/m^2. The upper limits of normal RV long axis is 83 mm and this value is the same for both sexes (see **Table 30.3**).

19. **Answer: E.** Mean PA pressure is derived from the peak velocity of the pulmonary regurgitation (PR) signal as 4(V^2) + RAP. Since the peak velocity is 3.5 m/s corresponding to 49 mm Hg, mean PA pressure is 59 mm Hg. PR end-diastolic velocity is used to estimate PA diastolic pressure.

20. **Answer: E.** A peak TR velocity of 2.7 m/s corresponds to an RV and PA systolic pressure of at least 29 mm Hg and thus by itself does not indicate the presence of pulmonary hypertension. A peak PR velocity of 1.9 m/s corresponds to mean PA pressure of at least 14 mm Hg and by itself is not diagnostic of pulmonary hypertension. PR end-diastolic velocity of 1.5 m/s corresponds to PA diastolic pressure of at least 9 mm Hg and by itself is not indicative of pulmonary hypertension. Isovolumic relaxation time is not used to estimate PA pressures. An acceleration time of 55 ms corresponds to mean PA pressure of 54 mm Hg, using the regression equation where mean PA pressure is given by 79 − (0.45 multiplied by acceleration time).

21. **Answer: D.** An IVC diameter with 80% inspiratory collapse is consistent with RAP at 0 to 5 mm Hg. Likewise, a tricuspid E/A ratio of 0.7 and RA end-systolic area of 10 cm² are seen in patients with normal RAP. In patients with chronic elevation of RAP, RA end-systolic area exceeds the upper limits of normal, which is 18 cm². A tricuspid E/A ratio >2 supports the presence of elevated mean RAP. For hepatic vein flow, systolic velocity–to–diastolic velocity ratio <0.5 is seen with increased mean RAP. Tricuspid E/e' ratio >6 is seen with increased mean RAP.

22. **Answer: D.** RV dP/dt can be obtained from the TR jet based on the expression: change in pressure/change in time. TR peak velocity of 2 m/s corresponds to RV-RA pressure gradient of 16 mm Hg, whereas peak TR velocity of 0.5 m/s corresponds to RV-RA pressure gradient of 1 mm Hg (using the simplified Bernoulli equation). Thus, in the question provided, the numerator is given by 16 − 1 or 15 mm Hg. The denominator is 0.03 seconds since units of dP/dt are in mm Hg/s. Therefore, dP/dt is equal to 15/0.03 or 500 mm Hg/s.

23. **Answer: E.** Peak TR velocity is dependent on the RV-RA pressure gradient and not the severity of TR. TR jet area more than 10 cm² is seen with severe TR. ERO of at least 0.4 cm² and RV of at least 45 mL support the conclusion of severe TR when Nyquist velocity is at least 50 cm/s. Likewise, vena contracta diameter of at least 0.7 cm is consistent with severe TR.

24. **Answer: E.** Neither pericardial constriction nor tricuspid stenosis cause systolic reversal. Severe TR causes systolic reversal in each cardiac cycle. Likewise, junctional rhythm with regular simultaneous depolarization and contraction of RA and RV leads to systolic reversal with each cardiac cycle. On the other hand, electronic RV pacing with lack of synchrony between RA and RV contraction leads to intermittent and irregularly occurring systolic reversal signals in the hepatic veins as they occur only in the cycles when the RA contracts against a closed tricuspid valve.

25. **Answer: C.** The hepatic venous flow shows holosystolic reversal compatible with severe TR, as in the setting of infective endocarditis of the tricuspid valve. A patient with controlled blood pressure has normal RA pressure and predominant forward systolic flow, not systolic reversal. In the setting of RV infarction and acute inferior wall MI, RV filling pressures are increased and there is predominant forward diastolic flow in the hepatic veins. Systolic flow is reduced, but not reversed in atrial fibrillation.

26. **Answer: D.** The hepatic venous flow shows a large Ar signal compatible with normal RA systolic function in the presence of increased RVEDP. In early stages of RV diastolic dysfunction, RVEDP is increased, whereas mean RAP is normal. This hemodynamic finding is compatible with option D. Systemic congestion occurs with increased RA mean pressure and predominant forward diastolic flow in all other choices.

27. **Answer: D.** RV dilatation with or without RV dysfunction is often noted on echocardiography done in symptomatic and asymptomatic patients. The differential diagnosis is broad and includes (1) shunts such as ASDs and anomalous pulmonary return; (2) myocardial conditions such as RV cardiomyopathy, RV infarction, and many biventricular cardiomyopathies; (3) pulmonary hypertension, both primary and secondary etiologies; (4) pulmonary and tricuspid regurgitation, both primary and secondary etiologies; (5) congenital abnormalities such as congenital absence of the pericardium; and (6) physiologic states associated with high output such as athlete's heart. VSDs and PDAs generally cause left ventricular not right ventricular enlargement.

28. **Answer: E.** TAPSE assumes that the tricuspid annulus displacement represents RV global systolic function. In reality, TAPSE reflects best longitudinal as opposed to global RV systolic function. The lower range for normal TAPSE is 17 mm.

29. **Answer: B.** The 4-chamber view demonstrates the presence of prominent thickening and retraction of septal and anterior tricuspid leaflets with annular dilatation, characteristic findings of carcinoid heart disease. Ebstein anomaly is characterized by apical displacement of the septal leaflet and an elongated anterior leaflet in that view. Rheumatic tricuspid valve disease is usually accompanied by mitral valve rheumatic disease in patients with a history of rheumatic fever. The pathologic characteristic is commissural fusion of the leaflets with diffuse thickening and resultant stenosis and regurgitation.

30. **Answer: B.** The PR signal is steep, indicating rapid equilibration of pressure between the PA and the RV. When RV stiffness is increased, RV diastolic pressure rises rapidly, leading to a PR signal that is similar to that seen in this case. This patient has increased RVEDP and RAP. Tricuspid inflow is characterized by predominant early filling with an E/A

ratio >1, and a steep deceleration time of tricuspid E velocity. Hepatic venous flow shows predominant forward flow in diastole (not systolic reversal).

31. **Answer: C.** The Doppler tracings show a mitral E/A ratio <1, a normal lateral e' velocity, and a reduced septal e' velocity. Collectively, these findings are seen in patients with pulmonary hypertension of a noncardiac etiology. The presence of a lateral E/e' ratio <8 is indicative of normal or reduced mean left atrial pressure. A mitral E/A ratio <1 is not due to impaired LV relaxation, but reduced LV filling due to pulmonary hypertension and dilated RV. With the reduction in pulmonary vascular resistance with bosentan, LV filling increases as well as mitral E/A ratio.

32. **Answer: B.** This patient has a pseudonormal LV filling pattern, and a lateral E/e' ratio >13 (grade II diastolic dysfunction). Collectively, the findings are consistent with pulmonary hypertension secondary to a cardiac etiology. LV relaxation is impaired given the reduction in lateral e' velocity. The increase in mitral E/e' ratio is consistent with increased LV filling pressures. Treatment with diuretics leads to a reduction in LV filling and the mitral E/A ratio.

33. **Answer: C.** The flow is obtained from a ventricular septal defect (VSD) signal showing flow between the LV and the RV during systole and diastole. This is compatible with a higher LVEDP than RVEDP, as well as a higher LV systolic pressure than RV systolic pressure. RV systolic pressure is the same as PA systolic pressure in the absence of pulmonary stenosis. Accordingly, PA systolic pressure can be computed as PA systolic pressure = LV systolic pressure $-4(V_{VSD})^2$, where V is in m/s and represents the peak velocity of the VSD jet by continuous-wave Doppler. In this case, PA systolic pressure = 150 − $4(5.5)^2$ = 29 mm Hg. This is not compatible with a TR jet of 3.5 m/s, which indicates an RV/PA systolic pressure of at least 49 mm Hg.

34. **Answer: E.** McConnell sign is a distinct echocardiographic finding in patients with acute pulmonary embolism. Echocardiography reveals akinesia of the mid RV free wall and a spared normally functioning RV apex. In a small cohort of 85 hospitalized patients with RV dysfunction, the overall diagnostic accuracy for acute pulmonary embolism was reported at 92%. Three mechanisms have been proposed to explain this abnormality. The first mechanism is tethering of the RV apex to a normal contracting and often hyperdynamic left ventricle. A second mechanism is that the RV assumes a more spherical shape to equalize wall stress to accommodate the acute increase in afterload. Finally, a third mechanism proposed that the RV dysfunction results from localized ischemia of the RV free wall due to increased wall stress. However, other causes of acute afterload increase may have similar findings. See **Table 30.4** with echocardiographic findings of pulmonary embolism.

Table 30.4. Echocardiographic Findings Seen With Pulmonary Embolism

- RV dilatation/dysfunction
- Small LV size/normal or hyperdynamic function
- Increased RV/LV size ratio
- Reduced LV stroke volume
- Reduced mitral E wave (due to decreased preload)
- McConnell sign
- Interventricular septal flattening in systole/paradoxical septal motion
- Tricuspid and pulmonary regurgitation (nonsevere)
- Increased pulmonary artery systolic pressure (<60 mm Hg with normal RV)
- 60/60 sign (pulmonary acceleration time <60 ms and TR pressure gradient <60 mm Hg)
- Early systolic notching of the RV outflow tract Doppler profile
- Increased RA pressure
- Thrombus in IVC, RA, RV, or PA

IVC, inferior vena cava; LV, left ventricle; PA, pulmonary artery; RA, right atrial; RV, right ventricle.

35. **Answer: C.** The PA systolic pressure is given by $4v^2$ + RA pressure, where v is the peak velocity of the TR jet. The patient with predominant forward diastolic flow is compatible with an RA pressure of 10 to 15 mm Hg. Accordingly, the PA systolic pressure is given by $4(2.8)^2$ + 10 to 15 mm Hg, or 41 to 46 mm Hg.

36. **Answer: A.** Onset of inspiration is confirmed by an augmentation in forward flow velocities, while onset of expiration is confirmed by a decrease in forward flow velocities with an increase in diastolic flow reversal velocity (although not seen in this example).

37. **Answer: D.** RV longitudinal strain obtained with speckle tracking echocardiography is an emerging measure of RV function. It can be obtained as 3-segment (free wall) or a 6-segment measurement (interventricular septum + free wall) in the apical 4-chamber view similar to obtaining LV chamber longitudinal strain measurement. It is not yet well-established which measure is most clinically useful. Although, RV strain is only available on recent cardiac ultrasound software updates, it can be adapted from LV strain–specific software. Abnormal values of RV longitudinal strain are >−20%. RV strain should be obtained in the RV-focused view. RV longitudinal strain is a useful prognostic marker in many disease states including heart failure, pulmonary HTN, valvular heart disease, cardiomyopathies, and congenital heart disease.

38. **Answer: D.** A semiautomated software for border detection volume measurements is recommended for 3D RVEF determination obtained from the composite of the basal and mid short-axis and 4-chamber view. 3D RVEF volumes underestimate those obtained by cardiac MRI, but EF measurements correlate well. A normal RVEF is >45% and therefore this patient has

a normal RVEF. Although 3D echo RVEF is a good measure of cardiac contractility, it is affected by load dependency, septal motion, and other factors like image quality and heart rhythm. It is expected that with newer echocardiographic machines 3D RVEF will become an easily and rapidly obtained parameter to use in the assessment of RV function.

39. **Answer: D.** The image is an apical 4-chamber view obtained in systole (the mitral valve is closed). There is no tricuspid leaflet coaptation and there is blue laminar flow (away from the transducer) from the RV to the RA. This represents "free TR" or torrential TR where there is equalization of pressures in the RA and RV. Because of this, the CW Doppler TR profile is low velocity (usually triangular) and cannot be used to determine RVSP.

40. **Answer: C.** The parasternal long-axis view shows an LV with reduced end-diastolic dimension, but increased wall thickness. While LV fractional shortening is normal, there is almost no change during the cardiac cycle in the RV area seen in ▶ **Video 30.3**. The latter observation is indicative of a severely depressed RV systolic function. Because of severe RV systolic dysfunction, LV filling and stroke volume are reduced, as can be inferred from the reduced aortic valve leaflet separation in this view. Since LV function is normal, and the patient has an intra-aortic balloon pump already (seen in ▶ **Video 30.3**, the descending aorta posterior to the left atrium), option D is wrong.

41. **Answer: C. Figure 30.14** shows the TR jet by CW Doppler recorded from a low left parasternal position. The signal is dense, triangular in shape and shows early peaking with a peak velocity of only 160 cm/s. These findings are consistent with severe TR, and an RV pressure that is very similar to RA "V" wave pressure. The patient would be expected to have holosystolic, and not just midsystolic, reversal in the hepatic venous flow. In this patient, the correct estimation of PA systolic pressure is challenging and is highly dependent on the accurate assessment of RAP, and not the TR jet peak velocity. In patients with longstanding ASD, secondary pulmonary hypertension develops with a much higher peak velocity of TR by CW Doppler.

KEY POINTS

- RV systolic dysfunction can be diagnosed by the change in RV dimensions and area by 2D echocardiography.
- Severe TR by CW Doppler is characterized by a dense signal with early peaking.
- In patients with severe TR and a small systolic transvalvular pressure gradient, the accurate assessment of PA systolic pressure is highly dependent on the correct estimation of RAP.

42. **Answer: D.** The apical 4-chamber views were obtained from a patient with Ebstein anomaly. The tricuspid valve leaflets are seen close to the RV apex, and color Doppler shows severe TR. LVEF appears normal, though additional views are needed for confirmation. RA, but not RV, size is increased because of the apical displacement of tricuspid valve leaflets in this condition. Because of reduced pulmonary blood flow, PA pressures are reduced to low normal, unless coexisting disease is present, which can lead to pulmonary hypertension. Therefore, the patient would not show a D-shaped septum during systole.

43. **Answer: D.** Patients with Ebstein disease frequently have interatrial shunting. This can result in systemic embolic events, which may manifest with recurrent transient ischemic attacks and silent strokes that can be identified by brain MRI studies. Likewise, shunting is usually the cause of exertional hypoxemia, and not LV diastolic dysfunction. Further evaluation with saline contrast is needed to identify the site of shunting.

KEY POINTS

- Ebstein anomaly is characterized by apical displacement of tricuspid valve leaflets. As a result, RA volume is increased and anatomic RV size is reduced.
- Tricuspid regurgitation of varying severity is frequently present in this condition.
- Interatrial shunting via PFO or ASD can occur and lead to transient ischemic attacks and systemic embolic events.

44. **Answer: A.** TEE shows a large RA with predominantly right-to-left shunting across the interatrial septum. The PFO shown in the TEE can be closed percutaneously. The presence of an RA to LA shunt supports the conclusion that RAP is higher than LA pressure.

45. **Answer: B.** The TR jet has a peak velocity close to 4 m/s. The estimated PA systolic pressure is 67 mm Hg. Pulmonary venous flow shows predominant systolic flow and small atrial reversal velocity with LA contraction. The pulmonary venous flow pattern is consistent with normal LV filling pressures, and the absence of significant MR (which would have led to systolic reversal). Patients with pulmonary hypertension have increased pulmonary vascular resistance. The increased RV afterload (and RV systolic dysfunction later on) leads to reduced RV systolic velocities that can be recorded at the interventricular septum as the septal systolic velocity, and the RV free wall.

KEY POINTS
- Color Doppler can be used to identify the presence of a shunt across the interatrial septum.
- In patients with a noncardiac etiology of pulmonary hypertension and reduced LV filling, pulmonary venous flow shows predominant forward systolic flow and a small atrial reversal (Ar) signal.

---

46. **Answer: A.** The short-axis view shows a D-shaped interventricular septum in systole and diastole, consistent with increased RV systolic pressure. See **Figure 30.20** with septal curvature with RV pressure and volume overload. Color Doppler shows flow acceleration across the pulmonic valve consistent with pulmonary stenosis. Therefore, PA systolic pressure is possibly normal. Color Doppler shows mild PR, whereas 2D imaging shows a hyperdynamic LVEF that is >70%. There is RV hypertrophy, and free wall thickness cannot be normal in this patient.

47. **Answer: C.** The CW Doppler signal indicates the presence of severe pulmonary stenosis with a peak velocity >6 m/s. TR peak velocity should therefore be closer to that value. The patient does not have pulmonary hypertension and pulmonary vascular resistance is not increased. With RV hypertrophy, RV stiffness and late-diastolic pressures are increased, which lead to a prominent Ar signal in hepatic venous flow with RA contraction. Percutaneous commissurotomy can be used to treat pulmonary valve stenosis with good results.

KEY POINTS
- Patients with significant pulmonary stenosis have increased RV systolic pressure and RV hypertrophy. Therefore, a D-shaped septum would be noticed in systole and diastole.
- RV hypertrophy is associated with increased RV stiffness and late-diastolic RV pressures. RV diastolic dysfunction can be identified by increased Ar velocity and duration in hepatic venous flow.
- Pulmonary stenosis can be diagnosed by CW Doppler using the peak velocity and the contour of the spectral envelope.

---

48. **Answer: D.** The parasternal long-axis view shows a LV with normal size and function but a dilated RV. Color Doppler shows some acceleration across the pulmonic valve in systole, indicating increased systolic flow across the valve. However, the most important finding by color Doppler is the presence of severe PR. This lesion is common after surgery for the repair of tetralogy of Fallot and does not lead to increased RV systolic pressure.

49. **Answer: D.** The CW Doppler signal is indicative of severe PR. Patients with severe PR have a steep rise in RV diastolic pressure that leads to the rapid equalization of the pressure gradient between the PA and the RV in early diastole, and therefore a PR signal with steep deceleration/short pressure halftime and early termination of diastolic flow along with brief forward flow across the pulmonary valve in end-diastole due to a high RV end-diastolic pressure. Severe PR leads to increased RV diastolic, not systolic, pressures. Therefore, a flat septum would be noted only in diastole, and not in systole (See **Table 30.5**).

KEY POINTS
- Patients with significant PR have a dilated RV with eccentric hypertrophy.
- Interventricular septal motion is characterized by an RV volume overload pattern, with a flat septum only in diastole.
- Color Doppler can be used to assess the severity of PR.
- Severe PR by CW Doppler shows rapid deceleration with short pressure halftime.

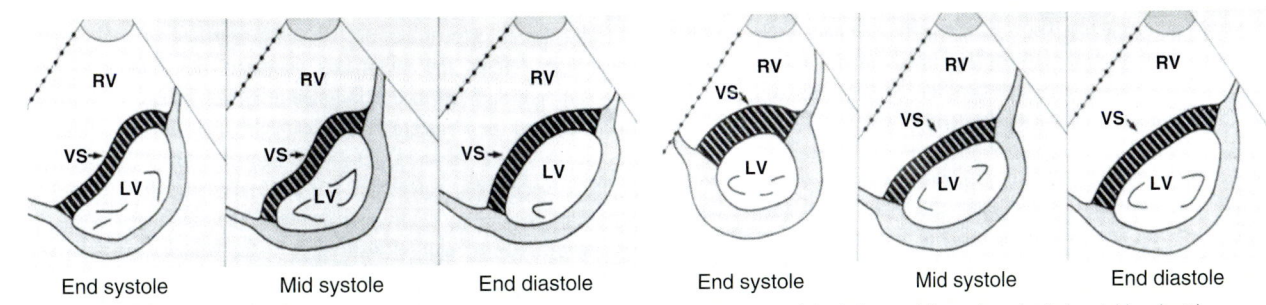

Figure 30.20. Serial stop-frame short-axis two-dimensional echocardiographic images of the left ventricle at the mitral chordal level with diagrams from a patient with isolated right ventricular (RV) pressure overload due to primary pulmonary hypertension *(left)* and from a patient with isolated RV volume overload due to tricuspid valve resection *(right)*. Whereas the left ventricular (LV) cavity maintains a circular profile throughout the cardiac cycle in normal subjects, in RV pressure overload, there is leftward ventricular septal (VS) shift and reversal of septal curvature present throughout the cardiac cycle with the most marked distortion of the left ventricle at end-systole. In the patient with RV volume overload, the septal shift and flattening of VS curvature occurs predominantly in mid to late diastole with relative sparing of LV deformation at end-systole. (Reprinted from Louie EK, Rich S, Levitsky S, Brundage BH. Doppler echocardiographic demonstration of the differential effects of right ventricular pressure and volume overload on left ventricular geometry and filling. *J Am Coll Cardiol*. 1992;19(1):84-90. Figures 1 and 2. Copyright © 1992 by the American College of Cardiology. With permission.)

Table 30.5. Echocardiographic and Doppler Parameters Useful in Grading PR Severity

Parameter	Mild	Moderate	Severe
Pulmonic valve	Normal	Normal or abnormal	Abnormal and may not be visible
RV size	Normal*	Normal or dilated	Dilated[†]
Jet size, color Doppler[‡]	Thin (usually <10 mm in length) with a narrow origin	Intermediate	Broad origin; variable depth of penetration
Ratio of PR jet width/pulmonary annulus			>0.7[§]
Jet density and contour (CW)	Soft	Dense	Dense; early termination of diastolic flow
Deceleration time of the PR spectral Doppler signal			Short, <260 ms[§]
Pressure halftime of PR jet			<100 ms[ǁ]
PR index[l]		<0.77	<0.77
Diastolic flow reversal in the main or branch PAs (PW)			Prominent
Pulmonic systolic flow (VTI) compared to systemic flow (LVOT VTI) by PW[#]	Slightly increased	Intermediate	Greatly increased
RF**	<20%	20%-40%	>40%

CW, continuous wave; LVOT, left ventricular outflow tract; PA, pulmonary artery; PR, pulmonary regurgitation; PW, pulsed wave; RF, regurgitant fraction; RV, right ventricular; VTI, velocity-time integral.
*Unless there are other reasons for RV enlargement.
[†]Exception: acute PR.
[‡]At a Nyquist limit of 50 to 70 cm/s.
[§]Identifies a cardiovascular magnetic resonance (CMR)-derived PR fraction ≥40%.
[l]Defined as the duration of the PR signal divided by the total duration of diastole, with this cutoff identifying a CMR-derived PR fraction >25%.
[ǁ]Not reliable in the presence of high RV end-diastolic pressure.
[#]Cutoff values for RVol and fraction are not well validated.
[§]Steep deceleration is not specific for severe PR.
**RF data primarily derived from CMR with limited application with echocardiography.
Reprinted from Zoghbi WA, Adams D, Bonow RO, et al. Recommendations for noninvasive evaluation of native valvular regurgitation: a report from the American Society of Echocardiography developed in collaboration with the society for cardiovascular magnetic resonance. J Am Soc Echocardiogr. 2017;30(4):303-371. Copyright © 2017 by the American Society of Echocardiography. With permission.

SUGGESTED READINGS

Appleton CP, Hatle LK, Popp RL. Superior vena cava and hepatic vein Doppler echocardiography in healthy adults. *J Am Coll Cardiol*. 1987;10(5):1032-1039.

Bhattacharyya S, Toumpanakis C, Burke M, Taylor AM, Caplin ME, Davar J. Features of carcinoid heart disease identified by 2- and 3-dimensional echocardiography and cardiac MRI. *Circ Cardiovasc Imaging*. 2010;3(1):103-111.

Lang RM, Badano LP, Mor-Avi V, et al. Recommendations for cardiac chamber quantification by echocardiography in adults: an update from the american society of echocardiography and the European association of cardiovascular imaging. *J Am Soc Echocardiogr*. 2015;16(3):233-270.

McConnell MV, Solomon SD, Rayan ME, Come PC, Goldhaber SZ, Lee RT. Regional right ventricular dysfunction detected by echocardiography in acute pulmonary embolism. *Am J Cardiol*. 1996;78(4):469-473.

Nagueh SF, Kopelen HA, Zoghbi WA. Relation of mean right atrial pressure to echocardiographic and Doppler parameters of right atrial and right ventricular function. *Circulation*. 1996;93(6):1160-1169.

Nagueh SF, Smiseth OA, Appleton CP, et al. Recommendations for the evaluation of left ventricular diastolic function by echocardiography: an update from the American Society of Echocardiography and the European Association of Cardiovascular Imaging. *Eur Heart J Cardiovasc Imaging*. 2016;17(12):1321-1360.

Rudski LG, Lai WW, Afilalo J, et al. Guidelines for the echocardiographic assessment of the right heart in adults: a report from the American Society of Echocardiography endorsed by the European Association of Echocardiography, a registered branch of the European Society of Cardiology, and the Canadian Society of Echocardiography. *J Am Soc Echocardiogr*. 2010;23(7):685-788.

Zoghbi et al., 2017 Zoghbi WA, Adams D, Bonow RO, et al. Recommendations for noninvasive evaluation of native valvular regurgitation: a report from the American Society of Echocardiography developed in collaboration with the society for cardiovascular magnetic resonance. *J Am Soc Echocardiogr*. 2017;30(4):303-371.

CHAPTER 31

Tumors, Masses, and Source of Emboli

Mohamed Al-Kazaz, Madeline Jankowski, and Kameswari Maganti

QUESTIONS

1. A structure found in the left atrium that can be misinterpreted as a pathologic mass is:
   A. Eustachian valve.
   B. Crista terminalis.
   C. Moderator band.
   D. Chiari network.
   E. Suture line following transplant.

2. The following are recommendations to perform echocardiography in patients with cardiac masses or tumors. Which of the following statements is correct?
   A. Contrast echocardiography using ultrasound-enhancing agents does not help differentiate vascular tumors from avascular masses such as thrombus.
   B. Follow-up or surveillance studies after surgical removal of masses is known to have a low likelihood of recurrence.
   C. Transthoracic echocardiography is superior to transesophageal echocardiography in evaluating cardiac tumors, especially papillary fibroelastoma.
   D. Complete transthoracic echocardiography is recommended on all patients with suspected cardiac mass.

3. This tumor is a benign cardiac tumor.
   A. Angiosarcoma.
   B. Rhabdomyoma.
   C. Lymphoma.
   D. Mesothelioma.
   E. Prominent ventricular trabeculations.

4. It is uncommon for this tumor to metastasize to the heart.
   A. Renal cell carcinoma.
   B. Breast.
   C. Thyroid.
   D. Lung.
   E. Melanoma.

5. Cardiac tumors are characterized by which of the following?
   A. Primary cardiac tumors are a common cardiac condition.
   B. Cardiac tumors are almost always symptomatic.
   C. Echocardiography is a costly and inconvenient test to evaluate a cardiac tumor.
   D. Embolization is a mechanism by which cardiac tumors cause symptoms.

6. Lipomatous hypertrophy of the atrial septum:
   A. Does not commonly cause symptoms.
   B. Is caused by fibrosis.
   C. Has the same histological patterns as lipomas.
   D. Can be seen on transthoracic echocardiography and is an indication for the performance of transesophageal echocardiography.
   E. None of the above.

7. The transesophageal echocardiographic evaluation of valvular vegetations:
   A. Always allows for the distinction between other cardiac masses.
   B. Can provide predictive information about embolic risk.
   C. Has shown that vegetations are more likely to be on the "downstream" side of the valve.
   D. Has not been used to determine the natural history of vegetations.
   E. Is not influenced by pretest expectations.

8. Which of the following statements about a patent foramen ovale is **CORRECT**?
   A. Patent foramen ovale is a rare congenital cardiac lesion that is estimated to occur in 1% of the population.
   B. The prevalence of patent foramen ovale is three times more frequent in females compared to males.
   C. Most individuals with patent foramen ovale are symptomatic.
   D. An incidentally detected patent foramen ovale requires surgical or percutaneous closure.
   E. Early saline contrast appearance in the left heart (within three beats of contrast appearance in the right heart) on transthoracic echocardiography with agitated saline contrast injection is suggestive of a patent foramen ovale.

9. The clinical manifestations of the Carney complex include:
   A. Papillary fibroelastoma.
   B. Hemangioma.
   C. Epilepsy.
   D. Cardiac myxoma.
   E. Nevoid basal cell carcinoma.

10. The following are symptoms associated with cardiac myxoma.
    A. Palpitations and diarrhea.
    B. Syncope and diarrhea.
    C. Dyspnea and fever.
    D. Dyspnea and dysphagia.
    E. None of the above.

11. Which of the following statements about tuberous sclerosis is **TRUE**?
    A. Tuberous sclerosis is a syndrome characterized by hamartomas in several organs, epilepsy, cognitive impairment, and adenoma sebaceum.
    B. The genetic defect for tuberous sclerosis has not been identified.
    C. Only a minority of patients with cardiac rhabdomyomas have tuberous sclerosis.
    D. Surgical resection of the cardiac tumors is recommended in asymptomatic patients with tuberous sclerosis.
    E. None of the above.

12. Papillary fibroelastomas:
    A. Cannot occur on the pulmonic valve.
    B. Are usually single rather than multiple.
    C. Exclusively occur on cardiac valves.
    D. Commonly result in valvular regurgitation.
    E. None of the above.

13. The most common malignant tumor of the heart is:
    A. Angiosarcoma.
    B. Lymphoma.
    C. Metastatic disease.
    D. Leiomyosarcoma.
    E. Myxoma.

14. A characteristic feature of a cardiac myxoma on two-dimensional echocardiography is:
    A. An associated pericardial effusion.
    B. A narrow stalk connected to the fossa ovalis.
    C. An intramural hyperechoic mass.
    D. A mobile mass with a short pedicle attached to a cardiac valve.
    E. None of the above.

15. In patients with human immunodeficiency virus (HIV) infection and acquired immunodeficiency syndrome (AIDS), this tumor has been described to affect the heart.
    A. Lipoma.
    B. Kaposi sarcoma.
    C. Rhabdomyosarcoma.
    D. Angiosarcoma.
    E. Hemangioma.

16. A 37-year-old patient was noted to have a mass in the left atrium. An astute sonographers administered ultrasound enhancing agent (UEA) at very low MI (<0.2), utilized a high-MI "flash" impulse over three frames to clear contrast from the myocardium, and demonstrated rapid replenishment of UEA within the mass. Which of the following statements is correct?
   A. The left atrial mass is most consistent with a thrombus.
   B. The left atrial mass is most consistent with a myxoma.
   C. The left atrial mass is most consistent with a sarcoma.
   D. The left atrial mass is most consistent with a papillary fibroelastoma.
   E. None of the above.

17. A 36-year-old woman was diagnosed with leiomyosarcoma (**Figure 31.1** of a zoomed view of the left atrium on the parasternal long axis). Which of the following statements about leiomyosarcoma is **CORRECT**?
   A. Treatment of cardiac leiomyosarcomas consists solely of chemotherapy and radiation.
   B. Leiomyosarcomas, like other malignant cardiac tumors, occur preferentially in the right heart.
   C. Leiomyosarcomas typically present in patients' seventh decade.
   D. Leiomyosarcomas are derived from smooth muscle cells.
   E. None of the above.

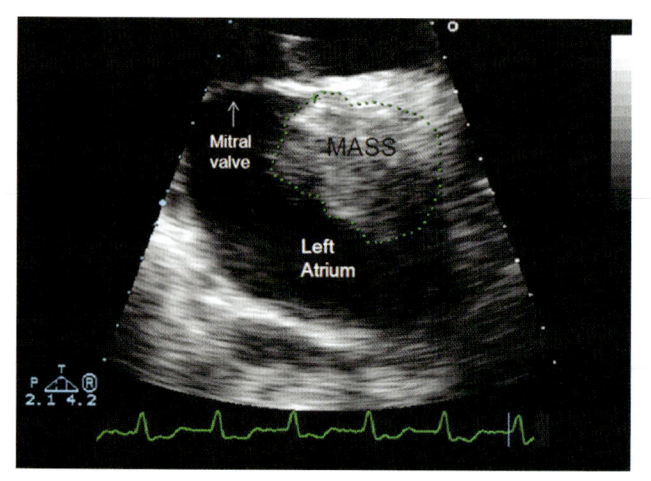

Figure 31.1

18. A 21-year-old college student in good health seeks medical clearance to travel abroad. She has no family history of heart disease and no symptoms. She has no history of rheumatic fever, night sweats, or chills and has had all childhood and youth vaccinations. On examination, palpitations are noted, and an echocardiogram is ordered. The left ventricular (LV) chamber size is normal and the ejection fraction (EF) is low normal. A large echodensity is noted on the parasternal long- and short-axis LV images (**Figure 31.2A** and **31.2B**). This abnormality is most likely a(n):
   A. Large pericardial mass.
   B. Large LV cavity tumor.
   C. LV aneurysm filled with thrombus.
   D. Mass embedded within the LV walls.
   E. None of the above.

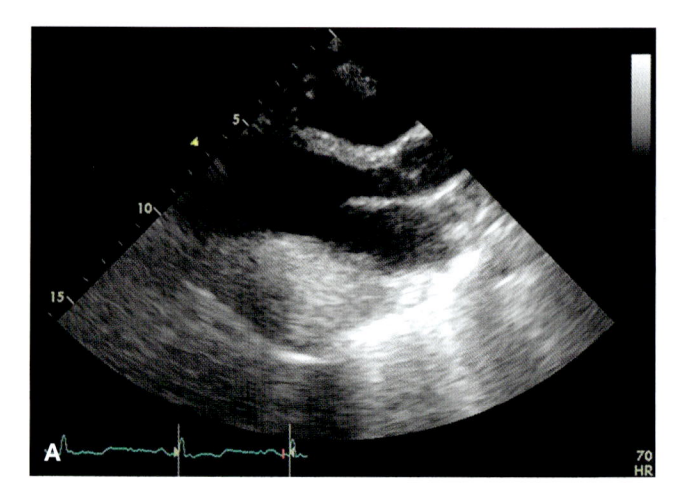

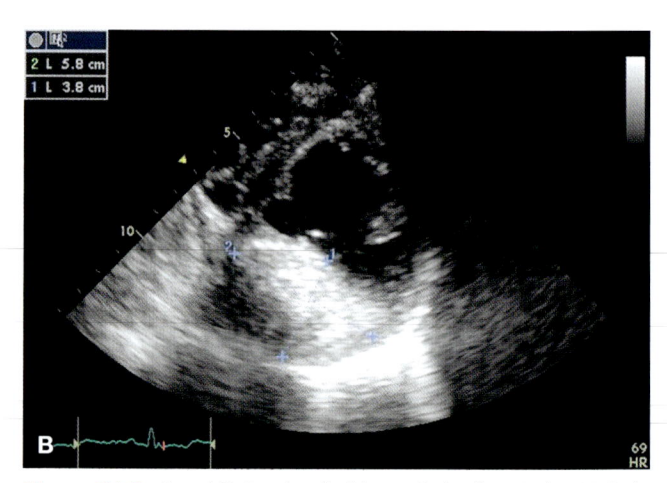

Figure 31.2. A and **B:** Reprinted with permission from Park MM, Park SH. Tumors, masses, and sources of emboli. In: Anderson B, Park MM, eds. *Basic to Advanced Clinical Echocardiography*. Wolters Kluwer; 2021:416-431. Figure 24.2AB.

19. A 65-year-old man with dyspnea is found to have a mass on transthoracic echocardiography (**Figure 31.3** of the right ventricular outflow tract view from parasternal long axis, and ▶ **Video 31.1A** and parasternal short axis view close to the pulmonic valve, ▶ **Video 31.1B**). Pathology at the time of surgery revealed an angiosarcoma. Which of the following accurately describes angiosarcomas?
   A. Angiosarcomas usually are discovered late and typically have grown to be large or metastasized at the time of diagnosis.
   B. Like other cardiac sarcomas, the gender distribution is equal (1:1).
   C. Angiosarcomas most often occur in the left ventricle.
   D. Patients usually present with tachyarrhythmias.
   E. None of the above.

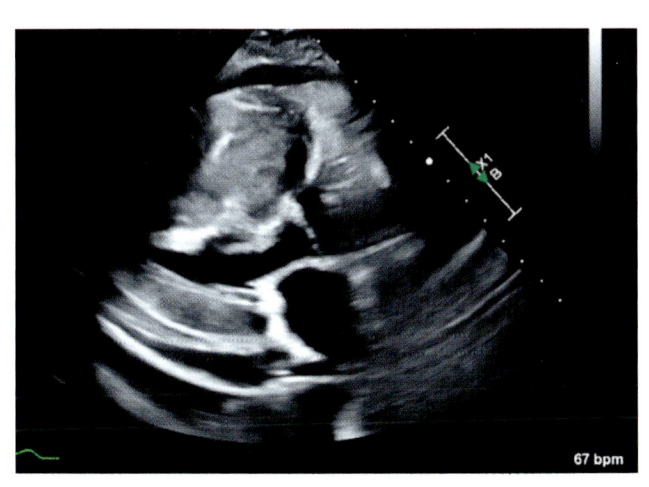

Figure 31.3

20. A 52-year-old woman presented with right flank pain and weight loss. Renal cell carcinoma was diagnosed. A transthoracic echocardiogram was performed (**Figure 31.4** of the parasternal long axis). Arrow points to a mass in the right ventricle. Which of the following statements about renal cell carcinoma is **CORRECT**?
   A. Intravascular extension of the tumor is not a common manifestation of renal cell carcinoma.
   B. Pulmonary embolization is not seen with metastatic renal cell carcinoma.
   C. Metastatic renal cell carcinoma is rarely confused with thrombus on echocardiography.
   D. The initial diagnosis of renal cell carcinoma can be made by the detection of an intracardiac mass on echocardiography in some cases.
   E. None of the above.

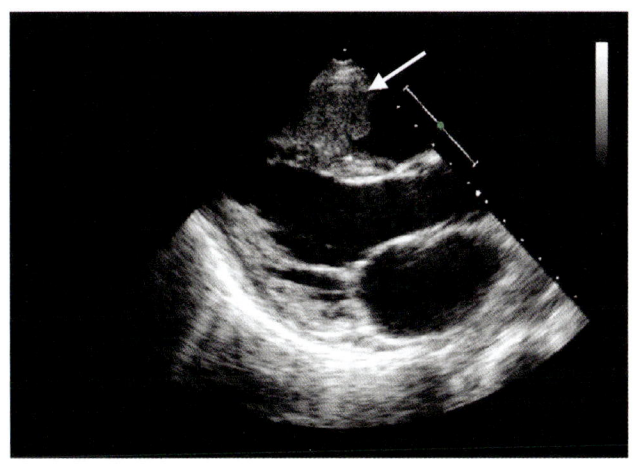

Figure 31.4

21. A 24-year-old man with synovial sarcoma had a transthoracic echocardiogram performed (**Figure 31.5** of the apical 4-chamber view demonstrating a large pericardial effusion and mass abutting the lateral left atrial wall and ▶ **Video 31.2**). Which of the following accurately characterizes synovial sarcomas?
   A. Synovial sarcoma is caused by a translocation between chromosome 18 and the X chromosome.
   B. Synovial sarcoma is not a malignant primary cardiac tumor.
   C. Synovial sarcoma is a common type of cardiac tumor.
   D. Synovial sarcoma has an excellent prognosis.
   E. None of the above.

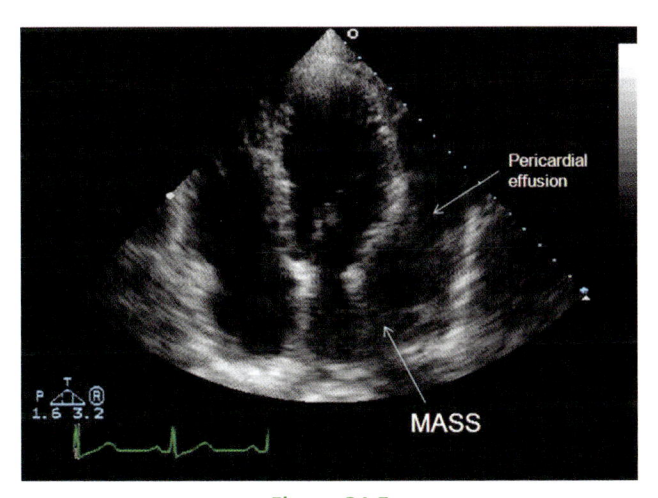

Figure 31.5

656 / Clinical Echocardiography Review

22. A 60-year-old woman with antiphospholipid syndrome presented with L MCA stroke. A 0.2-mL bolus of perflutren lipid microspheres was injected intravenously followed by a saline flush. A 4-apical chamber view on a transthoracic echocardiogram without an ultrasound-enhancing agent is shown in **Figure 31.6** and ▶ **Video 31.3A** and with an ultrasound-enhancing agent in **Video 31.3B**. Based on these images, which of the following conclusions is true about this patient's condition?
    A. The structure seen in the left ventricle close to the anterolateral wall is likely to be an angiosarcoma.
    B. The structure seen in the left ventricle close to the anterolateral wall is likely to be an avascular structure (eg, vegetation, thrombus, or aberrant structure).
    C. The structure seen in the left ventricle close to the anterolateral wall is likely to be rhabdomyosarcoma.
    D. The structure seen in the left ventricle close to the anterolateral wall is likely to be vascular fibroma.
    E. None of the above.

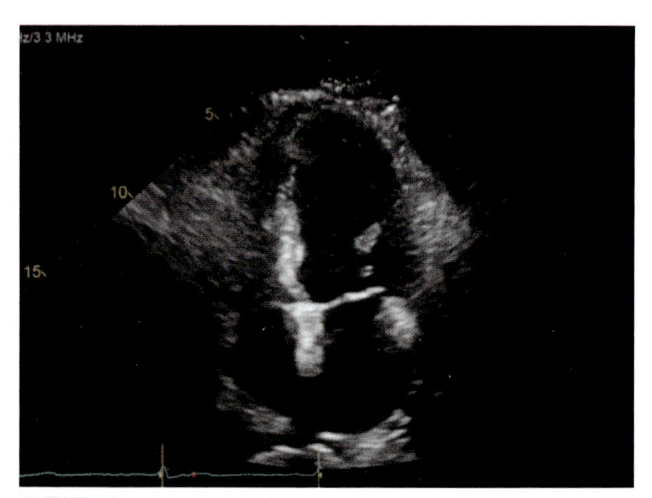

Figure 31.6

23. An apical view from a transthoracic echocardiogram is shown in **Figure 31.7** and ▶ **Video 31.4A** and **Video 31.4B**. A prominent Chiari network is seen in the right atrium. Based on these images, which of the following statements is **CORRECT**?

    A. A Chiari network is present in 20% to 30% of normal hearts.
    B. A Chiari network is associated with an increased risk of sudden cardiac death.
    C. A Chiari network is a congenital remnant of the right valve of the sinus venosus.
    D. A Chiari network is another name for crista terminalis.
    E. None of the above.

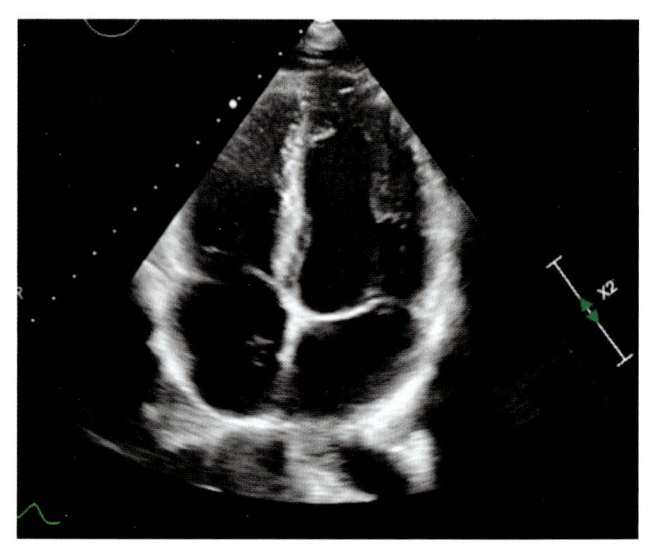

Figure 31.7

24. A 62-year-old woman presented with worsening dyspnea on exertion and chest pain that began 4 months earlier. A transthoracic echocardiogram revealed a fluid-filled cyst adjacent and partially compressing the right atrium (**Figure 31.8A** and **Figure 31.8B,** subcostal view with arrow pointing to pericardial cyst). This structure was evaluated by CT and cardiac MRI and it seems consistent with a pericardial cyst. Which of the following statements about pericardial cysts is **CORRECT**?
    A. The diagnosis of pericardial cysts can sometimes be suggested on chest radiograph by the identification of a rounded mass along the right heart border.
    B. Pericardial cysts are the most common anterior mediastinal mass lesion.
    C. Cysts are considered to be true neoplasms.
    D. It is common for pericardial cysts to become large enough to cause compressive symptoms.
    E. None of the above.

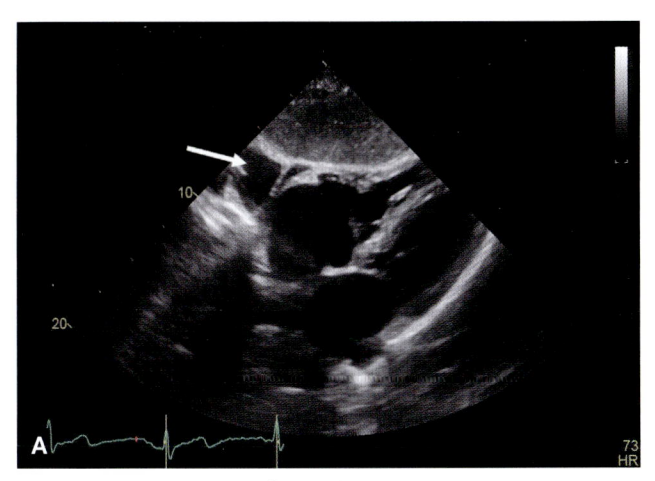

Figure 31.8A

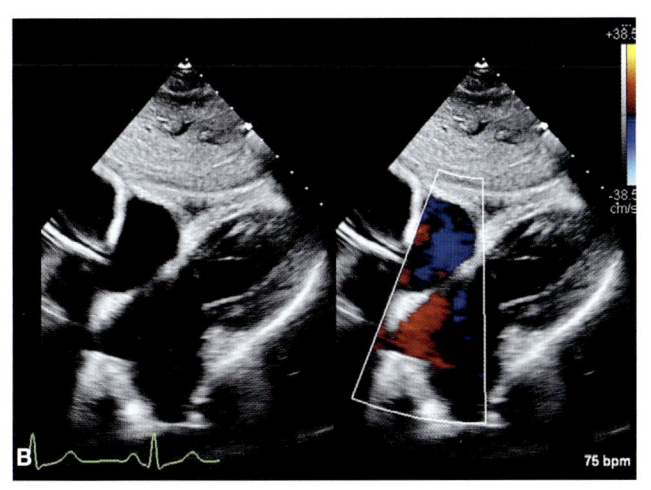

Figure 31.8B

B. There is a high occurrence of unsuccessful surgical left atrial appendage closure reported in the literature with suture closure.
C. Transesophageal echocardiography is not helpful in assessing the results of a surgical left atrial appendage closure procedure.
D. Residual communication between an incompletely closed left atrial appendage and the body of the left atrium is not a potential mechanism for thrombus formation and embolic events.
E. None of the above.

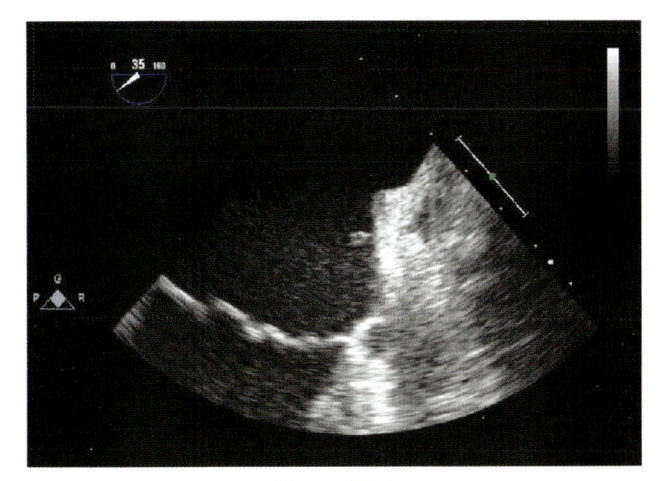

Figure 31.9

25. A 56-year-old man with persistent atrial fibrillation underwent a minimally invasive modified surgical Maze procedure with suture closure of the left atrial appendage. A transesophageal echocardiogram was performed 1 month later. **Figure 31.9** and ▶ **Video 31.5** show the left atrium at 35° with a small mobile echodensity that appears to be attached to the left atrial wall. Color Doppler showed contiguous flow between the left atrium and left atrial appendage and the pulsed Doppler tracing was consistent with a left atrial appendage flow pattern (not shown). Which of the following statements is **CORRECT**?
   A. The interpretation of masses found on echocardiography is not dependent on the clinical context in which it occurs.

26. A 77-year-old man with a past history of an anterolateral wall ST-segment elevation myocardial infarction had a transthoracic echocardiogram performed. A large left ventricular apical mass was seen (**Figure 31.10A** of the apical 4-chamber view and **Figure 31.10B** with an ultrasound-enhancing agent) and the anterior wall, anterolateral wall, and apex were akinetic. This mass most likely represents a:
   A. Myxoma.
   B. Rhabdomyosarcoma.
   C. Thrombus.
   D. Vegetation.
   E. None of the above.

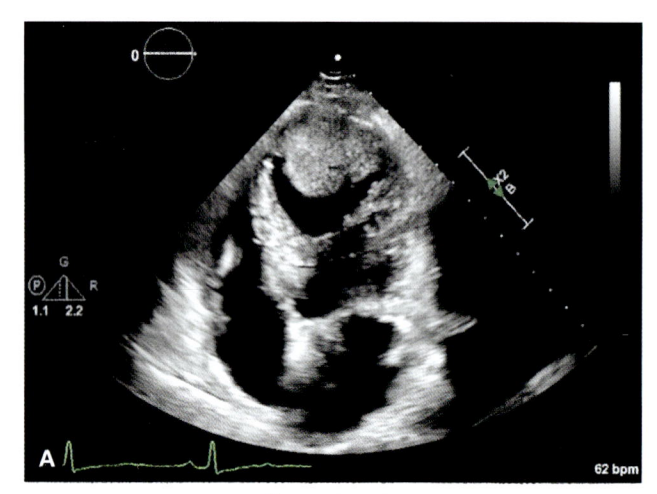

Figure 31.10A

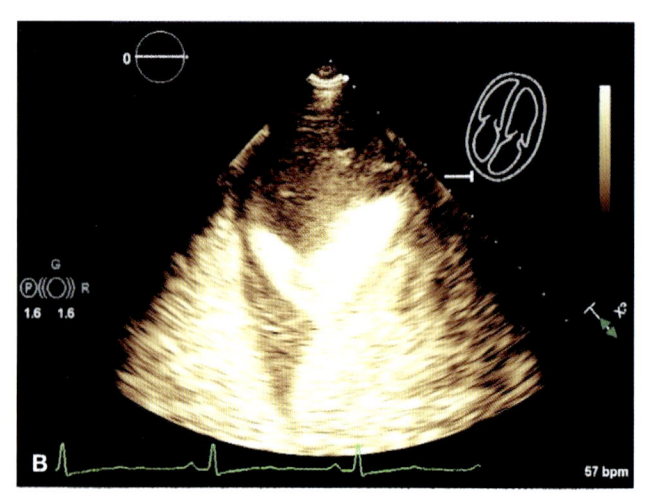

Figure 31.10B

27. A 16-year-old boy was diagnosed with a single rhabdomyoma during his first year of life. He is asymptomatic. ▶ **Video 31.6** is taken from his most recent transthoracic echocardiogram. Which of the following conclusions is **TRUE** about this patient's condition?
   A. The presence of a rhabdomyoma cannot be diagnosed before birth with fetal echocardiography.
   B. The ventricular wall is a typical location for rhabdomyomas.
   C. This patient should be referred to a cardiothoracic surgeon for the removal of rhabdomyoma.
   D. This patient meets diagnostic criteria for tuberous sclerosis.
   E. None of the above.

28. A 62-year-old woman with a history of end-stage interstitial lung disease who underwent bilateral orthotopic lung transplantation (BOLT) 2 weeks ago presents with shortness of breath for 2 days. She is hypotensive requiring vasopressors. Her echocardiogram 1 week ago was normal. **Figure 31.11,** ▶ **Video 31.7A, Video 31.7B,** and **Video 31.7C** are taken from her bedside transthoracic echocardiogram in the emergency room. It shows a mass lesion in the mediastinum compressing the right ventricle and the inferior vena cava is dilated. Her mitral inflow PW Doppler interrogation show >25% decrease in E wave with inspiration. Her Computed Tomography (CT) chest imaging is scheduled. Which of the following statements accurately characterizes the most likely reason for shock state in this patient based on the echocardiographic findings?
   A. Right ventricular failure related to pulmonary embolism.
   B. New diagnosis of lymphoma.
   C. Anterior mediastinal hematoma.
   D. Cystic tumor.
   E. None of the above.

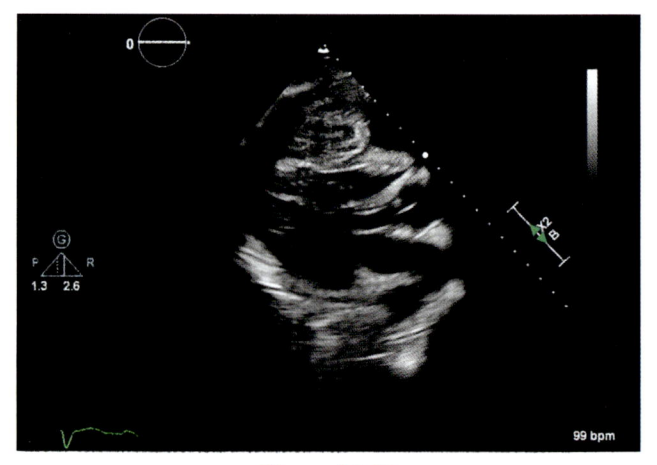

Figure 31.11

29. A 73-year-old man presents with right middle cerebral artery (MCA) stroke. He is undergoing mechanical thrombectomy with resolution of his neurological symptoms. He has no history of atrial fibrillation and his work up did not detect occult atrial fibrillation. **Figure 31.12**, and ▶ **Video 31.8** are taken from his most transesophageal echocardiogram looking at the thoracic aorta. Which of the following conclusions is **TRUE** about this patient's condition?
   A. Aortic atherosclerotic plaques are not an important potential source of emboli.
   B. The risk of embolism with aortic plaque is higher when the thickness >4 mm.
   C. Aortic plaque ulceration is not a high risk finding for thromboembolic events.
   D. The presence of mobile component on aortic plaques is not associated with higher risk of embolic events.

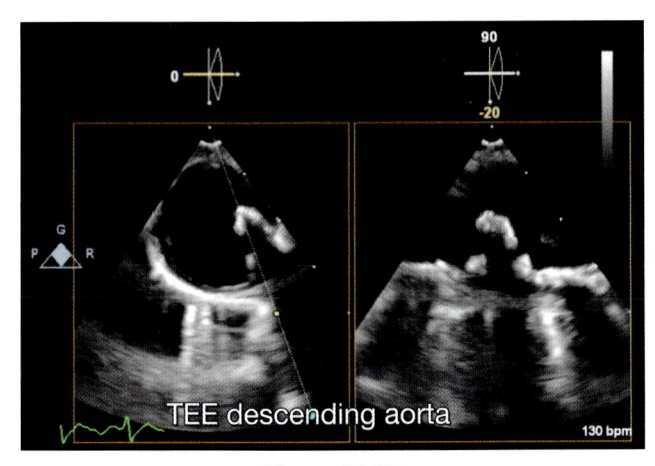

Figure 31.12

CASE 1

A 55-year-old man with diabetes mellitus and hypertension is undergoing an evaluation for exertional dyspnea. An exercise echocardiogram is ordered. The baseline transthoracic echocardiogram is reported to reveal an intracardiac mass. The exercise portion of the examination is not completed and the patient is referred for a transesophageal echocardiogram. ▶ *Video 31.9 shows a zoomed-in view of the left atrium at zero degree.* **Figure 31.13** *demonstrates the mass using real-time three-dimensional imaging.*

30. In regard to the patient in **Case 1** and ▶ **Video 31.9**, which of the following statements is **CORRECT**?
   A. The size of the mass makes it most likely to be a metastatic tumor to the heart rather than a primary cardiac tumor.
   B. The left atrial location of this tumor and its attachment to the midportion of the atrial septum make it most likely a myxoma.
   C. This tumor may be found as part of a multisystem disease called tuberous sclerosis complex.
   D. This tumor type accounts for approximately 10% of all primary cardiac tumors.
   E. This tumor is characterized by infiltration of the atrial septum by lipomatous material.

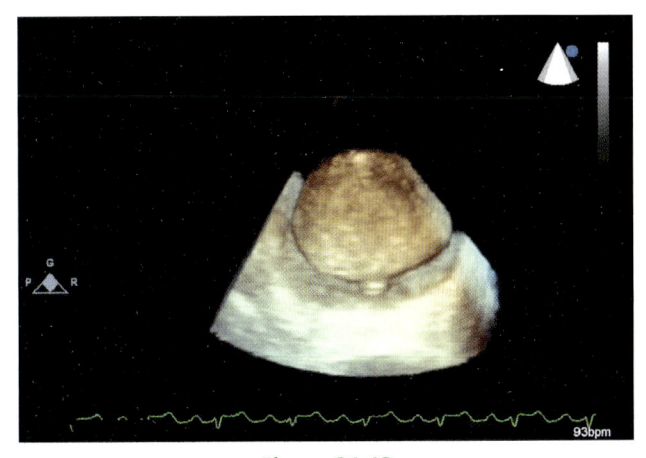

Figure 31.13

31. Which statement accurately describes the tumor shown in the echocardiogram from **Case 1**?
   A. It is typically recommended to surgically excise this tumor even if the patient is asymptomatic.
   B. This mass always prolapses through the mitral orifice in diastole.
   C. This tumor most commonly presents in the elderly (greater than 65 years of age).
   D. A pericardial effusion is often associated with this tumor.
   E. This patient would be expected to have severely reduced left ventricular systolic function.

CASE 2

A 66-year-old man presented with a transient ischemic attack. A transthoracic echocardiogram was performed. ▶ *Video 31.10A shows the parasternal long-axis view.* ▶ *Video 31.10B shows the long-axis view at 129° on the transesophageal echocardiogram. A diagnosis of papillary fibroelastoma is made.*

660 / Clinical Echocardiography Review

32. For the patient in **Case 2**, which of the following statements about papillary fibroelastomas is **CORRECT**?
   A. Papillary fibroelastomas are usually easily distinguishable from vegetations.
   B. Papillary fibroelastomas are typically associated with significant valvular regurgitation.
   C. Papillary fibroelastomas usually attach to the upstream side of the valve.
   D. Papillary fibroelastomas account for the majority of valve-associated tumors.
   E. The major risk associated with papillary fibroelastomas is cardiac tamponade.

33. Which of the following statements about the treatment of papillary fibroelastomas is **CORRECT**?
   A. After surgical resection, patients should be monitored closely with surveillance echocardiography performed every year, since the recurrence of papillary fibroelastomas is a common phenomenon.
   B. Tumor mobility does not impact the treatment decision for papillary fibroelastomas.
   C. Asymptomatic patients with immobile, small (<0.5 cm) papillary fibroelastomas should have surgical resection performed immediately.
   D. There is no role for anticoagulation in patients with symptomatic papillary fibroelastoma who are not surgical candidates.
   E. Symptomatic patients should be treated surgically because a successful and complete resection of papillary fibroelastomas is curative and the long-term postoperative prognosis is excellent.

34. Which statement accurately describes papillary fibroelastomas?
   A. Papillary fibroelastomas are the most common primary cardiac tumor in adults.
   B. The most commonly involved valve is the aortic valve, followed by the mitral valve.
   C. Papillary fibroelastomas are generally not visible by transthoracic echocardiography if they are less than 1 cm.
   D. The right ventricle is the predominant nonvalvular site involved.
   E. Multiple papillary fibroelastomas have been reported to be present in 50% of patients.

CASE 3

A 71-year-old woman presented with fatigue and dyspnea in the setting of diarrhea and flushing for 5 months. ▶ Video 31.11A shows the tricuspid valve in the right ventricular inflow view. ▶ Video 31.11B is the same view with the addition of color flow imaging.

35. For the patient in **Case 3,** which of the following statements about carcinoid heart disease is **CORRECT**?
   A. Carcinoid affecting the tricuspid valve frequently results in tricuspid stenosis as the dominant lesion.
   B. Involvement of the left-sided valves usually occurs without a patent foramen ovale or high tumor activity.
   C. The valve pathology of carcinoid involves fibrosis, smooth muscle proliferation, and endocardial thickening, which give the echocardiographic appearance of a thickened, retracted, and immobile valve.
   D. Treatment of carcinoid heart disease usually provides a cure with modern antitumor therapy and surgical intervention.
   E. Carcinoid heart disease typically causes severe symptoms shortly after the onset of the disease.

36. Which statement accurately describes carcinoid heart disease?
   A. Patients with carcinoid syndrome can have right-sided cardiac metastases without the involvement of the liver.
   B. If valve replacement surgery is indicated and feasible, a mechanical prosthetic valve is always the preferred choice.
   C. On echocardiographic evaluation, right ventricular size in patients with carcinoid heart disease is usually normal.
   D. Octreotide can be safely discontinued during the perioperative period.
   E. If there is pulmonic valve involvement, a continuous-wave Doppler signal through the pulmonary valve is an important part of the echocardiographic evaluation.

CASE 4

A 30-year-old woman was diagnosed with malignant melanoma and underwent complete surgical excision with adequate margins. Given the depth of the melanoma, it was considered high risk and the patient was treated with adjuvant high-dose interferon. Two months later, the patient developed shortness of breath. ▶ **Video 31.12A** *shows a right ventricular inflow view and* ▶ **Video 31.12B** *shows the apical view of the mass seen on transthoracic echocardiogram.*

37. Based on the patient from **Case 4,** which of the following is **TRUE** about metastatic melanoma?
    A. It is uncommon for melanoma to metastasize to the heart.
    B. There is no role for surgery in patients with metastatic melanoma to palliate symptoms or prevent death from cardiac complications.
    C. The history of primary melanoma can be remote, occurring years prior to the discovery of the cardiac mass in some cases.
    D. Melanoma has a high propensity for metastasizing to the myocardium but not the pericardium.
    E. None of the above

38. Which statement accurately describes metastatic melanoma?
    A. "Charcoal" heart is the most common cardiac extension of melanoma.
    B. Melanoma accounts for the majority of metastatic cardiac tumors.
    C. The development of dyspnea in a patient with a history of melanoma is not a concerning symptom.
    D. The incidence of metastatic tumors to the heart has decreased during the last 2 decades.
    E. None of the above.

CASE 5

A 73-year-old woman with a history of hypertension presents for further evaluation of palpitations. This symptom has been present for 1 week and is persisting. An ECG is performed which demonstrates atrial fibrillation with a ventricular rate of 120 beats/min. She starts treatment with metoprolol and rivaroxaban. She agrees to proceed with a treatment strategy that includes direct current cardioversion. Two days later she returns for a transesophageal echocardiogram prior to the cardioversion. ▶ **Video 31.13** *is taken from the transesophageal echocardiogram.*

39. Which of the following statements relating to **Case 5** and ▶ **Video 31.13** is **CORRECT**?
    A. This video shows a thrombus in the right atrial appendage.
    B. It is estimated that intracardiac sources of embolism account for 2% to 5% of the strokes that occur each year in the United States.
    C. This patient should proceed with direct current cardioversion after the transesophageal echocardiogram as it is scheduled.
    D. The sensitivity and specificity of transesophageal echocardiography for detection of left atrial/left atrial appendage thrombi is much higher than transthoracic echocardiography around 100% and 99% respectively.
    E. Spontaneous echo contrast or "smoke" is not commonly seen in echocardiograms where a left atrial appendage thrombus is detected.

40. Which of the following statements accurately characterizes the left atrium/left atrial appendage?
    A. Volume estimates are preferred for evaluating the size of the left atrium.
    B. The left atrium cannot dilate under normal physiological conditions.
    C. Atrial thrombi are frequently detected in the left atrium/left atrial appendage in the setting of sinus rhythm.
    D. The left atrial appendage is typically a blunt and shallow structure.
    E. There is no evidence to suggest that left atrial appendage flow velocity predicts the likelihood of maintaining sinus rhythm after cardioversion.

ANSWERS

1. **Answer: E.** There are many normal variants and benign conditions that can be misinterpreted on two-dimensional echocardiography as pathologic entities. A suture line following transplant is an example of a structure found in the left atrium that can be misinterpreted as a mass. The eustachian valve, crista terminalis, and Chiari network are all normal structures found in the right atrium. The moderator band is a normal structure present in the right ventricle.

2. **Answer: D.** Complete TTE is recommended in all patients suspected of having cardiac tumors. It is needed to evaluate location, size, mobility, and appearance as well as determining hemodynamic consequences. Echocardiography is recommended in patients with masses in several situations and are summarized in **Table 31.1**.

3. **Answer: B.** Rhabdomyoma is a benign cardiac tumor. Rhabdomyomas are usually small and lobulated with diameters in the range of 2 mm to 2 cm. Rhabdomyomas are most often multiple and are strongly associated with tuberous sclerosis. Angiosarcoma, lymphoma, and mesothelioma are all malignant cardiac tumors. Prominent ventricular trabeculations can also be seen on echocardiography and represent either a normal variant or if severe enough, may indicate noncompaction.

4. **Answer: C.** It is uncommon for thyroid cancer to metastasize to the heart. Renal cell carcinoma, breast cancer, lung cancer, and melanoma all are known to metastasize to the heart. **Table 31.2** lists the primary cancers that metastasize to the heart. Renal cell carcinoma spreads hematogenously to the inferior vena cava and right side of the heart. Breast cancer spreads to the heart by either hematogenous or lymphatic means. Lung cancer usually metastasizes to the heart via direct extension. Lymphoma spreads through the lymphatic system. Metastatic melanoma can result in intracavitary or myocardial involvement.

5. **Answer: D.** Cardiac tumors may cause symptoms through a variety of mechanisms. Embolization is one mechanism, which is usually in the systemic circulation but can also occur in the pulmonic circulation. Aortic valve and left atrial tumors are associated with the greatest risk of embolization. Other mechanisms of symptom production include obstruction, interference with valves causing regurgitation, direct invasion of the myocardium and/or conduction system (leading to impaired contractility, arrhythmias, heart block, or pericardial effusion), and constitutional or systemic symptoms. Primary cardiac tumors are rare. Incidence has been estimated to be at <1% (closer to 0.1%) based on autopsy studies. Cardiac tumors may be symptomatic or found incidentally during evaluation for an unrelated problem or physical findings. Echocardiography is the simplest technique for evaluating a cardiac tumor, although at times a cardiac MRI or CT scan may be needed to provide more detailed information.

6. **Answer: A.** Lipomatous hypertrophy of the atrial septum does not commonly cause symptoms. This condition is thought to be benign, although there is a reported association with atrial arrhythmias and superior vena cava obstruction if there is massive lipomatous hypertrophy. The atrial septum is infiltrated by lipomatous material that results in the thickening of the inferior and superior portions. The fossa ovalis is spared and results in a "dumbbell-shaped" appearance on two-dimensional

Table 31.1. Echocardiography Indications for Mass Evaluation

Echocardiography is recommended	• Complete transthoracic echocardiography is recommended in all patients suspected of having cardiac tumors. • For surveillance after surgical removal of masses known to have high recurrence rates (eg, myxomas). • Evaluating patients with clinical syndromes suggesting an underlying cardiac mass • Transesophageal echocardiography is possibly superior to transthoracic echocardiography evaluating cardiac tumor such as papillary fibroelastoma or myxoma. • Transesophageal echocardiography can be useful in the evaluation of infective endocarditis if it was on the differential diagnosis of mass. • Assessing patients with known primary malignancies where surveillance for cardiac involvement is part of the disease staging process.
Echocardiography is probably useful	• Using ultrasound-enhancing agents may help differentiate vascular tumors from thrombi or vegetations. • 3D echocardiography might improve diagnostic accuracy
Echocardiography is not recommended	• Evaluating patients where treatment plans will not be changed based on the results of echocardiography.

Table 31.2. Tumors That Metastasize to the Heart

Primary Cancer	Route of Spread and/or Cardiac Manifestation
Renal cell carcinoma	Inferior vena cava to the right side of the heart
Breast	Hematogenous or lymphatic spread; pericardial effusion common
Lung	Direct extension; pericardial effusion common
Melanoma	Intracavitary or myocardial involvement
Lymphoma	Lymphatic spread
Carcinoid	Tricuspid and pulmonic valve thickening

Adapted with permission from Armstrong WF, Ryan T, eds. *Feigenbaum's Echocardiography*. 7th ed. Philadelphia, PA: Lippincott Williams & Wilkins, 2010.

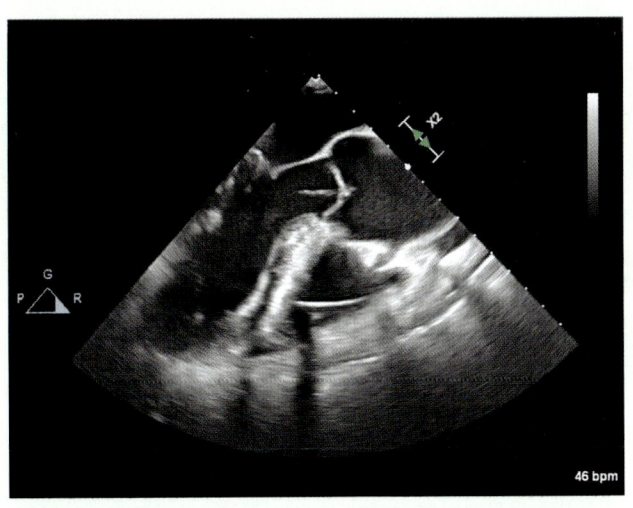

Figure 31.14. Transesophageal echocardiographic long-axis view showing Lambl excrescence attached to the aortic valve ventricular side.

echocardiography. Lipomatous hypertrophy of the atrial septum is usually distinguishable by the highly refractile echogenic quality of fat. Although no absolute diagnostic criteria have been established, a septal thickness of 20 mm is often quoted. Lipomatous hypertrophy of the atrial septum represents a hamartoma. Pathologically, in contrast to true lipomas, lipomatous hypertrophy consists of a nonencapsulated accumulation of mature and fetal adipose tissue and atypical cardiac myocytes within the interatrial septum. The term hypertrophy is a misnomer since the condition is due to an increased number rather than an increased size of adipocytes. This condition can be seen on transthoracic echocardiography and its presence alone is not an indication for transesophageal echocardiography.

7. **Answer: B.** Although some data are conflicting, in general, larger vegetation size on transesophageal echocardiography appears to be predictive of embolic risk. Patients with a vegetation diameter above 10 mm have been shown to have a significantly higher incidence of embolic events than those with smaller vegetations. This association has been shown to be strongest in patients with mitral valve endocarditis. The sensitivity and specificity of transesophageal echocardiography for detecting vegetations is 92% and 96%, respectively. False-positive findings on transesophageal echocardiograms may occur due to small irregularities and degenerative processes. For example, mobile strands are frequently encountered on valves that probably represent a normal degenerative process; these strands are known as Lambl excrescences (**Figure 31.14**). Valvular vegetations are usually on the "upstream" side of the valve and characteristically prolapse into the upstream chamber (ie, mitral vegetations into the atrium in systole and aortic vegetations in the left ventricular outflow tract during diastole). Echocardiography has been used to determine the natural history of vegetations. An increase in size suggests active disease. Pretest expectations for endocarditis should lead to an expanded scrutiny of the valves with extra images. However, as sensitivity rises, specificity may be reduced, and this must also be taken into consideration.

8. **Answer: E.** The timing of the appearance of agitated saline contrast (bubbles) in the left heart on echocardiography can help distinguish intracardiac shunting (via patent foramen ovale or atrial septal defect) from pulmonary arteriovenous shunting. Early contrast appearance in the left heart (within 3 to 6 beats of contrast appearance in the right heart) suggests intracardiac shunting, while late shunting (after 3 to 6 beats) is more consistent with pulmonary arteriovenous shunting. However, exceptions to this timing construct do occur; and ideally, it will be good to visualize the anatomy and location of the bubbles crossing to the left side of the heart (eg, pulmonic veins or interatrial septum) if feasible. Patent foramen ovale is a congenital cardiac lesion that frequently persists into adulthood. Patent foramen ovale has been found to be present in 25% to 30% of individuals in autopsy studies. The prevalence and size of patent foramen ovale is similar in females and males. Most individuals with patent foramen ovale are asymptomatic. An incidentally detected patent foramen ovale generally requires no follow-up or treatment. If a patent foramen ovale is deemed likely to be causally related to an embolic event, therapeutic options for secondary stroke or other embolic event prevention are controversial and include medical therapy with antiplatelet agents or anticoagulation, and surgical or percutaneous closure of the defect in certain

9. **Answer: D.** The diagnostic criteria for the Carney complex include having 2 of 12 recognized clinical manifestations or one clinical manifestation plus one of the two genetic criteria (**Table 31.3**). Cardiac myxoma is a diagnostic clinical criterion for the Carney complex. The other clinical manifestations relate to either pigmented skin lesions or endocrine neoplasia. Familial myxomas, such as those seen in the Carney complex, account for a small percentage of all myxomas. Patients with familial myxomas tend to present earlier, are more likely to have myxomas in atypical locations, may have multiple myxomas, and are more likely to develop recurrent tumors. Epilepsy is associated with tuberous sclerosis. Nevoid basal cell carcinoma is associated with cardiac fibroma in the Gorlin syndrome.

10. **Answer: C.** Myxomas present with symptoms resulting from intracardiac obstruction, systemic embolization, or constitutional symptoms. Dyspnea is the most common symptom. Syncope and palpitations are also seen. Constitutional symptoms, such as fever and weight loss, are seen in approximately 15% to 20% of patients. The association of constitutional symptoms with cardiac myxoma is likely due to the tumor's synthesis and secretion of interleukin (IL)-6. IL-6 is a proinflammatory cytokine that induces the acute phase response. Increased levels of IL-6 have been found in the myxoma tissue and the constitutional symptoms resolve after the removal of the myxoma. Diarrhea is seen in the carcinoid syndrome.

11. **Answer: A.** Histologic evidence suggests that cardiac rhabdomyomas are actually myocardial hamartomas or malformations that are composed of myocytes rather than true neoplasms. The microscopic hallmark is a large (<80 μm diameter) cell containing a central cytoplasmic mass that is suspended by myofibrillar processes, termed the spider cell. Tuberous sclerosis is an autosomal-dominant hamartoma syndrome whose causative genes (TSC-1 and TSC-2) are tumor suppressor genes that encode a protein complex that regulates cell size. At least 80% of patients with cardiac rhabdomyomas have tuberous sclerosis. Fifty percent or more of cardiac rhabdomyomas regress spontaneously after infancy. Therefore, in the absence of symptoms, surgery is not indicated.

12. **Answer: B.** More than 90% of papillary fibroelastomas are single. Papillary fibroelastomas can occur on any valve. The aortic and mitral valves are most commonly involved in adults. Despite their valvular attachment, valve dysfunction is rare. Much less commonly, papillary fibroelastomas can occur on papillary muscle, chordae tendineae, or in the atria. The median diameter of papillary fibroelastomas is 8 mm and the largest reported is 40 mm. A short pedicle is seen approximately 50% of the time.

13. **Answer: C.** Primary malignant tumors of the heart are much less common than metastatic tumors of the heart. Incidence rate of primary tumors is very low. It is estimated to be 1.38 of 100,000 person per year. The relative incidence of primary tumors of the heart (both benign and malignant) is shown in **Table 31.4**.

14. **Answer: B.** Cardiac myxomas typically have a narrow stalk connected to the fossa ovalis. Approximately 75% of cardiac myxomas occur in the left atrium, where the site of attachment is almost always in the region of the fossa ovalis of the interatrial septum. Cardiac myxomas may occasionally be found on the posterior wall of the left atrium. However, this location within the left atrium should raise the suspicion for a malignant cardiac tumor. Approximately 15% to 20% of cardiac myxomas occur in the right atrium and less often they can be seen in the right or left ventricle. There are case reports of myxomas originating from the atrioventricular valves. Pericardial effusions are usually found in the setting of malignant cardiac tumors. Lipomas appear as an

Table 31.3. Carney Complex Diagnostic Criteria

Clinical Criteria

1. Spotty skin pigmentation involving lips, conjunctiva, and genital mucosa
2. Myxoma (cutaneous and mucosal)
3. Cardiac myxoma
4. Breast myxomatosis
5. Primary pigmented nodular adrenocortical disease
6. Acromegaly
7. Sertoli cell tumor (or characteristic calcification on testicular ultrasound)
8. Thyroid carcinoma
9. Psammomatous melanotic schwannoma
10. Multiple epithelioid blue nevi
11. Multiple breast ductal adenoma
12. Osteochondromyxoma

Genetic Criteria

1. Affected first-degree relative
2. Inactivating mutation of PRKAR1 alpha gene

Adapted from Stratakis CA, Kirschner LS, Carney JA. Clinical and molecular features of the Carney complex: diagnostic criteria and recommendations for patient evaluation. *J Clin Endocrinol Metab*. 2001;86:4041-4046. Reproduced by permission of The Endocrine Society.

Table 31.4. Relative Incidence of Primary Cardiac Tumors

Type of Tumor	Percent
BENIGN	~90%
Myxoma	45%
Lipoma	20%
Papillary fibroelastoma	15%
Other benign (eg, angioma, hemangioma, rhabdomyoma, fibroma)	20%
MALIGNANT (eg, angiosarcoma, mesothelioma, rhabdomyosarcoma)	~10%

Data from Tyebally S, Chen D, Bhattacharyya S, et al. Cardiac tumors: JACC CardioOncology state-of-the-art review. *JACC CardioOncol*. 2020;2(2):293-311.

intramural hyperechoic mass. A mobile mass with a short pedicle attached to a cardiac valve is a papillary fibroelastoma.

15. **Answer: B.** Kaposi sarcoma, as well as malignant lymphoma, is recognized to occur in the setting of AIDS. Cardiac involvement with Kaposi sarcoma usually occurs as part of a disseminated Kaposi sarcoma. The incidence of Kaposi sarcoma involving the heart has been estimated to be 12% to 28% according to autopsy studies.

16. **Answer: C.** To differentiate a thrombus from an intracardiac tumor, real time very low MI perfusion imaging with high-MI flash should be used. Thrombi are avascular and show no contrast enhancement after a high-MI flash impulse, as opposed to tumors, which may be either poorly (benign stromal tumors, such as myxoma or papillary fibroelastoma) or highly (malignant tumors) vascularized and will demonstrate proportional degrees of perfusion by flash replenishment using optimal enhancement software.

17. **Answer: D.** Leiomyosarcomas are derived from smooth muscle cells and may originate from the smooth muscle cells lining the pulmonary veins. Although chemotherapy and radiation are part of the treatment plan, they are adjuncts to radical surgical resection. However, cardiac leiomyosarcomas have a poor prognosis, with a mean survival after surgery of less than 7 months. The majority of malignant tumors occur preferentially in the right side of the heart, with the exception of leiomyosarcoma, which often occurs in the left atrium. The preferential left atrial location and the frequently myxoid appearance of leiomyosarcomas makes them difficult to differentiate preoperatively from atrial myxomas. Unlike myxomas, leiomyosarcomas may originate from the posterior wall of the left atrium and involve the pulmonary veins. Patients with leiomyosarcoma typically present in their 30s, a decade younger than with other types of sarcomas.

18. **Answer: D.** This mass appears to be embedded within the LV intramural layers of the inferolateral and inferior LV walls. This mass is possibly an intramural tumor such as a fibroma or rhabdomyoma. On the echocardiogram, a fibroma usually appears as a distinct, well-demarcated, noncontractile and solid, highly echogenic mass within the myocardium. The most common locations for fibromas are the LV lateral wall and right ventricular free wall or the interventricular septum. A rhabdomyoma can occur within a cavity as a pedunculated mass or may be embedded within the myocardium. These tumors usually involve the LV free wall and are associated with ventricular arrhythmias. On echocardiography, rhabdomyomas appear as well circumscribed, homogeneous masses with acoustic properties similar to the myocardium. The distinction between fibromas and rhabdomyomas can be made via computed tomography and/or cardiac magnetic resonance imaging.

    Answer A is not correct since the mass clearly appears to be located within the LV myocardium and not outside the heart. Answer B is incorrect as this mass does not protrude into the LV cavity. Answer C is unlikely as there is no history of previous cardiac disease and the LV size and function are normal.

19. **Answer: A.** Angiosarcomas usually are large or have metastasized at the time of diagnosis. Angiosarcomas often are not amenable to complete resection and have a very poor prognosis, even compared to the other cardiac sarcomas. Unlike other sarcomas, which have a 1:1, gender ratio, there appears to be a 3:1 male-to-female ratio among patients with angiosarcoma. Angiosarcomas have a strong predilection for the right heart, particularly the right atrium. They can be either intracavitary or diffuse and infiltrative. The common presentation is right-sided heart failure or cardiac tamponade as well as constitutional symptoms.

20. **Answer: D.** Some patients with renal cell carcinoma may present with symptoms related to cardiac metastases. The diagnosis of renal cell carcinoma may be first recognized by echocardiogram. Intravascular extension of tumors is a common manifestation of renal cell carcinoma. Since vena cava and right heart involvement is known to occur with metastatic renal cell carcinoma, pulmonary embolism, either from the tumor or thrombus, can be seen. The appearance of metastatic renal cell carcinoma itself can be confused with thrombus on echocardiography and sometimes cardiac magnetic resonance imaging is helpful to distinguish these entities.

21. **Answer: A.** Synovial sarcoma is caused by a translocation between chromosome 18 and the X chromosome. Synovial sarcoma is one of the malignant primary cardiac sarcomas. Synovial sarcoma is an extremely rare cardiac tumor. Like most cardiac sarcomas, the prognosis of synovial sarcoma is poor.

22. **Answer: B.** The use of myocardial contrast echocardiography to identify intracardiac tumors based on masses with vascularization has been described for both transthoracic echocardiography and transesophageal echocardiography. The mass shown in **Figure 31.6** does not opacify with the administration of perflutren lipid microspheres. This lack of uptake indicates a lack of vascularity. Benign tumors, such as a myxoma or papillary fibroelastoma, typically have partial enhancement. The differential diagnosis will include cyst, vegetation, and thrombus and clinical correlation is usually needed. Given further workup with cardiac MRI and PET scan, it was deemed to be an avascular metabolically inactive structure that has decreased in size on the serial MRI with empiric anticoagulation being consistent with most likely a thrombus.

23. **Answer: C.** The Chiari network is a congenital remnant of the right valve of the sinus venosus. It consists of a network of fibers in the right atrium that originates from the region of the eustachian valve at the orifice of the inferior vena cava with attachments to the upper wall of the right atrium or atrial septum. Chiari networks are present in 2% to 3% of normal hearts. Chiari networks are usually not clinically significant although their role in cryptogenic stroke, in association with a patent foramen ovale or atrial septal aneurysm, is controversial.

24. **Answer: A.** The diagnosis of pericardial cyst can sometimes be suggested on chest radiograph by the identification of a rounded mass along the right heart border. Echocardiography or chest computed tomography is recommended to follow up this finding to better establish the diagnosis. Primary cysts of the mediastinum account for approximately 20% of all mediastinal lesions. This group includes pericardial cysts, bronchogenic cysts, enteric cysts, thymic cysts, and thoracic duct cysts. Cysts are not considered to be true neoplasms. Cysts lack malignant potential, although the examination of tissue either by open, thoracoscopic, or percutaneous means may be necessary to definitively exclude a neoplasm. However, conservative management of asymptomatic patients in whom noninvasive imaging is strongly suggestive of a pericardial cyst is a common approach. It is rare for pericardial cysts to become large enough to cause compressive symptoms and hemodynamic alterations.

25. **Answer: B.** In a series of multicenter studies in North and South America, only 46 of 72 (64%) surgical left atrial appendage exclusion had complete closure. Successful left atrial appendage closure occurred more often with excision than suture exclusion and stapler exclusion. Recent data shows efficacy rates of epicardial left atrial appendage closure of >90%. This clinical vignette highlights the importance of clinical correlation when interpreting echocardiographic images. In this case, the echodensity most likely represents suture material given the patient's history. Transesophageal echocardiography is an excellent method for assessing the success of left atrial appendage closure procedures. Evidence suggests that the residual communication between an incompletely closed left atrial appendage and the body of the left atrium is a potential mechanism for thrombus formation and embolic events.

26. **Answer: C.** The development of a left ventricular thrombus is one of the more common complications of myocardial infarction. Thrombi are important clinically because they can lead to embolic complications. The likelihood of developing a left ventricular thrombus after an acute myocardial infarction varies with infarct location and size. Left ventricular thrombus is most often seen in patients with large anterior ST elevation infarctions with aneurysm formation and akinesis or dyskinesis. Transthoracic echocardiography has been the standard procedure for the diagnosis of left ventricular thrombus after acute myocardial infarction. Echocardiography can help identify those patients at high risk of thromboembolism. The two major echocardiographic risk factors for clinical thromboembolism are mobile thrombi and protruding thrombi. Echocardiography can also be used to monitor the resolution of thrombus with anticoagulation. In patients with suboptimal acoustic windows or prominent trabeculations, the use of an ultrasound-enhancing agent to opacify the left ventricular apex can sometimes be used to improve the sensitivity and specificity of thrombus detection. Alternatively, cardiac magnetic resonance imaging could be performed.

27. **Answer: B.** Rhabdomyomas are usually found in the ventricular walls or in the right or left, atrial or ventricular cavities. The presence of a rhabdomyoma can be diagnosed before birth with fetal echocardiography. There is no evidence that these tumors undergo malignant transformation and no treatment is required for asymptomatic tumors. Although 80% to 90% of rhabdomyomas are associated with tuberous sclerosis, cardiac rhabdomyomas can occur as an isolated finding as it has in this case.

28. **Answer: C.** Mediastinal masses can include benign or malignant etiologies. The differential diagnosis for anterior mediastinal tumor includes thymic mass, lymphoma, germ cell tumor, thyroid tissue or hematoma related to trauma or thoracic surgery. It could be found incidentally on imaging or part of symptoms evaluation. Therefore, it is

very important to follow a systematic approach to reading echocardiograms to include extracardiac structures. They can have direct involvement or compression of mediastinal structures. They can compress the great vessels and right ventricle (as seen in this case) leading to hemodynamic compromise. This is related to obstructive shock and cardiac tamponade physiology. Prompt recognition is key and CT imaging provides more detailed information regarding location, size, tissue characteristics and relationship to other structures. In cases of anterior mediastinal hematoma leading to hemodynamic effects, urgent surgical intervention and wash out is critical. In ▶ Video 31.14, the right ventricle is no longer compressed after the surgical removal of hematoma.

29. **Answer: B.** Aortic atherosclerosis is part of a systemic process, and it is common in patients with cardiovascular risk factors such as hypertension, hypercholesteremia, diabetes mellitus, and smoking. It is important to recognize that thoracic aortic atherosclerosis is an important cause of thromboembolic events (eg, stroke and limb ischemia). Aortic plaques are strongly associated with stroke even in the presence of atrial fibrillation. The risk of thromboembolic events is higher in patients with complex plaques that is defined as a marked increase in thickness >4 mm and/or ulcerated plaque with or without a mobile component (eg, thrombus).

30. **Answer: B.** The most common location for cardiac myxomas is the left atrium with the attachment site at the atrial septum. Size is not a reliable way to distinguish between primary cardiac tumors and metastases. Cardiac myxoma may be found as part of a multisystem disease called the Carney complex. Cardiac myxoma is the most common primary cardiac tumor accounting for near 40% of intracardiac tumors. Lipomatous hypertrophy is characterized by fatty infiltration of the atrial septum.

31. **Answer: A.** Once the likely diagnosis of cardiac myxoma is made based on echocardiography, resection is recommended because of the risk of embolization or cardiovascular complications. Perioperative mortality is reported to be low and postoperative recovery is generally uneventful. Left atrial cardiac myxomas that are large enough may prolapse through the mitral orifice during diastole resulting in obstruction. This can result in the classically described auscultatory finding of the tumor "plop." The mean age at presentation for cardiac myxomas is 50 years of age. Pericardial effusion is not commonly seen in the setting of cardiac myxoma. Cardiac myxomas are not specifically associated with impairment in left ventricular dysfunction.

> **KEY POINTS**
> - Cardiac myxomas are the most common primary cardiac tumors.
> - Cardiac myxomas usually occur in the left atrium, with the attachment site at the atrial septum.

32. **Answer: D.** Papillary fibroelastomas account for approximately 85% of valve-associated tumors. Papillary fibroelastomas are not easily distinguishable from vegetations. Papillary fibroelastomas are small, generally 0.5 to 2.0 cm in diameter (**Figure 31.15**) and are often confused with vegetations. The distinction between papillary fibroelastomas and vegetations can be difficult using echocardiography. Therefore, the correct diagnosis often depends on the clinical context. Although papillary fibroelastomas occur on valves, they usually do not result in significant valvular regurgitation. Papillary fibroelastomas most often attach to the arterial side of semilunar valves and the atrial surface of the atrioventricular valves. Symptoms of papillary fibroelastoma are usually caused by embolization, either of the tumor itself or an associated thrombus. The most common clinical presentation is cerebrovascular accident or transient ischemic attack.

33. **Answer: E.** Surgical resection is indicated for papillary fibroelastomas in patients who have had embolic events, complications that are directly related to tumor mobility (ie, coronary ostial occlusion), and those with highly mobile or large (>1 cm) tumors. The recurrence of papillary fibroelastomas after surgical resection has not been reported. Asymptomatic patients with immobile, small (<0.5 cm) papillary fibroelastomas could be followed up closely with periodic clinical evaluation

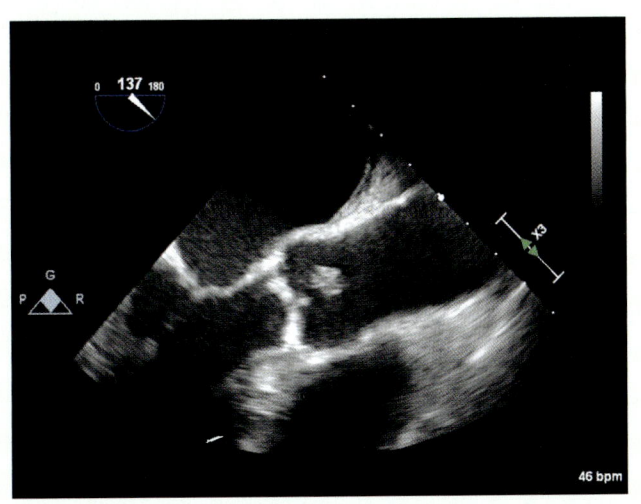

Figure 31.15. Transesophageal echocardiogram 137° showing fibroelastoma attached to aortic side of aortic valve.

and echocardiography. Surgical intervention should be considered when symptoms develop or the tumor becomes mobile, as tumor mobility is the independent predictor of nonfatal embolization. Symptomatic patients who are not surgical candidates could be offered long-term oral anticoagulation, although no randomized controlled data are available on its efficacy.

34. **Answer: B.** Papillary fibroelastomas most commonly involve the aortic valve followed by the mitral valve. Papillary fibroelastomas are the third most common primary cardiac tumors in adults, following cardiac myxomas and lipomas. Papillary fibroelastomas are generally not visible with transthoracic echocardiography if they are less than 0.2 cm. The left ventricle is the predominant nonvalvular site of involvement. Multiple papillary fibroelastomas have been reported to be present in 9% to 10% of patients.

KEY POINTS
- Papillary fibroelastomas account for approximately 85% of valve-associated tumors.
- Papillary fibroelastomas most often attach to the arterial side of semilunar valves and the atrial surface of the atrioventricular valves.
- The most common clinical manifestation of a papillary fibroelastoma is a cerebrovascular accident or transient ischemic attack.

35. **Answer: C.** The valve pathology of carcinoid involves fibrosis, smooth muscle proliferation, and endocardial thickening, which give the echocardiographic appearance of a thickened, retracted, and immobile valve. Appearances of the affected valve are pathognomonic for carcinoid in the absence of exposure to the appetite suppressants fenfluramine and phentermine, ergot-derived dopamine agonists, and ergot alkaloid agents such as methysergide and ergotamine. In carcinoid heart disease, the tricuspid valve becomes nearly fixed in a partially open position resulting in severe tricuspid regurgitation. A "dagger-shaped" continuous-wave Doppler profile results from severe tricuspid regurgitation, which causes early peak pressure and rapid decline, representing equalization of right atrial and ventricular pressures. Involvement of the left-sided valves occurs in less than 10% to 15% of cases and raises the likelihood of a concomitant patent foramen ovale, bronchial carcinoid, or high levels of circulating vasoactive substances. Left-sided valve disease is usually less severe than right-sided valvular lesions. Serotonin is thought to be inactivated as it passes through lung parenchyma. Although there has been significant progress in the treatment of carcinoid heart disease and many patients survive for years, cure is rarely achieved. Carcinoid heart disease is remarkably well-tolerated initially despite severe right-sided valve lesions. Eventually, dyspnea on exertion, lower extremity edema, and fatigue (signs and symptoms of right heart failure) develop.

36. **Answer: E.** If there is pulmonic valve involvement, a continuous-wave Doppler signal through the pulmonic valve typically shows increased systolic peak velocity consistent with stenosis and evidence of pulmonary insufficiency. There usually is rapid dampening of the regurgitant signal with late diastolic reversal of flow consistent with pulmonary stenosis and elevated right ventricular pressure. Only carcinoid patients with liver metastases develop the distinctive lesions of the right-sided heart valves. When the primary carcinoid tumor is of a pulmonary bronchus, the carcinoid valvular lesions may be limited to the left-sided valves. Initial reports favored the use of mechanical prosthesis given the concern for bioprosthetic valve degeneration in the setting of damage by vasoactive substances. However, improvements in medical therapy with somastatin analogs may be more protective for bioprosthetic valves. Additionally, these patients usually have multiple liver metastases and associated coagulopathies making bioprostheses more appealing. Mechanical prostheses may also be less than ideal since subsequent tumor resections are often required and may be complicated by the need for full anticoagulation. The choice of prosthesis should be tailored to the individual patient risk of bleeding, life expectancy, and future interventions. It is important to note that several series report high perioperative mortality, although the operative risk has declined from >20% in the 1980s to around 5% to 6% in more recent studies. Since the tricuspid valve (**Figure 29.16**), with or without pulmonary valve involvement, is affected in most cases of carcinoid heart disease, the right ventricle typically enlarges. As the right ventricle becomes volume-overloaded, paradoxical motion of the interventricular septum occurs. Right ventricular function seems to remain intact until later in the disease course. Carcinoid crisis characterized by hypotension, bronchospasm, and flushing can be precipitated by surgery. During the perioperative period, it may be difficult to make the distinction between carcinoid crisis and hypotension secondary to myocardial dysfunction. Perioperative octreotide, aimed at reducing serotonin release, is the most effective treatment for preventing carcinoid crisis during surgery. Intravenous octreotide (50-100 µg/h) should be started before surgery and the infusion should continue for 48 hours after surgery. Patients may require subcutaneous octreotide after this 48-hour period.

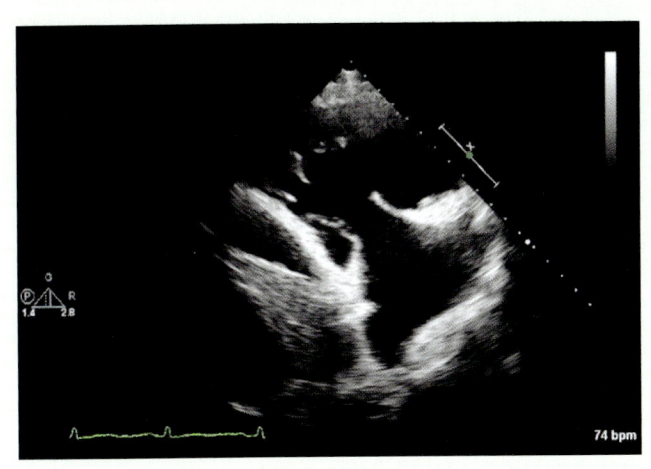

Figure 31.16

KEY POINTS
- Only carcinoid patients with liver metastases develop right-sided carcinoid heart disease.
- In carcinoid heart disease, the tricuspid valve becomes nearly fixed in a partially open position resulting in severe tricuspid regurgitation.
- Involvement of the left-sided valves occurs in less than 10% to 15% of cases and raises the likelihood of a concomitant patent foramen ovale, bronchial carcinoid, or high levels of circulating vasoactive substances.

37. **Answer: C.** Malignant melanoma can be diagnosed and initially treated years prior to the development and discovery of cardiac metastases. Metastatic melanoma involves the heart in more than 50% of cases. In select patients, there may be a role for surgery in patients with metastatic melanoma to palliate symptoms or prevent death from cardiac complications. Malignant melanoma may metastasize to the myocardium and/or pericardium.

38. **Answer: A.** "Charcoal" heart is the most common cardiac extension of melanoma. Although solid intracardiac metastasis from melanoma is well described and evident in this clinical vignette, most commonly cardiac extension of melanoma is subclinical and manifests as "charcoal" heart with tumor studding the pericardial surface. More common malignancies, such as breast and lung cancer, account for the greatest percentages of metastatic cardiac tumors. Even with a remote history of melanoma, there is concern for the subsequent development of cardiac metastasis and echocardiography should be performed for further evaluation. The incidence of metastatic tumors to the heart has increased over the last several decades due to advances in oncological treatment and improvement in cancer patient outcomes.

KEY POINT
- Malignant melanoma may metastasize to the myocardium and/or pericardium.

39. **Answer: D.** The sensitivity and specificity of transesophageal echocardiography for the detection of left atrial/left atrial appendage thrombi is both 95% to 100%. This was demonstrated in an intraoperative study where transesophageal echocardiography was compared with direct visualization of the left atrium/left atrial appendage at surgery. In comparison, conventional two-dimensional transthoracic echocardiography has a sensitivity of only 40% to 65% for left atrial thrombi due to poor visualization of the left atrial appendage. The left atrium, and specifically the left atrial appendage, is the most common location for atrial thrombus formation. Intracardiac sources of embolism may account for 15% to 20% of the 500,000 strokes that occur annually in the United States, in addition to other embolic issues such as organ infarction (eg, renal infarct or splenic infarct). Since there is a left atrial appendage thrombus seen on the transesophageal echocardiogram, the patient should not proceed with the direct current cardioversion. Spontaneous echo contrast or "smoke" is commonly seen within the left atrium/left atrial appendage among patients referred for the evaluation of a possible cardiac source of embolism. There is a strong association between left atrial spontaneous echo contrast and left atrial appendage thrombus as spontaneous echo contrast is seen in approximately 80% of cases.

40. **Answer: A.** Because of the irregular shape of the left atrium and the single and largely unrepresentative dimension represented by the M-mode image, volume estimates are preferred for evaluating the left atrium. These measurements require two-dimensional images, preferably two orthogonal apical planes. The volume estimations using an area–length algorithm as well as the biplane method of discs have been validated using angiography and contrast-enhanced cardiac computed tomography. Physiologic left atrial enlargement may occur in association with increased stroke volume. This can be seen with pregnancy and "athlete's heart." Atrial thrombi infrequently occur in the setting of sinus rhythm. In one series of over 20,000 transesophageal echocardiogram examinations, a left atrial thrombus during sinus rhythm was detected in 0.1% of the studies. The left atrial appendage is long and thin with a relatively narrow point of origin from the body of the left atrium. Thrombi have a predilection to form in the dysfunctional left atrial appendage

likely because of its shape and the presence of trabeculations. The evaluation of left atrial appendage morphology has become increasingly important with the development of percutaneous closure devices. A pulsed-wave Doppler sample, placed within the left atrial appendage, reveals a characteristic pattern that is dependent on the patient's underlying rhythm and atrial function. In patients with atrial fibrillation, studies have suggested that a left atrial appendage emptying velocity of >40 cm/s, measured precardioversion, was predictive of 1-year maintenance of sinus rhythm.

> **KEY POINT**
> - The sensitivity and specificity of transesophageal echocardiography for the detection of left atrial/left atrial appendage thrombi have been shown to both be 95% to 100%.

SUGGESTED READINGS

Armstrong WF, Ryan T, eds. *Feigenbaum's Echocardiography*. 8th ed. Lippincott Williams & Wilkins; 2019.

Aryana A, Singh SK, Singh SM, et al. Association between incomplete surgical ligation of left atrial appendage and stroke and systemic embolization. *Heart Rhythm*. 2015;12(7):1431-1437.

Bhattacharyya S, Davar J, Dreyfus G, Caplin ME. Carcinoid heart disease. *Circulation*. 2007;116(24):2860-2865.

Griborio-Guzman AG, Aseyev OI, Shah H, Sadreddini M. Cardiac myxomas: clinical presentation, diagnosis and management. *Heart*. 2022;108(11):827-833.

Kurfirst V, Mokracek A, Canádyová J, Frána R, Zeman P. Epicardial clip occlusion of the left atrial appendage during cardiac surgery provides optimal surgical results and long-term stability. *Interact Cardiovasc Thorac Surg*. 2017;25(1):37-40.

Ngyuen A, Schaff HV, Abel MD, et al. Improving outcomes of valve replacement for carcinoid heart disease. *J Thorac Cardiovasc Surg*. 2019;158(1):99-197.e2.

Oh JK, Kane GC, Seward JB, Jamil Tajik A. *The Echo Manual*. 4th ed. Lippincott Williams & Wilkins; 2019.

Peters PJ, Reinhardt S. The echocardiographic evaluation of intracardiac masses: a review. *J Am Soc Echocardiogr*. 2006;19(2):230-240.

Romero J, Husain SA, Kelesidis I, Sanz J, Medina HM, Garcia MJ. Detection of left atrial appendage thrombus by cardiac computed tomography in patients with atrial fibrillation: a meta-analysis. *Circ Cardiovasc Imaging*. 2013;6(2):185-194.

Saric M, Armour AC, Arnaout MS, et al. Guidelines for the use of echocardiography in the evaluation of a cardiac source of embolism. *J Am Soc Echocardiogr*. 2016;29(1):1-42.

Sun JP, Asher CR, Yang XS, et al. Clinical and echocardiographic characteristics of papillary fibroelastomas: a retrospective and prospective study in 162 patients. *Circulation*. 2001;103(22):2687-2693.

Tyebally S, Chen D, Bhattacharyya S, et al. Cardiac tumors: *JACC CardioOncology* state-of-the-art review. *JACC CardioOncol*. 2020;2(2):293-311.

CHAPTER 32

Noncyanotic Congenital Heart Disease

Benjamin W. Eidem

QUESTIONS

1. Which echocardiographic scan plane is most optimal to define a secundum atrial septal defect (ASD)?
   A. Suprasternal long-axis view.
   B. Parasternal long-axis view.
   C. Parasternal short-axis view.
   D. Subcostal 4-chamber view.
   E. Apical 4-chamber view.

2. Which of the following is the most common associated anatomic lesion found with a sinus venosus ASD?
   A. Anomalous right pulmonary venous connection.
   B. Inlet ventricular septal defect (VSD).
   C. Bicuspid aortic valve (AV).
   D. Persistent left superior vena cava.
   E. Coarctation of the aorta.

3. Which of the following associated congenital heart defects is most common in a patient with Down syndrome and an atrioventricular septal defect (AVSD)?
   A. Coarctation of the aorta.
   B. Total anomalous pulmonary venous connection.
   C. Aortic valve stenosis.
   D. Tetralogy of Fallot.
   E. Left ventricular (LV) hypoplasia.

4. Which of the following is the most common anatomic finding in a complete AVSD?
   A. Cleft in posterior leaflet of left atrioventricular valve.
   B. Medial rotation of LV papillary muscles.
   C. Ratio of LV inlet to outlet distance >1.0.
   D. Left ventricular outflow tract (LVOT) is "sprung" anteriorly.
   E. Left and right atrioventricular valve attachments are present at different levels.

5. The best echocardiographic view to delineate an outlet ventricular septal defect (VSD) is:
   A. Parasternal long-axis view.
   B. Apical 4-chamber view.
   C. Suprasternal long-axis view.
   D. Parasternal short-axis view.
   E. Apical 5-chamber view.

6. Which of the following is the most characteristic acquired lesion resulting from a subpulmonary (supracristal) VSD?
   A. Aortic insufficiency.
   B. LVOT obstruction.
   C. Right ventricular (RV) outflow tract obstruction.
   D. Pulmonary valve stenosis.
   E. Aortic valve stenosis.

7. Which of the following is the most characteristic physiologic effect of a large VSD?
   A. RV volume overload.
   B. Low pulmonary arterial pressure.
   C. Equal RV and LV pressure.
   D. Increased systemic blood flow.
   E. Decreased pulmonary blood flow.

8. The most common anatomic type of subaortic stenosis is:
   A. Tunnel type.
   B. Discrete membrane.
   C. Asymmetric septal hypertrophy.
   D. Systolic anterior motion of mitral valve.
   E. Anomalous mitral chordal insertion within the LVOT.

9. Which of the following congenital heart defects is demonstrated in **Figure 32.1** and ▶ **Videos 32.1A-C**.
   A. Partial AVSD.
   B. Sinus venosus atrial septal defect.
   C. Complete AVSD.
   D. Total anomalous pulmonary venous connection.
   E. Large inlet ventricular septal defect.

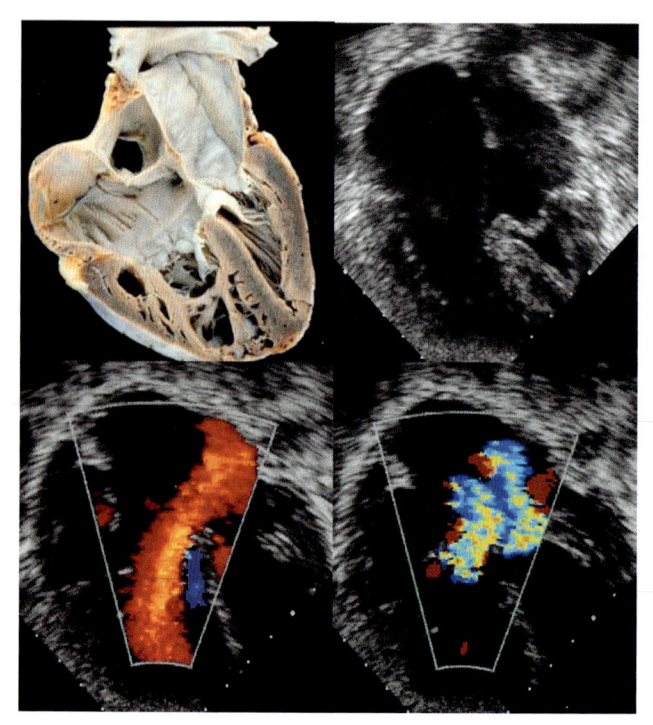

Figure 32.1

10. The most common associated cardiac abnormality in a patient with coarctation of the aorta is:
    A. Bicuspid aortic valve.
    B. VSD.
    C. ASD.
    D. Pulmonary valve stenosis.
    E. Coronary artery anomaly.

11. In patients with coarctation of the aorta, systemic arterial pressure begins to be significantly affected when the overall aortic lumen is narrowed by:
    A. 20%.
    B. 30%.
    C. 50%.
    D. 75%.
    E. 90%.

12. The most common type of VSD that is associated with coarctation of the aorta is:
    A. Apical muscular.
    B. Anterior malalignment.
    C. Perimembranous.
    D. Inlet.
    E. Subpulmonary (supracristal).

13. The Doppler phenomenon often seen in patients with supravalvar aortic stenosis has been demonstrated to be a high-velocity poststenotic jet that hugs the aortic wall and preferentially transfers kinetic energy into the right innominate artery. Which of the following best describes this Doppler finding?
    A. Coanda effect.
    B. Ohm's law.
    C. Continuity equation.
    D. Poiseuille's law.
    E. Bernoulli equation.

14. Interruption of the aortic arch is most common in which syndrome?
    A. DiGeorge.
    B. Down.
    C. Turner.
    D. Alagille.
    E. Holt–Oram.

15. A type A interruption of the aortic arch occurs:
   A. Between the right innominate and left common carotid arteries.
   B. Proximal to the right innominate artery.
   C. Between the left common carotid and left subclavian arteries.
   D. Distal to the left subclavian artery.
   E. Just distal to the sinotubular junction in the ascending aorta.

16. An echocardiogram is obtained on a 3-month-old infant with a loud cardiac murmur. The parasternal short-axis scan in **Figure 32.2** is obtained. Which of the following **BEST** describes the cardiac defect?
   A. Large membranous VSD.
   B. Large muscular VSD.
   C. Aneurysm of membranous septum.
   D. Severe valvar pulmonary stenosis.
   E. Severe aortic valve insufficiency.

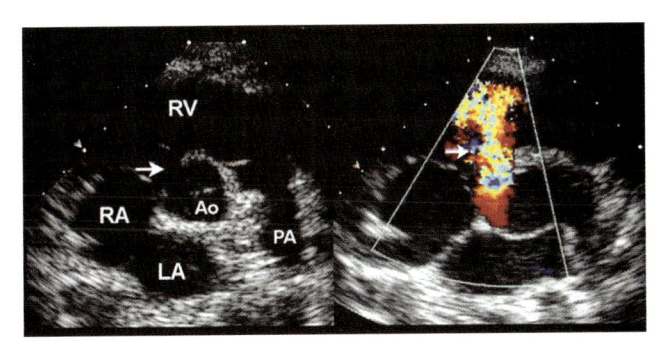

Figure 32.2

17. An echocardiogram is obtained after interventional device closure of a VSD (**Figure 32.3**). What anatomic type of VSD has been closed with this procedure?
   A. Membranous.
   B. Inlet.
   C. Subpulmonary (supracristal).
   D. Trabecular muscular.
   E. Anterior malalignment.

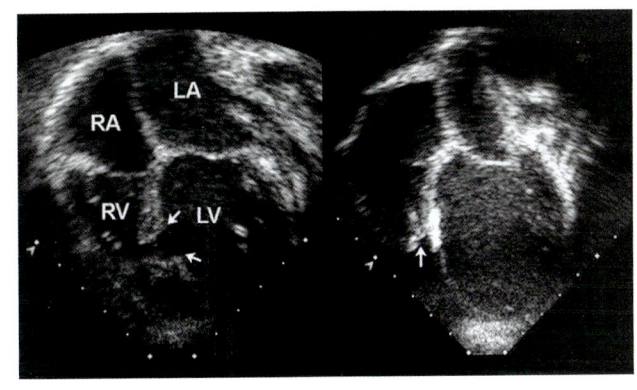

Figure 32.3

18. What anatomic type of VSD is demonstrated in the parasternal short-axis image in **Figure 32.4**?
   A. Membranous.
   B. Inlet.
   C. Subpulmonary (supracristal).
   D. Trabecular muscular.
   E. Anterior malalignment.

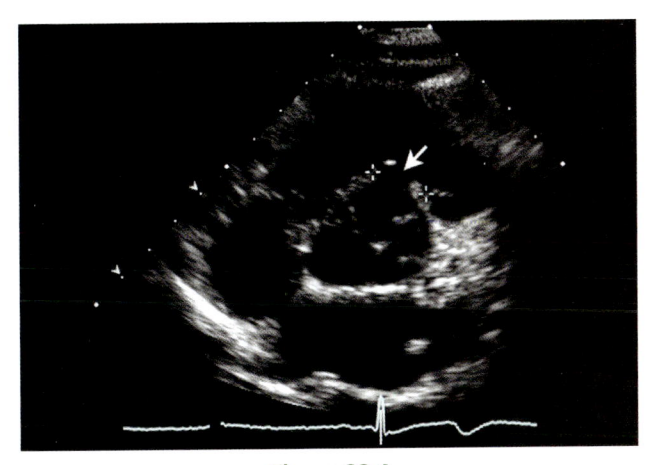

Figure 32.4

19. A 1-month-old infant undergoes an echocardiogram secondary to a cardiac murmur. What aortic to pulmonary artery peak pressure gradient is predicted by Doppler tracing in **Figure 32.5**?
   A. 16 mm Hg.
   B. 36 mm Hg.
   C. 48 mm Hg.
   D. 64 mm Hg.
   E. The peak aorta to pulmonary artery gradient cannot be calculated.

674 / Clinical Echocardiography Review

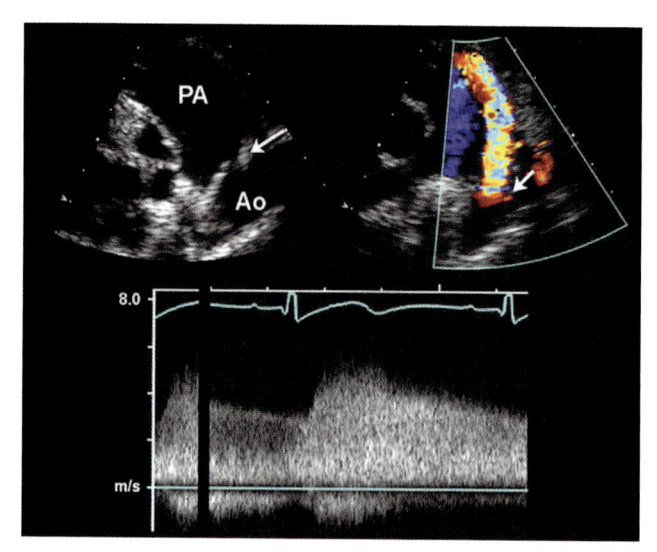

Figure 32.5

20. A 2-day-old infant undergoes an echocardiogram because of respiratory distress. What anatomic lesion and hemodynamic physiology is demonstrated in **Figure 32.6**?
    A. Patent ductus arteriosus (PDA) with exclusive left-to-right shunting.
    B. Aortopulmonary window with bidirectional shunting.
    C. Severe coarctation of the aorta with exclusive right-to-left shunting through the ductus arteriosus.
    D. PDA with bidirectional shunting.
    E. Aortopulmonary collateral vessel with exclusive right-to-left shunting.

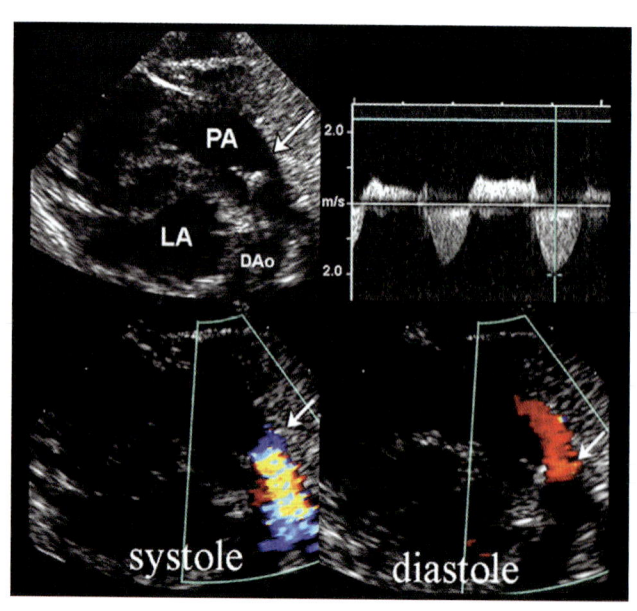

Figure 32.6

21. The parasternal long-axis image in **Figure 32.7** is obtained in a 12-year-old child with a new-onset cardiac murmur. Which of the following cardiac diagnoses **BEST** describes this image?
    A. Severe aortic valve stenosis.
    B. Subaortic membrane with moderate stenosis.
    C. Systolic anterior motion of the mitral valve with mild stenosis.
    D. Cardiac rhabdomyoma within the LVOT with moderate obstruction.
    E. Anomalous mitral valve chordal insertion with severe LVOT obstruction.

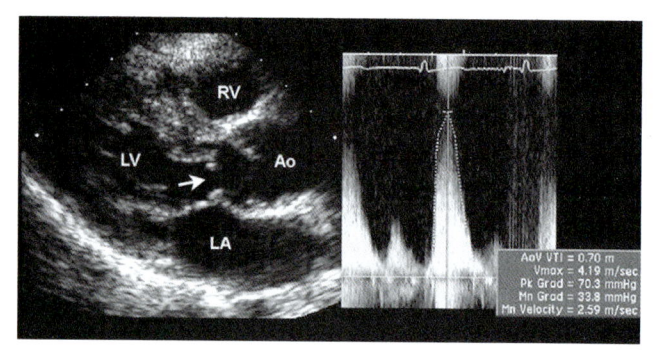

Figure 32.7

22. A 2-year-old child with Down syndrome presents for cardiac evaluation. The echocardiographic images in **Figure 32.8** are obtained. What cardiac defect is **BEST** demonstrated by color Doppler (arrow)?
    A. Primum ASD.
    B. Inlet VSD.
    C. Sinus venosus ASD.
    D. Persistent left superior vena cava to dilated coronary sinus.
    E. Malalignment outlet VSD.

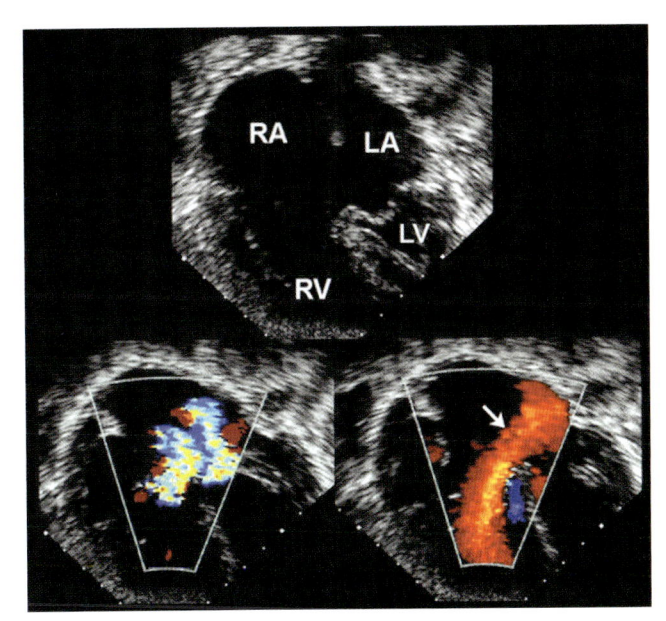

Chapter 32 Noncyanotic Congenital Heart Disease / 675

Figure 32.8

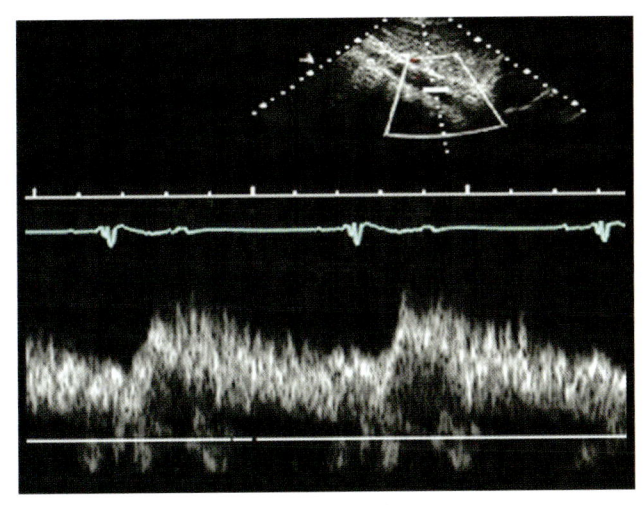

Figure 32.10

23. A previously healthy 6-year-old girl presents due to a recent episode of syncope with exercise. The suprasternal images in **Figure 32.9** are obtained. Which of the following **BEST** describes her cardiac diagnosis?
   A. Left pulmonary artery stenosis.
   B. PDA.
   C. Coarctation of the aorta.
   D. Interruption of the aortic arch.
   E. Transposition of the great arteries.

25. A 15-year-old teen presents for evaluation due to the presence of a cardiac murmur on auscultation. The echocardiographic images in **Figure 32.11** are most compatible with which of the following diagnoses?
   A. Pulmonary valve stenosis.
   B. Left pulmonary artery stenosis.
   C. Dynamic right ventricle (RV) infundibular obstruction.
   D. Tetralogy of Fallot with absent pulmonary valve.
   E. Double-chambered RV.

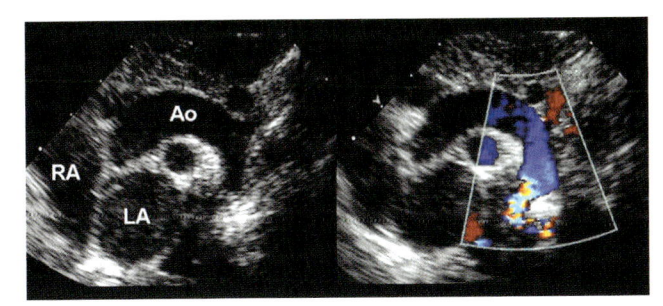

Figure 32.9

24. The Doppler pattern in **Figure 32.10**, in the abdominal aorta, is most consistent with:
   A. Severe aortic insufficiency.
   B. Large PDA.
   C. Normal aortic flow pattern.
   D. Coarctation of aorta.
   E. Mesenteric arterial flow.

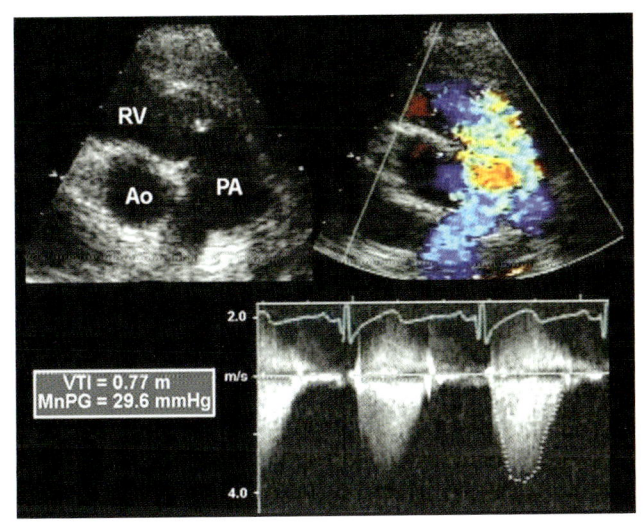

Figure 32.11

CASE 1

A neonate presents for evaluation secondary to a new cardiac murmur heard at his 2-week well-child outpatient visit. An echocardiogram was performed and the images in **Figure 32.12** were obtained.

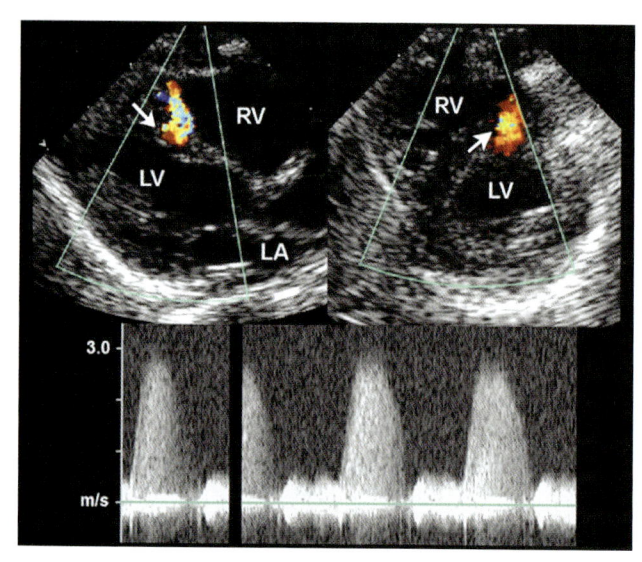

Figure 32.12

26. Which of the following diagnoses are most consistent with the images from **Case 1**?
   A. Small anterior muscular VSD with left-to-right shunting.
   B. Small posterior inlet VSD with left-to-right shunting.
   C. Large nonrestrictive muscular VSD with bidirectional shunting.
   D. Multiple "swiss cheese" VSDs with right-to-left shunting.
   E. Small outlet VSD with left-to-right shunting.

27. What is the peak LV to RV pressure gradient based upon the Doppler velocity displayed from **Case 1**?
   A. 16 mm Hg.
   B. 36 mm Hg.
   C. 64 mm Hg.
   D. 100 mm Hg.
   E. The peak pressure gradient cannot be calculated.

28. What is the likelihood of spontaneous closure of this defect during childhood?
   A. 5% to 10%.
   B. 20% to 30%.
   C. 40% to 50%.
   D. 60% to 70%.
   E. 80% to 90%.

CASE 2

A 7-year-old boy presents to your office with exercise intolerance. You note a 3/6 systolic ejection murmur at the left upper sternal border with a widely split S2 and a soft mid-diastolic rumble. The echocardiographic image in **Figure 32.13** is obtained.

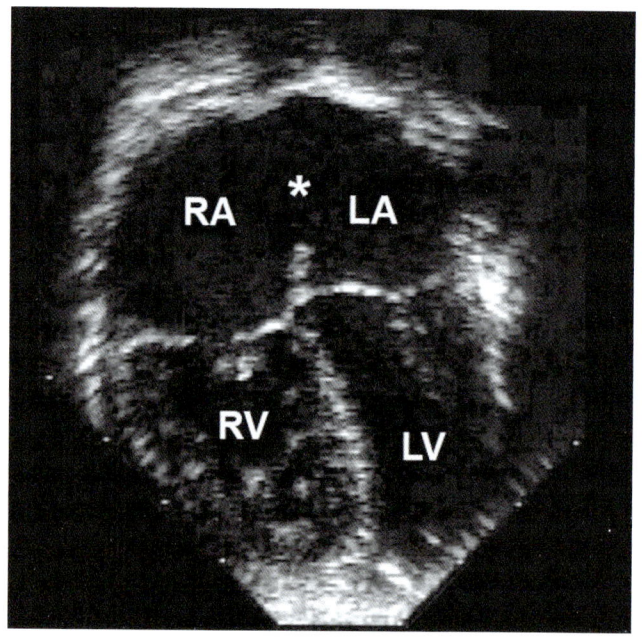

Figure 32.13

29. Which of the following diagnoses is **CORRECT** for the patient in **Case 2**?
   A. Primum ASD.
   B. Secundum ASD.
   C. Sinus venosus ASD.
   D. Coronary sinus ASD.
   E. Atrial septal aneurysm.

30. The direction in which blood flows across an ASD is primarily related to which of the following anatomic or hemodynamic factors?
   A. Relative compliances of the ventricles.
   B. Pulmonary vascular resistance.
   C. Systemic vascular resistance.
   D. Relative atrial pressures.
   E. Size and morphology of the ASD.

31. The family of the patient in **Case 2** is interested in repair of this defect but does not want him to undergo surgical repair. In your discussion with this family, which of the following defects would you tell them would be amenable to interventional device closure?
   A. Primum ASD.
   B. Secundum ASD.
   C. Sinus venosus ASD.
   D. Coronary sinus ASD.
   E. AVSD.

CASE 3

A 3-week-old infant presents to the emergency department with tachypnea and a cardiac murmur. These echocardiographic images in **Figure 32.14A** *and* ▶ **Video 32.2A-C** *are obtained.*

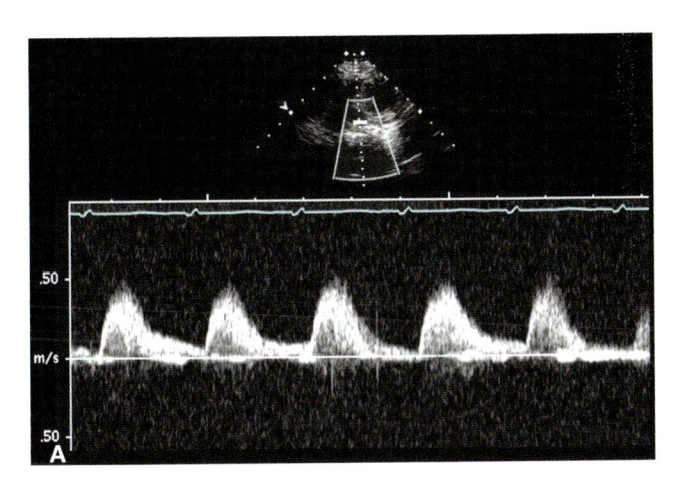

Figure 32.14A

32. What is the most likely diagnosis for the patient in **Case 3**?
   A. Coarctation of the aorta.
   B. Interruption of the aortic arch type A.
   C. Supravalvar aortic stenosis.
   D. Valvar aortic stenosis.
   E. Subaortic stenosis.

33. After the echocardiogram is completed for the patient in **Case 3**, the on-call resident performs four-extremity blood pressure measurements. The findings are as follows:
   Right leg: 40/25 mm Hg.
   Left leg: 42/22 mm Hg.
   Right arm: 48/27 mm Hg.
   Left arm: 72/35 mm Hg.

Which of the following is the most likely diagnosis?
   A. Interruption of the aortic arch with restrictive PDA.
   B. Coarctation of the aorta with VSD.
   C. Coarctation of the aorta with aberrant right subclavian artery.
   D. Truncus arteriosus with pulmonary artery ostial stenosis.
   E. Normal aortic arch with stenosis of the left subclavian artery.

34. Which of the following statements regarding coarctation of the aorta is **CORRECT**?
   A. It is caused by the formation of an anterior ledge of thickened aortic wall media tissue.
   B. The most common site of coarctation is opposite the ductal insertion.
   C. Involvement of the left subclavian artery is very common.
   D. It commonly presents in the neonatal period with systemic hypertension and LV hypertrophy.
   E. It is rarely associated with other congenital heart abnormalities.

35. The patient from **Case 3** undergoes a follow-up echocardiogram following the initiation of prostaglandin E. The Doppler profile in **Figure 32.14B** is obtained. What is the most likely explanation?
   A. Significant aortic insufficiency is present.
   B. The patent ductus arteriosus (PDA) is now open.
   C. The cardiac output is extremely low.
   D. Pulmonary hypertension is present.
   E. Thrombus is present in the descending aorta.

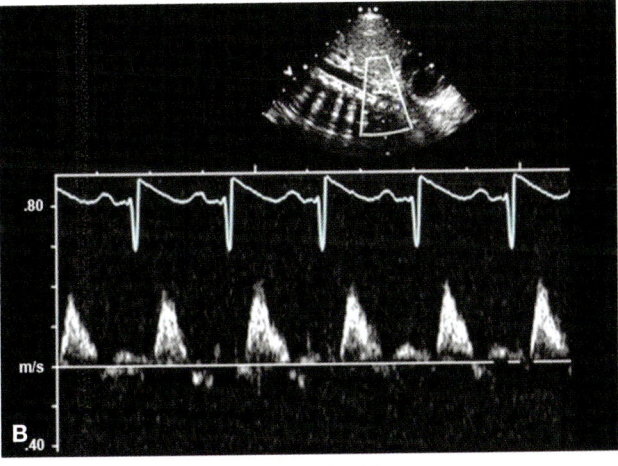

Figure 32.14B

CASE 4

A 27-year-old woman presents at 20 weeks of gestation with palpitations and a cardiac murmur. The echocardiographic images in ▶ Video 32.3A-C are obtained.

36. What is the underlying cardiac diagnosis for the patient in **Case 4**?
    A. Complete AVSD with large primum ASD and large inlet VSD.
    B. Large secundum ASD.
    C. Large primum ASD.
    D. Large sinus venosus ASD.
    E. Large malalignment outlet VSD.

37. The image of the left atrioventricular valve in ▶ **Video 32.3D** is obtained for the patient in **Case 4**. What abnormality is demonstrated?
    A. Double-orifice mitral valve.
    B. Mitral arcade.
    C. Cleft mitral valve.
    D. Mitral valve prolapse.
    E. Normal mitral valve anatomy.

38. The offspring of the patient in **Case 4** is born at term. The images in ▶ **Video 32.3E,F** are obtained shortly after delivery. What is the cardiac abnormality demonstrated in this newborn?
    A. Complete AVSD.
    B. Sinus venosus ASD.
    C. Secundum ASD.
    D. Tetralogy of Fallot.
    E. Large outlet muscular VSD.

CASE 5

A 6-year-old boy presents to you for evaluation of a cardiac murmur. His mom says that he has had the murmur "all his life" but it was felt to be functional. The patient does not complain of any symptoms but he is not very active. The only sport he seems interested in is basketball but he is too short. When you ask about the family history, they mention that there were a paternal uncle, grandfather, and great grandfather who had a very "thick heart muscle." On examination, you note short stature, a triangular face, an obvious chest deformity, a webbed neck, an RV lift, and a soft short systolic ejection murmur at the left upper sternal border without a click. He has normal distal pulses.

39. For the patient in **Case 5,** what is the finding demonstrated on echocardiography (▶ **Video 32.4A-E**)?
    A. Bicuspid aortic valve with coarctation of the aorta.
    B. Discrete supravalvular aortic stenosis.
    C. Thickened pulmonary valve with hypoplastic annulus.
    D. Severe branch pulmonary artery stenosis.
    E. Large PDA.

40. Which of the following would be the most expected cardiac abnormality in Noonan syndrome?
    A. Pulmonary valve stenosis.
    B. Dilated cardiomyopathy.
    C. Supravalvar aortic stenosis.
    D. Coarctation of the aorta.
    E. Aortic valve stenosis.

41. Percutaneous pulmonary valvotomy was performed for the patient in **Case 5** (▶ **Video 32.4F-I**). Cardiac hemodynamics obtained during catheterization are shown in **Table 32.1** (mm Hg): After the procedure, you note a grade 4/6 late-peaking harsh systolic murmur at the left upper sternal border, which has increased in intensity since his admission examination, and a new, soft diastolic murmur. His systemic blood pressure is 80/60 mm Hg. On echocardiography, the predicted RV systolic pressure is 60 mm Hg. The post-catheterization angiogram is shown in ▶ **Video 32.4H,I**. Which of the following is the most likely underlying cause of these findings?
    A. Significant residual pulmonary valve stenosis.
    B. RV infundibular obstruction.
    C. Hypovolemia with systemic hypotension.
    D. Distal pulmonary artery branch stenosis.
    E. Severe pulmonary regurgitation.

Table 32.1 Cardiac Catheterization Data

	Prevalvotomy	Postvalvotomy
RA (mean)	10	9
RV (systolic/EDP)	125/10	62/11
MPA	15/7	13/7
Systemic BP	86/60	80/60

BP, blood pressure; EDP, end diastolic pressure; MPA, main pulmonary artery; RA, right artery; RV, right ventricular.

CASE 6

A 7-year-old girl presents with a 3-month history of sudden random chest pain which is "squeezing" in character. The pain occurs with activities and sports participation and lasts for a few minutes with each episode. She has not had syncope or any other cardiovascular symptoms. At presentation, her vital signs, cardiovascular examination, and ECG are normal. Her chest pain is not reproducible.

42. What is the next BEST step in the management of the patient in **Case 6**?
    A. Treatment with a tapering dose of NSAIDs.
    B. Restriction from sports participation until chest pain resolves.
    C. Order an echocardiogram to rule out any cardiac abnormality as an etiology for chest pain.
    D. Order a CXR to rule out any pulmonary etiology for chest pain.
    E. Reassure the patient and family that chest pain is very common in children and is always benign.

43. You decide to order an echocardiogram for the patient in **Case 6** and the following images are obtained (**Figure 32.15A** and **B**, ▶ Video 32.5A-E). What is your diagnosis?
    A. Anomalous origin of left coronary artery from right sinus of Valsalva.
    B. Anomalous origin of the left coronary artery from the pulmonary artery.
    C. Hypertrophic cardiomyopathy.
    D. Anomalous origin of the right coronary artery from the left sinus of Valsalva.
    E. Recent history of Kawasaki disease.

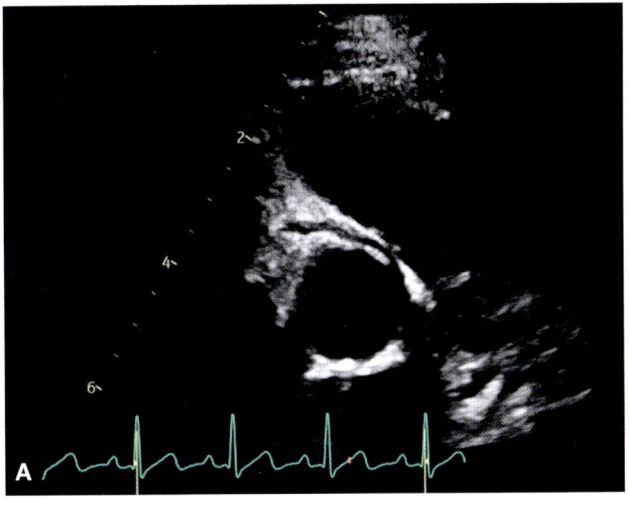

Figure 32.15A

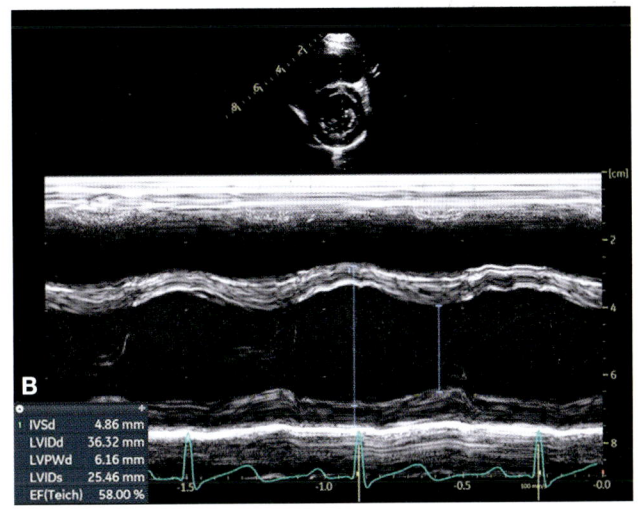

Figure 32.15B

44. What is the next BEST course of action in the care of the patient from **Case 6**?
    A. Surgical unroofing of the anomalous right coronary artery.
    B. Permanent restriction from competitive sports participation.
    C. Close clinical follow-up every 6 months.
    D. No clinical follow-up is indicated since the risk of sudden cardiac death is very low in children with anomalous right coronary artery origin versus those with anomalous left coronary artery origin.
    E. Perform cardiac catheterization to more comprehensively evaluate coronary artery origin.

ANSWERS

1. **Answer: D.** The subcostal imaging window is optimal to demonstrate the atrial septum and any associated ASDs that may be present. To visualize the atrial septum without potential dropout, the imaging plane of sound should be perpendicular to the cardiac structure of interest. With respect to the atrial septum, the imaging planes that are optimally perpendicular are the subcostal 4-chamber and sagittal views. ASDs can be demonstrated in other imaging windows, including the parasternal short-axis, apical 4-chamber, and high right parasternal views, but care must be taken not to diagnose an ASD when the plane of sound is more parallel to the atrial septum creating the potential for a false dropout in the two-dimensional image. The addition of color Doppler and spectral Doppler interrogation in these views may also facilitate the diagnosis of an ASD.

2. **Answer: A.** Sinus venosus ASDs are most commonly associated with an anomalous connection of the right pulmonary veins. Either a single right upper pulmonary vein or the right upper and middle pulmonary veins typically insert anomalously to the superior vena cava (SVC) or the SVC-right atrial junction. Sinus venosus defects are found most commonly superiorly adjacent to the entrance of the SVC. These defects can also be located inferiorly near the entrance of the inferior vena cava into the right atrium. Inlet VSDs are most commonly associated with atrioventricular septal defects. Bicuspid AV can be an isolated anomaly or is frequently seen in patients with coarctation of the aorta. A persistent left superior vena cava is seen in approximately 10% of patients with congenital heart disease but is not frequently associated with a sinus venosus ASD. Coarctation of the aorta is seen commonly with other left-sided obstructive lesions but not commonly with a sinus venosus ASD.

3. **Answer: D.** Patients with Down syndrome (trisomy 21) have an almost 50% incidence of congenital heart disease, with AVSDs being the most common cardiac anomaly in this cohort. AVSD in association with tetralogy of Fallot is a common constellation of cardiac anomalies in patients with Down syndrome. Obstruction of the LVOT and coarctation of the aorta are also common cardiac abnormalities in patients with AVSD but are not as common in Down syndrome patients. LV hypoplasia can occur in the setting of AVSD ("unbalanced AVSD with right ventricular [RV] dominance") but is less commonly seen in this cohort. Aortic valve stenosis and anomalous pulmonary venous connections are uncommon.

4. **Answer: D.** Anatomic hallmarks of AVSDs include a cleft in the anterior leaflet of the left atrioventricular valve, lateral rotation of the LV papillary muscles, and attachments of the left and right atrioventricular valves at the same level at the cardiac crux. In addition, due to the absence of the atrioventricular septum in these defects, the LV inflow is shortened and the LV outflow is elongated ("goose-neck deformity") creating a ratio of LV inlet to LV outlet ratio <1. Due to the presence of a common atrioventricular valve, the aortic valve is no longer "wedged" between the tricuspid and mitral valves and is pushed anteriorly ("sprung").

5. **Answer: D.** Outlet VSDs (**Figure 32.16A**, ▶ **Video 32.6**) are located in the region of the infundibular septum between the pulmonary and aortic valves (**Figure 32.16B**). These defects can be optimally demonstrated in the parasternal short-axis scan plane but can also be demonstrated from the subcostal and apical windows with appropriate angulation.

6. **Answer: A.** Aortic insufficiency is the most common associated abnormality because of prolapse of the aortic cusp into a subpulmonary VSD. While this associated prolapse of aortic tissue limits the size of the VSD and can lessen the left-to-right shunt, the progression of aortic insufficiency due to distortion of the aortic valve is well recognized. If this regurgitation is significant and progresses, then surgical closure is indicated (and is not dependent upon the size of the left-to-right shunt). LVOT obstruction is more characteristically present in patients with a posteriorly malaligned VSD or an atrioventricular septal defect while RV outflow tract obstruction is the hallmark of anterior malalignment VSDs in tetralogy of Fallot. Pulmonary stenosis and aortic stenosis are not characteristic findings in a patient with a subpulmonary VSD.

7. **Answer: C.** Large VSDs result in the equalization of right and left ventricular pressures as well as elevated pulmonary arterial pressure. Left-to-right shunting at the ventricular level results in a substantial increase in pulmonary blood flow with left

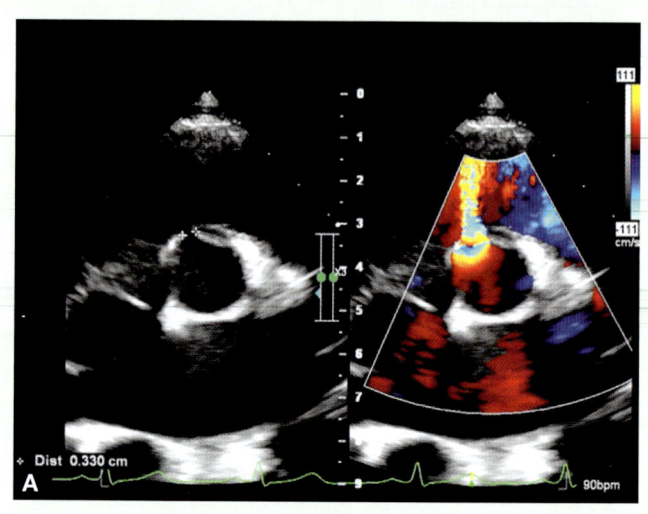

Figure 32.16A

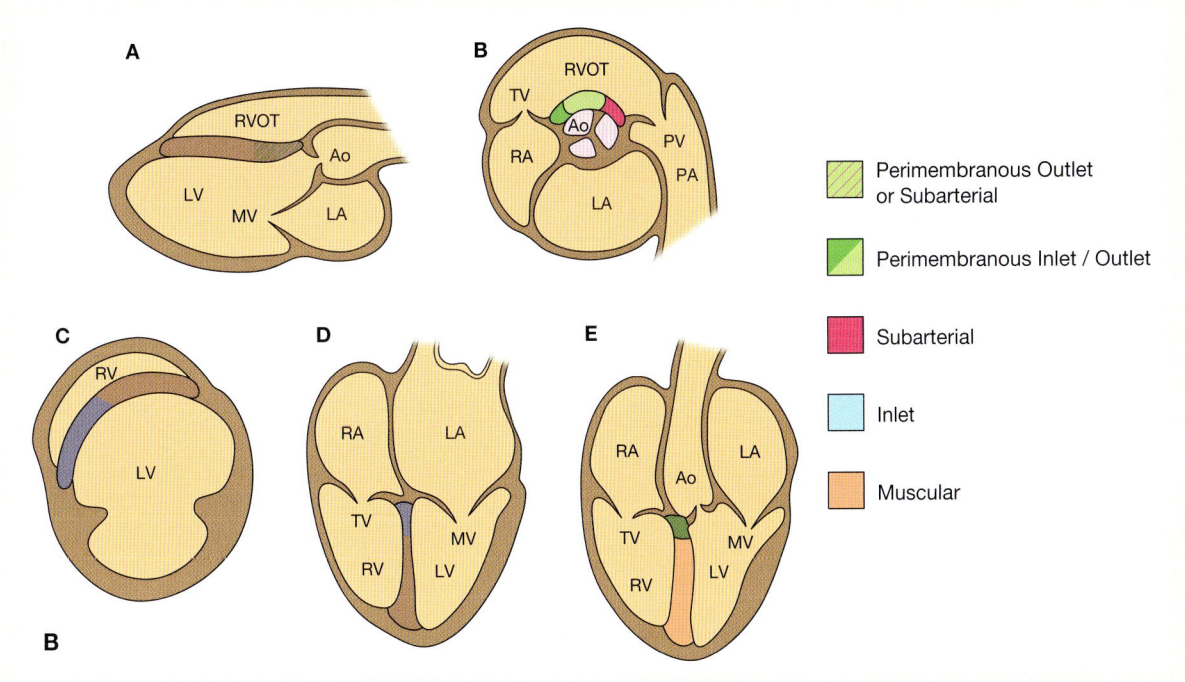

Figure 32.16B. Reprinted with permission from Gelehrter S, Thorsson T, Ensing G. Ventricular septal defects. In: Eidem BW, Johnson JN, Lopez L, Cetta F, eds. *Echocardiography in Pediatric and Adult Congenital Heart Disease.* 3rd ed. Wolters Kluwer; 2021:231-252. Figure 12.3.

atrial and left ventricular volume overload. Systemic blood flow is not significantly increased in this setting.

8. **Answer: B.** The most common type of subaortic stenosis is related to a discrete membrane proximal to the aortic valve within the LVOT. This membrane is most often circumferential and can be adherent to both the aortic valve as well as the anterior leaflet of the mitral valve. The other potential answers are not anatomic subtypes of subaortic stenosis. LVOT obstruction in the setting of hypertrophic cardiomyopathy is often related to asymmetric septal hypertrophy in combination with systolic anterior motion of the mitral valve chordal and leaflet tissue. Anomalous mitral chordal insertions within the LVOT can be isolated or found in association with congenital heart disease and may result in obstruction but are not as common as discrete membranes.

9. **Answer: A.** These images demonstrate the classic features of a partial AVSD (**Figure 32.1**, **Videos 32.1A-C**). There is a large primum atrial septal defect with a large left-to-right atrial level shunt. Owing to lack of the atrioventricular septum, both atrioventricular valves are inserted at the same level at the cardiac crux. The inlet ventricular septum is intact. Color Doppler also demonstrates significant mitral regurgitation, most likely related to a cleft in the anterior leaflet as well as tricuspid regurgitation.

10. **Answer: A.** Bicuspid aortic valve is the most commonly associated cardiac finding in patients with simple coarctation with some studies showing as high as an 80% occurrence in patients with coarctation. ASDs and VSDs are also common in patients with coarctation. Pulmonary valve stenosis and coronary arterial anomalies are much less frequent in this cohort.

11. **Answer: C.** The aortic lumen must be narrowed by at least 50% to significantly affect systemic arterial pressure.

12. **Answer: C.** The most common VSD associated with coarctation is a perimembranous defect. While less common, a posterior malalignment VSD often results in severe coarctation or interruption of the aortic arch. Muscular VSD as well as inlet VSD can also occur in the setting of coarctation, in particular with an unbalanced RV-dominant AVSD. Anterior malalignment VSDs are more commonly associated with RV outflow obstruction, most notably tetralogy of Fallot.

13. **Answer: A.** The systolic jet in patients with supravalvar aortic stenosis propagates further than the jet originating with aortic valvar stenosis and has a tendency to be entrained along the aortic wall thereby transferring its kinetic energy into the right innominate artery. This physical principle, termed the Coanda effect, is often expressed clinically in these patients by marked discrepancy in upper arm blood pressures, with the right arm pressure higher than the left arm blood pressure.

14. **Answer: A.** Interruption of the aortic arch is most commonly found in DiGeorge syndrome and is a deletion in chromosome 22q11. This chromosome deletion results in conotruncal defects, with interruption of the aortic arch type B being the most frequent cardiac abnormality. Down syndrome

(trisomy 21) is frequently associated with congenital heart disease, most commonly atrioventricular canal defects and VSDs. Turner syndrome (45 XO) has coarctation and bicuspid aortic valve as hallmark lesions while Holt–Oram is associated with secundum ASDs. Alagille syndrome is most characteristically associated with pulmonary branch stenosis or RVOT obstruction.

15. **Answer: D.** Type A interruption of the aortic arch occurs distal to the origin of the left subclavian artery. Type B interruption occurs between the left common carotid and left subclavian arteries. Type C interruption occurs between the right innominate and left common carotid arteries.

16. **Answer: A.** The parasternal short-axis image in **Figure 32.2** is a classic demonstration of a membranous VSD adjacent to the tricuspid valve. Color Doppler demonstrates a high-velocity mosaic jet from the left ventricle to the right ventricle. Muscular VSDs in the trabecular septum are best demonstrated in the apical 4-chamber and parasternal long- and short-axis views. Aneurysmal septal tricuspid leaflet tissue that obliterates a membranous VSD resulting in the absence of a left to right shunt is termed as a membranous septal aneurysm. While aortic insufficiency can rarely be associated with a membranous VSD, it is not demonstrated in this figure. Pulmonary valve stenosis can also be present in the setting of a VSD but is also less common.

17. **Answer: D.** The apical 4-chamber image in **Figure 32.3** demonstrates the muscular ventricular septum with a midmuscular defect occluded using a closure device. The apical 4-chamber view demonstrates the inlet portion of the ventricular septum (near the atrioventricular valves) and the mid and apical muscular septum. Membranous VSDs can also be closed with these types of devices and would be best visualized in the apical and parasternal short-axis imaging planes. Due to their proximity to either the atrioventricular valves (inlet VSD) or semilunar valves (supracristal VSD), these VSDs are not candidates for device closure in the cardiac catheterization laboratory.

18. **Answer: C.** The parasternal short-axis image in **Figure 32.4** demonstrates a defect in the subpulmonary region (supracristal) of the ventricular septum adjacent to the pulmonary valve. This defect has also been termed as an infundibular or conal VSD due to the defect's position within the infundibular muscular septum. Membranous VSDs are also demonstrated best in the parasternal short-axis scan plane but are adjacent to the tricuspid valve (within the membranous septum) instead of the pulmonary valve (within the infundibular septum). Inlet VSDs are best imaged in the apical 4-chamber plane and are adjacent to the atrioventricular valves. Trabecular muscular VSDs can be imaged in multiple imaging planes including the parasternal long- and short-axis, subcostal, and apical views. Anterior malalignment VSDs are the hallmark of tetralogy of Fallot and are optimally imaged in the parasternal short- and long axis as well as the subcostal imaging planes.

19. **Answer: D.** The high left parasternal short-axis image in **Figure 32.5** demonstrates a patent ductus arteriosus. Color Doppler is consistent with a left-to-right shunt from the aorta to the pulmonary artery (red color flow). Continuous-wave Doppler confirms an exclusive left-to-right shunt in both systole and diastole. The peak Doppler velocity is approximately 4.0 m/s predicting a peak instantaneous pressure gradient of 64 mm Hg utilizing the simplified Bernoulli equation.

20. **Answer: D.** The high left parasternal short-axis image in **Figure 32.6** demonstrates a PDA. Color Doppler is consistent with a bidirectional shunt from the aorta to the pulmonary artery (right-to-left shunting in systole and left-to-right shunting in diastole). Continuous-wave Doppler confirms bidirectional low-velocity shunting consistent with pulmonary hypertension.

21. **Answer: B.** The parasternal long-axis image in **Figure 32.7** demonstrates a circumferential subaortic membrane within the LVOT (see arrow). Note the significant narrowing of the LVOT and the association of the membrane with the anterior leaflet of the mitral valve. The peak Doppler velocity obtained from a high right parasternal location predicts a mean gradient of ~34 mm Hg (moderate stenosis). While aortic stenosis cannot be excluded from this still frame image, the major obstruction appears to be the membrane within the LV outflow tract. No systolic anterior motion (SAM) or anomalous mitral valve chord is demonstrated within the LVOT. Cardiac rhabdomyomas can rarely be present within the cardiac chambers or be adherent to cardiac valves, including the aortic valve; however, the majority of rhabdomyomas are intramyocardial, most typically within the LV or RV myocardium.

22. **Answer: A.** The apical 4-chamber image in **Figure 32.8** demonstrates a large primum ASD. The large left-to-right shunt is demonstrated across this defect by color flow imaging (arrow). Both atrioventricular valves are inserted at the same level at the cardiac crux consistent with an AVSD with a large primum component. No shunt is evident at the ventricular level. Significant atrioventricular valve regurgitation is also demonstrated by color Doppler. Sinus venosus ASDs are uncommon in the setting of an atrioventricular VSD and would be best demonstrated in the subcostal sagittal imaging plane. Malalignment outlet VSDs (posterior malalignment with LVOT obstruction or anterior malalignment with RVOT obstruction) are best imaged in the parasternal long- and short-axis imaging planes or anteriorly in the apical 4-chamber orientation. A persistent left SVC is also imaged optimally in the apical 4-chamber view with the plane of sound angled posteriorly demonstrating the dilated coronary sinus emptying into the right atrium. A left SVC can also be imaged

well from the parasternal long axis and high left parasternal windows.

23. **Answer: C.** The suprasternal long-axis image of the aortic arch in **Figure 32.9** demonstrates a juxtaductal coarctation of the aorta. Note the posterior shelf present in the descending aorta in the two-dimensional image and the area of coarctation demonstrated with color Doppler. Both LPA branch stenosis and PDA would be best imaged in the parasternal short-axis or high left parasternal imaging planes. D-TGA, with a parallel relationship of the great arteries, would be best visualized in the parasternal long axis, subcostal, and suprasternal short-axis windows. Interruption of the aortic arch can be imaged in the suprasternal and subcostal windows but has lack of continuity between the aortic segments with supply to the distal arch via the PDA.

24. **Answer: D.** Pulsed-wave Doppler interrogation is demonstrated in the descending aorta. The Doppler pattern in **Figure 32.10** and **Figure 32.17B** demonstrates classic findings in coarctation of the aorta with delayed arterial upstroke and prominent diastolic runoff. Also note the absence of an early-diastolic Doppler flow reversal, another hallmark of significant aortic obstruction. The normal Doppler pattern in the abdominal aorta consists of a rapid arterial upstroke in systole with a brisk return to the Doppler baseline in early diastole followed by an early brief diastolic flow reversal (**Figure 32.17A**). Both severe aortic insufficiency and a large PDA would characteristically have holodiastolic Doppler flow reversal in the abdominal aorta (**Figure 32.17C**). Arterial flow in branches from the abdominal aorta will often have a brisk systolic upstroke and downstroke in the arterial pulse followed by low-velocity continuous forward flow in diastole into the low-resistance gastrointestinal circulation (**Figure 32.17D**).

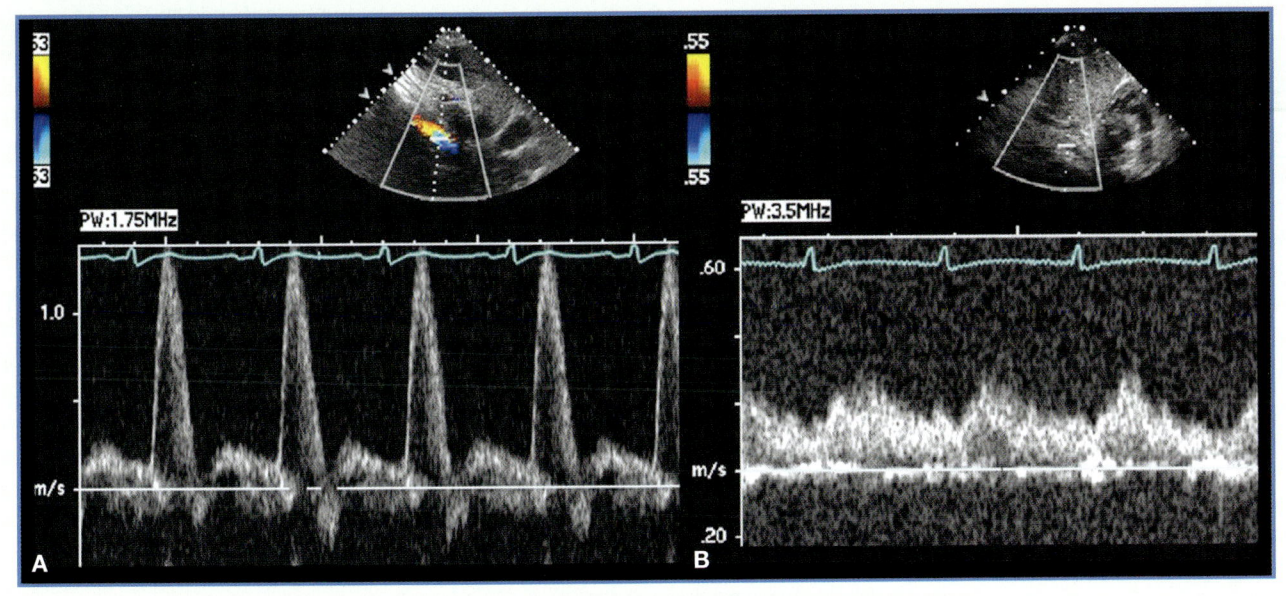

Figure 32.17A and B

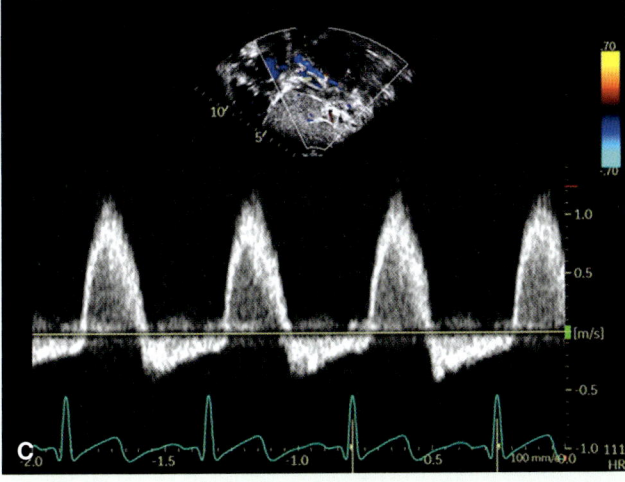

Figure 32.17C

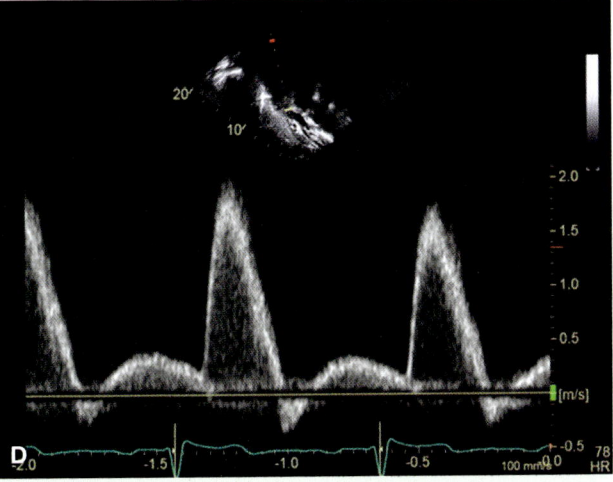

Figure 32.17D

25. **Answer: A.** The parasternal short-axis images in **Figure 32.11** demonstrate a thickened pulmonary valve with prominent color flow acceleration originating at the pulmonary valve consistent with valvar stenosis. Continuous-wave Doppler predicts a mean gradient of ~30 mm Hg suggesting a moderate degree of stenosis. LPA branch stenosis originates distal to the pulmonary valve in the branch pulmonary arteries and is best demonstrated in the parasternal short axis and high left parasternal views. Dynamic RV infundibular obstruction originates within the RVOT with a classic late peaking (dagger-shaped) Doppler signal. Double-chambered RV (DCRV) is an anomaly characterized by hypertrophied anomalous muscle bundles within the RVOT with more of a fixed pattern of obstruction demonstrated by spectral Doppler. DCRV is also commonly associated with membranous VSDs. Tetralogy of Fallot with absent pulmonary valve has a characteristic to and fro Doppler pattern of significant pulmonary stenosis and severe pulmonary regurgitation with massive dilatation of the main and branch pulmonary arteries on two-dimensional imaging.

26. **Answer: A.** The parasternal long-axis and short-axis scans in **Figure 32.12** demonstrate a small anterior muscular VSD in the midmuscular septum (arrow). The continuous-wave Doppler velocity of ~3 m/s suggests a restrictive defect. Remember, pulmonary vascular resistance in the neonate does not fall completely until 2 to 3 months of age so it would be expected with this small defect that the Doppler velocity will increase over the first few months of life consistent with a hemodynamically small defect. No additional VSDs are demonstrated by color Doppler imaging; however, the ventricular septum should be imaged in many different scan planes (parasternal long axis, parasternal short axis, apical 4-chamber, and subcostal views) to assure no additional defects are present.

27. **Answer: B.** Utilizing the simplified Bernoulli equation to obtain the peak instantaneous gradient across the VSD, $4 \times [velocity]^2$, then $4 \times [3.0]^2 = 36$ mm Hg.

28. **Answer: E.** Small trabecular muscular VSDs have a very high likelihood of spontaneous closure, typically 80%–90%. The majority will close within the first few years of life but spontaneous closure with these muscular defects can occur later in childhood and even in adulthood.

KEY POINTS
- Muscular VSDs can be characterized as restrictive if the Doppler velocity through the defect is elevated consistent with a large pressure gradient and small-sized defect.
- Most (80%-90%) muscular VSDs close spontaneously by late childhood.

29. **Answer: B.** The clinical examination in this patient suggests a large ASD. The apical 4-chamber image in **Figure 32.13** demonstrates an enlarged right atrium and right ventricle consistent with a significant left-to-right atrial shunt. While it is not the optimal echocardiographic view to evaluate the entire atrial septum (this scan plane is more parallel than perpendicular to the atrial septum), it does appear that there is a large dropout in the atrial septum consistent with a secundum ASD (*). The primum septum is intact inferiorly and is confirmed by noting that the atrioventricular valves are inserted at different levels at the cardiac crux (atrioventricular septum is present). This apical view is not optimal to demonstrate a sinus venosus ASD. Lack of dilatation of the coronary sinus does not exclude a coronary sinus ASD but makes it much less likely. No atrial septal aneurysm is demonstrated in this image.

30. **Answer: A.** The direction of atrial level shunting is primarily related to the compliance of the ventricles. The right ventricle is typically more compliant than the left ventricle with characteristic left-to-right shunting being most common. These other factors noted in the question also contribute to the degree and direction of atrial level shunting but ventricular compliance is most important.

31. **Answer: B.** Interventional device closure is performed in secundum ASDs of appropriate size and with adequate tissue rims. Sinus venosus, primum, and coronary sinus defects are not amenable to device closure due to their proximity to other cardiac structures (most notably the atrioventricular valves and the systemic and pulmonary veins).

KEY POINTS
- A secundum ASD will have an intact atrioventricular septum with normal insertion of the atrioventricular valves at different levels at the cardiac crux.
- The direction of atrial shunting is largely dependent on the relative compliance of the ventricles.
- Only the secundum-type ASD is amenable to interventional device closure.

32. **Answer: A.** The images presented are consistent with coarctation of the aorta. The suprasternal long-axis views demonstrate a juxtaductal coarctation of the aorta in the proximal descending aorta. Aliased color flow is demonstrated at the area of discrete narrowing. The parasternal long-axis images do not demonstrate any evidence of subaortic, valvar, or supravalvar aortic stenosis. A midmuscular VSD, however, is seen in this video. The pulsed-wave Doppler image from the descending aorta demonstrates diastolic runoff consistent with significant proximal obstruction (ie, coarctation).

33. **Answer: C.** In patients with coarctation of the aorta, the brachiocephalic vessels proximal to the coarctation typically have normal or increased systemic blood pressure while those vessels distal to the obstruction have decreased blood pressure. In a patient with a typical juxtaductal coarctation, the blood pressure in the arms is significantly higher than blood pressures recorded in the lower extremities. The blood pressures in the patient listed in this question are decreased in the right and left legs (as one would expect in coarctation) but the right arm also has decreased pressure. This is most likely due to an aberrant right subclavian artery that originates distal to the coarctation from the descending aorta.
34. **Answer: B.** The most common site of coarctation of the aorta in infants and children is juxtaductal—the narrowing is opposite the insertion site of the ductus arteriosus. This is accompanied by a posterior infolding ("ledge") of thickened aortic wall media tissue. The left subclavian artery is most often not involved in the narrowing but can be in some cases. The typical neonatal presentation of severe coarctation is cardiovascular collapse when the patent ductus closes. Systemic hypertension and LV hypertrophy often present later in childhood with coarctation. Coarctation is often associated with other congenital heart lesions including bicuspid aortic valves, VSDs, and additional left heart obstructive lesions.
35. **Answer: B.** With the initiation of prostaglandin E, the ductus arteriosus has reopened allowing pulsatile flow to the descending aorta (from the pulmonary artery). In the presence of a large PDA, the classic Doppler findings of "coarctation" in the abdominal aortic Doppler tracings will be absent because pulsatile flow can bypass the juxtaductal area of obstruction.

KEY POINTS
- The most common site of coarctation of the aorta is in the juxtaductal region.
- Other associated congenital heart lesions with coarctation of the aorta include bicuspid aortic valves, VSDs, and additional left heart obstructive lesions.
- The presence of a large PDA will eliminate the classic findings on the abdominal aortic Doppler tracing of coarctation of the aorta.

36. **Answer: C.** The apical 4-chamber images in ▶ **Video 32.3A-C** demonstrate a large primum ASD. Note that the atrioventricular valves are inserted at the same level at the cardiac crux consistent with the absence of the atrioventricular septum resulting in a large ASD. While there appears to be a small inlet VSD, there is no ventricular level shunt demonstrated by color Doppler. This potential area of shunting has been obliterated by atrioventricular valve leaflet and chordal tissue.
37. **Answer: C.** This parasternal short-axis image demonstrates a cleft in the anterior leaflet of the mitral valve. This defect is characteristic in patients with primum ASDs. Other mitral valve anomalies, such as a double-orifice mitral valve or mitral arcade, can occur in the setting of a primum ASD but are rare.
38. **Answer: A.** The apical 4-chamber view demonstrates a large primum ASD and a large inlet VSD. The subcostal view nicely demonstrates the common atrioventricular valve in this complete AVSD.

KEY POINTS
- A typical characteristic of a primum ASD is the insertion of the atrioventricular valves at the same level consistent with the absence of the atrioventricular septum.
- Primum ASD is associated with mitral valve anomalies, most notably a mitral valve cleft.

39. **Answer: C.** This patient has a physical examination and family history suggestive of Noonan syndrome. This autosomal dominant syndrome has phenotypic features including short stature, webbed neck, pectus excavatum, and triangular facies. Cardiovascular abnormalities are common in this syndrome and include pulmonary valve stenosis, hypertrophic cardiomyopathy, and ASDs. The patient's family history is suggestive of hypertrophic cardiomyopathy. The patient's physical examination is consistent with pulmonary valve stenosis.

    Common echocardiographic features of pulmonary valve stenosis are included in ▶ **Video 32.4A-E**. The subcostal (A and B) and parasternal short-axis scans (C and D) demonstrate thickening and restricted mobility of the pulmonary valve with color Doppler aliasing at the valve level consistent with stenosis. The apical 4-chamber scan (E) demonstrates the marked hypertrophy in this child with severe valvar pulmonary stenosis.
40. **Answer: A.** The cardiovascular anomaly characteristic of Noonan syndrome is valvar pulmonary stenosis. Other cardiac abnormalities common in this syndrome include hypertrophic cardiomyopathy and ASDs. Supravalvar stenosis is commonly found in patients with Williams syndrome. Coarctation of the aorta and valvar aortic stenosis are common in Turner syndrome. Dilated cardiomyopathies are common in the muscular dystrophies, such as Duchenne muscular dystrophy, and in other metabolic disorders.
41. **Answer: B.** This patient's preprocedure (▶ **Video 32.4F,G**) and postprocedure angiograms (▶ **Video 32.4H,I**) are included. The postangiography

cines demonstrate significant dynamic RVOT obstruction after the relief of valvar pulmonary stenosis. The patient's physical examination is consistent with dynamic RVOT obstruction as well, demonstrating a loud late-peaking systolic murmur as well as the murmur of pulmonary regurgitation after the balloon dilatation of the pulmonary valve. Treatment with beta blockade and eventual regression of RV hypertrophy will often significantly decrease the degree of dynamic obstruction in these patients with successful relief of pulmonary valve obstruction.

> **KEY POINTS**
> - Clinical features of Noonan syndrome include short stature, webbed neck, pectus excavatum, and triangular facies.
> - Cardiovascular features of Noonan syndrome include pulmonary valve stenosis, hypertrophic cardiomyopathy, and ASDs.

42. **Answer: C.** This patient's clinical presentation does not fit the common diagnosis of musculoskeletal chest wall pain in this age group. The nature of the pain ("squeezing") and its occurrence during active sports participation are red flags that require additional investigation. The performance of an echocardiogram to exclude any cardiomyopathy or coronary artery anomaly is indicated in this case. While a CXR may be helpful to rule out any underlying skeletal abnormality that may predispose to this chest pain is reasonable, it is unlikely to be abnormal considering her normal physical examination and lack of reproducible palpational chest pain. Treatment with NSAIDs, restriction from sports participation, or simple benign neglect are not indicated until an underlying cardiovascular etiology for her chest pain is excluded.

43. **Answer: D.** The echocardiogram images and video clips demonstrate an anomalous origin of the right coronary artery (RCA) from the left sinus of Valsalva with a proximal intramural course (**Figure 32.15A**, ▶ **Video 32.5A**). The RCA then travels between the aorta and main pulmonary artery (▶ **Video 32.5A**). The left main coronary artery has a normal origin from the left sinus of Valsalva (▶ **Video 32.5B and C**). There are no proximal coronary artery aneurysms in either coronary artery to suggest a diagnosis of Kawasaki disease. Similarly, there is no evidence on the echocardiogram of hypertrophic cardiomyopathy (HCM) (**Figure 32.15B**, ▶ **Videos 32.5D and E**).

44. **Answer: A.** Both the proximal intramural origin of the RCA from the left sinus of Valsalva as well as its course between the great arteries are significant risk factors for sudden death with this coronary anomaly. Surgical unroofing of the RCA ostia is the treatment of choice in this clinical scenario. While the risk of sudden cardiac death is higher in patients with an anomalous origin of the left coronary artery from the right sinus of Valsalva, those patients with an inter-arterial course of the anomalous right coronary artery are at significant risk and surgical intervention is indicated. Permanent restriction from sports participation is not an optimal management strategy, especially with the long-term success and minimal surgical risk that has been reported in these patients. Close serial follow-up, without surgical intervention, is also not a recommended strategy as these patients often present with sudden death as their initial clinical symptom. Finally, cardiac catheterization is seldom needed to diagnose an anomalous origin of a coronary artery, especially in children. Cardiac CT is ideal if additional information is required prior to surgery.

> **KEY POINTS**
> - Exertional chest pain in children is a red flag and a cardiac etiology should be sought.
> - Coronary artery anomalies can be visualized by TTE.
> - Anomalous origin of the RCA from the left sinus of Valsalva with an intramural course can be corrected with surgical unroofing.

SUGGESTED READINGS

Cabalka AK, Thompson AJ. Abnormalities of atria and atrial septation. In: Eidem BW, Johnson J, Lopez L, Cetta F, eds. *Echocardiography in Pediatric and Adult Congenital Heart Disease.* 3rd ed. Lippincott, Williams, and Wilkins; 2021:135-158.

Cetta F, Poderucha JT, Maleszewski JJ, O'Leary PW. Atrioventricular septal defects. In: Eidem BW, Johnson J, Lopez L, Cetta F, eds. *Echocardiography in Pediatric and Adult Congenital Heart Disease.* 3rd ed. Lippincott, Williams, and Wilkins; 2021:159-173.

Cohen MS, Lopez L. Ventricular septal defects. In: Shaddy RE, Penny D, Feltes TF, et al., eds. *Moss and Adams Heart Disease in Infants, Children, and Adolescents.* 10th ed. Lippincott, Williams, and Wilkins; 2021:746-764.

Eidem BW, O'Leary PW. Quantitative methods in echocardiography—basic techniques. In: Eidem BW, Johnson J, Lopez L, Cetta F, eds. *Echocardiography in Pediatric and Adult Congenital Heart Disease.* 3rd ed. Lippincott, Williams, and Wilkins; 2021:42-66.

Gelehrter S, Thorsson T, Ensing G. Ventricular septal defects. In: Eidem BW, Johnson J, Lopez L, Cetta F, eds. *Echocardiography in Pediatric and Adult Congenital Heart Disease*. 3rd ed. Lippincott, Williams, and Wilkins; 2021:231-252.

Lopez L, Saurers DL, Barker PCA, et al. Guidelines for performing a comprehensive pediatric transthoracic echocardiogram: recommendations from the American Society of Echocardiography. *J Am Soc Echocardiogr*. 2024;37:119-170.

Mahgerefteh J, Lopez L. Abnormalities of left ventricular outflow. In: Eidem BW, Johnson J, Lopez L, Cetta F, eds. *Echocardiography in Pediatric and Adult Congenital Heart Disease*. 3rd ed. Lippincott, Williams, and Wilkins; 2021:305-337.

Mitchell C, Rahko PS, Blauwet LA, et al. Guidelines for performing a comprehensive transthoracic echocardiographic examination in adults: recommendations from the American Society of Echocardiography. *J Am Soc Echocardiogr*. 2019;32:1-64.

Parthiban A, Sachdeva R. Atrial septal defects. In: Shaddy RE, Penny D, Feltes TF, et al., eds. *Moss and Adams Heart Disease in Infants, Children, and Adolescents*. 10th ed. Lippincott, Williams, and Wilkins; 2021:703-720.

Silvestry FE, Cohen MS, Armsby LB, et al. Guidelines for the echocardiographic assessment of atrial septal defect and patent foramen ovale: from the American Society of Echocardiography and Society for Cardiac Angiography and Interventions. *J Am Soc Echocardiogr*. 2015;28(8):910-958.

Truong D, Minich LL, Maleszewski JJ, et al. Atrioventricular septal defects. In: Shaddy RE, Penny D, Feltes TF, et al., eds. *Moss and Adams Heart Disease in Infants, Children, and Adolescents*. 10th ed. Lippincott, Williams, and Wilkins; 2021:721-725.

Wasserman MA, Shea E, Cassidy C, et al. Recommendations for the adult cardiac sonographer performing echocardiography to screen for critical congenital heart disease in the newborn: from the American Society of Echocardiography. *J Am Soc Echocardiogr*. 2021;34(3):207-222.

CHAPTER 33

Cyanotic Congenital Heart Disease

Pooja Gupta and James M. Galas

QUESTIONS

1. Which is the most common **CYANOTIC** congenital heart disease?
   A. d-Transposition of great arteries (TGA).
   B. Total anomalous pulmonary venous return (TAPVR).
   C. Truncus arteriosus.
   D. Tetralogy of Fallot (TOF).
   E. Tricuspid atresia.

2. A 21-year-old young man with Down syndrome and an unrepaired complete atrioventricular septal defect (AVSD) presents for echocardiographic evaluation. A right-to-left shunt is demonstrated at the ventricular level. Which of the following is the most likely explanation?
   A. Eisenmenger syndrome.
   B. Restriction of blood flow at the ventricular septal defect (VSD).
   C. Mild atrio-ventricular valve regurgitation.
   D. Partial anomalous pulmonary venous connections (PAPVCs).
   E. Goosencck deformity of the left ventricular outflow tract (LVOT).

3. A newborn infant is evaluated because of a heart murmur. The echocardiogram reveals a large VSD with an overriding great vessel and a single large great artery giving rise to the aorta and the pulmonary artery. Which is a **TRUE** statement about this congenital heart defect?
   A. There is a higher incidence of chromosomal abnormalities.
   B. Survival is dependent upon a PDA.
   C. Survival is dependent upon an ASD.
   D. The oxygen saturation is normal.
   E. Surgical repair may be deferred for up to 2 years.

4. An echocardiogram is done on a 4-year-old patient with unrepaired tetralogy of Fallot. He has a loud heart murmur at the upper left sternal border. The parasternal long-axis view reveals a typical large VSD with an overriding great aorta. The pulmonary arteries appear to be confluent and normal in size. There is right-to-left shunting at the ventricular level with no turbulence seen. Doppler interrogation of the tricuspid regurgitant signal reveals a velocity of 4.5 m/s. What can be said about this patient's heart disease?
   A. He has developed pulmonary hypertension.
   B. A tricuspid valve problem has developed.
   C. This is an expected finding of no concern.
   D. The VSD is becoming restrictive with time.
   E. The Doppler signal from the tricuspid valve is incorrect.

5. An echocardiogram is done on an infant with cyanosis and no heart murmur. The parasternal long-axis view reveals a large VSD with right-to-left shunt. The posterior great artery appears to bifurcate into two arteries. There is a patent foramen ovale with a small left-to-right shunt. A large patent ductus arteriosus is seen with bidirectional shunt. What is the most likely cause of the cyanosis?
   A. d-Transposition of the great arteries.
   B. Truncus arteriosus.
   C. Coarctation of the aorta.
   D. Pulmonary atresia.
   E. Total anomalous pulmonary venous return.

6. Which of the following cyanotic congenital heart defects is **MOST** likely to escape detection in childhood?
   A. Tetralogy of Fallot.
   B. Total anomalous pulmonary venous return.
   C. Transposition of the great arteries.
   D. Tricuspid valve atresia.
   E. Ebstein anomaly of the tricuspid valve.

7. In cyanotic congenital heart disease what is the **MOST** frequent hemodynamic abnormality?
   A. Abnormal great artery position.
   B. Pulmonary venous anomaly.
   C. Abnormal arteriovenous connection.
   D. Pulmonary hypertension.
   E. Decreased pulmonary blood flow and right-to-left intracardiac shunting.

8. Agitated saline (contrast) injection into the left antecubital vein reveals early appearance of bubbles in the left atrium, in a patient with a pulse oximetry reading of 90%. What is the most likely anatomic abnormality?
   A. Bilateral SVC with bridging vein.
   B. Bilateral SVC with absent bridging vein.
   C. Persistent left SVC to unroofed coronary sinus.
   D. Total anomalous pulmonary venous connections to the coronary sinus.
   E. Total anomalous pulmonary venous connections to the inferior vena cava.

9. Which of the following pulmonary venous connections is **NOT** abnormal?
   (Not a form of TAPVR)
   A. Connection to the innominate vein.
   B. Connection to the right atrium.
   C. Connection to the hepatic veins.
   D. Connection to the coronary sinus.
   E. Connection to the left atrium.

10. An echocardiogram is done on an infant with a heart murmur. The parasternal long-axis view reveals a large VSD with an overriding great vessel. The differential diagnosis includes all the following **EXCEPT**:
    A. D-TGA with VSD.
    B. TOF.
    C. Double outlet right ventricle (DORV).
    D. Truncus arteriosus.
    E. Coarctation.

11. A 2-month-old infant is seen for a heart murmur. The child is doing clinically well. The oxygen saturation is 90% by pulse oximetry. Echocardiography reveals tricuspid valve atresia. Which is a **TRUE** statement about this congenital heart defect?
    A. An ASD or PFO is always present.
    B. A PDA must be present for survival.
    C. The great arteries are transposed.
    D. The great arteries are normally related.
    E. A right aortic arch is usually present.

12. A 40-year-old man with D-transposition of the great arteries has previously undergone an atrial switch (Mustard) operation in childhood, and now presents with tachypnea and cough. The adult congenital cardiologist suspects pulmonary venous hypertension. What is the most likely finding on echocardiogram to explain this clinical presentation?
    A. Obstruction of the systemic venous baffle.
    B. Obstruction of the pulmonary venous baffle.
    C. Obstruction of the branch pulmonary artery.
    D. Obstruction of the right ventricular to pulmonary artery conduit (RV-PA).
    E. Obstruction in the coronary artery.

13. A 21-year-old patient with truncus arteriosus s/p surgical repair presents with a harsh systolic murmur at the left sternal border. Saturations are 97%. He is found to have a tricuspid regurgitation jet velocity of 4 m/s on echocardiogram. A previous echocardiogram done 2 years ago demonstrated tricuspid regurgitation jet velocity of 3 m/s. What is the most likely explanation for this finding?
    A. Primary pulmonary hypertension.
    B. Truncal valve stenosis.
    C. Modified Blalock-Taussig shunt stenosis.
    D. Worsening RV-PA conduit stenosis.
    E. Worsening pulmonary venous stenosis.

14. A newborn infant is found to have saturations of 60%. Echocardiogram demonstrates a large patent ductus arteriosus (PDA) and a patent foramen ovale (PFO) with otherwise normal intracardiac anatomy. The infant's blood pressure is 70/50 mm Hg. Right ventricular systolic pressure is estimated to be 90 mm Hg, based on tricuspid regurgitation jet velocities. What shunting pattern would you expect to find at the ductus arteriosus?
    A. Continuous left to right.
    B. Continuous right to left.
    C. Bidirectional, predominantly left to right.
    D. Bidirectional, predominantly right to left.
    E. The direction of PDA shunt in this patient cannot be predicted.

15. An infant is born with transposition of the great arteries with intact ventricular septum. A PDA is present and the baby is placed on prostaglandin E1 to maintain this. The infant remains cyanotic with an arterial saturation of 60%–63%. Which area of the heart should be studied thoroughly with echocardiography since it is most likely to account for this problem?
    A. The pulmonary venous return.
    B. The ductus arteriosus.
    C. The aortic arch.
    D. The systemic venous return.
    E. The atrial septum.

16. A 2-week-old newborn is being evaluated for cyanosis and a murmur. Echocardiography was performed as shown in **Figure 33.1A** (apical 4-chamber view) and **Figure 33.1B** (parasternal short-axis view in systole). The diagnosis of congenital heart disease was made. Based on these echocardiographic findings, what is the best estimate of right ventricular systolic pressure?
    A. ½ systemic.
    B. ¾ systemic.
    C. Near systemic.
    D. Systemic.
    E. Suprasystemic.

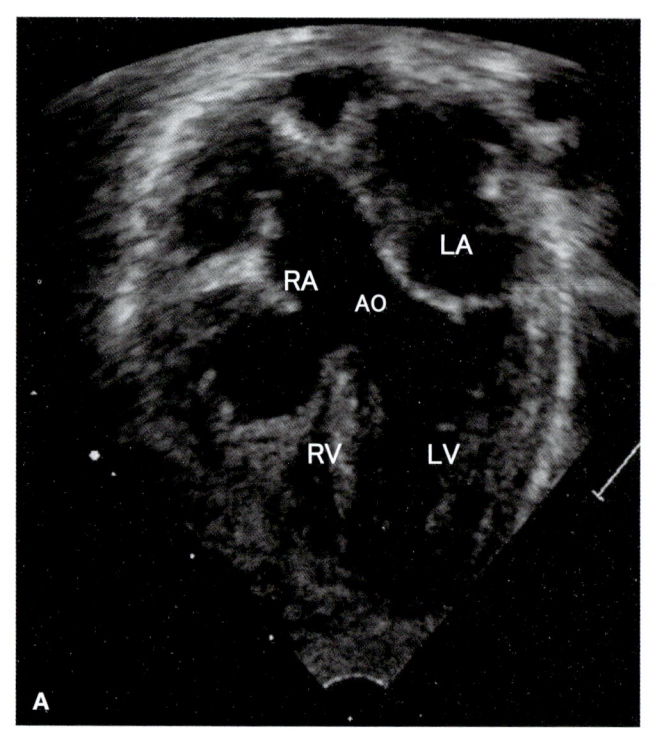

Figure 33.1A

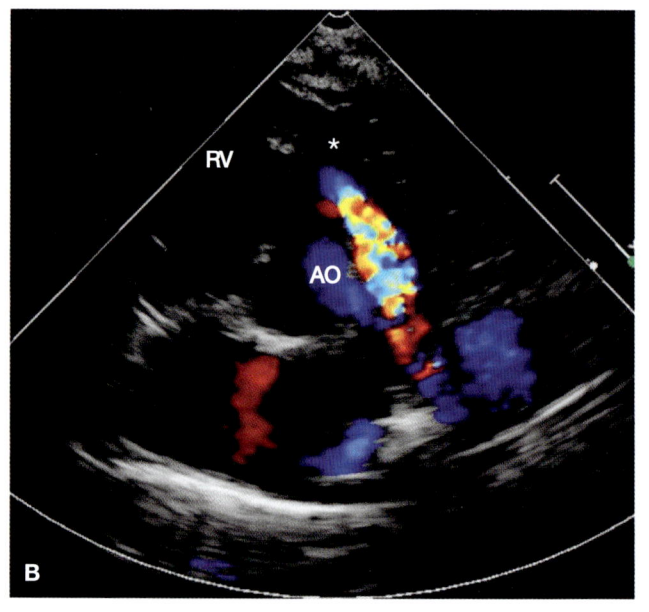

Figure 33.1B

17. A newborn infant presents with a saturation of 90% and tachypnea. An echocardiogram was performed as shown in **Figures 33.2A** and **33.2B**. Which of the following statements regarding this lesion is **TRUE**?
   A. This is a ductal-dependent lesion.
   B. This patient will benefit from 100% FiO$_2$ with mechanical ventilation.
   C. Atrial level shunting is not required in this condition.
   D. The patient is likely to have Down syndrome.
   E. A right aortic arch is commonly seen.

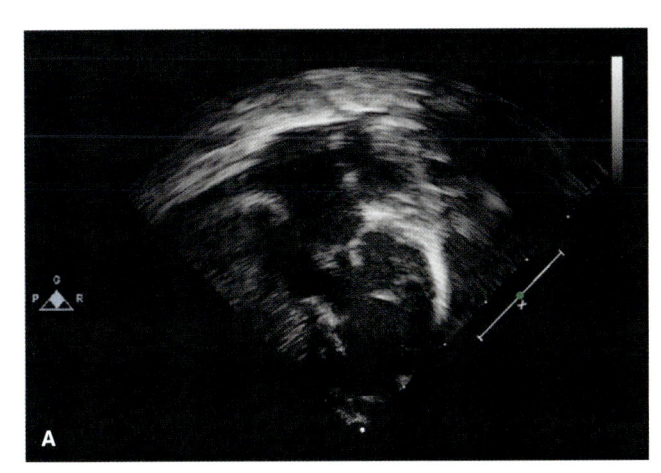

Figure 33.2A

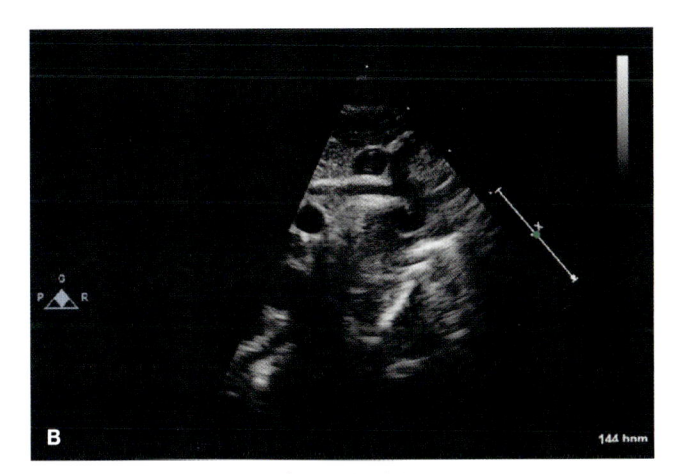

Figure 33.2B

18. A young adult was found to have an abnormal echocardiogram during evaluation of palpitations. The area marked with stars in **Figure 33.3** demonstrates:
   A. Dilated coronary sinus.
   B. Atrialized portion of RV.
   C. Tricuspid valve atresia.
   D. Hypoplastic RV.
   E. Dilated LV.

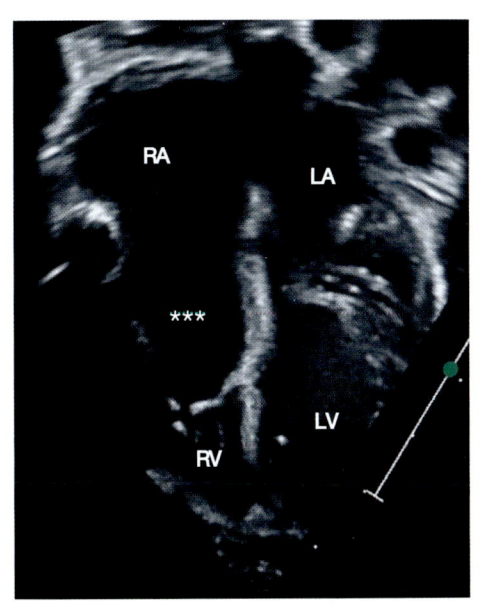

Figure 33.3

19. A 1-day-old newborn is transferred from the newborn nursery to the NICU because of cyanosis. His oxygen saturation is 75% and does not improve with 100% FiO$_2$. Echocardiography is as shown in **Figure 33.4A** (parasternal long-axis view) and **Figure 33.4B** (parasternal short-axis view). A = LV, B = RV, C = Pulmonary valve, D = Aorta. Which of the following choices is true for this condition? (AV = atrioventricular, VA = ventriculoarterial)
   A. AV concordance, VA concordance.
   B. AV discordance, VA discordance.
   C. AV concordance, VA discordance.
   D. AV discordance, VA concordance.

692 / Clinical Echocardiography Review

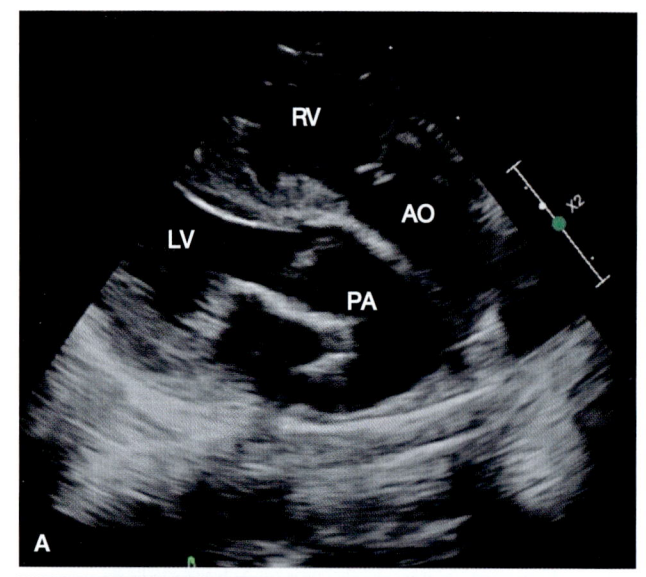

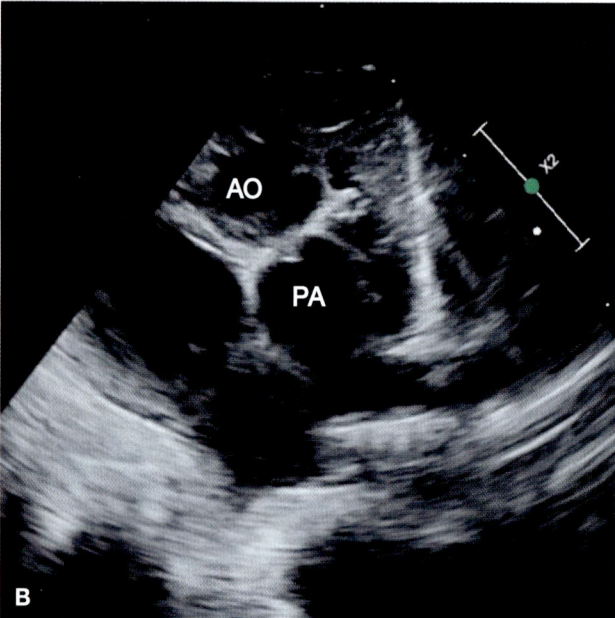

Figure 33.4

20. A 4-week-old girl presents to her primary care physician with cyanosis particularly with crying. On evaluation, her saturation is high 70s to low 80s. Cardiac exam reveals an ejection systolic murmur. Echocardiography was performed as shown in **Figure 33.5A** (parasternal long-axis) and **Figure 33.5B** (parasternal short-axis). Echocardiogram reveals pulmonary stenosis with overriding aorta. Which finding determines this girl's oxygen saturation?
   A. Severity of right ventricular outflow tract obstruction.
   B. Size of the VSD.
   C. Degree of overriding of aorta.
   D. Size of the ASD.

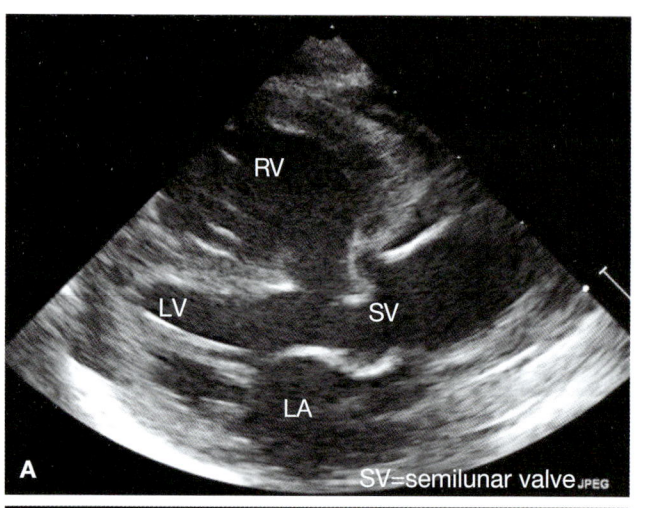

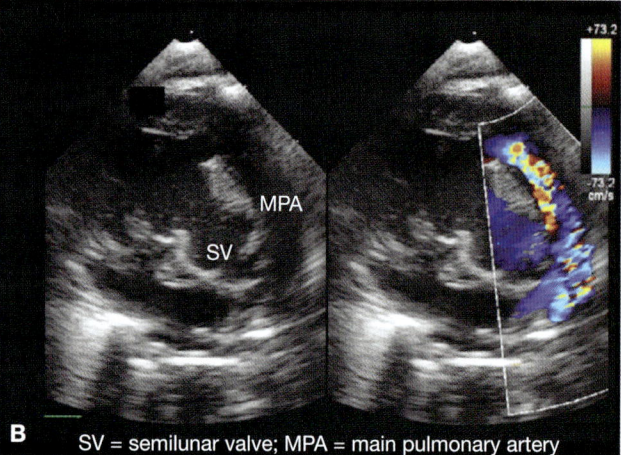

Figure 33.5

21. A 19-year-old young man was referred to a cardiology clinic for easy fatigability with sports and exercise. His vitals were within normal limits except oxygen saturation of 86%. Apical 4-chamber view on echocardiography is shown in **Figure 33.6**. What is the diagnosis?
   A. Tricuspid atresia.
   B. Pulmonary hypertension.
   C. Uhl anomaly.
   D. Ebstein anomaly.
   E. Large ASD.

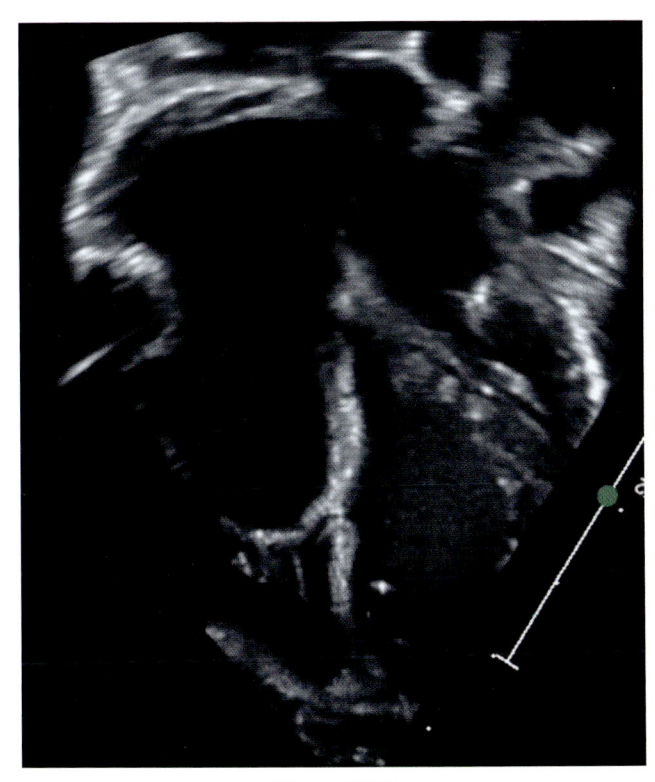

Chapter 33 Cyanotic Congenital Heart Disease / 693

Figure 33.6

22. An infant is born with an abnormal fetal echocardiogram. An echocardiogram performed shortly after birth is as shown in **Figure 33.7** (parasternal long-axis view). Which diagnosis can be excluded from this image?
   A. Interrupted aortic arch with posterior malaligned VSD.
   B. D-TGA with VSD
   C. Pulmonary atresia with VSD
   D. TOF.
   E. Truncus arteriosus.

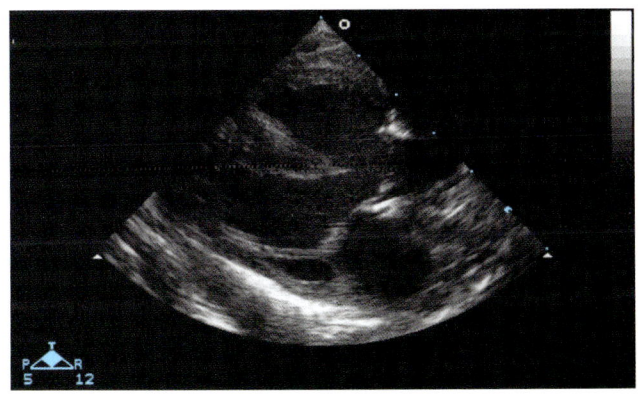

Figure 33.7

23. A 6-week-old infant was admitted to the PICU with poor feeding, respiratory distress, and mild cyanosis. Chest x-ray showed pulmonary congestion. Echocardiography is shown in **Figure 33.8A** (parasternal long-axis view) and **Figure 33.8B** (apical view). Which of the following describes best this child's condition?
   A. TOF.
   B. DORV (double outlet right ventricle).
   C. Truncus arteriosus.
   D. This patient has trisomy 21.
   E. TAPVR.

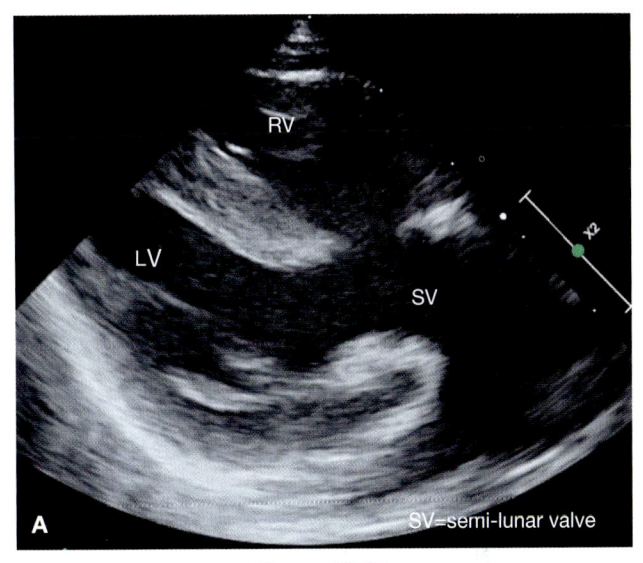

Figure 33.8A

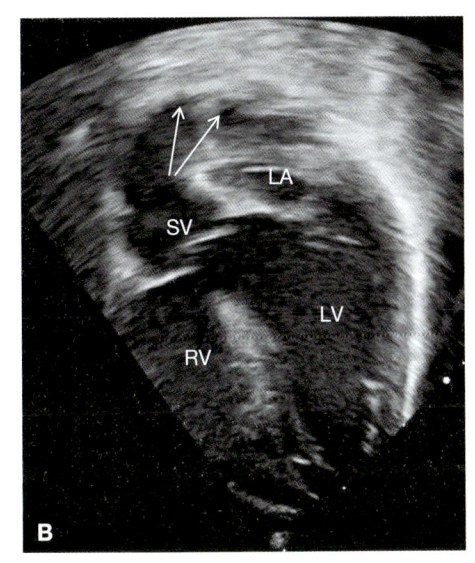

Figure 33.8B

24. You are called for an echocardiogram in the NICU on a newborn infant whose saturation is 80% at room air. Parasternal short-axis views were performed as shown in **Figures 33.9A** and **33.9B** (systole and diastole, respectively) and demonstrates a pulmonary valve that does not open. What is the next most important piece of information you would like to find out in this patient that will define proper diagnosis of this condition, natural history of this lesion, and future surgical management?

   A. Determine if an ASD is present.
   B. Determine if a VSD is present.
   C. Determine the size of the LV.
   D. Determine if a coarctation is present.
   E. Determine if abnormal pulmonary venous drainage is present.

   A. Right atrial thrombus.
   B. Redundant eustachian valve.
   C. A cast in the right atrium from a previous intracardiac line placement.
   D. Lateral tunnel/Fontan.
   E. Calcified RV to PA conduit.

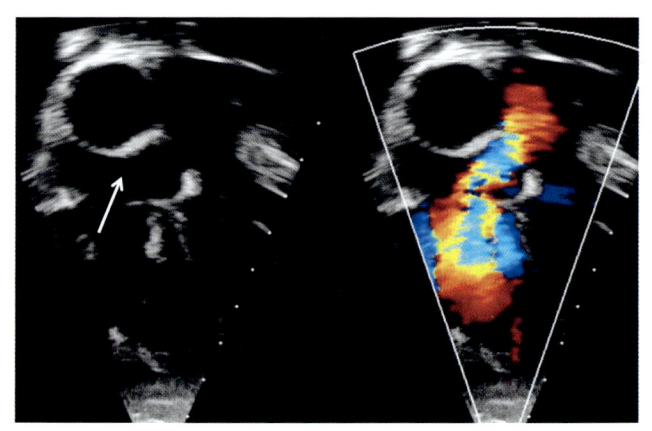

Figure 33.10

26. A 3-week-old female infant presents to her physician with respiratory distress. Her oxygen saturation is in the 80's. Echocardiography was performed. A subcostal picture is shown in **Figure 33.11**. The arrows in **Figure 33.11** are suggestive of:

   A. Localized posterior pericardial effusion.
   B. Truncus arteriosus.
   C. Pulmonary venous confluence/TAPVR.
   D. A mediastinal mass.
   E. Aortic aneurysm.

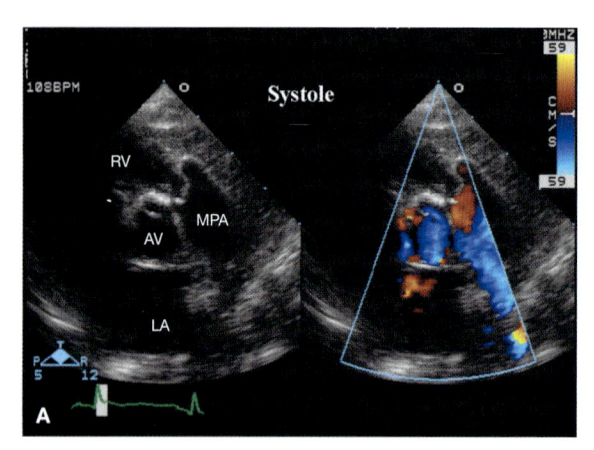

Figure 33.9A

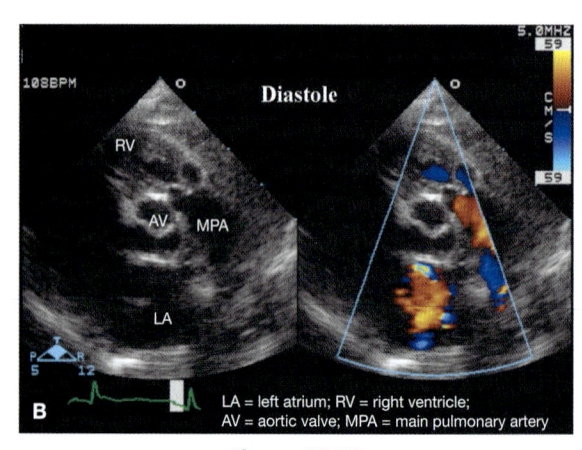

Figure 33.9B

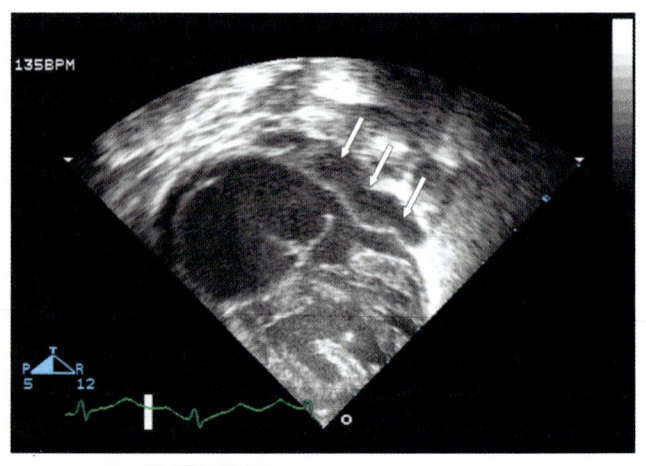

Figure 33.11

25. **Figure 33.10** is an apical 4-chamber view obtained in a patient with tricuspid atresia following surgical palliation. The circular structure shown by the arrow represents what structure?

CASE 1

*A 4-week-old male infant was referred to a pediatric cardiology clinic for a murmur found during a routine clinic visit at the pediatrician's office and mild cyanosis (oxygen saturation—86%). His echocardiography is shown in ▶ **Video 33.1A** (apical) and **Video 33.1B** (parasternal short-axis).*

27. Based on the clinical presentation and echocardiography shown in **Case 1**, the most likely diagnosis is:
    A. Truncus arteriosus.
    B. TOF.
    C. D-TGA with VSD.
    D. VSD.
    E. Pulmonary stenosis.

28. As the infant in **Case 1**, grew older (3 months of age), parents reported frequent episodes of bluish discoloration when the child was crying. According to the parents, there is no history suggestive of any lethargy, tiredness, or respiratory distress. He was brought to his pediatrician's office where his saturation is now 75% as compared to 86% at 4 weeks of life. Other than that, he was playful and active in the doctor's office. Echocardiography is shown ▶ **Video 33.1C**. Which of the following will be the most likely finding on his echocardiogram?
    A. Decreased blood flow across the pulmonary valve.
    B. Dynamic RVOT obstruction suggestive of TET spells.
    C. Decreased right-to-left shunting across the VSD.
    D. Decreased LV function.
    E. Increased blood flow across the pulmonary valve.

29. This infant is now 5 months of age and he has increasing cyanosis. He has moderate to severe RVOT obstruction along with a hypoplastic pulmonary valve. He is scheduled for surgery which includes relief of RVOT obstruction, transannular patch, and closure of VSD. Which of the following associated conditions play a major role in the above mentioned surgery?
    A. Right aortic arch.
    B. ASD.
    C. Coronary anomalies.
    D. Additional muscular VSD.
    E. Size of the VSD.

30. The single anatomic hallmark responsible for each of the anatomic components in this condition is:
    A. Hypertrophy of RV.
    B. Anterior deviation of the outlet septum.
    C. Hypoplasia of the pulmonary valve.
    D. Posterior deviation of the outlet septum.
    E. Hypoplasia of the branch pulmonary arteries.

CASE 2

*A 2-day-old baby boy is transferred to a tertiary care center for decreased oxygen saturation (80%) at discharge. Saturations did not improve with 100% O_2. ▶ **Video 33.2A** (parasternal long-axis view) and **Video 33.2B** (parasternal short axis view).*

31. What is the diagnosis of the patient in **Case 2**?
    A. DORV.
    B. Anomalous origin of coronary arteries.
    C. L-TGA.
    D. D-TGA.
    E. Truncus arteriosus.

32. What is the most common associated anomaly with this condition?
    A. LVOT obstruction.
    B. Coarctation of the aorta.
    C. VSD.
    D. ASD.
    E. Coronary anomalies.

33. In this condition in **Case 2**, which is the **TRUE** statement about the best source of intracardiac mixing?
    A. At the atrial level.
    B. At the ventricular level.
    C. At the PDA level.
    D. The degree of mixing does not matter.
    E. None the above

CASE 3

*A 12-year-old boy is seen at the cardiology clinic for shortness of breath with exertion. In the clinic, his saturation is 79%. Echocardiography is shown in ▶ **Video 33.3A,B**.*

34. What is the diagnosis of the patient in **Case 3**?
A. TAPVR.
B. Ebstein anomaly of the tricuspid valve.
C. Hypoplastic left heart syndrome (HLHS).
D. Truncus arteriosus.
E. None of the above

35. The most diagnostic echocardiographic feature of this condition is:
A. Displacement index >8 mm/m².
B. Sail like anterior tricuspid leaflet.
C. Posterior leaflet tethering to RV free wall.
D. Dilated tricuspid valve annulus.
E. RV dilatation.

36. What is the most common associated abnormality?
A. Accessory conduction pathway.
B. VSD.
C. Pulmonary stenosis.
D. Presence of left superior vena cava.
E. ASD/PFO.

CASE 4

A 24-year-old, insulin-dependent diabetic woman is referred for fetal echocardiography. The following images are obtained (Video 33.4A–C).

37. The fetal echocardiographic images from **Case 4** (Video 33.4A-C) are consistent with which of the following diagnoses?
A. Tricuspid atresia.
B. D-TGA.
C. Ebstein anomaly of the tricuspid valve.
D. Truncus arteriosus.
E. TOF.

38. For the patient in **Case 4**, immediately after birth, recommended therapy would be:
A. Emergency Blalock-Taussig shunt.
B. Starting prostaglandin E1 infusion.
C. Balloon atrial septostomy.
D. Observation.
E. Intubation and ventilation.

39. Which of the following is the most likely surgical option for the patient in **Case 4**?
A. Two ventricle repair at 6 months of age.
B. Bilateral Glenn operation at 6 months of age followed by Fontan operation at 2–3 years of age.
C. Norwood operation at 1 week of age.
D. Heart transplant.
E. No surgical option.

CASE 5

A 2-month-old baby with mild cyanosis and cardiomegaly on chest x-ray has an echocardiogram that shows four chambers and four valves with a normal great artery relationship. TAPVR is suspected due to right heart enlargement and a right-to-left atrial shunt.

40. Which is a **TRUE** statement about the type of TAPVR shown in this suprasternal view in **Video 33.5** from the patient in **Case 5**?
A. Never associated with obstruction.
B. Almost always associated with obstruction.
C. Associated with an intact atrial septum.
D. Most common form of TAPVR.
E. Produces profound cyanosis of the newborn.

41. In **Case 5**, which of the following echocardiographic features describes this condition?
A. The left atrium is usually normal in size.
B. The RV is dilated.
C. The atrial and ventricular septum bow into the right side of the heart.
D. Doppler is usually not helpful to establish pulmonary venous connection.
E. The pulmonary artery is often hypoplastic.

42. With TAPVR, in order to identify the location of the pulmonary veins, the echocardiographer needs to examine:
A. The RV.
B. The LV.
C. The systemic veins.
D. The aorta.
E. The ductus arteriosus.

ANSWERS

1. **Answer: D.** Tetralogy of Fallot is the most common form of cyanotic congenital heart disease.

   Common congenital cyanotic heart defects can be remembered using the pneumonic "5 Ts" and a miscellaneous category. The 5 Ts include: (1) Tetralogy of Fallot (10%); (2) Transposition of great arteries (5%); (3) Truncus arteriosus (1%); (4) Tricuspid atresia (1%); and (5) Total anomalous pulmonary venous return (1%).

   Other important groups of cyanotic heart disease include single ventricle such as hypoplastic left heart syndrome, double inlet left ventricle and other univentricular heart variants, Ebstein anomaly, pulmonary atresia with intact ventricular septum, and double outlet right ventricle. Occasionally, L-transposition of great arteries may present with cyanosis due to associated lesions (**Table 33.1**). The incidence of congenital heart defects ranges between 0.5% and 0.8% of live births.

   Table 33.1. Cyanotic Congenital Heart Disease

   5 Ts
   - Tetralogy of Fallot (TOF)
   - Transposition of great arteries (d-TGA)
   - Truncus arteriosus
   - Tricuspid atresia (TA)
   - Total anomalous pulmonary venous return (TAPVR)

   Other Defects
   - Hypoplastic left heart syndrome (HLHS)
   - Other single ventricle variants
   - Pulmonary atresia/intact ventricular septum (PA/IVS)
   - Critical pulmonary stenosis
   - Double outlet right ventricle (DORV)

2. **Answer: A.** Eisenmenger syndrome is referred to severe pulmonary hypertension and reversal of shunt from right to left resulting in cyanosis in patients. This is seen in patients with a shunt lesion such as ventricular septal defect, patent ductus arteriosus, or atrioventricular canal defect as in this case. It results from irreversible changes in the pulmonary vascular bed also referred to as pulmonary vascular obstructive disease. The timing for onset of these irreversible changes varies anytime between infancy to adulthood. Patients exposed to similar amounts of increased pulmonary blood flow with atrial septal defect tend to develop these changes less often or later compared to those who are exposed to increased pulmonary blood flow under higher pressures such as with VSD, PDA, or TGA. Patients with Down syndrome/trisomy 21 with a shunt lesion also have a predilection toward developing pulmonary vascular occlusive disease compared to their normal counterparts. Answer B is incorrect as the restriction of blood flow at the ventricle septal defect should protect the pulmonary vascular bed and hence the shunt should remain left to right. Answer C which is mild AV valve regurgitation may be seen through the cleft present in the mitral valve with an AVSD but should not contribute toward right-to-left shunting at the ventricular level. Answer D, PAPVC should not impact ventricular level shunting. Gooseneck deformity of the left ventricular outflow tract is a feature of an AV canal defect; however, this would not affect shunting at the ventricular level. Importantly, Eisenmenger syndrome is a sequence of events where (1) there is development of pulmonary vascular occlusive disease; (2) a shunt lesion (usually a large VSD, PDA, AV canal defect, unrepaired truncus arteriosus, and rarely ASD); and (3) shunt reversal with right to left flow with resulting cyanosis and erythrocytosis.

3. **Answer: A.** This patient has truncus arteriosus in which a single arterial vessel (truncus) gives rise to aorta, pulmonary arteries, and coronary arteries. A large VSD is always present. One-third of patients with truncus will have DiGeorge syndrome. Seventy percent of patients with DiGeorge syndrome have microdeletions of chromosome 22q11.2. Answer B is incorrect because this lesion is not ductal dependent as there is no restriction to pulmonary blood flow. Answer C is incorrect as there is no dependence on ASD which tends to be seen in AV valve atresia such as tricuspid atresia or mitral atresia. Answer D is incorrect as there is mixing of oxygenated and deoxygenated blood in truncus lowering the saturation to less than 100%. Truncus arteriosus may not be associated with profound cyanosis. Answer E is incorrect as surgical repair is often carried out in the newborn due to a high incidence of development of pulmonary vascular disease/ Eisenmenger syndrome. Surgical repair includes closure of the VSD and placement of a right ventricle to pulmonary artery conduit.

4. **Answer: C.** The correct answer is C because patients with TOF have systemic right ventricular systolic pressure due to the presence of a large VSD and equalization of pressures. The simplified Bernoulli equation ($P = 4V^2$) would predict a right ventricular systolic pressure of 90 mm Hg which would be same as systemic pressure. Answer A is incorrect as patients with TOF have pulmonary stenosis protecting their pulmonary vascular beds and therefore are unlikely to develop pulmonary hypertension. Answer B is incorrect as high right ventricular

pressure does not imply a tricuspid valve problem. Answer D is incorrect as VSD in TOF patients does not close or get restricted over time. Answer E is incorrect as patients with TOF can have systemic RV pressure and there is no reason to suspect that tricuspid valve Doppler signal is in incorrect.

5. **Answer: A.** This patient has d-transposition of great arteries as the posterior great artery arising from the morphologic LV bifurcates. TGA can be D or L malposed. In D-TGA, the morphologic RV gives rise to aorta and morphologic LV gives rise to pulmonary artery. There is atrioventricular (AV) concordance and ventricular arterial (VA) discordance. The aortic valve is anterior and to the right of pulmonary valve, an arrangement clearly seen in parasternal short-axis view. In L-TGA, the right atrium is connected to the morphologic LV which gives rise to the pulmonary artery and the left atrium is connected to the morphologic RV which gives rise to aorta. There is AV discordance and VA discordance. The aortic valve is anterior and to the left of the pulmonary valve in parasternal short-axis view. Answers B, C, D, and E are incorrect because the patient does not have a single arterial trunk giving rise to the aorta and pulmonary arteries; as in truncus arteriosus, there is no information to suggest coarctation of the aorta, pulmonary atresia, or anomalous pulmonary drainage.

6. **Answer: E.** Ebstein anomaly is the most likely defect to go unnoticed during childhood and be diagnosed for the first time in adulthood. This anomaly consists of downward displacement of the septal and posterior leaflets of the tricuspid valve into the RV cavity such that a portion of the RV is incorporated in the right atrium/atrialized RV. An interatrial communication is often present with right-to-left shunting. Some patients with mild displacement, mild AV valve regurgitation, and no atrial communication may go unnoticed until later in life or never get diagnosed. Answers A, B, C, and D are incorrect as tetralogy of Fallot will get attention due to a heart murmur, and TAPVR, TGA, and tricuspid atresia will get attention due to a heart murmur and/or cyanosis.

7. **Answer: E.** Clinical cyanosis occurs when the amount of reduced hemoglobin reaches 5 g/100 mL. Cyanosis can be due to desaturation of arterial blood or increased extraction of oxygen by peripheral tissue. Cyanosis secondary to desaturation of arterial blood is central cyanosis; the latter is peripheral cyanosis. Of note, cyanosis will be recognized at a higher level of oxygen saturation in patients with polycythemia and at lower level of oxygen saturation in patients with anemia. In cyanotic CHD, the primary physiologic abnormality can be: (1) arterial desaturation due to a right-to-left intracardiac shunt; (2) mixing of pulmonary and systemic venous return or; (3) secondary to a parallel circulation like TGA. The magnitude of arterial desaturation will be dependent on the severity of right ventricular outflow tract obstruction hence the right-to-left shunting or degree of intracardiac mixing. The correct answer is decreased pulmonary blood flow and right-to-left intracardiac shunting. TOF is the most common cyanotic heart disease where cyanosis is due to pulmonary stenosis, decreased pulmonary flow, and increased right-to-left shunting.

8. **Answer: C.** This patient has arterial desaturation based on pulse oximetry and early appearance of bubbles (saline contrast) in the left atrium which is suggestive of a right-to-left shunt. Based on all the choices available, answer C is the only one where there is a systemic venous to systemic arterial shunt. The coronary sinus runs along the posterior wall of the left atrium and unroofing brings the blue blood in the coronary sinus in direct connection with the left atrium. Bilateral superior vena cava with or without a bridging vein will drain into the right atrium and will not allow the saline contrast to appear in the left atrium immediately after injection. A total anomalous pulmonary venous connection may have a right-to-left shunt at the atrial level but will not result in detection of bubbles immediately on saline contrast injection.

9. **Answer: E.** In TAPVR, all pulmonary veins drain into a common pulmonary vein which then drains abnormally into either the left innominate vein, SVC, coronary sinus, portal vein, or other rare sites. When the pulmonary veins drain into structures above the heart such as left innominate vein or SVC, it is referred to a *supracardiac* TAPVR. When the pulmonary veins drain into the coronary sinus, it is called *cardiac* TAPVR. When the pulmonary veins drain below the diaphragm into the portal vein or other rare sites it is called *infracardiac* TAPVR. Infracardiac TAPVR is most likely to be obstructed. There can be a mixed type where some pulmonary veins drain above, at, or below the heart level. Pulmonary veins draining into the left atrium are normal and not a form of TAPVR. Answer E is correct.

10. **Answer: E.** The correct answer is coarctation of aorta which can be diagnosed on arch images and cannot be diagnosed on parasternal images. The differential diagnosis for a large VSD with an overriding great vessel includes: (1) TOF; (2) DORV; (3) Truncus arteriosus; (4) Pulmonary atresia with VSD; and (5) D-TGA with VSD. In each case, the parasternal view may be similar but the great vessel may not always be the aorta. The key is to identify the aorta from the pulmonary artery and its relative position/origin.

11. **Answer: A.** In tricuspid atresia, there is a plate-like structure in the region of the tricuspid valve and no valve. The right atrium is enlarged. An atrial

communication is always present. There is an obligatory right-to-left shunt. Tricuspid atresia is classified on the basis of associated defects. Type I: Normally related great vessels (75%); type II: D-transposition of great arteries; type III: malposition of the great arteries other than D-transposition. A VSD may be absent, small or large. The correct answer is A since an atrial communication is always present. B, C, D, and E are incorrect. A PDA may or may not be needed for survival based on the associated defects. The great arteries may or may not be transposed. A right aortic arch is rarely seen with tricuspid atresia.

12. **Answer: B.** This patient has pulmonary venous hypertension as a result of obstruction in the pulmonary venous baffle. Answer A is incorrect because obstruction in the systemic venous baffle would result in right heart failure/right-sided congestion including hepatomegaly, ascites, and lower extremity edema. Answer C is incorrect as this patient did not have a LeCompte maneuver. The LeCompte maneuver is performed when an arterial switch operation is performed for D-TGA. This patient underwent an atrial switch operation described below. Answer D is incorrect as the question does not mention that the patient had a RV to PA conduit. Answer E is incorrect as patients with an atrial switch operation are not at any higher risk for coronary artery issues.

In D-TGA, the pathway of blood flow is as follows: IVC and SVC--> RA--> tricuspid valve--> RV--> aorta. Pulmonary veins--> LA--> mitral valve--> LV--> pulmonary artery. The pulmonary and systemic circulation are parallel as opposed to being in series in the normal heart (see **Figure 33.12A,B**).

In the 1960s, D-TGA was corrected by switching the atria (atrial switch operation) also referred to as a Mustard or Senning procedure. A systemic venous baffle was created between the IVC and SVC to the mitral valve draining blue blood into the LV and out to the lungs through the pulmonary artery to get oxygenated. A pulmonary venous baffle was created draining the oxygenated blood from the pulmonary veins to the right-sided tricuspid valve, RV, and out to the body through the aorta (see **Figure 33.12C,D**).

In 1976, the first arterial switch operation also referred to as the Jatene operation was performed where instead of switching the atria, the great arteries were switched (**Figure 33.12E**). Starting in the late 1980s, the atrial switch operation was abandoned and D-TGA was repaired solely by switching the aorta and the pulmonary artery in the newborn (arterial switch procedure/Jatene). This involved some manipulation/repositioning of the branch pulmonary arteries referred to as the LeCompte maneuver which predisposed the pulmonary arteries to a variable degree of stenosis. In the arterial switch operation, the coronary arteries were also relocated to the neo-aorta (previous pulmonary valve) with a button around them predisposing them to stenosis/obstruction in the future.

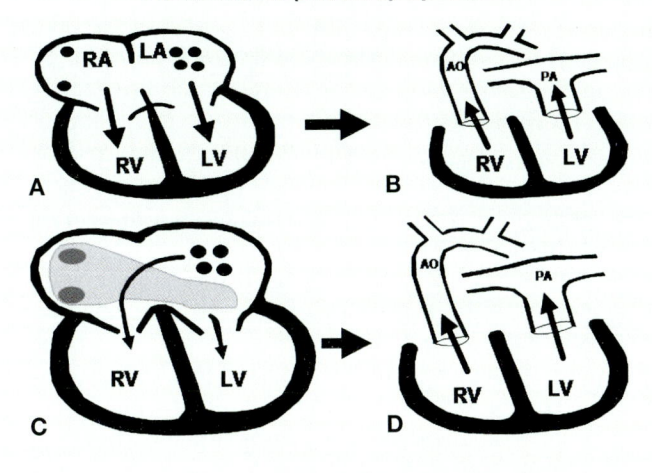

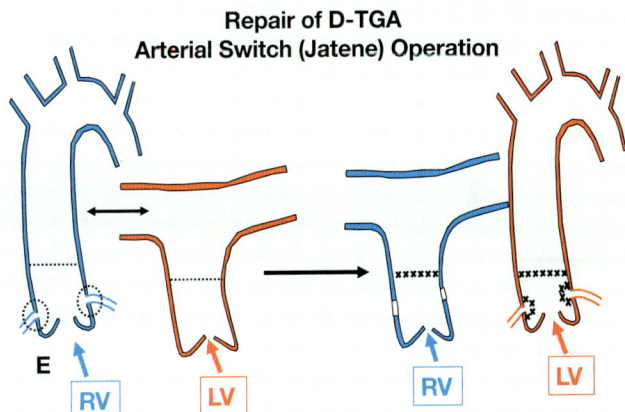

Figure 33.12. **A:** There is atrio-ventricular concordance and hence RA is connected to RV and LA to LV. **B:** There is ventriculo arterial discordance and hence RV is connected to AO and LV is connected to PA. **C:** After an atrial switch operation, the blood from the inferior and superior vena cavae, entering the RA, is directed, via an atrial baffle, toward the mitral valve and LV. Pulmonary venous blood travels anterior to this baffle to the RV. **D:** The redirected blood travels from RV to AO and LV to PA as before but oxygenation is now normal due to switched atria. **E:** In arterial switch operation, the great arteries are switched. RV is now connected to PA and LV to AO. RA, right atrium; LA, left atrium; RV, right ventricle; LV, left ventricle; AO, aorta; PA, pulmonary artery.

13. **Answer: D.** Truncus arteriosus is a lesion in which the aorta and the pulmonary arteries arise from a common arterial trunk, which overrides a large ventricular septal defect (VSD). Surgery is performed within the first few weeks of life and consists of separating the pulmonary arteries from the aorta, placing a RV to PA conduit, and patch closure of the VSD. This conduit does not grow with the patient and is subject to calcifications. A patient may require multiple replacements throughout a lifetime. Conduit stenosis is often first detected echocardiographically on spectral Doppler interrogation of the conduit itself or by estimating elevated right ventricular systolic pressures via tricuspid regurgitation jet velocities (choice D). Patients with unrepaired truncus arteriosus or delayed repairs may develop pulmonary hypertension, but unlikely given the time course in

this patient, making answer A incorrect. Answer B is incorrect as truncal valve stenosis is a known complication but will not raise right ventricular pressures and can be detected echocardiographically. A modified Blalock-Taussig (BT) shunt is a palliative surgery not needed in patients with truncus arteriosus. Hence, answer C is incorrect. Answer E is also incorrect as worsening pulmonary vein stenosis is unlikely given that the pulmonary veins are not involved in surgical management of this condition.

14. **Answer: B.** There is profound hypoxia with saturations of 60% suggestive of continuous right-to-left shunting across the PDA (Answer B). Pulmonary artery pressures can be high/systemic in the presence of a large PDA; however, this patient likely has pulmonary hypertension, based on the supra-systemic right ventricular systolic pressures. It would also be typical to see right-to-left shunting at the atrial level under these conditions. This situation actually occurs relatively frequently in newborn nurseries and may be provoked by severe respiratory problems such as meconium aspiration. A continuous left-to-right shunt would be expected in a patient with a PDA in whom the pulmonary vascular resistance has begun to fall, which usually occurs normally in the first few hours of life. Bidirectional shunts may occur with a large PDA, and the predominance of flow in one direction or the other is dictated by the relative pulmonary or systemic vascular resistance at that time. However, bidirectional shunting would not produce the profound hypoxemia seen here.

15. **Answer: E.** The echocardiogram must be focused to image the atrial septum. In patients with D-TGA, systemic and pulmonary circulations are in parallel and for survival, mixing between oxygenated and deoxygenated blood has to occur at the atrial, ventricular and or ductal level. The atrial septum is by far the most effective place for mixing of saturated and desaturated blood to take place. If the atrial communication/mixing is inadequate, pronounced cyanosis will occur, even if the ductus arteriosus is widely patent. Answer A is incorrect as it is not likely for pulmonary venous issues to present with severe cyanosis. Answer B is incorrect as in this case, prostaglandin E1 is running and hence the PDA is less likely to be an issue. Answer C is incorrect as aortic arch issues may present with poor perfusion but not particularly cyanotic. Answer D is incorrect as systemic venous issues are not commonly seen in DTGA and will not account for this presentation.

16. **Answer: D.** This patient has tetralogy of Fallot (TOF). **Figure 33.1A** shows a malaligned ventricular septal defect and overriding of aorta. **Figure 33.1B** shows right ventricular outflow tract obstruction in the form of infundibular (subpulmonary) narrowing (*). TOF (**Figure 33.13**) is a conotruncal anomaly consisting of: (1) VSD; (2) pulmonary stenosis; (3) overriding aorta; and (4) right ventricular hypertrophy. The VSD in TOF is usually large and nonrestrictive. This will result in equalization of pressure between the two ventricles. RV pressure will be same as LV/systemic.

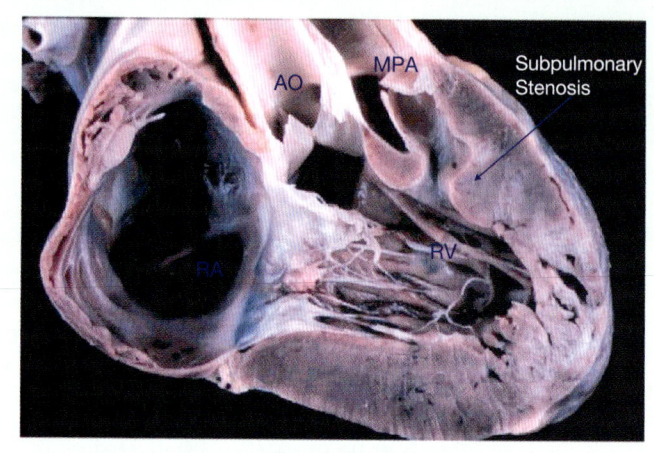

Figure 33.13

17. **Answer: A.** The patient has hypoplastic left heart syndrome (HLHS), which is a ductal-dependent lesion. The image in **Figure 33.2A** shows HLHS in an apical 4-chamber view which demonstrates two atria with a single ventricle and single AV valve. The left atrium is small and there is no obvious second AV valve. **Figure 33.2B** HLHS in a suprasternal view showing a diminutive ascending aorta. **Figure 33.14** is the same image with three arrows outlining the extremely hypoplastic ascending aorta and the aortic arch. HLHS consists of varying degrees of aortic stenosis or atresia, mitral stenosis or atresia, coarctation of the aorta, and hypoplasia of the LV and aortic arch. The ductus arteriosus must be kept open to supply blood to the systemic circulation, until a Norwood (stage I) palliative surgery can be performed. Answer B is incorrect as initiation of 100% FiO$_2$ is not recommended, as it will increase pulmonary blood flow and decrease systemic blood flow further in the face of systemic (aortic arch) obstruction. Cardiac output is maintained in this

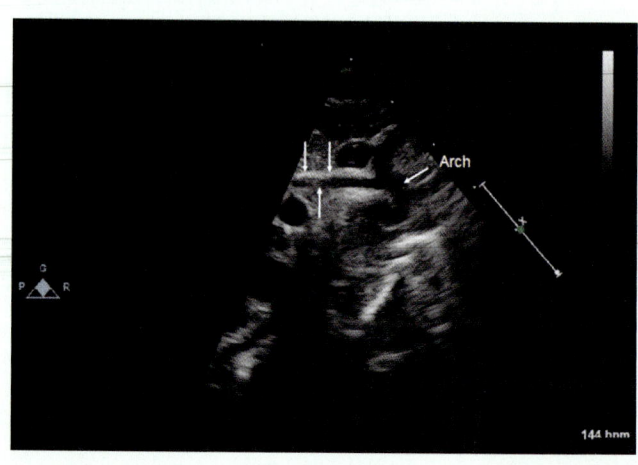

Figure 33.14

case as follows: oxygenated blood from pulmonary veins into LA, crossing the atrial septum through PFO/ASD, reaching RA, into RV through tricuspid valve, entering main PA, ductus arteriosus and then descending aorta bypassing the coarctation and hypoplastic aortic arch. Answer C is incorrect as *a left-to-right* atrial level shunt is essential to maintaining cardiac output. Answer D is incorrect as Down syndrome is not associated with HLHS. It is commonly seen in patients with AV canal defects and vice versa. Answer E is incorrect as a right aortic arch is very rare with this condition.

18. **Answer: B.** This patient has Ebstein anomaly of the tricuspid valve. Characteristic findings include apical (downward) displacement of the septal and posterior leaflets of the tricuspid valve into the RV to varying degrees. The arrows in **Figure 33.15** show the tricuspid valve annulus. The portion of the right ventricle between the true valve annulus and the displaced valve leaflets constitutes "atrialized" portion of the RV (marked with stars in **Figure 33.3**) that is continuous with the true RA. WPW syndrome/pre-excitation may be present in 20% of the patients with this condition leading to palpitations. Answers A, C, D, and E are incorrect.

In Ebstein anomaly, the effective RV size is reduced depending upon the severity of the tricuspid valve displacement. However, it is not associated with hypoplasia of right ventricle.

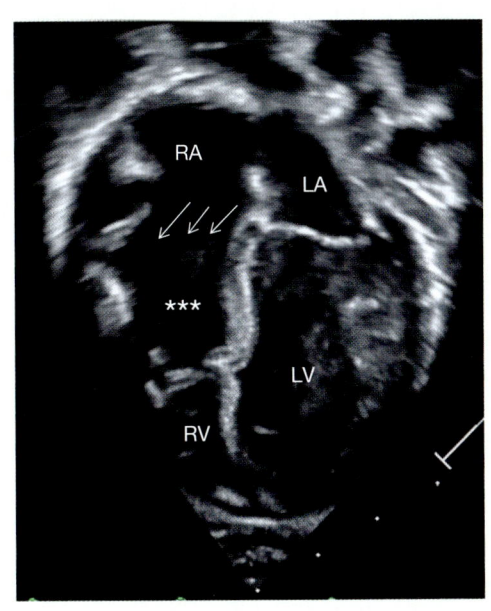

Figure 33.15

19. **Answer: C.** This patient has D-TGA defined as a connection of the RV→ aorta and LV→ pulmonary artery as described above. This abnormal ventricular arterial connection is also termed "ventriculoarterial discordance," a result of abnormal conotruncal septation. The atria are connected to the respective ventricles in D-TGA (atrioventricular concordance). Great artery position is a key to identify the type of transposition (D vs L). In transposition, the two great arteries course parallel to one another with the aorta being anterior, a distinctly different arrangement from the normal anteriorly placed pulmonary valve/artery crossing over the aortic root (**Figures 33.4A and 33.16B**). Normally, the pulmonary artery wraps in the front of the aorta as it courses posteriorly. In D-TGA, the aorta arises from the RV and is anterior and rightward of the pulmonary valve (**Figures 33.4B and 33.16A**). In L-TGA, the great arteries are again parallel, and the aorta is anterior but now leftward to the pulmonary valve (**Figure 33.16C**).

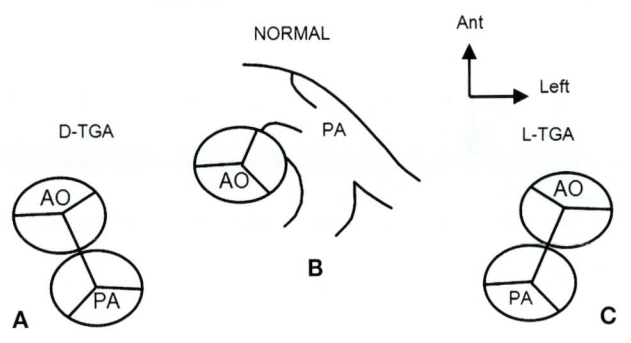

Figure 33.16

20. **Answer: A.** The oxygen saturation is determined by the severity of RVOT obstruction or how much blood goes across the RVOT. **Figure 33.5A** shows a parasternal long-axis view with a large VSD with overriding aorta. **Figure 33.5B** shows a parasternal short-axis view with narrowing of the RVOT, hypoplastic pulmonary valve, and hypoplastic main pulmonary artery. This is consistent with the diagnosis of TOF. It is important to note that in TOF, RVOT obstruction can be at any level and can be at multiple levels—subvalvar, valvar, and/or supravalvar. The degree of aortic override is usually about 50% but has been observed to range from 15% to 95% in one echocardiographic study. Answers B, C, D are incorrect as the size of the VSD, degree of overriding aorta, and size of the ASD have nothing to do with the degree of cyanosis. Cyanosis is a result of less pulmonary blood flow and more right-to-left shunt based on severity of the RVOT obstruction. Based on the severity of RVOT obstruction, TOF can be classified as (shown in **Figure 33.17**): (A) "Pink" tetralogy, (B) Classic tetralogy, and (C) Pulmonary atresia/VSD (TOF with pulmonary atresia).

In the "pink" form of TOF, there is minimal narrowing/RVOT obstruction. These infants will

"Pink tetralogy"
Mild pulmonary stenosis
A

Classic tetralogy
B

Severe tetralogy or pulmonary atresia
C

Figure 33.17

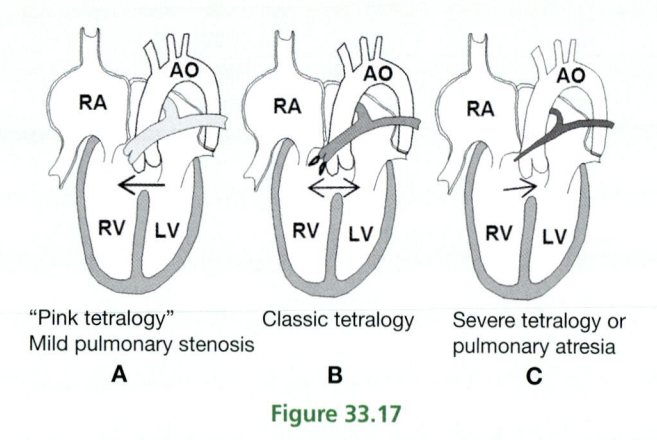

have very little or no cyanosis at all and will behave like a large VSD with breathing symptoms due to pulmonary overcirculation. In the classic TOF, there is significant amount of RVOT obstruction and these patients may need a palliative shunt surgery (Blalock-Taussig shunt) in the early period of their life to provide adequate pulmonary blood flow and then a complete repair. Patients may start life "pink" and progress to a cyanotic stage with time. Patients with pulmonary atresia/TOF have extreme right ventricular outflow tract obstruction with no forward flow across the pulmonary valve and are ductal dependent. They will need prostaglandin and then a palliative shunt in the immediate newborn to provide pulmonary blood flow (**Tables 33.2-33.4**).

21. **Answer: D.** In Ebstein anomaly, the apical displacement of the valve reduces the effective volume of the right ventricle available for pumping function and the valve itself may be regurgitant to a varying degree. Tricuspid regurgitation and poor forward flow results in right-to-left shunt at the atrial level. Right-to-left shunting can be worse during exertion leading to symptoms of exercise intolerance. Answers A, B, C, and E are incorrect as we see a displaced tricuspid valve not consistent with tricuspid atresia, pulmonary hypertension, Uhl anomaly, or ASD. Uhl anomaly, first described in 1980, is an extremely rare (less than 100 cases reported so far) congenital heart defect characterized by an almost total absence of the right ventricular myocardium and a normal tricuspid valve.

22. **Answer: A.** The image shows a large VSD with an overriding great vessel. The differential diagnosis for this image includes defects with an anterior malalignment VSD (Answers B, C, and D) and truncus arteriosus (Answer E). This image is not consistent with a diagnosis of interrupted aortic arch which is associated with posterior malalignment of the ventricular septum. Parasternal long-axis views

Table 33.3. Operative Concepts: Congenital Heart Disease

Holes, shunts	Close them (patch, suture)
Obstruction	Open it up (resection, conduit)
Decreased pulmonary flow	Add some (shunt)
Increased pulmonary flow	Restrict it (band)
One pump	Use it for systemic flow (Fontan)
Conduits, artificial valves do not grow and do not last forever	Anything in this category will likely need to be redone

Table 33.4. Cyanotic Congenital Heart Disease Surgical Repairs

	Surgical Repair
Tetralogy of Fallot	Palliative procedure: Blalock–Taussig shunt Complete repair: closure of VSD, relief of right ventricular outflow tract obstruction
Transposition of great arteries (d-TGA)	Palliative procedure: Balloon atrial septostomy Complete repair: arterial switch operation/Jatene operation Previously performed: atrial switch operation/Mustard or Senning procedure
Tricuspid atresia	Staged Fontan palliation
Total anomalous pulmonary venous return	Rerouting of pulmonary veins to left atrium
Truncus arteriosus	Complete repair: VSD closure, RV to pulmonary artery conduit

Table 33.2. Cyanotic Congenital Heart Disease

Increased Pulmonary Blood Flow	Decreased Pulmonary Blood Flow
Truncus arteriosus	Tetralogy of Fallot
Total anomalous pulmonary venous return	Tricuspid atresia
Transposition of great arteries (sometimes)	Pulmonary atresia/intact ventricular septum
	Critical pulmonary stenosis

of an interrupted aortic arch would most commonly demonstrate subaortic stenosis and aortic valve hypoplasia along with the VSD.

23. **Answer: C.** This infant has truncus arteriosus. The parasternal long-axis view shows the malalignment VSD and overriding great vessel, similar to many other conotruncal abnormalities. In **Figure 33.18A**, we see a common truncal valve (TV), single trunk/vessel (SV) dividing into ascending aorta (AA) and main pulmonary artery (MPA). In **Figure 33.18B,C** color flow Doppler confirmed division of the SV into AA and MPA (two arrows).

Answers A and B are incorrect, as even though the parasternal long-axis view can look similar, the apical outflow view (**Figure 33.8A**) reveals a common trunk giving rise to both aorta and pulmonary artery. Answer D is incorrect as truncus arteriosus is associated with DiGeorge (22q11 del) syndrome not with trisomy 21. VSD and complete atrioventricular canal defect are associated with trisomy 21. Answer E is incorrect as the echo images in TAPVR will not reveal large VSD/overriding great vessel.

24. **Answer: B.** This patient has pulmonary valve atresia. Even though there is a valve like structure, it never opens and there is no forward flow or regurgitation across the pulmonary valve, establishing the atresia. Pulmonary atresia is divided into two broad categories based on the presence or absence of a VSD. These two categories actually describe very different anatomic entities. These are: (1) pulmonary atresia with intact ventricular septum (PA/IVS) and (2) pulmonary atresia with VSD (PA/VSD). PA/IVS is commonly referred to as the "hypoplastic right heart syndrome." PA/IVS will have varying degrees of right ventricular hypoplasia and may frequently need to be repaired as a single ventricle. PA/VSD is a severe form of TOF. The correct answer is B as once we establish that there is pulmonary atresia, we need to know if there is a VSD or not. Answer A is incorrect as presence or absence of an ASD will not change the surgical management. Answer C is incorrect as size of the LV would not matter and are normal in both forms of pulmonary atresia. Answers D and E are incorrect as this condition is not associated with arch anomalies or pulmonary vein anomalies.

25. **Answer: D.** Patients with tricuspid atresia eventually get Fontan surgery using a lateral tunnel or extracardiac conduit. This patient has a lateral tunnel as seen in **Figure 33.10**. This is a typical echocardiographic appearance of a lateral tunnel traveling through the right atrium and connecting the IVC to the pulmonary arteries. Answer A is incorrect as a right atrial thrombus would be expected to have a homogeneous, echogenic appearance. Answer B is incorrect as a redundant eustachian valve typically connects to the atrial septum and does not have a circular appearance. Answer C is incorrect as the appearance of a cast from a previous intracardiac line does not have similar appearance. Answer E is incorrect as RV to PA conduit will not be seen in the region of right atrium.

26. **Answer: C. Figure 33.11** is highly suspicious of TAPVR, where the pulmonary veins come together as a confluence, posterior and superior to the left atrium. This is called a pulmonary venous confluence. In 1/3 of cases, the confluence drains into the heart by an ascending vein that joins the innominate vein or SVC and then to the right atrium (supracardiac type, most common); in approximately 16%, the confluence drains directly to the coronary sinus (coronary sinus

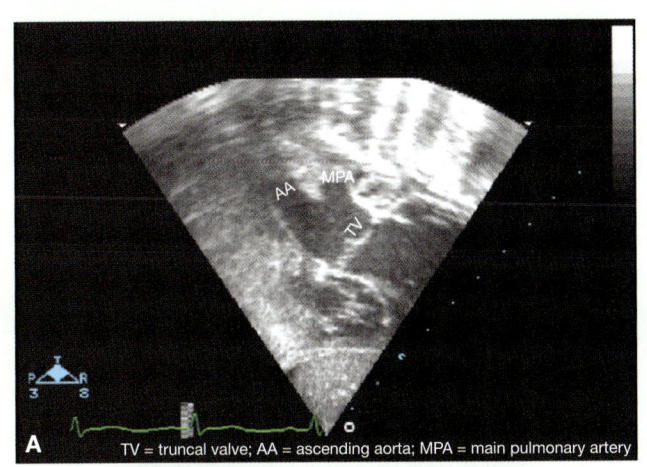

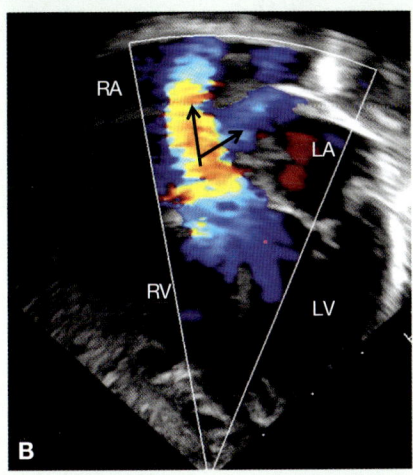

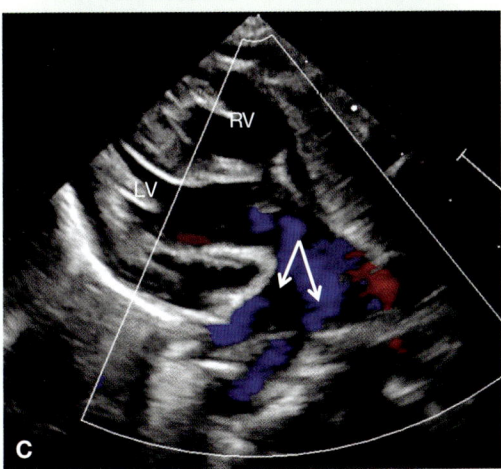

Figure 33.18

type) and in 15%, the veins connect directly to the right atrium (cardiac type); in approximately 13%, the confluence drains by way of a descending vein, below the diaphragm, to the portal vein, hepatic vein, inferior vena cava, or ductus venosus (infracardiac type). TAPVR has an obligatory right-to-left shunt at the atrial level, and in the echo image, we see the atrial septum pushed into the left atrium.

Answer A is not correct as there is no reason to suspect effusion and it would have no association with cyanosis. Answer B is not correct as truncus arteriosus is an anterior structure arising from the ventricles. Answer D is incorrect as a mediastinal mass would usually appear as a bright echogenic area. Answer E is not correct as descending aorta would be seen as a circular structure behind the left atrium and would have no association with leftward shift of the atrial septum, enlarged right atrium, and right ventricle.

27. **Answer: B.** Video 33.1A shows an overriding of aorta with malaligned VSD. Video 33.1B shows an infundibular narrowing along with a hypoplastic pulmonary valve and pulmonary artery. This combination of findings is diagnostic of TOF.

28. **Answer: A.** In TOF, cyanosis can progress secondary to hypertrophy of the infundibular septum and increase in RVOT obstruction. This is due to a decrease in pulmonary blood flow and increased right-to-left shunting at the ventricular level. Worsening of cyanosis can be a major determinant of the timing of surgical repair. Cyanosis can be more pronounced when the child cries.

Answer B is incorrect as the patient does not have "Tet spells." Episodes of increased cyanosis due to hypoxemia are called "Tet spells," during which time the child is breathing fast (hyperpneic). These occur due to an acute increase in right-to-left shunting through the VSD; hence, answer B is incorrect. Various etiologies have been proposed, such as dynamic obstruction at the infundibular level, increase in pulmonary vascular resistance, and decrease in systemic vascular resistance. Severe and often prolonged decrease in arterial saturation occurs which may lead to metabolic acidosis. Prolonged episodes may be life threatening. During the spell, the murmur of pulmonary stenosis may become diminished or completely disappear suggesting diminished blood flow to the pulmonary arteries. The child may have irritability and or lethargy. This patient had no lethargy and cyanosis with crying and no hyperpnea reported. Answer C is incorrect as the right-to-left shunt increases resulting in bluish discoloration. Answer D is incorrect as LV function remains unchanged until a very late stage where it can become compromised secondary due to severe metabolic acidosis. Answer E is incorrect as there is a decrease and not increase in flow across the pulmonary valve.

29. **Answer: C.** The associated anomalies in TOF are:
    - Valvular pulmonary stenosis (50%-60%).
    - Right aortic arch (25%)—usually mirror image branching.
    - ASD (15%).
    - Coronary anomalies (5%).
    - Additional muscular VSD (2%).
    - Unilateral absent pulmonary artery (rare).

    In current practice, TOF repair includes relieving the RVOT obstruction and patching the VSD (**Figure 33.19A**). The RVOT obstruction is relieved with a transannular patch or with just resection of the muscle bundles in those with adequate sized pulmonary valve. All patients with transannular patch will inevitably develop free pulmonary insufficiency.

    Coronary abnormalities include:

    1. A large conal branch or accessory LAD (10%-15%).
    2. LAD from RCA (5%).
    3. Single coronary artery (4%).
    4. Two coronary ostia arising from the same truncal sinus.
    5. High ostial origin.

    From a surgical perspective, the most important coronary anomaly is the origin of the LAD from RCA as it crosses the RVOT and will interfere with incision required for a transannular patch. To avoid transection of this vessel, surgeons may use a RV to PA conduit. Videos 33.1C and 33.6 show an

Figure 33.19A

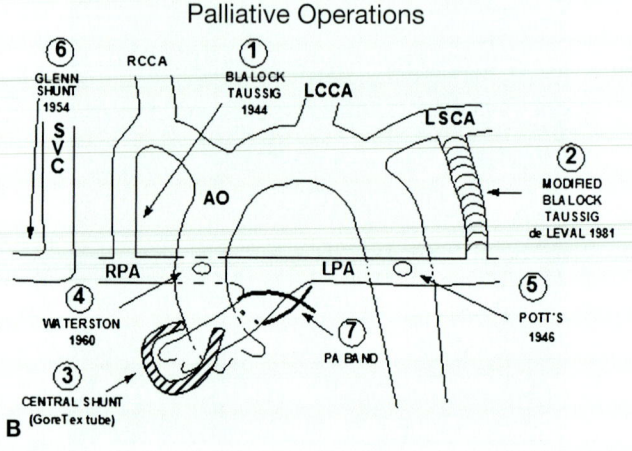

Figure 33.19B

example of an LAD from the RCA. Hence, C is the right answer.

In a small group of patients, a modified Blalock-Taussig (BT) shunt is performed by placing a Goretex tube between the subclavian artery and the ipsilateral pulmonary artery (**Figure 33.19B**). A right aortic arch is seen approximately in 25% of TOF cases. Answer A is incorrect as arch sidedness can affect the side the BT shunt is performed but does not play a role in the final surgery. Answer B is incorrect as presence of an ASD will not change surgical planning. Answer D and E are also incorrect as VSD needs to be closed but does not change surgical planning.

30. **Answer: B.** The infundibular obstruction found in TOF has been postulated to be a result of the anterior displacement of the bulbotruncal ridges with unequal separation of the developing outflow tracts and anterior deviation of the outlet septum. Anterior deviation of this septum results in misalignment of the outlet and trabecular portion of the ventricular septum causing a malaligned VSD and subsequent straddling of the aorta over the malaligned ventricular septum. Answer A is incorrect as RVH is secondary to RVOT obstruction which has resulted from anterior displacement of the outlet septum.

When stenosis or obstruction occurs at one level (in this case at the right ventricular infundibular level), hypoplasia is often present downstream or in the path of blood flow. In this case, it is common to have hypoplasia of the pulmonary valve and pulmonary arteries; hence, Answers C and E are incorrect. Answer D is incorrect as posterior deviation of the outlet septum is seen in the Taussig-Bing variety of double-outlet right ventricle and interrupted aortic arch and not in TOF.

KEY POINTS
Tetralogy of Fallot
(*See also* **Tables 33.1, 33.2, 33.4**; **Figure 33.19**)
- Most common cyanotic defect.
- Primary abnormality is a malaligned VSD (anterior deviation of outlet septum).
- Associated frequently with DiGeorge syndrome or 22q11 deletion (conotruncal anomaly).
- Degree of cyanosis is dependent on degree of RVOT obstruction.
- Three types: "Pink tet," "Classic tet," and pulmonary atresia/VSD.
- Initial repair may be a palliative systemic-pulmonary shunt.
- Corrective repair: relief of RVOT obstruction and VSD closure.
- Pulmonary insufficiency is the most common sequelae after repair.
- May need pulmonary valve replacement in adolescents/adults.

31. **Answer: D.** This patient has D-TGA as we see parallel relationship of the great arteries on the parasternal long-axis view (**Video 33.2A**) and the aorta/aortic valve is anterior and to the right of the pulmonary valve in the parasternal short-axis view (**Video 33.2B**).

32. **Answer: C.** VSD is common and present in about half of cases (40%–45%) of D-TGA. There are basically two forms of D-TGA: (1) with intact ventricular septum and (2) with VSD (usually perimembranous) (**Figure 33.20A,B**). PDA and PFO may be seen in all patients with D-TGA and not necessarily accounted for as associated defects.

Other associated anomalies:
- LVOT obstruction (5% and 10% cases of D-TGA with intact ventricular septum and D-TGA with VSD, respectively).
- Coronary abnormalities: circumflex from the right coronary artery, single coronary artery, or inverted arrangement of coronary arteries (in decreasing frequency).
- ASD.
- Pulmonary stenosis.

D-Transposition of the great arteries

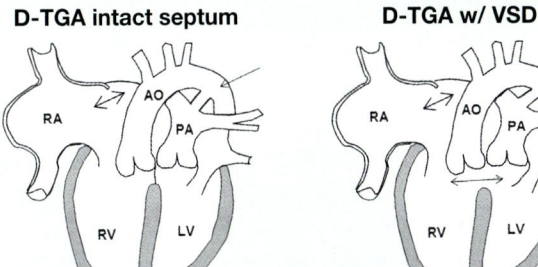

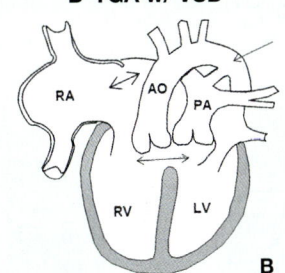

D-TGA intact septum   D-TGA w/ VSD

A   B

Figure 33.20

33. **Answer: A.** In D-TGA, due to parallel circulation, desaturated blood entering the RV reaches the aorta and the systemic circulation and oxygenated blood entering the left atrium/LV goes back to the lungs through the pulmonary arteries. This causes severe systemic desaturation (cyanosis) as deoxygenated blood does not reach the lungs and oxygenated blood does not reach the body. Without intracardiac mixing of systemic and pulmonary venous blood, the neonate will not survive. Survival depends on adequate mixing at the atrial and or PDA level. The best level of mixing is at the atrial level with an unrestricted communication. Hence, the correct answer is A. It is very important to evaluate the size of the atrial communication. In the case of a restrictive atrial septal communication, the child may need emergency balloon atrial septostomy to establish an area of adequate mixing and thereby adequate saturation. ▶ **Video 33.7A** shows balloon septostomy done for a restricted atrial septal

communication. After balloon septostomy, an adequate ASD is seen without any flow acceleration (▶ **Video 33.7B**). Answers B and C are incorrect as the mixing at those levels may be beneficial but still the atrial level is the best site. Answer D is incorrect as degree of mixing contributes toward improved oxygenation.

> **KEY POINTS**
>
> **D-TGA (Transposition of the Great Arteries)**
> (See also **Tables 33.1, 33.2, 33.4; Figures 33.12A-E, 33.16, 33.20, 33.21A,B**)
> - Produces profound early cyanosis.
> - There is AV concordance and VA discordance.
> - The anterior great artery is the aorta arising from the RV.
> - The posterior great artery is the pulmonary artery arising from the LV.
> - VSD is a common associated anomaly.
> - Areas of potential mixing of oxygenated/deoxygenated blood: atrial, ductal, and ventricular levels.
> - The atrium is the most important site for mixing.
> - The original repair was an atrial switch/Mustard/Senning procedure.
> - Current repair includes: arterial switch/Jatene procedure with LeCompte maneuver and coronary reimplantation.
>
> **Figure 33.21**

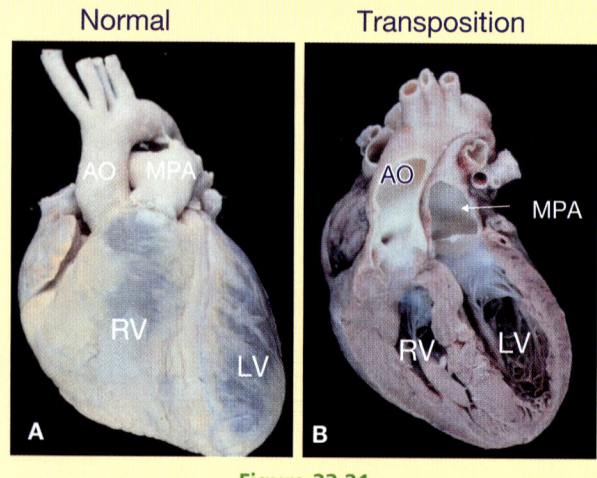

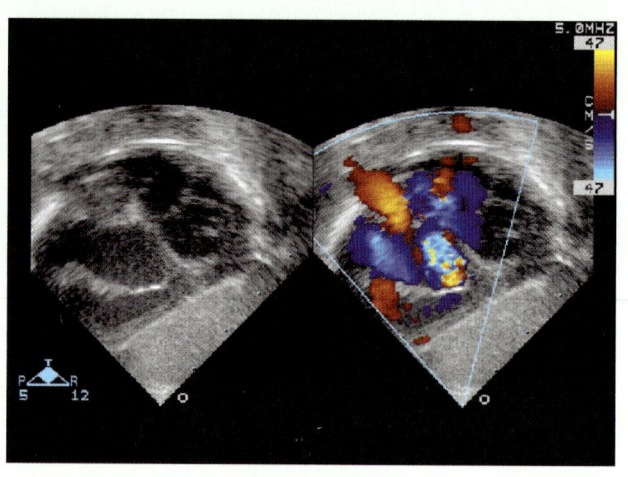

Figure 33.22

Ebstein anomaly is apical displacement of the septal leaflet more than 8 mm/m^2 and this helps make the distinction between true Ebstein and Ebstein like (Ebstenoid) anomaly of the tricuspid valve. This distance is measured along the septum from the insertion point of the mitral valve annulus (presumed insertion of a normal TV) to the actual insertion of the septal leaflet to be diagnostic.

Other echocardiographic findings include:

M-mode
- Paradoxical ventricular septal motion.
- Delayed closure of tricuspid valve leaflets more than 65 ms after mitral valve closure.

Two-dimensional
- Tethering of the posterior leaflet.
- Abnormal morphology of the tricuspid valve leaflet.
- ASD.
- Dilated right atrium.
- Dilated tricuspid valve annulus.
- Dilated RV.
- Left-sided cardiac abnormality in 25% of cases.

Doppler studies
- Varying degrees of tricuspid regurgitation.
- Varying degrees of tricuspid stenosis.
- Right-to-left/bidirectional shunting at atrial level.

34. **Answer: B.** This patient has Ebstein anomaly of the tricuspid valve. The desaturation results primarily from a right-to-left shunt at the atrial level shown in **Figure 33.22**. Answers A, C, and D are incorrect as we see the apically displaced tricuspid valve in **Video 33.3A,B**.

35. **Answer: A.** All the listed choices are features seen in Ebstein anomaly. The criterion to diagnose

36. **Answer: E.** All the listed choices are seen with this condition. An interatrial communication (ASD/PFO) is almost always present in patients with Ebstein anomaly hence the most common associated abnormality. Other choices A, B, and C are not as common. An accessory conduction pathway may be seen in approximately 25% of cases. Pulmonary stenosis and VSD may be seen but not as frequently as ASD/PFO. Answer D is incorrect as left superior vena cava is not associated with Ebstein anomaly.

> **KEY POINTS**
> **Ebstein Anomaly**
> (See also **Figures 33.3** and **Figure 33.6**)
> - A rare anomaly of the tricuspid valve.
> - Diagnostic criteria: Apical displacement of the tricuspid valve annulus >8 mm/m^2.
> - ASD is most common associated finding.
> - Shunting is usually right to left at the atrial level.
> - Significant tricuspid regurgitation may be present.
> - WPW/pre-excitation is seen in 25% of cases.
> - Morphology of the anterior leaflet should be studied for surgical repair.

37. **Answer: A.** Video 33.4A is an equivalent view to a parasternal long-axis view. The aorta and the MPA are shown. However, there is essentially no RV seen. Video 33.4B is a 4-chamber view which reveals a single AV valve and a membrane of tissue where the tricuspid valve should be and no RV. Video 33.4C shows color flow of the outflows. The larger (blue) outflow is the aorta. The smaller (blue) outflow is actually flow through a VSD which will eventually get to the main pulmonary artery. Most importantly, the right AV valve is atretic, consistent with tricuspid atresia. Answers B-E are incorrect. D-TGA can be a challenging fetal diagnosis in that the 4-chamber view often appears to be normal with all four chambers seen. The key is the examination of the outflow tracts. In a normal great artery relationship, the great arteries will "cross" as the pulmonary artery draping anteriorly over the ascending aorta. In D-TGA, the arteries assume a parallel course. Careful investigation can establish that the aorta arises from the RV and the pulmonary artery arises from the LV. Ebstein anomaly of the tricuspid valve would be diagnosed by an apically displaced tricuspid valve, seen in a 4-chamber view, not shown in these clips. This finding is often accompanied by tricuspid valve regurgitation and an enlarged right atrium. Truncus arteriosus is suspected when both the pulmonary and systemic outflows arise from a common arterial trunk which overrides a VSD. TOF is diagnosed by identifying an anterior malalignment VSD, resulting in an overriding aorta and RVOT obstruction.

38. **Answer: D.** In most cases of tricuspid atresia, there is adequate pulmonary and aortic blood flow. The correct answer to this question is based on an impression of the amount of flow through the VSD, which seems adequate in Video 33.4C. Many children with this problem are reasonably well saturated at birth and require little initial intervention. There is an obligatory right-to-left atrial level shunt, but there is almost always a VSD which allows blood to get to the pulmonary arteries, if they are normally related. The size of the VSD is key, as it controls blood flow to the artery arising from the RV. If the VSD is small or nonexistent, then a Blalock-Taussig shunt (subclavian artery to pulmonary artery) might be required to supply additional pulmonary blood flow, but this is rarely emergent. Prostaglandin therapy would be used to keep the ductus arteriosus patent, if pulmonary blood flow was inadequate. It is a possible therapy, but the ductus generally stays open for many hours and allows time for an adequate assessment of blood flow, presuming that the child was delivered at a center where this level of evaluation and care can be delivered—a good plan with this anatomy. While an adequate ASD is needed in tricuspid atresia, balloon atrial septostomy is rarely required as babies are born with it. Intubation and ventilation may be required for respiratory disease, but has no beneficial effect in cyanotic congenital heart disease.

39. **Answer: B.** This patient has tricuspid atresia, a single ventricle anomaly. Because there is no RV inflow, the RV cannot be used as a pump, making a two-ventricle repair impossible at any age. Hence, answer A is incorrect. Depending upon the degree of pulmonary outflow obstruction (at the VSD, subpulmonary or pulmonary valvar level), patients with tricuspid atresia often possess a "balanced" circulation in which a restricted, yet adequate amount of pulmonary blood flow exists for a time prior to single ventricle palliation. Answer B is correct as this patient's single ventricle palliation will consist of bilateral Glenn operation (SVC to pulmonary artery anastomosis) performed at about 6 months of age followed by Fontan operation at 2 to 3 years of age. During a Fontan operation, the inferior vena caval blood is directed to the pulmonary arteries by a variety of different techniques. Answer C is incorrect as Norwood operation is performed for HLHS and consists of an aortic arch reconstruction utilizing the main pulmonary artery as the "neo" aorta, resection of the atrial septum, and placement of a modified Blalock-Taussig shunt. Answer D and E are incorrect as surgical palliation exists for tricuspid atresia, and cardiac transplant is not the most likely method of management.

KEY POINTS: TRICUSPID ATRESIA
(See also **Table 33.4**; **Figure 33.23A,B**)
- A single ventricle anomaly.
- Great arteries could be normally related or transposed.
- Variable size of the ventricular septal defect.
- PDA may or may not be needed depending on the pulmonary blood flow.
- Ultimate repair will be Fontan operation with complete separation of pulmonary and systemic circulation.

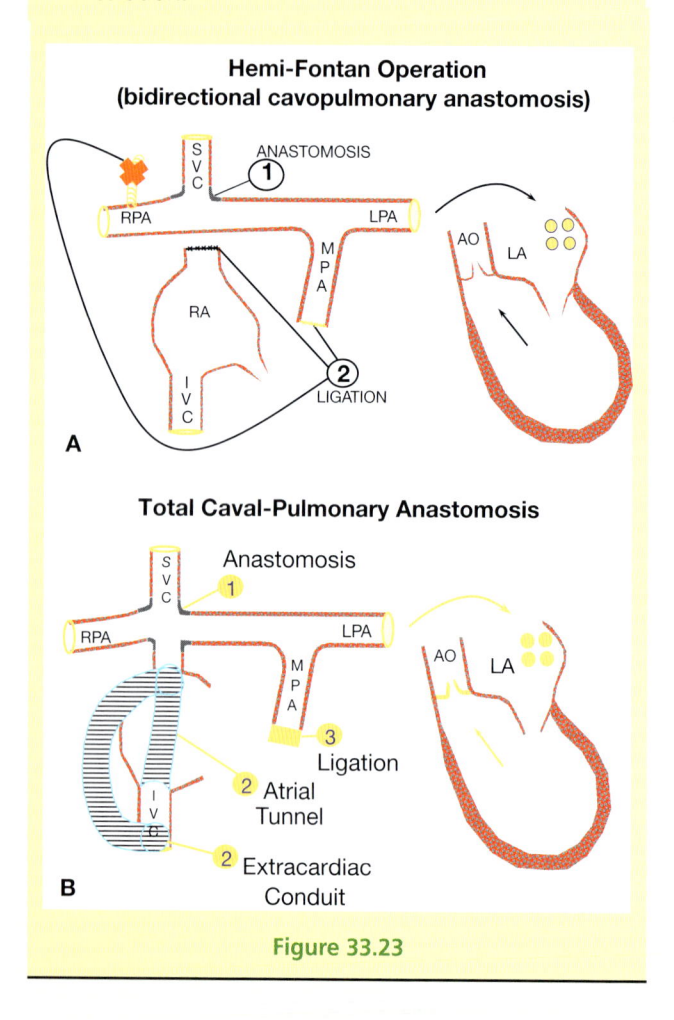

Figure 33.23

40. **Answer: D.** Echocardiography shows TAPVR of the supracardiac type.

In supracardiac TAPVR, the pulmonary venous confluence drains to the heart by way of an ascending vein to the innominate vein or SVC and then to the right atrium. Supracardiac is the most common form of TAPVR. Obstruction of venous return is virtually always present when the pulmonary venous return is below the diaphragm or infracardiac. In the supracardiac type, some form of obstruction is present in 50% of cases, but it is often mild. Obstruction is rarely seen in the cardiac type of TAPVR. In all forms of TAPVR, some form of atrial communication is almost always present. Profound cyanosis is unusual at any age. Some forms of TAPVR may go undetected until later in life.

41. **Answer: B.** In TAPVR, the right atrium receives all the systemic and pulmonary venous return leading to right-sided volume overload. This is true for all types of TAPVR. In obstructed TAPVR, development of pulmonary hypertension can also lead to RVH. On the contrary, left-sided structures, left atrium and/or LV are often smaller in size. Also, remember that a part of the left atrium is formed by absorption of the pulmonary veins which does not happen in TAPVR, resulting in a smaller left atrium. The atrial and ventricular septum bow to the left side because of volume and/or pressure overload on the right side. Doppler, particularly color flow Doppler, is very useful to establish the connection of pulmonary veins in normal hearts as well as in cases of TAPVR.

42. **Answer: C.** The scenario presented here is typical of a case of TAPVR. The first thing which needs to occur is an index of suspicion. In the case of small left heart or enlarged right heart or both, TAPVR should be suspected. When this is combined with right-to-left atrial shunting, a very strong suspicion for this entity should be present. The next phase of the echocardiographic evaluation involves a search of the systemic venous system for sources of abnormal flow. This includes the superior caval system and innominate vein, the coronary sinus, the liver, and hepatic veins and the right atrium. Color flow Doppler interrogation of the flows in these areas is essential to identifying the abnormal veins. Often the abnormal flow will produce very turbulent flow in some of these areas as well as unusually large venous structures. An example of infradiaphragmatic TAPVR is shown in ▶ **Video 33.8A,B** with an unusual, obstructed flow signal in the liver and hepatic veins which eventually drains into the IVC. Spectral Doppler interrogation is also important when obstruction is suspected from the color flow examination.

KEY POINTS: TAPVR
- Pulmonary veins end up draining into the systemic veins, which should be the focus of the echo examination.
- There is right atrial and RV dilation: since it receives both pulmonary and systemic venous return.
- Shunt flow at the atrial level is right to left.
- The atrial septum bows into the left atrium which is hypoplastic.
- Types of TAPVR: supracardiac, cardiac, infracardiac, and mixed.

- There may be obstruction to the drainage of the pulmonary veins into the heart.
- Infradiaphragmatic type is most likely to be obstructed.

Acknowledgments: We gratefully acknowledge the contributions of the previous edition author, Dr. Richard A. Humes, as portions of their chapter have been retained in this revision.

SUGGESTED READINGS

Gupta P, Sanil Y, Humes R. *Systemic Approach to Adult Congenital Heart Disease. ASE Comprehensive Echocardiography.* 3rd ed. Elsevier; 2021.

Humes R, Sanil Y, Gupta P. *Adult Congenital Heart Disease with Prior Surgical Repair. ASE Comprehensive Echocardiography.* 3rd ed. Elsevier; 2021.

Misra A, Gupta P, Aggarwal S, Singh G. *Multimodality Imaging for Repaired Tetralogy of Fallot.* Vessel Plus; 2021.

Misra A, Sriram C, Gupta P, Humes R. *The Adult with Post-operative Congenital Heart Disease: A Systematic Echocardiographic Approach.* Curr Cardiol Reports. Springer; 2019.

Stout KK, Daniel CJ, Aboulhosn JA, et al. 2018 AHA/ACC guideline for the management of adults with congenital heart disease. *J Am Coll Cardiol.* 2018;8:1029.

CHAPTER 34

Cardiovascular Point-of-Care Ultrasound for the Noncardiologist

Amer M. Johri, Braeden Hill, and Benjamin T. Galen

QUESTIONS

1. What is an appropriate definition of cardiac point-of-care-ultrasound (POCUS)?
   A. The application of POCUS to the heart and its vessels to replace the cardiac physical examination.
   B. The application of cardiovascular ultrasound, to assess the heart and its vessels by a medical provider at the bedside, to answer and immediate question.
   C. A formal, requisition-based referral service in which a sonographer acquires images assessing the heart and vessels following a defined protocol, with interpretation by a trained physician.
   D. The application of cardiovascular ultrasound by a specialist to provide a comprehensive assessment of the heart and its vessels during a scheduled outpatient appointment.

2. Which of the following is **NOT** a characteristic of cardiac POCUS?
   A. Must always involve a detailed archiving protocol and reporting structure.
   B. Ability to perform at the patient's bedside.
   C. Performed by the treating physician.
   D. Involves a limited examination that can answer an immediate clinical question.

3. Which of the following is a limitation of POCUS in the diagnosis of cardiac pathology?
   A. Inadequate sensitivity and specificity.
   B. Difficulty in obtaining adequate views in obese patients.
   C. Limited ability to evaluate cardiac function.
   D. Inability to detect structural abnormalities.

4. What was the primary advantage of cardiac POCUS in the context of the COVID-19 pandemic?
   A. It reduces the need for personal protective equipment (PPE).
   B. It is a more sensitive and specific test for COVID-19 than traditional laboratory testing.
   C. It eliminates the need for radiology departments and their staff, reducing healthcare costs.
   D. It provides real-time diagnostic information at the bedside, reducing patient movement and exposure.

5. Which of the following is an appropriate application of cardiac POCUS in the physical examination of a patient with suspected cardiac disease?
   A. Diagnosis of coronary artery disease.
   B. Quantification of left ventricular ejection fraction.
   C. Identification of pericardial effusion.
   D. Detection of dysrhythmias.

6. Practitioners of both cardiac POCUS and echocardiography should have knowledge to:
   A. Identify normal structures and artifacts from all acoustic windows.
   B. Understand basic ultrasound physics.
   C. Identify incidental and associated findings.
   D. Use quantitative techniques such as myocardial strain.
   E. Use advanced ultrasound techniques such as tissue Doppler and three-dimensional echocardiography.

7. Which of the following cardiac assessments is not an appropriate "target" for cardiac POCUS imaging?
   A. LV thrombus.
   B. LV systolic function.
   C. Left atrial (LA) size.
   D. Pericardial effusion.

8. Which of the following cardiac POCUS targets have proven useful in the serial (daily) evaluation of hospitalized patients?
   A. LV hypertrophy.
   B. LV systolic function.
   C. Pericardial effusion.
   D. Inferior vena cava (IVC) size and collapsibility.
   E. LA size.

9. Which of the following clinical tools has been useful to screen for cardiac disease?
   A. Physical examination to detect LV systolic dysfunction.
   B. Comprehensive echocardiography to detect LV systolic dysfunction.
   C. Bedside cardiac POCUS imaging to detect LV systolic dysfunction.
   D. ECG to detect LV systolic dysfunction.
   E. BNP to detect LV systolic dysfunction.

10. Which of the following is not a consideration when designing a cardiac POCUS imaging protocol?
    A. Limited functionality of small/pocket-sized ultrasound platforms.
    B. Image acquisition abilities of the practitioner.
    C. Interpretation ability of practitioner.
    D. Gender and body mass index of patient.
    E. Specialty of the practitioner.

11. Which of the following is true about cardiac POCUS training?
    A. A universal training protocol is preferred.
    B. It should be reserved for physicians trained in critical care and emergency medicine.
    C. It should include didactic training, hands-on training, and case interpretation training.
    D. The number of studies performed in training is an excellent predictor of clinical competence.
    E. Didactic training should all be performed in a lecture format.

12. Cardiac POCUS can be invaluable in the rapid assessment of a hypotensive patient. Based on Video 34.1, what would be the most likely cause of this patient's hypotension?
    A. Cardiogenic shock.
    B. Hypovolemia.
    C. Cardiac tamponade.
    D. RV dysfunction.

13. Based on Video 34.2A,B, what would be the most likely cause of this patient's hypotension?
    A. Cardiogenic shock.
    B. Hypovolemia.
    C. Cardiac tamponade.
    D. RV dysfunction.

14. Based on Video 34.3, what would be the most likely cause of this patient's hypotension?
    A. Cardiogenic shock.
    B. Hypovolemia.
    C. Pericardial tamponade.
    D. RV dysfunction.

15. While patients with significant murmurs should have complete comprehensive echocardiographic evaluation, cardiac POCUS can provide preliminary evaluation before an echocardiographic examination can be performed. What is the likely cause of this patient's loud systolic murmur (Video 34.4)?
    A. Mitral regurgitation.
    B. Aortic stenosis.
    C. Hyperdynamic LV function (flow murmur).
    D. Ventricular septal defect.

16. Cardiac POCUS can be invaluable in the rapid assessment of a patient with shortness of breath. Based on Video 34.5A,B, what would be the most likely cause of this patient's dyspnea?
    A. LV systolic heart failure.
    B. Acute RV syndrome.
    C. Diastolic heart failure.
    D. Cardiac tamponade.

17. Based on ▶ **Video 34.6**, what would be the most likely cause of this patient's dyspnea?
   A. LV systolic heart failure.
   B. Acute RV syndrome.
   C. Diastolic heart failure.
   D. Cardiac tamponade.

18. This is a cardiac POCUS in a patient hospitalized with acutely decompensated congestive heart failure on day 4 of their admission and after several liters of diuresis. What does ▶ **Video 34.7** of the IVC suggest?
   A. Adequate diuresis has been obtained and further diuresis should be avoided to prevent azotemia.
   B. Continued diuresis is needed, but the patient could be discharged without an increased risk of readmission.
   C. Continued diuresis is needed and if discharged, the patient has an elevated risk of readmission.
   D. The patient has been over-diuresed and needs fluid therapy.

19. This patient is short of breath, what procedure is potentially indicated for relief of symptoms based on ▶ **Video 34.8**?
   A. Pericardiocentesis.
   B. Paracentesis.
   C. Left-sided thoracentesis.
   D. Right-sided thoracentesis.

20. Does this patient have a pericardial effusion (▶ **Video 34.9**)?
   A. Yes.
   B. No.
   C. No, with exceptions.
   D. There is not enough information to answer the question.

CASE 1

An 84-year-old woman with hypertension and hyperlipidemia presents with persistent midthoracic pain radiating to her neck. ECG showed sinus rhythm at 61 beats/min, with ST segment elevation in leads II, aVF, V3, V4, V5, and V6, and troponin I level of 3832 ng/L. She tested positive for myocardial injury biomarkers, indicating anterolateral infarction in the subacute phase. ASA, clopidogrel, and low-molecular-weight heparin were started. Upon admission to ICU, physical examination revealed a systolic heart murmur radiating to the neck, but the patient remained asymptomatic with stable sinus rhythm. A cardiac POCUS was performed (▶ Video 10.10A), after which anticoagulants, antiplatelets, and beta-blockers were initiated. A follow-up cardiac POCUS examination was conducted 24 hours later (▶ Video 10.10B), with the patient on beta-blocker therapy. The next morning, coronary angiography did not reveal any significant coronary lesions, although the left anterior descending artery was abnormally elongated, wrapping around the apex and diaphragmatic surface.

21. What are the findings on cardiac POCUS in ▶ **Video 34.10A**, at admission for the patient in **Case 1**?
   A. Subcostal four-chamber view of the heart showing partial right atrial collapse.
   B. Apical five-chamber view of the heart showing dynamic left ventricular outflow tract obstructions and systolic anterior motion of the mitral valve.
   C. Subcostal view of the heart showing a dilated inferior vena cava.
   D. Parasternal long-axis view of the heart showing reduced left ventricular contractility.

22. What are the findings on cardiac POCUS(▶ **Video 34.10B**) of the patient in **Case 1**, at 24 hours with beta-blocker treatment?
   A. Apical four-chamber view of the heart showing a decrease in left atrial size.
   B. Parasternal short-axis view of the heart showing mitral valve prolapse.
   C. Subcostal four-chamber view of the heart showing a small and collapsible inferior vena cava, suggesting low right atrial pressure.
   D. Apical five-chamber view of the heart showing a decrease in dynamic systolic gradient and absence of systolic anterior motion of the mitral valve.

23. What is the most likely diagnosis for the patient in **Case 1**?
   A. Hypertrophic cardiomyopathy.
   B. Takotsubo syndrome.
   C. Spontaneous coronary artery dissection.
   D. Acute myocardial infarction.

CASE 2

A 35-year-old man with end-stage kidney disease and chronic pericardial effusion on hemodialysis presented to the emergency department with flulike symptoms and pleuritic chest pain. His blood pressure measured 108/67 mm Hg and heart rate 133 beats/min, with stable vitals otherwise. Pulsus paradoxus was absent. Jugular venous pulsation was not visible, heart sounds were soft, and no pericardial rub was detected. ECG revealed sinus rhythm with low voltages, and an enlarged cardiac silhouette was visible on chest x-ray. A cardiac POCUS exam was conducted to assess for pericardial effusion. Two sets of subcostal images were obtained 3 hours apart: one set before volume repletion (▶ Video 34.11A,B) and another set afterward (▶ Video 34.11C,D). The patient's blood pressure and heart rate during the second set of images were 137/75 mm Hg and 88 beats/min, respectively. A formal echocardiogram confirmed a 3-cm circumferential pericardial effusion that had increased from a baseline of 1.5 cm.

24. What are the cardiac POCUS findings indicated by ▶ Video 34.11A,B for the patient in **Case 2**?
    A. Subcostal view showing partial right atrial collapse and a small and collapsible inferior vena cava.
    B. Subcostal view showing right atrial enlargement and a dilated and noncollapsible inferior vena cava.
    C. Subcostal view showing left atrial collapse and a small and collapsible inferior vena cava.
    D. Subcostal view showing partial right atrial collapse and a dilated RV.

25. What intervention was likely performed between the 2 sets of images (**Video 34.11A,B** and **Video 34.11C,D**) for the patient in **Case 2**?
    A. Pericardiocentesis with removal of 500 mL of pericardial fluid.
    B. ASA 650 mg and colchicine 0.5 mg PO.
    C. 500 mL bolus of NS.
    D. Lasix 40 mg IV with 500 mL of diuresis.

26. What is the most likely diagnosis for the patient in **Case 2**?
    A. Cardiac tamponade.
    B. Type A aortic dissection with extension into the pericardium.
    C. Tension pneumothorax.
    D. Myocardial infarction.

CASE 3

A 61-year-old man with a history of systolic congestive heart failure and advanced renal failure who was admitted with dyspnea on exertion and acute hypoxemic respiration failure. A cardiac POCUS was performed, assessing LV function and size, RV function and size, presence of pericardial effusion, and inferior vena cava size and collapsibility (▶ Video 34.12A-E).

A chest POCUS was also performed, identifying a bilateral B-line pattern. Lung sliding is seen bilaterally (no pneumothorax), and large bilateral pleural effusions with associated consolidation, likely passive atelectasis (▶ Video 34.12F-M). Example lung views of a chest POCUS assessment are provided in **Figure 34.1**.

27. What were the cardiac POCUS findings concerning the left heart for the patient in **Case 3**?
    A. Severely reduced LV function; LV dilation.
    B. Severe LV dilation; no reduction in LV function.
    C. No significant LV abnormalities detected.
    D. Large pericardial effusion.

28. What were the cardiac POCUS findings concerning the right heart for the patient in **Case 3**?
    A. Reduced RV function; elevated RA pressure.
    B. No significant reduction of RV function; nor elevation of RA pressure.
    C. No significant right heart abnormalities detected.
    D. Moderate effusion adjacent to right ventricle.

29. Is a pericardial effusion present on this cardiac POCUS examination for the patient in **Case 3**?
    A. Yes, significant pericardial effusion is present.
    B. Yes, trace pericardial effusion is present (physiologic).
    C. No, pericardial effusion is not present.
    D. Pericardial effusion cannot be assessed based on the given cardiac POCUS exam.

30. What is the most likely diagnosis for the patient in **Case 3**?
    A. Acute decompensated congestive heart failure.
    B. Acute respiratory distress syndrome.
    C. COPD exacerbation.
    D. Pulmonary embolism.

Cardiopulmonary protocol	Structure imaged	Assessment	Example of disease associations
Lung	8 or 12 point exam	B lines (A lines, pleural sliding are normal)	Edema or pneumonia
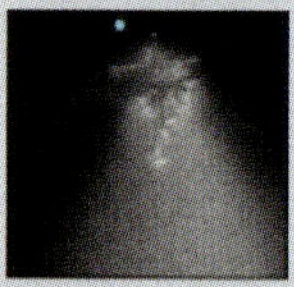		Subpleural consolidation Thickened pleura	Pneumonia ARDS
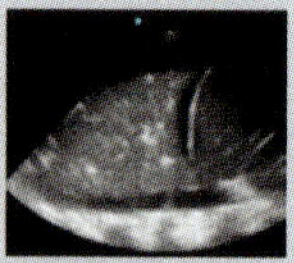		Lobar consolidation with air bronchograms	Pneumonia ARDS
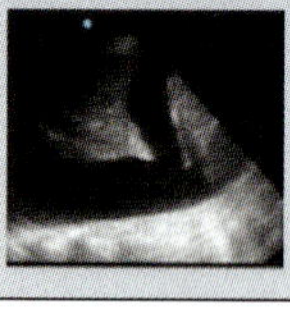		Effusion	CHF

Figure 34.1. ARDS, acute respiratory distress syndrome; CHF, congestive heart failure.

CASE 4

A 46-year-old obese man (BMI 51.9 kg/m^2) with type 2 diabetes and diagnosed COVID-19 was admitted with dry cough, hemoptysis, and a ratio of arterial oxygen partial pressure to fractional inspired oxygen (PaO$_2$/FiO$_2$) of 64. His heart rate was 70 beats/min, respiratory rate 15 breaths/min, and blood pressure 129/75 mm Hg. Cardiopulmonary auscultation found no significant abnormalities. Cardiac POCUS could not fully visualize the inferior vena cava due to gas interference. In the parasternal long-axis view, abnormal interventricular septum movement and reduced left ventricular function were noted (▶ **Video 34.13**). The short-axis view showed an enlarged right ventricle, septum flattening, and a hyperechoic image in the pulmonary artery. Chest POCUS revealed multiple B lines, mainly in the right anterior quadrants, with basal consolidation and superior multiple B lines posteriorly, and no pleural effusion. The ASE POCUS protocol for imaging COVID-19 patients is shown in **Figure 34.2**.

31. Based on the cardiac POCUS exam of the patient from **Case 4**, which of the following findings is suggestive of right ventricular dysfunction?
    A. Inferior vena cava not fully visualized due to gas interposition.
    B. Abnormal movement of the interventricular septum.
    C. Dilated right ventricle and flattening of the interventricular septum.
    D. Hyperechoic image in pulmonary artery.

32. What is the most likely diagnosis for the patient in **Case 4**?
    A. Acute respiratory distress syndrome.
    B. Pneumothorax.
    C. Acute myocardial infarction.
    D. Right heart thrombus.

CASE 5

A 42-year-old woman with no history of diabetes or hypertension and not taking any medications presented to the emergency department experiencing tachycardia for the first time, lasting 2 hours. Her blood pressure measured 120/70 mm Hg, with a heart rate of 120 beats/min and an irregular rhythm. During the chest examination, right ventricular heaving and a soft systolic murmur were noted in three of six of the left parasternal line of the intercostal space. An ECG indicated a right axis deviation accompanied by rapid atrial fibrillation. To manage her elevated heart rate, the patient received

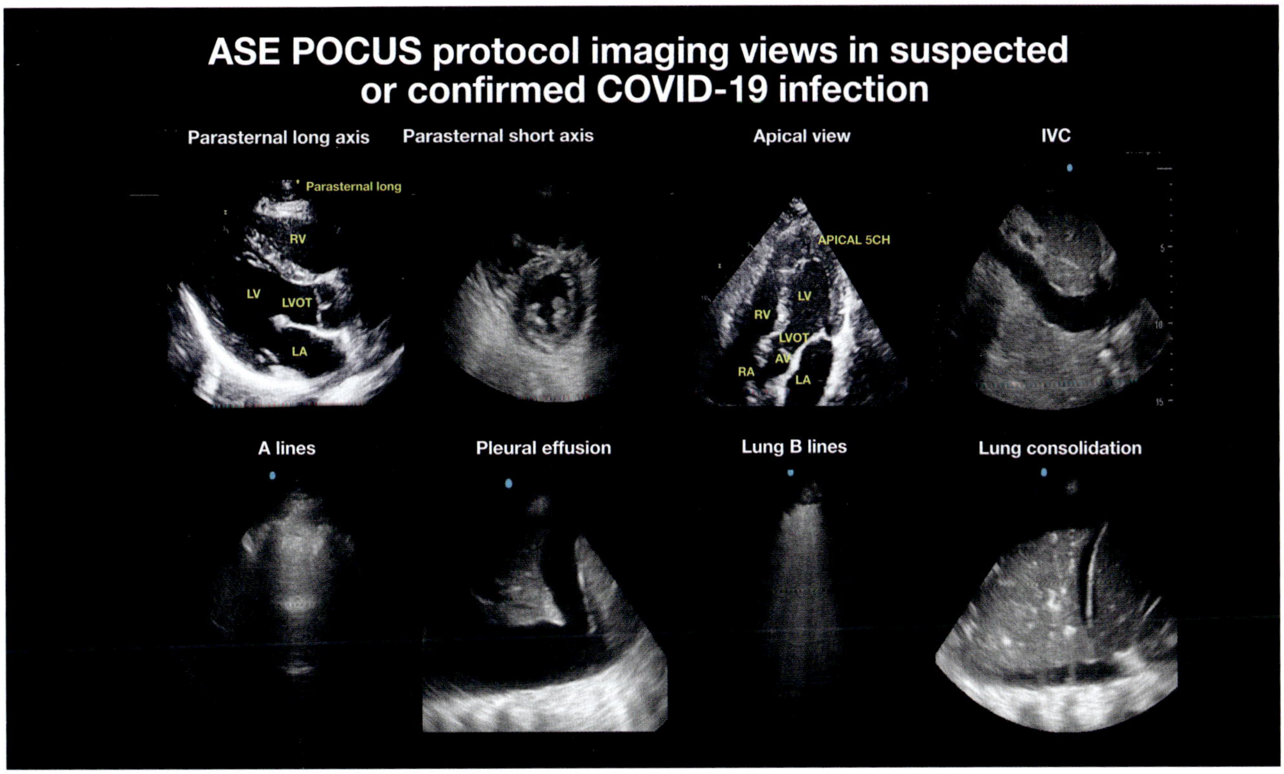

Figure 34.2

an intravenous administration of 5 mg verapamil, and her heart rhythm spontaneously returned to normal sinus rhythm after 4 hours. A cardiac POCUS was conducted (▶ Video 34.14A), followed by an agitated saline contrast cardiac POCUS (▶ Video 34.14B).

33. What did the bedside cardiac POCUS examination find in ▶ Video 34.14A for the patient in **Case 5**?
    A. Left heart thrombus.
    B. Sinus of Valsalva aneurysm.
    C. Dilated coronary sinus.
    D. Right atrial hypertension.

34. Based on the agitated saline contrast POCUS (▶ Video 34.14B) findings, which of the following is observed in **Case 5**?
    A. Saline bubbles from the left cubital vein entering the left atrium.
    B. Saline bubbles from the left cubital vein entering the coronary sinus and right ventricle.
    C. Saline bubbles from the left cubital vein entering the left ventricle.
    D. Saline bubbles from the left cubital vein entering the pulmonary artery.

CASE 6

A 29-year-old woman with shortness of breath presents to the emergency department after delivering at home 2 days prior to presentation. As per the patient and family, her shortness of breath was present at the time of delivery and has worsened since. As per the family's report, the delivery was uncomplicated and the child is healthy.

On physical examination, the patient is in moderate distress. Her respiratory rate is 30/min, heart rate is 125 beats/min, and she is saturating 86% on room air. Blood pressure is 80/60 mm Hg and temperature is 37.7 °C. Jugular venous pulsation is difficult to visualize. Heart sounds are without murmurs, rubs, or gallops. Abdomen is mildly tender in the lower quadrants with a distended uterus. 1+ lower extremity edema is present to the knees bilaterally.

Cardiac POCUS was performed at the bedside on presentation (▶ Video 34.15A,B).

35. What is the most likely cause of the patient's presentation in **Case 6**?
    A. Peripartum cardiomyopathy.
    B. Amniotic fluid embolism.
    C. Pneumonia complicated by septic shock.
    D. Pericardial effusion causing tamponade.

CASE 7

A 34-year-old man with a history of HIV presents to clinic complaining of fatigue and shortness of breath. He was in his usual state of health prior to 2 months ago, when he began to experience increasing dyspnea with activity, eventually progressing to shortness of breath with rest. Review of systems is positive for decreased appetite, paroxysmal nocturnal dyspnea, night sweats, and lower extremity swelling. He is not receiving antiretroviral therapy. Per his family, he has a long history of alcohol use.

Physical examination reveals a thin man in no distress. His respiratory rate is 18/min and heart rate is 110 beats/min, and he is saturating 90% on room air. He is without fever; blood pressure is 90/60 mm Hg. Neck veins are distended. Heart sounds are without murmurs, rubs, or gallops. Lower extremities demonstrate 2+ pitting edema to the midthigh region. CXR and comprehensive echocardiography have been ordered.

Cardiac POCUS was performed at the bedside on presentation (▶ Video 34.16A-C).

36. What is the most likely diagnosis for the patient in **Case 7**?
    A. HIV cardiomyopathy.
    B. Pericardial effusion causing cardiac tamponade.
    C. Pneumocystis pneumonia.
    D. Alcoholic cardiomyopathy.

CASE 8

A 55-year-old man with a history of stroke presents with shortness of breath, lower extremity edema, and chest pain with activity. The patient states that his symptoms began 1 month prior and have become progressively worse. He currently does not take medications. He smokes 10 cigarettes a day and has been smoking for 25 years.

Physical examination reveals a tired man in no distress. His respirations are 18/min with oxygen saturations at 92% on no supplemental oxygen. Blood pressure is 150/90 mm Hg. Cardiac examination reveals an elevated jugular venous pulsation, normal heart sounds, and crackles at the lung bases. Trace edema is present to the knee.

Cardiac POCUS was performed at the bedside (▶ Video 34.17A,B).

37. What is the most likely cause of the patient's symptoms in **Case 8**?
    A. Ischemic cardiomyopathy.
    B. Recurrent pulmonary embolism.
    C. Hypertensive heart disease.
    D. Rheumatic heart disease.

CASE 9

An 18-year-old man presents to your clinic, complaining of fevers, mild shortness of breath, and night sweats for several weeks. Prior to these symptoms, he felt healthy with no complaints. He has an uncle who was diagnosed with pulmonary tuberculosis 2 months ago whom he has seen often. Earlier this month, he had a tooth pulled after having pain from a cavity. He also states several years ago he was told he had a heart murmur.

Physical examination reveals an ill-appearing man in no distress. He has a heart rate of 110 beats/min and a respiratory rate of 18/min. Oxygen saturation is 94% and temperature is 38 °C. Lung examination is unremarkable. Cardiac examination reveals no rubs or gallops, and a grade 2/6 holosystolic murmur loudest at the apex. Blood cultures are in process.

Cardiac POCUS was performed at the bedside (▶ Video 34.18A,B).

38. Which is the next appropriate step in management for the patient in **Case 9**?
    A. Sputum acid fast stain × 3.
    B. Observation, return to clinic in 1 week if symptoms persist.
    C. Oral amoxicillin for 7 days.
    D. Intravenous antibiotics.

CASE 10

A 54-year-old man presents with shortness of breath and chest pain to the local health center. He states the pain started 2 months prior and is worse with activity. He has a history of hypertension and lung cancer for which he has been receiving treatment for 1 month.

Blood pressure is 140/90 mm Hg, and heart rate is 80 beats/min. Heart examination is without murmurs, rubs, or gallops. Lung examination reveals rales in the bases bilaterally. Trace edema is present to the knees.

Cardiac POCUS was performed at the bedside (▶ Video 34.19A,B).

39. What is the most likely cause of this patient's chest pain in **Case 10**?
    A. Ischemic heart disease.
    B. Malignant pericardial effusion.
    C. Cor pulmonale.
    D. Heart failure with preserved ejection fraction.

CASE 11

A 22-year-old woman with sickle cell disease presents with worsening shortness of breath for the past year. She has had several episodes of pain crisis in the past year, managed with fluids and pain control. She has received numerous blood transfusions. A year ago, she had no functional limitations, but currently can walk only 50 steps before becoming short of breath.

Physical examination reveals an ill-appearing woman. Blood pressure is 90/60 mm Hg with pulse oximetry of 90% on room air and a heart rate of 100 beats/min. Pulmonary examination demonstrates decreased breath sounds at the bases bilaterally with dullness to percussion. Heart examination is positive for a loud P2, with no murmurs.

Cardiac POCUS was performed at the bedside (▶ **Video 34.20A-C**).

40. What is the most likely etiology of the patient's shortness of breath in **Case 11**?
    A. Congestive heart failure secondary to iron overload.
    B. Severe anemia.
    C. Progressive pulmonary hypertension.
    D. Pneumonia.

CASE 12

A 65-year-old man presents with chest pain to his primary care physician. He was in his usual state of health until 1 month ago when he began to develop substernal chest pain made worse with exertion. He also states that he has mild shortness of breath also worse with activity.

Blood pressure is 130/90 mm Hg with a heart rate of 80 beats/min. Jugular venous pulsation is not elevated. Heart examination reveals a grade 3/6 systolic murmur. Lungs are clear to auscultation bilaterally.

Cardiac POCUS was performed at the bedside (▶ **Video 34.21A-C**).

Electrocardiography reveals T-wave inversions in V4–V6 and criteria for left ventricular hypertrophy.

41. What is the most likely etiology of the patient's chest pain from **Case 12**?
    A. LV systolic dysfunction with secondary mitral regurgitation.
    B. Mitral valve stenosis.
    C. Idiopathic pericarditis.
    D. Aortic valve stenosis.

ANSWERS

1. **Answer: B.** Cardiac POCUS does not replace the cardiac physical examination. Instead, it serves as an adjunct to the physical examination, providing additional information to help medical providers make more accurate and rapid diagnoses (Answer A is incorrect). Cardiac POCUS is performed at the bedside by the treating physician and is intended to answer specific clinical questions quickly rather than follow a formal, requisition-based echocardiography protocol (Answer C is incorrect). While cardiac POCUS is indeed used to assess the heart and its vessels, it is not intended for comprehensive assessments on a scheduled outpatient basis (Answer D is incorrect). Cardiac POCUS is used to quickly assess cardiac and vascular issues and answer clinical questions in a point-of-care setting, allowing providers to make timely decisions in the management of their patients (Answer B is correct).

2. **Answer: A.** A cardiac POCUS is a limited cardiovascular ultrasound performed by the treating physician at the bedside, facilitating immediate clinical decision-making and management (Answers B, C, and D are incorrect). Cardiac POCUS examinations do not follow a detailed archiving and reporting structure characteristic of a formal echocardiography service (Answer A is correct). Refer to **Table 34.1** for a comparison between the characteristics of cardiac POCUS and full-scale transthoracic echocardiography (TTE).

3. **Answer: B.** Although POCUS is not as comprehensive as a standard echocardiogram, it generally demonstrates good sensitivity and specificity for the detection of specific cardiac pathologies when performed by adequately trained practitioners (Answer A is incorrect). Cardiac POCUS can be used effectively to evaluate cardiac function, including ventricular function, valvular abnormalities, and certain structural abnormalities. While it may not provide a complete assessment like a standard echocardiogram, POCUS can still provide valuable information to guide clinical decision-making (Answers C and D are incorrect). Obtaining adequate views in obese patients can be challenging due to increased adipose tissue, which may hinder the visualization of certain cardiac structures and reduce the image quality on cardiac POCUS examinations (Answer B is correct).

Table 34.1. Characteristics of Cardiac POCUS Compared to TTE

	Cardiac POCUS	**TTE**
Operators	• Nonsonographer • Nonradiologist	• Level II, level III (physician) • ARDMS (sonographer) • Credentialed lab
Indications	• Valves (gross) • Pericardial effusion/tamponade • LV and RV function/thickness • IVC	• Wide spectrum • Published guidelines
Technological Capabilities	• Usually portable (<15 lbs) • 2D imaging • Color Doppler	• Full-service machine • 3D, strain • Pulsed-wave and continuous-wave Doppler • Telemetry, respirometer • Contrast-enhanced ultrasound
Advantages	• Portability • Accessibility • Relatively inexpensive • Immediacy of results	• "Gold standard" imaging quality • Standardized exam and reporting • Multiple techniques • Training benchmarks, guidelines • Advancing technology • Archiving
Disadvantages	• Lack of formal training benchmarks • Paucity of guidelines • Technological limitations	• Portability • Access • Cost

ARDMS, American Registry for Diagnostic Medical Sonography; IVC, inferior vena cava; LV, left ventricle; POCUS, point-of-care ultrasound; RV, right ventricle; TTE, transthoracic echocardiography.

4. Answer: D. PPE is still required for healthcare providers performing cardiac POCUS on COVID-19 patients to ensure their safety (Answer A is incorrect). Although cardiac POCUS is useful to assess cardiac function and identify potential complications related to COVID-19, such as myocardial injury or pericardial effusion, traditional laboratory testing, such as PCR or antigen tests, remains the standard for diagnosing COVID-19 (Answer B is incorrect). Although POCUS can provide valuable bedside diagnostic information, more comprehensive imaging modalities, such as standard echocardiography or computed tomography, may still be necessary for detailed assessment and management of specific conditions (Answer C is incorrect). Cardiac POCUS provides real-time diagnostic information at the patient's bedside, which is especially valuable during the COVID-19 pandemic as it reduces the need to transport patients to radiology departments for imaging. Thus, POCUS minimizes the risk of spreading the virus to other patients or healthcare staff, limiting exposure and potential cross-contamination (Answer D is correct).

5. Answer: C. As cardiac POCUS cannot visualize the coronary arteries directly, diagnosis of coronary artery disease typically requires more advanced imaging modalities, such as coronary angiography, computed tomography coronary angiography, or stress testing (Answer A is incorrect). Although cardiac POCUS can provide a qualitative assessment of left ventricular function, it is not intended for the precise quantification of left ventricular ejection fraction. Comprehensive echocardiography or other imaging modalities are better suited for accurately quantifying ejection fraction (Answer B is incorrect). Detection of dysrhythmias is primarily the domain of electrocardiograms, not cardiac POCUS. While POCUS can provide valuable information about cardiac function and structure, it is not designed to detect electrical abnormalities such as dysrhythmias (Answer D is incorrect). Cardiac POCUS is an appropriate tool for the identification of pericardial effusion during the physical examination of a patient with suspected cardiac disease, as the parasternal long-axis view, the parasternal short-axis view, the apical four-chamber view, and the subxiphoid view can allow the operator to assess the presence and extent of pericardial effusion by directly visualizing the space between the heart and the pericardium (Answer C is correct). **Figure 34.3** presents the common cardiac POCUS views used to assess cardiac function and pathology.

Cardiopulmonary protocol	Structure imaged	Assessment	Example of disease associations
Cardiac 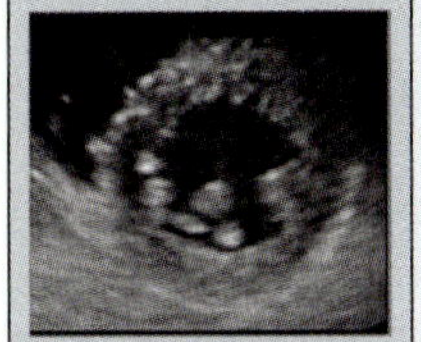	Left ventricle	Size, global and regional function	Myocarditis ACS Cardiomyopathy Shock
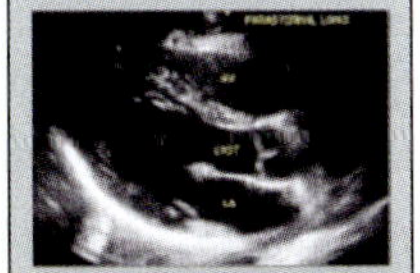	Right ventricle	Size and function; TR for PASP if available	PE Cardiomyopathy
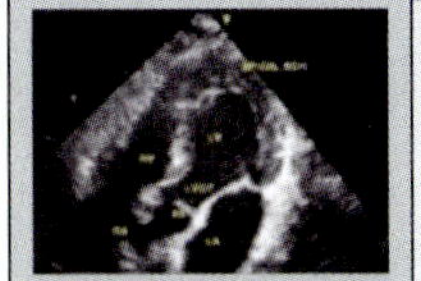	Pericardium	Effusion	Tamponade
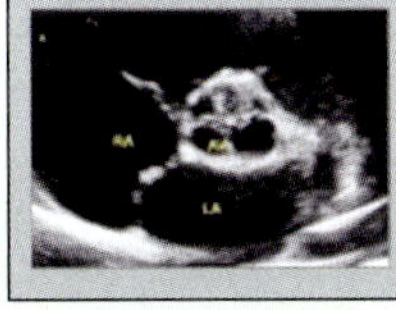	Valves	Gross regurgitation or stenosis	Preexisting CV disease

Figure 34.3. ACS, acute coronary syndrome; CV, cardiovascular; PASP, pulmonary artery systolic pressure; PE, pulmonary embolism; TR, tricuspid regurgitation.

6. **Answer: B.** All users of cardiac ultrasound need to understand the fundamentals of cardiac ultrasound physics. With cardiac POCUS, the goal is to gain expertise to acquire reliable images from a limited number of views and subjectively interpret these images for prechosen targets. Subsequent referral for echocardiography is usually indicated to delineate and quantify all findings, including incidental or associated findings, that may go unrecognized by cardiac POCUS. A physician with cardiac POCUS expertise does not have the image acquisition or interpretation training to identify all structures, image from all acoustic windows, or use advanced ultrasound techniques.

7. **Answer: A.** Assessment of LV systolic function, LA size, RV size, and pericardial effusion have all been validated as assessable by a practitioner with cardiac POCUS level image acquisition and interpretation training. Pathologies that are complex or unusual should not be expected to be diagnosed by a physician solely trained in cardiac POCUS. In addition, some pathologies are subtle and are difficult to recognize (aortic dissection, hypertrophic cardiomyopathy, LV regional wall motion abnormalities, cardiac masses, RV hypertrophy, LV thrombus, and valvular vegetations). Other abnormalities require assimilation of data from multiple views to correctly define (RV systolic function).

8. **Answer: D.** It would be impractical to use traditional echocardiography to assess a patient at the bedside every day or multiple times a day for a period of time, such as during hospitalization. In addition, there are few ultrasound parameters that would be useful to follow on such a frequent basis. Although a pericardial effusion may need serial assessment, repeated evaluation of this is best reserved for those with echocardiographic training to assess the hemodynamic effects of the effusion and serially compare images, which may be difficult with cardiac POCUS systems. Knowledge of patient volume status (at least as measured by RA pressure) is frequently assessed by physical examination and, therefore, suitable for cardiac POCUS. Cardiac POCUS assessment of the IVC is both more feasible and accurate than physical examination for detecting elevated central venous pressure. LV systolic function may need reassessment by cardiac POCUS if a patient's hemodynamic status changes but rarely requires frequent serial evaluation.

9. **Answer: C.** LV systolic dysfunction is an ideal target for screening. It is somewhat prevalent, even in a population of asymptomatic subjects, and has effective therapy even in the preclinical stage. BNP and EKG, while having good sensitivity, have very poor specificity to screen for LV systolic dysfunction (Answers D and E are incorrect). While comprehensive echocardiography has excellent accuracy, its costs make it impractical as a screening tool. Cardiac POCUS, which can be performed rapidly at the bedside, has very good sensitivity and specificity for identifying reduced LVEF, even when performed by practitioners with limited training. Cardiac POCUS is clearly superior to physical examination for detecting low LV ejection fraction (Answer A is incorrect).

10. **Answer: D.** Successful implementation of a cardiac POCUS practice must consider the abilities of the imager to acquire the required images and their training to interpret the findings (Answers B and C are incorrect). As with any clinical tool, inappropriate use of cardiac POCUS beyond a defined scope of training may have adverse consequences on patient care. The risk of a false-negative cardiac POCUS examination that leads to delayed treatment or a false-positive examination that results in unnecessary treatment must be recognized. Although easier to use, the simplified, miniaturized devices often used for cardiac POCUS have reduced imaging abilities and may simply be inadequate to detect certain abnormalities (Answer A is incorrect). Physician specialty will strongly affect cardiac POCUS protocols. Depending on the type of patients and clinical scenarios encountered, the ultrasound targets of the cardiac POCUS examination may vary significantly (Answer E is incorrect). While patient gender and body size may affect the ability to acquire useable images, the protocol will not vary as the goals of the examination remain unchanged (Answer D is correct).

11. **Answer: C.** While emergency and critical care physicians have been early adopters of cardiac POCUS, it is expected that physicians with diverse training backgrounds and specialties will find cardiac POCUS useful (Answer B is incorrect). Depending on the physician's scope of practice, the data they require when evaluating their patients may vary. This means that cardiac POCUS protocols may vary by specialty (Answer A is incorrect). Although frequently used as a surrogate measure, the relationship between the number of studies performed and clinical competency has a weak relationship (Answer D is incorrect). Cardiac POCUS courses should include three core components—didactic, hands-on imaging, and case-based image interpretation. Didactic training can be delivered in any number of formats (lecture, online, DVD) (Answer E is incorrect).

12. **Answer: C.** This subcostal image demonstrates a large pericardial effusion with collapse of the RV consistent with cardiac tamponade.

13. **Answer: B.** LV and RV systolic functions are preserved and there is no significant pericardial effusion. Cardiac POCUS assessment of the IVC from the subcostal window demonstrates a normal sized IVC with complete collapsibility with respiration, suggesting a right atrial pressure lower than 5 mm Hg. While cardiac POCUS findings need to be used in conjunction with history, and physical examination in the evaluation of patients, these data strongly suggest that hypovolemia (Answer B) is more likely than the other causes listed as the etiology of hypotension.

14. **Answer: D.** Rapid bedside assessment of this hypotensive patient with cardiac POCUS demonstrates no significant pericardial fluid, a small hyperdynamic LV, and a very enlarged poorly contractile RV. While not enough to be used in isolation, when combined with the clinical picture, this is consistent with an acute RV syndrome, in this case pulmonary embolism. Recognition of this may not direct immediate therapy, but it can dramatically change the subsequent testing, away from left-sided congestive heart failure to a cause of acute RV injury.

15. **Answer: B.** The parasternal long-axis image demonstrates preserved LVEF and marked calcification of the aortic valve with impaired leaflet motion, all consistent with aortic stenosis. Comprehensive transthoracic echocardiography (TTE) is indicated for assessment of stenosis severity and evaluation for concomitant valvular heart disease.

16. **Answer: C.** Parasternal long- and short-axis images demonstrate preserved LV systolic function, no significant pericardial effusion with significant concentric hypertrophy, and left atrial enlargement. These findings make diastolic heart failure likely. Comprehensive TTE is indicated for comprehensive evaluation of diastolic function and filling pressures, but these bedside images may allow more targeted therapy before the results of TTE are available.

17. **Answer: A.** While many findings on physical examination may suggest LV systolic dysfunction, cardiac POCUS in 20 to 60 seconds performed at the bedside definitively determines that this patient has serious LV systolic dysfunction. Determination of LVEF at this point is not required to guide therapy; simply a determination of LV systolic function as clearly normal, reduced, or very reduced allows targeted management decisions.

18. **Answer: C.** Cardiac POCUS imaging of the IVC demonstrates a dilated IVC with minimal respirophasic variation. This strongly suggests significant elevation of right atrial pressure (>15 mm Hg). This suggests that continued diuresis is needed. Studies have shown that patients with acutely decompensated CHF who are discharged with such a plethoric IVC have an elevated risk of readmission to the hospital.

19. **Answer: C.** The parasternal long-axis image demonstrates a minimal pericardial effusion, so there is no indication for a pericardial tap. There is a left pleural effusion. Although the cardiac POCUS from this window does not provide enough data to assess whether the effusion can be tapped, it is critical to recognize that in this view the fluid visualized outside of the heart is pleural, not pericardial. The most reliable feature to distinguish pleural from pericardial effusion is the descending thoracic aorta. Pericardial effusion will be anterior to the descending thoracic aorta in this view and left pleural effusions will be posterior. Ascites and right pleural effusion would typically not be seen from this imaging view.

20. **Answer: B.** The relatively echolucent layer anterior to the RV is epicardial fat. This is fairly common. This can be distinguished from pericardial fluid by using a number of features: (1) the layer is not completely echolucent like most effusions and (2) there is no significant posterior pericardial effusion, which one might expect as effusions are dependent and most patients are in supine position.

21. **Answer: B.** This is not a subcostal view and there is no indication of RA collapse or visualization of the inferior vena cava on this cardiac POCUS examination (Answers A and C are incorrect). Although there is reduced LV contractility seen on the cardiac POCUS, this is not a parasternal view (Answer D is incorrect). This cardiac POCUS examination shows an apical five-chamber view indicating dynamic left ventricular outflow obstruction and systolic anterior motion of the mitral valve (Answer B is correct). There are some contractility issues as well, which are further highlighted below.

22. **Answer: D.** This is not an apical 4-chamber, parasternal, or subcostal cardiac POCUS view (Answers A, B, C are incorrect). The cardiac POCUS clip shows an apical five-chamber view indicating a substantial decrease in dynamic systolic gradient at the left ventricular outflow tract and an absence of systolic anterior motion of the mitral valve (Answer D is correct).

23. **Answer: B.** Hypertrophic cardiomyopathy typically presents with a thickened and enlarged heart muscle, which was not clearly seen in this case (Answer A is incorrect). Measurements were not made, but with experience, the POCUS operator should know that the walls generally look normal thickness in this case. One may argue that there could be abnormal thickness that cannot be ruled out with caliper measurements; however, this answer is still not the best given the more obvious contractile abnormality as further described below. Coronary angiography did not reveal any coronary lesions, which would be expected in spontaneous coronary artery dissection (Answer C is incorrect). Although the patient presented with chest pain, ECG changes, and elevated markers of myocardial injury, the coronary angiography did not show any significant coronary lesions, which would be expected in acute myocardial infarction (Answer D is incorrect). The patient's most likely diagnosis is takotsubo syndrome, also known as stress-induced cardiomyopathy or broken heart syndrome. This condition is characterized by transient left ventricular dysfunction, often triggered by emotional or physical stress. The POCUS shows a dilated and akinetic LV apex with a hyperdynamic base. The patient's presentation, including chest pain, ECG changes, and elevated markers of myocardial injury without coronary lesions on angiography, is consistent with this diagnosis.

> **KEY POINTS**
> - Cardiac POCUS may be useful in the initial assessment of cardiomyopathy.
> - Apical akinesis with hyperdynamicity at the base of the LV may suggest takotsubo cardiomyopathy on cardiac POCUS.
> - Cardiac POCUS may also potentially detect hypertrophic cardiomyopathy if there is obvious thickening of the ventricular walls seen.

24. **Answer: A.** In this cardiac POCUS examination, the RA does not look particularly dilated and the inferior vena cava is seen to clearly collapse in the second video (Answer B is incorrect). The left atrium (bottom of screen) is not collapsing (Answer C is incorrect). The RV does not appear dilated in this view (Answer D is incorrect). This cardiac POCUS examination indicates partial right atrial collapse and a small (<2 cm) and collapsing inferior vena cava (>50% collapse on respiration) (Answer A is correct).

25. **Answer: C.** A pericardiocentesis is unlikely to have been performed on this patient since the amount of pericardial fluid has not changed. A removal of 500 mL would be expected to have seen a significant decrease in the size of the effusion (Answer A is incorrect). Although high-dose ASA and colchicine are used to treat pericarditis, and may reduce inflammation and accelerate resorption of the pericardial fluid, 3 hours is too early to begin seeing a hemodynamic response to these drugs (Answer B is incorrect). The diuretic effect would be expected to reduce intravascular volume and lower right atrial pressure. The expected response would be to increase the degree of right atrial collapse (Answer D is incorrect). The intervention most likely performed between the two sets of images is a 500 mL bolus of normal saline (NS). The administration of the fluid bolus would increase intravascular volume, which could subsequently raise right atrial pressure. This would counteract the partial early systolic right atrial collapse seen in the first set of images. The fact that there is no significant change in the size of the pericardial effusion between the two sets of images further supports this conclusion (Answer C is correct).

26. **Answer: A.** The patient's presentation and imaging findings do not suggest an aortic dissection, which would typically present with severe chest pain and characteristic findings on imaging such as an intimal

---

Case 1 was adapted from López Libano J, Alomar Lladó L, Zarraga López L. The Takotsubo Syndrome: clinical diagnosis using POCUS. *POCUS J.* 2022;7(1):137-139, licensed under a Creative Commons Attribution 4.0 International License.

Case 2 was adapted from Cenkowski M, Johri AM, Pal R, Hutchison J. Case report: early signs of tamponade may be detected by cardiac point-of-care ultrasound. *POCUS J.* 2017; 2(3):24-25, licensed under a Creative Commons Attribution 4.0 International License.

flap or a false lumen (Answer B is incorrect). The patient's presentation and imaging findings are not consistent with a tension pneumothorax, which would typically present with sudden onset of shortness of breath, hypoxia, and unilateral absence of lung sliding on lung POCUS (Answer C is incorrect). The patient's presentation and imaging findings do not suggest a myocardial infarction. An ECG showed sinus rhythm with low voltages, which is more consistent with a pericardial effusion, and there were no specific findings on imaging to suggest a myocardial infarction (Answer D is incorrect). The most likely diagnosis for this patient is cardiac tamponade. This is supported by the patient's blood pressure, history of end-stage renal disease on hemodialysis and a chronic pericardial effusion, the presence of a large pericardial effusion on POCUS, and the finding of partial early systolic right atrial collapse on a formal transthoracic echocardiogram. Although there were no other echo features of cardiac tamponade, the clinical presentation and imaging findings are most consistent with this diagnosis (Answer A is correct). It is important to remember that tamponade is a clinical diagnosis. In this case, the patient has somewhat low blood pressure, suggesting early tamponade. There are some important findings to reiterate from the set of images taken before and after volume repletion. In ▶ **Video 34.11A,B**, we can see right atrial collapse and a small and collapsible IVC. In ▶ **Video 34.11C,D**, we see that after volume repletion, right atrial collapse is no longer visible, though the IVC remains relatively small and collapsible.

KEY POINTS

- In an urgent situation, cardiac POCUS may help detect the presence of pericardial effusion and tamponade, based on findings including chamber collapse and IVC size.
- In such situations, cardiac POCUS may expedite management such as volume repletion and guide further testing and management.
- Lung ultrasound may compliment cardiac POCUS findings to help differentiate the etiology of cardiopulmonary symptoms.

27. **Answer: A.** The parasternal long-axis, parasternal short-axis, and 4-chamber views clearly show poor global contraction of the left ventricle. Though POCUS does not typically provide a quantified LVEF, a visual estimate, especially in the case where LV function is severely reduced, can and should be discerned by most operators. In this case, LVEF is probably in the 30% range based upon *visual* estimation. LV dilatation can be more difficult to assess by POCUS, especially in the absence of caliper measurements; however, Answer A remains the best answer even if one is unsure of whether LV dilatation is present or not (Answer A is correct). There clearly is reduction in LV function and LV abnormalities are present as described, with severe global reduction in LVEF (Answers B and C are incorrect). No significant pericardial effusion is seen. There is trace effusion seen posterior to the LV in the parasternal long-axis view only (Answer D is incorrect).

28. **Answer: A.** In both the parasternal long-axis views and 4-chamber views, the RV size is approaching the size of the LV. In the case of LV dilatation, using this comparison benchmark to determine RV dilatation may be challenging and may require expertise. The RV is particularly difficult to image, and the POCUS operator must be careful to not overcall or undercall findings for this challenging chamber. In this case, the inferior vena cava is clearly dilated and does not appear to collapse, suggesting increased right atrial pressure. Taken together, these findings suggest increased right-sided pressures that can occur in biventricular systolic dysfunction with group II pulmonary hypertension and so Answer A is the best option (Answer A is correct). Note that pulmonary hypertension was not estimated on this scan and requires slightly more advanced quantification typically conducted by a full-service echo machine. The RV is clearly reduced in function and the inferior vena cava dilatation does suggest increased RA pressure, and RV abnormalities are present as explained above (Answers B and C are incorrect). There is no pericardial effusion seen adjacent to the RV. The subcostal view is often the best view to see if there is an effusion next to the heart (Answer D is incorrect).

29. **Answer: B.** There is a trace effusion seen in the parasternal long-axis view. This sliver of an effusion is physiologic (Answer B is correct). The cardiac POCUS examination does not show significant pericardial effusion (Answer A is incorrect). This cardiac POCUS examination includes views that can detect pericardial effusion, and a degree of pericardial effusion is viewable on this examination (Answers C and D are incorrect).

30. **Answer: A.** Acute decompensated congestive heart failure is the most likely diagnosis after cardiac POCUS examination. This is clearly seen by the biventricular systolic dysfunction, dilated IVC without >50% respirophasic variation, the presence of a bilateral B-line pattern on lung ultrasound (an alveolar interstitial syndrome, pulmonary edema in this case), and significant bilateral pleural effusion (Answer A is correct). Acute respiratory distress syndrome can have B-line pattern on lung ultrasound, but the large pleural effusions are not typical. COPD flare is expected to have an A-line pattern on lung ultrasound, not substantial lung water as in this case. Acute pulmonary embolism is not expected to

cause pulmonary edema or bilateral large effusions (Answers B, C, and D are incorrect).

> **KEY POINTS**
> - Visually estimating LV function is an important and useful skill.
> - Chest ultrasound includes evaluating the pleural interface for lung sliding (to rule out pneumothorax), evaluating the pleural space for effusion, and evaluating the lung parenchyma for A lines (normal lung aeration) or B lines (alveolar-interstitial syndrome such as pulmonary edema).
> - Integrating chest with cardiac POCUS is important for the rapid assessment of dyspnea and respiratory failure at the bedside.

31. **Answer: C.** The inferior vena cava was not fully visualized and could not help in suggesting whether there was right ventricular dysfunction (Answer A is incorrect). Abnormal movement of the interventricular septum is a cardiac POCUS finding that is not definitively suggestive of right ventricular dysfunction (Answer B is incorrect). A hyperechoic image in the pulmonary artery may suggest pathology related to the RV, although this finding does not definitively indicate RV dysfunction and thus is not the best answer option (Answer D is incorrect). In the cardiac POCUS exam, a dilated right ventricle and flattening of the interventricular septum are suggestive of right ventricular dysfunction. These findings indicate that the right ventricle is under increased pressure and is struggling to maintain adequate output (Answer C is correct).

32. **Answer: D.** While the patient's PaO₂/FiO₂ ratio is low, the specific findings on the cardiac POCUS exam point more toward a right heart thrombus than acute respiratory distress syndrome (Answer A is incorrect). There are no specific findings on the cardiac POCUS exam or the chest POCUS that indicate a pneumothorax (Answer B is incorrect). The cardiac POCUS exam findings do not suggest an acute myocardial infarction; instead, they point toward right ventricular dysfunction likely due to a right heart thrombus (Answer C is incorrect). Based on the cardiac POCUS exam findings, the most likely diagnosis is a right heart thrombus. The presence of a hyperechoic image in the right ventricle, along with dilated right ventricle and flattening of the interventricular septum, suggests right ventricular dysfunction due to a potential clot (Answer D is correct).

Case 4 was adapted from Velasco Malagón S, Moreno Ladino J, Ruiz HA. Three cases of right heart thrombus: using POCUS for the diagnosis of thromboembolism in COVID-19. *POCUS J.* 2022;7(2):197-200, licensed under a Creative Commons Attribution 4.0 International License.

For additional explanation, the emphasis of this case was upon the right ventricular findings on cardiac POCUS to highlight the probable cause of the patient's main symptoms. However, an astute reader may also notice that there were some findings on the lung POCUS including confluent B lines and basal consolidation. Examples of these findings, as well as additional lung ultrasound findings, are presented in **Table 34.1** and **Figure 34.2**. These findings can be obtained via an 8-point or 12-point lung POCUS exam. The full performance of lung POCUS is beyond the scope of this particular case, although further resources are available as an educational module at https://pocusjournal.com/education/introduction-to-lung-pocus/. This module is highly comprehensive and discusses normal and pathological findings related to B lines, pleural sliding, consolidation, effusions, and A lines with and without lung point.

> **KEY POINTS**
> - Cardiac POCUS may be useful in the assessment of cardiopulmonary symptoms in patients with COVID-19.
> - Lung POCUS findings including B lines, consolidation, and pleural effusion may point to either edema or pneumonia.
> - Cardiac POCUS may be used for the detection of RV pathology.

33. **Answer: C.** A left heart thrombus would typically appear as an echogenic mass within the left atrium or left ventricle, usually attached to the walls or valves. In some cases, it can be mobile and may cause a risk of embolization. Cardiac POCUS did not reveal any such echogenic mass or structure, suggesting that there was no left heart thrombus present in this patient (Answer A is incorrect). On a cardiac POCUS examination, a sinus of Valsalva aneurysm would appear as a dilated, saccular, or fusiform structure arising from one of the aortic sinuses, usually in the parasternal long-axis or short-axis views. Cardiac POCUS did not show any such dilation or outpouching, indicating that a sinus of Valsalva aneurysm was not present in this patient (Answer B is incorrect). The cardiac POCUS examination reveals a dilated coronary sinus. A dilated coronary sinus can indicate increased pressure or volume in the right atrium, or it can be caused by an abnormal connection between the systemic and pulmonary venous systems. The cardiac POCUS examination found a dilated coronary sinus, which could suggest increased right atrial pressure, but it did not directly find right atrial hypertension (Answer C is correct, Answer D is incorrect).

34. Answer: B. Based on the agitated saline contrast cardiac POCUS findings, saline bubbles from the left cubital vein can be observed entering the coronary sinus and then the right ventricle. This finding indicates the presence of a persistent left SVC, in which the left upper extremity venous drainage enters the coronary sinus, resulting in dilation (Answer B is correct). The agitated saline contrast cardiac POCUS did not show saline bubbles entering the left atrium, left ventricle, or pulmonary artery (Answers A, C, and D are incorrect).

> **KEY POINTS**
> - Cardiac POCUS may be useful for the initial detection of some simple congenital heart disease lesions.
> - In the hands of experienced operators, cardiac POCUS with contrast may aid in the detection of simple congenital lesions.

35. Answer: A. The patient has a peripartum cardiomyopathy. This young woman appears quite ill, tachycardic, hypotensive, and hypoxic. Rapid bedside evaluation is critical. All of the diagnoses listed are possible and certainly have different management strategies. While she has peripheral edema that may steer the clinician toward CHF, edema has very poor specificity for cardiac involvement and is not uncommon in a postpartum patient. With the bedside cardiac POCUS images, both the parasternal long and short axes rapidly exclude a significant pericardial effusion and clearly demonstrate severe LV systolic dysfunction. While the patient may need further testing and should have comprehensive echocardiography as soon as possible, her immediate management could proceed using the information obtained from the cardiac POCUS.

> **KEY POINTS**
> - Cardiac POCUS can be useful as a binary assessment of pericardial effusion or LV dysfunction.

36. Answer: B. The patient has cardiac tamponade. Dyspnea in an immunocompromised patient has a broad differential. There are clues from the physical examination that he is in heart failure, leading away from pneumonia, but after physical examination, the differential still includes disorders with very different management strategies. The cardiac POCUS images obtained by a user with basic cardiac POCUS training demonstrate within minutes of arriving at the bedside that LV systolic function is preserved and there is a significant pericardial effusion. As the diagnosis of tamponade is clinical, seeing an effusion on cardiac POCUS should prompt the clinician to check for a pulsus paradoxus, which they may have not done initially without suspecting a pericardial effusion. While the ultrasound assessment of tamponade is complex and involves several modalities/views, looking for obvious compression of the RV (seen in the subcostal view) should be noted by a cardiac POCUS practitioner.

> **KEY POINTS**
> - Cardiac POCUS may be useful in the initial assessment of clinical tamponade; findings such as effusion and chamber collapse may expedite diagnosis and management.

37. Answer: C. Within minutes at the bedside, the differential of this patient is quickly narrowed. Both views clearly show normal LV systolic function (Answer A is incorrect). The RV size is normal, while normal RV size and function should never be used to exclude acute pulmonary embolism, it does lower the likelihood that recurrent pulmonary embolism is the correct diagnosis. Although the aortic valve is mildly calcified, there is nothing to suggest rheumatic involvement of the mitral valve. The parasternal views show LV hypertrophy (wall thickness at end diastole >1.1 cm) with preserved systolic function and an enlarged LA most consistent with hypertensive heart disease.

> **KEY POINTS**
> - Cardiac POCUS may help rule out significant pathology related to LV and RV dysfunction.

38. Answer: D. Cardiac POCUS performed from the parasternal view shows normal LV systolic function, no pericardial effusion, no LV hypertrophy, and a nondilated LA and RV. Valvular heart disease requires significant training to appropriately image and interpret so it is not in the purview of a typical cardiac POCUS examination. However, after evaluating the typical cardiac POCUS targets from the parasternal views, the mitral and aortic valves should be looked at for obvious abnormalities. Any suspected valvular abnormalities should prompt referral for comprehensive echocardiography. There is an obvious mass attached to the LA

Case 5 was adapted from Bitar ZI, Abdelfatah M, Maadarani OS, Alanbaei M, Al Hamdan RJ. Point-of-care ultrasound to detect dilated coronary sinus in adults. *POCUS J*. 2022;7(2):208-211, licensed under a Creative Commons Attribution 4.0 International License.

surface of the mitral valve consistent with vegetation. While awaiting complete TTE or TEE evaluation, this is certainly enough to start intravenous antibiotics as blood cultures have already been collected.

> **KEY POINTS**
> - Cardiac POCUS may be useful in the initial assessment of valvular disease; comprehensive echocardiography is often required for full assessment.

39. Answer: A. Cardiac POCUS images acquired from the parasternal views show that LV systolic function is not preserved (Answer D is incorrect). There is no pericardial effusion (Answer B is incorrect). While cor pulmonale cannot be excluded with cardiac POCUS, the normal size of the RV makes it less likely. Complete analysis of wall motion is a difficult interpretive skill and belongs in the scope of practice of an echocardiographer. However, a practitioner performing cardiac POCUS should note obvious wall motion abnormalities such as that present in this example. The parasternal long-axis view shows significant hypokinesis of the posterior wall and the short-axis view shows hypokinesis of the inferior-posterior segments. This cardiac POCUS study is in no way definitive, but it helps steer the initial management and next diagnostic set of tests toward ischemic heart disease.

> **KEY POINTS**
> - Cardiac POCUS may be able to detect wall motion abnormality and LV dysfunction, helping to guide initial diagnosis and management of ischemic disease.

40. Answer: C. While all of these diagnoses are clinically possible, the cardiac POCUS examination, which can be performed in less than 5 minutes, helps quickly narrow the differential. LV systolic dysfunction is excluded by noting the preserved contraction of the LV. Both the parasternal and subcostal views demonstrate severe RV enlargement and dysfunction. While this has a differential of its own, it strongly points to pulmonary hypertension as a potential diagnosis. Comprehensive TTE and further evaluation are indicated.

> **KEY POINTS**
> - Cardiac POCUS may be useful as an initial screening tool in the assessment of pulmonary hypertension.

41. Answer: D. An older man with dyspnea and chest pain has a broad differential. Cardiac POCUS certainly does not confirm any specific etiology. However, these views have rapidly excluded LV systolic dysfunction and a significant pericardial effusion. Assessment of valvular heart disease requires a comprehensive echocardiogram; however, while imaging a patient from the parasternal view, quick inspection of the aortic and mitral valve is reasonable. The significant reduction in aortic valve excursion along with its calcification and murmur on physical examination makes aortic stenosis a distinct possibility and would certainly alter the diagnostic and initial management of this patient while awaiting definitive testing.

> **KEY POINTS**
> - Cardiac POCUS can be useful in the initial assessment of aortic valve disease.

SUGGESTED READINGS

Díaz-Gómez JL, Mayo PH, Koenig SJ. Point-of-care ultrasonography. *N Engl J Med.* 2021;385(17):1593-1602.

Gianstefani S, Catibog N, Whittaker AR, et al. Pocket-size imaging device: effectiveness for ward-based transthoracic studies. *Eur Heart J Cardiovasc Imaging.* 2013;14(12):1132-1139.

Johri AM, Durbin J, Newbigging J, et al. Cardiac point-of-care ultrasound: state-of-the-art in medical school education. *J Am Soc Echocardiogr.* 2018;31(7):749-760.

Johri AM, Galen B, Kirkpatrick JN, Lanspa M, Mulvagh S, Thamman R. ASE statement on point-of-care ultrasound during the 2019 Novel Coronavirus Pandemic. *J Am Soc Echocardiogr.* 2020;33(6):670-673.

Johri AM, Glass C, Hill B, et al. The evolution of cardiovascular ultrasound: a review of cardiac point-of-care ultrasound (POCUS) across specialties. *Am J Med.* 2023;136(7):621-628.

Kovell LC, Ali MT, Hays AG, et al. Defining the role of point-of-care ultrasound in cardiovascular disease [published correction appears in *Am J Cardiol.* 2019;123(4):706-707]. *Am J Cardiol.* 2018;122(8):1443-1450.

Kirkpatrick JN, Grimm R, Johri AM, et al. Recommendations for echocardiography laboratories participating in cardiac point of care cardiac ultrasound (POCUS) and critical care echocardiography training: report from the American Society of Echocardiography. *J Am Soc Echocardiogr.* 2020;33(4):409-422.e4.

Lu JC, Riley A, Conlon T, et al. Recommendations for cardiac point-of-care ultrasound in children: a report from the American Society of Echocardiography. *J Am Soc Echocardiogr*. 2023;36(3):265-277.

Muhame RM, Dragulescu A, Nadimpalli A, et al. Cardiac point of care ultrasound in resource limited settings to manage children with congenital and acquired heart disease. *Cardiol Young*. 2021;31(10):1651-1657.

Zanza C, Longhitano Y, Artico M, et al. Bedside cardiac pocus in emergency setting: a practice review. *Rev Recent Clin Trials*. 2020;15(4):269-277.

CHAPTER 35

New Technologies and Expanding Utility of Ultrasound

Sasha-ann East and Partho P. Sengupta

QUESTIONS

1. In comparison with conventional cardiac ultrasound imaging, which of the following statements is **TRUE** regarding ultrafast ultrasound imaging?
   A. Temporal resolution is higher compared to conventional ultrasound imaging.
   B. Speed of image transmission to archiving is faster than conventional ultrasound imaging.
   C. Speed of the image displayed on the screen is higher than conventional ultrasound imaging.
   D. Axial resolution is higher compared to conventional ultrasound imaging.

2. In ultrafast ultrasound, beam transmission is:
   A. Narrow.
   B. Unfocused.
   C. Convergent.
   D. Focused.

3. Which of the following is characteristic of plane-wave transmission?
   A. Imaging a narrow field of view over multiple emissions.
   B. Imaging a narrow field of view in a phased array.
   C. Imaging a wide field of view with a single emission.
   D. Imaging a wide field of view in a linear array.

4. Plane-wave imaging can achieve frame rates up to:
   A. 10 to 20 frames per second.
   B. 40 to 80 frames per second.
   C. 250 to 500 frames per second.
   D. 2500 – 5000 frames per second.

5. Which of the following best describes the spatial resolution of a plane-wave image?
   A. Spatial resolution is high.
   B. Spatial resolution is not affected in plane-wave imaging.
   C. Spatial resolution is poor.
   D. Spatial resolution is superior to conventional imaging.

6. Which of the following is a potential benefit of ultrafast Doppler imaging?
   A. Better discrimination between blood flow and tissue movement.
   B. Evaluation of high continuous-wave velocities.
   C. Better evaluation of ejection fraction.
   D. Better evaluation of early diastolic annular motion.

7. Which of the following best describes vector flow imaging?
   A. Technique used to measure the direction of blood flow velocity.
   B. Technique used to measure the direction and magnitude of blood flow velocity.
   C. Technique used to measure the magnitude of blood flow velocity.
   D. Technique used to measure the magnitude of tissue movement.

8. Which of the following best describes shear wave imaging?
   A. Technique to measure myocardial viability.
   B. Technique to measure coronary flow.
   C. Technique to measure myocardial contractility.
   D. Technique to measure myocardial stiffness.

9. Natural shear wave imaging uses:
   A. Myocardial mechanical waves that occur with valve closure.
   B. Pulsed-wave features of coronary flow.
   C. Color flow waves due to average trace amounts of valvular regurgitation.
   D. Myocardial mechanical waves that occur from an external radiofrequency pulse.

10. Which of the following is not related to the concept of sonothrombolysis?
    A. Contrast ultrasound can be utilized to facilitate thrombus disintegration.
    B. Acoustic cavitation can be utilized to facilitate thrombus disintegration.
    C. Ultrasound can create shear stress to facilitate thrombus disintegration.
    D. Ultrasound can be used to track the efficacy of thrombolytics.

11. Which of the following best describes the concept of artificial intelligence?
    A. A computational program that efficiently collects data.
    B. A computational program that can mimic human intelligence when performing a task.
    C. A computational program that facilitates connectivity and data exchange between digital entities.
    D. A computational program that follows a defined set of rules.

12. Which of the following is not a definition of "big data"?
    A. The volume of data received.
    B. The variety of data available.
    C. The velocity of data processed.
    D. The vehicle of data transmission.

13. Which of the following statements does not belong to the description of machine learning?
    A. A computational technique that enables systems to learn without explicit programming.
    B. A computational technique that allows for the analysis of big data.
    C. A computational technique that can provide pattern recognition.
    D. A computational technique that creates rules without data.

14. Which of the following best describes the concept of supervised machine learning?
    A. The machine is trained using unlabeled data.
    B. The machine is given a defined set of rules to follow.
    C. The machine is trained using labeled data.
    D. None of the above.

15. Which of the following describes unsupervised machine learning?
    A. Pattern recognition develops freely without external input or outcome of interest.
    B. Algorithms powered by a defined set of rules.
    C. The use of labeled data to train models.
    D. None of the above.

16. Deep learning is best described as:
    A. A machine learning algorithm that uses multiple sets of labeled data.
    B. A machine learning algorithm that uses multiple layers of neural networks.
    C. A machine learning algorithm that uses multiple unstructured data feeds.
    D. None of the above.

17. Which of the following statements is **TRUE** regarding cluster analysis?
    A. Grouping of labeled data.
    B. A supervised learning technique.
    C. Grouping of unlabeled data.
    D. None of the above.

18. Which of the following is not a clinical application of machine learning to echocardiography?
    A. Image acquisition.
    B. Quantitative analysis.
    C. Prediction of patient outcomes.
    D. Promoting equity in patient care.

19. Which of the following is **CORRECT** regarding external validation of a machine learning model?
   A. The data used for training can be used to validate the algorithm externally.
   B. The data used for training cannot be used to validate the algorithm externally.
   C. If the model performs well on the dataset used for its training, it does not need to be externally validated.
   D. The dataset can be partitioned into data for training the algorithm and data for testing the algorithm.

20. Which of the following best describes the concept of overfitting?
   A. High variance and high bias.
   B. High variance and low bias.
   C. Low variance and low bias.
   D. Low variance and high bias.

21. Which of the following best describes the concept of underfitting?
   A. High variance and high bias.
   B. High variance and low bias.
   C. Low variance and low bias.
   D. Low variance and high bias.

22. Which of the following can lead to spectrum bias in a machine learning algorithm?
   A. The study population has a different disease spectrum than the target population.
   B. Experts cannot easily interpret the algorithm's decision.
   C. The algorithm was validated using the training dataset.
   D. The training dataset was too small.

23. Which scenario best describes a "black box" in artificial intelligence?
   A. A machine learning model that is not generalizable.
   B. A machine leaning model has a systemic bias.
   C. The output of a machine learning model cannot be explained by researchers.
   D. A supervised machine learning model that was developed using inaccurate inputs.

24. Explainable AI aims to **CORRECT** which of the following limitations of machine learning?
   A. Overfitting.
   B. Black box.
   C. Spectrum bias.
   D. Validation.

25. Which of the following best describes virtual reality?
   A. Artificial intelligence.
   B. Machine learning.
   C. A simulated immersive environment.
   D. Big data.

26. Which of the following is a clinical application of augmented reality in clinical echocardiography?
   A. Fusion imaging during cardiac interventions.
   B. Planning of interventional procedure.
   C. Remote assistance during interventions.
   D. All of the above.

ANSWERS

1. Answer: A. Conventional ultrasound imaging uses line-per-line focused beam transmission to generate images. It requires multiple sequential transmission events to image a region of interest. For example, a standard plane covering a 90° angle requires about 200 image lines with an imaging depth of 130 mm. This limits the temporal resolution. In ultrafast ultrasound imaging, the full aperture of the transducer is used to generate plane/diverging waves that can reconstruct an entire region of interest with one transmission event. This technique allows for a higher number of frames developed in one second (**Figure 35.1**). The speed of image transmission to archiving and display over the screen is similar to standard imaging. Axial resolution sees the two side-by-side structures as separate and distinct when parallel to the beam. So higher frequency and short pulse length will provide a better axial image. Both these features are not specific to ultrafast ultrasound imaging.

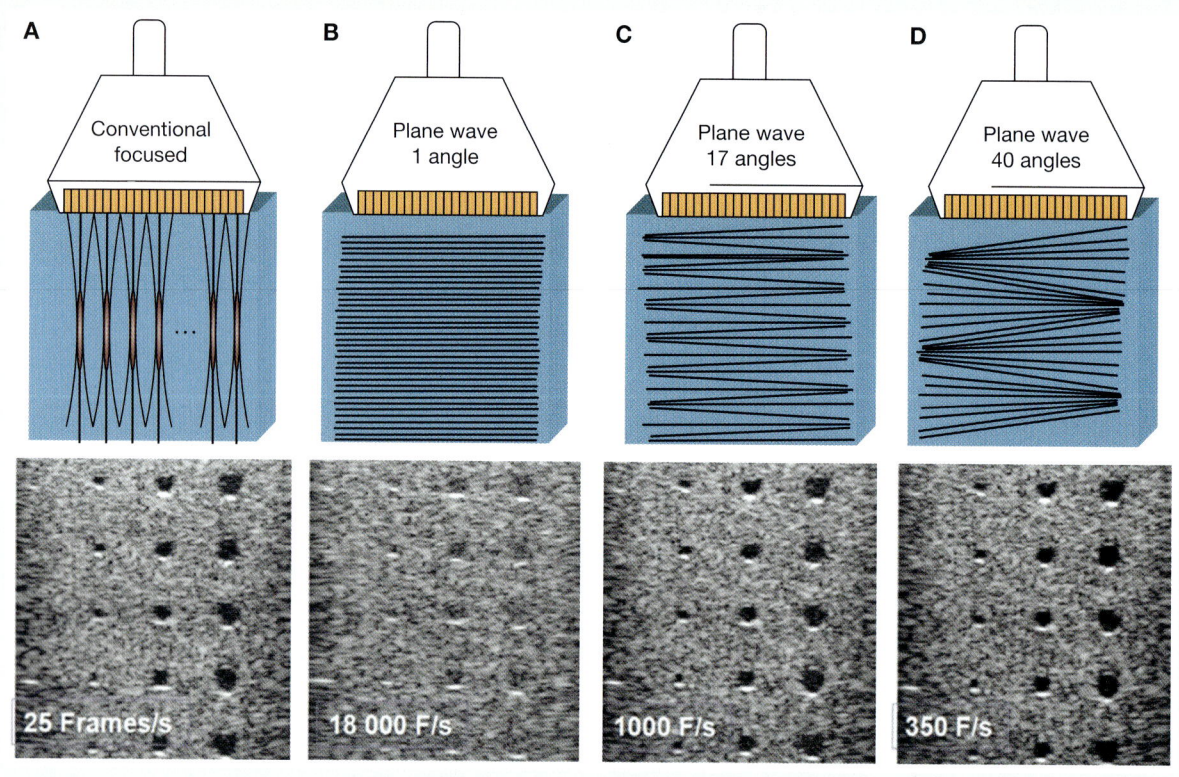

Figure 35.1. Conventional focused and ultrafast ultrasound imaging. **A:** Conventional focused imaging (128 focused beams leading to ~25fps), **B:** plane-wave imaging (~18,000 fps), **C:** plane-wave compounding with 17 angles (~1000 fps), and **D:** plane-wave compounding with 40 angles (~350 fps). (Reprinted with permission from Tanter M, Fink M. Ultrafast imaging in biomedical ultrasound. *IEEE Trans Ultrason Ferroelectr Freq Control.* 2014;61(1):102-119. Figure 2. Copyright © 2014 IEEE.)

2. **Answer: B.** Ultrasound beams can be focused or unfocused (**Figure 35.2**). The length of a focused beam consists of three components: near field, focal point, and far field. A mechanical method of focusing (ie, an acoustic lens) or electronic focusing is applied to the crystal elements, which narrows the beam's focal point, improving the axial resolution. Unfocused beams span the width of the transducer aperture and gradually diverge as the ultrasound waves spread outward from the surface of the transducer.

3. **Answer: C.** Focused beams image a narrow field of view. The transducer sends a pulse and receives returning echoes along the transmission line. The region of interest is insonified line-per-line in sequence, and the entire image is generated when all the transmission events are complete. In ultrafast ultrasound, all the crystal elements of the probe pulse simultaneously to form a flat wavefront that scans the whole region of interest in a single shot (**Figure 35.3**).

4. **Answer: D.** Ultrafast ultrasound can achieve frame rates up to 2500-5000 frames per second. Conventional echocardiographic imaging with multiline acquisition achieves a frame rate of up to 40 to 80 frames per second.

5. **Answer: C.** Beam focusing converges ultrasound waves to a narrow point, named the focal point. Spatial resolution is most significant at this point. Past the focal point, the waves diverge, and spatial resolution degrades. Plane-wave imaging uses unfocused waves to scan a wide region of interest in one emission. The broad transmit beams significantly degrade the spatial resolution. Plane-wave compounding is used to overcome this. In this technique, plane waves pulse the region of interest in slightly different directions, and the final image is the average of all acquisitions.

6. **Answer: A.** Continuous-wave Doppler imaging requires a signal filter to distinguish blood flow from the surrounding moving tissues. Pulsed-wave and color-flow Doppler imaging are required to localize the blood flow. These techniques must be used together to overcome limitations and require significant technical expertise to generate accurate information. Furthermore, even with optimal strategies, only a narrow region of interest can be scanned at a time to maintain an excellent temporal resolution. Plane-wave imaging allows for the discrimination of blood and tissue movement and the concurrent quantification and localization of blood due to its ability to image a wide field of view at a high frame rate. Plane-wave compounding can also be utilized to improve the spatial resolution of the image. Studies have demonstrated the ability of ultrafast Doppler to image small blood flow velocities, allowing flow detection in small structures such as coronary vasculature. This could assist in noninvasive intramural perfusion and coronary flow reserve assessment (**Table 35.1**). Conventional 2D/3D and

Chapter 35 New Technologies and Expanding Utility of Ultrasound / 731

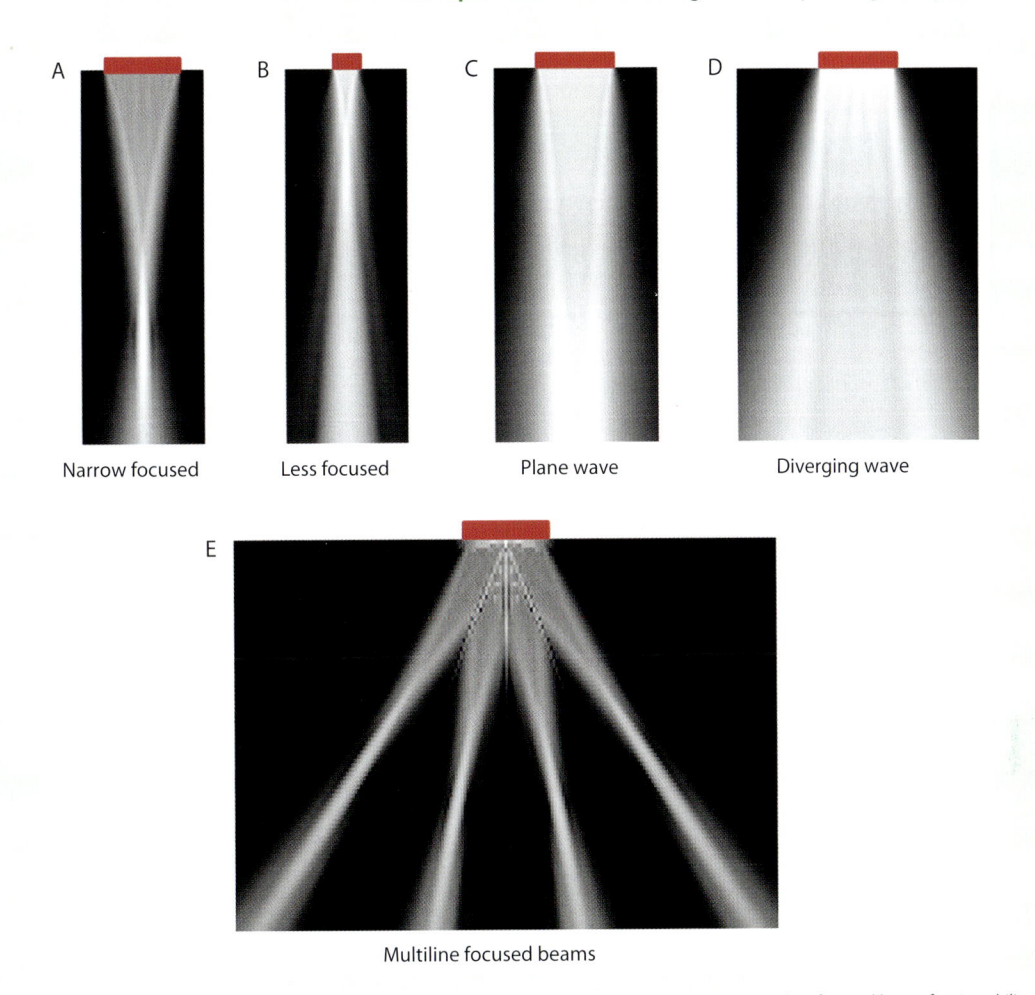

Figure 35.2. Different Kinds of ultrasound transmit beams. **A:** Narrow focused beam for single line transmission; **B:** less focused beam for 4-multiline transmission; **C:** unfocused plane wave and **D:** diverging wave for massive multiline acquisition; and **E:** 4-multiline narrow focused transmit beams. The red bar on top of the beams indicates the transducer aperture size. (Reprinted from Cikes M, Tong L, Sutherland GR, D'hooge J. Ultrafast cardiac ultrasound imaging: technical principles, applications, and clinical benefits. *JACC Cardiovasc Imaging.* 2014;7(8):812-823. Figure 2. Copyright © 2014 American College of Cardiology Foundation. With permission.)

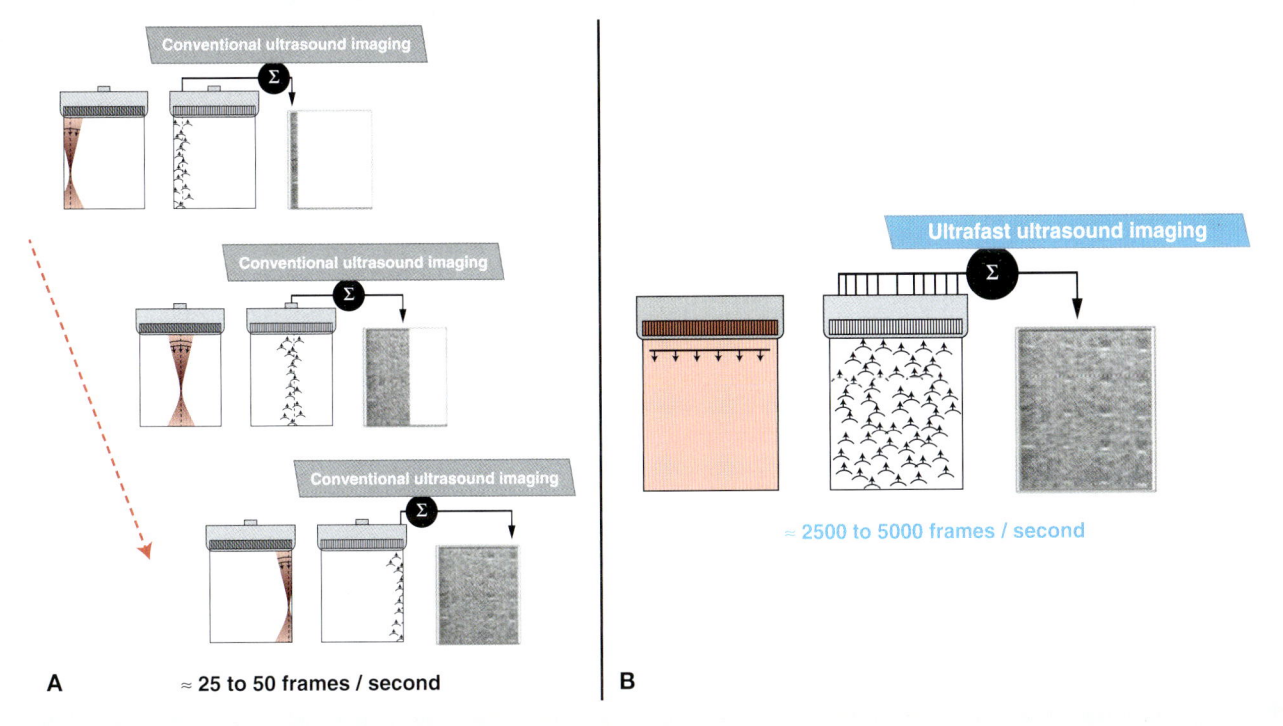

Figure 35.3. Conventional and ultrafast ultrasound imaging. **A:** Conventional imaging shows focused beams scanning the region of interest line-per-line, and **B:** ultrafast ultrasound imaging shows an unfocused plane wave scanning the entire region of interest with one plane. (Reprinted from Villemain O, Baranger J, Friedberg MK, et al. Ultrafast ultrasound imaging in pediatric and adult cardiology: techniques, applications, and perspectives. *JACC Cardiovasc Img.* 2020;13(8):1771-1791. Figure 1. Copyright © 2020 by the American College of Cardiology Foundation. With permission.)

Table 35.1. Summary of New Technologies in Echocardiography

Technology	Description	Potential Clinical Application	Limitations
Blood Flow Imaging using conventional 2D and Doppler Imaging			
Vector flow mapping	• Resolves color Doppler data using a complex equation to determine 2D flow and generate 2D vectors of blood flow. • Can resolve blood flow at conventional color Doppler flow rates (30-50 frames/s).	• Currently clinically available and can be used to assess 2D flow characteristics like vortex formation, energy dissipation, and pressure gradients.	• Cannot be applied to estimate blood flow velocities beyond the Nyquist limit. • Uses complex assumptions in resolving flow vectors.
Contrast particle imaging velocimetry	• Tracks motion of contrast bubbles used in LV flow opacification for generating 2D vectors of blood flow.	• Can be used to characterize blood flow during different phases of cardiac cycle.	• Technically challenging. Requires higher frame rates (>100 frames/s). • Underestimates peak blood flow velocities. • Clinically not available.
Ultrafast Doppler Imaging—Blood Flow			
Blood Speckle imaging	• Tracks blood speckles using high frame rate imaging for intracardiac blood flow analysis.	• Can be used to assess blood flow using a transthoracic probe in the pediatric population or using a transesophageal probe in the adult population.	• Requires high-frequency ultrasound probe. • Assessment is qualitative. • Not available in the United States.
High Frame Rate Echo-Particle Image Velocimetry	• Uses high frame rate ultrasound imaging with contrast agents to track microbubble speckles for intracardiac blood flow analysis.	• Clinical application not well established.	• Technically challenging as this technique requires contrast administration. • Requires high-frequency ultrasound probe. • Clinically not available.
Coronary Doppler Angiography	• Uses ultrafast doppler techniques for detection of coronary flow in epicardial and intramyocardial vessels.	• Evaluation of intramural coronary perfusion and coronary flow reserve.	• Clinically not available. • Requires high-frequency ultrasound probe.
Ultrafast Doppler Imaging—Tissue Motion			
Shear Wave Imaging	• Assesses mechanical shear wave propagation after an external acoustic radiation force to estimate myocardial stiffness.	• Can be used as a part of diastolic function assessment.	• Requires dedicated hardware and software. • Technically challenging. • Visualization of myocardial tissue motion phenomenon is short lived. • Clinically not available.
Natural Wave Imaging	• Assesses mechanical shear wave propagation after a natural event such as valve closure to estimate myocardial stiffness.	• Can be used as a part of diastolic function.	
Electromechanical Wave Imaging	• Assesses myocardial mechanical waves that occur as a result of electromechanical coupling to map the timing of electromechanical activation.	• Can be used to detect abnormal electrical activation in rhythm disorders and cardiac dyssynchrony assessment.	

Table 35.1. Summary of New Technologies in Echocardiography (Continued)

Technology	Description	Potential Clinical Application	Limitations
Ultrafast Doppler Imaging—Tissue Structure			
Backscatter Tensor Imaging	• Assesses myocardial tissue structure by evaluating the spatial coherence of speckle echoes in a volume.	• Alternative to cardiac magnetic resonance–based diffusion tensor imaging.	• Currently only in research and not clinically available.
Elastic Tensor Imaging	• Assesses myocardial fiber orientation using shear waves. Shear waves transmit more rapidly in the direction of the fibers.	• Alternative to cardiac magnetic resonance–based diffusion tensor imaging.	
Therapeutic Cardiac Ultrasound			
Sonothrombolysis	• Use of ultrasound to create contrast microbubble cavitation at the site of vascular thrombi, facilitating thrombus dissolution.	• Being assessed in clinical trials, improves thrombus dissolution in acute thrombotic vascular syndromes.	• Potential adverse effect on endothelial cell integrity and paradoxical vasoconstriction with too frequent high mechanical index pulses.

tissue Doppler imaging can readily appreciate ejection fraction and cardiac annular motion.

7. **Answer: B.** Conventional imaging measures blood flow along the transducer scan line. As a result, blood flow measurement is limited to the axial direction only (ie, blood moving toward and away from the probe). However, plane-wave imaging can visualize the movement and velocities of blood flow in different directions from any angle, facilitating the detection of more complex flow patterns (**Figure 35.4**). In addition, vector flow imaging overcomes the limitation of Doppler angle dependence characteristic of conventional imaging.

8. **Answer: D.** Higher frame rates facilitate the visualization of transient myocardial vibrations that is imperceptible with conventional imaging. In shear wave imaging, an external acoustic impulse from a high-intensity focused ultrasound beam generates shear waves. These waves propagate through myocardial tissue, and the propagation speed can be evaluated using ultrafast ultrasound techniques. Measurement of the propagation speeds helps determine the stiffness of myocardial tissue (**Figure 35.5**). This technique can be utilized for more complex domains, such as assessing the myocardial structure and quantifying cardiac systolic and diastolic function. For example, in patients with acute decompensated heart failure, shear wave elastography can be used to quantitatively measure liver stiffness, which has been utilized as a surrogate for central venous pressure.

9. **Answer: A.** Mechanical cardiac events create low-frequency shear waves in tissue. Natural shear wave imaging uses ultrafast Doppler ultrasound's temporal advantage to track the myocardium's transient velocities in response to natural mechanical events such as valve closure. For example, the closure of the heart valves creates shear waves that propagate across the tissue near the valve. The shear waves cause deformation based on the stiffness of the myocardial tissue. Using the shear modulus equation, the shear wave propagation velocity can be used to calculate the myocardial stiffness.

The shear equation is as follows:

$$Vc = \sqrt{\frac{\mu}{\rho}}$$

where Vc is the shear wave speed, μ is the shear modulus, and ρ is the local density which is essentially constant in tissue ($\rho \approx 1000$ kg/m³).

10. **Answer: D.** The acoustic force of ultrasound waves can initiate fluid motion by oscillating microbubbles (acoustic cavitation), enhancing thrombolysis. Under the pressure of ultrasound waves, contrast microbubbles expand, compress, and collapse. The microbubble oscillations create small streams of rapid flow around surrounding endothelial cells. These microstreams can cause shear stress and erosion of a thrombus, allowing fluid to mix in and increase the penetration of lytic enzymes to facilitate dissolution (**Figure 35.6**). Studies have shown

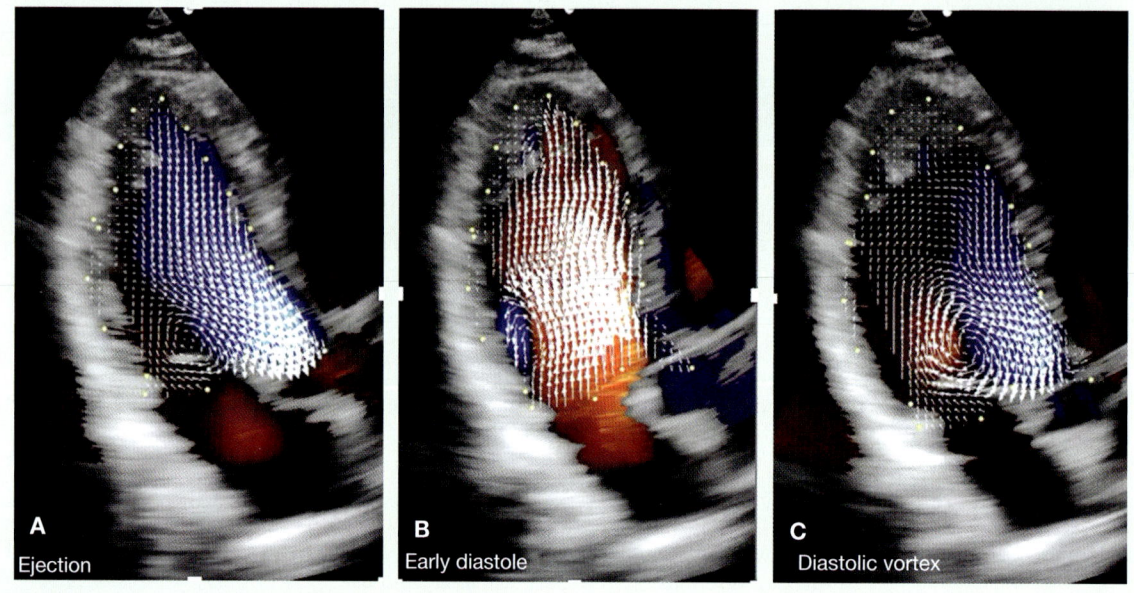

Figure 35.4. Vector flow mapping. Two-dimensional blood flow vectors mapped using vector flow mapping. The images show the blood flow field during ejection **(A)**, early diastolic filling **(B)**, followed by vortex formation during the deceleration phase, and diastasis **(C)**.

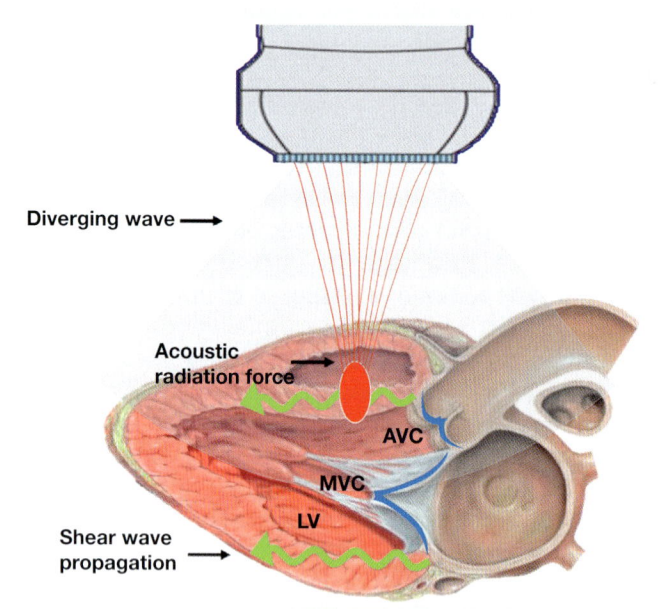

Figure 35.5. Shear wave imaging with intrinsic or external stimulus. External excitation by a strong focused ultrasound impulse (red) induces a shear wave (green) that propagates along the myocardium. The propagation of the wave is then visualized by high frame rate imaging. The propagation velocity of a shear wave is directly related to the stiffness of the tissue. Physiologic events, such as aortic or mitral valve closure (blue), can also generate a shear wave. AVC, aortic valve closure; LV, left ventricle; MVC, mitral valve closure. (From Petrescu A, D'hooge J, Voight J-U. Concepts and applications of ultrafast cardiac ultrasound imaging. *Echocardiography*. 2021;38:7-15. Figure 1. Copyright © 2021 Wiley Periodicals LLC. Reprinted by permission of John Wiley & Sons, Inc.)

promising results in using sonothrombolysis in acute ischemic events (see **Table 35.1**).

11. **Answer: B.** In artificial intelligence (AI), the machine makes autonomous decisions based on the data it collects. Artificially intelligent programs can perform tasks characteristic of human intelligence, such as pattern recognition, object identification, understanding language, and problem-solving.

12. **Answer: D.** Big data are defined by the 3 Vs: volume, variety, and velocity, independent of how the data were generated. It describes high-volume data, comes in multiple types, and is frequently produced. The application of artificial intelligence to big data has been essential for data management. Large datasets are broken down into individual pieces of information described as features. The features can then be used as datapoints within computational algorithms. For example, in cardiac imaging, data such as pixel density or measurement on an image can be used as features for machine learning.

13. **Answer: D.** Machine learning (ML) is a technique used to give artificial intelligence the capability to learn. The technique allows algorithms to analyze data for patterns, learn from that data, and apply that knowledge to make informed predictions without explicit human input (**Table 35.2**). As the model learns from the data, its predictions progressively improve over time. In health systems, for example, health records can be analyzed by machine learning algorithms to predict a likely disease based on the patterns that it recognizes within the data.

14. **Answer: C.** In this form of machine learning, the program is supervised to look for data patterns that fit an outcome of interest. There is an iterative analysis of labeled data with features selected and weighted based on the intended outcome. Regression analysis is a common, simple form of supervised machine learning that uses stepwise models.

15. **Answer: A.** Unsupervised machine learning focuses on identifying any potential patterns within an

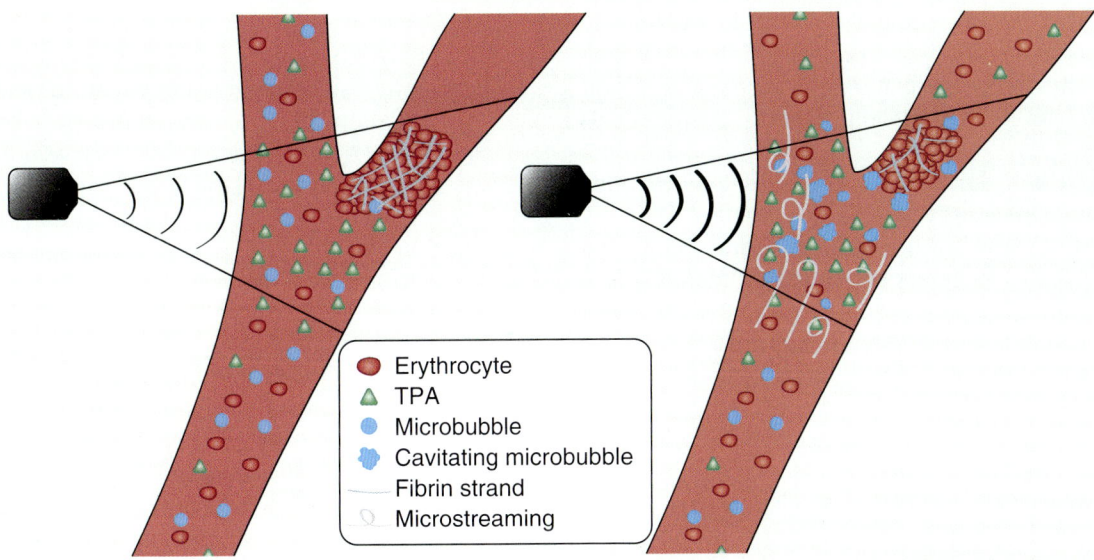

Figure 35.6. Sonothrombolysis. Increasing acoustic pressure creates microbubble oscillations (acoustic cavitation) and microstreaming, allowing for thrombus erosion and lytic therapy penetration. (Reprinted with permission from Roos S, Juffermans L, Slikkerveer J, Unger EC, Porter TR, Kamp O. Sonothrombolysis in acute stroke and myocardial infarction: a systematic review. *IJC Heart & Vessels*. 2014;4:1-6. Figure 1.)

Table 35.2. Summary of Artificial Intelligence in Echocardiography

Artificial Intelligence Methods	Definitions	Clinical Applications	Techniques
Machine Learning	A field in artificial intelligence that focuses on the use of algorithms that mimic human learning		
Unsupervised Learning	Pattern recognition develops from a dataset without explicit input or outcomes of interest	Disease phenotyping	Hierarchical clustering analysis (helpful for recognizing hidden patterns in cardiac diseases that are heterogeneous)
Supervised Learning	Pattern recognition that develops under supervision to fit data to an outcome of interest	Assistance with cardiac image acquisition and automated echo measurements	Regression analysis
Reinforcement Learning	Machine learning technique that learns to make decisions based on positive and negative reinforcement	Automation of medical diagnoses from clinical data	Q-learning
Deep Learning	A special field of machine learning that mimics human cognition with the use of multiple layers of neural networks and feature learning. Able to process highly dimensional unstructured data	Image segmentation to define heart chambers and vasculature	Convolutional neural networks

unlabeled dataset without trying to fit the data to any particular outcome of interest. The model typically learns through mimicry of the data and self-organizes as it uses its output errors to correct its biases.

16. **Answer: B.** Deep learning is a subset of machine learning that uses multilayered neural network techniques with feature learning (**Figure 35.7**). The model learns to detect and represent features from raw data automatically and uses multiple layers of interconnected nodes to progressively extract higher-level features. The network of nodes defines the rules for how the data are filtered, mimicking human neuronal circuit processing. Deep learning models can use labeled data (supervised learning) or unlabeled data (unsupervised learning).

17. **Answer: C.** Cluster analysis is an unsupervised learning technique designed to autonomously find hidden patterns in unlabeled data and group them based on similar (and different) features. This can be an effective tool for discovering new connections relevant to various disease phenotypes and classifications. For example, studies have used cluster analysis to aggregate left ventricular strain data into clusters of patients with different severities of diastolic dysfunction.

    The grouping of labeled data is termed classification, which is a form of supervised learning.

18. **Answer: D.** The ability to extract content from unlabeled imaging data is foundational to applying AI techniques to medical imaging. Machine learning algorithms can localize anatomical landmarks and delineate shapes, such as the contours of cardiac structures. Current applications of AI include a) recognition of standard imaging planes to guide probe manipulation in the acquisition of high-quality images; b) quantitative analysis such as automation of ejection fraction, strain, and velocity measurements; and c) detection of hidden trends between the imaging data and patient variables (eg, age, sex, BMI) to enhance prediction of disease. However, machine learning cannot define rules of equity and diversity and, for these reasons, can propagate current biases in healthcare utilization.

19. **Answer: B.** External validation is the most rigorous way to evaluate the performance of an algorithm. After a computational model has been trained, its prognostic accuracy must be tested by feeding new data into the model. External validation requires using a completely different dataset to test the prediction. For example, if a model was trained using a specific hospital dataset, the validation cohort may come from another hospital or region.

20. **Answer: B.** The accuracy of an AI model depends on the model fit: a well-performing model balances flexibility (variance) and a tendency toward an incorrect assumption (bias). Overfitting occurs when a model performs well on the training data but poorly on testing data. In this case, the model is too flexible and does not distinguish true signals from the noise within the training dataset (**Figure 35.8**). Therefore, the model learns irrelevant features unique to the training dataset that is not generalizable to new data.

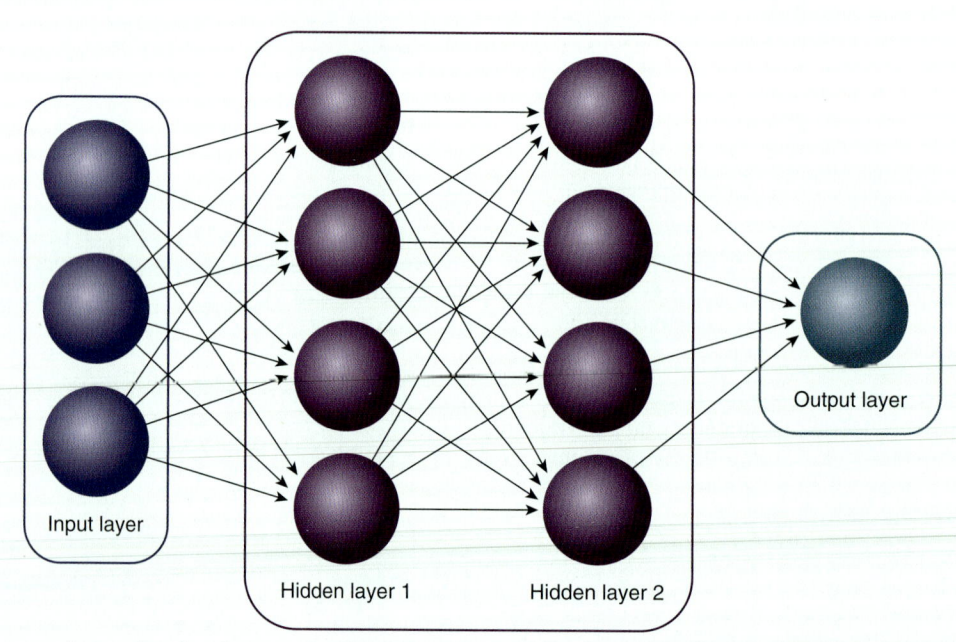

Figure 35.7. Deep neural network. A deep learning algorithm consists of an input layer that brings initial data into the system, multiple hidden layers that extract the inputs' features, and an output layer where desired predictions are obtained. (Reprinted from Davis A, Billick K, Horton K, et al. Artificial intelligence and echocardiography: a primer for cardiac sonographers. *J Am Soc Echocardiogr*. 2020;33:1061-1066. Figure 2. Copyright © 2020 by the American Society of Echocardiography. With permission.)

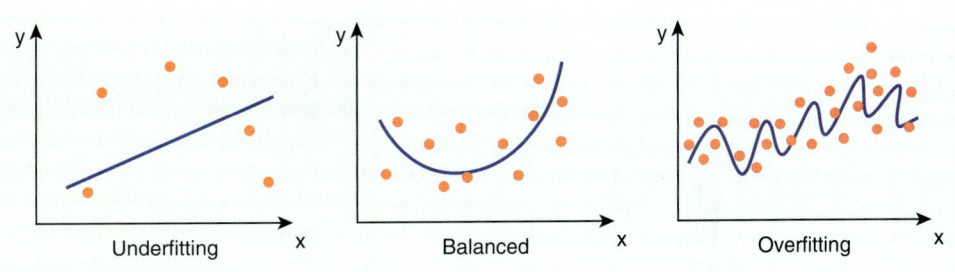

Figure 35.8. Underfitting versus overfitting.

21. **Answer: D.** Underfitting occurs when a model performs poorly on training data. In this case, the model is not flexible enough (low variance) to capture the relationship trends within the training dataset nor generalize new data (see **Figure 35.8**). In addition, it tends to make incorrect assumptions (high bias) about the training data and performs poorly.
22. **Answer: A.** Using extreme spectrums of a patient cohort (ie, all wholly healthy and categorically severe diseases) to train and validate an ML model can lead to spectrum bias. Even though the model may have been trained and validated using both extreme spectrums of a disease, there may be poor generalizability in real-world scenarios where the full spectrum of disease exists (eg, mild disease, equivocal disease).
23. **Answer: C.** Black box AI is a type of AI that is so complex that researchers cannot easily understand the prediction process. A lack of interpretability can undermine trust in the ML model when making decisions based on ML predictions. Deep learning techniques are prone to black box limitations due to using multilayered neural networks to filter data. Depending on the complexity of the network, it may not be readily apparent why the algorithm chose to represent the data in a particular way.
24. **Answer: B.** Explainable AI research has increased significantly in response to the challenges black box models pose. The research focuses on creating intelligible explanations of how a model works by identifying variables driving model predictions and translating the model into a design that resembles evidence-based clinical reasoning.
25. **Answer: C.** Virtual reality (VR) is a computer-generated environment that immerses the user. A head-mounted display masks the field of view and simulates the visual senses. Virtual reality technology is expanding in cardiovascular care due to its potential to assist in planning and performing complex cardiovascular interventions. For example, VR has displayed 3-dimensional (3D) cardiac anatomy in a virtual space.
26. **Answer: D.** Augmented reality (AR) overlays virtual elements in a real-world environment. In cardiovascular imaging, imaging modalities can be fused or integrated with reality to improve procedural success. For example, translucent displays can be used to generate superimposed images. In clinical practice, interventionalists use VR and AR to simulate optimal landing zones before TAVR procedures, fuse fluoroscopy and 3D CT images periprocedurally, and assist remotely during structural interventions.

SUGGESTED READINGS

Cikes M, Tong L, Sutherland G, D'hooge J. Ultrafast cardiac ultrasound imaging: technical Principles, applications, and clinical benefits. *J Am Coll Cardiol Img*. 2014;7(8):812-823.

Davis A, Billick K, Horton K, et al. Artificial intelligence and echocardiography: a primer for cardiac sonographers. *J Am Soc Echocardiogr*. 2020;33(9):1061-1066.

Dey D, Slomka P, Leeson P, et al. Artificial intelligence in cardiovascular imaging: JACC State-of-the-Art review. *J Am Coll Cardiol*. 2019;73(11):1317-1335.

El Kadi S, Porter T, Verouden N, van Rossum AC, Kamp O. Contrast ultrasound, sonothrombolysis and sonoperfusion in cardiovascular disease: shifting to theragnostic clinical trials. *J Am Coll Cardiol Img*. 2022;15(2):345-360.

Jung C, Wolff G, Wernly B, et al. Virtual and augmented reality in cardiovascular care: State-of-the-Art and future perspectives. *J Am Coll Cardiol Img*. 2022;15(3):519-532.

Narula S, Shameer K, Salem Omar A, Dudley J, Sengupta P. Machine-learning algorithms to automate morphological and functional assessments in 2D echocardiography. *J Am Coll Cardiol*. 2016;68(21):2287-2295.

Roos S, Juffermans L, Slikkerveer J, et al. Sonothrombolysis in acute stroke and myocardial infarction: a systematic review. *IJC Heart & Vessels*. 2014;4:1-6.

Tanter M, Fink M. Ultrafast imaging in biomedical ultrasound. *IEEE Trans Ultrason Ferroelectr Freq Control*. 2014;61(1):102-119.

Villemain O, Baranger J, Friedberg M, et al. Ultrafast ultrasound imaging in pediatric and adult cardiology: techniques, applications, and perspectives. *J Am Coll Cardiol Img*. 2020;13(8):1771-1791.

APPENDIX

Equations and Formulas

Dipan Uppal, Michael Chetrit, and Craig R. Asher

Table A.1. Hemodynamics and Physics

Doppler equation	$\Delta F = \dfrac{v \times 2(f_t) \times \cos\theta}{c}$
Doppler equation (rewritten)	$v = \dfrac{\Delta F \times c}{2(f_t) \times \cos\theta}$
	(ΔF = Doppler shift; f_t = transmission frequency; v = velocity of moving object; θ = angle of incidence; c = velocity of sound in tissue, 1,540 m/s)
Pressure gradient (ΔP)	ΔP = flow rate (Q) × resistance (R)
Poiseuille's law	$\Delta P = 8 \times \eta \times L \times Q / \pi r^4$
	$Q = \pi r^4 \times \Delta P / 8 \times \eta \times L$
	η(viscosity); L(length); Q = flow rate; r = radius
Pulse repetition frequency (PRF) (Hz)	77,000 cm/s / imaging depth (cm)
Pulse repetition period (PRP) (μs)	imaging depth (cm) × 13 μs/cm
Nyquist limit (Hz)	PRF/2
Duty factor (%)	pulse duration (μs) / pulse repetition period (μs)
Acoustic impedance (Z)	density of medium (ρ) × speed of sound in medium (c)
Pulse duration (s)	#cycles × period (s)
Spatial pulse length (mm)	#cycles × λ (wavelength, mm)
Snell's law: reflected sound	$\dfrac{\sin(\theta_1, \text{incident angle})}{\sin(\theta_2, \text{refraction angle})} = \dfrac{V_1}{V_2}$
Intensity (W/cm²)	power (W) / beam area (cm²)
Wavelength (mm)	1540 (m/sec) / frequency (MHz)

Appendix Equations and Formulas / 739

Table A.1. Hemodynamics and Physics *(Continued)*

Propagation speed (mm/μs)	frequency (MHz) × wavelength (λ) (mm)
Mechanical index (MI)	peak negative pressure (MPa) / $\sqrt{\text{frequency (MHz)}}$
Cardiac output (CO) (mL/min)	SV (mL) × HR (beats/min)
Cardiac index (CI) (L/min/m²)	CO (mL/min) / body surface area (m²)
Stroke volume (SV) (mL)	CSA (cm²) × VTI (cm)
	$\pi \times r^2 \times$ VTI (cm)
	$\pi \times (d/2)^2 \times$ VTI (cm)
	$0.785 \times d^2 \times$ VTI (cm)
	EDV (mL) − ESV (mL)
SV index (mL/m²)	SV (mL) / BSA (m²)
Flow rate (mL/s)	CSA (cm²) × V (cm/s)
Ohm's law	voltage = current × resistance
	pressure = flow × resistance
Continuity equation (conservation of mass)	flow (Q_1) = flow (Q_2)
	area$_1$ (cm²) × VTI$_1$ (cm) = area$_2$ (cm²) × VTI$_2$ (cm) or
	area$_2$ = area$_1$ × VTI$_1$ / VTI$_2$
	area$_1$ × V$_1$ = area$_2$ × V$_2$ or
	area$_2$ = area$_1$ × V$_1$ / V$_2$
Bernoulli equation (conservation of energy)	$\Delta P = \left[\frac{1}{2} \rho \left(V_2^2 - V_1^2 \right) \right] + \left[\rho \left(\int_1^2 dv/dt \right) ds \right] + [R(v)]$
	[convective acceleration] + [flow acceleration] + [viscous friction]
Modified Bernoulli equation	$\Delta P = 4 \left(V_2^2 - V_1^2 \right)$
	use if V$_1$ > 1.5 m/s
Simplified Bernoulli equation	$\Delta P = 4 V_2^2$

Table A.2. Left Ventricle

LVEF (%)	$(EDV\ (mL) - ESV\ (mL))/EDV\ (mL)$ or SV/EDV (Normal > 51% men, > 53% women)
LV systolic pressure (mm Hg)	$4(V_{MR\ max})^2 + LAP$
LV end diastolic pressure (mm Hg)	Diastolic BP $- 4(V_{AR\ end\ diastolic\ velocity})^2$ $4(V_{VSD\ end\ diastolic\ velocity})^2 + RAP_{(end\ diastolic)}$
LV mass (Cube formula, linear method)	$0.8 \times 1.04 \left[(LVID_d + PWT_d + IVS_d)^3 - (LVID_d)^3 \right] + 0.6\ g$ (Normal: men $\leq 115\ g/m^2$, women $\leq 95\ g/m^2$)
Relative wall thickness	$2 \times PWT_d/LVID_d$ (Normal ≤ 0.42)
LV MPI (Tei index)	$\dfrac{IVRT + IVCT}{LVET}$ $\dfrac{MCOT - LVET}{LVET}$
FS (%)	$(LVID_d - LVID_s)/LVID_d \times 100$
Lagrangian strain (%)	$\Delta L/L_1 = (L_2 - L_1)/L_1 \times 100$
GLS 2D echo (%)	$ML_s - ML_d/ML_d \times 100$
Strain rate (1/s)	$(V_1 - V_2)/distance$
LV dP/dt max	$(4V_2^2 - 4V_1^2)/time\ in\ sec$ (or simplified $32/time\ in\ sec \rightarrow$ where $V_2 = 3\ m/s$ and $V_1 = 1\ m/s$ velocity MR jet) Normal > 1,200 mm Hg/sec

Table A.3. Left Atrium

LA pressure (mm Hg)	$1.9 + 1.24 \times E/e'$ (or simplified $\rightarrow E/e' + 4$) $SBP - 4(V_{MR\ max})^2$ $4.6 + (5.27 \times E/V_p)$
LA volume (Area-Length)	$8/3\pi \left[(A_1 \times A_2/L) \right]$
(Disc summation)	$(\pi/4) h \times \Sigma (D_1)(D_2)$
LA volume index (mL/m²)	LA volume (mL)/BSA (m²) Normal <35 mL/m²

Table A.4. Right Ventricle

RV systolic pressure (mm Hg)	$4(V_{TR\,max})^2 + RAP$
	$SBP - 4(V_{VSD\,peak\,systolic\,velocity})^2$
RV end diastolic pressure (mm Hg)	$LVEDP - 4(V_{VSD\,peak\,diastolic\,velocity})^2$
RVEF 3D (%)	$(EDV\,(mL) - ESV\,(mL))/EDV\,(mL) \times 100$ (Normal ≥ 45%)
RV fractional area change (%)	$(ED_{area} - ES_{area})/ED_{area} \times 100$ (Normal ≥ 35%)
RV MPI (Tei index)	$\dfrac{IVRT + IVCT}{RVET}$ $\dfrac{TCOT - RVET}{RVET}$ (Normal PW Doppler ≤ 0.43; TDI ≤ 0.54)

Table A.5. Pulmonary Artery

PA systolic pressure (mm Hg)	$4(V_{TR\,max})^2 + RAP$
	$4(V_{TR\,max})^2 + RAP - PS\,gradient\,(if\,PS\,present)$
	$SBP - 4(V_{PDA\,peak\,systolic\,velocity})^2$
PA end diastolic pressure (mm Hg)	$4(V_{PR\,end\,diastolic\,velocity})^2 + RAP$
PAP mean (mm Hg)	$1/3(PASP - PADP) + PADP$
	$1/3(PASP) + 2/3(PADP)$
	$79 - (0.45 \times RVOT\,acceleration\,time)$
	$4(PR_{peak\,diastolic\,velocity})^2 + RAP$
	Mean gradient of $VTI_{TR\,jet}$ + RAP
	Mean arterial pressure − Mean gradient of PDA
PVR (WU)	$(V_{TR\,peak\,systolic\,velocity}/VTI_{RVOT}) \times 10 + 0.16$
	$(mean\,PAP - mean\,PCWP)/CO$

Table A.6. Aortic Stenosis

AVA (cm²) Continuity Equation	$VTI_{LVOT} \times \pi(d/2)^2 / VTI_{AV}$
	$VTI_{LVOT} \times 0.785 \, d^2 / VTI_{AV}$
	$VTI_{LVOT} \times CSA_{LVOT} / VTI_{AV}$
Simplified Continuity Equation	Peak Velocity$_{LVOT}$ × CSA$_{LVOT}$ / Peak Velocity$_{AV}$
AV peak systolic pressure (mm Hg)	$4(Vmax)^2$ if $V_1 \leq 1.5$ m/s
	$\Delta P = 4(V_2^2 - V_1^2)$ if $V_1 > 1.5$ m/s
Dimensionless index	VTI_{LVOT}/VTI_{AV} or Peak Velocity$_{LVOT}$/Peak Velocity$_{AV}$
Valvulo-arterial impedance (Z_{va}) mm Hg/mL/m²	Mean aortic pressure gradient + SBP/SV index
Transaortic flow rate (mL/s)	SV (mL/s)/LVET (s)
AT/ET ratio	Aortic transvalvular flow acceleration time (ms)/ejection time (ms)
Pressure recovery gradient (mm Hg)	$4V_{cw}^2 \times [2(EOA/AOA)] \times [1-(EOA/AOA)]$ (V_{cw} – continuous wave peak velocity at vena contracta, EOA – effective orifice area, AOA – ascending aortic cross-sectional area)
Projected AVA (cm²)	$AVA_{rest} + [(AVA_{peak} - AVA_{rest} / / Q_{peak} - Q_{rest}) \times (250 - Q_{rest})]$

Table A.7. Aortic Regurgitation

Regurgitant flow	$2\pi r^2 \times V_{aliasing}$
EROA (PISA method, cm²)	Regurgitant flow/$V_{AR\,max}$
	Regurgitant Volume$_{AR}$/VTI$_{AR}$
Regurgitant volume (mL)	EROA × VTI$_{AR}$
	$SV_{LVOT} - SV_{mitral}$ (if competent)
Regurgitant fraction (%)	$SV_{LVOT} - SV_{mitral}/SV_{LVOT}$
	Regurgitant Volume$_{AR}$/SV$_{LVOT}$

Table A.8. Mitral Stenosis

MVA (Pressure half-time, PHT, cm²)	220/PHT
	220/0.29 × DT
	759/DT
MVA (PISA method, cm²)	$2\pi r^2 \times V_{aliasing}/V_{max\,MS\,velocity} \times \alpha/180$ (α = angle of mitral orifice funnel shape)
MVA (continuity equation, cm²)	$(VTI_{LVOT} \times CSA_{LVOT})/VTI_{mitral}$

Table A.9. Mitral Regurgitation

Regurgitant flow	$2\pi r^2 \times V_{aliasing}$
EROA (PISA method, cm²)	Regurgitant flow/$V_{MR\,max}$
	Regurgitant Volume$_{MR}$/VTI$_{MR}$
EROA (simplified, cm²)	$r^2/2$
	if $V_{MR\,max} \sim 500$ cm/s and $V_{aliasing} = 40$ cm/s
Regurgitant volume (mL)	EROA × VTI$_{MR}$
	SV$_{mitral}$ − SV$_{aortic}$ (if competent)
Regurgitant fraction (%)	SV$_{mitral}$ − SV$_{aortic}$/SV$_{mitral}$
	Regurgitant Volume$_{MR}$/SV$_{mitral}$

Table A.10. Pulmonic Stenosis

PV gradient (mm Hg)	$4V^2$ (pulmonary valve peak systolic velocity)
PASP (when PS present, mm Hg)	RVSP − $4V^2$ (pulmonary valve peak systolic velocity)

Table A.11. Pulmonary Regurgitation

Regurgitant volume (mL)	SV$_{RVOT}$ − SV$_{LVOT}$
Regurgitant fraction (%)	Regurgitant Volume/SV$_{RVOT}$
PR$_{index}$	A/B
	(A-duration of PR signal, B-total duration of diastole)
	(< 0.77 = moderate to severe PR)

Table A.12. Tricuspid Stenosis

Tricuspid valve area (cm², ≤1 cm², hemodynamically significant TS)	
Pressure-half time (ms)	≥ 190 ms or 190/PHT
Continuity equation (cm²)	$\left(\text{VTI}_{LVOT\,or\,RVOT} \times \text{CSA}_{LVOT\,or\,RVOT}\right)/$ VTI$_{tricuspid}$ (more than mild TR reduces accuracy)

Table A.13. Tricuspid Regurgitation

Regurgitant flow	$2\pi r^2 \times V_{aliasing}$
EROA (PISA method, cm²)	Regurgitant flow$_{TR}$/$V_{TR\,max}$
Regurgitant volume (mL)	EROA × VTI$_{TR}$

Table A.14. Prosthetic Valves

EOA aortic prosthetic valve (cm²)	$(VTI_{LVOT} \times CSA_{LVOT})/VTI_{prosthetic\ aortic\ valve}$
EOA indexed aortic prosthetic valve (cm²/m²)	$EOA_{aortic\ prosthesis}/BSA$
Dimensionless index aortic prosthesis	$VTI_{LVOT}/VTI_{aortic\ prosthesis}$
Aortic prosthetic valve AT/ET ratio	Acceleration time (ms)/ejection time (ms) > 0.37 c/w prosthetic valve stenosis
EOA mitral prosthetic valve (cm²)	$(VTI_{LVOT} \times CSA_{LVOT})/VTI_{prosthetic\ mitral\ valve}$
Doppler VTI mitral ratio (for prosthetic dysfunction)	VTI prosthetic mitral/VTI_{LVOT} (normal < 2.2; significant stenosis > 2.5)
EOA indexed mitral prosthetic valve (cm²)	$EOA_{mitral\ prosthesis}/BSA$

Table A.15. Shunts

Q_p/Q_s (ASD, VSD)	$CSA_{pulmonary\ annulus} \times VTI_{RVOT}/CSA_{aortic\ annulus} \times VTI_{LVOT}$ ($Q_p/Q_s \geq 1.5$ consistent with hemodynamically significant left to right shunt)
Q_p/Q_s (PDA)	$CSA_{aortic\ annulus} \times VTI_{LVOT}/CSA_{pulmonary\ annulus} \times VTI_{RVOT}$

LEGEND

α—angle-width of the flow convergence hemisphere
AR EDP—aortic regurgitation end diastolic pressure
AVA—aortic valve area
BSA—body surface area
CI—cardiac index
CO—cardiac output
CSA—cross-sectional area
DBP—diastolic blood pressure
ED—end diastolic
EDV—end diastolic volume
EOA—effective orifice area
EROA—effective regurgitant orifice area
ES—end systolic
ESV—end systolic volume
ET—ejection time
FS—fractional shortening
GLS—global longitudinal strain
HR—heart rate
Hz—hertz
IVCT—isovolumetric contraction time
IVRT—isovolumetric relaxation time
IVS_d—interventricular septal wall thickness in diastole
LAP—left atrial pressure
L_1— original length
L_2— final length
ΔL—change in length
LVEDP—left ventricular end diastolic pressure
LVET—left ventricular ejection time
$LVID_d$—left ventricular internal diameter in diastole
LVIDs—left ventricular internal diameter in systole
LVOT—left ventricular outflow tract
MCOT—mitral valve closure to opening time
MI—mechanical index
ML_d—myocardial length end diastole
ML_s—myocardial length end systole
MPI—myocardial performance index
PADP—pulmonary artery diastolic pressure
PAP—pulmonary artery pressure
PASP—pulmonary artery systolic pressure
PCWP—pulmonary capillary wedge pressure
PDA—patent ductus arteriosus
PHT—pressure half-time

PRF—pulse repetition frequency
PS—pulmonic stenosis
PVR—pulmonary vascular resistance
PW—pulsed wave
PWT_d—posterior wall thickness in diastole
Q—flow
Q_p—pulmonary stroke volume
Q_s—systemic stroke volume
RAP—right atrial pressure
RVET—right ventricular ejection time
RVOT—right ventricular outflow tract
SBP—systolic blood pressure
SV—stroke volume
SWT—septal wall thickness in diastole
TAPSE—tricuspid annular plane systolic excursion
TCOT—tricuspid valve closure to opening time
V—velocity
V_p—color M-mode propagation velocity
VTI—velocity-time integral
WU—Woods units

INDEX

Note: Page numbers followed by f indicate figures and t indicate tables.

A

Abdominal ultrasound, 338
Acoustic impedance, 22
Acoustic shadowing, 7
Acquired immunodeficiency syndrome (AIDS), 568
Acromegaly, 570
Acute bacterial endocarditis, 530, 542
Acute decompensated congestive heart failure, 713, 722–723
Alcohol septal ablation (ASA)
    atrial arrhythmia, 478, 485
        effectiveness of, 477, 485
        myocardial contrast echocardiography, 477, 485
Amplatzer occluder devices, 122
Amyloid cardiac disease, 552, 566
Aneurysms, 571
Angiofibroma, 570
Angiokeratomas, 570
Angiosarcoma, 575, 580, 591
Angiosarcomas, 655, 655f, 665
AngioVac, 440, 450
Ankylosing spondylitis, 571
Annulus paradoxus, 210, 593
Annulus reversus, 590, 594
Anterior mediastinal hematoma, 658, 658f, 666–667
Anterior mitral annular calcification, 554, 567–568
Anterior mitral leaflet perforation, 441, 451
Anterior mitral valve aneurysm, 436, 436f, 448
Anterior mitral valve leaflet, 139
Anthracycline-based chemotherapeutic agents, 515
Anthracycline chemotherapy–related cardiac dysfunction, 207f
Anti-inflammatory drugs, 584, 594
Antiphospholipid antibody blood test, 561, 575
Antiphospholipid antibody (APLA) syndrome, 434, 446
Aortic aneurysms, 612
Aortic annular abscess, 435, 447
Aortic arch, type A interruption of, 673, 682
Aortic atherosclerosis, 600, 613t, 659, 659f, 667
Aortic bioprosthesis, 437, 448
Aortic diseases, 598–617
Aortic dissection, 351, 358
Aortic homografts, 418, 427
Aortic insufficiency, 671, 680
Aortic intramural hematoma, 616t
Aortic prosthetic paravalvular regurgitation, 458, 458f, 470–471
Aortic regurgitation, 144, 167, 421, 429, 429f, 440, 449, 602, 613–614
    aortic dissection, 351, 358
    aortic valve replacement, 346, 349, 352, 356
    effective regurgitant orifice area (EROA), 348, 350, 355
    grading of, 353t
    holodiastolic flow reversal, 351, 359
    left ventricular ejection fraction (LVEF), 346, 352
    modified Carpentier classification, 358
    proximal isovelocity surface area (PISA), 346, 352–353, 357
    regurgitant fraction, 359
    regurgitant jet, 353–354
    severe aortic regurgitation, 359
Aortic (pulmonary autograft) regurgitation, 416, 426
Aortic root
    abscess, 437, 437f, 448
    pathology, 437, 448
    transgastric long-axis view of, 445, 454, 455f
Aortic root dilation, 93
Aortic sinus of Valsalva aneurysms, 614
Aortic stenosis (AS), 248, 261, 323–345, 393, 619, 626, 711, 720
    intervention, 340t
    severity, 339t
Aortic thrombi, 612
Aortic valve (AV), 142, 163, 174
    calcification, 344
    endocarditis, 436, 436f, 448
    repair, 135
    replacement, 346, 349, 352, 356
    stenosis, 717, 725
Aortic valve replacement (AVR), 628
Aorto-mitral curtain thickening, 497, 516
Apical aneurysms, 497, 516–517
Apical hypertrophy cardiomyopathy, 483, 483f–484f, 493, 573
Arrhythmogenic right ventricular cardiomyopathy (ARVC), 565
Arrhythmogenic RV dysplasia (ARVD), 632, 642
Artificial intelligence (AI), 728, 734
    "black box" in, 729, 737
Ascending aorta, 598, 608
    aneurysm of, 599, 609
ASE guidelines, 98, 258, 272
Asymmetric septal hypertrophy, 506, 525–526, 526f
Atherosclerotic coronary artery disease, 568
Atrial arrhythmia, 478, 485
Atrial fibrillation (AF), 133, 378, 386, 396, 619–630
    hypertrophic cardiomyopathy, 620, 627
    left ventricular filling pressures, 619, 626
    lower forward flow, 619, 626
    reservoir phase, 621, 627, 627f
    sinus rhythm, 620, 627
Atrial reversal (AR), 248, 262
Atrial septal aneurysms (ASA), 484, 493
Atrial septal defect (ASD), 138, 145, 169, 579, 587
    large primum, 678, 685
    primum, 677, 684
    relative compliances of the ventricles, 676, 684
    secundum, 482, 491–492, 671, 680
    sinus venosus, 671, 680
Atrial septum, 690, 700
    lipomatous hypertrophy of, 652, 662–663
Atrioventricular dyssynchrony, 321
Atrioventricular (AV) optimization, 228, 239, 239f, 298–321
Atrioventricular septal defect (AVSD)
    anatomic hallmarks of, 671, 680
    complete, 678, 685
Attenuation, 3, 13, 23
    artifact, 37, 53
Augmented reality (AR), 729, 737
Axial resolution (AR), 23, 24

B

Balloon mitral valvuloplasty (BMV), clinical outcomes, 382, 387
Balloon valvuloplasty
    mitral and tricuspid valve, 403, 411
    planimetered valve areas, 458, 459f, 471
    pulmonary valve, 401, 401f, 410
Behçet disease, 435, 435f, 447
Benign cardiac tumor, 652, 662
Beriberi, 563
Bernoulli equation, 20, 28, 600, 601f, 613, 676, 684
Beta-blocking agents, 252, 268
Biatrial anastomosis, 547
Bicuspid aortic valves, 611, 612f, 672, 681
    aortopathy, 611, 611t
Big data, 728, 734
Bileaflet, 415, 424
    mechanical mitral valve replacement, 417, 417f, 427
Bioprosthetic valve stenosis, 420, 429, 460, 460f, 472
Bioprosthetic valve vegetation, 122
Blunt aortic trauma (BAT) classification, 608
Bovine aortic arch, 598, 607–608, 607f
Bronchus, 598, 608

C

Calcification, 497, 516
Calcific degeneration, 378
Calcific mitral stenosis (MS), 381, 386–387, 387f, 388f
Carcinoid heart disease, 562, 576, 637, 646, 660, 668, 669f
Carcinoid, valve pathology of, 660, 668
Cardiac amyloidosis, 232, 243–244, 527–528, 561, 570, 573–574
    diagnosis of, 498, 519
    echocardiographic findings, 520t
Cardiac catheterization, 270
Cardiac dyssynchrony, 312, 319, 321
Cardiac endomyocardial fibrosis, 521t
Cardiac hemochromatosis, 497, 517

Index / 747

Cardiac implantable electronic device (CIED), 452, 454t, 485, 494
Cardiac myxoma, 653, 664
    characteristic feature of, 653, 664–665
    symptoms, 653, 664
Cardiac point-of-care-ultrasound (POCUS), 710–725
    apical five-chamber view of, 712, 721
    cardiac tamponade, 711, 720
    characteristics of, 710, 717, 718t
    continued diuresis, 712, 720
    COVID-19 pandemic, 710, 718
    definition of, 710, 717
    diastolic heart failure, 711, 720
    dilated coronary sinus, 715, 723
    elevated RA pressure, 713, 722
    gender and body mass index of patient, 711, 720
    inferior vena cava (IVC) size and collapsibility, 711, 719
    interventricular septum, dilated right ventricle and flattening of, 714, 723
    limitation of, 710, 717
    LV systolic dysfunction, 711, 719
    LV thrombus, 711, 719
    pericardial effusion, identification of, 710, 718, 719f
    reduced RV function, 713, 722
    training, 711, 720
Cardiac sarcoidosis, 515, 515t, 552, 552f, 553f, 567
Cardiac tamponade, 561, 574, 711, 713, 720, 721–722
    vs. constrictive pericarditis (CP), 588t
    features of, 579, 587, 587t
    M-mode echocardiographic features, 582, 582f, 592
    pulmonary hypertension in cor pulmonale, 579, 589
    test performance characteristics, 592t
Cardiac tumors, 652, 662
Cardiac ultrasound artifacts, 34–56
Cardiomyopathies (CMs), 496–528
    dilated left ventricle, 550, 564
    peripartum, 496, 514–515
Cardioprotective therapy (CPT), 200, 208
Carney complex, 653, 664, 664t
Carney syndrome, 575
Carnitine deficiency, 550, 563
$CHA_2DS_2\text{-}VAS_C$ score, 477, 485
Chagas cardiomyopathy, 523t
Chamber quantification assessment, 76–103
Charcoal heart, 661, 669
Chiari network, 406, 482, 491, 656, 656f, 666
Chromosomal abnormalities, 688, 697
Chronic obstructive pulmonary disease (COPD), 580, 591, 591f
Chronic renal failure, 565
Chronotropic incompetence, permanent pacemaker for, 70–71
Cleft mitral valve, 678, 685
Cluster analysis, 728, 736
Coanda effect, 672, 681
Coarctation of the aorta, 339t, 672, 675, 677, 681, 683, 683f, 684
Coarctation repair, 615
Color Doppler artifact, 39, 53, 53t
Color Doppler imaging (CDI), 27, 28

Color Doppler M-mode (CMM) echocardiography, 250, 266
Color Doppler splay, 41, 55
Comet-tail artifacts, 34, 46
Commissural calcifications, 387
Commissural ratio, 390
Complete transthoracic echocardiography (TTE), 652, 662, 662t
Complex aortic atheromas, 598, 608
Comprehensive valve center (CVC), 390, 391f
Concentric hypertrophy, 229, 242
Congenital abnormality, 230, 243
Congenital heart defects, 672, 672f, 681
Congenital heart disease, 99
Congenital mitral stenosis (MS), causes of, 385, 392–393
Constrictive pericarditis (CP), 182, 196, 253, 269, 558, 559f, 572, 580, 588t, 589–590
    abnormal hemodynamics, 580, 591
    abnormal interventricular septal motion, 580, 590–591, 590f
    chronic, 582, 583f, 593
    chronic obstructive pulmonary disease (COPD), 580, 591, 591f
    echocardiographic findings in, 588t
    expiratory diastolic flow reversals, 583, 583f, 593
    intrathoracic and intracardiac pressures, 580, 590
    left ventricular mechanics, 586, 596
    myocardial mechanics in, 596t
    occult effusive, 585, 594–595
    radiation-induced, 586, 596, 596f
    respiration-related ventricular septal shift, 583, 593, 594f
    restrictive cardiomyopathy (RCM), 584, 594
Continuous Doppler interrogation, 340
Continuous spectral Doppler image, 15
Continuous-wave (CW) Doppler imaging, 41, 55–56, 394, 727, 730
    transvalvular aortic flow, 419, 419f, 427
Continuous wave spectral Doppler tracing, 176
Contractile reserve loss, 244
Contractility, 227, 237
Contrast-enhanced ultrasound imaging, 212–226
Conventional ultrasound imaging, temporal resolution, 727, 729, 730f
Coronary anomalies, 695, 704–705, 704f
Coronary artery graft vasculopathy (CAV), 539, 548
Coronary sinus (CS), 136, 139
Coronary vasospasm, 568
Coupling gel, 1, 11
COVID-19 pandemic, 710, 718
Cross sectional area (CSA), 169
Cyanotic congenital heart disease, 688–708, 702t
    operative concepts, 702t
    surgical repairs, 702t

D

3D echocardiography, 99, 228, 241
    amplatzer occluder devices, 122
    bioprosthetic valve vegetation, 122
    2D images, 104, 115
    interatrial septum, 118–119
    magnetic resonance imaging (MRI), 116
    mitral regurgitation, 120
    multiplanar reconstruction, 121
    multisegmental prolapse, 118

    stitch artifact, 115
    systolic phase, 121
    tricuspid septal leaflet, 118
Deep learning, 728, 736, 736f
Deep neural network, 736f
Deformation analysis, 228, 241
Dehisced mitral ring, 419, 419f, 427
Device-related thrombus (DRT), 625, 630
Diabetes, 496, 514
Diastolic blood pressure (DBP), 168
Diastolic dysfunction, 210
    grade of, 510, 528
Diastolic heart failure, 711, 720
Diastolic stress test, 249, 263
Diastology
    aortic stenosis, 248, 261
    ASE 2016 guidelines, 258, 272
    atrial reversal (AR), 248, 262
    beta-blocking agents, 252, 268
    cardiac catheterization, 270
    color Doppler M-mode (CMM) echocardiography, 250, 266
    constrictive pericarditis, 253, 269
    diastolic stress test, 249, 263
    dilated cardiomyopathy, pulsed-wave Doppler mitral flow velocity, 250, 267
    Doppler findings, 269
    Doppler recording, 250, 268
    early diastolic mitral annular velocity, 248, 261
    E-wave deceleration time, 250, 266
    first-degree AV block, 250, 265
    hypertension, 248, 261
    left atrial pressure, 259, 272
    left atrial reservoir function loss, 249, 265
    left atrial reservoir strain (LASr), 259, 272
    left ventricular end diastolic pressure (LVEDP), 269
    left ventricular function (LVEF), 253, 269
    left ventricular (LV) systolic function, 250, 251, 268
    maximum predicted heart rate (MPHR), 249
    mitral inflow pattern, 253, 269
    pulmonary capillary wedge pressure (PCWP), 248, 263
    pulmonary hypertension, 248, 261
    pulsed-wave Doppler imaging, 249, 265
    restrictive cardiomyopathy with apical sparing, 255, 270
    severe mitral annular calcification (MAC), 260, 273
    systolic velocities, 248, 262
    TTR cardiac amyloidosis, 255, 270
    Valsalva maneuver, 250, 268
DiGeorge syndrome, 672, 681–682
Dilated cardiomyopathy, pulsed-wave Doppler mitral flow velocity, 250, 267
Dilated coronary sinus, 715, 723
Dilute myocardial contrast, 478, 479f, 486
Dimensionless index (DI), 424
Direct current cardioversion (DCCV), 624, 629
Discrete membrane, 672, 681
Dobutamine, 293
    echocardiography, 275, 290, 292
    infusion, 289
Doppler angle, 2, 11
Doppler echocardiography, 338, 339, 340
Doppler effect, 2, 11, 142–196
Doppler findings, 269

Doppler recording, 250, 268
Doppler shift, 2, 12, 26
Doppler signals, 225
Doppler velocity index (DVI), 423–424
    calculation of, 416, 426
Double outlet mitral valve, 385, 392–393
Down syndrome, 599, 610, 671, 680
Doxorubicin cardiotoxicity, 551, 564–565
2D speckle tracking echocardiography, 315
3D transesophageal echocardiography (TEE), 382, 387
    mid-esophageal volumes, 428f
    mitral valve in, 457, 457f, 469
D-transposition, 610
d-Transposition of the great arteries, 688, 698
3D volume measurements, 228, 242
Dynamic outflow tract obstruction, 69–70
Dyssynchrony evaluation, 298–321

E

Early diastolic mitral annular velocity, 248, 261
Early phenotypic hypertrophic cardiomyopathy, 522t
Ebstein anomaly, 399, 408, 410, 692, 702
    tricuspid valve, 689, 696, 698, 706, 706f
Ebstein disease, 648
Echocardiographic contrast agents, 7
Echocardiographic optimization, 318
Echocardiography
    artificial intelligence (AI), 735t
    machine learning, 728, 736
    new technologies in, 727, 732t
Echoes, dynamic range of, 3, 13
Effective orifice area (EOA)
    calculation of, 415, 424–425
    patient-prosthesis mismatch (PPM), 414, 423
Effective regurgitant orifice area (EROA), 20, 29, 30f, 348, 350, 352, 355, 357
Eisenmenger syndrome, 688, 697
Electrocardiogram (EKG), 496, 498, 518, 552, 565
Electronic RV pacing, 634, 646
Elevated pulmonary artery pressure, 400, 400f, 409
Embolization, 136, 652, 662
Endocarditis, 433–455
Endomyocardial fibrosis, 521f
Enterococcus faecalis bacteremia, 436, 448
Eosinophilic endomyocardial disease, 559, 572–573
E-point septal separation (EPSS), 72
Equations
    aortic regurgitation, 742t
    aortic stenosis, 742t
    hemodynamics and physics, 738t–739t
    left atrium, 740t
    left ventricle, 740t
    mitral regurgitation, 743t
    mitral stenosis, 742t
    prosthetic valves, 744t
    pulmonary artery, 741t
    pulmonary regurgitation, 743t
    pulmonic stenosis, 743t
    right ventricle, 741t
    shunts, 744t
    tricuspid regurgitation, 743t
    tricuspid stenosis, 743t
Ergot-alkaloid use, 570
Ergot-associated valvular disease, 563, 577
Escherichia coli bacteremia, 434, 446
EVEREST trial, 456, 468
E-wave deceleration time, 250, 266

Exercise, 289–290
    stress echocardiography, 294
Extra-adrenal catecholamine-secreting paraganglioma, 572

F

Fabry disease, 522t, 556, 556f, 570, 573
FBN1 gene, 599, 609
Fibroelastoma, 398, 401, 401f, 406–407, 410
Folate deficiency, 550, 563
Formulas
    aortic regurgitation, 742t
    aortic stenosis, 742t
    hemodynamics and physics, 738t–739t
    left atrium, 740t
    left ventricle, 740t
    mitral regurgitation, 743t
    mitral stenosis, 742t
    prosthetic valves, 744t
    pulmonary artery, 741t
    pulmonary regurgitation, 743t
    pulmonic stenosis, 743t
    right ventricle, 741t
    shunts, 744t
    tricuspid regurgitation, 743t
    tricuspid stenosis, 743t
Fractional area change (FAC), 66
Fractional shortening, 98
Frame rate (FR), 25
Frequency
    resolution, 3, 12
    wave, 1, 10
Friedreich ataxia, 551, 551f, 565
Functional mitral regurgitation, 319

G

Gaucher disease, 573
Gel, 1, 11
Gerbode defect, 397, 406
Gerbode-type shunt, 445, 455
Ghosting, 39, 53
Global longitudinal strain (GLS), 101, 500, 522–523
    regional and global reduction, 507, 526
Globotriaosylceramide, 570
Granulomatosis, 566

H

Harmonic imaging, 212, 221
Heart failure (HF), 228, 240
Heart failure with preserved ejection fraction (HFpEF), 500, 522
Heart, malignant tumor of, 653, 664, 665t
HeartMate II outflow graft velocities, 537, 546
HeartMate 3 outflow graft velocities, 539, 540f, 548
Hemochromatosis, 552, 563, 566
    cardiac involvement in, 497, 517
Hemodynamics, 142–196
Hepatic vein diastolic flow reversal, 593
Hepatic vein late-systolic reversal velocity (Vr), 633, 643, 643t
Hepatic venous flow, 636, 646
Hereditary hemochromatosis, 550, 563
Human immunodeficiency virus (HIV)
    myocarditis, 551, 565
    with symptomatic pericardial effusion, 554, 554f, 568
Hydroxychloroquine cardiotoxicity, 550, 550f, 564

Hypertension, 93, 248, 261
Hypertensive heart disease, 527–528
Hypertrophic cardiomyopathy (HCM), 477–494, 483, 485, 493, 497, 499, 510, 516–517, 518t, 520, 527–528, 574, 712, 721
    classic M-mode tracings for, 525
    diagnosis of, 498, 518
    left ventricular outflow tract (LVOT) obstruction, 501, 523, 523f
Hypertrophic obstructive cardiomyopathy (HOCM), 192–193, 229, 242–243
Hypoplastic left heart syndrome (HLHS), 691, 691f, 700–701
Hypothyroidism, 561, 574

I

Iatrogenic atrial septal defect (iASD), 463, 474
Idiopathic dilated cardiomyopathy, 66
IE. *See* Infective endocarditis (IE)
Impella cannula, 40, 54
Infective endocarditis (IE)
    abscess, patients, 433, 445–446
    diagnosis of, 433, 445
    incidence of, 449
    modified Duke criteria, 452t
    native aorticvalve, 433, 446
    procedural risk factors for, 448
    recurrence of, 435, 448
    right-sided, 450t
    valvular mass, 433, 446
Inferior vena cava (IVC), 94, 165, 579, 587–588
Infundibular pulmonic stenosis, 398, 407–408
Interagency Registry for Mechanically Assisted Circulatory Support (INTERMACS), 542
Interatrial septum, 118–119
Interventional echocardiography
    hypertrophic cardiomyopathy, 477–494
    left atrial appendage, 477–494
    mitral, aortic, and prosthetic valve interventions, 456–475
    septum, 477–494
    tricuspid valve, 477–494
Intra-aortic balloon pump (IABP), 463, 474–475
Intracardiac echocardiography (ICE), 620, 627
Intraoperative echocardiography, 124–140
Intravenous ultrasound enhancing agents, 224
Ischemic cardiomyopathy, 274–297, 563
Ischemic heart disease, 716, 725
Isolated annular enlargement, 374
Isovolumic contraction time (IVCT), 184, 561, 574–575, 634, 645
Isovolumic relaxation time (IVRT), 634, 645

J

Jet lesion, 140, 337, 453
Jugular venous distension, 154
JUSTICE (Japanese ultrasound speckle tracking of left ventricle study), 199

K

Kaposi sarcoma, 568, 653, 665
Keshan disease, 563

L

Lambl excrescences, 653, 663, 663f
LAMP-2 gene mutation, 504, 524
Large "v" waves, in jugular venous profile, 400, 409, 409f

Index / 749

Left anterior descending artery territory, 231, 235, 243, 245
Left atrial appendage (LAA), 457, 468, 477–494
  anatomy, 620, 626, 626f
  chicken wing, 481, 481f, 491, 491f
  decreased velocities, 623, 623f, 629
  Doppler assessment of, 620, 626
  emptying velocity, 620, 620f, 626
  occlusion device, 479, 480f, 486, 486f
  pericardial effusion, 477, 485
  thrombi, 619, 626
  valvular atrial fibrillation (AF), 477, 485
Left atrial appendage occlusion (LAAO), 625, 630
Left atrial pressure (LAP), 259, 272, 389, 389f
Left atrial reservoir function loss, 249, 265
Left atrial reservoir strain (LASr), 259, 272
Left atrial volume (LAV), 194
Left atrium, 37, 53
Left-sided thoracentesis, 712, 720
Left ventricle outflow tract (LVOT)
  definition of, 477, 485
  gradient, 477, 485
  outflow obstruction, 478, 478f, 486
  stroke volume, 457, 468–469
Left ventricular assist device (LVAD), 530, 542
  acute bacterial endocarditis, 530, 542
  aortic valve replacement, with mechanical valve, 530, 542
  blood pressure (BP), 532, 544
  impeller thrombosis, 532, 544
  inflow cannula orientation, 535, 535f, 545
  mitral E velocity, 533, 544
  moderate to severe AR, 532, 544
  optimization echocardiography, 533, 544–545
  patent foramen ovale (PFO), 531, 543
  pump thrombosis, 531, 543
  right heart failure (RHF), 530, 542
  right-to-left shunt, 531, 543
  RV dysfunction, 532, 544
  secondary mitral regurgitation (MR), 530, 542
  suction, 532, 544, 547
  valvular lesions, 530, 542
Left ventricular (LV) diastolic pressure, 236, 246
Left ventricular ejection fraction (LVEF), 346, 352, 499, 520
Left ventricular end diastolic pressure (LVEDP), 66, 168, 269
Left ventricular function (LVEF), 253, 269
Left ventricular hypertrophy (LVH), 98, 497, 516
Left ventricular mass, 98
Left ventricular (LV) noncompaction, 237, 246
Left ventricular outflow tract (LVOT), 99, 142, 163, 169, 505, 507, 525, 526, 671, 680
  aortic prosthesis, dehiscence of, 438, 449
  obstruction, 416, 417f, 426
Left ventricular outflow tract obstruction (LVOTO), 30, 236, 246
Left ventricular pressure (LVP), 30, 389, 389f
Left ventricular systolic pressure (LVSP), 168, 169, 173, 250, 251, 268
Left ventricular (LV) torsion, 198, 206
Leiomyosarcomas, 654, 654f, 665
Libman-Sacks endocarditis, 555, 556f, 570
Lipomatous hypertrophy, 482, 491
  atrial septum, 652, 662–663
Loeffler disease, 521t
Longitudinal/circumferential strain, 228, 241
Longitudinal function loss, 234, 244

Low-flow state conditions, 341
Low left atrial compliance, 443, 452–453
L-transposition, 611
Lutembacher syndrome, 396
LV ejection fraction (LVEF), 342
LV end-diastolic diameter (LVEDD), 342
Lymphoma, 652, 662

M

Machine learning, 728, 734, 735t
  clinical application of, 728, 736
  echocardiography, 728, 736
  external validation of, 729, 736
  limitations of, 729, 737
  spectrum bias, 729, 737
  supervised, 728, 734
  unsupervised, 728, 734–736
Magnetic resonance imaging (MRI), 116
Malignant melanoma, 661, 669
Malignant mitral valve prolapse (MVP), 232, 243
Marfan syndrome, 571, 599, 609
Maximal inferior vena cava diameter, 99
Maximum predicted heart rate (MPHR), 249
McConnell sign, 637, 647
Mechanical index, 212, 221
Mechanical prosthetic mitral valve, 39, 53
Mechanical valves, 428f
Medtronic-Hall single disc valve, 416, 425–426
Metastatic carcinoid tumor, 558, 558f, 572
Metastatic melanoma, 661, 669
  charcoal heart, 661, 669
Methemoglobinemia, 133
Microvascular dysfunction, 292
Microvascular perfusion defect, 215, 224
Midesophageal 5-chamber view, 133
Mid-systolic signal void, 504, 524, 525f
Midventricular short-axis images, 318
Mirror-image artifact, 54
MitraClip, 456, 468
Mitral annular calcification, 387, 387f
Mitral-aortic intervalvular fibrosa, 393
Mitral arcade, 385, 392–393
Mitral balloon valvuloplasty
  clinical outcomes of, 382, 390
  mitral stenosis patients, 383, 390
  percutaneous, 385, 392
Mitral bioprosthesis, tricuspid ring dehiscence, 417f, 418, 427, 427f
Mitral inflow pattern, 253, 269
Mitral inflow signal, 381, 386
  pressure half-time of, 383, 390
Mitral paravalvular leak (PVL), 462, 473–474
Mitral prosthetic thrombosis, 420, 420f, 427
Mitral regurgitant jet, 441, 451
Mitral regurgitation, 20, 28, 120, 174, 188, 188t, 236, 246, 360–380
  severe, 442, 452
Mitral regurgitation (MR), 484, 494
  left ventricle outflow tract (LVOT) stroke volume, 457, 468–469
  left ventricular assist device (LVAD), 530, 542
  pulmonary vein flow, improvement/normalization of, 457, 468–469
  transient demand–associated, 620, 627
Mitral ring, 385, 393
Mitral stenosis (MS), 57, 65, 173, 381–396, 403, 411
  calcific, 387, 387f
  congenital, 385, 392–393

  etiologies of, 393t
  during pregnancy, 392, 392t
  radiation-induced heart disease, 385, 393, 393t, 394f
  rheumatic vs. calcific, 382, 387
  severity, 383, 390
    grading, 382, 387
  stages of, 387, 388t
  stress testing, 382, 388
Mitral valve, 73–74
  aneurysm, 434, 446
  atresia, 392
  congenital malformations of, 392
  en face view of, 382, 387
  hypoplasia, 392
  planimetry of, 381, 386
  posterior mitral valve leaflet, 439, 449
Mitral valve area (MVA), 142, 163–164, 387–388, 388f
  PISA method, 385, 394, 394f
  planimetry, 463, 474
  pressure half-time assessment of, 385, 395–396
Mitral valve prolapse (MVP), 378, 569
Mitral valve repair, 443, 453
M-mode echocardiography, 6f, 15, 45, 72–73, 73f, 312
  chronotropic incompetence, permanent pacemaker for, 70–71
  dynamic outflow tract obstruction, 69–70
  E-point septal separation (EPSS), 72
  idiopathic dilated cardiomyopathy, 66
  left ventricular (LV), 57, 64–65
  mitral stenosis, 57, 65
  mitral valve, 73–74
  recording, 69, 70f
  rheumatic mitral stenosis, 71
  right-sided heart failure, 72
  right ventricular diastolic collapse, 58, 65
  systolic function, 57, 65
  temporal resolution of, 58, 65
  transducers, 58, 65
  transesophageal echocardiography (TEE), 72–73, 73f
M-mode tissue Doppler, 211
Moderate ischemia, 296
Molecular weight (MW) gases, 212, 221
Multiplanar reconstruction, 121
Multisegmental prolapse, 118
Myocardial contrast echocardiography, 222, 477, 485, 656, 656f, 666
Myocardial deformation, 228, 242
Myocardial infarction (MI), 199, 208
Myocardial mechanical waves, 728, 733
Myocardial performance index, 634, 645, 645f
Myocardial perfusion imaging, 214, 222
Myxoma, 401, 401f, 410, 562, 575–576, 630

N

Native valve endocarditis (NVE), 447f
Near-field clutter, 36f, 52
Nonbacterial thrombotic endocarditis (NBTE), 575
Noncoronary cusp (NCC), 124, 133, 439, 449
Noncyanotic congenital heart disease, 671–686
Nonimaging probes, 336
Nonischemic cardiomyopathy, 274–297
Noonan syndrome, 678, 685
Nyquist limit, 27

O

Oral amoxicillin, 716, 724–725
Orthotopic heart transplant (OHT), 547
Overfitting, 729, 736, 737f

P

Pacing lead–induced tricuspid regurgitation, 400, 400f, 409
Papillary fibroelastomas, 653, 660, 664, 667, 667f
    surgical resection, 667–668
Papillary muscle rupture, 378
Parachute mitral valve, 385, 392–393
Paradoxical low flow, 342
Paravalvular mitral regurgitation, bioprosthesis with, 416, 416f, 426
Paravalvular regurgitation (PVR), 456, 466
Paravalvular regurgitation leak (PVL), 456, 466–467
Patent ductus arteriosus (PDA), 31, 143, 164, 614–615, 636, 646, 677, 685, 690, 700
    with bidirectional shunting, 674, 674f, 682
Patent foramen ovale (PFO), 137, 531, 543, 690, 700
Patient-prosthesis mismatch (PPM)
    diagnosis of, 414, 423
    effective orifice area (EOA), 414, 423
Peak longitudinal strain, 294
Peak prosthetic aortic jet velocity, 415, 424, 424f
Percutaneous left atrial appendage, 481, 490–491
Percutaneous mitral balloon commissurotomy (PMBV), 390, 391f
    Wilkins score, 385, 394–395
Percutaneous mitral balloon valvuloplasty, 385, 392
    contraindications to, 386, 396
Percutaneous pulmonary valvotomy, 678, 685–686
Pericardial constriction, 579, 587
Pericardial cysts, 580, 591
    diagnosis of, 656, 657f, 666
Pericardial diseases, 579–596
    diagnosis and management of, 579, 587
    hemodynamically significant, 579, 587
    loculated pericardial effusions, 580, 591
Pericardial effusion, 563, 712, 721
    cardiac tamponade, 716, 724
    normal pattern, 582, 582f, 592–593
Pericardial metastasis, 583, 583f, 593
Pericardiocentesis, 713, 721
Pericardium, absence of, 580, 591
Peripartum cardiomyopathy, 496, 514–515, 715, 724
Periprosthetic regurgitation, 135
Persistent left superior vena cava, 434, 434f, 446–447
Phenylephrine, 560, 573
Pheochromocytoma, 554, 568–569
Physics, 17–33
Pickelhaube sign, 232, 243
Piezoelectric crystals, 11
Plane-wave transmission, 727, 731, 732f
Planimetry, 381, 386, 463, 464f, 474
Polyangiitis, 566
Post endomyocardial biopsy complication, 403, 411
Posterior mitral leaflet restriction, 236, 246
Posterior mitral valve annulus, 442, 452
Posterior mitral valve leaflet, 441, 451
PPM. *See* Patient-prosthesis mismatch (PPM)

Pregnancy
    mitral stenosis (MS), 392, 392t
    percutaneous intervention, 385, 392
Pressure half-time (PHT), 142, 163–164, 382, 389–390
    atrial fibrillation, 386, 396
Pressure recovery, 414, 423, 423f
    bileaflet, 415, 424
Primary melanoma, 661, 669
Primary restrictive cardiomyopathy, 496, 505, 514, 524–525
Progressive pulmonary hypertension, 717, 725
Prolonged pressure halftime (PHT), 632, 642
Prosthesis, obstruction of, 462, 473
Prosthetic function, 415, 424
Prosthetic mitral stenosis, 421, 430, 431t
Prosthetic mitral valve function, 431t
Prosthetic valve endocarditis (PVE), 447f
Prosthetic valves, 414–431
    dehiscence of, 438, 448
    Doppler parameters of, 425t
    leaflets, vegetation on, 436, 436f, 448
    stenosis, diagnosis of, 415, 425
PROTECT AF trial, 477, 485
Proximal coronary arteries, 136
Proximal isovelocity surface area (PISA) method, 29, 30f, 346, 352–353, 357, 385, 394, 394f
Pseudoaneurysm, aortic root, 438, 449
Pseudodyskinesis, 68
Pseudomitral regurgitation, 36, 51
Pulmonary arterial hypertension, 564
Pulmonary artery diastolic pressure (PADP), 165
Pulmonary artery pressure, 94, 191
Pulmonary artery systolic pressure (PASP), 31, 32, 170, 180, 398, 406, 633, 643
Pulmonary artery wedge pressure (PAWP), 143, 166
Pulmonary capillary wedge pressure (PCWP), 210, 248, 263, 583, 583f, 593, 593f, 619, 626
Pulmonary embolism, 637, 647, 647t
Pulmonary hypertension, 248, 261, 401, 402f, 410, 572, 632–650
    cor pulmonale, 579, 589
    LV diastolic function, 637, 637f, 647
Pulmonary insufficiency, 398, 406, 408t
Pulmonary regurgitation (PR), 31, 399, 408–409, 636, 646–647
    end-diastolic velocity, 633, 643–644
    severity, 650t
Pulmonary valve, 134, 134f
    balloon valvuloplasty, 401, 401f, 410
    cusps, 398, 407
    regurgitation, 558, 558f, 571–572
    stenosis, 572, 675, 675f, 678, 684, 685
    systolic doming of, 398, 406
Pulmonary vascular resistance (PVR), 633, 643
Pulmonary veins, 136
    stenosis, 624, 624f, 629
Pulmonary venous baffle, obstruction of, 689, 699, 699f
Pulmonary venous confluence, 694, 694f, 703–704
Pulmonary venous connections, 689, 698
Pulmonic and tricuspid valvular disease, 397–412
Pulmonic stenosis
    acquired, 407t
    congenital, 407t

    diagnosis of, 398, 406
    infundibular, 398, 407–408
Pulsed-wave Doppler (PWD), 27–28, 249, 265
Pulsed-wave Doppler mitral inflow, 230, 243
Pulsed-wave spectral Doppler recordings, 177
PVR. *See* Paravalvular regurgitation (PVR)

Q

Quadricuspid aortic valves, 613

R

Radiation heart disease, 496, 497, 500, 514, 516, 517t, 521–522
Radiation-induced valvular disease, 385, 393, 393t, 394f
Radiation therapy, 572
Range ambiguity, 49–50, 49f
Range-ambiguity artifact, 51
Real-time myocardial contrast echocardiography (RTMCE), 222, 225
Reflectors, 35, 47
Refraction artifacts, 35, 42, 48, 49f, 55–56
Regional wall motion abnormalities, 552, 566
    noncoronary territories, 500, 522
Regurgitant jet, 353–354
Relative wall thickness (RWT), 497, 509, 516, 527
Renal cell carcinoma, 655, 655f, 665
Residual mitral regurgitation (MR), 457, 468
Restrictive cardiomyopathy (RCM), 498, 519, 560, 573, 584, 594
    apical sparing, 255, 270
    myocardial mechanics in, 596t
Restrictive filling pattern, 237, 247
Reverberation artifact, 34, 37, 45–46, 52, 53
Rhabdomyomas, 571, 658, 666
Rheumatic heart disease, 481, 488–489, 716, 724
Rheumatic mitral stenosis (MS), 71, 392
    medical therapy, 388, 389t
Rheumatic nodules, 569
Rheumatoid arthritis, 569
Right aortic arch, 599, 609, 610f
Right atrial appendage (RAA)
    thrombus, 619, 626
    width, 619, 626
Right atrial pressure (RAP), 165, 398, 406, 632, 642
Right coronary artery (RCA), 135, 678, 686
Right coronary cusp (RCC), 439, 449
Right heart failure (RHF), 530, 542
Right heart thrombus, 714, 723
Right-sided heart failure, 72
Right-sided infective endocarditis
    mortality, 441, 450–451
    surgical indications, 450t
Right ventricular diastolic collapse, 58, 65
Right ventricular disease, 632–650
    cardiac amyloidosis, 633, 643
    chamber size, 645t
    moderator band, 634, 644, 644f
Right ventricular ejection fraction, 95
Right ventricular end-diastolic pressure (RVEDP), 170
Right ventricular hypertrophy, 502, 524, 524f
Right ventricular index of myocardial performance (RIMP), 96f
Right ventricular outflow tract (RVOT), 143, 164, 169, 531, 543
Right ventricular systolic pressure (RVSP), 32, 100, 170, 180
Ross procedure, 416, 426

S

Sarcoidosis, 502, 523–524, 552, 566
Schwannomas, 625, 625f, 630
Scleroderma, 555, 555f, 569–570
Secondary pulmonary hypertension, 384, 391, 398, 406
Secundum atrial septal defect (ASD), 482, 491–492
  abnormality, 483, 493
  right ventricular enlargement, 482, 492
Selenium deficiency, 550, 563
Self-expanding transcatheter aortic valve replacement, 422, 422f, 430
Severe aortic regurgitation, 359
Severely dilated left ventricle, 350, 358
Severe mitral annular calcification (MAC), 260, 273
Severe tricuspid prosthetic stenosis, 417, 426
Severe tricuspid regurgitation, 632, 642
Shear wave imaging, 728, 733
Shone complex, 599, 610
Shone syndrome, 385, 393
Side lobe artifact, 35, 37, 47–48, 53
Sinus venosus defect, 138
Slice thickness artifacts, 36, 50–51
Smoothing, 16
Snell's law, 35, 47
Sound waves, 1, 3, 10, 13, 16
Spatial pulse length (SPL), 23
Spatial resolution, 3, 12, 24, 212, 221, 727, 730
Speckle tracking strain, 321
Spectral Doppler artifacts, 15, 35, 50, 55t
Spontaneous echo contrast (SEC), 619, 626
Standard Doppler, 198, 206
Staphylococcal infection, 402, 410
Staphylococcus aureus bacteremia, 433, 445
Stenotic/prosthetic valve, 29
Stented bioprosthesis replacement, 419, 419f, 427
Stitch artifact, 115
Strain rate, 198–211, 227, 237
Stress (takotsubo) cardiomyopathy, 236, 246
Stress echocardiography, 274–297, 291
  noncoronary indications for, 292t
Stress-induced cardiomyopathy, 567
Stroke volume (SV), 32, 342
Subaortic membrane, moderate stenosis, 674, 674f, 682
Subaortic stenosis, 337, 672, 681
Sudden cardiac death (SCD), 497, 516–517
Supervised machine learning, 728, 734
Supramitral ring, 385, 393
Supravalvular mitral ring, 385, 392–393, 393f
Surgical aortic valve replacement (SAVR), 436, 436f, 448
Suspected pacemaker endocarditis, 397, 404
Synovial sarcoma, 655, 655f, 666
Systemic disease, 550–577
  aortic valve abnormalities, 565t
  mitral valve abnormalities, 566t
Systemic lupus erythematosus (SLE), 575
Systemic sclerosis, 496, 514
Systolic anterior motion (SAM), 137, 137f, 525t
Systolic function assessment, 57, 65
  atrioventricular (AV) optimization, 228, 239, 239f
  cardiac amyloidosis, 232, 243–244
  concentric hypertrophy, 229, 242
  congenital abnormality, 230, 243
  contractile reserve loss, 244
  contractility, 227, 237
  3D echocardiography, 228, 241
  deformation analysis, 228, 241
  3D volume measurements, 228, 242
  extensive late contraction, 235, 245
  heart failure (HF), 228, 240
  hypertrophic obstructive cardiomyopathy (HOCM), 229, 242–243
  left anterior descending artery territory, 235, 245
  left anterior descending artery territory, stunned myocardium in, 231, 243
  left ventricular (LV) diastolic pressure, 236, 246
  left ventricular (LV) noncompaction, 237, 246
  left ventricular (LV) outflow tract obstruction, 236, 246
  left ventricular (LV) strain, 228, 241
  longitudinal and circumferential strain, 228, 241
  longitudinal function loss, 234, 244
  malignant mitral valve prolapse (MVP), 232, 243
  medical therapy, 229, 242–243
  mitral regurgitation, 236, 246
  multiple vessels, 233, 244
  myocardial deformation, 228, 242
  posterior mitral leaflet restriction, 236, 246
  pulsed-wave Doppler mitral inflow, 230, 243
  restrictive filling pattern, 237, 247
  strain rate, 227, 237
  stress (takotsubo) cardiomyopathy, 236, 246
  three-dimensional (3D) echocardiography RV ejection fraction (EF), 227
  tissue Doppler profile, 232, 243
  tissue velocity, 228, 242
  visual assessment of ejection fraction, 227, 238–239
  wall motion abnormalities, 227, 239
  wall stress, 227, 238
Systolic phase, 121
Systolic velocities, 248, 262

T

Tachycardia-induced cardiomyopathy (T-CMP), 551, 564
Takayasu arteritis, 557, 557f, 571
Takotsubo cardiomyopathy, 567, 569
Takotsubo syndrome, 712, 721
Tamponade/constrictive pericarditis, 184
Temporal resolution, 3, 13, 16, 727, 729, 730f
  M-mode echocardiography, 58, 65
Tetralogy of Fallot (TOF), 397, 406, 671, 680, 688, 695, 697, 704
Thebesian valve, 136
Thiamine deficiency, 550, 563
Thoracic aorta, 612t
Thoracic endovascular aortic repair (TEVAR), 604, 615
Three-dimensional echocardiography, 94
Three-dimensional (3D) echocardiography RV ejection fraction (EF), 227
Thromboembolism, 621, 628
Thrombus, 657, 658f, 666
Thyroid, 652, 662, 663t
Tiger stripes, 54
Tissue Doppler, 198–211, 232, 243
Tissue velocity, 228, 242
Total anomalous pulmonary venous return (TAPVR), 694, 694f, 703–704
  cardiac, 689, 698
  infracardiac, 689, 698
  supracardiac, 689, 696, 698, 708
Trachea, 598, 608
Transcatheter aortic valve implantation (TAVI)
  aortic regurgitation, 457, 468
  calcium location and burden, 456, 466
  female sex, 456, 467–468
  implantation depth, 456, 466
  left coronary ostium, 457, 469
  mitral regurgitation, 457, 468
  new wall motion abnormalities, 457, 468
  paravalvular leak, 456, 466–467, 467f
  transcatheter edge-to-edge repair (TEER), 457, 468
  valve under sizing, 456, 466
Transcatheter aortic valve replacement (TAVR), 436, 448
  chronic renal failure, 459, 460f, 471–472
  risk factor for, 436, 448
Transcatheter edge-to-edge repair (TEER), 456, 468
  adequate leaflet insertion and stable tissue bridge, 457, 468
  device orientation, 457, 469
  guide catheter positioning, 457, 469
  mitral regurgitation (MR) severity, 457, 468–469
  mitral valve (MV), 458, 469
  residual mitral regurgitation (MR), 457, 468
  severe mitral annular calcification, 458, 469–470
  transmitral diastolic gradients, 457, 468
  transseptal puncture, 457, 469
Transcatheter mitral edge-to-edge repair, 421, 430, 430f
Transcatheter vacuum-assisted aspiration, 440, 450, 450f
Transducer sound, 34, 42
Transseptal puncture, 135–136
Transesophageal echocardiography (TEE), 34, 45, 336, 397, 404, 579, 588, 589f
  anterior mitral valve leaflet, 139
  aortic ulcer, 605, 616
  aortic valve repair, 135
  atrial fibrillation, 133, 600, 612–613
  atrial septal defects, 138
  Behçet disease, 435, 435f, 447
  bronchus, 598, 608
  contraindications, 134, 134t
  coronary sinus (CS), 136, 139
  coronary sinus, vegetation, 442, 451, 452f
  descending thoracic aorta, 603, 615, 615f
  embolism, 136
  "ghost," 435, 447
  infective endocarditis (IE), 433, 445
  intraoperative, 135, 399, 409
  intraoperative echo, 135
  large pedunculated aortic thrombus, 612
  left ventricular assist device (LVAD), 530, 532, 542, 543
  Libman-Sacks endocarditis, 555, 556f, 570
  lipomatous hypertrophy, 482, 491

Transesophageal echocardiography (TEE) (*Continued*)
  methemoglobinemia, 133
  midesophageal 5-chamber view, 133
  mid-systolic closure of the aortic valve, 483, 483f, 493, 493f
  M-mode echocardiography, 72–73, 73f
  noncoronary cusp, 124, 133
  paravalvular regurgitation, 416, 426
  patent foramen ovale (PFO), 137
  periprosthetic regurgitation, 135
  proximal coronary arteries, 136
  pulmonary valve, 134, 134f
  pulmonary veins, 136
  rheumatic disease, 481, 488–489
  rheumatic mitral stenosis, 384, 391
  right coronary artery, 135
  secundum atrial septal defect (ASD), 482, 491–492
  septal, 480, 487, 488f
  single tilting disc, 418, 418f, 427
  sinus venosus defect, 138
  superior and posterior of the fossa ovalis, 458, 470
  systolic anterior motion (SAM), 137, 137f
  Thebesian valve, 136
  trachea, 598, 608
  transcatheter aortic valve replacement, 456, 467
  transseptal puncture, 135–136
  traumatic thoracic aortic deceleration injury, 598, 608, 608f
  tricuspid valve, 480, 487
  unicuspid aortic valve, 136
  valvular vegetations, 653, 663, 663f
Transient constrictive pericarditis, 584, 594
Transmitted waves, 5, 14
Transthoracic echocardiography (TTE), 91, 397, 404
  ascending aorta, 598, 606–607, 606t, 607f, 614
  basal anterior septal wall, thinning of, 496, 515, 515f
  chest pain, 599, 609–610
  LAMP-2 gene mutation, 504, 524
  regional wall motion abnormalities, noncoronary territories, 500, 522
  suprasternal notch image, 601, 601f, 613
Traumatic aortic injuries, 608f
Traumatic ventricular septal defect (VSD), 479, 486, 486f
Tricuspid annular plane systolic excursion (TAPSE), 67, 636, 646
Tricuspid atresia, 689, 698–699

Tricuspid mechanical valve stenosis, 632, 642
Tricuspid regurgitation (TR), 32, 94, 397, 406
  cardiac implantable electronic device (CIED), 409
  cause of, 398, 406
  etiology of, 398, 407t
  severe, 402, 410, 638, 648
  severity, 443, 453, 481, 489, 489t, 490f
  systole consistent, 403, 411–412, 412f
Tricuspid septal leaflet, 118
Tricuspid stenosis (TS), 397, 403, 406, 411
  Doppler echocardiographic assessment of, 398, 406
Tricuspid valve, 477–494
  deep esophageal and gastric views, 480, 487
  leaflets, 397, 404, 404f–405f
    posterior, 481, 488–489, 488f, 490f
  vegetation, 440, 450
  vegetations on, 443, 453
Truncus arteriosus, 689, 693, 693f, 695, 699–700, 703, 703f, 705
  pulmonary artery ostial stenosis, 677, 685
TS. *See* Tricuspid stenosis (TS)
TTR cardiac amyloidosis, 255, 270
Tuberous sclerosis, 570, 653, 664
Turner syndrome, 599, 610
Two-dimensional imaging artifacts, 43t–44t

U

Ultrafast ultrasound, 727, 730–731, 731f
Ultrasound, 727–737
  acoustic impedance, 22
  anatomy, 17, 22, 22f
  attenuation, 3, 13
  coupling gel, 1, 11
  Doppler effect, 2, 11
  Doppler shift, 26
  dynamic range of echoes, 3, 13
  frequency resolution, 3, 12
  frequency, wave, 1, 10
  human hearing range, 1, 10
  image resolution, 12t
  piezoelectric crystals, 11
  sound waves, 1, 3, 10, 13
  spatial resolution, 3, 12, 24
  speckle appearance, 18, 24
  temporal resolution, 3, 13
  thrombolytics, 728, 733, 735f
  transmitted waves, 5, 14
  unfocused, 727, 730
  wavelength, 1, 11
Ultrasound enhancing agent (UEA), 212, 220, 220t

Underfitting, 729, 737, 737f
Unicuspid aortic valve, 136
Unsupervised machine learning, 728, 734–736
Urinary 5-hydroxyindole acetic acid, 562, 576–577

V

Valsalva maneuver, 250, 268
Valvular aortic stenosis, 599, 610
Valvular atrial fibrillation (AF), 477, 485
Valvular heart disease, staging, 383, 390
Valvular perforation, 444, 453
Valvular stenosis, 420, 429
Valvular tissue destruction, 434, 446
Ventricular interdependence, 593
Ventricular septal defect (VSD), 22, 32, 145, 170, 637, 647, 695, 705, 705f
  aortic insufficiency, 671, 680
  coarctation, 689, 698
  large membranous, 673, 673f, 682
  parasternal short-axis view, 671, 680, 680f
  perimembranous, 494, 672, 681
  physiologic effect of, 672, 680–681
  posterior malaligned, 693, 693f, 702–703
  primum, 674, 675f, 682–683
  secundum, 676, 684
  small anterior muscular, 676, 684
  subpulmonary (supracristal), 673, 673f, 682
  trabecular muscular, 673, 673f, 682
  traumatic, 479, 486, 486f
Very-low-mechanical index (MI) imaging techniques, 212, 214, 221, 222–223
Violated assumptions producing artifact, 43t
Virtual reality (VR), 729, 737
Visual assessment of ejection fraction, 227, 238–239
Vitamin B_{12} deficiency, 550, 563
Volumetric 3D acquisition, 386, 386f

W

Wall motion abnormalities, 227, 239
Wall stress, 227, 238
Wall thickening, 289–290
Warfarin anticoagulation, 561, 575
Warfarin therapy, 622, 628
WASE Normal Values Study, 198, 205
Wavelength, 1, 11
Wilkins score, 385, 394–396

Z

Zoom function, 25